Handbook of
Immigrant Health

Handbook of Immigrant Health

Edited by

Sana Loue
Case Western Reserve University
Cleveland, Ohio

Plenum Press • New York and London

Library of Congress Cataloging-in-Publication Data

Handbook of immigrant health / edited by Sana Loue.
        p.   cm.
    Includes bibliographical references and index.
    ISBN 0-306-45959-0
    1. Immigrants--Health and hygiene--United States--Handbooks,
manuals, etc. 2. Minorities--Health and hygiene--United States-
-Handbooks, manuals, etc. 3. Medical care--United States--Cross
-cultural studies--Handbooks, manuals, etc. 4. Emmigration and
immigration--Health aspects--United States--Handbooks, manuals, etc.
5. Immigrants--Services for--United States--Handbooks, manuals, etc.
I. Loue, Sana.
    RA448.5.I44H36   1998
    362.1'086'91--dc21

                                                        98-34164
                                                           CIP

ISBN 0-306-45959-0

© 1998 Plenum Press, New York
A Division of Plenum Publishing Corporation
233 Spring Street, New York, N. Y. 10013

http://www.plenum.com

10 9 8 7 6 5 4 3 2 1

Printed in the United States of America

Contributors

Benjamin C. Amick III • The Health Institute, New England Medical Center, Boston, Massachusetts 02111

J. Xavier Apodaca • SDSU–UCSD Joint Doctoral Program, Clinical Psychology, San Diego State University, San Diego, California 92123

Keith B. Armitage • Division of Infectious Diseases, University Hospitals of Cleveland, Cleveland, Ohio 44106-5083

Roberta D. Baer • Department of Anthropology, University of South Florida, Tampa, Florida 33620-9951

Nadia Campbell • Graduate School of Public Health, Center for Behavioral and Community Health Studies, San Diego State University, San Diego, California 92123

Jeanette Candelaria • Graduate School of Public Health, Center for Behavioral and Community Health Studies, San Diego State University, San Diego, California 92123

Irma Castañeda • School of Social Work, University of Southern California, Los Angeles, California 90089

Lauren Clark • School of Nursing, University of Colorado Health Sciences Center, Denver, Colorado 80262

Margaret C. Cooney • Department of Anthropology, Case Western Reserve University, Cleveland, Ohio 44106

Lydia DeSantis • School of Nursing, University of Miami, Coral Gables, Florida 33124-3850

John P. Elder • Graduate School of Public Health, Center for Behavioral and Community Health Studies, San Diego State University, San Diego, California 92123

Kathleen Ell • School of Social Work, University of Southern California, Los Angeles, California 90089

Marlene Faust • School of Medicine, Case Western Reserve University, Cleveland, Ohio 44106–4945

Judy M. Ford • Alliance Healthcare Foundation, San Diego, California 92123

Atwood D. Gaines • Departments of Anthropology, Psychiatry, and Biomedical Ethics, Case Western Reserve University and School of Medicine, Cleveland, Ohio 44106

Bruce W. Goldberg • School of Medicine, Oregon Health Sciences University, Portland, Oregon 97201

Nahida H. Gordon • Department of Epidemiology and Biostatistics, School of Medicine, Case Western Reserve University, Cleveland, Ohio 44106-4945

Paul Grifhorst • European Research Center on Migration and Ethnic Relations, Utrecht University, Utrecht 3584CS, The Netherlands

Sylvia Guendelman • School of Public Health, University of California, Berkeley, California 94720-7360

Lisa Hofsess • School of Nursing, University of Colorado Health Sciences Center, Denver, Colorado 80262

Carol R. Horowitz • Departments of Health Policy and Medicine, Mount Sinai Medical Center, New York, New York 10029

Charlotte Ikels • Department of Anthropology, Case Western Reserve University, Cleveland, Ohio 44106

Carey Jackson • Division of General Internal Medicine, University of Washington, Seattle, Washington 98104

Barbara A. Koenig • Center for Biomedical Ethics, Stanford University, Palo Alto, California 94304

Jess F. Kraus • Department of Epidemiology, School of Public Health, and Center for Occupational and Environmental Health, University of California at Los Angeles, and Southern California Injury Prevention Research Center, Los Angeles, California 90095-1772

Amy S. Lightstone • Department of Epidemiology, School of Public Health, University of California at Los Angeles, and Southern California Injury Prevention Research Center, Los Angeles, California 90095-1772

Linda S. Lloyd • Alliance Healthcare Foundation, San Diego, California 92123

Sana Loue • Department of Epidemiology and Biostatistics, School of Medicine, Case Western Reserve University, Cleveland, Ohio 44106-4945

Geanne Lyons • Graduate School of Public Health, Center for Behavioral and Community Health Studies, San Diego State University, San Diego, California 92123

Patricia A. Marshall • Medical Humanities Program, Loyola University Chicago, Maywood, Illinois 60153

David L. McArthur • Department of Epidemiology, School of Public Health, University of California at Los Angeles, and Southern California Injury Prevention Research Center, Los Angeles, California 90095-1772

Marie Napolitano • Department of Primary Care, School of Nursing, Oregon Health Sciences University, Portland, Oregon 97201

Bonnie B. O'Connor • Department of Community and Preventive Medicine, MCP ♦ Hahnemann School of Medicine, Allegheny University of the Health Sciences, Philadelphia, Pennsylvania 19102

Karen N. Olness • Rainbow Babies and Children's Hospital, Cleveland, Ohio 44106

Deborah Parra-Medina • Graduate School of Public Health, Center for Behavioral and Community Health Studies, San Diego State University, San Diego, California 92123

Caroline Peterson • Department of Anthropology, University of South Florida, Tampa, Florida 33620-9951

L. A. Rebhun • Department of Anthropology, Yale University, New Haven, Connecticut 06511

Xinhua S. Ren • Center for Health Quality, Outcomes, and Economic Research, Health Services Research and Development Field Program, VA Medical Center, Bedford, Massachusetts 01730

Ruth Lyn Riedel • Alliance Healthcare Foundation, San Diego, California 92123

Robert A. Salata • Division of Infectious Diseases, University Hospitals of Cleveland, Cleveland, Ohio 44106-5083

Haikang Shen • School of Public Health, University of California at Los Angeles, Los Angeles, California 90095-1772

Susan B. Sorenson • School of Public Health, University of California at Los Angeles, Los Angeles, California 90095-1772

James C. Spilsbury • Department of Anthropology, Case Western Reserve University, Cleveland, Ohio 44106

Erika Takada • Division of Health Promotion, Graduate School of Public Health, San Diego State University, San Diego, California 92182

Mirjam van Ewijk • European Research Center on Migration and Ethnic Relations, Utrecht University, Utrecht 3584CS, The Netherlands

Adriana Villaseñor • Graduate School of Public Health, Center for Behavioral and Community Health Studies, San Diego State University, San Diego, California 92123

Bill Waddell • San Diego, California 92101

Maria Luisa Zuñiga de Nuncio • Graduate School of Public Health, Center for Behavioral and Community Health Studies, San Diego State University, San Diego, California 92123

Preface

This book represents the efforts of professionals across a multitude of disciplines (anthropology, epidemiology, ethics, health promotion, law, medicine, nursing, and social work) to examine the current health situation of our nation's immigrant populations. The scope of that inquiry ranges from attention to the most basic of questions, such as who is an immigrant, to an analysis of the health issues confronting specific immigrant subgroups, an examination of specific diseases that have impacted immigrant populations, and an exploration of health promotion and disease prevention strategies and public health policies that have and will continue to impact immigrant populations well into the future. This text represents one of the few efforts to integrate into a single source the vast literature across disciplines that pertains to U.S. immigrants and their health.

This effort is in no way intended to trivialize the differences that exist between and within groups or to subvert the importance of any individual immigrant's experience to that of the group. Rather, it is an attempt to explore the richness and diversity of our immigrant population and to foster a greater understanding of the nuances that exist between and within groups in their understandings of disease and illness; their search for healing and health; their susceptibility to disease; their ability to access health care, however it is defined; and the context in which this occurs. It serves as a guide for health care providers, health researchers, and health educators.

In addition, this text provides a blueprint for where we must go in the future in order to address the health needs of our immigrant populations: areas that lack adequate research for the identification and development of appropriate health promotion and disease prevention strategies, the absence of effective means of communication for the provision of information to many immigrant communities, and the relative scarcity of culturally appropriate services. This path cannot be so easily ignored or dismissed, for our attention to the health of our immigrant populations provides a mirror of our humanity, our understanding, and, ultimately, our own health.

Contents

Handbook of
Immigrant Health

1

United States Immigration

A Historical Perspective

BILL WADDELL

Introduction

United States immigration policy has once again become the subject of intense national debate. In 1994, California voters passed Proposition 187, the so-called "Save Our State" initiative, by a vote of 59% to 41%. The initiative attempts to bar undocumented immigrants from receiving public education and most government-funded social services, and to require educational, health care, and social service providers to verify the legal status of those suspected of being in the United States without documentation. Those unable to do so are to be reported to the Immigration and Naturalization Service.

Although the constitutionality of the proposition is currently being challenged in the courts, similar measures are being attempted in other states, and its passage ensured that immigration policy would remain a critical topic on the federal political agenda. Pat Buchanan, a contender for the Republican presidential nomination in 1996, called for a 5-year moratorium on immigration. He complained: "Hispanics, Asians and Africans will increase their present number of 65 million by at least 100 million in 60 years," and warned that south Texas and southern Califor-

nia may become "almost exclusively Hispanic" ("Presidential Candidates Hold Range of Views on Immigration," 1996).

A recently published book by the American Immigration Control Foundation warns of the "cultural dispossession" and "political subjugation" of European Americans (Nelson, 1994, p. 115). As will be seen, such anti-immigrant sentiment has occurred throughout American history.

Reference is made to the grounds of exclusion and deportation found in the Immigration and Nationality Act. Exclusion grounds were created by Congress to specify the types of persons that could be barred from admission to the United States if they were not citizens. They also apply to noncitizens in the United States who are applying for legal immigration status.

When the government wants to expel a noncitizen from the United States, then the deportation grounds are used. It should be noted that when Congress passed the Illegal Immigration Reform and Immigrant Responsibility Act of 1996 (U.S. Statutes at Large, September 30, 1996), it changed the terminology used for the exclusion grounds. They are now referred to as grounds of inadmissibility. In this historical perspective, the term *exclusion* is used throughout.

Although many deportation grounds mirror the exclusion grounds there are also differences. For example, noncitizens may be

BILL WADDELL • San Diego, California 92101.

Handbook of Immigrant Health, edited by Loue. Plenum Press, New York, 1998.

denied admission to the United States because they are infected with the human immunodeficiency virus (HIV), although immigrants who become infected with the HIV virus after admission cannot be deported for that reason. However, one who is determined to be a drug abuser or drug addict is both excludable and deportable.

Immigration Policy Prior to 1875

Although immigration to the United States was generally unrestricted by the federal government before 1875, voices advocating restrictions on immigration were heard even in colonial times. The predominant immigrant group residing in colonial America were the English. A number of Blacks also resided in the colonies, although they had been involuntarily brought as slaves beginning in Virginia in 1619. From 1619 until the end of the slave trade in 1807, 350,000 slaves were brought from Africa (Fuchs & Forbes, 1981, p. 42).

The immigration of hundreds of thousands of Germans and Scotch-Irish during the 1700s resulted in the first major debate on immigration policy (Seller, 1983). Germans arrived primarily because of political and religious persecution, while the Scotch-Irish fled because of religious restrictions and a rapid rise in rents (Seller, 1983, p. 140).

The British government had encouraged Protestant immigration to the colonies to enlarge the labor force and increase the market for British exports (Seller, 1983, p. 140). Criminals and debtors were also sent to the colonies with promises of pardons and free transportation, although not all immigrated by choice. The state of Georgia was originally founded as a penal colony for those unable to pay their debts (Dixon & Galan, 1990, p. 22).

Opposition to German and Scotch-Irish immigration was primarily due to concerns about the assimilation of immigrants from different cultures, although economics played a role in 1718 when Bostonians blamed Scotch-Irish immigrants for food shortages and the rising cost of grain (Seller, 1983, p. 141).

In 1738, George Washington said of the Germans, "I really think they [seem] to be as ignorant a Set of People as the Indians. [T]hey would never speak English but when spoken to they speak all Dutch" (quoted in Seller, 1983, p. 142). Benjamin Franklin considered the German immigrants to be "the most stupid of their own nation" (quoted in Seller, 1983, p. 142). He and others were offended by the "habits and peculiarities" of the new immigrants (Hull, 1985, p. 9). The Scotch-Irish were characterized at the time as being prone to disorder and violence (Seller, 1983, p. 142).

Attempts by the colonial assemblies to restrict the flow of German and Scotch-Irish immigrants by imposing a head tax on each immigrant or requiring the ship captains to post bonds for each passenger were rejected by the royal governors (Seller, 1983, p. 143). However, anti-Catholic legislation which resulted in special taxes, land restrictions, and religion-based voting qualifications being imposed on the Catholic population were upheld by the British authorities (Seller, 1983, p. 143).

For the most part, the attitudes of the colonists changed by the time of the American Revolution. British authorities had begun to limit immigration after 1763 because of fears that settlement of the West would make the colonies harder to defend, and they cut off immigration entirely in 1774. (Seller, 1983, p. 143). When Thomas Jefferson stated the offenses of King George III in the Declaration of Independence, the refusal of the Crown to grant the colonists a more liberal immigration policy was one of the complaints (Dixon & Galan, 1990, pp. 23–24). The colonists realized the importance of immigration to the growth of the new nation.

After the American Revolution, the federal government did not become directly involved in regulating immigration to the United States until 1875. However, the Federalist party passed the Alien Act of 1798 (U.S. Statutes at Large, June 25, 1798) which allowed the president to expel from the country any alien considered dangerous to the public peace or safety, or whom the president believed to be plotting against the country. It has been termed "the first effort of the American government to deport aliens" (Konvitz, 1953, p. 94). It was very unpopular, since it denied the accused the right to a trial by jury, and gave the president judicial powers (Konvitz, 1953, p. 96). The legislation expired after 2 years, and no one was expelled during its term.

During the same year, Congress passed the Alien Enemies Act (U.S. Statutes at Large, July 6, 1798). During a declared war between the United States and a foreign nation or an invasion, the government was given the authority to apprehend, restrain, secure, and remove all male resident aliens 14 years or older of the enemy nation who had not become citizens of the United States. In 1918, the legislation was revised to include women (U.S. Statutes at Large, 1918). The law is still on the books today.

From the end of the American revolution until 1830, approximately 375,000 immigrants arrived in the United States, primarily from England and northwestern Europe (Dixon & Galan, 1990, p. 28). However, the number of immigrants increased dramatically from 1830 to 1860, when approximately 4.5 million immigrants from Europe entered the country (Dixon & Galan, 1990, p. 28).

Economic conditions in the European countries were responsible for much of the immigration during this period. Irish people left their country when a plant disease destroyed Ireland's potato crop resulting in potato famines. The Irish had been the largest immigrant group during the period from 1841 to 1860, when 1,694,838 arrived according to statistics of the Immigration and Naturalization Service (INS) (cited in Harper, 1975, p. 663). Germans also left their country in huge numbers due to a depressed economy, and they were the second largest group during this period, with 1,386,293 immigrating to the United States (cited in Harper, 1975, p. 663).

What distinguished the Irish and German immigrants from previous arrivals was their religion. Practically all of the Irish and most of the new German arrivals were Catholic (Seller, 1983, p. 145). The centuries-old struggle between Protestants and Catholics in Europe led to anti-Catholic sentiment in the United States. From 1810 to 1860, the Catholic population increased from 75,000 to 3 million; rising from 1% of the nation's people to 10% (Seller, 1983, pp. 146–147). Many Protestant Americans believed that the Catholics were agents of the pope, sent over to colonize the United States (Dixon & Galan, 1990, p. 28). Anti-Catholic riots against the Irish occurred in New York, Philadelphia, and Boston, and convents and Catholic churches were burned (Fuchs & Forbes, 1981, p. 46).

Negative feelings toward immigrants led to the rise of nativism. The Know-Nothing party called for immigration reductions and became an important force during the 1850s (Hull, 1985, p. 10). While they were successful in winning governorships in some states and electing members of the party to Congress and state legislatures, they were unable to affect federal immigration policy. In fact, in 1864, Congress passed An Act to Encourage Immigration (U.S. Statutes at Large, 1864). The law established the U.S. Immigration Bureau whose purpose was to increase immigration so that American industries would have an adequate labor supply to meet production needs during the Civil War (Calavita, 1994).

Some states sought to restrict immigration, particularly the admission of criminals and the poor. Several states adopted laws forbidding the entrance of convicts into their state (Salyer, 1995, p. 4). New York and Massachusetts required shipmasters to post bonds guaranteeing that the state would not have to support indigent immigrants (Salyer, 1995, p. 4). Some states collected a head tax for each immigrant, which was then placed into a fund to help immigrants in need (Salyer, 1995, p. 4). The head taxes were declared unconstitutional in the *Passenger Cases,* 48 U.S. 283

(1849), with the majority ruling that the state laws infringed on the federal government's right to regulate foreign commerce. State attempts to regulate immigration were again found unconstitutional by the Supreme Court in *Henderson v. City of New York,* 92 U.S. 259 (1875).

After the Supreme Court rulings, states receiving large numbers of immigrants worried that local governments would have to support indigent immigrants. The New York Board of Emigration Commissioners and New York Board of Charities lobbied Congress to enact head taxes and exclude criminals and the indigent (Salyer, 1995, p. 5).

The Beginnings of Federal Immigration Legislation

Congress responded to the states' concerns by passing the first federal legislation restricting immigration to the United States (U.S. Statutes at Large, 1875). The law excluded certain criminals and prostitutes from admission. The primary concern was over the importation of Chinese prostitutes and European criminals (Hutchinson, 1981, p. 66). Regulation of immigration had become a federal responsibility.

In 1879, health concerns led to the passage of "An Act to Prevent the Introduction of Contagious or Infectious Diseases into the United States," (U.S. Statutes at Large, 1879). The law gave the National Board of Health authority to enforce regulations designed to prevent the introduction of such diseases to the United States. The president was authorized to appoint medical officers to serve at foreign ports and inspect vessels and crew. A ship sailing from a foreign post where such diseases existed had to obtain a bill of health from the medical officer, or a consular officer where no medical officer had been appointed, showing compliance with health regulations. Diseases of concern at the time were Asiatic cholera, yellow fever, plague, smallpox, typhus fever, and relapsing fever (Druhot, 1986, p. 88).

The first general immigration statute was passed in 1882 (U.S. Statutes at Large, August 3, 1882). The bill excluded "idiots," "lunatics," convicts, and those likely to become a public charge. It also imposed a head tax of 50 cents per immigrant. Authority was delegated to the secretary of the Treasury to enforce the new law.

The Chinese Exclusion Act

One author has concluded that "[t]he United States is ideologically a White country not by accident, but by design at least in part affected through naturalization and immigration laws" (I.F.H. Lopez, 1996, p. 117). Racial exclusion from the United States made its appearance in 1882 with the passage of the Chinese Exclusion Act (U.S. Statutes at Large, May 6, 1882). The law prohibited entry of all Chinese laborers for a period of 10 years.

Anti-Chinese sentiment was rampant on the West Coast, where approximately 100,000 Chinese had settled by 1880 (Hull, 1985). By 1870, Chinese comprised 25% of California wage earners (Salyer, 1995, p. 10). Many had been recruited by the Central Pacific Railroad Company to complete the transcontinental railroad. Chinese labor comprised 90% of the company's workforce (Salyer, 1995, p. 8). Like other immigrants, many Chinese left their native country to escape economic and social instability. The discovery of gold in California also led many to come and work the mines.

With the completion of the construction of the transcontinental railroad and the economic depression of the 1870s, Chinese were accused of taking jobs that "belonged" to White Americans (U.S. Commission on Civil Rights, 1980, p. 8). Chinese were also accused of bringing prostitution and gambling to the Pacific Coast (Fuchs and Forbes, 1981, p. 48), and were considered by much of the American public to be responsible for the spread of disease. In 1862, Dr. Arthur Stout published a book entitled *Chinese Immigration and the Physiological Causes of the*

Decay of the Nation, and the American Medical Association considered Chinese prostitutes to be of special health concern and sponsored an 1875 study of their effect on the "nation's bloodstream" (Salyer, 1995, pp. 11–12).

In 1854, an opinion of the Supreme Court of California called the Chinese a "race of people whom nature has marked as inferior, and who are incapable of progress or intellectual development beyond a certain point" (cited in Knapp, 1996, p. 415). The mood at the time resulted in many states passing laws prohibiting Chinese from owning property or holding certain occupations, and in 1876 led to the California Senate's passing a resolution which stated that "[t]he Chinese are inferior to any race God ever made" (cited in Hull, 1985, p. 11).

In 1884, the law was expanded to include all Chinese and was extended indefinitely in 1904 (U.S. Statutes at Large, 1904). The law remained in effect until 1943. The law's constitutionality was upheld in *Chae Chang Ping v. United States,* 130 U.S. 581 (1889), also known as the Chinese Exclusion Case, with the Court stating that Congress has the right to exclude the "presence of foreigners of a different race." The Chinese Exclusion Case was never overruled and remains valid law.

Congress Responds to Labor's Protests against Foreign Workers

A common practice during the 1800s was for American employers to recruit foreign workers, who would sign a contract to work for a specific period of time, and in return the company would pay their transportation costs to the states. Companies would pay the foreign workers less than their American counterparts, and the influx of cheap foreign workers led to protests by the American labor movement (Dixon & Galan, 1990, p. 43).

In response, Congress passed what became known as the contract-labor laws in 1885 and 1887 (U.S. Statutes at Large, 1885, 1887). The law prohibited companies from import-ing most foreign laborers under contract. Exceptions were made for artists, lecturers, servants, and those immigrants working in an industry that had not yet been established in the United States. An 1888 amendment provided for the deportation within 1 year for those entering in violation of the contract-labor laws (U.S. Statutes at Large, 1888). It was the first deportation statute since the short-lived Alien Act of 1798.

1891–1917: Closing the Door on the Sick and Poor

Further qualitative restrictions on entry became law with the passage of new legislation in 1891 (U.S. Statutes at Large, 1891). Polygamists, "paupers," and those convicted of a moral turpitude offense were now excludable. The law also provided for the deportation within 1 year of any immigrant who entered the country illegally. Additional medical grounds of exclusion included those suffering from a "loathsome or dangerous contagious disease."

The 1891 law also provided for the medical inspection of immigrants at U.S. points of entry. Physical examinations were performed by officers of the Marine Hospital Service, which was the predecessor to the Public Health Service. Symptomatic immigrants were marked "T.D.," which stood for temporarily detained (Dixon & Galan, 1990, p. 15). Those who failed the examination were shipped home.

Legislation in 1903 barred epileptics, insane persons, beggars, and anarchists, including "persons who believe in, or advocate, the overthrow by force or violence of the Government of the United States, or of all government, or of all forms of law, or the assassination of public officials" (U.S. Statutes at Large, 1903). Prior to the 1903 legislation, no person was excluded from the United States because of his or her political opinion. The addition of political grounds for exclusion was a direct response to the assassination of President William McKinley in

1901 by Leon Czolgosz, whose parents were Polish immigrants.

Legislation in 1907 contained additional restrictions on who was entitled to admission. Added to the list of excludable immigrants were "imbeciles," "feeble-minded persons," persons likely to become a public charge, those suffering from a mental or physical defect that might affect their ability to earn a living, those who admit to having committed a crime of moral turpitude, and those coming to the United States for prostitution or "any other immoral purpose," (U.S. Statutes at Large, 1907).

Eugenics and Immigration: In Search of the Perfect Immigrant

The early 1900s saw increased concern with the growth in immigration, particularly because the new European immigrants who were arriving were primarily from southern and eastern Europe, rather than northern and western Europe which previously provided the majority of immigrants. By 1907, 80% of the immigrants had come from southern and eastern Europe (Seller, 1983, p. 148).

Proposals for further immigration restrictions were bolstered by the "science" of eugenics, which held that ethnic groups were biologically distinct races (Varma, 1996). In 1914, noted sociologist Edward A. Ross stated that "Slavs and Hebrews" were unique races inferior in "good looks, stature and physique, morality, vitality, and natural ability," (cited in Varma, 1996, p. 734). He described Italians as "lack[ing] the power to take rational care of themselves," because of low craniums (cited in Hull, 1985, p. 14). By 1916, eugenics was firmly established in the nation's universities (Varma, 1996).

In 1907, a commission consisting of members of Congress and presidential appointees was established to study immigration. It was known as the Dillingham commission, named after its chairman, William P. Dillingham. In 1911, the commission released a 42-volume study on the impact of immigration on the United States. The commission, influenced by eugenics research, concluded that the new wave of immigrants was inferior and less desirable than previous immigrant groups. Dillingham stated that the commission report proved that the new immigrants were of "inferior stock," and concluded that immigration from southern and eastern Europe should be substantially reduced (Hull, 1985, p. 15).

The commission proposed the establishment of a literacy test, which it believed would discriminate against immigrants from southern and eastern Europe where illiteracy was high. Senator Henry Cabot Lodge believed that the literacy test would affect primarily "the Italians, Russians, Hungarians, Greeks and Asiatics," groups which he believed "the English-speaking people have never hitherto assimilated, and who are most alien to the great body of people of the United States" (quoted in Hull, 1985, p. 16). It was thought that such a test would decrease immigration from that region by 25% (Jacobson, 1996, p. 47).

Although literacy test legislation was passed by Congress in 1897, 1913, 1915, it was vetoed each time by the president in office (Keely, 1993, p. 61). However, in 1917, Congress overrode President Woodrow Wilson's veto, and immigration legislation that contained a literacy test was passed (U.S. Statutes at Large, 1917). This success has been attributed to the United States's entry into World War I, which brought new concerns about the ability of the country to assimilate the foreign born, and raised questions as to their loyalty (Fuchs & Forbes, 1981, p. 51).

The law also created an "Asiatic Barred Zone," which excluded Orientals. Japan was not included in the Asiatic Barred Zone, since in 1907, the governments of the United States and Japan had reached a so-called "Gentleman's Agreement," to restrict the immigration of Japanese laborers to the United States (Harper, 1975, p. 8). The Japanese government agreed to issue passports for travel to the United States only for those of its laborers who were former U.S. residents, or to parents, wives, or children of residents of the United States and to settled agriculturalists (Chuman, 1976, p. 35). The Senate had also passed a bill during the same period to exclude "all members of the African or black race," but it was defeated in the House after intensive lobbying by the NAACP (I.F.H. Lopez, 1996, p. 38).

The literacy test did not meet the expectations of those who thought that it would substantially reduce immigration from southern and eastern Europe. Literacy rates were higher than thought. Italy had even established schools to teach its nationals to pass the exam (Fuchs & Forbes, 1981, p. 53). Efforts to ban all immigration gained support among labor organizations and a group known as the "100 percenters," believing themselves to be 100% American. Although it garnered approval among some members of the House of Representatives, the ban failed to pass the Senate Committee on Immigration, which was influenced by business interests and ethnic constituencies (Fuchs & Forbes, 1981, p. 53).

The Quota Law of 1921: Establishing Numerical Limitations

Instead, following World War I, the Quota Law of 1921 (U.S. Statutes at Large, 1921) established numerical limitations on the number of immigrants admitted to the United States and discriminated on the basis of national origin. The Quota Law would for the first time establish numerical limitations on those who could enter the United States.

A quota system was established that limited immigration to 3% of the number of foreign-born people of each European ethnic group in the country at the time of the 1910 census. The quotas discriminated against southern and eastern European immigrants, whose immigrant population was significantly lower in 1910.

Dr. Harry N. Laughlin, a eugenics consultant to the House Judiciary Committee on Immigration and Naturalization in the early 1920s stated: "We in this country have been so imbued with the idea of democracy, or the equality of all men, that we have left out of consideration the matter of blood or natural born hereditary mental and moral differences. No man who breeds pedigreed pets and animals can afford to neglect this thing" (quoted in Select Commission on Immigration and Refugee Policy [SCIRP], 1979, p. 8)

Fears that Bolshevik aliens would enter the country after World War I was also a factor in establishing the quotas (Jacobson, 1996, p. 47). Initially, the law was to expire in 1922, but was extended until 1924.

The quota system went from a temporary to a permanent measure with the passage of legislation in 1924 known as the National Origins Act (U.S. Statutes at Large, 1924). A yearly quota of 150,000 was established for the European countries. The quota was divided according to the proportion of foreign-born residents from each particular country residing in the United States in 1890. The use of the 1890 census discriminated against southern and eastern Europeans even more than the quota law of 1921. The Italian quota was reduced from 42,000 to 4,000, the Polish quota went from 31,000 to 6,000, and the Greek quota went from 3,000 to 100 (Fuchs & Forbes, 1981, p. 54). The same legislation provided for the use of 1920 census beginning July 1, 1927 (U.S. Statutes at Large, 1924). The system remained substantially unchanged until 1952.

Another provision in the 1924 act barred the immigration of those ineligible for citizenship. Up until 1870, only "free white persons" were eligible for citizenship. After the Civil War, Congress granted "persons of African nativity or descent" naturalization privileges. It was not until 1952 that race was no longer a factor in qualifying for naturalization. Foreign-born Japanese were therefore ineligible for citizenship, a ban that was upheld by the Supreme Court in *Ozawa v. United States,* 260 U.S. 178 (1922).

The 1924 bar was specifically aimed at the Japanese, and the law was unofficially known as the Japanese Exclusion Act (Chuman, 1976, p. 101). Anti-Japanese sentiment was prevalent in California, with organizations such as the Japanese Exclusion League pressuring Congress to further restrict Japanese immigration. A statement introduced into the Senate in 1921 referred to the "steadily growing menace" of the Japanese; an "unassimilable race," who were unfit "for the responsibilities and duties of American citizenship" (Chuman, 1976, p. 96). The statement had the endorsement of the California Congressional delegation, the American Legion, the State Federation of Labor, the California Farm Bureau, the Federation of Women's Clubs, the Veterans of Foreign Wars, and many other groups (Chuman, 1976, p. 96).

The Immigration and Nationality Act of 1952

In 1952, Congress codified all prior immigration legislation into the Immigration and Nationality Act of 1952, also named the Mc-Carren-Walter Act after its Congressional sponsors (U.S. Statutes at Large, 1952). The legislation was the result of study of the immigration laws by the Senate Judiciary Committee. It revised and codified the prior immigration legislation, and remains the basic framework of U.S. immigration law. With the exception of the Internal Revenue Code, it has been considered to be "the longest, most complicated, and certainly the most arcane piece of legislation in modern United States history" (Hull, 1985, p. 20).

The law retained the national origins quotas with some modifications. Cultural stability rather than racial superiority was the primary rationalization for retention of the quotas. The 1950 report of the Senate Judiciary Committee stated: "Without giving credence to any theory of Nordic superiority, the subcommittee believes that the adoption of the national origins quota formula was a rational and logical method of numerically restricting immigration in such a manner as to

best preserve the sociological and cultural balance in the population of the United States" (cited in SCIRP, 1979, p. 8).

President Truman vetoed the legislation, but the veto was overridden by Congress. The retention of the quota system was the primary factor in Truman's veto. He condemned the system for "discriminat[ing] deliberately and intentionally against many of the peoples of the world," and called it "insulting to large numbers of our finest citizens, irritating to our allies abroad, and foreign to our purposes and ideals" (quoted in Konvitz, 1953, p. 16).

As in prior legislation, immigrants who came from Western Hemisphere countries were exempt from the quotas. Asian countries were given small quotas. Spouses and children of American citizens were also exempt from the quotas as they had been in the past. The legislation gave preferences to those immigrants with special skills.

Detailed grounds of exclusion and deportation were listed, essentially codifying prior Congressional concerns. Excluded for health reasons were those considered to be feeble-minded, insane, narcotic drug addicts, or chronic alcoholics, those with epilepsy, psychopathic personality, a mental defect, tuberculosis, leprosy, or a dangerous contagious disease, and those whose physical defects affect their ability to earn a living.

Sensitivity to business interests was apparent with the addition of a proviso declaring that the employment of undocumented immigrants was not "harboring," an offense under the 1952 Act. An attempt in the Senate to penalize employers if they had reasonable grounds to believe that an employee was not authorized to work was defeated by a vote of 69–12 (SCIRP, 1979, p. 36).

The Act was passed during the Cold War period, and foreign policy concerns were reflected in the new legislation. The Senate Judiciary Committee report believed that the United States Communist movement was an "alien" movement controlled by European communists and the Soviet Union and that "[t]he severance of this connection and the destruction of the life line of communism becomes, therefore, substantially an immigration problem" (cited in SCIRP, 1979, p. 10).

The Internal Security Act of 1950 was incorporated into the 1952 Act, resulting in Communist party members and supporters of the doctrine of "world communism" barred from entry to the country. The allocation of quotas to Asian countries was said to be the result of fear of alienating the Asian countries during the conflict with the Communists (Jacobson, 1996, p. 48).

However, discrimination against Asians and Blacks was still apparent in the law. Asia and Africa were allotted 2,990 visas and 1,400 visas respectively, while the European quotas totaled 149,667 (Keely, 1993, p. 65). Also, while non-Asians were counted against the quota of the country of birth, Asians were counted against the country of their forebears (Hull, 1985, p. 21). Countries in the Western Hemisphere were not restricted by quotas, which continued past policy.

1965: The End of the Quota System

Although opposition to the quota system had been in the presidential platforms of both major parties since 1952, no significant changes occurred in the immigration laws until 1965. In 1963, President John F. Kennedy submitted an immigration bill to Congress whose primary reform was the abolition of the national-origins quota system. Kennedy stated that the system was "without basis in either logic or reason . . . it discriminates among applicants for admission into the United States on the basis of accident of birth" (quoted in Dixon & Galan, 1990, p. 62). After Kennedy's assassination, his proposals for immigration reform were adopted by President Johnson. In 1965 legislation abolished the national-origins quota system, effective June 30, 1968 (U.S. Statutes at Large, 1965).

A quota of 170,000 was established for the Eastern hemisphere, and no more than 20,000 of the visas could be allocated to any one country. For the first time, a quota of 120,000 was established for the Western hemisphere; however, no per-country limits were imposed. Greater emphasis was placed on family reunification, with parents of United States citizens age 21 and over joining spouses and children of United States citizens as immigrants not subject to the quotas.

The legislation also prohibited immigration discrimination based on race or sex. Epilepsy was deleted as a ground of exclusion, and the term "feebleminded" was changed to read "mentally retarded." "Sexual deviation" was added as a ground of exclusion.

The 1970s saw additional calls for immigration restriction. In its 1980 report on immigration, the U.S. Commission on Civil Rights concluded that Mexicans replaced Chinese as bearing the brunt of the attacks (U.S. Commission on Civil Rights, 1980, p. 12). In 1976, Congress amended the 1965 Act by imposing a 20,000 numerical limitation per country on Western hemisphere nations. The report concluded that this was a partial response to the demand for "stemming the tide" of Mexican immigration (U.S. Commission on Civil Rights, 1980, p. 12). At the time of the legislation, legal immigration from Mexico had been at over 40,000 per year and in 1976 was cut by over 50% (U.S. Commission on Civil Rights, 1980, p. 12). An amendment to the statute in 1978 abolished the separate Eastern and Western Hemisphere quotas, and combined them into a single worldwide quota of 290,000 (U.S. Statutes at Large, 1978).

Mexican Immigration: Sometimes We Need You, Sometimes We Don't

Both President Gerald Ford and President Jimmy Carter supported special legislation to increase the Mexican immigration quotas after the 1976 legislation because of the special relationship between the United States and Mexico as the result of shared borders (Fuchs & Forbes, 1981, p. 59). The idea, however, was never acted on.

The Mexicans have been considered a source of cheap labor by U.S. employers for many years. When the national quota system was instituted in 1921, immigration from southern and eastern Europe declined, and Mexicans were seen by employers as a substitute for European labor (Calavita, 1994, p. 59). In 1918, because of a wartime labor shortage, Mexican workers were specifically exempted from the head tax, the exclusion of contract laborers, and the literacy requirements of immigration legislation (G. Lopez, 1981, p. 631 n. 72).

Attempts to restrict Mexican immigration in the 1920s were defeated in Congress. Those against restrictions described the Mexicans as an economical, unskilled labor force that could easily be deported to their native country (Calavita, 1994, p. 59). During the 1920s, approximately 500,000 Mexicans entered the United States (Lopez, 1981, p. 660).

At the time of the Great Depression, signs appeared in the Southwest reading "Only White Labor Employed" and "No Niggers, Mexicans, or Dogs Allowed" (Meir & Ribera, 1993, p. 150). Hundreds of thousands of Mexicans were forced to leave the country during what was termed a "repatriation campaign" (U.S. Commission on Civil Rights, 1980, p. 10). Some were formally deported, others were forcibly removed, and many left "voluntarily" after threats of termination of relief assistance (Meir & Ribera, 1993, p. 155). The "repatriation campaign" resulted from organized efforts from both governmental and private agencies to convince the Mexicans to return. Some authorities estimate that more than half of the Mexicans "repatriated" were U.S. citizens (U.S. Commission on Civil Rights, 1980, p. 10).

The government decided once again that Mexican workers were needed due to a labor shortage, and negotiated a treaty with the Mexican government, commonly known as the Bracero Program. The treaty permitted the temporary admission of male Mexican farm workers under contract with U.S. employers. The contracts were guaranteed by the U.S. government and included minimum guarantees regarding wages and working conditions, although these were often not followed (Lopez, 1981, pp. 664–665). The program continued under various legal authorizations for 22 years and involved in total approximately 5 million Mexican workers (SCIRP, 1979, p. 27).

The program has been identified as a primary cause of the increase in illegal entries beginning in 1944 (SCIRP, 1979, p. 35). During the 10-year period from 1934–1943, INS apprehensions averaged under 12,000 per year (SCIRP, 1979, p. 33). From 1942 to 1952, the INS apprehended more than 2 million undocumented immigrants, the majority Mexican (Calavita, 1994, p. 60).

In 1954, in response to public outcry over the growing numbers of Mexican immigrants, the U.S. government launched "Operation Wetback." The paramilitary operation, under the direction of Attorney General Herbert Brownell, resulted in the expulsion of more than 1 million Mexicans from the country, one sixth of the Mexican population residing in the United States (Hull, 1985, p. 84). The operation involved wholesale civil rights violations, and led to the deportation of a number of American citizens.

U.S. Immigration Policy and Refugees

The passage of the Refugee Act of 1980 (U.S. Statutes at Large, 1980), was intended to bring United States refugee law into conformity with international treaty obligations. Prior to World War I, the United States had no refugee policy at all and it was not considered necessary since there were few impediments to immigration. However, with the implementation of the national-origin quota system, the need for a refugee policy became more important.

In deference to the quota system, the United States had refused to admit hundreds of thousands of Jewish refugees attempting to escape persecution by the Nazis (Hull, 1985, p. 116). In 1939, the U.S. Congress defeated a bill that would have allowed the rescue of 20,000 children from Nazi Germany who had families in the U.S. willing to sponsor them on the grounds that the children would exceed the German quota (Fuchs & Forbes, 1981, p. 55). The United States refused to sign international conventions after World War I to facilitate refugee resettlement fearing a substantial influx of southern and eastern Europeans which the quota system was designed to prevent (Hull, 1985, p. 117).

In 1948, following World War II, the Truman administration enacted the Displaced Persons Act (U.S. Statutes at Large, 1948), which was amended in 1950 (U.S. Statutes at Large, 1950). The program ultimately resulted in admitting more than 400,000 European refugees to the United States (Konvitz, 1953, p. 23).

The motive in passing the Displaced Persons Act was not exclusively humanitarian, however, but was enacted also to prevent Europe from succumbing to Communism after the war (Hull, 1985, p. 117). The refugees were admitted only upon assurance that they would have employment and housing and not become a public charge (Harper, 1975, p. 16). Congress also made it clear that any visas issued beyond a country's allotment would be counted against future quotas.

The 1952 act had given the attorney general authority to "parole" aliens into the country "for emergent reasons or for reasons deemed strictly in the public interest" (U.S. Statutes at Large, 1952). The parole authority enabled the government to admit refugees from overseas. President Eisenhower used the parole power in 1956 to admit more than 38,000 Hungarian refugees, and, prior to the passage of the Refugee Act of 1980, it was the principal means by which refugees entered the country (Hull, 1985, p. 117). It was used almost exclusively to admit those fleeing communism (Helton, 1984, p. 246).

Following the expiration of the Displaced Persons Act, Congress passed the Refugee Relief Act in 1953 (U.S. Statutes at Large, 1953) which authorized the admission of 214,000

refugees. Beneficiaries were refugees fleeing Iron Curtain countries.

A procedure enacted in 1965 known as conditional entry status allowed the admission of refugees from overseas if they could demonstrate that they had fled a communist or Middle Eastern country because of persecution on account of race, religion, or political opinion (U.S. Statutes at Large, 1965). The enactment was on its face ideologically and geographically biased.

In 1968, the United States became a party to the 1967 United Nations Protocol relating to the Status of Refugees. The protocol incorporated Articles 2–34 of the United Nations Convention Relating to the Status of Refugees. Under the convention, a *refugee* is defined as any person who,

> [o]wing to a well-founded fear of being persecuted for reasons of race, religion, nationality, membership of a particular social group or political opinion, is outside the country of his nationality and is unable, or, owing to such fear, is unwilling to avail himself of the protection of that country; or who, not having a nationality and being outside the country or his former habitual residence is unable or, owing to such fear, is unwilling to return to it. (1951 United Nations Convention Relating to the Status of Refugees, July 28, 1951, 189 U.N.T.S. 137, 19 U.S.T. 6259, T.I.A.S. No. 6577)

The Refugee Act of 1980 amended the Immigration and Nationality Act so as to incorporate the international definition of *refugee,* using virtually the same language as the convention. However, it became clear that even after passage of the Refugee Act, ideological bias entered into adjudication of political asylum claims, since refugees from countries considered "friendly" to the United States were much less likely to be granted asylum than those from "unfriendly countries." (Helton, 1984, p. 253).

Bias in asylum adjudications led to a class action suit on behalf of Salvadoran and Guatemalan asylum applicants. (*American Baptist Churches v. Thornburgh,* 706 F. Supp. 796 (N.D. Cal. 1991). The settlement required the government to readjudicate thousands of asylum applications from Guatemalans and

Salvadorans. Such bias should be reduced with regulations that went into effect on October 1, 1990. Affirmative asylum applications (those submitted from aliens not in deportation proceedings) are heard by a corps of asylum officers who have received special training in international relations and international law. The officers have access to a documentation center with information on human rights conditions. Applicants who file for asylum in deportation proceedings continue to have their applications heard by an immigration judge.

The United States continues to lead the world in the absolute number of refugees admitted and persons granted asylum. Between 1975 and 1993, a total of 1,859,901 persons were given refugee or asylee status (U.S. Committee for Refugees, 1995, p. 46). In 1993 alone, the figure was 128,811 (U.S. Committee for Refugees, 1995, p. 46). However, in terms of the ratio of resettled refugees and asylees to the total population, the United States is fifth, following Sweden, Canada, Australia, and Denmark (U.S. Committee for Refugees, 1995, p. 46).

The Immigration Reform and Control Act of 1986

The 1980s were a time of increased concern on the part of the media and government with immigration. The attention has been said to have stemmed primarily from the increase in illegal immigration (Jacobson, 1996, p. 53). Demographers estimated that at the time of the 1980 census, 2.5 million to 3.5 million undocumented immigrants resided in the United States (Jacobson, 1996, p. 54). Although these figures have been questioned (Passel & Woodward, 1989, pp. 12–14), data apprehension figures of the INS, resulting in arrests of about 1 million a year, add further weight to the conclusion that illegal entries increased dramatically during the 1970s and 1980s (Jacobson, 1996, pp. 53, 54).

In 1978, Congress established a Select Commission on Immigration and Refugee Policy, headed by the Reverend Theodore Hesburgh of Notre Dame University, to recommend immigration reform policies. The commission released its report on March 1, 1981. The report considered the reduction of illegal entries to be a top priority, concluding that "the toleration of large-scale undocumented/illegal immigration can have pernicious effects on U.S. society" (quoted in Jacobson, 1996, p. 57). The report recommended increased border control, legalization of the status of undocumented immigrants in the country prior to January 1, 1980, and the sanctioning of employers who hire undocumented immigrants (Jacobson, 1996, p. 57).

Efforts on Capitol Hill to implement the recommendations were unsuccessful until 1986 when Congress passed the Immigration Reform and Control Act (IRCA) (U.S.Statutes at Large, 1986). For the first time, employers were subject to sanctions for hiring employees without proper authorization to work. If one was not a U.S. citizen or legal resident, proof of employment authorization from the immigration service was necessary. Employers were now required to keep records certifying that they inspected the documents of their employees.

In response to concerns that the new legislation would lead to employment discrimination against qualified workers who sound or look foreign, Congress included a provision prohibiting discrimination on the basis of citizenship status or national origin. However, the law also states that an employer may favor a citizen over a noncitizen if both are equally qualified.

Congress also directed the General Accounting Office to prepare three annual reports to determine whether the new provisions resulted in discriminatory practices. The final report indicated that national origin discrimination existed at a level amounting to a "serious pattern of discrimination" (cited in Espenoza, 1994, p. 381). As a result of the report, Congress amended the antidiscrimination provision, by, among other things, forbidding employers from asking for more or different documents than are legally required. However, some have concluded that discrimination still occurs since employees of Hispanic and Asian descent are scrutinized more closely by employers, and that sanctions give employers an excuse to discriminate (Espenoza, 1994, p. 385).

After an initial success in reducing the flow of illegal immigration, recent figures have shown that IRCA has not resulted in a significant decline in the number of undocumented aliens. Between November 1986 and September 1988, apprehensions declined about 35% (Jacobson, 1996, p. 62). Fiscal year 1989 showed a 20% decline (Jacobson, 1996, p. 63). However, the 1990s showed a significant jump in the number of apprehensions to well over 1 million a year (Jacobson, 1996, p. 62). Some authorities have attributed this increase to a significant growth in forged documents, as well as the fact that employers do not have to verify the authenticity of the documents that they accept (Jacobson, 1996, p. 63).

IRCA also allowed the legalization of undocumented immigrants who could show that they had resided in the United States in an illegal status prior to January 1, 1982. The provision was necessary to garner the support for IRCA from advocates of immigrants' rights and members of Congress concerned with the effects of employer sanctions on the labor supply (Calavita, 1994, p. 66). Approximately 1.7 million applicants applied for this program, with an approval rate of nearly 98% (Calavita, 1994, p. 68). Of the applicants, 69.8% were Mexican nationals, with the majority of the rest from Central America and Asia (Calavita, 1994, p. 68).

Pressure from agricultural interests led to provisions in IRCA for the legalization of special agricultural workers who could show that they had worked at least 90 days in agriculture during the year ending May 1, 1986. Approximately 1.3 million undocumented immigrants applied for this program, with a 94% approval rate (Calavita, 1994, p. 68). Of the applicants, 81.9% were Mexican nationals, and, like the legalization applicants, the majority of the rest were from Central America and Asia (Calavita, 1994, p. 68).

The Immigration Act of 1990

The immigration law was extensively revised with the Immigration Act of 1990 (1990 Act; U.S. Statutes at Large, 1990). The 1990 act set an annual limit on immigration to 700,000 a year for the first 3 years, and 675,000 thereafter. Of the visas, 465,000 were made available to family-sponsored immigration and 140,000 were for employment-based immigration. The 1990 act also established a "diversity" program that set aside 40,000 immigrant visas per year in 1992, 1993, 1994 for natives of countries that were adversely affected by IRCA. Refugees and asylees were considered separately.

The bulk of the allotments going to family-sponsored immigration showed the importance Congress placed on the reunification of families. The employment-based immigration gives preference to those with high skills and educational achievement in areas in which there are shortages of qualified American workers. Congress believed that "immigration can and should be incorporated into an overall strategy that promotes the creation of the type of workforce needed in an increasingly competitive global economy without adversely impacting on the wages and working conditions of American workers" (cited in Lawson & Grin, 1992, p. 265).

Immigration Policy and Health

As we have seen, U.S. immigration policy has been concerned not only with the quantity but with the "quality" of intending immigrants. The health-related exclusion grounds are found in section 212(a)(1) of the Immigration and Nationality Act. They currently exclude (1) those who have a "communicable disease of public health significance"; (2) intending immigrants who are unable to document having been vaccinated against vaccine-preventable diseases; (3) those who have a physical or mental disorder that poses a threat to themselves or others; and (4) those who have been determined to be drug abusers or addicts.

The first immigration statute passed in 1882 excluded "idiots," and "lunatics." Legislation in 1891 excluded those suffering from a "loathsome or dangerous contagious disease." Legislation in 1903 added epileptics and insane persons. "Imbeciles," "feeble-minded persons," and those whose mental or physical defect might affect their ability to earn a living were added in 1907.

The 1952 Immigration Act which codified all prior immigration legislation kept these health-related exclusion grounds, although it eliminated some of the prior terminology used. "Chronic alcoholics" and "narcotic drug users" were added to the exclusion list, as were those determined to have a "psychopathic personality."

The psychopathic personality ground of exclusion was used to bar homosexuals from admission (Gordon, Mailman, & Yale-Loehr, 1997). Court rulings upheld the exclusion of homosexuals under this ground, and Congress added the term "sexual deviation" in the 1965 immigration legislation to clarify their intent that homosexuals be excluded (Gordon *et al.*, 1997).

The 1990 legislation substantially changed the health-related grounds of exclusion. Criticism from public health organizations resulted in the term "dangerous contagious disease" being replaced with "communicable disease of public health significance." (Gordon *et al.*, 1997) Such diseases include chancroid, gonorrhea, granuloma inguinale, human immunodeficiency virus (HIV infection), infectious leprosy, lymphogranuloma venereum, infectious syphilis, and active tuberculosis.

Sexual deviation and chronic alcoholism were eliminated as grounds of exclusion. There are no longer any specific references to mental retardation or insanity. Those with a physical or mental disorder are now excluded only if the behavior associated with that disorder poses a threat to themselves or others. Though a significant improvement over prior law, the specific reference to HIV infection in the health-related grounds of exclusion continues to be criticized.

Immigration policy, politics, and health concerns were heatedly debated in determining the response of the United States to intending immigrants infected with the HIV virus, the precursor to Acquired Immune Deficiency Syndrome (AIDS). In 1987, an amendment by Senator Jesse Helms calling on the president to add HIV to the list of contagious diseases passed the Senate 96–0, and was later approved by Congress as part of a supplemental appropriations bill (U.S. Statutes at Large, 1987). The government began testing intending immigrants and those nonimmigrants that they suspected might have the disease (Osuna, 1993, pp. 10–11).

U.S. policy was criticized by numerous domestic and international organizations, including the National Commission on AIDS which was created to advise the president on national AIDS policy (Osuna, 1993, p. 14). After the 1990 act changed the exclusion terminology from "dangerous contagious disease" to "communicable disease of public health significance," the Public Health Service announced that it would remove HIV infection from the list of excludable diseases after their determination that the removal would not significantly increase the risk of infection to the U.S. population. (Osuna, 1993, p. 19). However, a public outcry resulted in the ban on HIV-infected immigrants remaining in effect. Although waivers are available for intending immigrants with a close family relationship with a U.S. citizen or legal resident, they are not easily obtained.

The 1990s and Beyond: Immigrants Once Again Come under Fire

In his State of the Union speech on January 24, 1995, President Clinton promised an aggressive approach to significantly decrease illegal immigration. He stated that "[i]t is wrong and ultimately self-defeating for a nation of immigrants to permit the kind of abuse of our immigration laws we have seen in recent years, and we must do more to stop it." ("Clinton Vows More Immigration Enforcement, Bills Introduced in Congress," 1995). Widespread concern over both legal and illegal immigration resulted in intensive efforts by Congress to pass new immigration legislation.

Immigration policy was significantly affected, even in legislation in which the primary concern had little to do with immigration. The Anti-terrorism and Effective Death Penalty Act of 1996 (AEDPA) (U.S. Statutes at Large, April 24, 1996), was legislation initiated by Congress in response to the bombing of the federal building in Oklahoma City, Oklahoma, a year earlier. The legislation established separate removal proceedings for alien terrorists and allowed the government to designate an organization as "terrorist" and exclude members of the organization from the United States. However, the legislation contained numerous immigration provisions having nothing to do with fighting terrorism. The most severe immigration provisions of the law affect long-term legal residents with one or more criminal convictions, many of whom were previously eligible to apply for a discretionary waiver before an immigration judge which would allow them to remain in the country. The AEDPA eliminated this waiver for most legal residents with criminal convictions, without consideration of long-term residency or family ties in the United States.

The next significant piece of legislation passed in 1996 that affected immigrants was the Personal Responsibility and Work Opportunity Reconciliation Act of 1996 (Welfare Act) (U.S. Statutes at Large, August 22, 1996). Again, the legislation was not primarily an immigration bill, but it portends drastic consequences for many legal immigrants. With certain exceptions, the law bars most noncitizens from eligibility for federal benefit programs, such as Medicaid, food stamps, and Supplemental Security Income (SSI), and allows the states to similarly place restrictions on access to their programs (Wheeler, 1996). Congress's stated purpose

in barring immigrant access to federal and state benefits was to encourage self-sufficiency and remove an extra incentive in immigrating to the United States (Wheeler, 1996, p. 123).

The legislation resulted in panic among many elderly immigrants. Estimates were that 500,000 immigrants who received SSI would lose their benefits (Lindt, 1997, p. 103). The outcry over the likely result of many elderly immigrants losing their only source of income led Congress to restore SSI and derivative Medicaid eligibility to all legal immigrants who were receiving SSI benefits on August 22, 1996 ("Balanced Budget Act Restores Immigrant Eligibility for Certain Public Benefits," 1997).

Critics of the Welfare Act predict a potential public health crisis as the result of certain of its provisions. Section 434 of the Act prohibits state or local governments from restricting the exchange of information with the Immigration and Naturalization Service (INS). Government employees would be able to report to the INS undocumented immigrants who seek public services.

New York City mayor Rudolph W. Giuliani has stated that the provision was specifically meant to overturn an executive order prohibiting New York City employees from providing such information to the INS ("States' Early Response to Welfare Reform Reveals Variety, Confusion," 1996). He foresees a public health crisis if undocumented immigrants refuse to get treatment for fear of being turned over to the INS. A lawsuit against the act was filed by New York City on March 26, 1997.

The most significant piece of immigration legislation in decades is the Illegal Immigration Reform and Immigration Responsibility Act of 1996 (U.S. Statutes at Large, September 30, 1996). The law extensively revised the process for the exclusion and deportation of aliens. Exclusion and deportation proceedings are now consolidated as "removal proceedings." Some forms of relief from deportation previously available have been eliminated or restricted. The legislation eliminates judicial review by the federal courts in many cases where it was previously available.

The laws included additional restrictions on access to public benefits, and requires practically all family-based visa applicants to submit an affidavit of support from a sponsor at 125% of the poverty level. Health-related exclusion grounds are essentially the same. However, the 1996 act adds a new ground of inadmissability for failing to provide evidence of vaccination against "vaccine-preventable diseases," including mumps, measles, rubella, polio, tetanus and diphtheria toxoids, pertussis, influenza type B and hepatitis B, and any other vaccinations recommended by the Advisory Committee for Immunization Practices.

The emphasis of the 1996 legislation was on increased enforcement to prevent illegal immigration and to facilitate the deportation of criminal immigrants. Attempts to reduce legal immigration in the same bill failed. Most Congressional members wanted to deal with the issue of illegal immigration separately from that of legal immigration. Efforts to pass a bill with reductions in legal immigration will likely occur in the future.

Contrary to common belief, legal immigration actually declined in 1994, the largest drop in 15 years, according to an INS news release of June 29, 1995 ("Immigration's Waning Tides"). Although by 1994, the foreign-born population of the United States reached 22 million, the percentage of the population that is foreign born (8% in 1990) is much lower than its historical high, and considerably lower than in many other countries (Passel & Fix, 1994, p. 153). From 1870 to 1920, almost 15% of the U.S. population were immigrants, nearly double the current percentage (Passel & Fix, 1994, p. 153). Although immigrants have been accused of being a drain on U.S. tax dollars, substantial research has shown that immigrants have contributed in tax dollars more than they take out in benefits (Wheeler, 1996, p. 124).

Immigration will remain an issue in the foreseeable future. As of January 17, 1997, 19 immigration-related bills have been intro-duced in Congress, including a bill to deny citizenship to children born in the United States whose parents are not citizens or permanent resident aliens ("New Bills May Indicate an Active 105th Congress on Immigration," 1997). The history of immigration law has shown that Congress is often inclined to legislate as the result of public scapegoating of immigrants. Recent Congressional action is no exception.

References

Balanced Budget Act restores immigrant eligibility for certain public benefits. (1997). *Interpreter Releases, 74,* 1290.

Calavita, K. (1994). U.S. immigration and policy responses: The limits of legislation. In W. A. Cornelius, P. L. Martin, & J. F. Hollifield (Eds.), *Controlling immigration: A global perspective* (pp. 55–82). Stanford, CA: Stanford University Press.

Chuman, F. F. (1976). *The bamboo people: The law and Japanese-Americans.* Del Mar, CA: Publisher's.

Clinton vows more immigration enforcement, bills introduced in Congress. (1995). *Interpreter Releases, 72,* 169.

Dixon, E. H., & Galan, M. A. (1990). *The Immigration and Naturalization Service.* New York: Chelsea House.

Druhot, D. M. (1986). Immigration laws excluding aliens on the basis of health: A reassessment after AIDS. *Journal of Legal Medicine, 7,* 85–112.

Espenoza, C. M. (1994). The illusory promise of sanctions: The Immigration Reform and Control Act of 1986. *Georgetown Immigration Law Journal, 8,* 343–389.

Fuchs, L. H. & Forbes, S. S. (1981). Immigration and U.S. history—The evolution of the open society. In T. A. Aleinikoff, D. A. Martin, & H. Motomura (Eds.), *Immigration: Process and policy* (3rd ed., pp. 41–61). St. Paul, MN: West.

Gordon, C., Mailman, S., & Yale-Loehr, S. (1997). *Immigration Law and Procedure.* Albany, NY: Bender.

Harper, E. J. (1975). *Immigration laws of the United States.* Indianapolis, IN: Bobbs-Merrill.

Helton, A. C. (1984). Political asylum under the Refugee Act: An unfulfilled promise. *University of Michigan Journal of Law Reform, 17,* 243–264.

Hull, E. (1985). *Without justice for all.* Westport, CT: Greenwood.

Hutchinson, E. P. (1981). *Legislative history of American immigration policy, 1798–1965.* Philadelphia: University of Pennsylvania Press.

Immigration's waning tides. (1995). *Bender's Immigration Bulletin, 1,* 6.

Jacobson, D. (1996). *Rights across borders: Immigration and the decline of citizenship.* Baltimore: The Johns Hopkins University Press.

Keely, C. B. (1993). The United States of America: Retaining a fair immigration policy. In D. Kubat (Ed.), *The politics of migration policies: Settlement and integration, the first world in the 1990s* (pp. 60–84). New York: Center for Migration Studies.

Knapp, K. K. (1996). The rhetoric of exclusion: The art of drawing a line between aliens and citizens. *Georgetown Immigration Law Journal, 10,* 401–440.

Konvitz, M. R. (1953). *Civil rights in immigration.* Ithaca, NY: Cornell University Press.

Lawson, M. & Grin, M. (1992). The Immigration Act of 1990. *Harvard International Law Journal, 33,* 255–276.

Lindt, M. (1997). The 1996 Immigration Act: Public benefits restrictions, the elderly, and citizenship. *Interpreter Releases, 74,* 101–114.

Lopez, G. P. (1981). Undocumented Mexican immigration: In search of a just immigration policy. *UCLA Law Review, 28,* 615–714.

Lopez, I. F. H. (1996). *White by Law: The legal construction of race.* New York: New York University Press.

Meier, M. S. & Ribera, F. (1993). *Mexican Americans/American Mexicans: From conquistadors to Chicanos.* New York: Hill and Wang.

Nelson, B. A. (1994). *America balkanized: Immigration's challenge to government.* Monterey, VA: The American Immigration Control Foundation.

New bills may indicate an active 105th Congress on immigration. (1997). *Interpreter Releases, 74,* 147.

Osuna, J. P. (1993). The exclusion from the United States of aliens infected with the AIDS virus: Recent developments and prospects for the future. *Houston Journal of International Law, 16,* 1–41.

Passel, J., & Fix, M. (1994). Myths about immigrants. *Foreign Policy, 95,* 151–161.

Passel, J., & Woodward, K. (1989). *Immigration to the United States* (Rev. ed.). Washington, DC: U.S. Bureau of the Census.

Presidential candidates hold range of views on immigration. (1996). *Interpreter Releases, 73,* 264.

Salyer, L. E. (1995). *Laws harsh as tigers.* Chapel Hill: University of North Carolina Press.

Select Commission on Immigration and Refugee Policy (SCIRP). (1979). *U.S. immigration law and policy: 1952–1979.* Washington, DC: U.S. Government Printing Office.

Seller, M. S. (1983). Historical perspectives on American immigration policy: Case studies and current implications. *Law and Contemporary Problems, 45,* 137–162.

States' early response to welfare reform reveals variety, confusion. (1996). *Interpreter Releases, 73,* 1432.

U.S. Committee for Refugees. (1995). *1995 World Refugee Survey.* Washington, DC: Immigration and Refugee Services of America.

United States Statutes at Large:

Act of June 25, ch. 58, 1 Stat. 570 (1798).
Act of July 6, ch. 66, 1 Stat. 577 (1798).
Act of July 4, ch. 246, 13 Stat. 385 (1864).
Act of March 3, ch. 141, 18 Stat. 477 (1875).
Act of June 7, ch. 11, 21 Stat. 5 (1879).
Act of May 6, ch. 126, 22 Stat. 58 (1882).
Act of August 3, ch. 376, 22 Stat. 214 (1882).
Act of February 26, ch. 164, 23 Stat. 332 (1885).
Act of February 23, ch. 220, 24 Stat. 414 (1887).
Act of October 19, ch. 1210, 25 Stat. 565 (1888).
Act of March 3, ch. 551, 26 Stat. 1084 (1891).
Act of March 3, ch. 1012, 32 Stat. 1213 (1903).
Act of April 27, ch. 1630, 33 Stat. 394, 428 (1904).
Act of February 20, ch. 1134, 34 Stat. 898 (1907).
Act of February 5, ch. 29, 39 Stat. 874 (1917).
Act of April 16, ch. 55, 40 Stat. 531 (1918).
Act of May 19, ch. 8, 42 Stat. 5 (1921).
Act of May 26, ch. 190, 43 Stat. 153 (1924).
Act of June 25, ch. 647, 62 Stat. 1009 (1948).
Act of June 16, ch. 262, 64 Stat. 219 (1950).
Act of June 27, ch. 477, 66 Stat. 163 (1952).
Act of August 7, ch. 336, 67 Stat. 400 (1953).
Act of October 3, Pub. L. No. 89-236, 79 Stat. 911 (1965).
Act of October 5, Pub. L. No. 95-412, 92 Stat. 907 (1978).
Act of March 17, Pub. L. No. 96-212, 94 Stat. 102 (1980).
Act of November 6, Pub. L. No. 99-603, 100 Stat. 3359 (1986).
Act of July 11, Pub. L. No. 100-71, 101 Stat. 391, 475 (1987).
Act of November 29, Pub. L. No. 101-649, 104 Stat. 4978 (1990).
Act of April 24, Pub. L. No. 104-132, 110 Stat. 1214 (1996).
Act of August 22, Pub. L. No. 104-193, 110 Stat. 2105 (1996).
Act of September 30, Pub. L. No. 104-208, 110 Stat. 3009 (1996).

U.S. Commission on Civil Rights. (1980). *The tarnished golden door: Civil Rights issues in immigration.* Washington, DC: U.S. Government Printing Office.

Varma, J. K. (1996). Eugenics and immigration restriction: Lessons for tomorrow. *Journal of the American Medical Association, 275,* 734–737.

Wheeler, C. (1996). Immigrant sponsorship and public benefits. In R. Patrick Murphy and Associates (Eds.), *Introducing the 1996 Immigration Reform Act* (pp. 123–154). Washington DC: American Immigration Lawyers Association.

2

Defining the Immigrant

SANA LOUE

Introduction

A large literature has developed relating to immigrants' health status, their access to care, and their economic impact on systems of care. All too often, though, researchers have failed to define the people they are discussing. As an example, consider refugees. When speaking of refugees' health status and health services utilization in the United States, is one discussing individuals who self-identify as refugees? Individuals who have legally been admitted to the United States as refugees at the time of their entry? Individuals who have colorable status as refugees under international law, but may or may not qualify as refugees under the laws of the country that they have entered or to which they are destined?

This chapter considers the need for greater precision in our definitions of our study populations. It provides varying definitions of who is and who is not an immigrant in a number of different contexts. The chapter is intended primarily as a reference for researchers who are attempting to better define their study population and refine their hypotheses, but may also prove useful to clini-cians who must determine their patients' eligiblity for various publicly funded medical benefit programs.

Background

The Social Science Definition

The *International Encyclopedia of the Social Sciences* (Sills, 1968) has defined migration as "the relatively permanent movement of persons over a significant distance" (Vol. 10, p. 286). Various other definitions have been offered, including the following:

> We define migration as the physical transition of an individual, or a group from one society to another. This transition usually involves abandoning one social setting and entering a different one. (Eisenstadt, 1955, p. 1)

> Migration is a relatively permanent moving away of . . . migrants, from one geographical location to another, preceded by decision-making on the part of the migrants on the basis of a hierarchically ordered set of values or valued ends and resulting in changes in the interactional set of migrants. (Mangalam, 1968, p. 8)

> Migration is defined as a permanent or semipermanent change of residence. (Lee, 1966, p. 49)

What these definitions seem to indicate is that all individuals who have relocated across national boundaries, whether temporarily or permanently, whether voluntarily or involuntarily, whether repetitively or on a single oc-

SANA LOUE • Department of Epidemiology and Biostatistics, School of Medicine, Case Western Reserve University, Cleveland, Ohio 44106-4945.

Handbook of Immigrant Health, edited by Loue. Plenum Press, New York, 1998.

casion, and for whatever purpose, may be considered immigrants. Herein lies the root of our imprecision and lack of clarity.

It is difficult to distinguish between a temporary sojourn and a more permanent one. A Mexican tourist entering through San Ysidro, California, from Tijuana for a day of shopping is clearly a temporary sojourner. Someone who enters the United States intending to remain permanently and who does remain permanently clearly falls at the other end of this temporary–permanent spectrum. But what of the foreign student who enters for a few years only, intending all the while to return to his or her country? Is that student to be considered an immigrant in the context of research relating to "immigrants"? Once an individual is an "immigrant," is he or she always an "immigrant," regardless of the number of years of residence or the strength of attachment to one's new country of residence? Does status as an immigrant in one's new country ever end?

Similar difficulties attend the identification of the refugee. The *International Encyclopedia of the Social Sciences* (Sills, 1968) defines a refugee as

> an involuntary migrant, a victim of politics, war, or natural catastrophe. Every refugee is naturally a migrant, but not every migrant is a refugee. A migrant is one who leaves his residence (usually for economic reasons) in order to settle elsewhere, either in his own or in another country. A refugee movement results when the tensions leading to migration are so acute that what at first seemed to be a voluntary movement becomes virtually compulsory. The uprooted become either internal refugees, that is, "national refugees" (persons who have been displaced in their own country), or "international refugees" (persons outside of their country of origin).

At what point in this relocation process does an individual become a refugee, for example, at the point of departure from his or her native country, or at the point of entry into the new one, or at the decision-making phase, which preceded any actual physical movement? At what point does he or she cease to be a refugee? This is also unclear.

> There are no generally accepted criteria to determine when a refugee ceases to be a refugee. Proposed criteria include: when the refugee is earning a living and has found a permanent place to live; when he has acquired a new nationality and has obtained equal rights with the inhabitants of the country of asylum or resettlement; and both criteria together. (Sills, 1968, Vol. 13, p. 362).

These criteria bring us back to our starting point. What is permanent? Is permanency to be judged by a subjective or an objective standard, or by both, for example, whether the individual feels permanently resettled or whether he or she has been granted legal permission to remain in the country indefinitely?

The Legal Definition

Immigrants under Immigration Law

Legal definitions are equally confusing. Consider the United States's definition of "immigrant" pursuant to immigration law.

First, our laws essentially divide the world into two categories: citizens and aliens. Citizens are those individuals who were born in the United States, who derived citizenship from a parent, or who acquired citizenship through the process of naturalization. All who are not citizens are aliens.

Those who are aliens are further classified as immigrants and nonimmigrants. Immigrants are those individuals who have been granted permanent or conditional residence status based on specific familial relationships recognized in the law, such as the spouse of a U.S. citizen, or based on specific employment. "Nonimmigrant" encompasses those individuals who have entered the United States, in most cases, for a temporary period, and who intend to return to their countries of origin, such as journalists, professional athletes, and so on. A nonimmigrant within the legal definition of the term, such as a student or a guest worker, may, in fact, be classifiable as an immigrant in the social science definition. Tables 1 and 2 provide brief summaries of the categories of persons classified as immigrants and nonimmigrants under our current immigration laws.

Other situations exist in which an individual's status is not clearly defined. An individual may have entered the United States, for example, self-identifying as an asylee or refugee. However, he or she may not be a refugee or asylee within the legal definition. In the United States, status as a refugee requires that (1) the individual be physically outside of his or her country of nationality or of last habitual residence if he or she does not have a country of nationality; (2) the individual be unwilling or unable to return to that country or be unwilling or unable to avail him- or herself of the protection of that country because of persecution or a well-founded fear of persecution; and (3) the persecution or well-founded fear of persecution is based on race, religion, nationality, membership in a particular social group, or political opinion. Recent legislation provides that the following individuals are also to be considered refugees:

> [A] person who has been forced to abort a pregnancy or to undergo involuntary sterilization, or who has been persecuted for failure or refusal to undergo such procedure or other resistance to a coercive population program shall be deemed to have been persecuted on account of political opinion, and a person who has a well-founded fear that he or she will be forced to undergo such a procedure or subject to persecution for such failure, refusal or resistance shall be deemed to have a well-founded fear of persecution on account of political opinion. (Illegal Immigration Reform and Responsibility Act 1996, Section 601).

An individual who is successful with an application for refugee status is admitted to the United States as a refugee. An asylee

TABLE 1. Nonimmigrant Visa Categories

Category	General description
A	Diplomatic or consular officers, their family members and personal employees
B-1	Visitors for business
B-2	Visitors for pleasure
C	Aliens in continuous and immediate transit
D	Crewmen
E	Treaty traders, treaty investors, and their family members
F	Students, their spouses, and their minor children
G	Certain representatives of foreign governments, their immediate family members, and their personal servants and employees
H-1A	Registered nurses
H-1B	Specialty occupations
H-2A	Agricultural labor or services
H-2B	Temporary labor or services, excluding graduates of medical schools coming to the United States to perform services as members of the medical profession
H-3	Trainees, seeking other than graduate medical education or training
I	Media representatives
J	Exchange visitors, their spouses, and minor children
K	Fiancé(e) of a United States citizen and his or her minor children
L	Manager, executive of certain companies, or holder of specialized knowledge, with spouse and children
M	Vocational students, spouses, and minor children
N	Parents and children of certain special immigrants
O	Aliens with extraordinary ability in the sciences, arts, education, business or athletics, their assistants, and spouses and children
P	Certain athletes, artists, and entertainment groups, their spouses and children
Q	Participants in certain international cultural exchange programs
R	Religious workers and their spouses and children

TABLE 2. Immigrant Visa Categories

Category	Description
	Family-based immigration
Immediate relatives	Spouses, parents, and unmarried minor children of United States citizens; children born abroad to aliens lawfully admitted for permanent residence during a temporary visit abroad
First preference	Unmarried sons and daughters of U.S. citizens
Second preference	Unmarried sons and daughters and spouses of permanent resident aliens
Third preference	Married sons and daughters of U.S. citizens
Fourth preference	Brothers and sisters of U.S. citizens
	Employment-based immigration
First preference	Certain aliens with extraordinary ability in the sciences, arts, education, business, or athletics; outstanding professors and researchers; certain multinational executives and managers
Second preference	Members of the professions holding advanced degrees or aliens of exceptional ability
Third preference	Skilled workers, professionals, and other workers

must meet the same requirements as a refugee; the difference is that an asylee is in the United States at the time of his or her application and a person applying for refugee status is outside of the United States at the time of his or her application. An individual who has applied for asylum but has not yet been adjudicated an asylee by the Immigration and Naturalization Service or an immigration judge is not an immigrant within the legal definition. Nor, however, is he or she necessarily a nonimmigrant. He or she might, for instance, have entered the United States illegally.

It is also important to distinguish between those individuals who are documented and undocumented. Being documented is not synonymous with being in the United States legally. Individuals who have entered the United States illegally or who have violated the terms of their status, such as a tourist who engages in employment, are considered to be undocumented. In the case of an applicant for asylum, for example, an individual may be in the United States with documentation, but may not have legal status. The individual may have received authorization from the INS to remain in this country (documented presence) while awaiting a final determination on the application for asylum

(legal status). Attempts to distinguish between "legal" and "illegal" aliens are often misguided, in that the legality of an individual's presence in the United States may be determined only by an immigration judge or a judge of a higher court who is reviewing the original judicial determination (Loue, 1992). Table 3 summarizes categories of persons classified as citizens and as documented and undocumented aliens under current immigration law.

Clearly, an individual who may be considered an immigrant within the social science definition of the term, such as a long-term student or a self-identified refugee, may not be an immigrant in the legal meaning of the term. Public benefit law adds yet another level of complexity and confusion.

Immigrants under Public Benefit Law

Consider, now, the situation of noncitizens in the context of publicly funded medical care. Those who are considered "immigrants" for the purpose of benefit eligibility under public welfare laws are not necessarily considered "immigrants" under immigration law. In addition, categories of eligibility for public benefits, including publicly funded health care, have changed over time.

TABLE 3. Classification of Individuals as Citizens and as Documented or Undocumented Noncitizens of the United States[c]

United States citizens	Noncitizens of the United States	
	Documented	Undocumented
Persons born in the United States	Lawfully admitted permanent resident ("green card" holder)	Individuals who have entered the United States illegally
Persons born outside of the United States after 12/12/52 and before 11/14/86 to one U.S. citizen parent; second parent may be citizen or noncitizen; U.S. citizen parent resided in the U.S. for at least 10 years prior to birth of respondent, at least 5 of which were after parent was 14 years old.	Individuals admitted as refugees	Individuals who entered the United States legally, but violated the terms of their visa.[b] This can include employment without authorization, changing employers without authorization, failing to attend school if admitted as a student, committing a crime, or overstaying the length of time granted to stay in the U.S.
	Nonimmigrants who have not done anything to violate that status and who entered legally (e.g., tourists, students, journalists)	
Persons born outside of the United States after 11/14/86 to one U.S. citizen parent, second parent may be citizen or noncitizen of U.S.; U.S. citizen parent resided in U.S. for at least 5 years before birth of respondent, at least 2 of which were after parent was 14 years old.	Individuals granted an extraordinary administrative immigration remedy (parole, deferred action, extended voluntary departure)[a]	
	Individuals who have applied for legal status under the amnesty or special agricultural worker programs, whose applications are pending[a]	
Persons born outside of U.S. and its territories to parents both of whom are U.S. citizens; one parent resided in U.S. prior to respondent's birth.		
Individuals who obtained U.S. citizenship through the process of naturalization.		
Individuals who obtained citizenship through the naturalization of their parent(s).		

[a] Individuals in these categories may possess documentation of their status, but a determination regarding the legality of their presence may be pending. They could ultimately be found to be in the U.S. illegally.
[b] These individuals may appear to be both documented and legally present in the U.S. In fact, their documentation is no longer valid and their presence is no longer legal.
[c] Adapted from Loue, S., & Foerstel, J. (1966). Assessing immigration status and eligibility for publicly funded medical care: A questionnaire for public health professionals. *American Journal of Public Health, 86,* 1623–1625. Printed with the permission of the American Public Health Association.

Medicaid is a joint federal–state program that provides reimbursement for doctors' services, hospital care, and prescription drugs to qualifying providers for services rendered to eligible recipients (Social Security Act, 1988, as amended). Prior to the adoption of the Personal Responsibility and Work Opportunity Reconciliation Act of 1996, federal law provided for such reimbursements for otherwise eligible individuals who were categorically eligible, such as those receiving assistance under the former Aid to Families with Dependent Children (AFDC) program. Other persons, known as the medically needy, could receive benefits under Medicaid if they could meet the requirements imposed by their state. Medically needy individuals were those who could pay for life's basic necessities, but who could not afford the cost of required medical care (*DeJesus v. Perales,* 1985). However, federal law limited payments to states under Medicaid for nonemergency medical assistance to those aliens who were "lawfully admitted for permanent residence or otherwise permanently residing in the United States under color of law" (42 U.S.C. section 1396b(v)). Already, then, if we are doing a study on the financial impact of immigrants on the state publicly funded medical programs, we see that, depending on the specifics of the study, we may have to distinguish between these categories of immigrants and all others and between emergency and nonemergency medical services.

The statute further provided that payments would be made for the provision of emergency medical services to all otherwise eligible aliens, regardless of status, if the care provided was not related to an organ transplant. "Emergency medical condition" was defined as

> a medical condition (including emergency labor and delivery) manifesting itself by acute symptoms of sufficient severity (including severe pain) such that the absence of immediate medical attention could reasonably be expected to result in
>> (A) placing the patient's health in serious jeopardy.

> (B) serious impairment to bodily functions. or
> (C) serious dysfunction of any bodily part or organ. (42 U.S.C. section 1396b(v)(3))

The category of aliens "permanently residing in the United States under color of law" is not a recognized status within the context of immigration law, but is a construct of public benefit law. This "color of law" or PRUCOL category specifically excludes individuals classified as nonimmigrants under the immigration law, such as students and tourists. An individual may, however,

> be eligible for Medicaid if the individual is an alien residing in the United States with the knowledge and permission of the Immigration and Naturalization Service (INS) and the INS does not contemplate enforcing the alien's departure. The INS does not contemplate enforcing an alien's departure if it is the policy or practice of INS not to enforce the departure of aliens in the same category, or if from all the facts and circumstances in a particular case it appears that INS is otherwise permitting the alien to reside in the United States indefinitely, as determined by verifying the alien's status with the INS. (42 C.F.R.sections 435.408(a), 436.408(a))

The following categories of individuals were considered PRUCOL:

(1) refugees and conditional entrants;
(2) parolees, including Cuban/Haitian entrants;
(3) aliens whose residence in the United States had been permitted on the basis of an indefinite stay of deportation;
(4) aliens who received indefinite voluntary departure;
(5) aliens who were the beneficiaries of an immediate relative petition, who were entitled to voluntary departure, and whose departure the INS did not contemplate enforcing;
(6) aliens who "properly filed" an aplication for adjustment of status and whose departure the INS was not enforcing;
(7) aliens granted a stay of deportation, whether by court order, statute, regulation, or administrative action;
(8) aliens granted political asylum;
(9) aliens granted voluntary departure;
(10) aliens granted deferred status;
(11) aliens who resided in the United States pursuant to an order of supervision;
(12) aliens who were eligible for registry;
(13) aliens granted suspension of deportation and whose departure the INS was not enforcing;

(14) aliens who received withholding of deportation; and

(15) "[a]ny other alien living in the United States with the knowledge and permission of the Immigration and Naturalization service and whose departure that agency does not contemplate enforcing." (42 C.F.R. section 435.408(b))

A glossary defining each of these categories is provided at the end of this chapter.

Again, these categories of eligibility for Medicaid are not synonomous with classification as a documented or undocumented immigrant. Table 4 provides a listing of documented and undocumented classes of individuals entitled to Medicaid benefits under the laws that predated the Personal Responsibility and Work Opportunity Reconciliation Act of 1996.

The Personal Responsibility and Work Opportunity Reconciliation Act of 1996, however, changed eligibility criteria for publicly funded medical benefits substantially. This, again, has implications for studies relating to access to care, the fiscal impact of aliens' receipt of medical benefits, and health-seeking behavior, to name but a few areas. Table 5 summarizes which groups of aliens are eligible for emergency and nonemergency medicaid benefits under this legislation.

Federally funded medical benefits, with certain exceptions, are available only to "qualified aliens." The PRUCOL category has been eliminated. "Qualified" aliens are those who

(1) have been admitted to the United States for permanent residence;

(2) have been granted asylum status;

(3) have been admitted to the United States as refugees;

(4) have been paroled into the United States for 1 year or more;

(5) have received withholding of deportation; and

(6) have been granted conditional entry pursuant to the law in effect prior to April 1, 1980. (Personal Responsibility and Work Opportunity Reconciliation Act of 1996).

Certain battered spouses and children are also to be considered "qualified aliens."

If the medical assistance, however, constitutes a means-tested benefit whereby the alien is ineligible for assistance unless he or she establishes financial eligibility, for example, income or assets below a predesignated level, new "qualified aliens," with certain exceptions, are ineligible to receive that benefit for a period of 5 years from the date of entry into the United States. This applies to most aliens who entered the United States on or after August 22, 1996. An exception is provided for (1) aliens admitted as refugees; (2) aliens who have been granted asylum; (3) aliens who have received withholding of deportation; (4) aliens who are lawful residents in a state and are veterans who have been discharged with an honorable discharge; (5) aliens who are lawful residents in a state and are on active duty, other than for training, in the United States Armed Forces; and (6) aliens who are lawful residents in a state and are the spouse or unmarried dependent children of an individual in category (4) or (5) above (Personal Responsibility and Work Opportunity Reconciliation Act of 1996). The 5-year bar, then, will apply to certain parolees and to permanent resident aliens who are not veterans, service members, or their family members, and to permanent residents who were not asylees or refugees. The bar does not apply to emergency Medicaid, the immunization services described in the next paragraph, and short-term, noncash, in-kind, emergency relief.

The following services are available to any alien, regardless of his or immigration status:

(1) medical services required to treat an emergency medical condition that is not related to an organ transplant procedure and

(2) public health assistance for immunizations and for the testing and treatment of symptoms of communicable diseases, even if it is later found that these symptoms are not caused by the communicable disease. (Section 401(b)(1)(A))

The new legislation did not change the definition of "emergency." However, the House and the Senate conferees attempted to clarify its application by noting that such care was to encompass only "medical care that is strictly of an emergency nature, such as medical care administered in an emergency room, critical

TABLE 4. Listing of Documented and Undocumented Classes of Individuals Entitled by Law to Medicaid Benefits, if Otherwise Eligible, by Immigration Status, Prior to Effective Date of the Personal Responsibility and Work Opportunity Reconciliation Act of 1996[c]

U.S. citizens	Individuals entitled to full scope Medicaid		Individuals entitled to emergency/ labor and delivery services only	
	Documented	Undocumented	Documented	Undocumented
All	Lawfully permanent residents ("green card" holders) Asylees[a] Refugees[a] Grantees of deferred action[a] Recipients of extended voluntary departure[a,b] Grantees of suspension of deportation[a] Grantees of a stay of deportation[a,b] Individuals who have filed an application for adjustment of status and whose departure the INS does not contemplate enforcing[a,b] Individuals who are the beneficiaries of an approved immigration petition filed on their behalf by a U.S. citizen spouse, parent, or child over the age of 21 and whose departure is not being enforced by INS[a,b] Recipients of parole (special permission) to enter the U.S.[a]	All other individuals whose presence is known to the INS, who intend to reside in the U.S. permanently, and whose departure the INS does not contemplate enforcing[a,b]	Nonimmigrants, such as tourists, students, journalists, businesspersons	Individuals who entered the U.S. illegally Individuals who entered the U.S. legally but violated their immigration status

[a] Individuals who are not U.S. citizens or permanent residents but whose immigration status entitles them to full scope Medicaid coverage, if they are otherwise eligible for Medicaid, are known in public benefits law as individuals "permanently residing under color of law" (PRUCOL).

[b] Note that these classes of persons are documented. However, the ultimate legality of their continuing presence in the United States has yet to be determined.

[c] Adapted from Loue, S., & Foerstel, J. (1966). Assessing immigration status and eligibility for publicly funded medical care: A questionnaire for public health professionals. *American Journal of Public Health, 86,* 1623–1625. Printed with the permission of the American Public Health Association.

care unit, or intensive care unit" (Conference Report, 1996, 379–380).

The statute further grants states the authority to determine the eligibility for state public benefits of qualified aliens, nonimmigrants, and aliens paroled into the United States for less than a year. Qualified aliens, as defined previously, are eligible for any state publicly funded medical benefits. The exceptions established to the noneligibility under federally funded medical assistance programs apply, as well, in the context of state-funded medical assistance programs (Personal Responsibility and Work Opportunity Reconciliation Act of 1996).

Methodological Implications

The preferred definition of "immigrant" that the researcher uses necessarily depends on the nature and objectives of the study, the time period under study, and the specific target population. Changes in definitions of immigrants and public benefit criteria over time must be considered in any study evaluating trends, such as health care costs, or studies examining individual behavior, such as health care seeking. Consider reliance on databases as one example of situations in which these issues may arise.

Census data can provide the basis for studies of the relationship between wages and immigrant experience (Jasso & Rosenzweig, 1990), between English ability and time in the United States (Jasso & Rosenzweig, 1990), and between wages, English ability, and length of time in the United States (Chiswick & Miller, 1992). This is possible because each census enumerates all foreign-born residents in the United States on April 1 of the year for which the census is conducted and provides basic information that can be used to estimate the number of years that individuals have been in the United States, wages earned, and English language ability (Lindstrom & Massey, 1994).

Numerous difficulties, however, attend reliance on census data. The census data may seriously undercount individuals who are undocumented, that is, individuals who are immigrants in the social science context but are not immigrants in the legal meaning of the term and who have no legal authorization to be present in the United States. Passel's (1985) estimates of the 1980 census results indicate that 20%–40% of undocumented individuals were not counted in that census. Studies relying on that census data as inclusive of all "immigrants" would, consequently, be inaccurate.

Additionally, census data, not surprisingly, does not provide information relating to legal status. Consequently, all immigrants are treated as an homogenous group, when there may actually exist significant differences between groups, due to the nonrandom distribution of certain characteristics among immigrant groups, such as residence in multifamily households (de la Puente, 1992). This inability to control for immigration status through either restriction or analysis may result in seriously biased results, depending on the nature and design of the study.

Similar difficulties attend the use of records for studies related to refugees. Presumably, the potential sampling frame that can be constructed will be larger if the study is to focus on all individuals who are refugees within the social science meaning of the term, as compared with the legal meaning, that is, those who have been legally admitted with the legal status of refugee. The appropriateness of relying on either definition as the basis for constructing a sampling frame will depend, again, on the purpose of the study. A study focusing on the economic impact of refugee use of emergency medical care or health-seeking behaviors will more likely rely on the expansive definition of refugee, in view of the fact that all aliens, regardless of legal status, are potentially eligible under public benefit law for emergency medical assistance. In either of these studies, it would be advisable to control for legal status, as there may be significant differences related to delay in presentation and consequent cost and duration of care. Reliance on the legal definition of refugee, how-

TABLE 5. Listing of Documented and Undocumented Classes of Individuals Entitled by Law to Medicaid Benefits, if Otherwise Eligible, by Immigration Status, Pursuant to the Personal Responsibility and Work Opportunity Reconciliation Act of 1996 and the Illegal Immigration Reform and Immigrant Responsibility Act of 1996

| U.S. citizens | Individuals entitled to full scope Medicaid | | Individuals entitled to emergency/ labor and delivery services only | |
	Documented	Undocumented	Documented	Undocumented
All	Lawfully admitted permanent residents ("green card" holders)[a]	None	Lawfully admitted permanent residents ("green card" holders) who are subject to 5-year bar	Individuals who entered the U.S. illegally
	Asylees		Nonimmigrants, such as students and journalists	Individuals who entered the U.S. legally but violated their immigration status
	Refugees		Applicants for asylum	
	Parolees admitted for 1 year or more		Applicants for registry	
	Recipients of withholding of deportation		Applicants for adjustment of status	
	Conditional entrants pursuant to law prior to April 1, 1980		Recipients of deferred action	
	Certain battered spouses and children		Recipients of temporary protected status (TPS)	
			Individuals subject to an order of supervision	
			Recipients of status under family unit	

[a] Subject to 5-year bar from date of entry into the United States, except for certain veterans and active duty members of the armed services, and permanent residents who were refugees or asylees.

ever, may be more appropriate in constructing a sampling frame to examine refugee utilization of nonprofit community clinic mental health services, where such services are provided only to those with documented refugee status, and the clinic receives state or federal funding for services rendered to documented refugees. Any such study, of course, must be cognizant of changes in the legal definition of "refugee" that have occurred over time and must consider whether such changes are reflected in the agency's compilation of refugee patients.

Consequently, it is not surprising that agency records based on patient self-identification or screening by staff may yield a less than complete sample. Agencies often do not maintain lists of clients or patients with immigration status. An individual may be reluctant to self-identify as nonnative due to distrust of the investigators (Lipson & Meleis, 1989), fear of stigmatization, fear of the potential immigration consequences (Lipson & Meleis, 1989), or a feeling or belief that he or she is no longer an immigrant.

Glossary

Adjustment of status. Adjustment of status is a process whereby an individual already within the United States can change his or her status from one of the nonimmigrant categories to become a conditional or permanent resident of the United States. Specific procedures must be followed to effectuate this change.

Deferred status. Deferred status is an administrative remedy available through the Immigration and Naturalization Service to delay the removal from the United States of the individual granted the remedy. It is considered an extraordinary remedy. It is generally not available to individuals who have other remedies under immigration law. Applicants are generally required to demonstrate that extreme hardship would result if they were to be removed from the United States

and that they are persons of good moral character, i.e., no criminal record.

Immediate relative petition. Under immigration law, certain categories of individuals are considered "immediate relatives" for the purpose of becoming permanent residents. These individuals are not subject to a quota requirement. Immediate relatives include spouses and parents of United States citizens over the age of 21, and United States citizens' unmarried children who are under the age of 21.

Order of supervision. Under immigration law, an alien can be taken into custody following a determination that he or she is to be removed from the United States. If that removal (deportation) could not be effectuated within a 6-month period, the alien was required to be released under an order of supervision. The order set forth the conditions for reporting to a local officer of the Immigration and Naturalization Service.

Parole. Prior to the September 30, 1996, adoption of the Illegal Immigration Reform and Immigrant Responsibility Act of 1996, the Immigration and Naturalization Service had authority to grant entry to the United States to aliens not eligible for admission on other bases "for emergent reasons or for reasons deemed strictly in the public interest." This was a highly discretionary remedy. Effective September 30, 1996, such entry can be granted "only on a case-by-case basis for urgent humanitarian reasons or significant public benefit."

Asylum. An individual applying for asylee status must be within the United States at the time of his or her application for asylee status. If the application is successful, the applicant will be granted status as a political asylee. Status as a refugee requires that (1) the individual be physically outside of his or her country of nationality or of last habitual residence if he or she does not have a country of nationality; (2) the individual be unwilling or unable to return to that country or be unwilling or unable to avail him- or herself of the protection of that country because of persecution or a well-founded fear of persecution; and (3) the persecution or well-founded fear of persecution is based on race, religion, nationality, membership in a particular social group, or political opinion. Persons who have been forced to abort a pregnancy or to undergo involuntary sterilization, or who have been persecuted for failure or refusal to undergo such procedure or be other resistance to a coercive population program and persons who have a well-founded fear that they will be forced to undergo such a procedure or subject to persecution for such failure, refusal, or resistance are now considered refugees.

Refugee. An individual applying for refugee status must be outside of the United States at the time of his or her application for refugee status. If the application is successful, the applicant will be admitted as a refugee. Status as a refugee requires that (1) the individual be physically outside of his or her country of nationality or of last habitual residence if he or she does not have a country of nationality; (2) the individual be unwilling or unable to return to that country or be unwilling or unable to avail him- or herself of the protection of that country because of persecution or a well-founded fear of persecution; and (3) the persecution or well-founded fear of persecution is based on race, religion, nationality, membership in a particular social group, or political opinion. Persons who have been forced to abort a pregnancy or to undergo involuntary sterilization, or who have been persecuted for failure or refusal to undergo such procedure or other resistance to a coercive population program and persons who have a well-founded fear that they will be forced to undergo such a procedure or be subject to persecution for such failure, refusal, or resistance are now considered refugees.

Registry. Registry is a mechanism by which individuals who have been residing continuously in the United States since prior to January 1, 1972 can become permanent residents.

The individual must prove entry prior to that date, continuous residence since that date, and good moral character.

Stay of deportation. A stay of deportation is available either administratively through the Immigration and Naturalization Service or from an immigration judge. The remedy provides relief from expulsion from the United States for a short period only and is available in very limited circumstances.

Suspension of deportation. Suspension of deportation was a remedy available to eligible aliens prior to April 1, 1997. Suspension of deportation was available only in the context of a deportation hearing in front of an immigration judge. Eligibility required that the applicant demonstrate that (1) the applicant and/or a United States citizen or permanent resident spouse, parent, or child would suffer extreme hardship as the result of the alien's deportation; (2) the applicant had been continuously physically present in the United States for a period of at least 7 years; and (3) the applicant had maintained good moral character throughout this period of time.

Temporary protected status (TPS). TPS is an administrative remedy available from the Immigration and Naturalization Service to aliens in the United States who are from specific foreign states, as delineated by the attorney general. The attorney general may designate nationals of specific foreign states eligible for this remedy only if (1) there is an ongoing armed conflict within the foreign state and as a result of that conflict, the return of the foreign nationals to that state would seriously threaten their safety; (2) there has been a natural disaster in that foreign state which has temporarily, but substantially, disrupted living conditions and that foreign state, as a result, is unable to handle the return of its nationals, and the foreign state has requested that it be included within this designation; or (3) there are extraordinary and temporary conditions in the foreign state that prevent the foreign nationals from returning to that state in safety, in the opinion of the U.S. Attorney General.

Voluntary departure. Voluntary departure is a remedy available in the context of a hearing before an immigration judge or administratively from the Immigration and Naturalization Service. It allows the individual to leave the United States voluntarily within a designated period of time. Because the departure is voluntary, it does not preclude the individual's future admission to the United States.

Withholding of deportation. Withholding of deportation was a remedy available in the context of a deportation hearing in front of an immigration judge. Withholding of deportation withheld the deportation of an alien, otherwise deportable, because the alien's life or freedom would be threatened in the country to which he or she would be sent and that threat was due to the alien's race, religion, nationality, membership in a particular social group, or political opinion. The remedy was unavailable to aliens who had participated in the persecution of others, who had committed a particularly serious crime and were therefore considered dangerous, or those who were believed to be a threat to the security of the United States. The remedy became obsolete with the Illegal Imigration Reform and Immigrant Responsibility Act of 1996. A similar remedy, known as restriction on removal, is available instead.

Appendix

Assessment of Immigration Status and Health Benefit Eligibility

I. PLACE OF BIRTH

    A. In the United States

        1. Were you born in the United States?
        No . . . Go to question I.B.1.
        Yes . . . Go to question I.A.2.

        2. Did you give up your citizenship?

        No. . .
> United States citizen.
> Eligible for full-scope Medicaid; not subject to 5-year bar.
> Eligible for Medicare.

        Yes . . . Go to question I.B.1.

    B. Outside of the United States

        1. Were both parents United States citizens?
        No . . . Go to question I.B.3.
        Yes . . . Go to question I.B.2.

        2. Did one of your parents reside in the United States prior to your birth?
        No . . . Go to question I.B.3.

        Yes . . .
> United States citizen.
> Eligible for full-scope Medicaid; not subject to 5-year bar.
> Eligible for Medicare.

        3. Did both of your parents acquire citizenship through naturalization?
        No . . . Go to question I.B.5.
        Yes . . . Go to question I.B.4.

        4. Were you under the age of 18 and residing in the United States at the time that your parent was naturalized?
        No . . . Go to question I.B.5.

Yes . . . United States citizen.
Eligible for full-scope Medicaid; not subject to 5-year bar.
Eligible for Medicare.

5. Was one parent a United States citizen?
   No . . . Go to question II.A.1.
   Yes . . . Go to question I.B.6.

6. Were you born after 12/24/1952 and before 11/14/1986?
   No . . . Go to question I.B.8.
   Yes . . . Go to question I.B.7.

7. Did the United States parent live in the United States for at least 10 years before your birth, 5 of which were after the parent was 14 years old?
   No . . . Go to question II.A.1.

   Yes . . . United States citizen.
   Eligible for full-scope Medicaid; not subject to 5-year bar.
   Eligible for Medicare.

8. Were you born after 11/14/1986?
   No . . . Go to question II.A.1.
   Yes . . . Go to question I.B.9.

9. Did your United States parent live in the United States for at least 5 years prior to your birth, 2 of which were after the parent was 14 years old?
   No . . . Go to question I.B.10.

   Yes . . . United States citizen.
   Eligible for full-scope Medicaid; not subject to 5-year bar.
   Eligible for Medicare.

10. Were you a permanent resident who applied for and received citizenship ("naturalization") and a certificate showing that you are a United States citizen?
    No . . . Go to question I.A.11.

    Yes . . . United States citizen.
    Eligible for full-scope Medicaid; not subject to 5-year bar.
    Eligible for Medicare.

11. Were you a permanent resident who applied for and received citizenship through the Department of State and a United States passport showing that you are a United States citizen?
    No . . . Go to question II.A.1.

    Yes . . . United States citizen.
    Eligible for full-scope Medicaid; not subject to 5-year bar.
    Eligible for Medicare.

II. CURRENT STATUS

A. Permanent Residence

1. Do you have lawful permanent residence ("green card," "mica")?
   No . . . Go to question II.B.1.

   Yes . . . Documented (permanent resident).
   Eligible for full-scope Medicaid and Medicare.
   May be subject to 5-year bar on receipt of benefits under federal programs.

B. Other Status

    1. Have you been granted status in any of the following categories: asylum, withholding of deportation, or refugee?
        No . . . Go to question II.B.2.

        Yes . . . | Documented. "Qualified alien."
                   Eligible for full-scope Medicaid. Not subject to 5-year bar. |

    2. Have you been granted status in either of the following categories: parole for 1 year or more or conditional entry under the law in effect prior to April 1, 1980?
        No . . . Go to question II.B.3.

        Yes . . . | Documented. "Qualified alien." Eligible for full scope Medicaid; probably subject to 5-year bar on receipt of benefits under federal programs. |

    3. Have you or your child been battered or subjected to extreme cruelty by a United States citizen spouse/parent, or by a member of your spouse's family, residing in the same household, with the consent or acquiescence of your spouse?
        No . . . Go to question III.A.1.

        Yes . . . | Individual may be a qualified alien if certain other requirements have been met. If a qualified alien, documented. Eligible for full-scope Medicaid; not subject to 5-year bar. |

III. POTENTIAL REMEDIES

A. Asylum

    1. Are you afraid to return to your country of origin or your country of last habitual residence?
        No . . . Go to question III.B.1.
        Yes . . . Go to question III.A.2.

    2. Are you afraid of being persecuted or have you been persecuted in your country?
        No . . . Go to question III.B.1.
        Yes. . . Go to question III.A.3.

    3. Was the persecution based on race, religion, nationality, political opinion (including refusal to abort a child or to be sterilized), or membership in a particular social group (such as a labor union, or being a homosexual, or being HIV-positive)?
        No . . . Go to question III.B.1.
        Yes . . . Go to question III.A.4.

    4. Did you persecute other people?
        No . . . Go to question III.A.5.
        Yes . . . Go to question III.B.1.

    5. Have you been convicted of a very serious crime, such as murder or drug trafficking?
        No . . . Go to question III.A.6.

        Yes . . . | Probably undocumented. Probably no immigration remedy. Eligible for emergency Medicaid only. |

    6. Have you already filed an application for asylum, which was denied?
        No . . . Go to question III.A.7.
        Yes . . . Go to question III.B.1.

7. Have you been in the United States for less than one year?
No . . . Go to question III.B.1.

Yes . . . | Individual may be documented or undocumented depending on status at entry and current status. Potentially eligible for asylum but must apply within 1 year of date of entry into United States. If individual receives asylum, he/she will be "qualified alien" and eligible for receipt of full-scope Medicaid benefits; not subject to 5-year bar.

B. Registry

1. Have you been residing in the United States continuously since before January 1, 1972?
No . . . Go to question III.C.1.
Yes . . . Go to question III.B.2.

2. Have you ever violated narcotics laws, smuggled aliens into the United States, or committed a crime?
No . . . Go to question III.B.3.
Yes . . . Go to question III.C.1.

3. Have you been convicted since 1972 of anything other than a minor traffic violation?

No . . . | Undocumented or documented depending on status at entry and current status. Potentially eligible for registry. Currently eligible for emergency Medicaid only. If receives registry, eligible for full-scope Medicaid as "qualified alien;" probably subject to 5-year bar.

Yes . . . Go to question III.C.1.

C. Family Immigration

1. Do you have a United States citizen spouse, parent, child or sibling over the age of 21 who is willing and able to petition for you to immigrate?
No . . . Go to question III.C.2.

Yes . . . | Undocumented or documented depending on status at entry and since entry. Potentially eligible for permanent residence. Currently eligible for emergency Medicaid only. Classifiable as a "qualified alien" following receipt of permanent residence; probably subject to 5-year bar.

2. Do you have a spouse who is a lawfully admitted permanent resident ("green card holder") who is willing and able to petition for you to immigrate?
No . . . Go to question III.C.3.

Yes . . . | Undocumented or documented depending on status at entry and since entry. Potentially eligible for permanent residence. Currently eligible for emergency Medicaid only. Classifiable as a "qualified alien" following receipt of permanent residence; probably subject to 5-year bar.

3. Are you unmarried, with a parent who is a lawful permanent resident ("green card holder") who is willing and able to petition for you to immigrate?
No . . . Go to question III.D.1.

Yes . . . | Undocumented or documented depending on status at entry and since entry. Potentially eligible for permanent residence. Currently eligible for emergency Medicaid only. Classifiable as a "qualified alien" following receipt of permanent residence; probably subject to 5-year bar.

D. Special Immigrants—Juveniles

1. Have you been declared a dependent of a juvenile court in the United States?
   No . . . Go to question III.E.1.
   Yes . . . Go to question III.D.2.

2. Did the court find that you are eligible for long term care?
   No . . . Go to question III.E.1.
   Yes . . . Go to question III.D.3.

3. Has a court or administrative body found that it will not be in your best interest to be returned to your original country?
   No . . . Go to question III.E.1.
   Yes . . . Probably undocumented. Currently eligible for emergency Medicaid only. Potentially eligible for permanent residence as a special immigrant. If receives status as a permanent resident, eligible for full scope Medicaid as a "qualified alien"; may be subject to 5-year bar.

E. Employment Immigration

1. Do you have a potential employer in the United States who is willing to file a petition for you to immigrate to work for him/her?
   No . . . Go to question III.F.1.
   Yes . . . Go to question III.E.2.

2. Does the employer have a real job for you to fill?
   No . . . Go to question III.F.1.
   Yes . . . Go to question III.E.3.

3. Do you have the job skills required for the job?
   No . . . Go to question III.F.1.
   Yes . . . Go to question III.E.4.

4. Are there probably United States citizens or permanent residents who are qualified to do the job that the employer would offer you and who would be willing to do that job?
   No . . . Undocumented or documented depending on status at entry and current status. Currently eligible for emergency Medicaid only. Potentially eligible for permanent residence. If receives permanent residence, potentially eligible for full-scope Medicaid as a "qualified alien"; probably subject to 5-year bar.
   Yes . . . Go to question III.F.1.

F. Cancellation of Removal for Nonlawful Permanent Residents

1. Have you been continuously physically present in the United States for a period of at least 10 years?
   No . . . Go to question III.G.1.
   Yes . . . Go to question III.F.2.

2. Have you been convicted during this time for any offense other than a minor traffic violation?
   No . . . Go to question III.F.3.
   Yes . . . Go to question III.G.1.

3. Would your removal from the United States result in exceptional and extremely unusual hardship to your United States citizen or permanent resident spouse or child?

No . . . Go to question III.G.1.

Yes . . . | Probably undocumented. Currently eligible for emergency Medicaid only. Potentially eligible for cancellation of removal. If receives cancellation, eligible for full-scope Medicaid; subject to 5-year bar. |

G. Administrative Remedies (Deferred Action, Voluntary Departure)

1. Are there particularly sympathetic factors in your situation that might convince the INS to let you stay here temporarily, such as a serious illness or the serious illness of a close relative who is a United States citizen or permanent resident?

No . . . | Probably undocumented. Currently eligible for emergency Medicaid only. No obvious immigration remedy. |

Yes . . . Go to question III.G.2.

2. Have you done anything to make the United States not want you to be here, like commit a crime, or use drugs, or abuse a spouse or child?

No . . . | Probably undocumented. Currently eligible for emergency Medicaid only. Potentially eligible for administrative immigration remedy. |

Yes . . . | Probably undocumented. Currently eligible for emergency Medicaid only. No obvious immigration remedy. |

Note. This questionnaire has not been tested for reliability. However, it is similar to one developed for use prior to the enactment of the Illegal Immigration Reform and Immigrant Responsibility Act of 1996 and the Personal Responsibility and Work Opportunity Reconciliation Act of 1996 (Loue & Foerstel, 1996).

References

Chiswick, B. R. & Miller, P. W. (1992). Language in the labor market: The immigrant experience in Canada and the United States. In B. R. Chiswick (Ed.), *Immigration, language, and ethnic issues: Canada and the United States* (pp. 229–296). Washington, DC: American Enterprise Institute.

DeJesus v. Perales, 770 F.2d 316 (2d Cir.), *cert. denied,* 478 U.S. 1007 (1985).

Eisenstadt, S. N. (1955). *The absorption of immigrants.* Glencoe, IL: Free Press.

Illegal Immigration Reform and Immigrant Responsibility Act of 1996, Pub. L. No. 104–207, 110 Stat. 3008 (October 1, 1996).

Jasso, G., & Rosenzweig, M. R. (1990). *The new chosen people: Immigrants in the United States.* New York: Sage.

Lee, E. (1966). A theory of migration. *Demography, 3,* 47–57.

Lindstrom, D. P., Massey, D. S. (1994). Selective emigration, cohort quality, and models of immigrant assimilation. *Social Science Research, 23,* 315–349.

Lipson, J.G., & Meleis, A. I. (1989). Methodological issues in research with immigrants. *Medical Anthropology, 12,* 103–115.

Loue, S. (1992). Access to health care and the undocumented alien. *Journal of Legal Medicine, 13,* 271–332.

Loue, S., & Foerstel, J. (1996). Assessing immigration status and eligibility for publicly funded medical care: A questionnaire for public health professionals. *American Journal of Public Health, 86,* 1623–1625.

Mangalam, J. J. (1969). *Human migration: A guide to migration literature in English, 1955–1962.* Lexington: University Press of Kentucky.

Passel, J. S. (1985). Undocumented immigrants: How many. In *Proceedings of the Social Statistics Section of the American Statistical Association* (pp. 65–71). Washington, DC: American Statistical Association.

Personal Responsibility and Work Opportunity Reconciliation Act of 1996, Pub. L. No. 104–193, 110 Stat. 2105 (Aug. 11, 1996).

de la Puente, M. (1992). An analysis of the underenumeration of Hispanics: Evidence from Hispanic concentrated small area ethnographic studies. In *Proceedings of the 1992 annual research conference* (pp. 45–69). Washington, DC: U.S. Department of Commerce, Bureau of the Census.

Sills, D. L. (Ed.) (1968). *International encyclopedia of the social sciences* (Vols. 10, 13). New York: Macmillan and Free Press.

42 United States Code sections 1395i-2, 1395o, 1396b(v) (1992 and Suppl. 1996).

42 Code of Federal Regulations. Section 435. 408.

3

Acculturation

LAUREN CLARK AND LISA HOFSESS

Introduction

Experienced nurses and physicians report their clinical observations that acculturation affects both health behaviors and outcomes for immigrant patients. The co-authors have frequently heard comments from both health care providers and their Mexican-origin patients about infant health beliefs and child rearing practices among unacculturated women from Mexico, which are modified through long-term residence in the United States. Professional observations often are linked with musings about the acculturation process and its unfavorable influences on the health of Mexican women and children. Such comments, rather than being dismissed as ethnic stereotyping, can be used to heighten awareness of possible acculturative differences and their relationship to health.

Clinical observations about patients' acculturation and health can be transferred to the research world for scientific investigation. Before examining acculturation and health in detail, however, the theoretical underpinnings of the concept must be understood. Throughout this chapter, most examples are drawn from the literature on Latino health and the acculturation of Mexican-origin peoples, the population with which the co-authors work and are therefore most familiar. Coincidentally, most acculturation research to date has been conducted with Latino populations. In addition, as the largest immigrant group in the United States, Latinos are predicted to continue to grow in numbers and influence into the 21st century.

Theoretical Development of the Acculturation Concept

In 1954, the Social Science Research Council defined acculturation as "culture change that is initiated by the conjunction of two or more autonomous cultural systems," evidenced through the selective adaptation of value systems, as well as integration and differentiation of knowledge and behavior among the culture groups (Broom, Sigel, Vogt, Watson, & Barnett, 1954, p. 974). This definition acknowledges that acculturation is only one type of culture change, and the stimulus for change is continuous intercultural contact. Current definitions of acculturation describe it as "essentially a continuous, dynamic process" rather than a static event (Melville, 1983; Ramirez, 1984). Often considered a group-level variable, the concept of acculturation also identifies intracultural variation among individuals who have acculturated more or less to the host culture.

The Historical Roots of Acculturation: Race and Ethnicity

In attempting to classify and categorize, scientists and laypersons alike have variously

LAUREN CLARK AND LISA HOFSESS • School of Nursing, University of Colorado Health Sciences Center, Denver, Colorado 80262.

Handbook of Immigrant Health, edited by Loue. Plenum Press, New York, 1998.

used race, ethnicity, and, more recently, acculturation, to categorize people into groups and then describe them. The practice of distinguishing human groups into races extends back at least as far as the Greeks and Romans whose cosmology conceptualized a metropolis, "a mother city," surrounded by "lands of barbarians" who were "not quite human" (Wolf, 1994, p. 4). Nonwestern tribal groups also developed schemata involving "human" in-groups and a continuum of out-groups from hostile to nonhuman. "Christendom inherited the schemata of Classical antiquity and transformed them to fit its own logic and understanding . . . the trichotomy of civilized, barbarians, and monstrous humans was transformed into one of the faithful, the unredeemed, and the unredeemable" (Wolf, 1994, pp. 2–3).

Racial systems of human classification were promoted as science by botanist Carolus Linnaeus in the early 18th century. Linnean classification divided humans into four groups, defined primarily by the four geographic regions of conventional cartography: America, Europe, Asia, and Africa. In 1795, Johann Blumenbach, a German anatomist, naturalist, and student of Linnaeus, added a fifth geographic category: Malaysian to include Polynesians, Melanesians, and Australian aborigines. Blumenbach's classification introduced a hierarchy of worth based on perceived beauty, with Caucasians at the pinnacle. Blumenbach coined the term "Caucasian" in reference to the Caucasus mountains in what is now eastern European Georgia, where Noah's ark was believed to have come to rest. He considered Noah's descendants not only the most beautiful people in the world, but the original ancestors of all humans (Wolf, 1994). Other 18th-century scholars "believed that by sorting people into physical types one could gauge their temperamental and moral dispositions" (Wolf, 1994, p. 4). During the 19th-century's colonial expansion the European victors were portrayed as "energetic, [and] dynamic, and the vanquished as backward looking, . . . retarded, and regressive" (Wolf, 1994, p. 4).

An early anthropologist, Franz Boas, opposed racial bio-moral schemata, assailing "any attempt to explain cultural form on a purely biological basis [as] doomed to failure" (Boas, 1940, p. 165). Boas introduced into anthropology the idea that both environment and genetics influence human behavior and physiology. By demonstrating that morphological characteristics, then considered purely biological or racial, changed when groups immigrated into different environments, Boas proved morphology to be plastic and thus changeable (Boas, 1922). Genetic evidence also focused attention away from racial classifications when it was determined that race accounts for only 0.012% difference in human genetic material (Lewontin, 1972).

Racial classifications gave way to the similar concepts of ethnicity and ethnic identity, based on more subtle cultural and linguistic factors. While ethnicity is defined by both objective and subjective criteria, ethnic identity is determined purely subjectively. Like race, ethnicity can be observed and ascribed. Ethnic identity, on the other hand, is only self-identified.

Ethnicity has been defined several ways. Some consider ethnicity the "self-identification and the identification by others of membership in a distinct socio-cultural group based on specific national and/or biological characteristics" (Melville, 1988, p. 76). Another position describes ethnicity as a function of cultural history and psychological identity (Melville, 1988). A third position emphasizes both culture and class, stating "ethnicity does not occur where the socio-cultural environment is homogeneous" (Melville, 1988, p. 76). Thus, ethnicity addresses not only individual cultures, but also their interconnections with the larger socioeconomic and political systems.

The *Harvard Encyclopedia of American Ethnic Groups* (Thernstrom, 1980) lists more than 100 distinct ethnic groups based on the following shared characteristics: geographic origin; migratory status; race; language or dialect; religious faith; ties that transcend kinship, neighborhood, and community; traditions, values, and symbols; literature, folklore, and music; food preferences; settlement and employment patterns; special interest with regard to politics in the homeland and the United States; institutions that specifically serve and maintain the group; internal sense of distinctiveness; and external perception of distinctiveness. Despite the long list of possible commonalties among members of an ethnic group, shared language is considered by researchers and theorists alike the primary marker of ethnicity (Macías, 1993). By extension, many scales that measure acculturation are language based. (See sections titled "Differences Between Acculturation and Other Concepts" and "Language and Generation Proxies for Acculturation of Individuals" for further discussion.)

While ethnicity contains both subjective and objective components, ethnic identity is defined by wholly subjective personal knowledge about one's group and pride in membership (Aboud & Doyle, 1993). Aboud cited three psychological components of ethnic identification: identification of self, recognition of self as different from other ethnic groups, and the perception that ethnicity is constant (Aboud, 1988). Knight, Tein, Shell, and Roosa (1993) added the ideas of role behaviors (customs, traditions, and language), and ethnic preferences and feelings. Ethnic identity persists because of enculturation, meaning socialization into the ethnic culture. All children enculturate. Ethnic minority children also must acculturate to the dominant culture, which affects their ethnic identity (Knight *et al.,* 1993).

Practical Considerations in Using Ethnic Categories

Researchers using large data sets containing prescribed ethnic categories may need to grapple with the limitations of both assigned and self-selected ethnic classification. Often, the source of the data is unknown. In many cases, subjects cannot select a meaningful label for themselves from the choices available. Whether subjects are objectively assigned to a group by a rater or interviewer or subjects choose a label to match their ethnic identity in a forced-choice situation (Evinger 1995; Stanfield, 1993) is important. Forced-choice categories are neccessarily limited in number and scope. Individuals from mixed race or mixed ethnic backgrounds find the forced-choice format restrictive because choosing one category implies denial of other aspects of one's heritage.

Standardized ethnic categories established by the U.S. government may appeal to researchers and clinicians needing quick and easy categories to identify subgroups of patients or subjects. Unfortunately, the very ease of classification can be unreliable and misleading. For governmental surveys, respondents are requested to identify themselves as either American Indian or Alaskan Native, Asian or Pacific Islander, Black, White, Hispanic, or Other. These six categories have remained unrevised since 1977 when first coined by the Office of Management and Budget [OMB], 1977.

Data tied to these ethnic categories should be used with caution, since the ethnic labels were neither defined nor selected by the people whom they allegedly describe. For example, in the San Luis Valley of southern Colorado, 57% of the residents classified by researchers as Hispanic checked the box marked "Other" when asked to categorize their ethnicity. What motivated respondents to select "Other" instead of "Hispanic"? Follow-up research revealed that these respondents traced their ancestry to the early 17th-century Spanish colonists who settled in what are now New Mexico and Colorado. They consider themselves "Spanish," a category not listed (Pappas, 1993).

Problems with the validity and reliability of ethnic reporting are exemplified by Mexican-origin populations' responses to the ethnicity categories used by the U.S. Census Bureau. Under the category "Hispanic," the Mexican-origin population is provided with three separate cues: Mexican, Mexican American, and Chicano.

In a pilot-testing phase prior to the 1990 census, interviewers uncovered significant concern and discrepancy among Latinos around issues of ethnic labeling. The following list, presented by Estrada (1993) outlines major concerns with census categories:

1. Native-born Mexican-origin persons still react negatively to the "hyphenated American category" . . . feeling that it represents marginalization.
2. Older Mexican-origin persons still react strongly to the term "Chicano," and do not like to be associated with that term . . . based on the activist groups associated with the term and what some regard as a "street language" term.
3. "Mexican" and "Mexican American" are often used by Mexican-origin persons to distinguish between Mexico-born and U.S.-born persons, although that was not the intention of the item. Thus, Mexican-born parents self-identify as Mexican, but they list their children as Mexican American if they were born in the U.S.
4. Recent analysis of a [pretested and] expanded race item . . . showed that a number of Hispanics identified themselves and their children as Asian and Pacific Islanders, having mistakenly marked the item "Laotian" in the race item, obviously confusing it for "Latino." (pp. 175–176)

In addition to the ambiguity, unintended meanings, and aversions to particular ethnic labels, politically strategic selection of ethnic categories can also discredit their utility in research and practice. For Mexican-origin individuals, the selection of the "right" label for one's ethnicity can be crucial, as Margarita Melville (1988) eloquently explains:

What is so embarrassing about being Mexican? Why would anyone want to say they were Colombian or Spanish rather than Mexican? . . . The presumption is that if you are Colombian, you came to the U.S. by airplane, could pay your own way, were somewhat sophisticated, probably of middle- or upper-class. If you are Mexican, on the other hand, the presumption is that you or your ancestors swam across the Rio Grande or climbed over the fence in California, were penniless, and have been working as unskilled or farm laborers ever since. By saying that one is Colombian, rather than Mexican, one establishes social class rather than ethnic identity. (p. 75).

In an environment of heightened suspicion toward immigrants and open hostility to their use of health and social services, strategic uses of alternative identities should be expected.

Checking a box to identify one's ethnic identity is far from a dispassionate, bureaucratic response to a seemingly factual question. It is more akin to a creative process of self-invention, status preservation, or alliance formation. Ethnic identity is not based on a defined set of characteristics central to a group's identity, but a matter of negotiation at the group's margins, with distinctions made where one group's borders "bump" up against other groups (Velez-Ibánez, 1996). "By defining and claiming an ethnic identity, individuals try to place themselves in larger currents of life, try to find a sense of destiny and purpose, and try to get out, at least momentarily, from under the burden of being isolated individuals responsible for their own self-definition and direction at every moment" (Limerick, 1995, p. 27).

As vexing as these practical impediments to valid, reliable ethnic data may be, philosophical misgivings about the enterprise of ethnic classification pose problems, as well. Standard ethnic categories are criticized for being "grounded in folk beliefs derived from precolonial era thinking about the inherent superiority and inferiority of populations along phenotypic and genetic lines" (Stanfield, 1993, p. 17). The charge that entire groups of people are considered inferior based on their ethnic background surfaces at times in civic, social welfare, and educational discussions. For example, attempts to acculturate and assimilate children in racially integrated schools have been considered by some members of minority groups as a reformist attempt to "fix" minority children.

Beyond Race and Ethnicity: Development and Use of the Acculturation Concept

Over time, the historical fixation on dividing humans into racial, or ethnic, groups receded as a tide of interest in more subtle intragroup variations arose. The concept of acculturation evolved from the need to recognize and quantify both distinct and shared attributes of people living in multicultural environments. In those interstitial spaces between cultural groups in contact, individuals and subgroups assemble creative and selective combinations of language, cultural knowledge, values, attitudes, and practices to form mosaics rather than monoliths of culture. Though part of the race-ethnicity lineage, acculturation has the potential to unite human groups through the identification of similarities, shared characteristics, and strengths, rather than divide and stratify them based on differences. Attending to the concept of acculturation complicates, yet enriches, both health care practice and research. No longer are mutually exclusive and finite numbers of racial or ethnic categories tolerated. Now the public and professionals demand recognition of the complex cultural variation in real-world health behaviors and outcomes.

Gathering cultural data from patients or research subjects potentially overcomes the shortcomings of forced-choice, standardized racial reporting, thus increasing the validity of ethnic classification. Acculturation measurement may be useful to those interested in intercultural variation (similarities and differences between individuals from different cultural traditions), as well as intracultural variation (the range of possible expressions of cultural knowledge and behavior within any one cultural system). Understanding within-group variation is one way to conduct research "more in terms of self-definitions than in terms of . . . popular folk wisdom" (Stanfield, 1993, p. 24).

For health researchers, an acculturation measurement may help explain intracultural variability in health behaviors or outcomes.

For example, Mexicans, Mexican Americans, Cubans, Puerto Ricans, and immigrants from Central and South America perceive themselves as distinct peoples, yet are often described by a single category, "Hispanic." As a relatively recent, politically assigned label, "Hispanic" glosses over intercultural distinctions by lumping all Spanish-speaking peoples together into one undifferentiated group (Shorris, 1992). Since variation within and between different ethnic groups may make a difference in health processes and outcomes, and because differences are important to patients, detecting dimensions of both intracultural and intercultural variation among "Hispanic" groups is a challenge to health care providers.

Like the evolution of the theories and methods of human classification, definition and measurement of acculturation has changed over time. Although now considered multidimensional and fluid, the earliest models of acculturation depicted the process as linear (Figure 1). In its simplest form, acculturation is a continuum of acculturative possibilities, from the unacculturated to the fully acculturated, with the bicultural option somewhere in the middle (Keefe & Padilla, 1987). Linear models imply people who become acculturated "gain" something, moving from a state of having none of whatever it is, to a point of being somehow completely filled. All of this occurs in a smooth, one-way progression. One's prior culture (or presumed lack thereof) is overwritten by a new culture, and preexisting traits are replaced in their entirety. Keefe and Padilla reviewed numerous studies in which this linear model of acculturation was implicit (Brunner, 1956; Graves, 1967; Humphrey, 1943; Linton, 1940; Matthiasson, 1968; Samora & Deane, 1956; Spindler, 1955).

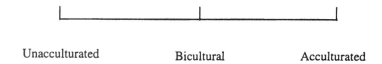

Unacculturated   Bicultural   Acculturated

FIGURE 1. Single continuum model of acculturation. From *Chicano Ethnicity* (p. 17), by S. Keefe and A. M. Padilla, 1987, Albuquerque: University of New Mexico Press. Copyright 1987 by University of New Mexico Press. Reprinted with permission.

A second model of acculturation—the two-culture matrix—has been represented graphically by McFee (1968) and described by Keefe and Padilla (1987, Figure 2). In this model, the immigrant's original culture is seen as one axis and the new culture as a cross-cutting second axis. The predictable cells of "unacculturated" and "acculturated" describe individuals who are highly affiliated with one or another culture, whereas the "marginal" individual is not accepted by or proficient in either culture. The "bicultural" category describes a situation of high acceptance and proficiency in both cultures. The two-culture matrix model allows for individual variation in acceptance of both native and new cultures, but assumes an individual will be best described by a particular box, as opposed to inhabiting different boxes in relation to different traits or settings. One is either "acculturated" or "not acculturated" in this model.

A third, more contemporary, model of acculturation introduces the idea of multidimensional acculturation in relation to specific traits (Figure 3). Milton Gordon (1964) was the first to suggest a multifaceted quality to acculturation, with the most important dimensions being structure and culture.

Gordon observed that even if an immigrant group adopts the host country's food, dress, customs, and language in a relatively short time (making them culturally indistinguishable from the host-country residents), they may maintain structural uniqueness within endogamous marriages, occupational specialties, and ghettoized neighborhoods. The concept of selective acculturation has been used to describe the common tendency for immigrants and ethnic minorities to adopt certain strategic traits (especially those likely to improve their economic status, such as learning the language of the host culture), while retaining other traditional cultural values and patterns, including child-rearing practices, family organization, native foods, and music preferences (Keefe & Padilla, 1987).

If one assumes acculturation is multidimensional, some new traits may be quickly embraced and incorporated into an immigrant's life, whereas other traits retained from the original culture may be emphasized. With a multidimensional acculturation process, a bicultural person will have a mix of new and traditional traits, selectively acquired over time. Ramirez and Castenada (1974) define a bicultural person as one "with extensive so-

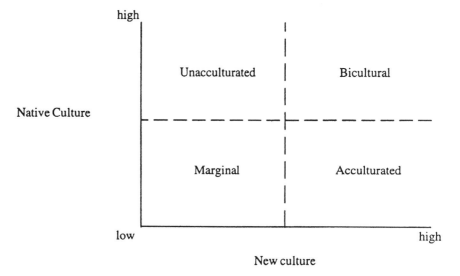

FIGURE 2. Two cultural matrix model of acculturation. From *Chicano Ethnicity* (p. 17), by S. Keefe and A. M. Padilla, 1987, Albuquerque: University of New Mexico Press. Copyright 1987 by University of New Mexico Press. Reprinted with permission.

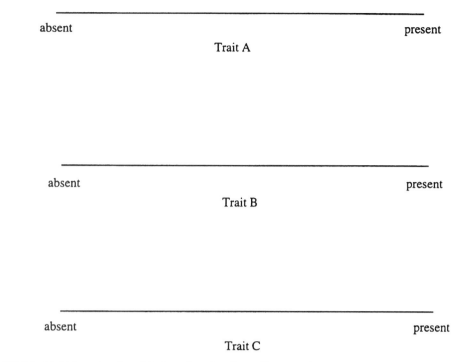

absent   present
Trait A

absent   present
Trait B

absent   present
Trait C

FIGURE 3. Multidimensional model of acculturation. From *Chicano Ethnicity* (p. 17), by S. Keefe and A. M. Padilla, 1987, Albuquerque: University of New Mexico Press. Copyright 1987 by University of New Mexico Press. Reprinted with permission.

cialization and life experience in two or more cultures and [who] participates actively in these cultures" (Ramirez & Castenada, 1974; cited in Ramirez, 1984, p. 81). Bicultural individuals develop "an expanded behavioral repertoire including skills and knowledge from both cultures" (Ramirez, 1984, p. 81).

Suggesting a multidimensional component in acculturation begs the question, *"How does one acculturate?"* What processes account for the ultimate incorporation of new cultural traits into one's life? Several types of acculturation have been suggested. Emphasizing the role of individual choice, a humanistic interaction model (Figure 4) suggests that individual acculturation depends on personality and choice, multicultural environments, socioecological variables (including socioeconomic status and other noncultural environmental factors), and social behaviors (Garza & Lipton, 1984). An important feature of this model is the allowance for differential individual acculturation outcomes

based on interaction among components of the model and mediated by individual choice.

Similarly, Ramirez (1984) described the acculturative as a "growth process" in different domains, providing flexibility, adaptability, and understanding of others with the "potential for . . . developing a multicultural orientation to life" (p. 92). A particular immigrant's pattern of acculturation, or selective integration of cultural traits, depends on his distinctive heritage as well as the value or desirability attached to new and old traits. Value and desirability determine whether an individual or group moves toward or away from traits in the dominant culture while preserving or rejecting traits in their own culture (Berry, 1993; Sowell, 1996; Tajfel, 1981).

The Social Science Research Council (SSRC) (Broom, Sigel, Vogt, Watson, & Barnett, 1954) described acculturation as taking the forms of (a) diffusion, (b) cultural creativity, (c) cultural disintegration, or (d) reactive adaptation. These processes of acculturation,

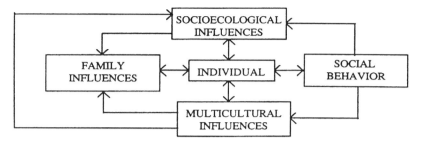

FIGURE 4. A model of environmental influences and personal choice in acculturation. From "Foundations for a Chicano Social Psychology," by R. T. Garza and J. P. Lipton. In J. L. Martinez, Jr. and R. H. Mendoza (Eds.), *Chicano Psychology* (2nd ed., pp. 335–336), 1984, New York: Academic Press. Copyright 1984 by Academic Press. Reprinted with permission.

devised nearly a half-century ago, prove useful in identifying acculturation processes in clinical and research settings. They continue to be discussed in the acculturation literature, sometimes with different labels. For example, Berry (1993) described four acculturation strategies used by minority groups: integration, assimilation, separation, and marginalization.

As described by the SSRC, *diffusion* refers to the process of selective adaptation of cultural materials (objects, traits, or ideas) between two systems. Pharmaceuticals, for example, are cultural artifacts of western medicine, yet they have been exported and marketed extensively in developing countries, where they are incorporated into local healing cosmologies (van der Geest & Whyte, 1989; Whyte, 1982, 1988). The use of pills has diffused, but the microbial theory of communicable disease has not.

Cultural creativity results in new combinations and possibilities in cultural constructions, sometimes called "syncretism" (see Crandon-Malamud, 1990, for extensive documentation of this process in Bolivia). In Arizona, one of the co-authors (L.C.) met a woman who described the traditional Mexican illness, *empacho,* and its associated cure using a modern metaphor: "*Empacho* is the clogging of the intestines. *Pamita* [tansy mustard] is a little granule, I give it in a bottle with milk, and what it does is, it's almost like Draino, you know, it'll flush all that stuff out of her."

Cultural disintegration is the third possible acculturative process described by the SSRC.

When traits from the native culture and the new culture cannot be selectively integrated, "differentiating alternatives . . . demand partisan commitments by the society's members." In this way, "factional struggles, such as those between 'progressives' and 'conservatives'" develop (Broom *et al.,* 1954, p. 986). In the United States, one cannot legally obtain a circumcision for a female child. One must either acculturate to the new norms of the host country, and presumably forgo a circumcision, or seek assistance outside the country or the dominant medical community. These types of acculturation decisions polarize immigrant families and communities. Cleavages may split generations of a family, men and women, or one class of people from another, with the possible result of cultural disintegration.

Reactive adaptation describes the overwhelming withdrawal and encysting of traditional values. Native traits are reaffirmed and reinforced, with acculturation proceeding away from assimilation and toward entrenchment. Ethnic rights groups such as the American Indian Movement (AIM) are sometimes cited as examples of reactive adaptation.

A frontier for theoretical development in acculturation is the consideration of bidirectional acculturation among groups in close proximity in which members of both cultures adopt and adapt traits introduced through their interactions. In many regions of the United States, Latin cultural practices have been incorporated into mainstream American life. Some "average" Americans now eat Mexican foods like tortillas and refried beans, listen to music with Tejano or Mexicano influences, and speak a little Spanish (if not more). Acculturation research, however, usually emphasizes the process of minority acculturation to Anglo culture, rather than the other way around. Given a multicultural society, the properties of bidirectionality and multidimensionality in the acculturation concept pose challenges to both theory and research (Padilla, 1995).

Acculturation Theory to Acculturation Measurement

Following increasingly sophisticated models of acculturation, refined methods for measuring acculturation have become available (for samples in the measurement of Hispanic acculturation, see Cuellar, Harris, & Jasso, 1980; Cuellar, Arnold & Maldonado, 1995; Deyo, Diehl, Hazuda, & Stern, 1985; Luna Solorzano, 1992; McFee, 1968; R. Mendoza & Martínez, 1981; Peréz-Stable, Marín, Marín, Brody, & Benowitz, 1990). Sample acculturation rating scales are described in Table 1. In most acculturation measurements, a person's relative position in the acculturative process is "translated into a score that is used as in indicator of type or degree of acculturation" (R. H. Mendoza, 1984, p. 63). Multidimensional models and the measurements patterned after them basically contain two dimensions of change within the minority culture: (1) maintenance or loss of traditional culture, and (2) gain of new culture traits.

Current multidimensional models include the concept of "selective acculturation" in which each aspect of culture change is measured independently (M. P. Clark, Kaufman, & Pierce, 1976; Keefe & Padilla, 1987; Olmedo & Padilla, 1978). Multidimensional models have focused on semantic meaning (Olmedo, Martínez, & Martínez, 1978); psychological models of self-reported behaviors and value dimensions (Szapocznik, Scopetta, & Kurtines, 1978); cultural awareness and ethnic identification (Padilla, 1980); language, social patterns, and country of origin (Burnam, Hough, Karno, Telles, & Escobar, 1987); and sociocultural adjustments (R. Mendoza & Martínez, 1981). Szapocznik and colleagues (1978) and Burnam and colleagues (1987) found acculturation directly related to the length of exposure to the host culture, with generation of residence in the United States highly correlated with acculturation scores.

TABLE 1. A Sample of Acculturation Rating Scales for Mexican-Origin Individuals

Authors	Instrument title	Geographic location of instrument development
Cuellar, Harris, & Jasso (1980)	Acculturation Rating Scale for Mexican Americans (ARSMA) (revised for use with H-HANES (in 1984)	San Antonio, TX
Cuellar, Arnold, & Maldonado (1995)	Revised Acculturation Rating Scale for Mexican Americans (ARSMA-II)	Edinburg, TX
Olmedo, Martinez, & Martinez (1978)	Acculturation for Adolescents	Los Angeles, CA
Deyo, Diehl, Hazuda, & Stern (1985)	Language-based Acculturation Scale (LAS)	San Antonio, TX
Burman, Hough, Telles, & Escobar, (1987)	Los Angeles Epidemiologic Catchment Area (LAECA)	Los Angeles, CA
Marín, Sabogal, Marín, Otero-Sabogal, & Perez-Stable (1987	Short Acculturation Scale for Hispanics	San Francisco, CA

Dimensions of acculturation identified in various acculturation instruments vary in both number and focus. Keefe and Padilla (1987) formulated six dimensions of acculturation: children's cultural heritage, parental cultural heritage, language preference, ethnic social orientation, ethnic pride and affiliation, and ethnic identity. The Biculturalism/Multiculturalism Experience Inventory (B/MEI; Ramirez & Castenada, 1974) posits three dimensions: demographic-linguistic, personal history, and bicultural participation. The Revised Acculturation Rating Scale for Mexican Americans (ARSMA-II) (Cuellar, Arnold, & Maldonado, 1995) taps the four factors of language, ethnic identity, reading-writing-cultural exposure, and ethnic interaction. The Los Angeles Epidemiological Catchment Area (LAECA) reports factors of language, social activities, and ethnic background (Burnam, Hough, Karno, Telles, & Escobar, 1987). (Reliability and validity for the ARSMA, ARSMA-II, and LAECA are described in Table 2).

Despite the attention given to multidimensional scales and multidimensional models of acculturation, a single item—language—appears to be one of the most frequently used assessments of acculturation. Since the linguistic factors in various acculturation scales generally account for over 70% of the variance in the total acculturation score, language-based scales claim to be both accurate and clinically useful (Deyo *et al.*, 1985). Using a strictly language-based measure of acculturation, however, violates the theoretical assumption that acculturation can unfold differentially across

TABLE 2. Acculturation Measurement Instruments for Mexican-Origin Individuals: Major Factors Measured, Number of Items, and Psychometric Properties[a]

Instrument	Factors measured	Number of items	Validity	Reliability
ARSMA	1) Language use and preference 2) Ethnic identity and classification 3) Cultural heritage and ethnic behaviors 4) Ethnic interaction	20 items	Criterion, convergent, construct (generation)	Test–retest $r = .72–.80$, interrater reliability, internal consistency Cronbach's $\alpha = .81–.88$
ARSMA-II	Identical to ARSMA	30 items: divided into 2 subscales	Correlation with original ARSMA $r = .89$	Test–retest coefficient Scale 1 $r = .96$ Scale 2 $r = .94$
Acculturation for adolescents	1) Nationality-language 2) Socioeconomic status 3) Semantic factor	127 items	Construct (based on factor loadings)	Test–retest $r = .89$
LAS	Language	4 items	Construct (natality and generation)	Coefficient of scalability (Guttman) = .81 Coefficient of reproducibility = .96
LAECA	1) Language use and skills, contact with Mexico 2) Social activities 3) Ethnic background	26 items	Criterion, construct (generation & years in U.S.)	Internal consistency Cronbach's $\alpha = .91–.97$
Short Acculturation Scale for Hispanics	1) Language use 2) Media preferences 3) Ethnic social relations	12 items	Criterion, construct (generation, length of residence, self-evaluation, age of arrival)	Internal consistency Cronbach's $\alpha = .92$

[a] See table 1 for complete information on instrument developers and geographic location of development.

various traits and reinforces the idea that minority groups adopt the dominant culture in a smooth, uniform progression from native culture to new culture. (Pros and cons of language as a proxy for acculturation are discussed in the section titled "Language and Generation Proxies for Acculturation of Individuals.")

Differences between Acculturation and Other Concepts

Acculturation is the culture change resulting from the contact of two or more cultural systems. As discussed earlier, one part of acculturation, *ethnic identity*, is self-identification as a member of a group sharing a common history and traditions (De Vos & Romanucci, 1975; see also Aboud, 1984, 1988, who talks about belonging to an ethnic group). This symbolic and subjective identity is conceptually distinct from acculturation, but sometimes confused with it.

Another similar concept, *assimilation,* describes the complete integration and absorption of individuals from one cultural system into another. When assimilated, an ethnic minority group participates fully and freely in the social, economic, and political life of the mainstream society (Gordon, 1964; Keefe & Padilla, 1987). Assimilation is preceded to some degree by acculturation, but it is not the sole or necessary endpoint in the acculturation process (Gordon, 1964). One type of assimilation is *homogenous assimilation,* typified by a "melting pot" where both minority and majority cultures blend equally. *Unidirectional* or *unilateral assimilation* occurs when the minority culture loses its distinctiveness and is absorbed completely into the dominant culture. In the United States, assimilation has been called Americanization or Anglo conformity (Jibou, 1988).

"Complete assimilation," the Social Science Research Council noted years ago, "is much less frequent in fact than is indicated by the frequency with which the term is used in the literature" (Broom *et al.,* 1954, p. 988). A California-based study of Latinos reinforced this observation, noting that accultur-

ation and assimilation increased dramatically from the first to the second generation, but leveled off thereafter. Second-generation Latinos became integrated into stable blue-collar jobs, but "white collar jobs continue to be out of reach for the vast majority of those from succeeding generations." Without continued economic and political assimilation, the "initial burst" of Americanization is followed by a long-term process of settling into an "ethnic community of Chicanos, a unique creation" born of the contact of Latino and Anglo cultures (Keefe & Padilla, 1987, p. 8).

Other concepts can also overlap with, or become confused with, the concept of acculturation. *Industrialization,* for example, refers to an intracultural change in the societal means of production, and not necessarily to cross-culturally introduced changes in cultural values, knowledge, or practices. *Socialization* and *enculturation* often refer to children's introduction and training in a cultural system, again with emphasis on an intracultural process of learning and adaptation on the part of individuals. *Urbanization* and *secularization,* too, describe cultural changes, but not those borne of contact between ethnic enclaves (Broom *et al.,* 1954). None of the related concepts described here capture the essence of acculturation.

In summary, theories of acculturation seek to refine systems of classification established initially as concepts of race and ethnicity. Acculturation has variously been considered a linear progression from native to new cultural systems, a matrix of acculturative possibilities, and a multidimensional growth process in which individuals creatively reassemble cultural traits from native and new sources into unique patterns. Acculturation differs from related concepts, in that acculturation is concerned with culture change resulting from the contact of cultural systems and the selective adaptation attributable to the intercultural contact. Following sections consider the association between acculturation and health, examples of health-related systems altered by acculturation, and issues related to the measurement of acculturation in research and practice.

Relationships among Acculturation and Health Variables

Clinical hunches suggesting relationships between acculturation and health dovetail with research verifying the importance of acculturation in health outcomes. Within the Latino population, acculturation (as measured by nativity) shows a striking effect. Immigrants from Mexico illustrate the "healthy migrant effect" by demonstrating lower levels of mortality, in general, than U.S.-born Mexican Americans (Sorlie, Backlund, Johnson, & Rogot, 1993). In specific health outcomes, too, acculturation can make a difference. The "Hispanic health paradox" describes the counterintuitive finding that Hispanics in the Southwest deviate from expected morbidity and mortality outcomes in positive ways (Markides & Coreil, 1986). For example, Mexican women give birth to a lower proportion of low-birthweight infants than one would expect given their poverty and low education levels. The lower low-birthweight statistic also shows a Mexican advantage in comparison with women from different ethnic backgrounds but similar socioeconomic status (Guendelman, Gould, Hudes, Eskenazi, 1990; Williams, Binkin & Clingman, 1986). Unfortunately, the favorable health status of approximately a quarter of those "paradoxically" healthy children born to Mexican immigrants of low acculturation status is eroded by social conditions during the first year of life (Guendelman, English, & Chavez, 1995).

The following sample of studies on Latino populations illustrates the importance of acculturation in relation to health. Taken as a collective, these studies also affirm the importance of including acculturation in general health assessments.

- Increasing levels of acculturation among Latinos is associated with early sexual initiation, higher rates of adolescent pregnancy, and more frequent use of commercial sex workers. For pregnant Latina adolescents, acculturation is associated with more smoking, drugs, and alcohol consumption (Amaro, Whitaker, Coffman, & Heeren, 1990; Balcazar, Peterson, & Cobas, 1996; Carrier & Magaña, 1991; B. V. Marín, Tschaun, Gomez, & Kegeles, 1993).

- Higher acculturation for Latinos is associated with deviant behavior and drug use (Gil, Vega, & Dimas, 1994; Vega & Amaro, 1994).

- Intrauterine Growth Retardation (<10% of weight for length given sex and gestational age) is lower among Mexican Americans than Anglos, but increases with increasing acculturation (Balcazar, 1993).

- Breastfeeding initiation for Hispanic mothers is 48.4%, compared to 23% for African American mothers and 58% for Anglo mothers (Balcazar, Trier, & Cobas, 1995). Low levels of acculturation for Hispanic mothers are associated with higher levels of breastfeeding initiation after the birth of an infant (Rassin et al., 1993).

- Highly acculturated female adolescents report greater levels of stress from the assimilation process, but also more coping strategies and greater social support (Balcazar et al., 1996).

- Low levels of acculturation for Hispanic adult males are associated with lower levels of self-rated health (Markides & Lee, 1991), and both male and female Hispanic adults provide lower self-rated health scores than Anglo adults with similar objective measures of health (Shetterly, Baxter, Mason, & Hamman, 1996).

- Acculturation is related to health care utilization in complex and subtle ways, with some studies showing a direct effect of acculturation on increased utilization of health services (e.g., Chesney, Chavira, Hall, & Gary, 1982), and others showing no direct effect and only limited indirect effect of acculturation on utilization (e.g., Markides, Levin, & Ray, 1985). Among Hispanics, low acculturation is related to a lower probability of outpatient care for mental health problems (Wells, Golding, Hough, Burnam, & Karno, 1989).

In summary, prior research on acculturation and health confirms clinical hunches. Health advantages associated with low acculturative status are demonstrated for Latinos from adolescence through pregnancy, birth, and breastfeeding initiation. However, perceived health status is lower for Latinos than Anglos even when objective measures of health are approximately equal. Perhaps standard "objective" measures of health fail to tap the dimensions of health on which Latinos base their subjective perceptions. Alternately, low perceived health status for Latinos may indicate that perceived health status is a metaphor for low social status and social discrimination. Nichter (1981) proposes bodily experiences and perceptions as an "idiom of distress" that communicates meta-physical experiences in patterned ways.

Organizing Knowledge of Community-Level Acculturation

In public health, learning about community-level acculturation and the suspected range of individual variation in the community is an essential prerequisite for effective aggregate-level health planning and implementation. Three background, community-level acculturation variables identified by Gordon (1964) are helpful in organizing data on the acculturative forces in communities and understanding the acculturation experiences of individuals. These three variables are discrimination and historical events of the immigrant group, socioeconomic and occupational experiences, and social life. Taken together, they provide an estimate of the structural difficulty or ease with which acculturation may be possible for an ethnic group and its members in a community.

First, *discrimination and historical events* of the immigrant group refer to the circum-stances that explain how a group of people came to be in a particular community at a given time. Did slavery bring them? Were the residents landowners in New Spain before the United States purchased the area? A refugee may invoke imagery of being "saved" by a host nation and its health care system. On the other hand, an indigenous person with a different sense of her collective history and a longer memory of discrimination may characterize her relationships to the nation and the health care system as abusive.

The Yaqui experience provides an example of the complexity of historical and discriminatory forces in acculturation. In the later 1800s, the Yaqui in southern Sonora, Mexico, retreated from official extermination campaigns by fleeing to the Sierra Madre mountains. Some members of the Yaqui tribe fled across the United States–Mexico border at the turn of the century, during and after the bloody Mexican Revolution, to establish communities in southern Arizona. For the next 60 years, the U.S. government did not recognize Yaqui as immigrants or indigenous peoples, consequently denying them services offered to other indigenous groups through the U.S. Public Health Service's Indian Health Service. In 1979 Congress declared the Yaqui eligible for Indian Health Services. Today, Yaqui communities and individuals construct ethnic identities using an array of historical identities originating from both native and host countries and traversing warrior to survivor, immigrant to native.

History is critical. The near-extermination and later discrimination experienced by immigrant Yaquis may stymie acculturation or render it an undesirable aim. Acculturation in this instance allows for multiple possibilities. A person of Yaqui ancestry potentially can acculturate in unique ways and at an individual rate, by selectively combining components from Yaqui, Mexican, or North American cultures. For the practitioner, understanding historical events and discrimination of the ethnic group sets the stage for an individualized assessment of personal experience. Without both the general picture of cultural group history and the fine-tuning of individual experience, practitioners will either fail to recognize individual variation in acculturation or overlook collective acculturation experiences.

A second community-level aspect of the structural environment in which acculturation occurs is the *socioeconomic and occupational experience* of ethnic groups in particular communities. Often, ethnic groups participate or specialize in occupations with particular health risks and hazards. Mexican-origin immigrants, for example, may participate heavily in the agricultural and meat-packing industries which, in addition to being among the most dangerous occupations, are characterized by low-paying employment and limited opportunity for career training or advancement. Neighborhoods often arise near workplaces, or workplaces may locate in lower-income, ethnic areas of cities to capitalize on the available workforce. Either way, ethnically segregated and self-contained neighborhoods often result. Structurally, opportunities for assimilation and acculturation are limited in ethnic workforces and neighborhoods segregated by socioeconomic and occupational status. The high level of correlation between socioeconomic status (and constituent factors of education and income) and acculturation has been borne out in research (Negy & Woods, 1992). Health care practitioners familiar with patterns of occupational concentration and socioeconomic opportunity in ethnic communities can infer information about health risks, economic disadvantages, and opportunities for acculturative experiences among members of an ethnic group.

Finally, *social life* may be either a structural barrier or predisposing factor to acculturation. The degree to which people mingle and socialize across ethnic boundaries and acculturation levels in social settings contribute to the rate of acculturation for ethnic group members. The degree of intermingling among ethnic groups relates to the rate of endogamous marriage. For example, one co-author (L.C.) asked a Mexican woman who

had lived in Denver most of her life if she had any opinions about Mexican compared with American men. She answered in fluent English, "I don't know. I've never dated, or even talked much, with men who aren't from Mexico." She met Mexican men at church, at local dances, and through friends. In her case, the social ties that bind the Mexican and Mexican American community together are strong and exclusive. Although she spoke both Spanish and English, had a U.S. high school diploma, and worked in an English-speaking environment, she had little informal social experience outside her ethnic group and would likely never enter into an exogamous marriage—the most potent acculturative force possible. Social life, then, shapes and limits acculturative opportunities.

Famous neighborhoods in major U.S. cities known as "Chinatown," "Little Italy," or "Little Mexico" attest to the historical precedent of ethnic community segregation and isolation. Immigrants and long-term residents may reside in a community vastly different from the surrounding city. While exploring a neighborhood in west Denver, shopping in *panaderías* (bakeries), *papelerías* (stationery stores), and *carnecerías* (butcher shops), one co-author (L.C.) spoke Spanish to workers who spoke no English, and listened to Mexican music while waiting in line. Two women ahead of her at the *panadería* who lived nearby described their neighborhood as "puro México" (pure Mexico)." Their exposure to middle-class, non-Mexican members of the larger community was limited, despite their combined length of residence in the area of over 7 years. They relied on stereotypes popularized by television when they asked L.C. about her life. Did she have a maid and a butler? Did a live-in nanny care for her children? Did she have a big yard? Although not unreasonable questions, these are not the kinds of questions one would ask after close contact with typical middle-class Anglo women. The structural isolation and segregation of these women in their ethnic community suggests that opportunities to acculturate have been limited.

Although Gordon's (1964) typology of structural variables related to community acculturation has been reviewed and illustrated in this section, the reason for using such a typology in practice may appear unclear. What are the benefits of assessing structural variables related to acculturation for immigrant groups? First, the typology can serve as an organizing framework for clinicians and researchers embarking on community-level assessments or interventions. At a minimum, a community assessment of these acculturation factors will situate knowledge about the community in the landscape of the surrounding area, historical events and experiences, and interactions of residents with other groups. The assessment will be contextualized to reflect the community as an entity through time and in relation to structural and social organizations outside the community. Second, community-level assessments of acculturation can redirect programs initially based on faulty or incomplete understandings of immigrant communities. Since community-level interventions arise from community assessments, inclusion of acculturation variables in preintervention assessments will improve the likelihood of program success. From selecting a title for a community intervention to choosing a logo or disseminating results in a local newspaper, there are numerous ways community-based researchers and program planners can unknowingly elicit apathy, disgust, or anger in communities by demonstrating their ignorance or insensitivity to the community's collective past and present.

Finally, using an acculturation typology at the community level helps clinicians working on the individual and family level. The backdrop of general community acculturation information prepares clinicians to adapt general plans of care to unique individuals from specific backgrounds. Mentioning to a client that one is familiar with current social or political issues affecting the community, and drawing parallels between current issues and historical events is more than showing off. Sharing an understanding of these issues can be a bridge between the medical work prompting the visit and the social and cultural worlds of meaning that connect clinicians, clients, and communities.

Language and Generation Proxies for Acculturation of Individuals

In clinical situations, individual acculturation is, at worst, haphazardly intuited, and at best measured with a brief (but valid and reliable) acculturation instrument. Somewhere between intuition and multidimensional measurement, language and generation are often used as proxy measures of acculturation. Neither language nor generation, however, replaces formal measurement of acculturation due to limitations in scope and sensitivity. Furthermore, from the standpoint of a multidimensional model of acculturation, neither of these single-item, unidimensional indicators is a sufficient substitute for a multidimensional measure.

Language is perhaps the most commonly used proxy indicator of acculturation. Clinically, "language spoken" questions quickly and efficiently identify the least acculturated patients. If a hospitalized patient speaks Russian, for example, the nurses and physicians must, by law, provide for medical interpretation to assure informed consent for treatment. As clinicians locate and coordinate interpretation, cultural issues naturally arise. Language differences suggest the possibility of differences in cognitive structuring of experiences of health and illness. Cued by language, expert clinicians spend additional time explaining or illustrating the organ systems involved, or surgical procedures recommended. Language barriers prompt greater attention to cultural aspects of care through the salient message that this patient is different and requires individualized health care attuned to cultural nuances.

On the positive side, a language proxy for acculturation is both efficient and defensible from a measurement standpoint. In the development of instruments to formally measure acculturation, investigators typically discover through factor analysis that language accounts for most of the variance in the entire acculturation scale (examples include Burnam *et al.*, 1987; Cuellar *et al.*, 1980; Cuellar *et al.*, 1995; Olmedo *et al.*, 1978). On the negative side, a language proxy for acculturation is theoretically indefensible in light of the prevailing idea that acculturation is multidimensional. Measuring one part of the entire acculturation experience cannot substitute for an assessment of other areas of acculturation. More concretely, assuming that an immigrant patient and provider share cultural assumptions about the body, health, and healing simply because they share a common language is untenable. Acculturation may be evident in the linguistic domain, but unrelated to acculturation in health-related knowledge structures and value systems.

Assessing the generation of residence of an immigrant in the host country is another common, but problematic, proxy measure of acculturation. Researchers and clinicians who ask patients if they are first-, second-, or third-generation residents of the host country make several assumptions. First, a generation proxy for acculturation assumes that over time, families acculturate to the host country and become assimilated. Given isolated ethnic neighborhoods, occupational segregation, and racism, this assumption is difficult to defend. Furthermore, even highly assimilated individuals are not necessarily highly acculturated. One study suggests the most assimilated Mexican-origin residents in the United States are also the most "adamant about preserving their ethnic distinctiveness," and retain and transmit to their children a distinctively ethnic identity (Hurtado, Rodríguez, Gurin, & Beals, 1993, p. 138).

Second, a generation question lacks reliability, since both patients and providers may define generation differently. Even researchers who specialize in acculturation offer different definitions of what "first" and "second" generation means (Cuellar *et al.*, 1980; Guendelman & Abrams, 1995).

A third assumption made when assessing acculturation generationally rather than multidimensionally is that generation suggests a

continuous presence in the host country. One might assume a third-generation resident has accumulated more family history in the host country than a first-generation resident has, and thus more opportunity for acculturation. Given the migratory patterns of many immigrant groups, and Mexican immigrants in particular, frequent moves over generations between the host and native country makes a conflation of generation and acculturation unwarranted. For many immigrants, determining one's generation in either country is confusing and difficult. "I was born *con un pie en cado lado*," states Carlos Velez-Ibañez. (1996) "That is, [I was] born with one foot on each side of the political border between Mexico and the United States. It is only by chance that I was not born in Sonora rather than Arizona" (p. 3). Given the flaws of generation as a proxy measurement for acculturation, it is interesting to observe how often generation is cited in the establishment of validity for new acculturation instruments (see G. Marín, Sabogal, Marín, Otero-Sabogal, & Peréz-Stable, 1987, as one example of generation as validation criterion). The wisdom of selecting dubious indicators of acculturation as a standard in developing instrumentation deserves further consideration.

Language and generation, although easy to elicit from a patient or research subject, fail to satisfy the criteria of multidimensional acculturation measurement. Both are proxies with questionable relationships to the concept of acculturation. Actual measurement of a broad spectrum of knowledge, values, and behavior is a far better method of obtaining valid and reliable information about an individual's acculturation.

The Measurement of Individual Acculturation

Usually, when intuition or proxy measurements of acculturation are unsuitable, researchers and clinicians embark on a search for an appropriate instrument to measure acculturation among individuals in the population of interest. To date, no universal acculturation rating scale is available to measure acculturation across many ethnic groups. Therefore, acculturation must be measured using a group-specific instrument. Using existing data to estimate acculturation and gathering self-reported information are the two most common methods of assessing acculturation of individuals. Each of these methods offers strengths and weaknesses.

Measurement of Acculturation Using Existing Data Sets

In retrospective studies involving chart reviews or other data sets collected for purposes unrelated to acculturation, selected items could be scored, weighted, and summed to yield an indicator of acculturation. Constructing an estimate of acculturation from an existing data set requires creativity. Availability and theoretical relevance of items contained in the data set may vary, but commonly accessible demographic, social, and linguistic information includes birthplace, location of education, first language, language spoken, and years of residence in the host country.

One often-used national data set is the Hispanic Health and Nutrition Examination Study (H-HANES). Conducted during 1982–1984 with a probability sample of Hispanics in the southwestern United States (National Center for Health Statistics [NCHS], 1985), the H-HANES is exceptional in that it contains self-reported measures of acculturation for adult subjects, in addition to a wide range of information on health and nutrition. The H-HANES acculturation scale is an 8-item acculturation scale derived from the 20-item ARSMA scale (Cuellar *et al.,* 1980). The H-HANES data have proven valuable due to the strength of the sampling plan and the inclusion of the acculturation scale, but not every research question related to acculturation can be answered using this particular data set. Researchers and clinicians who work with subjects and patients face-to-face can avoid the pitfalls of relying on a predetermined measure or constructing a composite indicator of acculturation by conducting a self-reported acculturation assessment.

Evaluating Self-Report Measures of Acculturation

For researchers and clinicians working with a particular ethnic group, several psychometrically sound acculturation rating scales based on self-report may be available. A sample of acculturation rating scales designed for Mexican and Mexican Americans illustrates how to select and potentially modify an instrument. As listed in Table 1, each of these acculturation rating scales was developed in a geographic location with a large Mexican-origin population, then subsequently used throughout the United States. Table 2 provides more information about each instrument, including measurement emphasis, length, and psychometric properties. Before selecting an acculturation index for a research or practice setting, one must consider at least four points that clarify the purpose and desired results of the measurement.

First, elucidating the purpose of acculturation assessment is essential. Throughout the process of selecting an acculturation rating scale, one should ask, "Why are we doing this?" Is the principal aim description, or associating acculturation with an important clinical outcome or set of health behaviors? In clinical situations, information on language preferences and reading abilities in English and Spanish may be more germane than a comprehensive acculturation measurement. Clarifying objectives prevents either over- or underidentification of salient acculturation issues.

Second, consider the implicit or overt conceptual definition of acculturation underlying each acculturation rating scale. Some scales may not elucidate the author's view of acculturation, but others are quite specific. One acculturation measurement system states in the introduction, "[A]cculturation involves more than becoming knowledgeable of the language, norms, and values of the new culture; it can involve a fundamental . . . relearning [of] the meaning of symbols, readjustment to a new system of values, and relinquishing old customs, beliefs and behavior" (Burnam *et al.*, 1987, p. 107). This definition differs from the description of acculturation implied in the preface to another instrument, which states: "[L]anguage ability is perhaps the aspect of acculturation which has the greatest direct impact on doctor-patient interaction and . . . is a strong marker for other aspects of acculturation" (Deyo *et al.*, 1985, p. 53).

Third, indicators contained in each acculturation rating scale can be examined for applicability to the *target subpopulation* and *geographic locale* of interest. For example the LAECA contains an item asking, "What language do you speak at school or work?" While this question may not apply with retirees or housewives, it could be adapted. Considering the literacy, age, developmental level, and suspected range of acculturation of the target sample may also limit the applicability of items contained in previously developed scales.

In considering the geographic locale, determining local applicability is important. Generic questions about food preferences and radio and TV viewing are common in many acculturation instruments, but lack specificity. For example, the LAECA and the ARSMA ask whether subjects view TV programs exclusively or mostly in Spanish or English or equally in Spanish and English. Questions about reading newspapers and magazines are similar. Yet subtle differences between Spanish-language radio, TV, and newspapers exist in particular geographic areas. In some areas, Spanish-language media may not be available at all. Instead of asking merely whether a respondent reads a Spanish newspaper, knowing which one and why yields richer data about their acculturation experience. Generic acculturation instruments can be enhanced through inclusion of more locally specific responses to items.

Fourth, the ideal precision of the acculturation measurement can be estimated. If the clinician needs only a rough estimate of acculturation among individuals, then a short acculturation scale may be adequate. An efficient alternative to a single-item proxy is Deyo and colleagues' (1985) 4-item language-based scale. When all short acculturation scales are inappropriate because acculturation level varies widely in the target group and identifiable gradations of acculturation can be discerned, then a more sensitive measure such as the 26-item LAECA may be more appropriate.

Another consideration in determining the desired level of precision relates to the anticipated relationship between acculturation and other variables of interest. Is acculturation a covariate, an independent variable, or an antecedent to an outcome of interest? Or are acculturation and concomitant acculturative stress the outcomes? Depending on the place of acculturation in the research design, the level of measurement precision may vary.

Modifying Self-Report Acculturation Instruments

The acculturation rating scales listed in Table 1 share a common weakness. None was developed to measure acculturation in Yuma, Arizona, or Las Cruces, New Mexico, or Greeley, Colorado. Assuming that the process of acculturation is similar among Mexicans in every state of the United States is neither logical nor theoretically sound. The alternative is tailoring existing instruments to provide valid and reliable data in a new location. Matching an existing instrument with a new measurement situation requires consideration of the following criteria:

- *Semantics of items*. Instruments developed in a different location should be examined in all language versions (e.g., English and Spanish) for appropriateness in the new study site. Slang and dialect differences exist across regions in the United States, and even within cities across acculturation level and age ranges. Importing an existing acculturation scale from one location to another requires a careful linguistic review by local speakers similar in demographic characteristics to the target population. Changes in words and phrasing may be required.

- *Specificity of items.* Items in an instrument that seem most transferable from the site of development to the new research site may prove too general and vague, yielding bland, decontextualized information about acculturation. The desired level of geographic specificity should be considered before importing an existing instrument to a new location. For example, in one ongoing ethnographic study in Denver, 46% of the Mexican-origin women interviewed reported reading books, magazines, and periodicals in Spanish only, mostly Spanish, or both English and Spanish (L. Clark, 1995). Knowing this, the researchers still do not know which of the three available Spanish newspapers are read, to what extent the respondents agree or disagree with the political and editorial flavor of the various newspapers, or whether newspaper preference is related to other variables, such as the cost of the newspapers, where respondents attend church, or recentness of immigration. Answering these more detailed questions would require open-ended interviewing about acculturation and language to supplement the general question about newspaper readership. To describe local patterns of acculturation, specificity of items may need to be increased by adding local examples, such as the names of the three available newspapers, for example. Increasing the specificity of items may be less important when a total score is sought for comparison across study locations and local examples of acculturation pathways are less relevant.
- *Emphasis of measurement.* Many acculturation rating scales focus on a few factors in acculturation, such as social interaction, ethnic identity, or language. Typically, language is the most salient

factor in acculturation rating scales. If a more performative, behavioral assessment of acculturation is required, an instrument with language-based emphasis may be inadequate or misleading.

- *Scoring.* Researchers and clinicians should bear in mind that similar scores on a standard acculturation instrument do not eliminate the possibility of identified subgroups maintaining strong differences in patterns of behavior and interaction. For example, two different individuals may achieve an identical score on a standard acculturation rating scale, yet differ in key ways. This is most evident with heavily or exclusively language-based instruments. Although two women may speak Spanish at home, one may have abandoned her Catholic religious heritage, eliminated herbal medications from her routine care of minor infant illnesses, and become accustomed to thinking of prenatal care as an important assurance of a healthy pregnancy. Another woman with the same score may have a strong cultural and religious link with Catholicism, use herbal remedies almost exclusively, and be more nonchalant about early prenatal care. Although some researchers think of these other variables as co-occurring with acculturation, they may be important indicators of acculturative differences. Language is only one facet of acculturation, and the practices that accompany, precede, or postdate acquisition of English may go completely undetected if language is assumed to be synonymous with acculturation.
- *Context of acculturation.* An acculturation instrument designed to yield a total acculturation score does not necessarily reflect the social, political, and interpersonal context in which the acculturation process proceeds and recedes for an individual over time. Scales will report *which* behaviors associated with acculturation an individual employs, but leave unanswered questions about *how long* and *with whom* the behaviors are em-

ployed. A pitfall in practice and research using acculturation instruments is the tendency to obsess on the indicators of acculturation while ignoring how people manifest acculturation within specific social settings. Perhaps more than other sociobehavioral variables amenable to measurement, acculturation can also be shaped by personal force of will as much as by accommodation, adjustment, or assimilation into a new culture.

Each of these considerations extends the discussion of acculturation measurement beyond the psychometric adequacy of a particular instrument. Acculturation measurement may require careful scrutiny of available instruments, revision of the language and geographic specificity, and, finally, consideration of the meaning and implications of the total score produced through measurement of individuals. When available instruments are not adequate or amenable to modification for the purpose of the clinical or research setting, a new instrument may need to be developed. Consulting instrument development and measurement texts prior to launching an acculturation measurement venture is recommended.

Summary

This chapter has reviewed the historical roots of acculturation, its relationship to other concepts, and a variety of models depicting acculturation. The multidimensional nature of acculturation and the role of individual choice and structural predisposing factors were emphasized. The process of adopting new knowledge, values, and behaviors (known as acculturation) is related to immigrant health. Depending on immigrants' ethnicity and specific health issues, groups may demonstrate health advantages or disadvantages as they relocate to a new area and adopt new values and behaviors. Whether immigrants are involved as groups or individuals in obtaining health care and participating in

research, professionals can assess the community-wide acculturation experience as well as the individual experience. As a critical variable in many health research and practice settings, acculturation must be conceptualized in relation to the setting, purpose, and target population, and then measured with the most appropriate, valid, and reliable instrument possible. Proxy measures of acculturation were discussed, and considerations in the selection of an acculturation measurement scale reviewed. Language is a well-documented component of acculturation, but the behavioral and performative aspects of acculturation have not been well described.

Acculturation and the related concepts of race and ethnicity have become entwined in discussion beyond individual health and illness. "Categories such as race and ethnicity have been and continue to be important determinants of access to societal resources" (Hahn & Stroup, 1994, p. 13). Scientific use of a social category such as race, ethnicity, or acculturation may be interpreted as endorsement of its validity. Using these social categories, therefore, becomes a matter of policy and ethics as much as scientific method (Marshall, 1968). Acculturation is a further refinement in the legacy of human classification. Careful and appropriate measurement of acculturation allows clinicians and researchers to better understand the cultural determinants and correlates of health.

Acknowledgments

Supported in part by a grant to Lauren Clark (principal investigator). Mexican-origin Children's Health in Cultural Context (NIH/NICHD R29 HD232366). The authors wish to thank Lorena Marquez, who provided assistance in manuscript preparation.

References

Aboud, F. (1984). Social and cognitive basis of ethnic identity constancy. *Journal of Genetic Psychology, 184,* 217–230.

Aboud, F. (1988). *Children and prejudice.* New York: Blackwell.

Aboud, F., & Doyle, A.-B. (1993). The early development of ethnic identity and attitudes. In M. Bernal & G. P. Knight (Eds.), *Ethnic Identity: Formation and transmission among Hispanics and other minorities* (pp. 47–59). Albany: State University of New York Press.

Amaro, H., Whitaker, R., Coffman, G., & Heeren, T. (1990). Acculturation and marijuana and cocaine use: Findings from H-HANES 1982–84. *American Journal of Public Health, 80* (Suppl.), 54–60.

Balcazar, H. (1993). Mexican Americans' intrauterine growth retardation and maternal risk factors. *Ethnicity and Disease, 3,* 169–175.

Balcazar, H., Trier, C. M., & Cobas, J. A. (1995). What predicts breastfeeding intention in Mexican-American and non-Hispanic white women? Evidence from a national survey. *Birth, 22*(2), 74–80.

Balcazar, H., Peterson, G., & Cobas, J. (1996). Acculturation and health-related risk behaviors among Mexican American pregnant youth. *American Journal of Health Behavior, 20*(6), 425–433.

Berry, J. (1993). Ethnic identity in plural societies. In M. Bernal & G. P. Knight (Eds.), *Ethnic identity: Formation and transmission among Hispanics and other minorities* (pp. 271–296). Albany: State University of New York Press.

Boas, F. (1922). Report on the anthropometric investigation of the population of the United States. *Journal of the American Statistical Association, 18,* 181–209.

Boas, F. (1940). *Race, language, and culture.* New York: Free Press.

Broom, L., Sigel, B. J., Vogt, E. Z., Watson, J. B., & Barnett, B. H. (1954). Acculturation: An exploratory formulation. *American Anthropologist, 56,* 973–1000.

Brunner, E. (1956). Primary group experience and the process of acculturation. *American Anthropologist, 58,* 605–623.

Burnam, A. M., Hough, R. L., Karno, M., Telles, C. A., & Escobar, J. I. (1987). Measurement of acculturation in a community population of Mexican Americans. *Hispanic Journal of Behavioral Sciences, 9*(2), 105–130.

Carrier, J. M., & Magaña, R. (1991). Use of ethnosexual data on men of Mexican origin for HIV/AIDs prevention programs. *Journal of Sex Research, 28,* 189–202.

Chesney, A. P., Chavira, J. A., Hall, R. P., & Gary, H. E. (1982). Barriers to medical care of Mexican-Americans: The role of social class, acculturation, and social isolation. *Medical Care, 20*(9), 883–891.

Clark, L. (1995). *Mexican-origin children's health in cultural context* (Grant funded by NICHD/NINR [R29 HD32366]). Denver: University of Colorado School of Nursing.

Clark, M. P., Kaufman, S., & Pierce, R. (1976). Explorations of acculturation: Toward a model of ethnic identity. *Human Organization, 35,* 2131–2138.

Crandon-Malamud, L. (1990). *From the fat of our souls: Social change, political process, and medical pluralism in Bolivia.* Berkeley: University of California Press.

Cuellar, I., Harris, L. C., & Jasso, R. (1980). An acculturation scale for Mexican American normal and clinical populations. *Hispanic Journal of Behavioral Sciences, 2*(3), 199–217.

Cuellar, I., Arnold, B., & Maldonado, R. (1995). Acculturation rating scale for Mexican Americans: II. a revision of the original ARSMA scale. *Hispanic Journal of Behavioral Sciences, 17*(3), 275–304.

De Vos, G., & Romanucci, L. (1975). Ethnicity: Vessel of meaning and emblem of contrast. In G. De Vos & L. Romanucci (Eds.), *Ethnic identity: Cultural continuities and change* (pp. 363–365). Palo Alto, CA: Mayfield.

Deyo, R. A., Diehl, A. K., Hazuda, H., & Stern, M. P. (1985). A simple language-based acculturation scale for Mexican Americans: Validation and application to health care research. *American Journal of Public Health, 75*(1), 51–55.

Estrada, L. F. (1993). Family influences on demographic trends in Hispanic ethnic identification and labeling. In M. Bernal & G. P. Knight (Eds.), *Ethnic identity: Formation and transmission among Hispanics and other minorities* (pp. 163–179). Albany: State University of New York Press.

Evinger, S. (1995). How shall we measure our nation's diversity? *Chance, 8*(1), 7–14.

Garza, R. T., & Lipton, J. P. (1984). Foundations for a Chicano social psychology. In J. L. Jr. Martinez, Jr. & R. H. Mendoza (Eds.), *Chicano Psychology* (2nd ed., pp. 335–365). New York: Academic Press.

Gil, A. G., Vega, W. A., & Dimas, J. M. (1994). Acculturative stress and personal adjustment among Hispanic adolescent boys. *Journal of Community Psychology, 22,* 43–54.

Gordon, M. M. (1964). *Assimilation in American life: The role of race, religion, and national origins.* New York: Oxford University Press.

Graves, D. T. (1967). Acculturation, access, and alcohol in a bi-ethnic community. *American Anthropologist, 69,* 306–321.

Guendelman, S., & Abrams, B. (1995). Dietary intake among Mexican-American women: Generational differences and a comparison with White and non-Hispanic women. *American Journal of Public Health, 85,* 20–25.

Guendelman, S., Gould, J., Hudes, M., & Eskenazi, B. (1990). Generational differences in perinatal health among the Mexican American population: Findings from H-HANES 1982–84. *American Journal of Public Health, 80* (Suppl.), 61–65.

Guendelman, S., English, P., & Chavez, G. (1995). The effects of maternal health behaviors and other risk factors on immunization status among Mexican-American infants. *Pediatrics, 95*(6), 823–828.

Hahn, R. A., & Stroup, D. F. (1994). Race and ethnicity in public health surveillance: Criteria for the scientific use of social categories. *Public Health Reports, 109*(1), 7–15.

Humphrey, N. D. (1943). On assimilation and acculturation. *Psychiatry, 6,* 343–345.

Hurtado, A., Rodríguez, J., Gurin, P., & Beals, J. L. (1993). The impact of Mexican descendants' social identity on the ethnic socialization of children. In M. E. Bernal & G. P. Knight (Eds.), *Ethnic identity: Formation and transmission among Hispanics and other minorities* (pp. 131–162). Albany: State University of New York Press.

Hurtado, A., Gurin, P., & Peng, T. (1994). Social identities—A framework for studying the adaptations of immigrants and ethnics: The adaptations of Mexicans in the United States. *Social Problems, 42*(1), 129–151.

Jibou, R. M. (1988). *Ethnicity and assimilation.* Albany: State University of New York Press.

Keefe, S., & Padilla, A. M. (1987). *Chicano ethnicity.* Albuquerque: University of New Mexico Press.

Knight, G. P., Tein, J. Y., Shell, R., & Roosa, M. (1993). Family socialization and Mexican American identity and behavior. In M. E. Bernal & G. P. Knight (Eds.), *Ethnic identity: Formation and transmission among Hispanics and other minorities* (pp. 105–129). Albany: State University of New York Press.

Lewontin, R. C. (1972). The apportionment of human diversity. *Evolutionary Biology, 6,* 381–398.

Limerick, P. N. (1995). Peace initiative: Using Mormons to rethink culture and ethnicity in American history. *Journal of Mormon History, 21*(2), 1–29.

Linton, R. (1940). *Acculturation in seven American Indian tribes.* New York: Appleton-Century.

Luna Solorzano, M. I. (1992). *The psychometric properties of the measurement of culture change in Mexican-American children and its contributions to the theory of acculturation.* Unpublished doctoral dissertation, University of Arizona, Tucson.

Macías, R. (1993). Language and ethnic classification of language minorities: Chicano and Latino students in the 1990s. *Hispanic Journal of Behavioral Sciences, 15*(2), 230–257.

Marín, B. V., Tschaun, J. M., Gomez, C., & Kegeles, S. M. (1993). Acculturation and gender differences in sexual attitudes and behaviors: Hispanic versus non-Hispanic white unmarried adults. *American Journal of Public Health, 83*(12), 1759–1766.

Marín, G., Sabogal, F., Marín, B., Otero-Sabogal, R., & Peréz-Stable, E. J. (1987). Development of a short acculturation scale for Hispanics. *Hispanic Journal of Behavioral Sciences, 9,* 183–205.

Markides, K. S., & Coreil, J. (1986). The health of Hispanics in the southwestern United States: An epidemiologic paradox. *Public Health Reports, 101*(3), 253–265.

Markides, K. S., & Lee, D. J. (1991). Predictors of health status in middle-aged and older Mexican Americans. *Journal of Gerontology, 46*(5), S243–249.

Markides, K. S., Levin, J. S., & Ray, L. A. (1985). Determinants of physician utilization among Mexican-Americans. *Medical Care, 23*(3), 236–246.

Marshall, G. A. (1968). Racial classifications: Popular and scientific. In M. Mead, T. Dobzhansky, E. Tobach, & R. E. Light (Eds.), *Science and the concept of race* (pp. 149–164). New York: Columbia University Press.

Matthiasson, C. W. (1968). *The acculturation of Mexican Americans in a midwestern industrial city.* Unpublished doctoral dissertation, Cornell University, Ithaca, NY.

McFee, M. (1968). The 150% man: A product of Blackfeet acculturation. *American Anthropologist, 70,* 1096–1103.

Melville, M. B. (1983). Ethnicity: An analysis of its dynamism and variablity focusing on the Mexican/Anglo/Mexican American interface. *American Ethnologist, 10,* 272–289.

Melville, M. B. (1988). Hispanics: Race, class, or ethnicity? *Journal of Ethnic Studies, 16*(1), 67–83.

Mendoza, R., & Martínez, J. L., Jr. (1981). The measurement of acculturation. In A. Baron, Jr. (Ed.), *Explorations in Chicano psychology* (pp. 71–82). New York: Praeger.

Mendoza, R. H. (1984). Acculturation and sociocultural variability. In J. L. Martinez, Jr. & R. H. Mendoza (Eds.), *Chicano Psychology* (2nd ed., pp. 61–76). Los Angeles: Academic Press.

National Center for Health Statistics. (1985). *Plan and operation of the Hispanic Health and Nutrition Examination Survey, 1982–1984.* Washington, DC: U.S. Government Printing Office, Public Health Service.

Negy, C., & Woods, D. (1992). A note on the relationship between acculturation and socioeconomic status. *Hispanic Journal of Behavioral Sciences, 14*(2), 248–251.

Nichter, M. (1981). Idioms of distress: Alternatives in the expression of psychosocial distress: A case study from South India. *Culture, Medicine, and Psychiatry, 5,* 5–24.

Office of Management and Budget. (1977). Directive No. 15: Race and Ethnic Standards for Federal Statistics and Administrative Reporting. U.S. Department of Commerce, Office of Federal Statistical and Policy Standards.

Olmedo, E. L., & Padilla, A. M. (1978). Empirical and construct validation of a measure of acculturation in Mexican Americans. *Journal of Social Psychology, 105*(2), 179–187.

Olmedo, E. L., Martínez, J. L., Jr., & Martínez, S. R. (1978). Measure of acculturation for Chicano adolescents. *Psychological Reports, 42,* 159–170.

Padilla, A. M. (1980). The role of cultural awareness and ethnic loyalty. In A. M. Padilla (Ed.), *Acculturation: Theory, models and some new findings* (pp. 47–84). Boulder, CO: Westview.

Padilla, A. M. (1995). *Hispanic psychology.* Thousand Oaks, CA: Sage.

Pappas, G. (1993). *La Raza—Identify yourselves!* Denver, CO: Latin American Research and Service Agency.

Perez-Stable, E. J., Marín, B. V., Marín, G., Brody, D. J., & Benowitz, N. L. (1990). Apparent underreporting of cigarette consumption among Mexican American smokers. *American Journal of Public Health, 80,* 1057–1061.

Ramirez, M. (1984). Assessing and understanding biculturalism-multiculturalism in Mexican-American adults. In J. L. Martinez & R. H. Mendoza (Eds.), *Chicano psychology* (2nd ed., pp. 77–94). New York: Academic Press.

Ramirez, M., & Castenada, A. (1974). *The psychodynamics of biculturalism: Systems and evaluations in education.* Arlington, VA: Office of Naval Research.

Rassin, D. K., Kyrizkos, M. S., Baranowski, T., Bee, D. E., Richardson, C. J., Mikrut, W. D., & Winkler, A. (1993). Acculturation and breastfeeding on the United States–Mexico border. *American Journal of the Medical Sciences, 306*(1), 28–34.

Samora, J., & Deane, W. N. (1956). Language usage as a possible index of acculturation. *Sociology and Social Research, 40,* 307–311.

Shetterly, S. M., Baxter, J., Mason, L., & Hamman, R. F. (1996). Self-rated health among Hispanics vs. non-Hispanic white adults: The San Luis Valley health and aging study. *American Journal of Public Health, 86*(12), 1798–1801.

Shorris, E. (1992). *Latinos.* New York: Norton.

Sorlie, P. D., Backlund, E., Johnson, N. J., & Rogot, E. (1993). Mortality by Hispanic status in the United States. *Journal of the American Medical Association, 270*(20), 2464–2468.

Sowell, T. (1996). *Migrations and cultures: A worldview.* New York: Basic Books.

Spindler, G. D. (1955). *Sociocultural and psychological processes in Menomini acculturation* (Arnold and Caroline Rose Monograph Series in Sociology). Berkeley: University of California Press.

Stanfield, J. H., II. (1993). Epistemological considerations. In J. H. Stanfield, II & R. M. Dennis (Eds.), *Race and ethnicity in research methods* (pp. 16–36). Newbury Park, CA: Sage.

Szapocznik, J., Scopetta, M. A., & Kurtines, W. (1978). Theory and measurement of acculturation. *Interamerican Journal of Psychology, 12,* 113–130.

Tajfel, H. (1981). *Human groups and social categories: Studies in social psychology.* London: Cambridge University Press.

Thernstrom, S. (Ed.). (1980). *Harvard Encyclopedia of American Ethnic Groups.* Cambridge, MA: Belknap.

van der Geest, S., & Whyte, S. R. (1989). The charm of medicines: Metaphors and metonyms. *Medical Anthropology, 3*(4), 545–567.

Vega, W. A., & Amaro, H. (1994). Latino outlook: Good health, uncertain prognosis. *Annual Review of Public Health, 15,* 39–67.

Velez-Ibánez, C. (1996). *Border visions.* Tucson: University of Arizona Press.

Wells, K. B., Golding, J. M., Hough, R. L., Burnam, M. A., & Karno, M. (1989). Acculturation and the probability of use of health services by Mexican Americans. *Health Services Research, 24*(1), 237–257.

Whyte, S. R. (1982). Penicillin, battery acid and sacrifice. *Social Science and Medicine, 16,* 2055–2064.

Whyte, S. R. (1988). The power of medicines in East Africa. In S. van der Geest & S. R. Whyte (Eds.), *The context of medicines in developing countries* (pp. 217–234). Dordrecht: Kluwer Academic.

Williams, R. L., Binkin, N. J., & Clingman, R. J. (1986). Pregnancy outcomes among Spanish surname women in California. *American Journal of Public Health, 76*(4), 387–391.

Wolf, E. (1994). Perilous ideas: Race, culture, people. *Current Anthropology, 35*(1), 1–12.

4

Medical Interpretation

An Essential Clinical Service for Non-English-Speaking Immigrants

CAREY JACKSON

Introduction

The most pervasive need of non-English-speaking immigrants and refugees is interpretation for every English transaction. Interpretation is needed in stores, schools, and job training, and it is of critical importance in health care. If medical interpretation is unavailable or mismanaged, the costs can be enormous; these costs include human costs such as unnecessary pain and suffering and the substantial financial consequences of care for patients who present at late stages of an illness or who are unable to give a clear and meaningful history. While the potential cost savings of having skilled interpretation has never been adequately assessed, the assumption is that physicians will err on the conservative side, and will rely on technology to answer questions if they suspect the patient is not able to provide a clear history. Consequently, blood tests, X rays, and CT scans are ordered unnecessarily, or conversely, tests may be needed but not ordered when physicians are unsure of the true nature

of the complaint. These are high stakes, both in human terms and health system dollars.

In this chapter I provide an overview of features of medical interpretation pertinent for health care delivery to recently arrived immigrants. I direct my comments especially toward immigrants unfamiliar with Western biomedical care. First, I discuss how interpreting needs are influenced by a community. I then turn my attention to the inner workings of interpreted encounters, considering the agenda of patients, physicians, and interpreters during the encounters. Each partner in a medical encounter presents specific linguistic issues that must be addressed. Any attempt at successful resolution must address the needs of each sector. I conclude with a discussion of models for providing interpreter services, and the training required. The unique challenges of translated written health education materials are touched on, but are not the focus of this chapter. The important technical issues in translating and developing cross-cultural instruments for research deserve special consideration and are the topic of Chapter 5.

The Triadic Relationships: Patient, Clinician, Interpreter

Complicated dynamics in medical encounters have been described in a number of ex-

CAREY JACKSON • Division of General Internal Medicine, University of Washington, Seattle, Washington 98104.

Handbook of Immigrant Health, edited by Loue. Plenum Press, New York, 1998.

cellent articles (Chavez, 1993; Kaufert, 1984; O'Neil, Koolage, & Kaufert, 1988; Putsch, 1985, 1990;) describing several common issues that arise during bilingual clinical encounters: Bad paraphrasing, impatience, the lack of linguistic equivalence, interpreter beliefs, ethnocentrism, and role conflicts are just a few of the complexities that can impact interpreted communication. The problem of role conflicts is especially important as interpreters assume expanding roles as advocates and cultural brokers (Kaufert & Koolage, 1984; Kaufert, O'Neil, & Koolage, 1985). Each member of the triad has a unique agenda and set of challenges. It is useful to consider each point of view as we analyze the work to be done.

The Patient's Experience

Immigrant Communities in a Nation of Immigrants

With the exception of Native Americans, this is a country of immigrants and refugees fleeing from persecution. Each arriving group came driven by oppression, called by opportunity, or both. Religious persecution in England prompted the flight of the Puritans and Quakers to form small religious colonies. The most traumatic immigration occurred when Africans were forced to relocate as slaves. In the 1870s, new opportunity and a severe famine brought the Irish. Jews fleeing pogroms in Eastern Europe arrived in the late 1800s and through the turn of the century.

The current era in immigration from Asia began following the Southeast Asian wars in Cambodia, Laos, and Vietnam (Meuecke, 1983; Office of Refugee Resettlement, 1990). In 1975, the initial waves of what would later total more than a million Vietnamese refugees began to hit the United States. While the Vietnamese were resettled in urban and rural communities across the country, they often relocated to areas where older, established Asian-American communities had an organized presence, cities such as Honolulu, Los Angeles, Oakland, San Francisco, Seattle, and New York. The distinct identity of the Vietnamese community grafted itself to these well-established Chinese and Japanese communities before branching out into new locations, such as Garden Grove, California, Houston, Texas, St. Paul, Minnesota, and Washington, D.C. The Vietnamese identity is historically and socially distinct from the Chinese, yet there are shared Confucian filial values, Buddhist precepts, and historical origins that facilitated early relocation efforts.

Other Southeast Asian immigrants have less in common with the older established Chinese communities. Cambodians, for example, began to arrive shortly after the Vietnamese, and their numbers grew considerably during the Khmer Rouge reign of terror (1975–1979). The origins of Khmer culture, however, are in India and the Khmer have an uneasy historical relationship with Vietnam, their neighbor to the east. Similarly, the hill tribes from the mountains of Southeast Asia are minorities who have long been neglected, at times persecuted, living in remote areas of China, Thailand, Laos, and Vietnam. Each of these groups have distinct cultural traditions, histories, and languages that affect their medical translation needs (Gilman et al., 1992; Hoang, 1985).

Political and social upheaval in Central Asia and Central America, East Africa, and Eastern Europe brought more recent waves of immigrants to U.S. cities in large numbers. In 1980, 23 million residents spoke little or no English. By 1990, another 38% or 8.8 million people spoke English as a second language (Guillemin, Bombardier, & Beaton, 1993). In inner-city neighborhoods and in suburbs, Afghans, Eritreans, Ethiopians, Haitians, Ukrainians, Salvadorans, Somalis, and Tibetans establish their businesses, mosques, churches, temples, restaurants, and stores. Distinctly different languages, cultures, historical experiences, and relationships with neighboring groups are reestablished in these settings. While the non-English-speaking members of immigrant communities share a common reliance on interpretation, their unique cultures, colonial histories, familiarity with Western medicine, educational experiences, healing traditions, and the organization of scientific health care in their countries further modify their expectations and the dynamics of interpretation during medical encounters (Haffner, 1992).

For example, the use of oral medicines to treat diabetes may be very familiar to a Ukranian patient, but the diagnosis and the treatment may be unheard of by a Mien patient from Laos. The Mien patient may require significant education about the symptoms, sequelae, and prognosis of the illness itself. In contrast, the Ukranian may understand diabetes, but require equal amounts of explanation to understand how the American medical system works differently from the old Soviet system. Both patients may elect to use herbal therapies with their hypoglycemic medication. For each patient, the linguistic and educational issues reflect their personal and community experience as immigrants with American medical care.

Physicians and health workers providing health care for immigrant communities need to consider the patient's origins, urban or rural, their socioeconomic status, especially their educational background, ethnic identity, relocation history, personal medical traditions, and experience with Western colonial institutions, especially medical systems in their home countries. The technical skills needed in an industrialized economy may be a challenge for a relocated rural farmer. Adjusting to loss of privilege and responsibility may be among the challenges for a resettled aristocrat. The assistance of a knowledgeable interpreter is invaluable in making these assessments. The relevance of a patient's gender, family role, ethnicity, education, previous contact with industrialized society, and familiarity with Western medicine to the level and intensity of interpretation required cannot be stressed enough. This fact constantly reemerges through this chapter.

Linguistic Access

Recent arrivals get information by word of mouth from sponsors, friends, or relatives who direct them to known sources of care. Getting an appointment, understanding directions, registering with an HMO, community or public health clinic requires the non-English speaker to have interpretation available in the form of a friend or family member, if the institution does not provide it. Once registered and the appointment made, the patient faces obstacles including making sense of parking instructions, navigating the facility, greeting the receptionist, and filling out intake forms at the front desk of the clinic.

It is impossible for hospitals and clinics to provide signs in all of the languages of its patient population. At Harborview Medical Center in Seattle, patients need interpretation in more than 60 languages. A cafeteria sign in 60 languages would be absurd. There are only 10 commonly spoken languages, but this is not much better. Pictograms may be the most useful visual aid for illiterate patients and non-English speakers alike. Although not every activity or department lends itself to representation in the form of an icon, many do. Colored icons and other visual aids can help people pathfind. Finding the clinic is not the central issue in access. The heart of the matter is to make health needs clear, and in turn, to receive a meaningful response from the caregiver.

The Semantics of Illness

In a now classic paper entitled "The Heart of What's the Matter: The Semantics of Illness in Iran," Byron Good and Mary Jo Delvechio Good outline what this author considers the central interpretation issue for patients and physicians from different cultures (B. Good & Good, 1977). During a survey of health issues for rural Iranian women in a village where "heart distress" was a frequently encountered complaint, physicians were often frustrated by their inability to find an "organic" basis for this routine complaint. Iranian women readily described the symptoms of heart distress and its numerous causes: poverty, nerves, anxiety, worry, old age, contraception, too little blood, cold, and dampness. The anatomical heart was identified as a cause by only 6% of the women. Not surprisingly, the physicians' concerns to exclude cardiovascular sources of pain were doomed from the outset since they did not understand the real nature of "heart distress."

B. Good and Good (1977) concluded that complaints such as "heart distress" are part of a semantic network of terms such as worry, poverty, pollution, and cold. These authors defined the term *semantic network* to mean that disease categories are more than a constellation of symptoms, but form a "syndrome of typical experiences, a set of words, experiences, and feelings which typically run together for the members of a society. Such a syndrome is not merely a reflection of symptoms linked with each other in natural reality, but a set of experiences associated through networks of meaning and social interactions in a society" (p. 27). This definition can be applied to both folk illnesses such as "heart distress" and biomedical diagnoses like "influenza" or "epilepsy." Because symptoms and illnesses are linked with other concepts of illness and treatment for both patients and physicians, the semantics of illness are critical junctures of communication that must be managed appropriately and meaningfully by medical interpreters.

Consider this example: A rural Cambodian woman of 50 resettles in Los Angeles and presents to the local community clinic complaining of *"loan sboan." Loan sboan,* in Khmer, is literally "noisy womb," and means that this woman is experiencing a moderate amount of uterine prolapse. For older Cambodian women, uterine prolapse is considered a worrisome experience; if not controlled, it might progress to *tloeak sboan,* which is a severely prolapsed uterus. *Tloeak sboan* and *roliak sboan* (inflammation) are considered a precursor to *sboan tom,* a grave

condition where the uterus is inflamed and has a foul-smelling discharge. *Sboan tom* is considered a condition similar to cancer, *mahareak sboan;* it is generally felt that there is no treatment for *mahareak* or *sboan tom* and the patient will die. This woman has identified a potentially life-threatening condition which in her opinion could become severe if not treated.

The gynecologist who sees her is told by the interpreter that she is complaining about her prolapsed uterus and in response the gynecologist asks about accompanying symptoms. There is no urinary incontinence, no discharge, no pelvic pain, no significant uterine descent, and currently no embarrassment. The gynecologist does a pelvic examination, a urine culture, and urodynamics. Everything is fine. She reassures the patient that the problem is mild and surgery is not necessary, and she recommends Kegel exercises. The woman is glad not to need surgery but she is not consoled; her mother died of *sboan tom* in Cambodia and she wants a medicine, or massage therapy, a device, something to prevent *tloeak sboan,* so she goes to another provider in another clinic and begins again.

The cultural significance of the semantics of illness for this woman were not understood and therefore not discussed by the gynecologist. The patient and the gynecologist used terms from their respective semantic networks. For the gynecologist, mild to moderate uterine prolapse suggests conservative therapy, beginning with exercises, perhaps hormone replacement if appropriate, or surgery if the problem progresses. However, uterine prolapse itself is not a precursor to cancer, and is not a life-threatening illness. The gynecologist has no suspicion that uterine prolapse might have a familial and cultural significance for Cambodian women. In stark contrast, the patient has memories of her mother's prolapsed uterus, her discomfort, embarrassment, and slow death. Pap testing means nothing to her. Her personal story is nested in a cultural model of reproductive health signified by the terms she uses for uterine prolapse.

The point here is not only that the semantics of illness are different in modern medicine and in traditional non-Western cultures, but that these networks of meaning tie linguistic communities together. Words represent things, but they also are used in specific contexts to suggest appropriate behaviors. This is true in professional and in lay cultures alike. Bridging the distance between the semantic networks of physicians and immigrant communities is at times impossible, but it is the demanding and critical work of medical interpreters.

Constant change while preserving continuity is characteristic of culture and language. Add to the previous discussion of semantic networks the fact that these networks are constantly modified by and adapted to new experiences, yet are preserved to ensure a common meaningful linguistic framework. Traditional models of health and illness can change with acculturation to biomedical notions of disease. Change occurs through new experiences with neighbors and with healers from diverse places. Misinformation and personal experience also add to cultural change in the use of terms. In a clinical setting, one must wonder if it is possible to keep track of these moving semantic targets. Yet on a daily basis, people have meaningful conversations, navigating networks of meaning as they adapt the new to the old.

The Clinician's Perspective

Language is medicine's most essential technology, its principal instrument for conducting its work. This dual role of language in medicine as both a social tie and technical instrument routinely contributes to misunderstandings between physicians and patients. Consider as an example information about the risk of disease transmission from unprotected intercourse. In a clinical context, questions about sexual activity are technical questions to help the clinician decide about risks of pregnancy and sexually transmitted diseases. These are also highly personal, revealing, and potentially embarrassing ques-

tions about social relationships. Unless they handled these questions carefully, clinicians can easily offend patients in a sincere effort to help them determine their risk of disease.

The translation of medical speech is a daily clinical event in cities and towns across the country. Information about symptoms, diagnoses, prognoses, and treatment are routinely interpreted for non-English-speaking patients with little critical attention paid to the quality of the translations. Misunderstandings routinely occur even when patient and provider speak a common language. The uterine prolapse example shows that misunderstandings can be even more dramatic when the interaction is cross-cultural and must be negotiated through an interpreter.

The Origins of Medical Language

Physicians themselves may not appreciate the unique language they speak and how it facilitates their work. Greek and Latin roots are used in medicine today for historical reasons with origins in the medieval scholastic tradition (Skinner, 1949). Greco-Roman medicine was preserved in Byzantium and Alexandria in Greek and was translated into Arabic and then passed on to European scholars by Islamic and Jewish scholars. In the thirteenth century, medicine became a university subject and was taught in Latin. Through the Middle Ages into the Renaissance, classical languages conveyed the learning of clerics and scholars (Jonsen, 1997).

Classical languages provided a common tongue for clerics to debate and refine church dogma throughout early church history. Although Greek and Latin terms had their origins in scholasticism, they persist because the structure of these languages allows for easy recombination of suffixes and prefixes making subtle distinctions possible. Newly coined medical words are intended to be part of a universal language of medicine that refers to universal biological processes. As in antiquity, this classical lingua franca is intended to tie scientists and clinicians together with common linguistic forms and semantic networks, a way of thinking that now circles the globe. The sanctifying and mystifying effect of medical speech may be an unintended consequence that unites clinicians but divides them from lay people. While this separate form of speech can be exploited to reinforce status and power, in general, it is an obstacle that is constantly negotiated in physician–patient interactions.

In the West, since the thirteenth century, clinicians have learned the practice of medicine by first learning the language of medicine. Once learned, medical language becomes an invisible technology, but an essential linguistic tool for sorting. For example, it is central for the medical history and review of systems. While taking a history, physicians silently restructure patient experience into symptom complexes by means of this specialized language, employing Latin and Greek words such as *orthopnea, angina,* and *paroxysmal nocturnal dyspnea.* These words are conceptually linked with the words of diagnosis and treatment in a semantic network that is the linguistic basis of clinical activity. Without losing track of the person, physicians attempt to deconstruct an individual experience of illness and give precedence to well-recognized expressions consistent with known disease processes over idiosyncratic experiences incongruent with clinical reasoning. Once the patient's experience has been reconfigured according to a medical paradigm, as one word evokes another, a physician can find his or her way along the semantic pathways to the implied evaluation and treatment algorithms.

For laypeople, language and behaviors are linked in entirely different ways. Consider the Cambodian woman in the previous example. Cambodian illness terms are linked to an intricate web of natural forces, supernatural beings, family life, social obligation, and karmic law. For example, illness terms associated with the accumulation of wind, or *kyol,* imply dermabrasive coining to release wind. Other illnesses evoke the performances for ancestor care, the behaviors to ward off witchcraft, charitable actions to address the laws of

karma, or, as in the case of *sboan tom,* the use of herbs and massage. It is the culturally defined knowledge and social practices of Cambodian people that links experience through language to an implied set of behaviors.

Medical language gives expression to the allopathic process of order to experience and set the structural features of a disease apart from the particular person who has experienced that disease. Meaning, certainty, and authority lie in the scientific features of the disease that stand apart and supersede the personalized experiential features of illness. The process of sorting the subjective from the objective through the use of medical terms has the unintended effect of deciding what is "important" and what is "superfluous" in an individual's (and culture's) experience of illness, decisions that do not necessarily coincide with what that patient or group of patients thinks is important about the illness.

Most clinicians are keenly aware that the technical paradigms of science and lay paradigms of illness are incongruent, and they struggle to adapt the technical thinking of biomedicine to the individual and social contexts of their patients. When gender, class, and culture must be negotiated in addition to medical thinking, the struggle is complex and delicate. Physicians rely on input from interpreters to negotiate these differences. If the physician is uninformed about the common semantics of illness in the patient population, it is impossible to address the issue.

Diagnosis and Treatment

As physicians attempt to diagnose and treat illness, or as public health educators and program developers attempt to discuss risk, they move between medical thinking and socially specific contexts. Medical interpreters can be preoccupied with the precision of medical language and the sophisticated interpretation it requires, and then lose track of their audience. Similarly, clinicians who speak medical language fluently may rely on medical speech to express their thoughts. In so doing, they can lose track of which view of reality is being discussed, the biological reality or the socially situated reality of a patient's daily life. Medical words for clinicians may imply risk for the health of biological bodies, but may not acknowledge the relationships at risk for the social body. Consider the difference in the quality of the personal relationships acknowledged through the choice of the words "unprotected intercourse," compared with "making love spontaneously without a condom."

The responsibility for interpreting does not lie exclusively with physicians. Even simple phrases may require special consideration in translation. Thai, Buchwald, and Hooten (1993) surveyed five Southeast Asian immigrant communities seen for routine care in a primary care clinic in Seattle. He interviewed Cambodian, Vietnamese, Lao, Mien, and Chinese patients. Patients were asked about their knowledge and understanding of the causes of commonly translated medical terms: cold, high blood pressure, heart attack, TB, and seizures. For these immigrants routine medical terms were unrecognizable, even in translation. In another study of public health pamphlets assessing the comprehensibility of Hepatitis B for Cambodian patients, only 6 of the 34 respondents recognized the meaning of *rauk tlaam,* the Cambodian translation of hepatitis. In contrast, when Cambodians were presented with the symptoms of acute and chronic hepatitis all 34 immediately recognized the illness and identified it by several terms such as *khan leoung* or *tloeak andoek* (Jackson *et al.,* 1997). What accounts for the difficulty with translation? Is it physician insensitivity? Patient ignorance? Interpreter incompetence? The authors note that there may be something inherent in medical thinking about illness that does not translate into many cultural contexts.

Cambodian experiential and conceptual equivalents were not considered when initially translating hepatitis B information because of the importance of giving information of universal importance about the liver while assuming that the uniquely Cambodian experience of illness was

minimally important. . . . Khmer medical interpreters have expressed their frustration to us in trying to explain this "unseen, unperceived structure of disease to Khmer patients who identify an illness based on the experience of that illness. Diseases like hypertension, diabetes, and hepatitis B are especially difficult because they may be asymptomatic for long periods of time; during asymptomatic periods, when people feel fine, clinicians insist that disease and disorder are present when the patient has no experience of either." (pp. 297–298)

Treatment intentions are equally unrecognizable by immigrant patients who are operating according to traditional health concepts. Compliance is a challenge regardless of the population and clinical issue. In an interpreted setting the semantics of illness influence treatment decisions as well. Shimada, Jackson, Goldstein, and Buchwald (1995) surveyed Cambodian refugee patients in a primary care setting and found that 70% of the patients were noncompliant with prescribed therapy. In personal interviews, she discovered that patients were attempting to be compliant, but according to Cambodian paradigms of medicine. Patients were adjusting medications by alternating days, lowering doses, and refusing to combine medication in an effort to match perceived strength of medicine with perceived strength of illness, other illnesses, and personal history. Chart reviews suggested physicians were completely unaware of this behind-the-scenes manipulation of medications.

The Interpreter's Work

Bridging Worlds

Medical interpreters are presented with the challenge of bridging the cultures of patients and physicians. In the clinical encounter they must find bridging concepts and words between the semantic networks of patients and physicians. Equivalent words are easier to find if the language groups share a common linguistic base and cultural history, such as the Indo-Aryan-based European languages, but if linguistic structure and daily practices differ significantly, then equivalent words and experiences may not exist. If the interpretation takes place between languages with markedly different linguistic and cultural origins such as English and Navajo, or English and Mhung, the difficulty of the task is determined by the availability of common experiences in each speaker's world.

Translation has been described as a process of finding equivalent verbal structures, while recognizing significant cultural variations in their uses and meanings (Catford, 1965). Sechrest, Fay, and Hafeez-Zadi. (1972) distinguished between five types of equivalence in translation: Vocabulary, grammatical, idiomatic, conceptual, and experiential. *Vocabulary equivalence* entails finding the word with the equivalent nuances and connotations to carry the meaning. Often there are no vocabulary equivalents for concepts or items available in another language. English often adopts terms precisely because there are no vocabulary equivalents. Words such as *taboo, amok,* and *sitar* are words borrowed from languages to represent complicated ideas and things unfamiliar in English. The term *rauk tlaam* from the hepatitis B survey is a good example of Khmer translation focusing only on a vocabulary equivalent of hepatitis. Beginning with an organ-based model of illness, an attempt was made to convey this anatomic view of hepatitis to the Khmer by creating a verbal counterpart focused on the liver. The fact that very few Cambodian people could make sense of this term shows how limited this approach to translation is.

Grammatic equivalence refers to parts of speech present, absent, or problematic in certain languages. In some languages abstract terms such as "livestock" may not exist and people rely on concrete terms such as "cows, buffaloes, pigs, and chickens." Some languages lack subjunctive tenses so that hypothetical concepts easily expressed in English by the subjunctive pairing "if you could, would you _____" cannot be translated except through a carefully constructed contextual format.

There are *idiomatic equivalences* that can be found between languages, but in general idioms are so language-specific that it is not a surprise they do not readily translate.

Conceptual equivalence refers to the multiple linguistic associations of certain words. As in poetry, the values associated with a word, its linkage to other words, and the implications of its use in that culture are its conceptual associations. For example, in English, heart refers to an organ, the seat of emotion, a person's character (as in cold-hearted or lion-hearted), and the core of an issue (as in the heart of the matter). Because conceptual associations are steeped in history and usage, conceptual equivalence in translation, while ideal, is routinely impossible.

Experiential equivalence means that for a word or phrase to be meaningful it must refer to real things and real experiences that are familiar in both cultures. The association of a word with specific experiences links that word in socially and conceptually unique ways for the groups that share that language. In medical translation experiential equivalence can often, although not always, be found in bodily symptoms (Ots, 1990). This is usually the most productive place to focus the interpretive effort.

Linking concepts to experiences, and experiences to implied behaviors, requires that special attention be paid to both referential and performative values of words. The *referential value* of a word means that the word refers to some element or concept in the speaker's world. *Performative value* means that the use of a word will imply specific behaviors in a given context (Austin, 1965). For example, the sentence "there is a bear," may imply entertainment and education at the zoo with my children, and a move toward safety in the mountains with my children. In both contexts the referent may be the same, but the performative value is markedly different. This is a crucial observation about language relevant both to health education and interpretation. Keeping track of the reference and the actions implied by that reference in a given context are extremely difficult tasks when people do not share the same daily activities and realities.

The performative value of word choice comes up on a daily basis in communication across disciplines as well as across cultures. Peter Jucovy studied dermatopathologists in the Philadelphia area and found that among the group of pathologists interviewed, the word *dysplasia* was a useful referential feature of cells used for descriptive purposes. These same pathologists were reluctant to use the word *dysplasia* with surgeons because of the dire performative consequences of that word in a surgical context (Jucovy, 1982).

In a cross-cultural context, where words connect to semantic networks with performative implications unknown to clinicians, interpreters must explore the intended meaning of words with patients, and help explain the conceptual linkages to clinicians. It is because simple vocabulary equivalence is not always possible that an interpreter's work is simultaneously critical and complex.

Community Expectations

Most of the discussion so far has focused on conceptual and linguistic demands of medical interpretation from the point of view of those people directly involved in the encounter. The interpreter is connected to a larger community through culture and language (O'Neil, Koolage, & Kaufert 1988). In addition to language and culture, the community influences clinical encounters in more subtle ways. In many towns and cities, interpreters come from relatively small communities; within these communities English speakers are important community figures. Interpreters play critical roles in these communities and are relied on for information and advice (J. Kaufert, 1984). Interpreters are well aware of their importance in the community and usually take the responsibility quite seriously, often volunteering uncompensated assistance.

Because of community and clinical roles, medical interpreters are privy to very confidential information. Professional ethics are taught in most interpreter training programs, but unless constantly reminded, interpreters can inadvertently violate patient or physician confidences. Patients may be unfamiliar with the notion of professional interpreter confidentiality and worry that sensitive information will leak back to the community. Given the small size of some communities, information travels through the grapevine quickly. One or two breaches of confidentiality may impede the free flow of interpreted information between physician and patient for significant periods of time, both for that patient and others who hear the report.

Beyond confidentiality, family and community members may expect favors or special consideration from interpreters. The etiquette of social engagement differs significantly between clinical and community settings. Community members may expect special consideration within the institution made possible by the interpreter.

Physicians may expect interpreters to understand the medical agenda and to represent the clinic or hospital in interpreted interactions. The social pressure experienced by interpreters can be considerable. Political factions can split small communities. The rippling effects of community politics are often felt in the clinic. The conflicting expectations, multiple roles, and privileged position of interpreters as trusted repositories of information in both communities and clinics can overwhelm and isolate interpreters. Competing expectations may become unmanageable and interpreters may inadvertently violate confidences or have irreconcilable conflicts of interest. If interpreters make culturally or politically unpopular decisions, they may become pariahs in their own communities.

The professional role and responsibilities of interpreters, the political and social pressures they experience, and the differences between the cultures of medical institutions and traditional communities create a rich and complicated subtext for even the most straightforward clinical encounter. As interpreters are negotiating the complexities of the semantics of illness, they are keeping an eye on the social implications of their work. The ability to interpret in clinical settings, to navigate this terrain, requires special training.

Organizing Interpreter Services

Who Should Interpret?

Medical interpreters have only recently been acknowledged as critical professionals in health care delivery to non-English-speaking patients (Ginsberg *et al.*, 1995). In years past, English-speaking family, friends, or bilingual staff were relied on to provide this service. In light of the conceptual and linguistic complexity of the work, it should be obvious why only trained professional interpreters have enough experience and understanding to bridge the semantic networks of medical culture and the targeted immigrant group. Only people adept at representing common health complaints in a clinical setting should be allowed to do this work. The subtleties of interpretation can be lost by the less skilled and the patient easily can be misrepresented and then misdiagnosed. Unless hired in this capacity, bilingual clinic staff have other responsibilities, and their loyalty to the clinic sometimes make it difficult for them to be patient advocates.

Graduates of foreign medical schools and nursing programs working as interpreters in this country may seem to be the ideal people to interpret in clinical settings. This is not always the case. Often medical professionals are from higher social classes or are young and unfamiliar with concepts and terms of traditional culture. They may understand medical culture better than they do aspects of their own culture and have little interest or patience in exploring the semantics of illness unfamiliar to them. Young interpreters raised in the United States may speak English well, but may not be very fluent in the language and concepts of their mother tongue. How and where to find adequately skilled medical professionals remains an evolving challenge in many cities across the country.

Accuracy versus Advocacy

There is considerable debate among professional interpreters about the appropriate roles and responsibilities of interpreters. Some policy makers feel that interpreters should say exactly what is said in the room between patient and provider and take no responsibility for additional contextual information. Others feel that non-English-speaking patients are in a position of vulnerability and they need advocates within the system to make their needs known (J. M. Kaufert & Koolage, 1984).

Given the preceeding linguistic discussion, it should be clear that unless there are easily identifiable equivalences between languages, interpreters will find themselves obscuring meanings by being very literal. If they choose to clarify meanings by going beyond strict interpreting, they are culture broking. There are without a doubt patients and settings that require nothing but careful literal interpretation, and others that need considerable advocacy and cultural interpretation. When the interpreters feel inadequate to provide the larger context, they should at least make it clear to the provider that such a context may exist and suggest clarifying questions or other resources for obtaining clarification.

Physician Training

The responsibility for obtaining medical history lies with the clinician, not the interpreter. Training interpreters how to work with physicians is important, but it is equally important to train physicians how to work with interpreters. Interpreters' skills are available to providers only if they know how to use them. Teaching physicians to work with interpreters is a critical practice rarely taught by most medical schools and residencies. While hours are spent teaching students how to obtain a medical history, virtually no attention is paid to the special skills needed to do this efficiently through interpretation. There are notable exceptions. Eric Hart and the group at Boston University have produced a set of teaching videotapes available from Boston University. Similarly, the University of Arizona has paid attention to this topic, providing tapes to demonstrate how physicians ought to address patients through interpreters. The Cross-Cultural Health Care Program in Seattle also addresses this issue through regional and national level attention to interpretation needs in medical institutions. Robert W. Putsch and Joel Kaufert, in particular, have written for physicians about the special dynamics of interpreted encounters and the role conflicts encountered by interpreters (J. M. Kaufert *et al.,* 1985; Putsch, 1985). No single set of tapes or articles can analyze the multitude of things that can be encountered or go wrong in an interpreted medical visit.

Role-playing is one way residents and students can simulate the common problems encountered in interpreted patient visits. In this exercise an interpreter speaking English presents as a typical patient with a common complaint. One resident acts as the physician while a second acts as an interpreter, trying to recall all that is said by both physician and patient, and then relaying the exact message, but in a culturally meaningful way, to the other party. The entire exercise is in English and residents critique both the interpreter and the physician on memory, accuracy, and conceptual clarity. It is an effective way to experience the difficulty of the interpreter's role. Residents and students learn how to work in synchrony with interpreters, and learn to identify how and why things can get confused. Unfortunately, these sessions are not routinely organized in all teaching programs and physicians are left to their own devices to develop a style of work through interpretation.

In addition to work with interpreters it is very helpful to have community leaders or interpreters provide didactic sessions for house staff on the expectations and attitudes of local communities toward biomedical care. Clearly this is most relevant when the discussions focus on immigrant communities that frequently use the medical center.

How to Interpret

The optimal medical interpreter is capable of a range of interpreting styles. Simultaneous word-for-word interpretation, as practiced in the United Nations, is difficult to do unless the content is known beforehand, or unless the content is very routine, such as simple instructions for dosing medication. Phrase-by-phrase interpretation is the interpretation of one or two sentences or ideas at a time. This style allows for efficient interpretation during most encounters. Complete ideas can be expressed and the interpreter can negotiate the semantics of both patients and providers a phrase at a time.

If stories are long and beside the point, or if the semantic fields require extensive explanation, then occasionally summary interpretation is helpful. Summary interpretation means that entire stories or complicated ideas are paraphrased with annotation to make them comprehensible.

> Patient: I awakened earlier than usual before dawn to pray, knowing that I would have to take my medication before the rising of the sun. Ramadan feels different in America in winter; the days are short and it is not so hard to keep the fast since the weather is cool. It is also not the same feeling since the whole city is not observing the fast. Many people are unaware of our holy month. It is often hard to adjust my medication during these times.

A simple summary might be:

> Interpreter: She is dosing her medication for Ramadan, awaking early to pray and take her pills before sunrise; she is finding it hard to adjust her medication.

In contrast, culture broking is the expansion of information to make it comprehensible. Consider the simple statement, "We will get a CAT scan of your lower back to see what is wrong." This requires culture broking to explain what a CT scan is, how it is different from an X ray, what the experience is like, and why it is generally done.

Many good interpreters speak in the first person, saying "I" instead of "he (or she) says," assuming that the patient and provider prefer to hear the expression as close to the original as possible. This verbal device can make it seem as though the interpreter is invisible. Some are so capable that they mimic the affect of the speakers when appropriate, simulating fatigue, animation, or sorrow.

Interpreter training should teach these difficult skills. In addition to interpretation skills, medical interpreter training programs should include medical terminology, a discussion of professional ethics, and an introduction to the basics of the medical and social services system in the region. Most importantly, *community members should assess the language skills and cultural knowledge of the professionals representing them.*

Organization and Efficiency

In 1995 the National Public Hospital Institute surveyed teaching hospitals about their interpreter services. Their findings are summarized in a report that notes that 33% of the responding hospitals reported that about 27% of their patients required interpreter services. Only one half of the surveyed hospitals had an identifiable department administering all interpreter services, and fewer than a quarter of the hospitals trained staff in interpretation services (Ginsberg *et al.,* 1995). The authors concluded that in institutions serving a large number of non-English-speaking patients, interpreter services requires centralization. In these departments the role of the interpreter should be clearly defined. Those authors also noted that cost considerations were not insubstantial and that third-party payers should consider paying for these services, in view of the cost of excess patient care costs from miscommunication. This report outlines how interpreter services are currently provided at representative institutions across the country and warrants close scrutiny by those involved in planning these services. In general, interpreter services in clinics and hospitals are organized by some combination of four interpreter models: institution-based interpreters, contract interpreters, bilingual staff, and case management.

Clinic- and Hospital-Based Interpreters

There are towns and city neighborhoods where one or two non-English-speaking communities predominate. In these settings, large numbers of immigrant patients from select communities may use a single facility, and so it may be cost-effective to hire interpreters to work as part of the staff. If permanent employee interpreters are not interpreting they can be involved in patient education, making written translations, or involved in telephone contact.

The presence of professional trusted interpreters can easily recruit patients to a clinic, and the converse is also true: their absence can keep people away. Efficient scheduling is the key to cost-effectiveness. If interpreters are not kept busy the efficiency is lost and what is an excellent service to an immigrant community becomes an unaffordable luxury. There are now a number of computerized scheduling programs that can assist with the scheduling of interpreters.

Contract Interpreters

In most large urban areas there are agencies that provide interpreter services through a contractual relationship with the hospital system or individual clinics. These services are usually a contract between the institution and agency in which the agency agrees to provide certified and professionally trained interpreters on a reliable basis in return for regular business. The advantage of this staffing model is apparent when it comes to the cost of paying regular salaries and benefits to employees who have limited, seasonal, or short-term utility to the institution. Many clinics see patients who speak a variety of languages such as Bosnian, Russian, Polish, Somali, Hindi, and Vietnamese. It is not cost-effective to employ an interpreter for a community if there are only a few visits a day, unless there are other tasks the interpreter can do in the clinic or hospital that do not conflict with the role as an interpreter. It is not realistic to rely on a single interpreter for a community if there are large numbers of simultaneous visits. For these reasons, contractually organized interpretation makes a great deal of sense for patients, institutions, and interpreters. The disadvantage of this model is the difficulty of planning for continuity of interpretation. The quality of interpreter skills is incumbent on the agency to guarantee and without careful communication between agency and institution, and scheduled monitoring, the quality of interpretation is difficult to assess.

Individual interpreters can also contract with clinics and hospitals. Here the interpreter is a "known quantity." There is more flexibility to provide continuity of interpretation, and the skills of the individual become well known. The advantages for the interpreter are visibility and familiarity with clinics and staff, but they do not have a guaranteed amount of work. The social influence of individual interpreters comes into play when two or three individually contracted interpreters find themselves in competition for the hourly interpreting work in an institution. Nevertheless, there are advantages to both models.

Bilingual Staff

In general the deployment of bilingual staff as interpreters is a bad idea. It sets up role conflicts for staff that are difficult to reconcile. Having said this, it is also true that in certain settings where there are no other options, a staff member who is compensated to work in two roles is better than no interpreter at all. In some clinics, staff work as both medical assistants and interpreters and this model can function within limitations. The use of front-desk staff, nurses, janitors, or phlebotomists as regular interpreters may create more problems than it solves, and should be avoided.

Case Management

Another model for interpreter services is the use of case managers (Ethnic Minorities and Health Centre, 1992; Jackson-Carroll, Graham, & Jackson, 1996; Vlaams, Centrum Integratie Migranten, 1994). The case management model is cost-effective in a setting where multiple family members use a clinic or related set of clinics so that the institution has an incentive to coordinate the care of the family to ensure access while managing resource utilization. An HMO, for example, would have a financial interest in this model of care. In this model the institution hires case managers as salaried employees and benefits by preventing unnecessary and expensive ER use and hospitalizations by capitated members. Case managers work with clinics to help encourage access of preventive services and primary care and limit unnecessary clinic visits of the individuals they manage. Families with multiple medical or social issues are the obvious high-risk families to be managed. By having continuity with families, interpreters are in excellent positions to explain the social context of illness and the semantic networks of their community to continuity care providers. Similarly, they can teach the semantics of biomedicine to patients with chronic illnesses, who will have long-term relationships with institutions and must learn some medical semantics to navigate the system.

There are added efficiencies with this model of care. Interpreters working with families in the targeted immigrant community can address broader public health education topics with the community on behalf of the medical system. Similarly, as institutional employees they have the position and familiarity with the clinics to explain community issues to the institution. Case managers become resources in both the community and hospital because of their familiarity with each arena. Because the institution supports case management they can be given time to produce written documents, audiotapes, or videos on a variety of topics. These will serve their client, other interpreters, and the general community. The diffusion of their knowledge to other community members and to the professional staff in the hospital is difficult to measure, but presumably improves understanding, establishes trust, and thereby improves efficiency in work done in the targeted community.

The Community House Calls Program at Harborview Medical Center in Seattle is an example of this kind of program (Jackson-Carroll, Graham, & Jackson, 1996). The Children's and Refugee Clinics in Seattle developed a model of interpretation focused on communities and families in these communities. The House Calls Program selected five of the neediest refugee groups that have resettled in the Seattle area. Refugee community leaders assisted the Medical Center in selecting interpreters and community members to develop the program together. The interpreters were chosen with the communities to represent their interests in the institution. The Medical Center pays their salaries and benefits, and provides them with pagers and office space. The interpreters work either half-time or full-time depending on the volume of patients from their community seen by physicians in the Medical Center.

The interpreters have multiple roles. They are known by the acronym ICM which stands for Interpreter/Case Manager or Interpreter/ Cultural Mediator, depending on the role they are playing. Interpreters provide continuity of interpretation and case management for select families. The families are chosen based on the burden of need determined by the number of social and health services needs each family has. The interpreters accompany the family members to clinic to provide interpretation. In this setting they can advocate for their clients and explain contextual issues for providers. The clinicians gain confidence with the families by knowing that they have a means of obtaining feedback about misunderstandings, following up on tests, assuring medication compliance, and tracking patients for missed appointments.

The interpreters go beyond culture broking, case management, and patient advo-

cacy; they also organize health education activities for the larger community to address commonly encountered clinical problems or public health issues. For example, the community may request a general discussion of parenting issues in intergenerational conflict, older people may want to learn more about diabetes and its management, and mothers may want sessions on breast feeding and immunizations.

The interpreters also teach physicians, residents, nurses, and medical staff. In this capacity they present at CME sessions and in-services, and teach individual clinicians during clinic conferences. In this way they serve as community advocates in the institution and as institutional resources for patient education and patient services.

For patients who are in managed care programs, case management provides access to clinic services and decreases the need for expensive hospital-based care while ensuring advocacy and linguistic assistance. This type of cultural mediation and case management contributes to the general health of the community, attracts that community to services in the medical center designed just for them, and then manages care in the institution by educating both patients and providers.

The disadvantage of this model is that the program is expensive, requires major institutional commitment, and needs skilled leadership to make it work. Patients may become dependent on ICMs rather than independent interpreters. The expense of the program is more than offset by the improved efficiency in clinical encounters, improved compliance, improved communication, and patient satisfaction. The cost is also offset by the decreased use of hourly interpreters for case-managed families.

The training of interpreters to work as case managers and cultural mediators demands time and attention to the context of their work. Each institution must move forward training their interpreters to address the context they work in. There is no single curriculum or formula; case management will be dictated by the dynamics of medicaid–managed care–low-income allowance reimbursement strategies of the state and institution. The central issues in cultural mediation will be determined by the target population, the region of the country, and the institutional culture (e.g., county hospital, teaching hospital, large HMO, community clinic). The essential elements in most programs should include listening and interpreting skills, medical terminology, basic knowledge of the specific clinic or hospital, general knowledge of health and human services programs in the area, and community support for linguistic and cultural variability in the target population. Each program will by design have to work out their training focus with "fear and trembling" in order to appropriately bridge the cultural groups they will be expected to serve.

Public Health Translations

The challenge of written translation deserves special attention. Interpretation is dynamic and relies on the presence of a bilingual-bicultural person who can adjust tone and affect to enhance communication. Written translations are static documents that do not allow one to check comprehension and address misunderstanding. As such, they demand special attention to determine the targeted audience of the document. Often professional interpreters are employed. If not given special instruction, interpreters may not adjust the sophistication of their translation to the educational level of the real target group. If this is the case the document may do little good (Jackson *et al.,* 1997).

If the document is intended for a community that has many classes and educational levels represented, then either multiple translation may be necessary or certain educational levels should not receive translated documents and should instead be taught in person (Erickson & Hoang, 1980; Meuecke, 1983). Clearly, this is the case for the illiterate. While audio- and videotape can address the needs of the illiterate, the issue of meaningful recordings is the same. The cultural, educational, economic, and gender issues of the target community must shape the written or recorded message for the message to be appropriately incorporated into the semantic network of the target group.

Specialized Interpretation

There are disciplines in medicine that require a special set of interpreting skills. Two good examples are mental health and speech pathology, but each discipline presents a special set of interpreting challenges. Most notable is mental health.

Mental Health Interpreting

Patients from different cultures are generally familiar with the idea that one goes to a healer and complains of bodily symptoms. The rhythm of complaint and inquiry is familiar. Although the semantics of illness and the meaning of symptoms can vary drastically, as we have seen, the general exchange is familiar. Mental health is an area that requires considerable explanation for immigrant patients from non-Western countries (Kleinman, 1980). In part, this is because of our own Western concepts of mental health; the semantics of mental illness penetrate deep into the sociocultural matrix and there have been rapid changes in the medical management of depression, bipolar disorder, and schizophrenia.

Many cultures from Asia and Africa have a high threshold for considering something a "mental illness." Psychotic disorders, autism, and retardation would be recognized as forms of "craziness," and distinct from possession states, ghost sickness, soul loss, and other severe non-Western illnesses. Dysphoria, depression, posttraumatic stress disorder, and personality disorders would not evoke a picture of madness in most immigrant communities. Until severe, affective disorders may simply be considered sadness, prolonged grief, or a spiritual problem. Any suggestion that prolonged depression and anxiety are mental illness could be construed as a misunderstanding, an ethnocentric judgment, or an insult.

Interpreters are likely to be the best source of information for professionals about cultural presentations and means of talking about mental illness and the social dynamics surrounding its care. They will also be familiar with many of the spiritual and cultural causes and treatments for varying degrees of mental illness. Interpreters are also the best means for explaining the therapeutic goals of counseling to a patient, family, or group. Interpreters require special education because they may share many of the prejudices and misunderstandings about depression and its treatment held by their community.

The notion of counseling is unfamiliar to many immigrants from rural developing countries. Until these patients experience some benefit, the process of discussing at length painful or humiliating memories, relationships with parents, and emotional struggles with friends and family will continue to strike many immigrants as an absurd and masochistic exercise. They will not have this opportunity if interpreters are not trained to function effectively in a mental health setting.

Mental health interpreting is particularly difficult because the interpreting is less routine and mechanical. The fabric of people's lives are discussed in some depth and many of the issues patients face are identical to those faced by interpreters and their families. The session can awaken painful memories or irreconcilable dilemmas for the interpreter. Unless interpreters are thoroughly professional and can contain their own emotional boundaries, they may lose focus. The sessions can be long and exhausting, and both therapist and interpreter need time to process the content of the session to assure accuracy. Most importantly, the interpreter needs to understand the goal of medication and of the talking sessions. If they do not appreciate the circuitous nature of the work, they will not be able to respond appropriately when patients ask, "Why are we talking about all these things? My problem is headache and sleeplessness."

Some interpreters are better at this kind of interpreting than others. Patients and therapists are wasting scarce resources if reluctant, unmotivated interpreters are working in mental health. If interpreters find the discussion of incest, rape, or domestic violence objectionable they may intentionally undermine the encounters. Knowledgeable and motivated interpreters can bridge the semantics of family and spiritual life from the target community to the therapeutic goals of psychotherapy. These interpreters have a special set of skills and should be compensated for the difficulty of this work. There should also be emotional support provided to interpreters who find themselves overwhelmed by the parallel nature of their own and their clients' struggles.

Speech Pathology and Speech Therapy

For immigrant victims of diseases such as stroke or gunshot, or for those who have had injuries affecting their ability to speak, the work of speech pathologists represents a specialized set of demands on interpreters. Providing the specialized feedback for patients about the sounds they are making, how to form those sounds, and how to develop the facial strength needed to make the words can only be done by a native speaker of the language. For example, to create tones in a tonal language is an acoustic subtlety only a native speaker can help with. Partnerships in disciplines like this increase the efficiency of the institution to provide rehabilitative assistance to patients and families. The need for these services is relatively infrequent, but interpreters who have a verifiable skill in this area will increase the efficiency of the therapist, and this should more than offset the additional compensation they merit for this skill.

Research Instruments

The development of new research instruments for a targeted linguistic group, or the modification of existing instruments for the same purpose, is another special case in translation and cross-cultural measurement (Guillemin, Bombardier, & Beaton, 1993). I refer the reader to Chapter 5. I will note here that the dynamics of back-translation or de-centering (depending on the purpose of the instrument) are separate issues that do not supplant the need for ethnographic work to build a solid bridge between the semantic networks.

Back-translation is an iterative method to assure that the translated document is in fact uniformly received as intended. The iterative cycle has more to do with the quality and appropriateness of the translation from English into the intended language than it does with the cultural content or context of that message. While some of these issues may come to light in the back-translation method, they will not necessarily be addressed. Ethnographic inquiry is a more direct means of addressing the semantic network of the targeted audience. The back-translation method can be used later to refine the success of translation.

The significance of semantic networks to cross-cultural research is beyond the focus of this chapter. It is important at least to raise this topic for later discussion and to remind researchers that "common sense" suggests "common values" and consensus. Therefore, measuring attitudes, opinions, or behaviors through commonsense translation means that nothing can be considered common or straightforward until validated as such.

EthnoMed

Electronic tools to aid interpretation may be helpful. EthnoMed is an experiment to address this possibility. This site on the World Wide Web was developed through a collaboration between the Health Sciences Library at the University of Washington and the Harborview Medical Center's Children's and Refugee Clinics (EthnoMed, 1996). The purpose of the website is to serve as a clinical tool for clinics providing services to several of the refugee communities living in Seattle. At present, EthnoMed is a pilot effort, largely unfunded, and has evolved in an effort to develop simple ethnographic documents for easy access by providers and community members.

The concept of semantic networks is central to the information in these documents. A brief perusal will reveal a growing number of documents written for clinicians addressing the concepts, context, linguistics, and meaning of symptoms, diseases, and social life for seven of Seattle's refugee populations. The internet allows providers in clinics across the city, who may not have the assistance of a skilled cultural mediator, to access information pertinent to the clinical care of community members. Each document is written in partnership with a community reader so that stereotypes and misinformation can be identified and corrected. The documents are brief and somewhat superficial by design since they are intended to be used quickly to identify commonly encountered problem areas for providers unfamiliar with the sociocultural dynamics affecting their care of patients. Anyone can add documents to this website if appropriate and produced according to the EthnoMed method.

The static nature of translated ideas and materials into English is a liability of written documents; this can be somewhat ameliorated by inviting feedback from the community and from users of the site through e-mail and a bulletin board intended for this purpose. As concepts and practices change with time and by region of the country, variances can be incorporated into revised documents.

Another feature of the website is patient education. The limitations of written patient education documents have been outlined previously. In spite of these limitations translated brochures are sometimes useful if patients are literate, providing the brochures are well developed, and especially when there is no better alternative. EthnoMed is being developed to contain documents in the script of targeted language groups written at appropriate literacy levels. While a goal would be to have documents written that incorporate the semantics of illness, this is not always possible.

The social dynamics of refugee and immigrant populations also impact their health care in unique ways. Immigration reform, welfare restrictions, local initiatives, acculturation, and poverty create anxiety and real constraints for patients and providers. Relevant information can be included in EthnoMed, as well as references to related websites of interest.

EthnoMed is without a doubt a work in progress, of limited real use at this time, but the hope is that with national and international contributions there will be a growing repository of useful clinical information to assist with interpreted cross-cultural care of a growing number of immigrant communities.

Conclusion

Interpretation is central for linguistic and cultural access to health care for recently arrived non-English-speaking groups in the United States. Interpretation is complicated by the internal dynamics of medical language as well as the linguistics of target languages. The culturally defined semantics of health and illness are central to understanding the very difficult work of medical interpreters as they attempt to bridge the culture of biomedicine and their own unique cultural communities. The unique needs of medical providers and patients have to be attended to by interpreters as they struggle to find equivalence between the two worlds.

Physicians and interpreters need special training to work together efficiently. As medical interpreters evolve as a professional group there will be growing recognition of varying roles of interpreters as culture brokers, case managers, community advocates, specialists, and document translators. Curricula to train interpreters to do medical interpretation depend on the scope and context of the work and reimbursement structure. Unfortunately, the training and support given to professional interpreters in this country is severely underdeveloped. The unique interpreting demands of specialties, such as mental health, should be acknowledged and supported.

References

Austin, J. L. (1965). Introduction. In J. O. Ormson (Ed.). *How to do things with words.* New York: Oxford University Press.

Buchwald, D., Panwala, S., & Hooton, T. M. (1992). Use of traditional health practices by Southeast Asian refugees in a primary care clinic. *Western Journal of Medicine, 61,* 508–511.

Catford, J. C. (1965). *A linguistic theory of translation: An essay in applied linguistics.* London: Oxford University Press.

Chavez, J. M. (1993, February). Breaking through the language barrier. *Urban Medicine,* pp. 9–10.

Erickson, R., & Hoang, G. (1980). Health problems among Indo-Chinese refugees. *American Journal of Public Health, 70*(9), 1003–1005.

Ethnic Minorities and Health Centre, Flanders Migrants' Integration Centre. (1992). *Project intercultural health mediators.* Brussels, Belgium: Author.

EthnoMed. (1996). www.hslib.washington.edu/clinical/ethnomed. Seattle: University of Washington, IAIMS Program and Health Sciences Libraries.

Gilman, S., Justice, J., Saephaen, K., & Charles, G. (1992). Use of traditional and modern health services by Loatian refugees. *Western Journal of Medicine, 157*(3), 213–390.

Ginsberg, C., Martin, V., Andrulis, D., Shaw-Taylor, Y., & McGregor, C. (1995, March). Interpretation and translation in health care: A survey of U.S. public and private teaching hospitals. *National Public Health and Hospital Institute Report,* 1–68.

Good, B., & Good, M. J. D. (1977). The heart of what's the matter: The semantics of illness in Iran. *Culture, Medicine and Psychiatry, 1,* 25–58.

Good, B. J. (1994). How medicine constructs its object. In *Medicine, rationality, and experience: An anthropological perspective* (pp. 65–88). Cambridge, England: Cambridge University Press.

Guillemin, F., Bombardier, C., & Beaton, D. (1993). Cross-cultural adaptation of health-related quality of life measures: Literature review and proposed guidelines. *Journal of Clinical Epidemiology, 46*(12), 1417–1432.

Haffner, L. (1992, September). Cross-cultural medicine a decade later: Translation is not enough, interpreting in a medical setting. *Western Journal of Medicine, 157,* 255–259.

Hoang, G. N., & Erickson, R. (1985). Cultural barriers to effective medical care among Indochinese patients. *Annual Review Medicine, 36,* 229–239.

Jackson, J. C., Rhodes, L. A., Inui, T. S., & Buchwald, D. (1997) Hepatitis B among the Khmer: Issues of translation and concepts of illness. *Journal of General Internal Medicine, 12,* 292–298.

Jackson-Carroll, L. M., Graham, E., & Jackson, J.C. (1996). Beyond medical interpretation: The role of interpreters cultural mediators. In *Building bridges between ethnic communities and health institutions.* HTTP:///www.hslib.washington.edu/clinical/ethnomed/ICM.

Johnson, T. M., & Kleinman, A. M. (1989). Cultural factors in the medical interview. In *Society for Research and Education in Primary Care Internal Medicine.* Task Force on the Medical Interview.

Jonsen, A. (1997). Personal communication, University of Washington, Department of Medical Ethics and History.

Jucovy, P. M. (1982). Developing a critical model for diagnostic language. In *Proceedings of the Medcomp '82—First IEEE Computer Society International Conference on Medical Computer Science/Computational Medicine* (pp. 465–489).

Kaufert, J. (1984). *A study of medical interpreters and health communication in Inuit communities* (No. 6607-1364-46). Ottawa, Ontario, Canada: National Health Research and Development Program, Health and Welfare.

Kaufert, J. M., & Koolage, W. W. (1984). Role conflict among culture brokers: The experience of Native Canadian medical interpreters. *Social Science and Medicine, 18*(3), 283–286.

Kaufert, J. M., Koolage, W. W., Kaufert, P. L., & O'Neil, J. D. (1984). The use of "trouble case" examples in teaching the impact of sociocultural and political factors in clinical communication. *Medical Anthropology, 8*(1), 36–45.

Kaufert, J. M., O'Neil, J. D., & Koolage, W. W. (1985). Culture brokerage and advocacy in urban hospitals: The impact of Native language interpreters. *Sante Culture Health, 2*(3), 3–9.

Kaufert, J. M., O'Neil, J. D., & Koolage, W. W. (1991). The cultural and political context of informed consent for Native Canadians. *Arctic Medical Research* (Suppl.), 181–184.

Kleinman, D. (1980). The cultural construction of illness experiences and behavior: Affects and symptoms in Chinese living. In *Patients and Healers in the Context of Culture* (pp. 119–136). Berkeley: University of California Press.

Meuecke, M. A. (1983). In search of healers—Southeast Asian refugees in the American health care system. *Western Journal of Medicine, 139*(6), 835–840.

Office of Refugee Resettlement. (1990). *Annual report FYI, 1990* (Report to Congress, pp. 1–17). Washington, DC: U.S. Department of Health and Human Services.

O'Neil, J. D., Koolage, W. W., & Kaufert, J. M. (1988). Health communication problems in Canadian Inuit communities. *Arctic Medical Research, 47*(1), 374–378.

Ots, T. (1990). The angry liver, the anxious heart and the melancholy spleen: The phenomenology of perceptions in Chinese culture. *Cultural Medicine Psychiatry, 14*(1), 21–28.

Putsch, R. W. (1985). General guidelines for monolingual providers in a cross-cultural environment. Cross-cultural communication: Special case of interpreters in health care. *Journal of American Medical Association, 254*(23), 3344–3348.

Putsch, R. W. (1990). Language in cross-cultural care. In H. K. Walker, W. D. Hall, & J. W. Hurst (Eds.), *Clinical methods* (3rd ed., pp. 1060–1065). Boston: Butterworths.

Putsch, R. W. & Joyce, M. (1990). Dealing with patients from other cultures. In H. K. Walker, W. D. Hall, & J. W. Hurst (Eds.), *Clinical methods* (3rd ed., pp. 1050–1065). Boston: Butterworth.

Sechrest, L., Fay, T. L., & Hafeez Zaidi, S. M. (1972). Problems of translation in cross-cultural research. *Journal of Cross-Cultural Psychiatry, 3*(1), 41–56.

Shimada, J., Jackson, C., Goldstein, E., & Buchwald, D. (1995). "Strong medicine": Cambodian views of medicine and medical compliance. *Journal of General Internal Medicine, 10,* 369–374.

Skinner, H. A. (1949). *The origin of medical terms.* Baltimore: Williams & Wilkens.

Stephenson, P. H. (1995). Vietnamese refugees in Victoria, B.C.: An overview of immigrant and refugee health care in a medium-sized Canadian urban centre. *Social Science Medicine, 40*(12), 1631–1642.

Thai D.-Q., Buchwald, D., & Hooton, T. M. (1993). *Medical knowledge and familiarity with western medicine among Southeast Asian refugees.* Unpublished medical thesis, University of Washington Medical Center, ISMS Project, Seattle.

Vlaams Centrum Integratie Migranten. (1994, October 12, 13). *Send me an angel or a devil's advocate?* Paper presented at the closing congress: Speaking for Ourselves. Houthalen, Flanders, Belgium: NOW project: New Opportunities for Women.

5

Cross-Cultural Use of Measurements

XINHUA S. REN AND BENJAMIN C. AMICK III

Introduction

In recent years, health-related quality of life (HRQoL) measures are rapidly becoming standard tools for evaluating clinical effectiveness in patients and for assessing health status in populations (Guillein, Bombardier, & Beaton, 1993; McDowell & Newell, 1987). As more people live longer with chronic diseases (Croog & Levine, 1989; Patrick & Erickson, 1993), the goal of health care is no longer focused on survival or curing the disease, but on optimizing individual's functional health and well-being (Ferguson & Cherniack, 1993). This shift in focus of health care suggests that health assessment will depend more heavily on an individual's participation, that is, his or her perception and accurate reporting of symptoms, functioning, and disabilities (Campen, Sixma, Friele, Kerssens, & Peters, 1995; Geigle & Jones, 1990; Till, Osoba, Oater, & Young 1994).

Despite a proliferation of new instruments and a burgeoning theoretical literature in the measurement of health-related quality of life (Berzon, Hays, & Shumaker, 1993; Guillein et al., 1993; Guyatt, 1993; Hunt et al., 1991; Mathias, Fifer, & Patrick, 1994; Orley & Kuyken, 1994), most health status measures have so far been developed in English. Few studies have gathered systematic information on functioning and well-being among immigrant populations in the United States. Since a large majority of these immigrants are not yet proficient in English, defining and assessing health-related quality of life among various immigrant populations thus requires the development of outcome measures in the non-English languages that are appropriate for cross-cultural or ethnic studies (Barker, 1992; Giachello, 1992; Hatton, 1992).

Demographic Transition and Cross-Cultural Use of Health Status Measures

Growing ethnic diversity has transformed America into a multicultural society. By the turn of the century, "minority" populations will comprise more than 25% of the U.S. population (U.S. Bureau of the Census, 1991); by the year 2050, non-Hispanic Whites will make up less than 50% of the population (U.S. Bureau of the Census, 1995). This demographic transition has tremendous ramifications for

XINHUA S. REN • Center for Health Quality, Outcomes, and Economic Research, Health Services Research and Development Field Program, VA Medical Center, Bedford, Massachusetts 01730. BENJAMIN C. AMICK III • The Health Institute, New England Medical Center, Boston, Massachusetts 02111.

Handbook of Immigrant Health, edited by Loue. Plenum Press, New York, 1998.

the nation's health care. Although health-related quality of life measures are increasingly used for evaluating clinical effectiveness in patients and for assessing health status in populations (Guillein *et al.,* 1993; McDowell & Newell, 1987), cross-cultural validation of these instruments has focused on international comparisons and not on ethnic diversity within a country.

Evidence in social and behavioral science literature suggests variability in the reporting of symptoms and the interpretation of health among different racial or ethnic groups (Krause & Jay, 1994; Meredith & Siu, 1995; Ren & Amick, 1996a, 1996b; Rogers, 1992; Zborowski, 1952). For instance, Lieu, Newacheck, and McManus (1993) found that compared with Whites and Hispanics, African Americans had a lower number of bed days and school-loss days, but they were more likely to report poor health. According to Gibson (1991), the subjective interpretation was a more valid measure of internal health state for African Americans than for Whites, whereas the disability interpretation was a less valid measure for African Americans than for Whites. Therefore, in cross-cultural use of health status measures, it is important to evaluate whether relevant health domains are covered for various ethnic groups with different cultural backgrounds.

Health services research often underrepresent ethnic minorities, especially recent immigrants, who do not speak English or are not yet proficient in English. Although there has been an increasing interest in providing culturally appropriate health care services, recent immigrants remain largely invisible to health service providers due to the lack of appropriate health status measures. The absence of information on the perceptions of health and well-being makes it extremely difficult for service providers to understand health care needs, to ascertain clinical effectiveness, and to evaluate health-related quality of life among these unique populations.

Thus, there is increasing demand for measurement tools to evaluate clinical effectiveness and assess health-related quality of life among various ethnic groups, especially recent immigrants to the United States. Continued neglect of this group's health problems and patterns of utilization of services will only lead to increases in morbidity, mortality, and health care costs for the nation. The measurement tools designed specifically for these populations (i.e., in their native languages) can be used not only to monitor their health-related quality of life and health care behaviors, but also to improve the quality of health care by encouraging participation and enhancing doctor–patient communication with the ultimate goal of improving their health status.

In this chapter, we address conceptual and methodological issues related to cross-cultural development and validation of health status instruments; that is, how best to design instruments both socially and culturally appropriate for different groups with which they are being used. To illustrate these issues we discuss the development of a Chinese version of the Medical Outcomes Study 36-Item Short-Form Health Survey (SF-36). First, we discuss issues concerning the choice of health status measures to be used among populations with varying cultural backgrounds. Second, we provide an example using the SF-36. Third, we illustrate the use of this new measure in an elderly immigrant population. Finally, we discuss future research directions.

Developing a Culturally Appropriate Health Status Measure

Strategies

There are two different strategies in constructing a culturally appropriate health status measure. The choice of one strategy over the other depends on the particular research question. Researchers may construct a new health status measure that incorporates culture-specific domains into the instrument. These instruments can best be used for research within a single cultural group. This class of instruments will maximize the health status variation observed within a population. They are best used for within–cultural-group comparisons. However, health status measures developed using this approach are not well suited for cross-cultural comparison due to the idiosyncratic nature of the instruments.

An alternative approach is to translate and adapt health status measures previously developed and validated in English or some other single language (Alonso, Prieto, & Anto, 1994; Badoux & Mendelsohn, 1994; Bullinger, 1995). Although this approach is less sensitive to cultural domains of health, these health status measures with adequate cultural adaptation are more appropriate for use in a multicultural society to compare cultural or ethnic disparities in health status because of their relative equivalence to the original language instruments.

Furthermore, while new measurement development is often the first option for cross-cultural research, such an approach requires extensive financial and human resources to conduct the required qualitative and quantitative studies for developing a valid and reliable measure. In addition, researchers concerned with clinical effectiveness evaluations must extend development to demonstrate the sensitivity of the measure to change in clinical status. Therefore, it is often advisable to select a measure to be translated where much of this work has been completed.

Approach of Translation and Adaptation

One fundamental issue in cross-cultural instrument development involves the approach of translation (Forsberg & Bjorvell, 1993; Sartorius & Kuyken, 1993). Across cultures there are differences in the levels of literacy, taboo subjects, and social desirability. Specific differences in health beliefs between cultures may challenge the adaptability of certain health status measures. Furthermore, certain features of the language, such as idioms, are very difficult to translate and make little sense in a different cultural context. For instance, the translation of Western health status measures into Chinese offers an unusual challenge due largely to contrasting cultural beliefs and practices about the body, health and illness, and social norms with regard to the reporting of disease and sickness (Hsu, 1976; Mo, 1992; Muller & Desmond, 1992). The reluctance of Chinese people to express or discuss their feelings of health-related quality of life, especially to persons outside the family, has raised concerns about whether any Western health status measures can be translated and used among Chinese (Lam, Weel, & Lauder, 1994). In this regard, two approaches are critical to a successful translation and adaptation of health status measures: (a) selecting appropriate health status measures to be translated and adapted, and (b) using a systematic approach to cross-cultural adaptation.

Selection of Health Status Measures

Three criteria are essential in selecting a health status measure to be translated and adapted: reliability, validity, and easy administration. Reliability refers to the extent to which a measure produces consistent results; validity refers to the extent to which an instrument measures what it is supposed to measure. Because both validity and reliability are key attributes of psychometric tests that are often required for health status measures, it is therefore recommended that researchers and clinicians should select those health status measures that have been previously validated and that possess high reliability estimates for cross-cultural adaptation.

In selecting health status measures, researchers and clinicians should also consider issues regarding the degree of difficulty in administering the instrument. For example, the amount of time required to complete a health status instrument (e.g., fewer number of items) is often critical in ensuring a successful cross-cultural adaptation of health status measures.

Of the numerous health status measures, we choose to translate the Medical Outcomes

Study Short-Form Health Survey (SF-36) (Ware, Snow, Kosinski, & Gandek, 1993) because of four considerations. First, the SF-36 is based on a multidimensional model of health. As summarized in Table 1, the SF-36 includes eight general health concepts: physical functioning (PF), role limitations due to physical health problems (RP), bodily pain (BP), general health perceptions (GH), vitality (VT), social functioning (SF), role limitations due to emotional problems (RE), and mental health (MH). The SF-36 items can also be aggregated into two summary scales, physical component summary (PCS) and mental component summary (MCS) (Ware, Kosinski, Bayliss, *et al.*, 1995; Ware, Kosinski, & Keller, 1995).

Second, the SF-36, especially the mental health dimension, also contains items that are relatively less sensitive and taboo to the Chinese. Previous studies have observed a tendency for Chinese to present somatic complaints in place of psychological symptoms (Kleinman, 1977; Kleinman, Eisenberg, & Good, 1978; Liang, Wu, Krause, Chiang, & Wu, 1992). Unlike measures of dysphoric symptoms, which often connote antisocial or bizarre behavior in Chinese culture, the SF-

TABLE 1. Summary of the MOS SF-36 Health Survey

SF-36 subscales	Item	Definitions of item content
Physical functioning (PF)	PF1	Vigorous activities, such as running, lifting heavy objects, strenuous sports
	PF2	Moderate activities, such as moving a table, vacuuming, bowling
	PF3	Lifting or carrying groceries
	PF4	Climbing several flights of stairs
	PF5	Climbing one flight of stairs
	PF6	Bending, kneeling, or stooping
	PF7	Walking more than a mile
	PF8	Walking several blocks
	PF9	Walking one block
	PF10	Bathing or dressing yourself
Role physical (RP)	RP1	Limited in the kind of work or other activities
	RP2	Cut down the amount of time spent on work or other activities
	RP3	Accomplished less than would like
	RP4	Difficulty performing the work or other activities
Bodily pain (BP)	BP1	Intensity of bodily pain
	BP2	Extent pain interfered with normal work
General health perceptions (GH)	GH1	Is your health: excellent, very good, good, fair, poor
	GH2	My health is excellent
	GH3	I am as healthy as anybody I know
	GH4	I seem to get sick a little easier than other people
	GH5	I expect my health to get worse
Vitality (VT)	VT1	Feel full of pep
	VT2	Have a lot of energy
	VT3	Feel worn out
	VT4	Feel tired
Social functioning (SF)	SF1	Frequency health problems interfered with social activities
	SF2	Extent health problems interfered with normal social activities
Role emotional (RE)	RE1	Cut down the amount of time spent on work or other activities
	RE2	Accomplished less than would like
	RE3	Didn't do work or other activities as carefully as usual
Mental health (MH)	MH1	Been a very nervous person
	MH2	Felt downhearted and blue
	MH3	Felt so down in the dumps nothing could cheer you up
	MH4	Been a happy person
	MH5	Felt calm and peaceful

36 mental health scale measures psychological well-being and life satisfaction. Because the measure touches on a subject matter that is close in meaning to vitality (Ren, Amick, Zhou, Gandek, & Ware, in press), Chinese have less trouble or fear in disclosing their feelings about them. Thus, the translated SF-36 is more likely to generate reliable and valid information from the Chinese about their mental health status.

Third, the SF-36 has been proven to be psychometrically sound. The instrument is currently regarded as one of the more promising generic health status measures and because the instrument is constructed for use in general population surveys, the SF-36 is suited for comparative studies involving diverse populations (McHorney, Ware, Lu, & Sherbourne, 1994; Ware & Sherbourne, 1992). The SF-36 has currently been translated into 14 languages, and the psychometric test results for the translated versions indicate that SF-36 is a reliable generic health survey instrument across different nations.*

Finally, compared with other health status measures, the SF-36 contains fewer questions. Because of its brevity, the SF-36 is less difficult to translate and is easy to administer.

Systematic Approach to Cross-Cultural Adaptation

A systematic approach is also a prerequisite to a successful translation and adaptation of health status measures into non-English languages. Four steps are recommended in the development of a health status measure for cross-cultural use: forward translation, committee review, backward translation, and committee review. The original English version of the instrument should be translated by three independent native speakers. The three independent translations should then be reviewed by a review committee to determine a common version to be back-translated into the original language. The back-translation should

again be reviewed by the review committee to evaluate the quality of the adapted instrument using two criteria: The adapted instrument has replicated the original instrument content to allow cross-cultural comparisons; it has identified culture-based items that make little sense in a different cultural context.

In translating and adapting the SF-36 into Chinese (Ren *et al.,* in press), we followed a systematic protocol, developed in the International Quality of Life Assessment (IQOLA) Project (Ware, Keller, *et al.,* 1995), to translate, adapt, and test the cross-cultural applicability of the SF-36. The original SF-36 was translated into Chinese by three independent native Chinese speakers with excellent knowledge of English and with multidisciplinary backgrounds—a social scientist, a physician, and a linguist. Together, these three translators also formed a review committee to evaluate the quality of three different versions of the translation. From these three translations, the review committee agreed on a common version of the Chinese SF-36. This common version was then back-translated into English by two other speakers bilingual in Chinese and English. The backward translations were reviewed by IQOLA Project researchers for conceptual equivalence with the original form. A final Chinese version of the SF-36 was developed by the review committee through discussion and comparisons among the original, the forward, and the backward translations.

This process ensures cross-cultural comparability. However, the translation process also reveals places in the instrument where adaptation is necessary. Unlike translation, adaptation requires knowledge of the local culture—its language and practices.

Adaptation of MOS SF-36

In capturing the content of the original SF-36, the Chinese translation of the SF-36 has made appropriate adaptations on several items that make little sense in the Chinese cultural context. Alterations were made to the wording of the idiomatic expressions in the

---

* The instrument has been largely translated into languages of industrialized Western European countries (e.g., French and German).

SF-36. For example, idiomatic equivalence cannot be reached in Chinese for expressions such as "full of pep," "down in the dumps," and "downhearted and blue." Instead, these idioms were translated into Chinese expressions that capture the closest possible meaning of the original, such as "liveliness" or "vigor," "low in mood," and "sadness."

Similarly, most Chinese immigrants are not familiar with the concept of "mile" to measure distance. In the Chinese translation, we converted "more than a mile" into "one kilometer." Further, the concept of "blocks" appear to be ambiguous. In Chinese, there is no equivalent expression of "blocks." The Chinese word "streets" varies in distance from less than a mile to more than several miles. Thus, in the Chinese translation, we changed "several blocks" into "several hundred meters," and "one block" into "one hundred meters."

There are also difficulties in translating the physical functioning scale item describing moderate activities (Ware, Keller, *et. al.,* 1995). For example, "playing golf" is not a common activity among Chinese immigrants. However, unaware of a salient descriptor of moderate activity among Chinese immigrants, we retained "playing golf" as a moderate activity in the initial translation. In the most recent revision, we have replaced "playing golf" with "playing shadow boxing (Tai Ji Quan)," which is a very popular moderate activity in mainland China.

This process of adaptation takes phrases or idiomatic expressions that are not common cross-culturally and replaces them with culturally relevant phrases. One concern may be that the adaptations have changed the meaning of the question or affected how a person will respond. Thus, to ensure that the adapted instrument captures the same domains of health it is necessary to examine its psychometric properties.

Testing the Reliability of the Translation

Once a health status measure has been translated and adapted, it is essential to test the reliability of the new instrument, that is, whether the instrument yields consistent results. There are four reliability tests that must be conducted.

1. *Item-Internal Consistency.* A basic assumption in developing scales is that an item chosen to measure a concept will have a substantial association with the scale representing the concept. This is reflected in the correlation between an item and its hypothesized scale. However, to avoid inflating the item–scale correlation coefficient it is important to remove the item from its hypothesized scale when calculating the correlation (remove overlap). To evaluate scale internal consistency, a correlation coefficient of 0.40 or above (corrected for overlap) between an item and its hypothesized scale is the standard for scaling success (Nunnally, 1978).

2. *Score Reliability.* This test examines the degree to which the items in a scale measure the same underlying concept. The internal consistency reliability, estimated by Cronbach's alpha, measures the extent of the variation in a score that is true as opposed to random error, or the proportion of observed variance that is reliable (Hays, Anderson, & Revicki, 1993). An alpha coefficient of 0.70 or greater is recommended for group-level cross-cultural comparisons (Nunnally, 1978).

3. *Test–Retest Reliability.* Test–retest reliability measures the relationship between scores obtained on two or more administrations of the instruments. This test assesses the temporal stability of responses. It is important that the second administration be close to the first administration (e.g., 2 weeks) to prevent significant events from potentially influencing the response. Test–retest reliability is estimated with Pearson product–moment correlation coefficients for each item or scale at both administration periods.

4. *Equivalent-Forms Reliability.* Equivalent-forms reliability refers to the agree-

ment between the scores on the original as well as the translated and adapted version of an instrument. The forms are presumed to be equivalent. If the Chinese translation of the SF-36 attempts to measure the same attribute as the original SF-36, then equivalent-forms reliability tends to be reflected by the high correlation coefficients between the items and scales. Therefore, to conduct an equivalent-forms test requires that a population of native- and English-speaking persons complete both the original and translated version of the instrument within a week. Equivalent-forms reliability is estimated using the Pearson product–moment correlation coefficients between the two instruments.

An alternative test of equivalence is to compare the ordering of item mean scores on the instrument for a Chinese immigrant sample and the U.S. general population sample (Ware, Keller, et al., 1995). The ordering of item means for the Chinese sample should not differ from U.S. norms, although the absolute value of the item means might differ due to population differences. In general, items measuring "good" health define a higher level of health and should have lower mean scores than "poor" health items.

While these tests are not the only tests that can be done, they provide evidence that the translation-adaptation is measuring the same concepts (there is conceptual equivalence) and that people answer questions similarly (measurement equivalence). Others may require more advanced tests such as latent variable modeling to demonstrate that the underlying measures are composed of the same items (Liang et al., 1992). To demonstrate the utility of these measures we present data from the development of the Chinese translation-adaptation of the SF-36.

Sample Characteristics. To date, two samples have been used to test the reliability and quality of the Chinese SF-36. The first sample, drawn from convenience samples in the Greater Boston area, included a total of 156 respondents (Ren et al., in press). In order to minimize possible biases resulting from a convenient sampling approach, we diversified the sample by selecting respondents from five different sources. Among the total sample, 65 (42%) were ambulatory patients at a local community health center with a mean age of 49; 16 (10%) were patients undergoing dialysis treatment at a local tertiary hospital (mean age = 66); 20 (13%) were college students (mean age = 31); 12 (8%) were drawn from the community (mean age = 39); and 43 (28%) were drawn from the elderly community (mean age = 71). Among the respondents, 70 (45%) were male and 86 (55%) were female.

The second sample came from a validation study of the Chinese SF-36 among Chinese nationals bilingual in Chinese and English living in Tucson, Arizona (Yu, 1995). A total of 321 subjects was selected through the convenience sampling method. The mean age of these subjects was 35 with a range of 20 to 64. About 54% of the respondents were male and 46% were female. The subjects were randomly assigned to four study groups, with about 75 in each study group. Group 1 completed the English SF-36 followed by the Chinese SF-36 on the same day, whereas Group 2 reversed the order: Chinese version, then English version. Group 3 completed the English version followed by the English version in a week, while Group 4 completed Chinese version twice in a week. The demographic profiles of the four study groups were very similar.

We use the first sample to test internal consistency reliability and the equivalence of the Chinese translation of the SF-36 with the original English language version. The second sample is used to evaluate test–retest reliability and equivalent-forms reliability of the Chinese SF-36.

Internal Consistency Reliability. In validating the internal consistency reliability of the Chinese SF-36, we employed the Multi-Trait Analysis Program (MAP) for the psychometric testing of scales (Hays & Hayashi,

1990; Hays, Hayashi, Carson, & Ware, 1988). In the multitrait scaling analyses, we evaluate score reliability and item–scale correlation (corrected for overlap).

The psychometric testing results indicate that each the Chinese SF-36 scale measures a distinct health construct, as demonstrated by higher item–scale correlations within each scale (that is, high internal consistency reliability), and lower correlations with other

scales, with the exception of social functioning (see Table 2). All items for each scale exceed the standard (.40) for item–internal consistency.

However, as Table 2 shows, there are a few exceptions. First, the correlation coefficient between item VT4, "did you feel tired," and hypothesized vitality scale was slightly below the accepted norm. The correlation of this item was higher with three other scales than

TABLE 2. Correlations[a] between SF-36 Items and Hypothesized Scales, Total Sample

Item	Mean	Standard deviation	PF	RP	BP	GH	VT	SF	RE	MH
PF1	1.87	.74	.53[b]	.27	.25	.40	.25	.22	.10	.08
PF2	2.44	.71	.71[b]	.36	.37	.35	.32	.32	.18	.16
PF3	2.67	.62	.77[b]	.22	.34	.35	.23	.17	.13	.05
PF4	2.50	.65	.81[b]	.27	.31	.36	.41	.29	.23	.23
PF5	2.83	.49	.77[b]	.09	.32	.19	.22	.26	.07	.08
PF6	2.59	.68	.70[b]	.14	.31	.36	.27	.23	.21	.08
PF7	2.57	.71	.63[b]	.33	.35	.33	.37	.42	.30	.14
PF8	2.67	.60	.69[b]	.18	.32	.25	.24	.22	.15	.10
PF9	2.86	.47	.75[b]	.12	.26	.19	.19	.29	.05	.01
PF10	2.89	.43	.68[b]	.06	.21	.13	.12	.28	.01	.03
RP1	1.73	.44	.26	.62[b]	.40	.37	.45	.44	.51	.34
RP2	1.63	.48	.18	.67[b]	.43	.49	.50	.45	.67	.46
RP3	1.76	.43	.23	.66[b]	.33	.37	.37	.36	.40	.31
RP4	1.64	.48	.25	.63[b]	.41	.44	.48	.35	.48	.38
BP1	4.19	1.30	.35	.40	.65[b]	.50	.34	.38	.32	.28
BP2	4.10	1.07	.39	.49	.65[b]	.49	.43	.46	.37	.40
GH1	3.13	.86	.23	.39	.39	.66[b]	.42	.35	.28	.34
GH2	3.73	1.22	.41	.47	.49	.56[b]	.47	.50	.42	.37
GH3	3.45	1.24	.27	.30	.26	.59[b]	.38	.27	.24	.33
GH4	3.36	1.23	.25	.30	.45	.53[b]	.38	.35	.30	.41
GH5	3.39	1.22	.35	.54	.50	.75[b]	.55	.45	.45	.51
VT1	3.65	1.47	.27	.44	.33	.38	.55[b]	.40	.37	.41
VT2	3.65	1.41	.31	.52	.41	.50	.64[b]	.46	.46	.51
VT3	4.50	1.20	.26	.35	.28	.41	.51[b]	.48	.46	.58[c]
VT4	4.12	1.31	.20	.34	.22	.41[c]	**.39**[b]	.34	.47[c]	.52[c]
SF1	4.42	.88	.22	.35	.40[c]	.34	.37	**.39**[b]	.43[c]	.39[c]
SF2	3.66	1.26	.35	.46	.37	.48[c]	.54[c]	**.39**[b]	.33	.50[c]
RE1	1.59	.49	.18	.58	.34	.42	.54	.41	.89[b]	.47
RE2	1.59	.49	.18	.58	.34	.42	.54	.41	.89[b]	.47
RE3	1.66	.47	.18	.56[c]	.34	.37	.50	.36	.56[b]	.42
MH1	4.26	1.35	.06	.26	.17	.29	.37	.31	.37	.49[b]
MH2	4.59	1.39	.18	.44	.25	.38	.52	.43	.47	.57[b]
MH3	4.06	1.43	.07	.29	.32	.26	.47[c]	.42[c]	.28	.42[b]
MH4	4.43	1.34	.07	.31	.26	.41	.44	.41	.35	.55[b]
MH5	3.94	1.57	.07	.34	.29	.47	.55[c]	.33	.31	.51[b]

[a] Item-total correlations corrected for overlap. Standard error = .08.
[b] Correlation between an item and its hypothesized scale.
[c] Correlation ≥ correlation between an item and its hypothesized scale.
Figures in bold and underscored represent correlations below the standard (0.40).

with vitality: general health perceptions, role limitations due to emotional problems, and mental health. Similarly, the two items of social functioning were below the norm and were highly correlated with several other scales. The correlation coefficients for item SF1, "during the past 4 weeks, to what extent has your physical health or emotional problems interfered with normal social activities with family, friends, neighbors, or groups," were .39 with mental health and above .40 with bodily pain and role limitations due to emotional problems. The correlation coefficients for item SF2, "during the past 4 weeks, how much of the time has your physical health or emotional problems interfered with your social activities (like visiting with friends, relatives, etc.)," were above .40 with general health perceptions, vitality, and mental health.

In addition, the correlation coefficient between item VT3, "did you feel worn out," and mental health was higher (.58) than that between item VT3 and the hypothesized vitality scale (.51). For items MH3, "have you felt calm and peaceful" and MH5, "have you been a happy person," both correlation coefficients were higher with vitality, role physical, and role emotion scales than with their hypothesized mental health scale.

Table 3 presents item means of the transformed scales. The means of the eight SF-36 scales for the total sample ranged from 59 for the general health perceptions and vitality to almost 80 for physical functioning. Floor effects were most salient for role limitations due to emotional problems, whereas ceiling effects were noteworthy for role limitations due to physical health problems, social functioning, and role limitations due to emotional problems. The scaling success rates (tests of item-discriminant validity) for the combined sample were perfect (100) for 4 scales (PF, RP, BP, GH), above 95 for 2 scales (RE, MH), 88 for vitality and 56 for social functioning. Most measures met the minimum reliability standard, that is, the internal consistency coefficients were above 0.70 for all but the social functioning scale.

Table 4 presents the mean scale scores for the four subsamples. As expected, the health status as measured by the eight SF-36 scales were generally superior among the healthy samples as compared with the unhealthy samples. For example, dialysis patients had lower scores in all health scales except the mental health scale. While the scaling success rates were consistently lower for all four subsamples than the overall sample (due to large standard errors of the correlation coefficients with small sample sizes), variations in the scaling success rates existed across different subgroups (results not shown). These differences were also nonsystematic in that no single subgroup achieved higher success rates on all eight scales. Similarly, the internal consistency coefficients also varied across groups; only social functioning scale was uniformly below .70 for all subgroups.

TABLE 3. SF-36 Subscale Psychometric Results ($N = 156$)

SF-36 subscales	Mean (0–100)	Standard deviation	Floor %	Ceiling %	Success %	Reliability
PF	79.4	23.4	3.5	16.8	100	.92
RP	67.5	37.3	14.0	49.0	100	.82
BP	62.3	21.9	1.4	0.0	100	.78
GH	58.8	22.7	1.4	1.4	100	.82
VT	59.0	20.3	0.0	2.1	88	.73
SF	75.1	22.7	1.4	27.3	56	.54
RE	61.2	43.7	26.6	52.4	96	.88
MH	63.9	20.4	0.0	4.9	95	.74

TABLE 4. SF-36 Subscale Means, by Subgroups

	Group 1[a] (n = 65)	Group 2[b] (n = 16)	Group 3[c] (n = 20)	Group 4[d] (n = 12)
PF	84.6 (16.4)	39.7 (32.7)	92.5 (8.8)	81.3 (27.6)
RP	62.7 (37.0)	45.3 (50.2)	78.8 (28.4)	85.4 (34.5)
BP	61.2 (23.6)	47.5 (24.4)	69.5 (21.9)	70.0 (16.5)
GH	57.0 (25.5)	46.3 (22.1)	69.5 (12.5)	71.7 (12.5)
VT	57.1 (20.6)	50.1 (24.7)	60.8 (18.1)	70.0 (17.3)
SF	77.1 (21.8)	60.2 (33.3)	73.8 (19.9)	72.9 (22.5)
RE	61.3 (44.4)	54.2 (48.5)	56.7 (43.4)	77.8 (35.7)
MH	61.2 (18.8)	68.0 (26.0)	60.2 (15.5)	76.3 (16.4)

Parentheses indicate standard deviations.
[a] Ambulatory patients (mean age = 49).
[b] Dialysis patients (mean age = 66).
[c] Students (mean age = 31).
[d] General community sample (mean age = 39).

TABLE 5.   One-Week Test–Retest for the Chinese SF-36

	Product-moment correlations	
SF-36	Chinese–Chinese (n = 77)[a]	English–English (n = 78)[b]
PF	0.90	0.81
RP	0.69	0.70
BP	0.68	0.83
GH	0.74	0.78
VT	0.83	0.79
SF	0.67	0.80
RE	0.78	0.84
MH	0.86	0.87

[a] Among respondents who were administered the Chinese SF-36 twice within a week.
[b] Among respondents who were administered the English SF-36 twice within a week.
Note. From *The Reliability of the U.S. Chinese-American Test Version of the SF-36 Health Survey* (Table 12, p. 84), by J. Yu, 1995, Master's Thesis, The University of Arizona, Tucson, AZ. Reprinted with permission of the author.

Test–Retest Reliability. Table 5 reports the test–retest correlation coefficients for the Chinese SF-36. All the test–retest reliability estimates exceeded the minimum standard of 0.50 for group comparison (Helmstadter, 1964), and all scales either exceed or are close to the standard of 0.70 (Nunnally, 1978). The highest value is for the physical functioning scale and the lowest for the social functioning scale. These results suggest that respondents who score high on one assessment also tend to score high on a repeat assessment. These results are also comparable with the test–retest reliability estimates for the English SF-36 with correlation coefficients ranging from .70 to .87.

Equivalent-Forms Reliability. Equivalent-forms reliability correlations between scores of two different forms will generate good reliability estimates if the forms are truly equivalent in terms of item content. Table 6 presents the correlation coefficients and z-statistics for the significance of difference between the equivalent-forms of the SF-36 in Groups 1 (English–Chinese) and 2 (Chinese–English). The equivalent-forms reliability estimates for both groups are comparable and satisfactory. Correlations range from .81 to .98 for Group 1 and from .82 to .95 for Group 2. For Group 1, the highest correlation is for the physical functioning scale and the lowest for the role-physical scale. For Group

TABLE 6. Correlation Coefficients and Z-Statistics for the Significance of Difference between the Equivalent Forms of the SF-36

SF-36	Group 1[a] (n = 75)	Group 2[b] (n = 79)	z-score
PF	0.98	0.82	6.936
RP	0.81	0.92	−2.809
BP	0.92	0.95	−1.476
GH	0.88	0.88	0.000
VT	0.97	0.88	4.357
SF	0.90	0.87	0.846
RE	0.94	0.99	−5.525
MH	0.95	0.92	1.476

[a] English version then Chinese version on the same day.
[b] Chinese version then English version on the same day.
Note. From *The Reliability of the U.S. Chinese-American Test Version of the SF-36 Health Survey* (Table 9, p. 78), by J. Yu, 1995, Master's Thesis, The University of Arizona, Tucson, AZ. Reprinted with permission of the author.

2, the highest correlation is for the role-emotional scale and lowest for the physical functioning scale.

The significance of the differences between independent correlations for the equivalent-forms of the SF-36 scales is tested by the z-statistics. As shown in Table 6, the z-statistics indicate that the correlations for the SF-36 scales are fairly similar for the English–Chinese administration order in Group 1 and the Chinese–English administration order in Group 2. Correlations for four of the SF-36 scales (BP, GH, SF, and MH) are not different significantly for one order versus the other order (z-score < 1.96). Correlations for the PF and VT scales are higher in the English–Chinese administration order than in the Chinese–English administration order, while the estimates for RP and RE scales are lower in the English–Chinese administration order than in the Chinese-English administration order. These results suggest that there is no systematic effect of administration order between the English and the Chinese version on the correlations of scale scores on the English–Chinese equivalent-forms. Therefore, the Chinese and English versions of the SF-36 are considered equivalent.

Quality of the Translation. It is also important to evaluate the quality of the translation by comparing the ordering of item mean scores within each scale of the Chinese sample with that of the U.S. general population (Ware, Keller, *et al.*, 1995). If the Chinese translation is of high quality, the ordering of item means of the Chinese sample should be similar to that of the U.S. norm, although the absolute value of the item means might be different due to differences in populations.

Table 7 presents means of the SF-36 for the Chinese sample and the U.S. general population. The results suggest that the Chinese translation of the SF-36 is satisfactory as indicated by a consistent ordering of item clusters within scales between the two samples. It is interesting to note that exceptions were found in both samples within role physical and general health perception scales. The only scale in which the Chinese sample deviated from the U.S. norm was within physical functioning. For example, the "moderate activities" had lower means than its previous item cluster, that is, "climb several flights," "bend and kneel," and "walk mile." This may be attributed to the fact that the "moderate activities," as discussed earlier, include "bowling" and "playing golf," two activities that are uncommon and considered difficult to perform among Chinese Americans.

Summary

In this chapter, we discussed the development of the Chinese SF-36. Despite concerns about the differences between the Chinese and Western cultures (Tseng & Wu, 1985), there seems little difficulty in applying the SF-36 Health Survey among various Chinese populations. This finding suggests that a systematic approach to translation and cultural adaption is a prerequisite to a successful development of health instruments into non-English cultures or languages. The SF-36 instrument discriminated relatively well between healthy populations and un-

TABLE 7. Means for SF-36 Items for the Chinese Sample and General U.S. Population

Scale	SF-36 Item	Mean	
		Chinese ($N = 156$)	U.S. ($N = 2224$)
Physical functioning (PF)	Vigorous activities	1.87	2.17
	Climb several flights	2.50	2.54
	Bend, kneel	2.59	2.59
	Walk mile	2.57	2.55
	Moderate activities	2.44	2.65
	Lift, carry groceries	2.67	2.72
	Walk several blocks	2.67	2.69
	Climb one flight	2.83	2.78
	Walk one block	2.86	2.82
	Bathe, dress	2.89	2.88
Role physical (RP)	Accomplish less	1.63	1.73
	Cut down time	1.73	1.83
	Limited in kind	1.76	1.78
	Had difficulty	1.64	1.77
Bodily pain (BP)	Pain-magnitude	4.19	4.79
	Pain-interfere	4.10	4.58
General health (GH)	General health	3.13	3.77
	As healthy	3.45	3.80
	Health excellent	3.39	3.72
	Health to get worse	3.36	3.66
	Sick easier	3.73	4.19
Vitality (VT)	Pep/life	3.65	3.82
	Energy	3.65	3.82
	Worn out	4.50	4.34
	Tired	4.12	4.02
Social functioning (SF)	Social-extent	4.42	4.35
	Social-time	3.66	4.25
Role emotional (RE)	Accomplish less	1.59	1.75
	Cut down time	1.59	1.84
	Not careful	1.66	1.82
Mental health (MH)	Peaceful	4.06	4.06
	Happy	3.94	4.43
	Nervous	4.26	4.85
	Down in dumps	4.59	5.33
	Blue/sad	4.43	4.98

healthy patients. These results are very encouraging, suggesting that the Chinese SF-36 may be appropriate in general population surveys as well as clinical practice or clinical trials.

Unlike previous studies which observed a tendency of Chinese to present somatic complaints in place of psychological symptoms (Kleinman, 1977; Kleinman *et al.,* 1978; Liang *et al.,* 1992), in our study this notion of somatization as a predominant symptom in Chinese was not supported. The correlations of mental health items were low with the physical health scale, but high with the hypothesized mental health scale. However, the mental health scale was also highly associated with the vitality scale. This finding seems to suggest that vitality is the essence of a healthy mental state for Chinese. In traditional Chinese medicine mental disorder simply refers to the loss of a vital substance or spirit (Veith, 1972), whereas "happiness," a healthy mental state, is a sign of possessing vitality. This close association between mental health and vitality is consistent with the expression of positive well-being, identified as one of the two major components of mental health among Chinese by Liang and colleagues (1992).

However, the psychometric testing results also indicate specific areas of the Chinese SF-36 in which further work will be required. Of the eight scales of the SF-36, social functioning is least satisfactory in terms of discriminant validity as well as reliability. For Chinese, the two social functioning items were correlated more highly with the vitality and mental health scales than with the hypothesized social functioning scale. This finding seems to point to the differences in the cultural interpretation of items. The concept of social functioning may be less clearcut for Chinese. Deeply ingrained in the Confucian ideology of collectivism, it is socially unacceptable for Chinese to use "sickness" as an excuse to avoid socialization with others. This denial of disturbances of emotions and physical health on social activities

is more palpable among Chinese men than women. This is likely attributable to the domineering status of males in the Chinese patriarchal culture.

Further work is also required to explore the meanings of social functioning among Chinese. Why do Chinese tend to associate the ability to engage in social activities more with vitality or mental health? The Chinese terms that focus on key metaphors about vitality and social activities may be central to how a person experiences, defines, and communicates his or her ability to engage in social activities.

Despite these concerns, the results of the study indicate that the Chinese SF-36 will serve very well as an instrument for measuring the health status among Chinese Americans who tend to manage self-recognized episodes of sickness exclusively outside the perimeter of the formal health care system (Kleinman, 1977). The instrument will be a valuable tool in clinical study; it will fill the vacuum in assisting doctors to better understand the feelings of their Chinese patients. The instrument will not only be a fundamental tool to assess the effectiveness of medical care among this underserved population, but also a valuable tool in social science research on determinants of health among Chinese Americans.

The study fills a major gap in the literature of health services research on Asian Americans. These results, as discussed earlier, strongly suggest that due to language barriers, Chinese Americans are largely understudied in health services research. The results of this work will benefit others around the United States who work with Chinese populations. It is our expectation that the results of this study will stimulate further research to establish the reliability, validity, and clinical application of the SF-36 among Chinese. The results of the study will also provide an invaluable experience for generating appropriate methods for developing health status survey measures across other underserved populations, in particular recent immigrants from Southeast Asia—Vietnam and Cambodia.

Applying the Chinese SF-36 in Assessing Health Status among Elderly Chinese

The psychometric testing results of the Chinese SF-36 are found to satisfy conventional psychometric criteria, which suggests that the translation of SF-36 into Chinese is successful. We applied this newly developed Chinese SF-36 to assessing the functional health status and well-being of elderly Chinese.

Limited Health Status Data for Elderly Chinese

The Chinese elderly represent a high-risk and high-needs population in the United States. Steeped in the traditional Chinese culture, many elderly Chinese are likely to resort to self-care in managing episodes of sickness (Kleinman *et al.*, 1978). Furthermore, because of language barriers, many elderly Chinese are often restricted to activities in Chinatowns in many U.S. cities. While Chinatowns provide these elderly people a cultural "enclave" that fosters their cultural heritage and protects them from feeling alienated by an unfamiliar American culture, Chinatowns nonetheless manifest many of the nation's worst social ills: congestion, substandard housing, and poor sanitation (Huang & Pilisuk, 1977; Ong & LEAP, 1993).

Elderly Chinese Americans, due to language barriers and unique cultural backgrounds, have remained largely invisible to health services surveys (F. J. S. Lin, 1991; Yu, 1991). Despite tremendous growth in the size of this population (U.S. Bureau of the Census, 1991), knowledge of the health status of elderly Chinese Americans remains grossly inadequate (Yu, 1986). Based on conventional mortality health statistics (e.g., mortality rates), Chinese Americans are often viewed as a "model" minority with no health problems (U.S. Department of Health and Human Services [USDHHS], 1985). This public image has concealed great variability in health status among Chinese Americans (Chinese Canadian Medical Society, 1990). More importantly, the general perception that Chinese have good health has masked the serious health problems among elderly Chinese Americans (Huang & Pilisuk, 1977).

Health Status of Chinese Elderly Persons as Measured by the SF-36

The data for this analysis came from the subsample of 43 Chinese elderly persons included in the first sample of the validation study of the Chinese translation of the MOS SF-36. The Chinese elderly subsample was drawn from the active members of a senior community service center in Massachusetts. This sampling procedure has one great advantage in that it is cost-effective. The senior center, located in Chinatown, has a primarily Chinese administrative-service staff and a comprehensive network of programs and services focusing on the social, economic, and physical well-being of Chinese elderly persons.

The SF-36 health profiles are contained in Table 8. Compared with the U.S. norm population (ages 65–74), these elderly Chinese Americans report similar health status in bodily pain (BP), general health (GH), vitality (VT), social functioning (SF), but they report better health in physical functioning (PF). They report worse health in role limitations due to emotional problems (RE) and in mental health (MH). This difference in physical versus mental health between the elderly Chinese and U.S norm becomes quite salient in the two SF-36 component summary scores. While Chinese elderly persons tend to have higher physical summary (PCS) scores, they report worse mental summary (MCS) scores. This trend persists even when we compare Chinese elderly persons with the U.S. norm (ages ≥ 75). Compared with this older U.S norm population, Chinese elderly persons again report worse mental compo-

TABLE 8. SF-36 Health Profiles for the Elderly Chinese and U.S. Norm

SF-36 subscales	Chinese elderly (mean age = 71) (N = 43)	U.S. norm (ages 65–74) (N = 442)	U.S. norm (ages ≥ 75) (N = 264)
Physical functioning	80.1 (15.8)	69.4 (26.3)[c]	53.2 (30.0)[d]
Role physical	72.6 (32.5)	64.5 (41.3)	45.3 (42.0)[d]
Bodily pain	67.0 (19.3)	68.5 (26.4)	60.9 (26.0)
General health	64.0 (20.9)	62.6 (22.4)	56.7 (21.2)[b]
Vitality	61.6 (18.4)	59.9 (22.1)	50.4 (23.6)[c]
Social functioning	81.7 (17.1)	80.6 (25.6)	73.9 (28.8)[a]
Role emotional	61.2 (43.6)	81.4 (34.6)[d]	63.2 (42.9)
Mental health	66.1 (20.7)	76.9 (18.1)[d]	74.0 (20.2)[c]
Physical summary score[a]	48.2 (6.2)	43.5 (11.2)[c]	38.0 (11.2)[d]
Mental summary score[a]	46.3 (10.8)	52.6 (9.3)[d]	50.8 (11.7)[c]

Parentheses indicate standard deviation.
[a] p < .10 level.
[b] p < .05 level.
[c] p < .01 level.
[d] p < .001 level.

nent summary (MCS) but better physical component summary (PCS) scores.

The finding of the discrepancy in physical and mental health observed in Table 8 could be a result of a selection bias; that is, the study selected physically healthy elderly Chinese subjects who came to the community service center for mental health–related services. If this is the case, we would then expect that this group of elderly Chinese would have better physical health and worse mental health scores. However, when we compared these elderly Chinese subjects with a more general Chinese population sample in Boston, we found that these elderly Chinese tended to have lower physical functioning and role limitations scores, but they fared better in the mental health domain (results not shown). This finding seems to point away from this selection bias.

In summary, the Chinese SF-36 can be used to provide a summary profile of functional health and well-being for Chinese elderly persons, an underserved immigrant population. Consistent with the notion of Chinese being a healthy minority, elderly Chinese Americans perceived better physical health than the American norm populations (ages 65–74; ages ≥ 75, respectively). How-

ever, this healthy minority model also concealed tremendous mental health problems among the elderly Chinese. Compared with the U.S. norm, Chinese elderly persons reported poorer mental health.

This finding underscores the appropriateness of using the Chinese version of the SF-36 in assessing health status, particularly mental health, among Chinese elderly persons. Conventional measures of mental health (e.g., those used in epidemiological surveys) often measure depressive symptoms or dysphoric conditions, which connote antisocial or bizarre behavior in Chinese culture. Therefore, there is a strong tendency among the Chinese elderly persons not to disclose their feelings about depressive symptoms that are pathognomonic in nature (Lin, 1985; Ying & Miller, 1992). Because the mental health domain of the SF-36 measures subjective assessments of the frequency and intensity of symptoms of psychological well-being and life satisfaction, the instrument is likely to generate reliable and valid information among Chinese elderly persons. Since mental health domain in the SF-36 touches on subject matter that is close in meaning to vitality (Ren et al., in press), the elderly Chinese have less trouble or fear in discussing their feelings about them.

This finding has important policy implications. There is a strong tendency among elderly Chinese, who are more likely to have poor understanding of Western medicine and still adhere to traditional Chinese medicine, not to seek help due to the stigmatization of mental problems and subsequent fear of spreading family disgrace (Lin, 1983). The technique of the "talking therapies" of American psychiatry is not always appreciated or even understood by Chinese elderly persons, who consider that discussion of mental health would provoke feelings of shame (Myers, Croake, & Singh, 1987). Coupled with the reluctance to seek mental health care, the prevalence of poor mental health identified in this study poses a particularly serious problem among elderly Chinese Americans. The study finding highlights the need to study mental health issues among this underserved Chinese population.

Future Directions

HRQoL measures that are reliable and valid (Curtis, Deyo, & Hudson, 1994; Ware, 1987) allow clinicians and researchers to easily collect patient information about functional health and well-being. Such measures can be used to evaluate differences in health plans or to describe the functional burden due to disease conditions in a population. Such measures can also be used to monitor the quality, efficiency, and effectiveness of patient care.

While the majority of health status measures have been developed in English, few have been developed to monitor the health status of immigrant populations not yet proficient in English. These immigrant populations are often excluded from research or evaluations due to language barriers. Consequently, the health status of immigrant populations is not represented in HRQoL statistics. The development of cross-cultural instruments allows for the inclusion of under-represented immigrant populations in HRQoL data. We have demonstrated this use in an elderly Chinese population in Boston.

To develop valid and reliable cross-cultural measures, we encourage the selection of currently available instruments over the development of new instruments. Like others (Orley & Kuyken, 1994), we single out the process of adaptive translation as a key methodology. In addition, we have suggested several psychometric tests necessary to assess the equivalence of instruments. Although this approach assumes a level of homogeneity within immigrant populations that may not exist (Guarnaccia, 1996), it provides a first step that will eventually bring information about all immigrant populations to the table.

One important future direction is to design methodological studies that result in measures that capture HRQoL variability within immigrant populations. For example, a researcher may choose first to administer a newly adapted translation to an immigrant population where there is variation in the degree of acculturation or in social status and then to ascertain through qualitative interviews whether strong differences exist in the interpretation of the questions or the meaning of the responses. Typically, qualitative research is completed prior to instrument development. This approach allows for the immigrants, rather than the researcher, to provide the interpretation of the quantitative results. To the degree that variability exists in meaning across levels of acculturation or social status, single HRQoL measures will need to be augmented with additional data to capture some of the heterogeneity.

A second important direction is the identification of a series of core health domains that can be measured within each immigrant group. Although such research will require large samples, a major component of this work will be the development of conceptual models for health and a consideration of cultural variation. This research is important because it then allows the development of measures that are unique to a single immigrant group.

In health care, there is certainly a place for cross-cultural measures, but measures that capture the unique HRQoL components within immigrant populations are just as necessary. These measures, when developed, could be used in conjunction with a strong set of core measures. The methodology for the development of these measures must first be qualitative allowing the immigrant group to identify and frame elements of HRQoL not included in a core instrument. Then quantitative measures could be developed and used to complement other measurement tools. Clearly, the future will require more creative integration of theory and diverse methods of data gathering and analysis to deepen our understanding of HRQoL in diverse immigrant populations in the United States (Levine, 1995). We have offered a methodological stepping-stone in the long walk to developing both cross-culturally valid and culturally appropriate measures of HRQoL.

Acknowledgments

We dedicate this work to the late Sol Levine, our mentor and friend, for his inspirational support and leadership. Preparation of this chapter is supported by a grant from the New England Medical Center through the auspices of the Henry J. Kaiser Family Foundation, and in part by a grant (R03 HS09352) from the Agency for Health Care and Policy Research to the first author. We are also grateful to Ms. Jung Yu for allowing us to use two tables from her master's thesis.

References

Alonso, J., Prieto, L., & Anto, J. M. (1994). The Spanish version of the Nottingham Health Profile: A review of adaptation and instrument characteristics. *Quality of Life Research, 3,* 385–393.

Badoux, A., & Mendelsohn G. A. (1994). Subjective well-being in French and American samples: Scale development and comparative data. *Quality of Life Research, 3,* 395–401.

Barker, J. C. (1992). Cultural diversity—Changing the context of medical practice. *Western Journal of Medicine, 157,* 248–254.

Berzon, R., Hays, R. D., & Shumaker, S. A. (1993). International use, application and performance of health-related quality of life instruments. *Quality of Life Research, 2,* 367–368.

Bullinger, M. (1995). German translation and psychometric testing of the SF-36 Health Survey: Preliminary results from the IQOLA project. *Social Science and Medicine, 41,* 1359–1366.

Campen, C. V., Sixma, H, Friele, R. D., Kerssens, J. J., & Peters, L. (1995). Quality of care and patient satisfaction: A review of measuring instruments. *Medical Care Research and Review, 52,* 109–133.

Chinese Canadian Medical Society. (1990). *Health problems related to the Chinese in North America.* Proceedings of the fifth conference, the Faculty of Medicine, University of Toronto, Ontario, Canada.

Croog, S. H., & Levine, S. (1989). Quality of life and health care intervention. In H. E. Freeman & S. Levine (Eds.), *Handbook of medical sociology* (pp. 508–528). Englewood Cliffs, NJ: Prentice-Hall.

Curtis, J. R., Deyo, R. A., & Hudson, L. D. (1994). Health-related quality of life among patients with chronic obstructive lung disease. *Thorax, 49,* 162–170.

Ferguson, G. T., & Cherniack R. M. (1993). Management of chronic obstructive pulmonary disease. *New England Journal of Medicine, 328,* 1017–1022.

Forsberg, C., & Bjorvell, H. (1993). Swedish population norms for the GHRI, HI and STAI-state. *Quality of Life Research, 2,* 349–356.

Geigle, R., & Jones, S. B. (1990). Outcomes measurement: A report from the front. *Enquiry, 27,* 7.

Giachello, A. L. (1992). Reconciling the multiple scientific and community needs. In *Health behavior research in minority populations: Access, design, and implementation* (pp. 237–239). Washington, DC: National Institute of Health.

Gibson, R. C. (1991). Race and the self-reported health of elderly persons. *Journal of Gerontology: Social Sciences, 46,* S235–242.

Guarnaccia, P. J. (1996). Anthropological perspective: The importance of culture in the assessment of quality of life. In B. Spilker (Ed.), *Quality of life and pharmacoeconomics in clinical trials* (2nd ed., pp. 523–528). New York: Raven.

Guillein, F., Bombardier, C., & Beaton, D. (1993). Cross-cultural adaptation of health-related quality of life measures: Literature review and proposed guidelines. *Journal of Clinical Epidemiology, 46,* 1417–1432.

Guyatt, G. H. (1993). The philosophy of health-related quality of life translation. *Quality of Life Research, 2,* 461–465.

Hatton, D. C. (1992). Information transmission in bilingual, bicultural contexts. *Journal of Community Health Nursing, 9,* 53–59.

Hays, R. D., & Hayashi, T. (1990). Beyond internal consistency: Rationale and user's guide for Multitrait Analysis Program on the microcomputer. *Behavioral Research Methods, Instruments and Computers, 22,* 167.

Hays, R. D., Hayashi, T., Carson, S., & Ware, J. E. (1988). *User's guide for the Multitrait Analysis Program (MAP)* (A Rand Note, N-2786-RC) Santa Monica, CA: Rand.

Hays, R. D., Anderson, R., & Revicki, D. (1993). Psychometric considerations in evaluating health-related quality of life measures. *Quality of Life Research, 2,* 441–449.

Helmstadter, G. C. (1964). *Principles of psychological measurement.* New York: Appleton-Century-Crafts.

Hsu, F. L. K. (1976). *Americans and Chinese: Passages of differences.* Honolulu: University of Hawaii Press.

Huang, K., & Pilisuk, M. (1977). At the threshold of the golden gate: Special problems of a neglected minority. *American Journal of Orthopsychiatry, 47,* 701–713.

Hunt, S. M., Alonso, J., Bucquet, D., Niero, M., Wiklund, I., & McKenna, S. (1991). Cross-cultural adaptation of health measures. *Health Policy, 19,* 33–44.

Kleinman, A., Eisenberg, L., & Good, B. (1978). Culture, illness, and care. *Annals of Internal Medicine, 88,* 251–258.

Kleinman, A. M. (1977). Depression, somatization, and the new "cross-cultural psychiatry." *Social Science and Medicine, 11,* 3–10.

Krause, N. M., & Jay, G. M. (1994). What do global self-rated health items measure? *Medical Care, 32,* 930–942.

Lam, C. L. K., Weel, C. V., & Lauder, I. J. (1994). Can the Dartmouth COOP/WONCA Charts be used to assess the functional status of Chinese patients? *Family Practice, 11,* 85–94.

Levine, S. (1995). Time for creative integration in medical sociology. *Journal of Health and Social Behavior* (extra issue), 1–4.

Liang, J., Wu, S. C., Krause, N. M., Chiang, T. L., & Wu, H. Y. (1992). The structure of the mental health inventory among Chinese in Taiwan. *Medical Care, 30,* 659–676.

Lieu, T. A., Newacheck, P. W., & McManus, M. A. (1993). Race, ethnicity, and access to ambulatory care among US adolescents. *American Journal of Public Health, 7,* 960–965.

Lin, F. J. S. (1991). Population characteristics and health care needs of Asian Pacific Americans. *American Journal of Public Health, 81,* 1423.

Lin, T. Y. (1983). Psychiatry and Chinese culture. *Western Journal of Medicine, 129,* 862.

Lin, T. Y. (1985). Mental disorders and psychiatry in Chinese culture: Characteristics features and major issues. In W. S. Tseng & Y. H. Wu (Eds.), *Chinese culture and mental health* (pp. 369–393). New York: Academic Press.

Mathias, S. D., Fifer, S. K., & Patrick, D. L. (1994). Rapid translation of quality of life measures for international clinical trials: Avoiding errors in the minimalist approach. *Quality of Life Research, 3,* 403–412.

McDowell, I., & Newell, C. (1987). *Measuring health: A guide to rating scales and questionnaires.* New York: Oxford University Press.

McHorney, C. A., Ware, J. E., Lu, J. F., & Sherbourne, C. D. (1994). The MOS 36-Item Short Form Health Survey (SF-36): III. Tests of data quality, scaling assumptions, and reliability across diverse patient groups. *Medical Care, 32,* 40–66.

Meredith, L. S., & Siu, A. L. (1995). Variation and quality of self-report health data: Asians and Pacific Islanders compared with other ethnic groups. *Medical Care, 33,* 1120–1131.

Mo, B. (1992). Modesty, sexuality, and breast health in Chinese-American women. *Western Journal of Medicine, 157,* 260–264.

Muller, J. H., & Desmond, B. (1992). Ethical dilemmas in a cross-cultural context: A Chinese example. *Western Journal of Medicine, 157,* 323–327.

Myers, K. M., Croake, J. W., & Singh, A. (1987). Adult fears of four ethnic groups: Whites, Chinese, Japanese and "Boat People." *International Journal of Social Psychiatry, 33,* 56–67.

Nunnally, J. C. (1978). *Psychometric theory* (2nd ed.). New York: McGraw-Hill.

Ong, P., & LEAP Asian Pacific American Public Policy Institute. (1993). Inner-city communities. In LEAP Asian Pacific American Public Policy Institute (Eds.), *Beyond Asian American poverty* (pp. 27–42). San Francisco, CA: LEAP Asian Pacific American Public Policy Institute.

Orley, J., & Kuyken, W. (1994). *Quality of life assessment: International perspectives.* New York: Springer-Verlag.

Patrick, D. L., & Erickson, P. (1993). *Health status and health policy: Allocating resources to health care.* New York: Oxford University Press.

Ren, X. S., & Amick, B. (1996a). Race and self assessed health status: The role of socioeconomic factors in the USA. *Journal of Epidemiology and Community Health, 50,* 269–273.

Ren, X. S., & Amick, B. (1996b). Racial and ethnic disparities in self-assessed health status: Evidence from the National Survey of Families and Households. *Ethnicity and Health, 1*(3), 293–303.

Ren, X. S., Amick, B., Zhou, L., & Gandek, B. (in press). Chinese version of the SF-36 Health Survey: Translation and report on the psychometric evaluation among Chinese Americans. *Journal of Clinical Epidemiology.*

Rogers, R. G. (1992). Living and dying in the U.S.A.: Sociodemographic determinants of death among Blacks and Whites. *Demography, 2,* 287–303.

Sartorius, N., & Kuyken, W. (1993). Translation of health status instruments. In J. Orley & W. Kuyken (Eds.), *Quality of life assessment: International perspective* (pp. 3–18). New York: Springer-Verlag.

Till, J. E., Osoba, D., Oater, L., & Young, J. R. (1994). Research on health-related quality of life: Dissemination into practical applications. *Quality of Life Research, 3,* 279–283.

Tseng, W. S., & Wu, D. Y. H. (1985). *Chinese culture and mental health.* New York: Academic Press.

U.S. Bureau of the Census. (1991). *1990 census of population and housing.* Summary Tape File 3. Washington, DC.

U.S. Bureau of the Census. (1995). *Statistical abstract of the United States.* Washington, DC: U.S. Government Printing Office.

U.S. Department of Health and Human Services. (1985). *Report of the Secretary's Task Force on Black and minority health: Vol. I. Executive Summary.* Washington, DC: U.S. Government Printing Office.

Veith, I. (1972). *The yellow emperor's classic of internal medicine.* Los Angeles: University of California Press.

Ware, J. E. (1987). Standards for validating health measures: Definition and content. *Journal of Chronic Disease, 40,* 473–480.

Ware, J. E., & Sherbourne, C. D. (1992). The MOS 36-item short-form health survey (SF-36): I. Conceptual framework and item selection. *Medical Care, 30,* 473–483.

Ware, J. E., Snow, K. K., Kosinski, M., & Gandek, B. (1993). *SF-36 Health Survey: Manual and interpretation guide.* Boston: New England Medical Center, Health Institute.

Ware, J. E., Keller, S. D., Gandek, B., Brazier, J. E., Sullivan, M., & the IQOLA Project Group. (1995). Evaluating translations of health status questionnaires: Methods from the IQOLA project. *International Journal of Technology Assessment in Health Care, 11,* 525–550.

Ware, J. E., Kosinski, M., Bayliss, M. S., McHorney, C. A., Rogers, W. H., & Raczek, A. (1995). Comparison of methods for scoring and statistical analysis of SF-36 health profile and summary measures: summary of results from the Medical Outcomes Study. *Medical Care, 33,* AS264–279.

Ware, J. E., Kosinski, M., & Keller, S. D. (1995). *SF-12: How to score the SF-12 Physical & Mental Health Summary scales.* Boston: New England Medical Center, Health Institute.

Ying, Y. W., & Miller, L. S. (1992). Help-seeking behavior and attitude of Chinese Americans regarding psychosocial problems. *American Journal of Community Psychology, 20,* 549.

Yu, E. (1986). Health of the Chinese elderly in America. *Research on Aging, 8,* 84–109.

Yu, E. (1991). The health risks of Asian Americans. *American Journal of Public Health, 81,* 1391–1393.

T. Yu, J. (1995). *The reliability of the U.S. Chinese-American test version of the SF-36 Health Survey* (Master's thesis, University of Arizona, Tucson).

Zborowski, M. (1952). Cultural components in responses to pain. *Journal of Social Issues, 8,* 16–30.

6

Access to Health Care

RUTH LYN RIEDEL

The anxious questions of yesterday's immigrants on Ellis Island and the anguished screams of today's newcomers at Guantanamo Bay suggest an all too familiar continuity. The double helix of health and fear remains encoded in American Society and culture, reappearing in patterns fresh but familiar.

Alan Kraut (1994), Silent Travelers: Germs, Genes and the "Immigrant Menace" (p. 9)

Introduction

For over 30 years, health policy makers, administrators, and consumers have voiced concern about access to health care and have exhaustively described the need for system reorganization and improvement. Innumerable programs have been funded, implemented, and evaluated. Most of these programs were intended to improve access to care for vulnerable populations.

Since the early 19th century, the United States has received wave after wave of immigrants. In search of better employment and better living conditions, these immigrants have suffered malnutrition, communicable diseases, losses of family members and social support systems, and feelings of social and cultural alienation (DeSantis & Halberstein, 1992). In the early years, when immigrants were supplying labor for a growing

economy, social disruption occurred but was resolved once new population groups learned the intricacies of American society (Kennedy, 1996). But, as Borjas (1996) points out, recent waves of immigrants lack the skills demanded by the U.S. economy, and economic assimilation is slow. Changes in immigration policy since the 1960s reflect the perception of the American populace that immigrants are substantially economically dependent on the states, counties, and cities that are most affected, and the struggle to manage overburdened health and welfare systems.

The literature on immigrant health clearly describes poor health outcomes associated with subsequent reduction in entitlements for immigrants and ethnic minorities. Despite all that is known about the need for a vigorous effort to reduce these disparities in health care (Bollini & Siem, 1995), America has entered "an era of 'compassion fatigue'"(Rumbaut, Chavez, Moser, Pickwell, & Wishik, 1988) from which it may never emerge. Poor access to health care for immigrants is a public health and public policy issue that has been designated as low priority by "a wary and weary public and its elected leaders" (Rumbaut *et al.,* 1988). Bollini and Siem (1995) emphasize that, in addition to "poor working and living conditions, which are per se determinants of poor health," today's migrants and ethnic minorities must also contend with "reduced access to health care for political, administrative and cultural reasons" (p. 821).

This chapter begins with a review of the traditional health services research approach

RUTH LYN RIEDEL • Alliance Healthcare Foundation, San Diego, California 92123.

Handbook of Immigrant Health, edited by Loue. Plenum Press, New York, 1998.

101

to access spanning 30 years, and focusing on access to services and public and private insurance coverage, as well as utilization of services. Regrettably, most of this work had minimal impact on policy makers at the federal level. The exception was research on the early years of the Medicaid program which did demonstrate improvements in access to care for eligible, low-income individuals and families. This exception was temporary, as a reversal of fortune occurred for these Medicaid enrollees and for the Medicaid eligibles who followed. The economic recession of the early 1980s fueled political reform that resembled a social movement. Health care cost containment became a "front-burner" issue, as the federal government pointed to the discipline of "the market" to correct inequities in the U.S. health care system.

The chapter proceeds with a detailed review of the 1993 Institute of Medicine (IOM) Report, *Access to Health Care in America,* which underscores the importance of "traditional" barriers to access (e.g., financial, organizational, cultural) and recommends carefully selected measures of access for improved program monitoring and policy development. A description of general and specific access problems of several larger immigrant groups and subgroups in the United States follows, with a description of access problems exacerbated by the implementation of the federal welfare reform law (H.R. 3734). Given that the responsibility and financial risk for health care for immigrants is being pushed down to the lowest level of organization (e.g., from the federal government to states, and from the states to the counties), most "promising" strategies are emerging at the community level. It is important to note that local solutions, without support from outside, are limited because they cannot address the fundamental issues which are social and political.

Background

When Aday and Andersen (1975) wrote the classic, *Development of Indices of Access*

to Medical Care, the concept of access required definition, both conceptually and empirically. In the early 1970s there were several schools of thought in health services research. One group of researchers viewed access according to characteristics of the population such as family income, insurance coverage, and attitudes toward the health care system. A second conceptual framework depicted access as characteristics of the delivery system or system-specific attributes. Yet a third school viewed access as a consumer's experience with the health care system which included utilization of services and satisfaction with the organization and delivery of health care.

In these early years of investigating access, researchers assumed that accessible care was care that was available whenever the patient was in need, that the point of entry into the health care system was well defined, and that individuals used services according to their need for care (Freeborn & Greenlick, 1973). Barriers to access were identified as the shortage of primary care physicians in the inner-city and rural areas (Rogers, 1973). Others considered the consumer's willingness to seek care (Mechanic, 1972), and financing or reimbursement (Fox, 1972) which currently seem to be the fundamental predictors of access.

Starting with health policy that guides financing, public education, manpower distribution, and organization, Aday and Andersen (1975) offered one of the first frameworks for conceptualizing access to medical care. Logically, characteristics of the system and characteristics of the "population-at-risk" affect the utilization of services. The relative importance of consumer satisfaction is less clear, but characteristics of the system and an individual's utilization experience are shown to affect satisfaction. Subsequently, Aday and Andersen separated indicators of access into two categories: process and outcome. Process indices were considered independent variables predictive of outcome. Process indicators include (1) having a regular source of care, (2) travel time to medical care, (3) having a specific appointment instead of dropping in, and (4) a reasonable waiting time for the appointment. Indicators of outcome were dependent variables, for example, the results or end products.

Two data sets used to test their model were a 1969 National Center for Health Statistics survey and a 1970 Center for Health Administration Studies (University of Chicago) national survey of health services utilization and expenditures. Aday and Andersen (1975) were successful in identifying population groups with reduced access according to both process and outcome indicators. They were individuals whose income was below the federal poverty level, ethnic minorities, and inner-city and farm residents. Because these people did not have a regular source of care, they were more likely to use the hospital emergency room or outpatient departments for all presenting problems. They were more likely to travel farther to reach the health care facility. They often walked in without an appointment and waited a long time to be seen.

By the time "poor" individuals accessed the system their problems were more severe, and more visits and resources were required to resolve them. Even though more resource consumption was needed to address more severe problems, the poor, ethnic minorities and farm residents still used fewer resources than expected. Of individuals with incomes below the federal poverty level, 52% saw physicians less frequently than other income groups, according to a panel of experts from the University of Chicago Medical School. When a medical severity index was used the same groups of individuals demonstrated the greatest and most urgent need for medical care.

One Step Forward, Two Steps Back

By the mid 1970s, the enactment of Medicaid temporarily reversed the trend portrayed in early survey data on use of physician services, and utilization rates for the poor were equivalent to or higher than individuals with incomes above the federal poverty level (Davis, 1991). In the mid 1970s researchers discovered the importance of controlling for differences in

health status, but results were mixed. Regrettably, there were no definitive answers for policy makers about the effectiveness of Medicaid in closing the gap in use of ambulatory care or other health services. Temporary gains that could be attributed to Medicaid were halted by a national recognition of spiraling health care costs and the economic recession of the early 1980s. Policy makers became concerned with a latent demand for publicly funded health care services that surfaced with improvements in health care financing. In the 1980s, America was obsessed with health care cost containment. Regulatory programs designed to constrain costs had failed, and conservative professional lobbies and business interests championed "market reform." William MacBeath (1991), a long-term president of the American Public Health Association, described the gradual "abrogation of governmental responsibility in public health" until the federal government went into a "broad scale retreat" on health policy issues.

In 1984 Aday, Fleming, and Andersen revisited their tried and true access paradigm by applying it to data from a 1982 National Survey of Access to Medical Care funded by the Robert Wood Johnson Foundation and conducted by Lou Harris and Associates. The representative sample for the 1982 telephone survey included 4,800 U.S. families; low-income families were oversampled by 1,800. The overall response rate was 60%. Several income groups reported losing insurance or losing benefits, resulting in reduced coverage; these included "37 percent of the poor, 52 percent of poor nonwhites, 39 percent of those with public insurance only, and 37 percent of the unemployed" (p. 106). Results showed that these groups were without a regular source of care, and had trouble obtaining ambulatory care for chronic disease management. Families headed by an unemployed earner, as well as those with public insurance or no insurance, were refused care twice as often as families with private insurance. While the investigators did not have the wherewithal to estimate the effects of a recent recession or of reductions in health care financing, it was clear that there had been an impact on millions of families. Of course, the unemployed, uninsured, and ethnic minorities had been disproportionately affected (Aday *et al.,* 1984).

Using data from the 1982 National Health Interview Survey, Newacheck (1988) looked at utilization differences in relation to Medicaid coverage using an adaptation of the familiar Aday and Andersen 1975 and Aday and colleagues 1984 model. He introduced independent variables estimated to improve the understanding of the impacts of poverty and Medicaid status on the annual number of physician contacts. After adjusting for health status, Newacheck's analyses showed that, overall, the nonpoor had a 45% higher use rate than the poor. However, poor persons with Medicaid coverage had the same or higher numbers of contacts with physicians. Newacheck also showed that, in 1982, poor persons in poor health were 62% more likely to have Medicaid coverage then poor persons reported in "excellent" health; however, fewer than half of poor persons in poor health were on Medicaid. In addition, Newacheck's study supported prior findings that poor individuals were less likely to use preventive services than nonpoor.

From the health services literature it was clear that, even though more work needed to be done on removing barriers to appropriate care, federal and state Medicaid eligibility policy exerted a great deal of influence on service use. Throughout the 1980s, researchers continued to focus on vulnerable population groups providing the rationale for "continued, modest expansions" in Medicaid and community health centers funding (Davis, 1991). In the main, policy makers' concerns with the rising costs of health care engendered state and federal cutbacks. Using data from the 1986 National Health Survey, Blendon, Aiken, Freeman, & Corey (1989) described widening gaps between the insured and uninsured, and between Blacks and Whites between 1982 and 1986, noting the "persistent disparity" in the use of health services, death rates, and health status between Black and White Americans.

In 1994, the Robert Wood Johnson Foundation funded yet a fourth National Access to Care Survey as a follow-up to the 1993 National Health Interview Survey. As in 1982, this survey focused on the family. Field methods were improved by adding face-to-face interviews with persons included in the National Health Survey who said they did not have a telephone. In addition to standard questions about medical and surgical services included in the three prior access surveys (1976, 1982, and 1986), respondents were questioned about dental care, eyeglasses, and mental health care; mental health was chosen because of the marked decreases in mental health benefits in both public and private sectors.

Berk, Schur, and Cantor (1995) described the results of analyses of the 1994 survey conducted by staff in the Center for Health Affairs at Project HOPE. Based on representation in the sample, more than 41 million people were unable to get the care they needed. Demographic characteristics, family income, and insurance coverage explained most of the variance in access to care. Approximately 24% of Blacks, 17.5% of Hispanics, and 21% of adult women reported access problems. One third of the uninsured described unmet needs for care. The authors concluded that their findings were "consistent with the long history of health services research that has shown the problems of access experienced by vulnerable populations. . . . The greatest barriers to care are experienced by the poor and the "uninsured" (p. 145). While there had been much speculation about the "creep" of access problems to the middle class, Berk and colleagues removed all reasonable doubt. Nearly half of respondents who described unmet need were middle class, with family annual incomes ranging from $20,000 to $50,000.

Access to Health Care in America, the 1993 IOM Study

A 1993 report, *Access to Health Care in America,* developed by a committee of the

National Academy of Sciences' Institute of Medicine (IOM), concluded that little progress had been made in increasing access to personal health services in the past decade. The Institute's committee of experts defined access as "the timely use of personal health services to achieve the best possible outcomes" (p. 33). The study had two overall objectives: (1) to propose a set of indicators to monitor access to health care nationally, and (2) to use the proposed indicators "to assess the current status of access." Investigators viewed the benchmarking provided by this study as a stimulus to continue monitoring access on a regular basis and to make crucial modifications in existing data sets that would provide better information for policy decisions.

The IOM access study begins with a "General Conclusions" section in which the authors describe the lack of progress in improving access to personal health care. Instead of progress, the committee described an insidious process of "stagnation," with growing discrepancies "between the haves and the have-nots in our society." Predictably, the evidence in this report suggests that people who are uninsured or underinsured, and who live in low-income neighborhoods, do not have timely access to appropriate care. African Americans and ethnic minorities are disproportionately represented in this population group.

Classification of Barriers to Care

Aware that "the number of uninsured, poor, and ethnic and racial minorities is growing" (p. 44), IOM experts explored the ways in which measures of access (i.e., utilization and outcome) varied according to measures of equity (i.e., financial, structural, personal, and cultural factors). *Structural barriers* were defined as "impediments to medical care directly related to the number, type, concentration, location, or organizational configuration of health care providers" (p. 39). *Financial barriers* restrict access by inhibiting patients' ability to pay for or reimburse providers for needed medical services; financial barriers also discourage physicians and hospitals from treating patients "of limited means." *Personal and cultural barriers* "may inhibit people who need medical attention from seeking it" (p. 39) or from following the recommendations of caregivers (IOM, 1993).

Structural and Institutional Barriers

After World War II there was a national movement to expand the capacity of the health care system. The Hill-Burton Act of 1946 is one example of programs that financed facilities' construction to increase hospital bed space in communities. New funding streams stimulated incredible growth in the pool of health care professionals. Legislation to create the National Health Service Corps and community health centers was also designed to improve public sector capacity at the local level (IOM, 1993). The committee optimistically viewed the 1990s as a period of restructuring and redistribution of health resources, a decade of quality improvement through the judicious use of health services by all. However, the inequities in the distribution of resources were acknowledged, and the authors lamented the interminable use of hospital emergency rooms and outpatient clinics as regular sources of care (IOM, 1993).

Financial Barriers

While market forces have contributed to a reduction in resources in low-income and rural areas of the country, they have not contained the cost of heath care. In 1997 there were an estimated 40.3 million uninsured Americans. More than half of individuals and families who were uninsured or underinsured were unable to pay for most health services, with annual incomes under $20,000. African Americans and ethnic minorities are disproportionately uninsured or underinsured. The IOM committee argued that "direct service delivery programs" should act as a safety net "when insurance fails" (IOM, 1993), but the public sector safety net has been stretched to the breaking point. Safety net organizations include community health centers, county health clinics and hospitals, and the Veterans Administration, all suffer constant cutbacks while being called on to serve more and more people.

Personal and Cultural Barriers

In 1993, nearly 9% of the U.S. population of 258 million was foreign-born (Hargraves, 1996). Virtually all immigrants require care that is culturally sensitive. Homogenized health care that ignores personal and ethnic differences magnifies the inequities in access. Migrant workers, refugees and asylees, and legal immigrants often need language assistance, targeted outreach, and health professionals who are trained to understand special cultural needs (IOM, 1993). Institutional and professional biases against the poor and foreign-born discourage patients from appropriately using health care systems, thereby jeopardizing successful outcomes achieved through appropriate treatment and patient education.

Indicators of Appropriate Access to Health Care

To guide its work, the committee chose five access objectives, and a set of utilization and outcome indicators for each. The selection of indicators was, to a large extent, based on available data that could be used as measures for each indicator of access to care. Used in this way, the indicators reflect societal values, demonstrating the extent to which the sociopolitical system is managing the delivery of health care to vulnerable social groups. With an understanding of the inherent problems with selected data sources, the committee chose an array of vital statistics, surveys, hospital discharge data, tumor registries, reportable diseases, and claims data for the first application of the measures.

The IOM Study objectives were the following:

1. Promoting successful birth outcomes
2. Reducing the incidence of vaccine-preventable childhood diseases
3. Early detection and diagnosis of treatable diseases
4. Reducing the effects of chronic disease and prolonging life
5. Reducing morbidity and pain through timely and appropriate treatment

Indicators for these objectives were all measurable with data from basic data sets that had been maintained from 1983 to 1990. The application of this framework showed disturbing trends for low-income subpopulations (IOM, 1993), and the relative position of Hispanic immigrants which was the same as or worse than that of African Americans.

Objective 1: Birth Outcome Indicators. Analyses showed that between 1979 and 1988, ethnic minorities were much more likely to have low or very low birth-weight babies. Very low birth-weight babies were born to African American women three times more often than to Caucasian women, and 80% more often than to Puerto Rican women. The mortality rate for Black infants grew substantially during the same period. Black women, Puerto Rican women, and women from Central and South America were using prenatal care sporadically. Also, the analyses demonstrated that between 1985 and 1988, the rate of congenital syphilis increased 132% among Blacks.

Objective 2: Vaccine-Preventable Childhood Diseases. Preschool immunization rates, a utilization measure selected by the committee, were much lower for children residing in the central-city sectors of metropolitan statistical areas (MSAs), than in other sectors of MSAs, the suburbs, or outside of MSAs. Preschool immunization was a special problem for undocumented immigrants and other low-income groups. In the 1987 measles outbreak, Hispanic children were four times more likely than Caucasian children to become infected.

Objective 3: Early Detection and Diagnosis of Treatable Illnesses. Breast and cervical cancer screening and the incidence of late-stage breast and cervical cancers were chosen as indicators. Overall, Black and Hispanic women were 11% more likely than Caucasians to have gone without a clinical breast exam. About half of Black and Hispanic women over the age of 70 had never experienced this procedure; 72% had never had a mammogram. Nearly 25% of Hispanic women over the age of 18 had never had a Pap test. Women with less than a high school education from low-income areas often have no regular source of care and use hospital outpatient departments and community clinics for all health services. It was assumed that providers were reluctant to encourage poor women to have a nonreimbursable procedure when they cannot afford food or rent.

The IOM's review of existing data from the American Cancer Society (1989) and the National Center for Health Statistics (1990) revealed that the age-adjusted death rate for Black women with breast cancer (27 per 100,000) was higher than it was for Whites (23 per 100,000). In addition, Whites had a higher 5-year survival rate, regardless of the invasiveness of the cancer.

Objective 4: Reducing the Effects of Chronic Disease and Prolonging Life. The committee selected physician contact within the past year as a proxy measure for follow-up care for identified chronic disease. Not surprisingly, the 1989 National Health Interview Survey showed that low-income, uninsured individuals were more than twice as likely not to have had contact with a physician during the measurement period.

A second indicator for chronic disease management was the use of high-cost discretionary care such as "referral-sensitive surgeries." A review of a 1988 analysis of data from 11 states on breast reconstruction and cardiovascular surgeries showed that individuals residing in low-income areas were less likely than individuals in high-income areas to undergo these discretionary procedures.

An analysis of the same data set for another indicator, "avoidable hospitalizations," yielded dramatic differences in admission rates between high- and low-income areas for chronic diseases that can be managed on an outpatient basis. Residents of low-income areas were approximately six times more likely to be hospitalized for congestive heart failure and asthma, and seven times more likely to be admitted for hypertension than residents of high-income areas. Also, poor and predominantly Black areas experienced higher admission rates, overall, than low-income White areas. These population groups also experienced higher mortality rates from chronic diseases, even when behavioral risk factors were removed statistically.

Objective 5: Reducing Morbidity and Pain Through Timely and Appropriate Treatment. Analyses were initiated highlighting the lack of dental care and the frequency of avoidable hospitalizations for residents of low-income zip codes with acute illnesses such as bacterial pneumonia, cellulitis (with and without skin grafts), and severe upper respiratory infections.

In an abbreviated summary and recommendations section, the committee pointed out the many advantages of national, state, and local monitoring systems, However, their expectation was that the costs of future iterations would be borne by the federal government and private foundations. This seems quite unrealistic given the lukewarm attention given to more dramatic public health problems such as the "new epidemic" of viruses and drug resistant bacterial infections.

The critical and continuing findings of the IOM's access research underscore prior findings illuminating the differences in access that exist between Caucasians and ethnic minorities. In closing, the IOM (1993) study identified emerging public domain problems that require special monitoring. These include HIV/AIDS, substance abusers waiting for treatment, and the health care access problems of the homeless and migrants, especially migrant farm workers. Migrants and the undocumented share many of the same problems experienced by the homeless because they have no entitlements, no unemployment benefits, and, usually, no health insurance.

Social Status and Legal Status

In the same year as the IOM Access and monitoring study (1993), Aday published *At Risk in America: The Health and Health Care Needs of Vulnerable Populations in the United States.* Vulnerable populations were defined as those "at risk" for "poor physical, psychological, and/or social health" (p. 5). In Aday's 1993 conceptual framework, individual risk varies as a function of "opportunities and resources" associated with the (1) demographic characteristics of the individual, or his or her *social status,* (2) the nature of interpersonal relationships with family, friends, and neighbors, or *social capital,* and (3) educational, vocational, and financial opportunities, resulting from investments in *human capital.* Aday (1993) argued that people "who are poorly educated, unemployed, and poorly housed have [fewer resources for dealing with] illness or other personal or economic adversities" (p. 7). In her exposition of physical, psychological, and social needs, Aday identifies nine population groups as most vulnerable; these include high-risk mothers and infants, the chronically ill and disabled, persons with HIV/AIDS, the mentally ill, the homeless, violence-prone and abusing families, and immigrants and refugees.

Using data from the Immigration and Naturalization Service (INS) and the U.S. Bureau of the Census, Aday (1993) noted that in the 1980s alone, more than 5.8 million people legally immigrated to the United States. Many were asylees, leaving untenable political conditions and even family behind, bringing psychological and health problems with them. Taking into consideration Aday's concepts of social status, social capital, and human capital into consideration, immigrants and refugees are clearly the most vulnerable, at-risk population groups in America.

From 1970 to 1990, the population of foreign-born residents in the United States increased dramatically, from 9.6 million to 19.8 million individuals (Thamer, Richard, Wald-man Casebeer, & Fox Ray, 1997). In 1990, the foreign-born included 26% from Central America, 5% from Asia, 22% from Europe, 9% from the Caribbean, and the remaining 18% from Africa and other parts of the world. Between 1990 and 1993, 5.2 million immigrants were granted permanent resident status in the United States; these data include the 2,191,154 individuals legalized under the Immigration Control and Reform Act (IRCA) in fiscal years 1990 through 1993 (Rumbaut, 1997). Thamer and colleagues (1997) reported that, in 1990, 90% of immigrants living in the United States were legal residents.

An analysis of sociodemographic characteristics of legal immigrants in aggregated data from the 1989–1990 National Health Interview Survey shows that they are younger, poorer, less educated, and have larger families than U.S.–born residents. More than 94% live within Metropolitan Statistical Areas, as compared with 76% of U.S.–born residents. Thamer and colleagues (1997) described the metropolitan immigrant population as 39% Hispanic, 34.1% White, 18.7% Asian–Pacific Islander, and 8.2% Black or other.

In the National Health Interview Survey, self-reported health status of foreign-born and U.S.–born residents did not differ significantly. However, about 6% of the foreign-born had not seen a physician in the past 2 years. Thamer and colleagues (1997) pointed out that the foreign-born were less likely to have Medicare coverage, and twice as likely to be uninsured. Considering Hispanics only, 40.8% of the foreign-born were uninsured, as compared with 24.8% of the U.S.–born. The difference in insurance status between U.S.– and foreign-born Asian–Pacific Islanders was approximately 11%. Analyses conducted by Thamer and colleagues strongly suggest that Hispanic immigrants are at highest risk for access problems, especially if they have been in America fewer than 15 years.

Categories of Immigrant Status

In an article describing the health needs of immigrants in Texas, Hargraves (1996) describes six categories of immigrants that exist both in the United States and other Western countries:

1. *Legal immigrants* are also known as "lawful permanent residents." They are legally permitted to live and work in the country permanently. Until 1997, all legal immigrants were eligible for all federal assistance programs including AFDC, food stamps, Medicaid, and unemployment insurance. As of August 22, 1997 (or until the law changes), legal immigrants must live and work in the United States for 10 years in order to be eligible for most entitlements. Legal immigrants are admitted because of valuable job skills or family ties (Hargraves, 1996).
2. *Refugees* are immigrants living outside of their countries of birth but not, as yet, in America. At entry, refugees are eligible to work in the United States for 1 year before their status is modified to permanent residence. Refugees are admitted while facing persecution because of race, religion, nationality, political persuasion, or social group.
3. *Asylees* are refugees who are already living in the United States when they apply for protected status. They are eligible for the same benefits as refugees. However, only 10,000 asylees can be granted refugee status in the Unikted States each year.
4. *Legalized aliens* are immigrants who were previously unauthorized or undocumented "aliens." These immigrants were given "amnesty" or legal status under the Immigration Reform and Control Act of 1986. This bill granted lawful permanent resident status to immigrants who could prove that they had resided in the United States since 1982, or that they were "qualified, special agricultural workers." This group is ineligible for federal assistance for 5 years past their legalization date.
5. *Parolees* are permitted to live in the United States for humanitarian, legal, or medical reasons. They are allowed to remain here only temporarily, and have no entitlements.
6. *Unauthorized immigrants* are also known as undocumented or illegal aliens. Generally this group includes persons who cross the border illegally or who remain in the United States after their immigration documents expire. The majority of unauthorized immigrants in the United States are Hispanic. The undocumented are eligible for emergency medical services only (Hargraves, 1996).

Access Problems Experienced by the Hispanic-Latino Population in the United States

As Hargraves (1996) points out, the term "Hispanic" is no more than an official term used to describe a nonhomogeneous group of people from different countries, with very different histories, cultures, and perspectives on health care. "Hispanic" is a term that may be used to describe Spanish-speaking people, those born in Spanish-speaking countries and their children. It may even be used to describe indigenous Americans from Mexico, Central America, or South America who are not Spanish-speaking (Ganey & De Bocanegra, 1996). Racial and ethnic categories such as this one combine waves of immigrants from different points in time. The category, Hispanic immigrant, includes "highly educated political asylees and illegal or recently amnestied agricultural workers"(Ladenheim, 1997). In the 1990 Census, the Census Bureau classified the 20 million Hispanics in the United States by country of origin, yielding the following population subgroups (*Statistical Abstract of U.S., 1990*):

Mexican American	62%
Puerto Rican	13%
Cuban	5%
Central and South American	12%
Other	8%

The "Other" category includes Native Americans and Hispanics of the Southwest.

In 1990, California was home to the largest Hispanic-Latino population of 7.7

million; 4.3 million resided in Texas, 2.2 million in New York, and 1.6 million in Florida. At the same time, states with the largest proportion of Hispanics were New Mexico (38.2%), California (25.8%), and Texas (25.5%). Other states with significant Hispanic presence in 1990 included Illinois and New Jersey.

Ginsberg (1991) suggested that the most important factors affecting access to care for Hispanics, now and in the future, are relatively low socioeconomic status, the heterogeneity of the Hispanic population, demographic and epidemiologic characteristics that create demand for services, underrepresentation of Hispanics in the health professions, and occupational and environmental health problems.

Mexican Americans. DeSantis and Halberstein (1992) observed that the Mexican American population, settling mostly in California, New Mexico, Texas, and Arizona, has experienced "virtually every possible barrier to adequate medical care." According to Treviño, Treviño, Medina, Ramirez, and Ramirez (1996), the two major factors affecting the health status of Mexican Americans are being uninsured, and low use of health services. Mexican Americans are the fastest growing segment of the U.S. immigrant population, and they are most likely to be uninsured. Treviño and colleagues (1996) reminded us that the absence of health insurance leads to unacceptable health outcomes. Mexican Americans who lack insurance coverage tend to be poor and less educated. Those affected with chronic disease suffer most, experiencing relatively higher rates of morbidity and mortality, relative to Whites.

However, the picture is more complex and interesting than Treviño and colleagues (1996) described. Hayes-Bautista (1996) pointed out that Mexican Americans born in Mexico have superior health status to those born in the United States for several reasons. Compared with other immigrant groups arriving in this country, Mexican Americans are healthy. Mexican immigrants in some

rural areas are still exposed to hepatitis A and typhoid; but, if new arrivals bring anything with them, tuberculosis and intestinal parasites are the most likely candidates. Once in the United States, Latino immigrants are subject to the extreme stresses of transition, and are exposed to new infectious diseases. Psychological stress which is high on entry, increases among the more acculturated (Kaplan & Marks, 1990). Some speculate that the relative economic deprivation experienced by a number of Mexican Americans born in this country may lead to heightened stress, depression, and substance abuse.

According to Hayes-Bautista, (1996) the relative good health of Mexican Americans improves the general health status in U.S. border counties, with the exception of San Diego. Overall, Latinos who live near the border have long life expectancies, "low mortality rates for most causes of death," healthy birth outcomes, and low infant mortality. Hayes-Bautista also observed low rates of insurance coverage and lower utilization rates than other ethnic groups. At the same time, he pointed out that the death rates for Latinos in border states for chronic liver disease, cirrhosis, and homicide are higher than state norms in California, Arizona, Texas, and New Mexico. After acculturation, dietary changes and a more sedentary lifestyle bring the threat of chronic disease to many, and the prevalence of cardiovascular disease, diabetes and diabetic complications, and cancer mimics rates in the Caucasian population.

Migrants from Puerto Rico. This group began to settle in the United States after World War II. Harwood (1981) described this population group as generally low-income, with minimal education and a low level of occupational skills. Although men are viewed as authority figures and the providers, many Puerto Rican American families have female heads of households. We know from the IOM 1993 report, *Access to Care,* that, even though low-income Puerto Rican women have large families, they use prenatal care infrequently and experience poor birth outcomes similar to African Americans. They are three times less likely than Whites to be screened for breast and cervical cancer, and their children are infrequently immunized against childhood diseases. Goldsmith (1990) describes the newly acculturated and first-generation Puerto Ricans as especially vulnerable to violence, substance abuse, and HIV/AIDS. Harwood (1981) suggested that the adaptation pattern of Puerto Ricans has been bicultural, with frequent movement between Puerto Rico and the U.S. mainland seeking employment. Thus, this Hispanic subgroup has been called "resistant" to assimilation. Men are the "traditional" providers and are expected to follow work in order to support the family.

Cuban Immigrants. The first exodus from Cuba in the lifetime of many of us occurred in the early 1950s when Fidel Castro and his supporters overthrew the dictator, Fulgencio Battista. At that time, immigrants from Cuba were the wealthy, the intelligentsia, and highly educated professionals, for example, physicians, attorneys, and scientists. This early wave of Cuban refugees was assimilated into U.S. society, often after a painful period of "retraining" in order to qualify for positions in U.S. professions.

The Cuban in-migration in the early 1980s was markedly different. The Mariel boatlift, alone, brought 125,000 Cubans to southern Florida, where they settled. Currently, 40% of the population of Dade County, Florida, consists of Cuban immigrants and refugees (DeSantis & Halberstein, 1992). Nearly 300 of the Mariel "boat people" died during their first year in the United States. Many of these deaths were violent; the Mariel refugees included individuals with known social and psychiatric problems. Many of these asylees were asthmatic, malnourished, and dehydrated on arrival. More importantly, the incidence of tuberculosis, hepatitis B, and sexually transmitted diseases among these refugees overwhelmed state and local health care systems, greatly reducing access to care (Gordon, 1982). Federal and voluntary re-

sources marshaled to deal with the entry of thousands of Cuban asylees were woefully inadequate for the needs of the "Marielitos." At approximately the same time, southern Florida received another 50,000 to 70,000 undocumented Haitian refugees. This wave of Haitian immigration brought the total of Haitian asylees to nearly 700,000. The group that coincided with the Mariel boatlift brought with them nearly 300 known cases of active pulmonary tuberculosis, and an epidemic of hemorrhagic conjunctivitis that spread to 18 Florida counties beyond Dade County (Gordon, 1982). The Haitians of southern Florida experience "high rates of chronic illness, poverty, illiteracy, and mental illness," problems that cannot be addressed by public sector health care, even in the 1990s (DeSantis & Halberstein, 1992, p. 225).

The majority of the asylees of the 1980s, including the Marielitos, the Haitian "boat people," and Nicaraguans who came after 1988, were designated as "entrants"; entrant status allowed them to live in the United States while immigrant status was pending (DeSantis & Halberstein, 1992). After 18 months in the United States, "entrants" lose eligibility for federal and state assistance, thereby losing access to health care and welfare.

Dade County: Where the Safety Net Is Torn. In 1989, the South Florida Hospital Association commissioned a study to assess the impact of two decades of "massive immigration" from the Caribbean and Central and Latin America on the health care delivery system of southern Florida. In this area, public sector health services are provided by a broad array of facilities and services that emerged in relation to need; these include public hospitals, general and specialized clinics (e.g., for prenatal care, maternal and child health, immunizations, and sexually transmitted diseases [STDs]). A large primary and urgent care center and a clinic for Mexican American farm workers is also a part of the "safety net."

Investigators engaged by the Florida State Hospital Association conducted a literature search and interviewed samples of providers and immigrant clients (DeSantis & Halberstein, 1992). Despite an apparently comprehensive array of facilities and services, clients did not have appropriate access to care. Findings showed a need for greatly increased maternal and child health and prenatal care services, including nutritional services and counseling, and culturally sensitive mental health services.

Migrant Farm Workers. Subgroups of Latinos have specialized needs stemming from their occupations. Latinos are well represented in the migrant and seasonal farm worker population; the size of this subgroup varies with the estimate, but ranges between 2.7 and 5 million people, depending on the data source and the time of year (IOM, 1993). Farm workers are routinely exposed to chemicals in fertilizers and pesticides, and to the elements. In border counties, farm workers often live in Spartan encampments. Many use contaminated water for cooking and washing. Skin rashes, eye problems, upper respiratory infections, and gastrointestinal disorders are frequent problems (Waterman, 1992). Studies of Latino farm workers in northern states show a decline in health status over time. Repeated exposure to occupational hazards and limited access to health care are the usual and customary culprits here, as elsewhere (Chi, 1985).

Even though the family income of 90% of migrant and seasonal farm workers is below the federal poverty level (FPL), and fewer than 2% have private insurance, they are least likely among all low-income groups to have Medicaid coverage (IOM, 1993). Problems obtaining and retaining Medicaid include the inability to establish residency, and the application process (e.g., time, amount of paperwork, cultural and linguistic barriers, distance to enrollment offices). While the IOM's 1993 Access to Care Committee provided recommendations for methods and data systems to assess and track health status, utilization of services, and barriers to access for this group, there are no funding sources that could be used for implementation.

Access Problems Experienced by Asians and Pacific Islanders

The term "Asian/Pacific Islander" or "AP/I" is used to describe people from many different regions, with very diverse cultures and languages. The A/PI designation can include Chinese, Japanese, Asian Indians, Koreans, Vietnamese, Hmong, Laotians, Thais, Filipinos, and the Pacific Islanders (such as Hawaiians, Samoans, Fijians, and Guamanians). The Hmong, Vietnamese, Laotians, and Cambodians (Khmer), are relatively recent immigrants to the United States. The total U.S. population of Asians and Pacific Islanders was 7.2 million (or 3% of the total U.S. population) at the 1990 census. Asians represented 6.9 million (95%), and Pacific Islanders the remaining 365,024 (5%). The western region of the United States is the predominant area of residence for the Asian and Pacific Islander population (59%). In 1991, the majority (94%) of Asians and Pacific Islanders lived in metropolitan statistical areas and half lived in the suburbs; the median age of this population group was 30.4, and 30% were younger than 18 years. Access issues for these groups are as frequent and varied as diseases and risk factors, but are much more difficult to address.

Diseases and Risk Factors Requiring Treatment and Prevention. Southeast Asian refugees are at risk for Hepatitis B and ensuing liver damage, sometimes culminating in cirrhosis or cancer (Hargraves, 1996). They are also at high risk for tuberculosis, with an overall infection rate of 40% to 50%. Other problems experienced by Southeast Asian refugees include intestinal parasites and other disorders, vision, hearing, and dental problems, causing them to seek outpatient services (Rumbaut *et al.,* 1988). Most of these illnesses are preventable or manageable in ambulatory settings if treated appropriately. While Indochinese in refugee camps may be screened and treated for some of these problems, treatment and follow-up in the United Sates is haphazard for many reasons.

While data on mental health problems of Southeast Asian refugees is not generally available, Hargraves (1996) described their extreme need for care. Many cases of post-traumatic stress disorder and depression have been cited in studies of both Vietnamese and Cambodian refugees. Pickwell (1989), noted that estimates of mental illness range from 17% for Vietnamese in Minnesota to 43% for Cambodians in California. Mental health problems are common among the Khmer and the Hmong. According to Rumbaut and colleagues (1988), more than 35% of the Khmer and 23.9% of Hmong respondents were classified in the "high depression" group. Many Khmer respondents had survived the genocidal period in Cambodia (1975–1979) and their depression scores were higher than any other group studied previously.

Financial Barriers to Access. Hargraves (1996), reported that, according to the 1990 census, 11% of Asian and Pacific Islander families lived below the FPL, as compared with 8% of White families. In 1990, the per capita income of the Asian and Pacific Islander population was $13,420 as compared with $15,270 for Whites. In 1989, the number of Vietnamese families in Texas with incomes below the poverty level was three times that of other Asian subgroups. High levels of unemployment are exhibited among Indochinese. According to Rumbaut and colleagues' research (1988), 45% of Indochinese men had not been employed since their arrival in the United States; the unemployment rate for women was 74.4% (Rumbaut *et al.*, 1988). The financial picture of this group of refugees suggests that in the 1970s and 1980s they were bouncing in and out of Medicaid. Those who had annual incomes slightly above the level of Medicaid eligibility could not afford individual insurance products

without sacrificing other basic needs, such as housing and transportation.

Language and Cultural Barriers. Stephenson (1995) reported language as the most commonly identified access problem reported by both the Vietnamese community and their service providers. Rumbaut and colleagues (1988) found that the level of English literacy was a principal predictor of health status of Indochinese in San Diego. Among Indochinese, health status was found to be highest for employed men, increasing with rising levels of English literacy, education, and income. Stephenson (1995), noted that "being misunderstood implies far more than simply confusion over the meaning of words or having a strong accent" (p. 1637) Being unable to understand the reasons for hospitalization, and the use of procedures and technical equipment, creates obvious fear and resistance. Language barriers virtually prohibit the appropriate use of diagnostic and treatment services for mental health problems in the United States. Even the use of antidepressant medications appropriate for survivors of physical and psychological trauma requires considerable verbal interaction.

The use of "traditional healing" methods is common for immigrant groups. Many Asian cultures use methods ranging from herbal remedies and teas to wearing amulets and rubbing coins. Natural healers may use a hot and cold classification system for food, diseases, and treatment; for example, hot food should be taken for "hot conditions" and cold food for "cold conditions" (Gany & De Bocanegra, 1996). The widespread use of these methods suggests the need for understanding and even incorporating "traditional" methods to improve utilization. Hargraves (1996), and Rumbaut and colleagues (1988) agreed that differing cultural norms and attitudes about health and Western medicine may result in noncompliance with medications or advice for all immigrant groups. However, cultural and linguistic isolation did not keep 80% of Vietnamese women in Texas from seeking out prenatal care in the first trimester (Hargraves, 1996). Deserved or not, the length of time spent in the United States was directly related to "trusting" the U.S. health care system. In any case, "trust" does not necessarily predict appropriate utilization (Jenkins *et al.*, 1995).

Structural and Institutional Barriers. Hargraves (1996) reminded us that, in the mid 1990s, Indochinese immigrants may use hospital emergency rooms and outpatient clinics because they have difficulty providing proof of residency or citizenship; these problems prolong waiting periods for appropriate, cost-effective treatment. However, in Hargraves's 1996 study of Hispanic and Asian populations in Texas, 53% of Vietnamese already had private health insurance while 45% had "government-assisted" insurance; 26% were medically indigent. The majority of Laotians (73%) had private health insurance provided by their employer or their spouse's employer; 23% had government-assisted health insurance, and 21% were without coverage. The improvement in health insurance coverage in 20 years is noteworthy.

Rumbaut and colleagues (1988) discovered that the Indochinese preferred to use community health centers near their homes or "private clinics of local Indochinese physicians" as regular sources of care. Then and now, the Hmong use health services less than any other refugee group; they wait longer to be treated and rely more on folk practices. A partial explanation for Hmong abstemiousness may be the Hmong's "innate value of independence and self-sufficiency" which inhibits adequate utilization (Jenkins *et al.*, 1995). Community-based interventions that provide encouraging education and outreach have been effective in some areas of the United States.

Access Problems Experienced by African Refugees

Diseases and Risk Factors. Leaving one's homeland to begin a new life in a new country, to learn a new language, and to start the process of cultural assimilation can be extremely stressful. Furthermore, many African refugees have experienced major trauma from the death of or extended separations from close family, and injuries from civil wars. They have faced the hardships of living in refugee camps where they may have contracted severe and chronic disease (Gany & De Bocanegra, 1996). In a 1996 survey conducted by the San Diego Urban League, HIV, tuberculosis, diabetes, and hypertension were all cited as common problems among African immigrants. HIV is a special problem for these "New Americans" because HIV is considered a death sentence, and infected individuals do not seek treatment (MacWilson, 1996).

On arrival, new problems emerge. Children and adolescents assimilate faster than their elders, leading to intergenerational conflict which may result in child abuse and violence. Irrespective of genesis, some have observed an increase in crime and substance abuse in African young people (McWilson, 1996). Gangs that were initially formed by youth to protect them from other ethnic groups also aggressively compete with each other.

Financial and Institutional Barriers. Many African refugees left countries with agrarian, subsistence economies. Without formal education in Africa, refugees may be illiterate prior to arrival in the United States. Few enter the competitive American job markets with desirable job skills or proficiency in English. Consequently, most African refugees qualify for employment that requires minimal language ability and training, and many may remain unemployed for long periods.

Special Problems of Immigrant Women, Children, and Elderly Persons

It has been demonstrated that access to health care is a problem for all immigrants, but, at times, women, children, and the elderly seem disproportionately affected. The burden of beginning life in a new country may be heavier for these groups. They appear to be less educated and less literate in English. Rumbaut and colleagues (1988) found that older Mexican women were less likely to speak or read English. They were more likely to be socially isolated and unemployed. In the Treviño and colleagues (1996) study of Mexican Americans, more women were uninsured or using public insurance; they were more likely to require health care and less likely to receive it. Preventive services such as prenatal care, Pap tests, and mammograms were not necessarily covered. Elderly persons were found to be at high risk for chronic disease and disability. Children were less likely to be immunized. Even Hispanic adolescents, 92% of whom reside in or near an MSA, portray poorer health status than non-Hispanic, White youth (Lieu, Newacheck, & McManus, 1993). However, these young people make fewer visits to medical providers even when they are insured. When uninsured, the disparity in visits to medical providers virtually doubles (Lieu *et al.,* 1993).

Devolution: The Public Sector Plays "Corporate"

Medi-Cal is a magnet for illegal aliens. [It] shields illegal aliens from [the] INS. [Its] design invites and promotes fraud.

Bob Brandenburg, Chair, San Diego County Social Services Advisory Board (May 15, 1997)

Though unsettling, it is no surprise that immigration policy is a central focus of national debate. David Kennedy (1996) reminded us that, according to economic theory, the "receiving" country benefits from immigration which adds workers to the labor pool. In the past most immigrants came to the United States in search of work and found jobs. Recent waves of immigrants include many "low-skill" workers who compete with "low-skill" natives for jobs (Kennedy, 1996). According to Borjas (1996), the education, skills, and earning capacity of "recent arrivals" are significantly reduced. Prior to

welfare reform legislation in 1996, "21% of immigrant households participated in some means-tested social assistance program (such as cash benefits, Medicaid or food stamps) as compared with 14% of native households" (p. 74). As noted earlier, the increased dependency on health and social services, and other public programs does create real financial and institutional burdens in affected areas such as California, the Southwest, and southern Florida. However, as Borjas pointed out, native business owners and consumers benefit from low-cost labor, and society benefits overall. The significant economic losses are borne by low-skilled native workers.

Fix and Passel (1993) perceived similar dynamics underneath the heated public debate surrounding immigrant policy. These include

- the ever increasing numbers: in the last decade, immigration has risen to an all-time high
- the decreasing numbers of "new" jobs in the U.S.
- the concentration of new immigrants in six states
- "inequitable cost distribution": the federal government benefits from taxes paid by immigrants (e.g., revenues are not equitably shared by states and counties)
- the inability to control illegal immigration

State and local governments, eager to "recover" some of the "costs" of immigration, publish reports in which the financial burdens of immigration are exaggerated. Service costs and job displacement costs are usually overstated, and the dollars in state taxes collected from immigrants is understated. In fact, only 2.3% of nonrefugee immigrants used public benefits in the 1980s (Fix & Zimmerman, 1995). In fact, the denial of federal public benefits creates new costs for state and local governments and further strains the safety net. Extending benefits to the undocumented is less costly in the long run. The cost-effectiveness of providing prenatal care to pregnant undocumented women is only one example. But these arguments are too little and too late.

In the United States the relationship between government and health care has always been precarious. Over the past two decades, all levels of government have tried to limit financial responsibility for the uninsured and underinsured. In recent months the federal government has kept busy in this area, passing legislation that shifts responsibility to the states. States such as New York and California, following suit, are using legislation and other pressure to try to shift fiscal responsibility to counties and to private sector health care systems. States, counties, and even institutions may try to fight back, arguing that immigration is a function of foreign policy, and, therefore, the federal government should be held responsible for financing immigrant health care (Rumbaut *et al.*, 1988). In 1993, Florida filed an unsuccessful suit against the federal government to recoup health care and other costs for undocumented immigrants. Florida attested that in 1993 alone, the cost of incarceration, education, and health care for illegal immigrants totaled $884 million (Siddarthan & Ahern, 1996). Another unsuccessful attempt to assist states with health care costs for the undocumented occurred in 1995 when the Clinton administration urged Congress to approve an additional $300 million to reimburse the states.

In 1994, two former INS commissioners wrote California's Proposition 187, the ballot initiative that prevented undocumented immigrants from receiving most government-funded health and social services, as well as public education. Support for "Prop. 187" came from Republican officials at the state level, and local and national anti-immigrant groups who wanted to send a message to Washington about "illegal" immigration (Nash, 1995). The initiative was passed by California voters, stimulating a series of proposals designed to deny benefits to both documented and undocumented immigrants. The culmination of this frenzy of denial occurred in the federal welfare reform law (H.R. 3734) which was signed into law in August 1996. As

written, H.R. 3734 created a new category of legal immigrants, known as "qualified aliens"; these are immigrants who have worked in the United States for at least 10 years, veterans and those honorably discharged, people on active duty and their dependents, and asylees (Ingram, 1996). In California, immigrants who are no longer "qualified" lose Aid to Families with Dependent Children (AFDC), Supplementary Security Income (SSI, which entails cash assistance for recipients of federal SSI), State Supplementary Payments (SSP, or cash assistance for federal SSI recipients), Medicaid, housing assistance, and food stamps. The only remaining benefit for the "unqualified" is Medicaid for emergency medical care.

Reflecting the concerns of a majority of native U.S. voters, H.R. 3734 eliminated all federal benefits and mandated the termination of state and local aid for undocumented immigrants, pending state legislation that might authorize assistance. California's Governor Wilson issued a subsequent executive order to state agencies, directing them to terminate benefits for "unqualified" immigrants as soon as possible. However, in June 1997, the California State Assembly approved a countermeasure to restore prior benefits to "legal" immigrants put at risk by H.R. 3734. Realizing that the diminution of federal funding puts more of a strain on states and counties, legislators in other states are introducing bills to restore entitlements. Currently, New York City and New York State stand to lose $1.4 billion over 5 years from the termination of SSI and food stamps. Republican Senator Alfonse D'Amato and Representative Peter King introduced a bill in the House to give more time for elderly and disabled immigrants to become citizens (*The Nation's Health*, May/June, 1997). But the occasional attempts to restore benefits are no cause for optimism, as public sentiment against immigrants and refugees burns hot. On the eve of the end of America's 62-year-old welfare system, "most states regard even a low-paying, dead-end job as preferable to the education and training programs" of the past (DeParle,

1997). Some states are setting stringent limitations. Texas set a limit of 12 months of benefits for those considered most able to work. Welfare recipients in Tennessee are limited to 18 consecutive months, and in Connecticut, to 21 months.

Seeing the handwriting on the wall, enlightened county policy makers in California and other states began to design "self-sufficiency programs" as early as 1992. Now it is clear that states and counties must transform the welfare system "from an entitlement system to one focused . . . on moving individuals into jobs and off the welfare rolls" (DeLapp, 1997). County governments that are driving welfare clients to self-sufficiency place themselves in a high-risk position, and must spread the financial risk to other sectors of the community. The planning and implementation of broad-based integrated services systems require collaboratives that include employers, community-based organizations (CBOs), religious organizations, and public and private agencies (see Chapter 30, "Public Health Planning and Policy Change"). Examples in California include the Healthy Start collaboratives and new mental health collaboratives that integrate services and revenue streams. Placer County's Children's System of Care offers child welfare, mental health, probation, special education, and health services to families with multiple needs; multidisciplinary teams work with families to tailor a development plan for each child.

Ku and Coughlin (1997) pointed to the significant changes in Medicaid from the Personal Responsibility and Work Opportunity Reconciliation Act of 1996 (PL 104-193) as

- de-coupling welfare and Medicaid eligibility
- narrowing Medicaid eligibility in the Medicaid SSI program
- terminating access to Medicaid for legal immigrants who lose SSI
- barring future legal immigrants from Medicaid

While some noncitizens terminated from SSI will be able to requalify for Medicaid be-

cause they are disabled, the elderly, who constitute the majority of this group will have the most difficulty requalifying.

With the new flexibility given to states, who must reduce spending to 80% or less of the 1994 block grant levels, dollars are being directed away from health care to corrections, schools, and other programs; New York has redirected $700 million, and California, $500 million, in this manner. Following the preferences of registered voters who are tired of "big government," devolution has turned out to be the process of reducing financial risk for the federal government (Van Lare, 1997). National polls have shown definitively that U.S. citizens have lost confidence in the federal government, and policy "wonks" are predicting even lower levels of expenditure on America's poor. The current, popular perception is based on sheer numbers showing that increases in federal spending did little more than increase the number of families who were dependent on the welfare system by 65% in 8 years. Other perceptions are based on some evidence that noncitizens are receiving larger SSI checks than citizens, a view espoused by the Subcommittee on Human Resources of the Committee on Ways and Means, U.S. House of Representatives (Haskins, 1997). Conservatives and moderates of both parties argue that welfare reform gives states an opportunity to rethink what they want to do, and a chance to create an improved system if they so desire.

"Promising" Program Strategies Are Community Based

With the federal government bent on shifting costs to states, and state and local governments lobbying to recover the costs of immigration, communities are left to their own devices to piece together programs for new immigrants, and for "working poor" immigrants who are not Medicaid eligible. Problems that immigrants face in obtaining appropriate care include legal, economic, and cultural barriers. They are complex, multisectorial problems that require complex solutions arrived at through the collaboration of public and private sector entities such as health care systems, unaffiliated providers, government, and other public sector agencies and organizations.

Programs that Work for New Immigrants

Gany and De Bocanegra (1996) argue that ensuring health care access for immigrant women benefits the entire community, immigrant or U.S.–born. Given that adult immigrant women are usually the health decision makers, they are often viewed as the conduits to the health care system for men and young people. The New York Task Force on Immigrant Health assembled a network of healthcare providers and administrators, community advocates, and social scientists to address the task of delivering culturally and linguistically sensitive services according to need. Programs that have worked for this task force include the integration of immigrant and practitioner perspectives and the use of bilingual, bicultural outreach workers based in the community. These successful programs "use the strengths of immigrant communities such as healthy behaviors and lifestyles from the home country" and community support in the "receiving" country (Gany & De Bocanegra, 1996, p. 159). The task force designed programs for providers and clinic staff to train them to understand immigrant cultures and the impacts on health seeking and health behaviors and on client–provider interaction. The training also addressed language barriers, working with interpreters, and common legal issues.

In Solana County, California, the Healthy Vacaville Task Force identified transportation as a major barrier to health care. First generation Hispanics in that area were unable to afford cars, and there was no public transportation available to them; health care services and facilities were located far away from major bus lines. The community health care coalition negotiated with the city transit authority which agreed to reroute buses to improve access to care. A sister coalition in Vallejo was developed to address the problem of Spanish-speaking residents not keeping appointments for prenatal and well-child care. When the issue was identified as one of language skills, the coalition turned a bus into a classroom for a course in using buses. Participants learned how to catch a bus, how to obtain and use a transfer, and how to choose the correct route to a health care facility. Coalition members included the KaiserHealth Plan, the Vallejo Transit Authority, and the Vallejo Adult School (American Hospital Association [AHA], 1997).

Programs for migrant workers include several low-cost approaches to provide primary and some specialty care to farm workers in different parts of the country. In West Virginia, the Shenandoah Community Health Center in a partnership with the Winchester Medical Center located in Virginia jointly operate a clinic within a migrant camp with a population of 1,700. The clinic, which is staffed by a coordinator, two nurses, and volunteer physicians, provides primary care, case management, and health education, and instructs clients in future use of available health services. The clinic offers evening hours two nights each week, and outreach to other camps. A Migrant Services Council that includes representatives of the state employment council, the growers, and a religious organization oversees the program (AHA, 1997).

A similar program, initially called the Canyon Healthcare Coalition, began in 1989 in northern San Diego County. Services included a van driven by an Hispanic physician who provided some primary care in migrant camps, and transported farm workers to community clinics for primary and specialty care. The physician used his time wisely, providing health education to patients en route. Funded for start-up by a local foundation, this program was absorbed by the Vista Community Clinic and continues today (Munoz, 1989).

Other programs in this area of the country include the training of camp residents in health promotion and illness prevention, recognizing health problems, and knowing whom to call. One program, initiated by a local foundation in partnership with the County Department of Health Services and the CDCs, also provided dollars and expertise for an epidemiological survey of major encampments, and the installation of potable water and sanitation facilities (Waterman, 1992).

Currently, Planned Parenthood of San Diego and Riverside counties is training male migrant workers to work as "Promotores Pro Salud," health promoters in reproductive health. Peer education through male and female health promoters has been used successfully in Mexico for over 20 years (Salo, 1997). The Tijuana Planned Parenthood reproductive health program successfully serves 30,000 residents along the border. In addition to the focus on reproductive health, the "promotores" will educate male farm workers to access health and social services and to care better for themselves through healthier lifestyles. All of these programs identify health problems before they reach critical stages. They also provide guided experience for clients who may be using the system for the first time, and advocacy to make sure that they receive timely and appropriate care.

In 1992, the prevalence of AIDS in the Asian and Pacific Islander communities in San Diego was still low relative to other communities of color, but the incidence of HIV was rising at an unparalleled rate (i.e., a 108% increase in 1 year). Initially designated as Project HAPI (Health for Asian–Pacific Islanders), the intervention provided HIV education to individuals and training for community-based organizations based on the findings of a carefully constructed epidemiological needs assessment. The survey provided data on attitudes, knowledge, and risk behaviors related to HIV. Target communities included Lao, Chinese, Filipino, Vietnamese, Thai, and Cambodian (Loue, 1994).

As described earlier in this chapter, southern California is an attractive entry point for African refugees. There are more than 25,000 of these "new Americans" living in San Diego County. With foundation funding, the San Diego Urban League is implementing a program that will centralize available health services, identify resources within the immigrant family, and help build self-sufficiency skills. Goals of the program include an epidemiologic needs assessment and improving health services so that they are sensitive to the unique health issues of over a dozen African refugee groups. The service system is staffed by members of the refugee community, and guided by providers who are sensitive to African cultures and values, as well as to the problems of resettlement. Staff conduct monthly cultural sensitivity trainings for local health care providers, and educational workshops for refugees that teach them how to seek health care in America (McWilson, 1996).

Programs for the Uninsured, "Working Poor"

Nationally, a few options are emerging for the "working poor," who do not qualify for Medicaid, Medicare, or other public sector health insurance coverage. Obviously, program strategies in this category benefit individuals, children, and families who have successfully addressed survival needs such as housing, food, and jobs. Many of these models are child focused because, in the words of one health policy pundit, "Kids are popular, and kids are cheap!" (Thompson, 1997).

New Hampshire Healthy Kids provides affordable health and dental benefits for uninsured children, ages 3 months to 18 years. For families to qualify, parents must not have been enrolled in employment-related group insurance programs for at least 3 months. New Hampshire Healthy Kids manages to keep premiums affordable through its partnerships with Blue Cross and Blue Shield of New Hampshire (with the assistance of an inspired CEO), Northeast Delta Dental, and the state's hospitals. Coverage is $77/month for babies (ages 3 months to 2 years), and for children over age 2. This is a rich benefits package that includes inpatient services and dental and vision care. The program is seeded with $240,000 annually by the state (Brooks, 1997).

The Florida Healthy Kids Corporation was created by the state legislature in 1990. The Healthy Kids nonprofit program began enrolling children in 1992, and offered the first children's benefit package in the United States to uninsured children not eligible for Medicaid or other public sector coverage. In an initial partnership with Health Options, Inc. (a Blue Cross HMO), Healthy Kids designed a comprehensive benefits package to keep children well. Healthy Kids also includes inpatient care, emergency room services and outpatient mental health. Averaged across 17 program sites in as many counties, the monthly premium is $51 per child. Local sites raise funds for insurance services such as medical premiums and third-party administrator costs (Florida Healthy Kids Corporation, 1997). In fiscal year 1996–97, they raised $3.6 million as a partial match for the state's $13 million appropriation from general revenue. Depending on annual income, families pay from $5 to $45 in premium costs. Services are decidedly multicultural, as there are 350 different languages spoken in Dade County alone (Naff, 1997).

There are other programs, like California's AIM program, for children up to age 2, that are fully or partially subsidized and base the amount of subsidization on family annual income. Hawaii, Vermont, Minnesota, Tennessee, and Rhode Island leverage their programs off federal dollars, charging a premium fee to families that are 100% or more of the federal poverty level (FPL). Below these income levels, the premiums are fully subsidized. There are more than 4.4 million uninsured children in U.S. working families earning from 100% to 250% of FPL (Gauthier & Schrodel, 1997).

CaliforniaKids is a nonprofit organization developed in 1992 that provides premium-subsidized primary and preventive health care services to 16,000 children ages 2 to 18.

A charitable spin-off of the California Blue Cross Plan, the core of the California Kids program is a partnership with Blue Cross of California, Delta Dental, Vision Service Plan, and Access Health to offer a rich package of outpatient benefits; there is no inpatient coverage. Plans in the partnership donate administrative expenses. The CaliforniaKids generates revenues each year by raising funds from other private donors to subsidize the program. The number of dollars raised annually determines the size of CaliforniaKids' enrollment. Parents are responsible only for co-payments of between $5 to $25, depending on the service provided. Like other partially subsidized programs described earlier, CaliforniaKids gets most of its referrals from schools. Currently, with funding from a foundation in southern California, "CalKids" is developing a sliding premium scale, so that working, uninsured parents with incomes above 150% FPL can assist with premium payments (Koch, 1997).

The Vista Community Clinic in northern San Diego County, in partnership with the local hospital (i.e., the Tri-City Medical Center), designed an effective prenatal care and delivery program that operated successfully for Medi-Cal eligible women. Working "poor" women were turned away until the clinic established a loan fund to cover the costs of prenatal care and delivery in a partnership with the Rancho Vista National Bank. The bank processed loans in the usual manner. In 7 years of operation, only seven women defaulted. Women who made all scheduled payments earned excellent credit ratings; they also gave birth to healthy babies (Mannino, 1991).

Conclusion

It is widely known and universally reflected in the last 30 years of health services research that, regardless of citizenship, "poor" individuals in the United States who do not have public insurance coverage experience significant problems obtaining needed health care. They see primary care providers less frequently than appropriate, and have no regular source of care. They use hospital emergency rooms and outpatient departments or clinics for primary care as well as urgent care. If they are hospitalized, uninsured, low-income patients are the recipients of fewer services and less specialty care. When controlling for health status on admission, hospital mortality rates are 1.2 to 3.2 times higher for the uninsured than for individuals with private health insurance (Hadley *et al.,* 1991).

With some exceptions, immigrants and refugees have the same experiences with the health care system, or worse. Newcomers and ethnic minorities have fewer entitlements in "receiving" countries. They are exposed to poor working and living conditions which predispose them to poor health. Political, administrative, and cultural barriers add to access problems encountered by immigrants. Language differences and different conceptualizations of sickness and health further complicate the transactions between ethnic minorities and providers and systems of care. Misunderstandings and suspicions on both sides are further exacerbated by individual and institutional expressions of racism (Bollini & Siem, 1995). If it is true that policies designed to reduce "health gaps" for immigrant groups and ethnic minorities must be "accompanied by a more general effort to promote integration and full participation . . . in the mainstream of society" (Bollini & Siem, 1995, p. 819), it is no surprise that three decades of research on access to care have done little more than stimulate public policy debate.

By and large immigrants receive substandard care because they are uninsured and because they underutilize health services. Hispanics, the largest immigrant group in the United States, are least likely to have insurance coverage and least likely to use sufficient services to maintain health status (Treviño *et al.,* 1996). Mexican Americans are the largest U.S. Hispanic subpopulation (60% of all Hispanics), and the immigrant group with the highest uninsured rates.

At this time it seems that health policy and immigrant policy are working in tandem, but to the disadvantage of new and unassimilated immigrants, a rapidly growing and extremely diverse group. With more years of residence in the United States and more exposure to the health care system, access to care appears to improve somewhat for the more adaptive ethnic groups (Leclare, Jensen, & Biddlecom, 1994). These tend to be English-speaking, literate immigrants who have marketable occupational skills and are able to find employment.

References

Aday, L. (1993). *At risk in America: The health and health care needs of vulnerable populations in the United States.* San Francisco: Jossey-Bass.

Aday, L., & Andersen, R. (1975). *Development of Indices of Access to medical care.* Ann Arbor, MI: Health Administration Press.

Aday, L., Fleming, G. V., & Andersen, R. (1984). *Access to medical care in the U.S.: Who has it, who doesn't.* Chicago: Pluribus.

American Public Health Association. (1997, May/June). Immigrants may benefit from fine-tuning welfare reform. *Nation's Health,* 4.

Berk, M., Schur, C. L., & Cantor, J. C. (1995). Ability to obtain health care: Recent estimates from the Robert Wood Johnson Foundation National Access to care survey. *Health Affairs, 14*(3), 139–145.

Blendon, R. J., Aiken, L. H., Freeman, H. E., & Corey, C. R. (1989). Access to medical care for Black and White Americans—A matter of continuing concern. *Journal of the American Medical Association, 261*(2), 278–281.

Bollini, P., & Siem, H. (1995). No real progress towards equity: Health of migrants and ethnic minorities on the eve of the year 2000. *Social Science and Medicine, 41*(6), 819–828.

Borjas, G. J. (1996, November). The new economics of immigration. *Atlantic Monthly,* 72–80.

Brandenburg, B. (1997, May 15). Illegal aliens and Medi-Cal. Paper presented to Joint Healthy San Diego Consumer and Professional Advisory Committee, San Diego, CA.

Brooks, T. (1997). The New Hampshire Healthy Kids Program. Presentation to the Alliance Healthcare Foundation, San Diego, CA.

Center for Health Care Leadership. (1997). Title of article. In *Health care access and coverage: Local initiatives* (pp. 1–50). Chicago: American Hospital Association.

Chi, P. S. K. (1995). Health care and health status of migrant farm workers in New York State. *Migration Today, 13*(1), 39–44.

Davis, K. (1991). Inequality and access to health care. *Milbank Quarterly, 69*(2), 253–273.

DeLapp, L. (1997, April). *Broadening the vision: Integrated services and welfare reform.* Sacramento, CA: Foundation Consortium for School-linked Services.

DeParle, J. (1997, June 30). U.S. welfare system dies as state programs emerge. *The New York Times,* pp. A1, A10.

DeSantis, L., & Halberstein, R. (1992). The effects of immigration on the health care system of south Florida. *Human Organization, 51*(3), 223–234.

Evans, C. A. (1995). Immigrants and health care: Mounting problems. *Annals of Internal Medicine, 122*(4), 309–310.

Fix, M., & Passel, J. S. (1993, Fall). *Immigrants and welfare.* Washington, DC: *Urban Institute, Policy and Research Report, 23*(3), 7–8.

Fix, M., & Zimmermann, W. (1995). Immigrant families and public policy: A deepening divide. *Urban Institute Policy and Research Report, 25*(3), 35–36.

Florida Healthy Kids Corporation. (1997). Title of article. In *Healthy Kids annual report* (pp. 1–20). Tallahassee, FL: Author.

Fox, P. D. (1972). Access to medical care for the poor: The federal perspective. *Medical Care, 10,* 272–277.

Freeborn, D. K., & Greenlick, M. R. (1973). Evaluation of the performance of ambulatory care systems: research equipments and opportunities. *Medical Care, 11* (Suppl.), 68–75.

Gany, F., & De Bocanegra, H. T. (1996). Overcoming barriers to improving the health of immigrant women. *Journal of American Women's Medical Association, 51*(4), 155–160.

Gardner, R. J. (1993). National health care reform and community and migrant health centers. *Journal of Health Care for the Poor and Underserved, 4*(3), 268–271.

Gauthier, A. K., & Schrodel, S. P. (1997). Expanding children's coverage: Lessons from state initiatives in health care reform. *State Initiatives in Health Care Reform, 19,* 29–35.

Ginsberg, E. (1991). Access to health care for Hispanics. *Journal of the American Medical Association, 265*(2), 238–241.

Goldsmith, M. F. (1990). Forum focuses on Hispanic-American Health. *Journal of the American Medical Association, 263,* 622–626.

Gordon, A. M. (1982). Caribbean basin refugees: The impact of Cubans and Haitians on health in south Florida. *Journal of the Florida Medical Association, 69*(7), 523–527.

Hadley, J., Steinberg, E. P., & Feder, J. (1991). Comparison of uninsured and privately insured hospital patients. *Journal of the American Medical Association, 265*(3), 374–379.

Hargraves, M. H. (1996, October). Immigrants needing health care in Texas. *Texas. Medicine,* 64–76.

Harwood, A. (1981). Mainland Puerto Ricans. In A. Harwood (Ed.), *Ethnicity and Medical Care* (pp. 397–481). Cambridge, Massachusetts: Harvard University Press.

Haskins, R. (1997, May 6). *Coping with welfare reform: A challenge for states and communities.* Paper presented at the annual conference of the Council on Foundations, Honolulu, HI.

Hayes-Bautista, D. E. (1996). *Work force issues and options in the border states.* Unpublished manuscript, University of California Center for the Study of Latino Health, Los Angeles.

Ingram, C. (1996, October 11). Welfare bill could cost state $7 billion, study says. *Los Angeles Times,* pp. A3–4.

Institute of Medicine. (1993). *Access to health care in America.* Washington, DC: National Academy Press.

Jenkins, C. N. H., Le, T., McPhee, S. J., Stewart, S., & Ha, N. T. (1995). Health care access and preventive care among Vietnamese immigrants: Do traditional beliefs and practices pose barriers? *Social Science and Medicine, 43*(7), 1049–1056.

Kaplan, M. S. & Marks, G. (1990). Adverse effects of acculturation: Psychological distress among Mexican American young adults. *Social Science & Medicine, 31,* 1313–1319.

Kennedy, D. M. (1996, November). Can we still afford to be a nation of immigrants? *Atlantic Monthly,* 52–68.

Koch, M. J. (1997). *Sliding Premium Scale for an Insurance Premiums Pilot Program.* Proposal to the Alliance Healthcare Foundation, San Diego, CA.

Kraut, A. M. (1994). *Silent travelers: Germs, genes and the "immigrant menace."* Baltimore: Johns Hopkins University Press.

Ku, L., & Coughlin, T. A. (1997, February). How the new welfare reform law affects Medicaid. *Urban Institute* (Series A, No. A–5), 1–4.

Ladenheim, K. (1997). Comment: Health insurance coverage of foreign-born U.S. residents—The implications of the new welfare reform law. *American Journal of Public Health, 87*(1), 12–14.

Leclere, F. B., Jensen, L., & Biddlecom, A. E. (1994). Health care utilization, family context, and adaptation among immigrants to the United States. *Journal of Health and Social Behavior, 35,* 370–384.

Lieu, T. A., Newacheck, P. W., & McManus, M. A. (1993). Race, ethnicity, and access to ambulatory care among U.S. adolescents. *American Journal of Public Health, 83*(7), 960–965.

Loue, S. (1994, January). *Child and adolescent health outreach project for Asian/Pacific Islander communities.* Proposal to the Alliance Healthcare Foundation, San Diego, CA.

Mannino, B. (1991, November). *North County perinatal program*. Proposal to the Alliance Healthcare Foundation, San Diego, CA.

McBeath, W. H. (1991). Health for all: a public health vision. *American Journal of Public Health, 81*(12), 1560–1565.

McWilson, J. (1996, October). *New Americans health-care initiative to serve the African refugee community in San Diego County*. Proposal to the Alliance Healthcare Foundation, San Diego, CA.

Mechanic, D. (1972). *Public expectations and health care: Essays on the changing organization of health services*. New York: Wiley.

Millman, M. (1993). *Access to health care in America*. Washington, DC: National Academy Press.

Munoz, G. (1989). *Health care access for migrant workers in North County*. Proposal to the Alliance Healthcare Foundation, San Diego, CA.

Naff, R. M. (1997, August 26). Presentation to Alliance Healthcare Foundation on Florida Healthy Kids, San Diego, CA.

Nash, P. T. (1995). *Reweaving our social fabric: challenges to the grantmaking community after Proposition 187* (pp. 1–22). San Francisco: MEJIDESIGN.

The Nation's Health. (1997, May/June). Immigrants may benefit from fine-tuning welfare reform, p. 4. Washington, DC: The American Public Health Association.

Newacheck, P. W. (1988). Access to ambulatory care for poor persons. *Health Services Research, 23*(3), 401–418.

Pickwell, S. (1989, June). The incorporation of family primary care for Southeast Asian refugees in a community-based mental health facility. *Archives of Psychiatric Nursing, 3,* 173–177.

Rogers, D. E. (1973, June 28). Shattuck lecture—The American health care scene. *Journal of the American Medical Association, 288,* 1377–1383.

Rosenberg, J. A., & Givens, S. S. (1986). Teaching child health-care concepts to Khmer mothers. *Journal of Community Health Nursing, 3*(3), 157–168.

Rumbaut, R. G. (1997, May 7). *Paths to success: Social capital, human capital, and political capital in the incorporation of immigrant families in the United States*. Paper presented at the annual conference of the Council on Foundations, Honolulu, HI.

Rumbaut, R. G., Chavez, L. R., Moser, R. J., Pickwell, S. M., & Wishik, S. M. (1988). The politics of mi-grant health care: A comparative study of Mexican immigrants and Indochinese refugees. *Research in the Sociology of Health Care, 7,* 143–202.

Salo, M. (1997, January). *Expansion of the "Promotores Pro Salud" program*. Proposal to the Alliance Healthcare Foundation, San Diego, CA.

Siddharthan, K. (1996). Inpatient utilization by undocumented immigrants without insurance. *Journal of Health Care for Poor and Underserved, 7*(4), 355–363.

Statistical Abstract of the United States, 1990. Washington, DC: U.S. Bureau of the Census, 1990.

Stephenson, P. H. (1995). Vietnamese refugees in Victoria, BC: An overview of immigrant and refugee health care in a medium-sized Canadian urban centre. *Social Science and Medicine, 40*(12), 1631–1642.

Thamer, M., Richard, C., Waldman Casebeer, A., & Fox Ray, N. (1997). Health insurance coverage among foreign-born U.S. residents: The impact of race, ethnicity, and length of residence. *American Journal of Public Health, 87*(1), 96–102.

Thompson, S. (1997, January 31). Paper presented at statewide conference, *Getting the uninsured insured: public and private efforts*. Sacramento, CA.

Treviño, R. P., Treviño, F. M., Medina, R., Ramirez, G., & Ramirez, R. R. (1996). Health care access among Mexican Americans with different health insurance coverage. *Journal of Health Care for the Poor and Underserved, 7*(2), 112–121.

Trude, S., & Colby, D. C. (1997). Monitoring the impact of the Medicare fee schedule on access to care for vulnerable populations. *Journal of Health Politics, Policy and Law, 22*(1), 67–71.

Van Lare, B. L. (1997, May 6). *Coping with welfare reform: A challenge for states and communities*. Paper presented at the annual conference of the Council on Foundations, Honolulu, HI.

Waterman, S. (1992). *North County safe water and sanitation project*. Proposal to the Alliance Healthcare Foundation, San Diego, CA.

Zane, N. W. S., Takeuchi, D. T., & Young, K. N. J. (1994). *Confronting critical health issues of Asian and Pacific Islander Americans*. Thousand Oaks, CA: Sage.

7

Health Care Seeking Behavior

KATHLEEN ELL AND IRMA CASTAÑEDA

Introduction

Illness-related human experience has long been the subject of literary, philosophical, and religious discourse. During the later half of the 20th century, scientific interest in better characterizing specific elements of illness behavior and health-related actions has increased dramatically (Gochman, 1988; McHugh & Vallis, 1985). Spurred by advances in preventive and curative medical care and by the desire to help ensure that all members of society would make optimal use of health care, medical and public health researchers and behavioral and social scientists have been increasingly drawn to the study of human behavior and illness. Included in this growing body of literature are studies of health care seeking behavior (Ostrove & Baum, 1983). Based on different theoretical and methodological traditions, medical practitioners, epidemiologists, economists, psychologists, sociologists, and anthropologists are studying the use of health care services, factors associated with utilization, and the ways in which people interpret health-related symptoms and take action to address these symptoms, including seeking help from a range of alternative sources to prevent, ame-

liorate, treat, or cope with the symptoms (Mechanic, 1985).

This chapter addresses two overarching questions. In what ways do cultural variations characterize health care seeking behavior among immigrant populations in the United States? In what ways does the use of health services by people who have immigrated to the United States vary from people born in the United States, and what factors best explain health service utilization within both groups? These questions have traditionally been of keen interest to anthropologists. Early anthropological studies of health care seeking behavior focused attention on the folk medicine practices of different cultural groups. Subsequent theoretical and empirical developments in anthropology focused on culturally grounded factors, such as health beliefs and culture-bound syndromes, that shape group members' illness behavior and choice of traditional therapies, folk healers, and biomedical practitioners (Good, 1985). This research began to shape an anthropological perspective on health care seeking behavior that rejects a normative view of health culture in favor of a more inclusive or holistic view, considers the full range of care seeking options, not solely the professional care sector, and seeks to understand the organization of culturally shaped illness meanings at the level of the individual before assuming the existence of universal health perceptions (Good, 1985). In recent years, the study of culture and related

KATHLEEN ELL AND IRMA CASTAÑEDA • School of Social Work, University of Southern California, Los Angeles, California 90089.

Handbook of Immigrant Health, edited by Loue. Plenum Press, New York, 1998.

concepts such as ethnicity and race, once considered to be solely the domain of anthropology, have become a prominent focus in epidemiological and social-psychological research (Weidman, 1988). Public health and medical practitioners have spurred research aimed at explaining variation in health service use, with the knowledge gained to be applied in designing interventions aimed at improving the delivery of health services to all people.

Four perspectives on care seeking behavior have dominated the literature to date: (a) a public health and medical care approach that is represented in epidemiological studies of health care utilization behavior and studies of preventive and curative care seeking practices; (b) an anthropological view that focuses on cultural influences and variations in symptom perception and expression, health beliefs, and help seeking behaviors; (c) a psychological perspective that examines cognitive and emotional processes in symptom response; and (d) a sociological view that draws attention to the interpersonal processes involved in care seeking behavior and the social-structural influences on individual care seeking behavior (such as access to care discussed in the preceding chapter). Many studies on care seeking behavior combine elements of each perspective.

Given the diverse research traditions represented in this growing body of research, it is not surprising that the umbrella concept of health care seeking behavior is applied to different types of care (e.g., primary and secondary preventive care, curative and rehabilitative care, disease management, maintenance, long-term care); physical and mental illness; actual care seeking practices and utilization of care; individual, health service organizational, and societal attributes assumed to influence individual care seeking behavior; and psychological and social processes involved in care seeking behavior.

Attempts to describe or explain health care seeking behavior across immigrant groups, between immigrant and nonimmigrant populations, and among immigrants at different levels of acculturation have been approached from each of these theoretical and observational perspectives. Two lines of scientific inquiry comprise sources of data on the health care seeking behavior of people who have immigrated to the United States. A relatively small group of studies focus specifically on immigrant populations (e.g., Mirales, 1989). The second and much larger body of research extrapolates knowledge about the behavior of immigrants from studies of the general population and comparative studies across racial-ethnic populations, albeit often without specific examination of immigrant subgroups or degree of acculturation.

Following a brief illustration of research perspectives on health care seeking behavior, selected research from both immigrant and racial-ethnic studies is reviewed. Utilization behaviors and factors that have been found to be related to service use, pathways and processes involved in seeking preventive and curative care for physical and psychological symptoms, and specific variables that are presumed to represent culturally determined influences on care seeking are examined. Finally, a future research agenda on the health care seeking behavior of immigrant populations is suggested.

Health Care Seeking Behavior: Public Health and Medical Care, Anthropological, Psychological, and Sociological Perspectives

Four approaches to scientific theory and research have contributed to our understanding of health care seeking behavior. While research on care seeking can be distinguished along disciplinary lines, each approach has been influenced by the contributions of investigators in differing fields (Cummings, Becker, & Maile, 1980). Increasingly, studies combine constructs and apply methodologies from different theoretical models (e.g., Chesney, Chavira, Hall, & Gary, 1982). Indeed, as is suggested in the following discussion, results from existing research and theoretical developments provide a strong basis for future interdisciplinary research aimed at refining and empirically testing conceptually integrated, dynamic, multidimensional models of health care seeking behavior among immigrant and nonimmigrant populations (Briones et al., 1990; Rogler & Cortes, 1993).

Public Health and Medical Care Research

Consistent with its practice-focused goals, public health and medical care research on health service use has addressed the broad spectrum of care seeking: preventive care use, such as immunization and health care screening and detection service use; curative care seeking practices, such as delay in seeking care; diagnostic follow-up; and adherence to recommended treatments and medical regimens.

Public health and medical care research on health care seeking behavior is characterized by large-scale epidemiological studies of the utilization of professional health care services (Howard et al., 1996), frequently correlating utilization with specific individual attributes, including predisposing factors, perceived need for care, and cultural indicators (Berkanovic, Hurwicz, & Landsverk, 1988), and personal and social enabling resources, such as health insurance and availability of health services (Hopkins, 1993). Indeed, attempts to explain variation in patterns of health service use (particularly underutilization of professional care), have spurred examination of racial-ethnic status as potential explanatory variables. To help explain utilization behavior, Andersen's model of predisposing, enabling, and need factors (Andersen & Aday, 1978; Andersen & Newman, 1973) is frequently applied in epidemiological research (e.g., Leaf et al., 1985). In a recent analysis using the 1990 National Health Interview Survey Supplement on Family Research, the model was revised to encompass specific elements of immigrant experience, including (a) duration of residence in the United States and (b) measures of immigrant adaptation, family characteristics and exposure to the health care system. Results indicated that duration of residence had a strong effect on health care utilization, in addition to socioeconomic status, access to health insurance, and differences in morbidity (Leclere, Jensen, & Biddlecom, 1994). Similarly, lower acculturation has been found to predict less timely follow-up and inadequate adherence following an abnormal cancer screen among Hispanic women (Harmon, Castro, & Coe, 1996).

Anthropological Models and Constructs

Based on its cross-cultural research base, anthropology has convincingly advanced the understanding of illness experience as reflecting basic cultural values and shared beliefs about dysfunction (Landrine & Klonoff, 1992). Broadly characterizing health beliefs, Landrine and Klonoff described Western cultural traditions as the basis on which White Americans view illness "as an episodic, intrapersonal deviation caused by microlevel, natural, etiological agents such as genes, viruses, bacteria, and stress" enabling White American laypersons and professionals to assume "that illness can be described and treated without reference to family, community, or the gods" (p. 267). In striking contrast to Western traditions, they suggested that "many ethnic-cultural minority groups in the United States, as well as many cultures around the world, view illness as a long-term, fluid, and continuous manifestation of long-term and changing relationships and dysfunctions in the family, the community, or nature as well as in the relationship between the individual and any of these" (p. 268), which, in turn, significantly influences care seeking behaviors.

Influenced by research in non-Western societies, anthropologists have identified culturally determined and culturally distinct normative patterns of physical and psychological symptom definition, response, and help seeking in all cultures (Lewis-Fernandez & Kleinman, 1995). Interest in health beliefs has led anthropologists to demonstrate empirically that the health beliefs of laypersons *and* health professionals are culturally informed, and that there is significant variation in beliefs *within* all cultural groups as well as *between* groups (Castro, Furth, & Karlow, 1985; Landrine & Klonoff, 1992; Weller, Pachter, Trotter, & Baer, 1993). Beliefs are thought to be critical antecedents of behavior, including health care seeking behavior.

Anthropologists have studied both the decision to seek care and the choice of care from available alternatives (Garro, 1985). Good (1985) suggested that two overarching but related paradigms of help seeking or care seeking have emerged in the anthropological literature. The first focuses on subjective individual decision making that assumes considerable individual autonomy and control. Shifting emphasis away from a primary focus on culturally determined behaviors, a second overarching paradigm on care seeking is based on political economic theories that focus on powerful social structural constraints on individual decision making (Good, 1985). From this viewpoint, it is argued that culturally patterned behavior is not independent of powerful structural constraints of poverty and oppression (Anderson, Blau, & Lau, 1991). This viewpoint is frequently represented in studies of racial and ethnic minority populations in the United States.

Attempts to integrate perspectives are also emerging. For example, anthropological research that is guided by what has been termed the decision modeling approach (which emphasizes cognitive processes in individual decision making) provides opportunity to evaluate the relative influence of cultural beliefs and external constraints on treatment choices (Garro, 1985). Proponents of this perspective argue that it is possible (and desirable) to identify the influence of cultural factors such as beliefs about illness, socioeconomic marginality, and local unavailability of services (Garro, 1985).

Psychological Theories

Two theoretical models have dominated psychologically focused research on health care seeking behavior: the health belief model and a self-regulation model of coping with health threats. Based on behaviorist theories, the health belief model was developed by social psychologists during the 1950s (Becker, 1974). The model assumes that health beliefs shape individuals' rational decision making about health actions. Emphasizing individual perceptions, the model specifically hypothesizes that before taking preventive health actions, adhering to prescribed regimens, or utilizing medical services, individuals will systematically appraise their perceived susceptibility to a disease, its perceived severity, the perceived benefits of preventive care, and the perceived barriers and costs associated with taking preventive health actions (Kirscht, 1988).

The health belief model has been used extensively to guide research on a variety of preventive health actions, including smoking behavior, dental care, immunization practices, cancer detection, and diagnostic care seeking (Janz & Becker, 1984). The model was originally posited to be a powerful predictor of preventive service use but numerous studies have demonstrated relatively modest predictive power (Good, 1985). Conceptual and methodological critique has suggested that little more can be learned from a simple application of the existing model (Janz & Becker, 1984). Particularly important to the study of care seeking behavior among immigrant populations is the criticism that the model mistakenly assumes both that all individuals are free to engage in rational health-related decision making and that they have the degree of knowledge about an illness and its treatment to act in a prescribed manner. The model fails to consider the interactive and dynamic interplay of culture and other relevant factors in all health actions (Good, 1985).

The self-regulation model of Leventhal (1985) and Leventhal, Zimmerman, and

Gutman (1984) assumes that individuals apply implicit theories about illness to understand the degree of threat posed by specific symptoms and to make decisions about subsequent health actions or ways of coping with the health threat. The model proposes three stages in the decision-making process: (1) the individual's cognitive perception and representation of the nature of the health threat; (2) the activation of a coping or action plan; and (3) an appraisal of the likely success of and barriers to reducing the health threat. Cultural influences are likely to occur at each of these stages, including the influence of significant others on the appraisal of the health threat (Croyle & Hunt, 1991). However, psychological research on culture, ethnicity, and race is relatively sparse (Betancourt & Lopez, 1993).

Sociological Theories

Sociological research has drawn attention to the powerful influences of social interactional and social structural processes on individual health care utilization and decision-making behavior. Particularly important to immigrant care seeking behavior is research on the role of family, kin, and friendship networks (Alonzo, 1986; Kang, Bloom, & Romano, 1994; McKinlay, 1973; Suarez, Lloyd, Weiss, Rainbolt, & Pulley, 1994). Examination of pathways to care have underscored the critical role of significant others in individuals' health care–related decision-making processes. Among immigrant and nonimmigrant populations, these studies have identified personal network influences on information about and attitudes toward the use of health and mental health care services (Pearlman et al., 1997; Rogler & Cortes, 1993).

Sociological research has also focused on the affects of interactions between recipients and professional providers of care on adherence to treatment recommendations (Seijo, Gomez, & Freidenberg, 1991; Sue, Fujino, Hu, Takeuchi, & Zane, 1991); social-structural influences on individual care seeking behavior (including status and power); societal perceptions about illness or dysfunction; and the role of community and residential neighborhood politics and resources (Bastida, 1989).

Social status and psychosocial stressors have also been found to affect care seeking behavior. For example, studies have highlighted the stressful daily lives and competing priorities for many low-income women (including immigrant women) as deterrents to optimal adherence (Formenti et al., 1995; Lacey, 1993).

Review of Literature

Evidence from research on health care seeking behavior among racial-ethnic minority populations can be broadly characterized along three types: (1) demographic, social-relational, and social-structural factors that have been found to be correlated with the use of preventive and curative health care services for physical and psychological symptoms; (2) culturally determined beliefs, perceptions, and expectations that have been found to vary among cultural groups and to be differentially associated with health care seeking behavior; and (3) differential pathways to care and decision-making processes. The majority of studies address questions about utilization patterns and static sociodemographic variables. Fewer studies examine culturally determined beliefs and perceptions and utilization of care. Research on pathways to care and the cognitive and emotional processes associated with the decision to seek care is particularly scant.

Results from studies on care seeking behaviors of immigrants and racial and ethnic minorities born in the United States, particularly that of individuals of Hispanic, Asian–Pacific Islander, and African heritage provide preliminary answers to the questions posed at the beginning of the chapter. The most striking variation in health service use among immigrant populations is underutilization of professional health care services when compared with the general population. However, similar factors influence health service utilization among immigrant and nonimmigrant groups, the most powerful being sociostructural factors or enabling factors, such as financial resources, health insurance, access to medical care (as discussed elsewhere), knowledge about the availability of care, and supportive personal and community resources. Culturally determined differences in utilization are most apparent in the pathways to care and in the presentation of symptoms and related health beliefs.

Utilization of Care

Differential prevalence and incidence rates of physical and mental illnesses among specific racial-ethnic groups, as well as higher rates of all illnesses among socioeconomically disadvantaged populations are well documented by an extensive body of research, much of which is presented throughout this handbook. This evidence has spurred a related series of studies on the frequency, type, and timing of the use of preventive and curative health care services within and across cultural groups. Unfortunately, only a handful of studies have specifically focused on immigrant populations; thus, conclusions are drawn primarily from studies of racial and ethnic minority populations.

Numerous studies have documented both underutilization and delayed utilization of formal health and mental health services among Asian American, African American, and Mexican American groups (Balcazar, Hartner & Cole, 1993; Becerra & Greenblatt, 1983; Braveman, Bennet, Lewis, Egerter, & Showstack, 1993; Cornelius, 1993a, 1993b; Escarce, Epstein, Colby, & Schwartz 1993; Schur, Bernstein, & Berk, 1987; Snowden & Cheung, 1990; Snowden, Storey, & Clancy, 1989; Sue et al., 1991; Sussman, Robins, & Earls, 1987; K. B. Wells, Golding, Hough, Burnam, & Karno, 1988; S. J. Williams, Diehr, Drucker, & Richardson, 1979). A smaller number of studies have reported overrepresentation of specific types of mental health service use

(hospitalization and outpatient care for adolescents) among African Americans (Broman, 1987; Snowden & Cheung, 1990; Sue, 1977; Sue et al., 1991). However, these data have been attributed to nonvoluntary mental health service use (McMiller & Weisz, 1996). Higher hospitalization rates for asthma among Hispanics and African Americans, however, is an indicator of poorer outcome among these groups (Carr, Zeital, & Weiss, 1992).

Delay in seeking care is the second most prominent characteristic of health care seeking behavior among minority cultural groups. Delay in obtaining prompt emergency care in the face of potentially life-threatening cardiac symptoms and in early care for cancer-related symptoms is particularly disturbing because prompt treatment and early diagnosis save lives and reduce morbidity (Hopkins & Hensley, 1993; Mandelblatt, Andrews, Kerner, Zauber, & Burnett, 1991; Richardson et al., 1992). Unfortunately, evidence indicates that African American and Hispanic populations are more likely to delay seeking care for each of these illnesses (Chin, Trapido, & Davis, 1994; Ell et al., 1995; Ell et al., 1994; Gregorio, Cummings, & Michalek, 1983; Loehrer et al., 1991) as well as for symptoms of depression and abnormal behavior (Greenley, Mechanic, & Cleary, 1987). Undiagnosed and thereby undertreated asthma has been found among urban minority children (Crain et al., 1994)

Preventive service use, including prenatal care, immunization, and screening and diagnostic follow-up, is also found to vary by cultural group. Again, underutilization by minority and immigrant populations is the primary finding (Balcazar et al., 1993; Braveman et al., 1993; Estrada, Trevino, & Ray, 1990; Solis, Marks, Garcia, & Shelton, 1990). Similarly, low rates of cancer screening have been found among African American and Hispanic women (Guerra, Mesa, Casner, & Moldes, 1994; Yancey & Walden, 1994), although recent evidence suggests that differences in screening behaviors between African American and Hispanic women and White women in urban communities are declining (Duelberg, 1992; Richardson *et al.*, 1987).

Treatment choice and adherence to prescribed treatment regimens have been shown to vary among minority and immigrant groups. For example, African Americans have been reported to be less likely to follow recommendations for cardiac surgery (Maynard, Fisher, Passamani, & Pullum, 1986), to have higher dropouts rates for hypertension treatment (C. A. Williams *et al.*, 1985), and to be less likely than non-Hispanic Whites to receive mammography follow-up for abnormal findings (Marcus *et al.*, 1992). A recent study of Latina immigrants with cervical cancer found inadequate adherence to a potentially life-saving radiation treatment protocol (Formenti *et al.*, 1995).

Factors Affecting Care Seeking

Studies of factors that are presumed to influence health care seeking behavior among all individuals repeatedly point to what is generally termed access to care. In the United States, access to health care services is primarily determined by whether an individual has adequate financial resources, particularly health insurance (Braveman *et al.*, 1993; Corn, Hamrung, Kalb, & Kalb, 1995; McManus & Newacheck, 1993; Rogers & Schiff, 1996; Weissman, Stern, Fielding, & Epstein, 1991; Wells *et al.*, 1988; Wells, Golding, Hough, & Burnam, 1989). Again, as described elsewhere in this book, there is convincing data of disadvantaged access to care among racial-ethnic and immigrant groups because they lack adequate health insurance (Butler, Winter, Singer, & Wenger, 1985; Fox & Roetzheim, 1994; Hopkins, 1993; Hubbell, Waitzkin, Mishra, Dombrink, & Chavez, 1991; Schur *et al.*, 1987). Taken together, numerous evidence suggests access to care, often determined by SES, is a stronger predictor of health care seeking behavior than racial-ethnic or immigrant status (Jenkins, Le, McPhee, Stewart, & Ha, 1996; Marks *et al.*, 1987; McPhee, Bird, Davis, Jenkins, & Le, 1997; Siddharthan & Ahern, 1996; Thamer, Richard, Casebeer, &

Ray, 1997). The future impact of the current reorganization of health care financing on access to care of all members of society, including minority populations and especially immigrant populations, is unknown.

Health provider behaviors and the organizational structure of health care delivery systems have also been identified as significant factors affecting health service use (Carr *et al.*, 1992). Particularly disturbing is evidence of differential treatment for members of racial and ethnic minority groups. For example, evidence indicates that economically disadvantaged minority populations are less likely to receive aggressive cancer therapy (Greenberg *et al.*, 1992) and less likely to be referred for cancer screening (McCoy, Nielson, & Chitwood, 1991). Similarly, African Americans have been shown to receive substantially less tertiary health care, as measured by coronary arteriography, angioplasty, and coronary artery bypass surgery rates (Ford, Cooper, Castaner, Simmons, & Mar, 1989; Goldberg, Hartz, Jacobsen, Krakauer, & Rimm, 1992; Wenneker & Epstein, 1989), and to be less likely than Whites to receive the most technologically advanced medical procedures and diagnostic tests (Diehr *et al.*, 1989; Escarce *et al.*, 1993; Javit *et al.*, 1991).

Characteristics of health delivery systems have also been shown to influence the utilization of care by minority and refugee populations. In a study of Hmong women seeking prenatal care, patients reported dissatisfaction with limited clinic hours, discontinuity in physician, and dissimilar communication styles (and interpersonal relations), including physician failure to fully explain medical procedures (Spring, Ross, Etkin, & Deinard, 1995). Language barriers have been found to negatively impact adherence to medication protocols and to be associated with higher use of emergency rooms among Hispanic patients (Manson, 1988). Failure to tailor health services and to target programs to make optimal use of health care services has also been linked with health care seeking behavior of minority and immigrant groups (e.g., Copeland, 1996; Lannon *et al.,* 1995; Suarez *et al.,* 1994; Tosomeen, Marquez, Panser, & Kottke, 1996).

Individual attributes such as gender, age, level of education, geographic location, and degree of acculturation have also been shown to influence care seeking behavior directly and through the interaction with race and ethnicity (Grau & Padgett, 1988; Hopper, 1993; Mechanic, Angel, & Davies, 1992). Acculturation is particularly relevant to a consideration of immigrant health behavior. Briefly, acculturation is the adoption of attitudes, values, and behaviors of the host society. It is often conceptualized as a process of change that immigrants undergo throughout their lifetime. This change is seen as movement from involvement with the culture of the country of origin to adoption of the host country's culture (Berry, 1980). Assessing the degree of acculturation of individuals and its association with the use of health care has helped to explain health behaviors of racial-ethnic minorities and immigrants. Acculturation has been measured by quantifying many factors including whether a particular language is used in a variety of situations and social relations, the consumption of particular ethnic foods, parental heritage, life experiences in one culture or another, cultural identification, exclusivity of association with similar immigrant peers, and even cultural pride (Cuellar, Harris, & Jasso, 1980; Rogler, Cortes, & Malgady, 1991). Unfortunately, existing measures of acculturation are confounded by the effects of education and social and economic conditions (Marin & Marin, 1991; Suarez & Pulley, 1995). For example, many past studies of cancer screening utilization have relied on language use alone as a measure for acculturation, but such studies have been criticized since they may also measure the even more powerful effects of education and SES on health behavior (Suarez & Pulley, 1995). (See Chapters 3 and 5 for an in-depth discussion of acculturation, its definition, and its measurement.)

Studies examining the effects of acculturation on health seeking behavior have shown inconsistent results. Studies have found acculturation levels to be correlated with psychological distress (Burnam, Hough, Karno, Escobar, & Telles, 1987), childhood immunization practices (Anderson, Wood, & Sherbourne, 1995), consumption of cigarettes (Marin, Perez-Stable, & Marin, 1989), and the use of preventive cancer screening practices (Elder *et al.,* 1991), whereas other studies have found little or no effect of acculturation on preventive health behavior (Marks *et al.,* 1987) and mental health service use (Vega, Kolody, & Valle, 1988).

Suarez and Pulley (1995) examined the independent relationship of various acculturation dimensions including language, traditional Mexican family attitudes, ethnic identity, generation in the United States, and Mexican cultural values. Only English-language proficiency and traditional Mexican family attitudes were significant predictors of Pap smear and mammography screening. Studies suggest that language acculturation has both direct effects on care seeking behavior (Solis *et al.,* 1990) and indirect effects insofar as language acculturation predicts media exposure which increases cancer screening and symptom knowledge (Ruiz, Marks, & Richardson, 1992).

Finally, there is evidence that competing life stress can influence health care seeking. For example, high stress on the immigrant version of the Hispanic Stress Inventory was recently found to be significantly correlated with poorer adherence to a potentially life-saving radiation treatment protocol for cervical cancer among Latina immigrants (Meyerowitz, Formenti, Ell, & Leedom, 1996) and high life stress was found to be associated with delayed use of pediatric emergency care among young immigrant Latina mothers (Zambrana, Ell, Dorrington, Wachsman, & Hodge, 1994) and with immunization among Mexican American infants (Guendelman, English, & Chavez, 1995). A multivariate analysis of readiness to use a mental health facility among a stratified random sample of 806 Anglo- and Mexican Americans and Mexican respondents in El

Paso, Texas, found life stress to exert both direct effects on service utilization readiness and an indirect effect through increasing depression (Briones *et al.,* 1990).

Pathways to Care and Decision Making

Rogler and Cortes (1993) have defined pathways to care to "mean the sequence of contacts with individuals and organizations prompted by the distressed person's efforts, and those of his or her significant others, to seek help as well as the help that is supplied in response to such efforts" (p. 555). It is important to note that studies of pathways to care frequently involve clinical samples. Consequently, far less is known about the pathways of those persons who do not receive formal health care (Ell *et al.,* 1995; Rogler & Cortes, 1993). Two distinct features characterize pathways to health care service use among minority and immigrant populations: (1) reliance on network member advice, information, actual provision of care, and decision making, and (2) use of folk healers and practices before seeking professional care, in lieu of seeking professional care, or in combination with professional care.

The supporting functions of network ties are multiple, including emotional nurturance (e.g., expressive support) and resource and information assistance (e.g., instrumental support). For example, social networks are prime pathways for transmitting cultural beliefs (Ritter, 1988). Extant research on the role of social networks in care seeking behavior highlights important elements to be considered in planning interventions to influence the health care seeking behavior of minority and immigrant populations.

Reliance on family caregiving is particularly evident among African American, Latino, and Asian families. Social networks also influence the sequence of care seeking behavior (Starrett, Bresler, Decker, Walters, & Rogers, 1990). For example, McMiller and Weisz (1996) found that in contrast to Anglo Americans, African American and Latino parents were unlikely to initially choose professional mental health services. Paths to care among the minority families included lengthier trials of informal help seeking and caregiving before seeking formal care. In this study, African American and Latino parents sought help from professionals and agencies only after initial help from family and community contacts was found to be inadequate. In contrast, the majority of Caucasian parents first sought care from mental health professionals and agencies. Similar results were found in a comparison among African American, Hispanic American, and European American families seeking help for mental health problems (Guarnaccia & Parra, 1996). The investigators attributed these results to differences in illness perceptions, suggesting that European Americans saw the problematic behaviors as medical problems, whereas minority families attributed the problems to a wider range of possible causes. Frequently, the care seeking paths taken by minority groups result in the tendency to present to health professionals at more severe stages of mental disorder (Uba, 1994). Social networks have also been found to influence preventive care seeking behaviors, including mammography (Suarez & Pulley, 1995; Suarez, Lloyd, Weiss, Rainbolt, & Pulley, 1994) and childhood immunizations (Anderson *et al.,* 1995) among Hispanics.

A few studies related to seeking care in the general population have attempted to describe the decision-making process in which individuals engage before seeking care and the resulting pathways to formal health care services (Dracup *et al.,* 1995). Other data highlight the interactive involvement of health care professionals and family members (Deimling, Smerglia, & Barresi, 1990; High, 1990). These studies have focused on the cognitive and emotional processes involved in symptom perception and subsequent coping processes. For example, comparing African Americans, Latinos, and Whites seeking emergency room care for acute chest pain, Ell and colleagues (1995) found significant within-group variation by socioeconomic status in patients' perceptions of symptom intensity and incapacitation, and in the motivations for seeking care and the specific care seeking paths to care. Of interest, few differences between foreign- and U.S.–born Latinos were found on the paths to care. Among all groups, the length of time patients spent in deciding to seek emergency care was longest among patients of lower socioeconomic status and those who lacked health insurance.

It is important to note that informal care providers can exert both positive and negative effects on care seeking behavior. Alonzo (1986) concluded from his study of care seeking for emergency cardiac conditions that family and lay others (e.g., friends) often provide coping resources, in terms of medications and travel for the individual, including corrective advice needed to avoid excessive self-treatment and extended symptom evaluation. However, inadequate assistance or misguided help from personal network members (and from professional care providers) can also deter optimal use of health services. For example, Ell and colleagues (1994, 1995) found that having consulted network members and medical professionals increased the duration between symptom onset and the decision to seek emergency care.

Of related interest are conflicting findings regarding the continued availability of social networks to some immigrants to the United States. It is unclear whether immigrants sustain serious deterioration of network support as a result of their immigration experience. For example, Golding and Baezconde-Garbanati (1990) found that Mexican immigrants received less emotional support from their social networks than non-Hispanic Whites. However, data from a large prospective study of Mexican immigrants revealed that (1) social networks, including both friends and family, were available to immigrants from the early stages of immigration; (2) friendship contacts were stable over time; and (3) family contacts increased with time (Vega, Kolody, Valle, & Weir, 1991).

Informal community, religious, and folk healers are frequently a significant presence in the care seeking paths of diverse cultural groups (Chung & Lin, 1994; Gilman, Justice, Saepharn, & Charles, 1992). For members of many ethnic groups, the range of options available for treating illness thus extends considerably beyond establishment and even marginal providers. Consequently, investigations of health service utilization must be much more broadly framed for these groups.

Many ethnic collectivities support alternative providers of health care, who may be used prior to, in conjunction with, or following mainstream services. Laotian refugees to the United States (Gilman et al., 1992) and Vietnamese, Hmong, and Cambodians routinely combine multiple healing systems, including private and public health care providers as well as traditional healing practices (Chung & Lin, 1994). *Curanderos* and other lay practitioners among Mexican Americans (Lopez-Rangel, 1996), *espiritistas* and *santiguadores* among Puerto Ricans (Harwood, 1977), herbalists and other curers among Chinese Americans (Jung, 1996) and Southeast Asians (Fisher & Lew, 1996), and various healers among urban African Americans (Snow, 1978) are examples of culturally prescribed health practices for a broad range of illnesses and health threats.

Knowledge, Health Beliefs, and Symptom Expression

Harwood (1981a) suggests three ways in which cultural background influences how people view disease and illness: (1) knowledge about illness, including biomedical categories of disease; (2) culturally patterned classification of symptoms into illness categories and symptoms expression (an example of this is the "culture-specific syndrome"); and (3) beliefs about the causes of disease and illness, such as punishment or God's will (Garcia & Lee, 1988), humoral imbalance among Laotian refugees (Gilman et al., 1992), "hot-cold" theories among Chinese (Gould-Martin & Ngin, 1981), and nonnatural or spiritual beliefs of Haitian refugees (Laguerre, 1981; Wilk, 1986). Each of these culturally determined characteristics influences health care seeking behavior and begins to explain the differential use of mainstream and nonmainstream health services, and differences in adherence to treatment regimens.

The challenge to health care professionals to make accurate diagnoses when symptoms are perceived and communicated in terms of folk beliefs is based on well-documented research (Alarcon, 1995; Lewis-Fernandez & Kleinman, 1995; S. M. Manson, 1995; Weidman, 1988). Reported misdiagnoses of minority psychiatric illness which raise questions about the validity of current diagnostic psychiatric nomenclature for minority populations (Lewis-Fernandez & Kleinman, 1995) and problems in accurate diagnosis for acute chest pain (Haywood, Ell, Sobel, deGuzman, & Blumfield, 1993) are examples of factors affecting adequate care among different cultural groups. Pointing to folk illnesses such as *susto* ("fright") (Marsh & Hentges, 1988) or *caida de mollera* ("fallen fontanel") in the Mexican American community (Marsh & Hentges, 1988), *ataques de nervios* ("attack of nerves") in the Puerto Rican community (Guarnaccia, Canino, Rubio-Stipec, Bravo, 1993; Harwood, 1981b), and *empacho* ("blocked intestines") among Hispanic populations in and outside of the United States (Weller *et al.,* 1993), anthropological research illustrates the logic of the use of culturally traditional care and cures among immigrant populations (Good, 1985).

Striking differences have been demonstrated in the culturally patterned ways in which symptoms are perceived, defined, and presented to health professionals (Low, 1985). Most frequently studied are variations in the presentations of pain and in seeking care for pain (Berkanovic & Telesky, 1985; Haywood *et al.,* 1993; Koopman, Eisenthal, & Stoeckles, 1984; Lipton & Marbach, 1984; Strogatz, 1990; Woodrow, Friedman, Siegelaub, & Collen, 1972; Zborowski, 1952) and psychological symptoms (Alarcon, 1995; Lewis-Fernandez & Kleinman, 1995; S. M. Manson, 1995). Ethnographic studies have

also uncovered shared meanings of symptoms and illness that exert a potent influence on individual response to and management of changing symptoms and illness course over time (Anderson *et al.,* 1991; Kleinman, 1985).

Somatic expression of psychological symptoms in care seeking behavior is particularly common among Asian and Hispanic groups. For example, data from comparative research on Hispanic subgroups of Peruvians (Mezzich & Raab, 1980), Colombians (Escobar, Gomez, & Tuason, 1983), and U.S. Hispanics suggest a tendency for depressed Peruvians and Colombians to somatize more than U.S. Hispanics, regardless of socioeconomic status. Somatic manifestations were also the most common symptoms reported among a sample of Cambodian female refugees in the United States (Davanzo, Frye, & Froman, 1994).

Chavez, Hubbell, McMullin, Martinez, and Mishra (1995) found that the perceptions of breast and cervical cancer risk factors varied according to the interviewees' immigrant or nonimmigrant status and ethnicity (Latino vs. Anglo women). Mexicans, Salvadorans, and to some extent Chicanas (U.S.–born women of Mexican descent), considered physical trauma–stress and behavioral–lifestyle choices as influencing both breast and cervical cancers. Anglo, and to some extent Chicana, women's perceptions were generally consistent with a biomedical model in which heredity, high stress, and environmental pollution are risk factors, presumably reflecting the attention that these factors have received in the popular media and culture. The Chicanas were more likely to maintain bicultural perceptions of cancer risks.

Culturally influenced beliefs about the cause and source of control over health and illness are also shown to influence health care seeking behavior (Bundek, Marks & Richardson,1993; Chavez *et al.,* 1995). For, example, Perez-Stable, Sabogal, Otero-Sebogal, Hiatt, and McPhee (1992) found that Hispanics are more likely to doubt that one can prevent cancer, or influence its outcome. Tortolero-Luna, Glober, Villareal, Palos, and Linares (1995) found that a higher proportion of Hispanic women, particularly those age 50 or older, were more likely to believe that becoming ill is a matter of chance or fate and that recovery from illness is a result of good luck. Hispanic respondents were more likely to fear cancer than were non-Hispanic women. Garcia and Lee (1988) found that Hispanics were more likely than Chinese and Vietnamese respondents to believe that cancer was "God's will" and that Vietnamese were most likely to view it as a form of punishment. These beliefs about disease and the fear of cancer among Hispanics are consistent with the cultural concept of fatalism, raising concerns about their influence on preventive and screening practices and delay in seeking curative care.

Unanswered Questions and Future Research

Despite increasing awareness of cultural influences on health care seeking behavior, research on care seeking behavior is in the early stages of development, particularly as it focuses on immigrant behavior. While much has been learned, critical questions remain to be addressed in future research. Based on the current state of knowledge development and research, it is possible to identify important next steps.

Studies vary as to whether cultural factors are assessed as static variables and then correlated with selected health care seeking behaviors or whether cultural factors and processes are of central focus or are examined from a dynamic perspective. Analyzing the status of research on illness behavior, Mechanic (1982) concluded that illness behavior and help seeking are processes that develop over time, yet much of the data on help seeking behavior come from cross-sectional studies. While cross-sectional studies allow data collection from large numbers of people on a variety of indicators and apply sophisticated quantitative

analyses to the data, longtitudinal studies that follow individuals over a period of time are needed to adequately describe the multiple interactions and transactions that occur among psychological, cognitive, sociocultural, and organizational variables.

Future qualitative studies are needed because this approach limits potential masking or distortion of cultural diversity caused by imposing quantitative measures developed primarily on Anglo American populations. Qualitative approaches are likely to advance knowledge about the dynamic processes in care seeking behavior over time and over the course of an illness and to highlight the cultural meanings of symptoms and illness that influence care seeking decisions.

Because little research has been conducted from an interdisciplinary framework, integrated theoretical models await future testing. Interdisciplinary research teams and approaches, including combining qualitative and quantitative methods are most likely to yield critical information about the relative contributions of biological, psychological, and social factors to care seeking behavior (Taylor, 1990). Particularly needed are theoretically driven studies to test hypotheses about the processes that predict utilization behavior among immigrants and racial ethnic minorities, with an emphasis on theory-driven intervention studies. For example, Dracup and colleagues (1995) have recently set forth a research agenda on the underlying cognitive and emotional processes in the decision to seek care and in the length of that decision process. Lauver (1994) has proposed examining the relative contribution of multiple variables. In a similar vein, Rogler and Cortes (1993) and Briones and colleagues (1990) have called for examination of multimodal models of the pathways to mental health care.

Finally, a critical weakness in much of the extant research results from the failure to examine potential within-group (racial-ethnic) variation attributable to differences in socioeconomic status, gender, age, and geographic location (Ell *et al.,* 1994, 1995).

Conclusion

The research on health care seeking behavior of racially and ethnically diverse groups has uncovered rich patterns and complexity in human illness-related behavior (Garro, 1985; Kleinman, 1985; Lewis-Fernandez & Kleinman, 1995; Mechanic, 1985). The research reviewed here is heuristic in identifying key factors and variables that are involved in health-related actions among different cultural groups, including highlighting relevant characteristics of health care seeking behavior among immigrant populations in the United States. The scientific knowledge base on health care seeking behavior available to health care providers and policy makers has been advanced dramatically in recent years. As a result, the opportunity and challenge to improve the health of all members of society, if the collective will of society can be mobilized to do so, has also been advanced.

References

Alarcon, R. D. (1995). Culture and psychiatric diagnosis: Impact on DSM-IV and ICD-10. *Psychiatric Clinics of North America, 18,* 449–465.

Alonzo, A. (1986). The impact of the family and lay others on care-seeking during life-threatening episodes of suspected coronary artery disease. *Social Science & Medicine, 22,* 1297–1311.

Andersen, R., & Aday, L. (1978). Access to medical care in the U.S.: Realized and potential. *Medical Care, 16,* 533–546.

Andersen, R., & Newman, J. F. (1973). Societal and individual determinants of medical care utilization in the United States. *Milbank Memorial Fund Quarterly, 51,* 95–124.

Anderson, J. M., Blau, C., & Lau, A. (1991). Women's perspectives on chronic illness: Ethnicity, ideology and restructuring of life. *Social Science & Medicine, 33,* 101–113.

Anderson, L. M., Wood, D. L., & Sherbourne, C. D. (1995). Maternal acculturation and childhood immunization practices among children in Latino families in Los Angeles. Unpublished manuscript.

Balcazar, H., Hartner, J., & Cole, G. (1993). The effects of prenatal care utilization and maternal risk factors on pregnancy outcome between Mexican Americans and non-Hispanic Whites. *Journal of the National Medical Association, 85,* 195–202.

Bastida, E. (1989). The increasing significance of the social context in the utilization of aging services by Mexican American and Black elderly. *California Sociologist, 12,* 22–43.

Becerra, R. M., & Greenblatt, M. (1983). *Hispanics seek health care: A study of 1,088 veterans of three war eras.* New York: University Press of America.

Becker, M. H. (Ed.). (1974). *The health belief model and personal health behavior.* Thorofare, NJ: Slack.

Berkanovic, E., & Telesky, C. (1985). Mexican-American, Black-American, and White-American differences in reporting illnesses, disability and physician visits for illness. *Social Science & Medicine, 20,* 567–577.

Berkanovic, E., Hurwicz, M., & Landsverk, J. (1988). Psychological distress and the decision to seek medical care. *Social Science & Medicine, 27,* 1215–1221.

Berry, J. W. (1980). Acculturation as varieties of adaptation. In A. M. Padilla (Ed.), *Acculturation: Theory, models, and some new findings* (pp. 9–25). Boulder, CO: Westview.

Betancourt, H., & Lopez, S. R. (1993). The study of culture, ethnicity, and race in American psychology. *American Psychologist, 48,* 629–637.

Blendon, R. J., Aikens, L. M., Freeman, H. E., & Corey, C. R. (1989). Access to medical care for Black and White Americans. *Journal of the American Medical Association, 261,* 278–281.

Braveman, P., Bennett, T., Lewis, C., Egerter, S., & Showstack, J. (1993). Access to prenatal care following major Medicaid eligibility expansions. *Journal of the American Medical Association, 269,* 1285–1289

Briones, D. F., Heller, P. L., Chalfant, H. P., Roberts, A. E., Aquirre-Hauchbaum, S. F., & Farr, W. F. (1990). Socioeconomic status, ethnicity, psychological distress, and readiness to utilize mental health facility. *American Journal of Psychiatry, 147,* 1333–1340.

Broman, C. (1987). Race differences in professional help-seeking. *American Journal of Community Psychology, 15,* 473–489.

Bundek, N., Marks, G., & Richardson, J. (1993). Role of health locus of control beliefs in cancer screening of elderly Hispanic women. *Health Psychology, 12,* 193–199.

Burnam, M. A., Hough, R. L., Karno, M., Escobar, J. I., & Telles, C. A. (1987). Acculturation and lifetime prevalence of psychiatric disorders among Mexican Americans in Los Angeles. *Journal of Health and Social Behavior, 28,* 89–102.

Butler, J. A., Winter, W. D., Singer, J. D., & Wenger, M. (1985). Medical care use and expenditure among children and youth in the United States: Analysis of a national probability sample. *Pediatrics, 76,* 495–507.

Carr, W., Zeital, L., & Weiss, K. (1992). Variations in asthma hospitalizations and deaths in New York

City. *American Journal of Public Health, 82,* 59–65.

Castro, F. G., Furth, P., & Karlow, H. (1985). The health beliefs of Mexican, Mexican American and Anglo American women. *Hispanic Journal of Behavioral Sciences, 6,* 365–383.

Chavez, L. R., Hubbell, F. A., McMullin, J. M., Martinez, J. M., & Mishra, S. I. (1995). Structure and meaning in models of breast and cervical cancer risk factors: A comparison of perceptions among Latinas, Anglo women, and physicians. *Medical Anthropology Quarterly, 9,* 40–74.

Chesney, A. P., Chavira, J. A., Hall, R. P., & Gary, H. E. (1982). Barriers to medical care of Mexican-Americans: The role of social class, acculturation, and social isolation. *Medical Care, 20,* 883–891.

Chin, F., Trapido, E., & Davis, K. (1994). Differences in stage at presentation of breast and gynecologic cancers among Whites, Blacks and Hispanics. *Cancer, 73,* 2838–2842.

• Chung, R. C., & Lin, K. (1994). Help-seeking behavior among Southeast Asian refugees. *Journal of Community Psychology, 22,* 109–120.

Copeland, V. C. (1996). Immunization among African-American children: Implications for social work. *Health & Social Work, 21,* 105–114.

Corn, B., Hamrung, G., Kalb, T., & Kalb, E. A. (1995). Patterns of asthma death and near-death in an inner-city tertiary care teaching hospital. *Journal of Asthma, 32,* 405–412.

Cornelius, L. (1993a). Barriers for White, Black, and Hispanic children. *Journal of the National Medical Association, 85,* 282–288.

Cornelius, L. (1993b). Ethnic minorities and access to medical care: Where do we stand? *Journal of the Association for Academic Minority Physicians, 4,* 16–25.

Crain, E. F., Weiss, K. B., Bijur, P. E., Hersh, M., Westbrook, L., & Stein, R. E. (1994). An estimate of the prevalence of asthma and wheezing among inner-city children. *Pediatrics, 94,* 356–362.

Croyle, R. T., & Hunt, J. R. (1991). Coping with health threat: Social influence processes in reactions to medical test results. *Journal of Personality and Social Psychology, 60,* 382–389.

Cuellar, I., Harris, L. C., & Jasso, R. (1980). An acculturation scale of Mexican American normal and clinical populations. *Hispanic Journal of Behavioral Sciences, 2,* 199–217.

Cummings, K. M., Becker, M. H., & Maile, M. C. (1980). Bring the models together: An empirical approach to combining variables used to explain health actions. *Journal of Behavioral Medicine, 3,* 123–145.

Davanzo, C. E., Frye, B., & Froman, R. (1994). Stress in Cambodian refugee families. *Image—The Journal of Nursing Scholarship, 26,* 101–105.

Deimling, G. T., Smerglia, V. L., & Barresi, C. M. (1990). Health care professionals and family involvement in care-related decisions concerning older patients. *Journal of Aging and Health, 2,* 310–325.

Diehr, P., Yergan, J., Chu, J., Feigl, P., Glaefke, G., Moe, R., Bergner, M., & Rodenbaugh, J. (1989). Treatment modality and quality differences for Black and White breast-cancer patients treated in community hospitals. *Medical Care, 27,* 942–958

Dracup, K., Moser, D. K. , Eisenberg, M., Meischke, H., Alonzo, A. A., & Braslow, A. (1995). Causes of delay in seeking treatment for heart attack symptoms. *Social Science Medicine, 40,* 379–392.

Duelberg, S. I. (1992). Preventive health behavior among Black and White women in urban and rural areas. *Social Science Medicine, 34,* 191–198.

Elder, J. P., Castro, F. G., de Moor, Mayer, J., Candelaria, J. I., Campbell, N., Talavera, G., & Ware, L. M. (1991). Differences in cancer risk-related behaviors in Latino and Anglo adults. *Preventive Medicine, 20,* 751–763.

Ell, K., Haywood, J., Sobel, E., deGuzman, M., Blumfield, D., & Ning, J. (1994). Acute chest pain in African Americans: Factors in the delay in seeking emergency care. *American Journal of Public Health, 84,* 965–970.

Ell, K., Haywood, J., deGuzman, M., Sobel, E., Norris, S., Blumfield, D., Ning, J., & Butts, E. (1995). Differential perceptions, behaviors, and motivations among African Americans, Latinos, and Whites suspected of heart attacks in two hospital populations. *Journal of the Association for Academic Minority Physicians, 6,* 60–69.

Escarce, J. J., Epstein, K. R., Colby, D. C., & Schwartz, J. S. (1993). Racial differences in the elderlys' use of medical procedures and diagnostic tests. *American Journal of Public Health, 83,* 948–954.

Escobar, J. I., Gomez, J., & Tuason, V. B. (1983). Depressive phenomenology in North and South American patients. *American Journal of Psychiatry, 140,* 47–51.

Estrada, A. L., Trevino, F. M., & Ray, L. A. (1990). Health care utilization barriers among Mexican Americans: Evidence from HHANES, 1982–84. *American Journal of Public Health, 80* (Suppl.), 27–31.

Fisher, N. L., & Lew, L. (1996). Culture of the countries of Southeast Asia. In N. L. Fisher (Ed.), *Cultural and ethnic diversity: A guide for genetics professionals* (pp. 113–128). Baltimore: Johns Hopkins University Press.

Ford, E., Cooper, R., Castaner, A., Simmons, M., & Mar, M. (1989). Coronary arteriography and coronary bypass surgery among Whites and other racial groups relative to hospital-based incidence rates for coronary artery disease: Findings from NHDS. *American Journal of Public Health, 79,* 437–440.

Formenti, S. C., Meyerowitz, B. E., Ell, K., Muderspach, L., Groshen, S., Leedham, B., Klement V., & Morrow, P. (1995). Inadequate adherence to radiotherapy in Latina immigrants with carcinoma of the cervix: Potential impact on disease-free survival. *Cancer, 75,* 1135–1140.

Fox, S., & Roetzheim, R. (1994). Screening mammography and older Hispanic women: Current status and issues. *Cancer, 74* (Suppl. 7), 2028–2033.

Garcia, H. B., & Lee, P. C. Y. (1988). Knowledge about cancer and use of health care services among Hispanic- and Asian-American older adults. *Journal of Psychosocial Oncology, 6,* 157–177.

Garro, L. (1985). Decision-making models of treatment choice. Explanatory models and care-seeking: A critical account. In S. McHugh & T. M. Vallis (Eds.), *Illness behavior: A multidisciplinary model* (pp. 173–188). New York: Plenum.

Gilman, S. C., Justice, J., Saepharn, S. K., & Charles, G. (1992). Cross-cultural medicine, a decade later: Use of traditional and modern health services by Laotian refugees. *Western Journal of Medicine, 157,* 310–315.

Gochman, D. S. (1988). Health behavior: Plural perspectives. In D. S. Gochman (Ed.), *Health behavior: Emerging research perspectives* (pp. 3–17). New York: Plenum.

Goldberg, K. C., Hartz, A. J., Jacobsen, S. J., Krakauer, H., & Rimm, A. A. (1992). Racial and community factors influencing coronary artery bypass graft surgery rates for all 1989 Medicare patients. *Journal of the American Medical Association, 267,* 1473–1477.

Golding, J. M., & Baezconde-Garbanati, L. A. (1990). Ethnicity, culture, and social resources. *American Journal of Community Psychology, 18,* 465–486.

Good, B. (1985). Explanatory models and care-seeking: A critical account. In S. McHugh & T. M. Vallis (Eds.), *Illness behavior: A multidisciplinary model* (pp. 161–172). New York: Plenum.

Gould-Martin, K., & Ngin, C. (1981). Chinese Americans. In A. Harwood (Ed.), *Ethnicity and medical care* (pp. 130–171). Cambridge, MA: Harvard University Press.

Grau, L., & Padgett, D. (1988). Somatic depression amoung the elderly: A sociocultural perspective. *International Journal of Geriatric Psychiatry, 3,* 201–207.

Greenberg, E. R., Chute, C. G., Stukel, T., Baron, J. A., Freeman, D. M., Yates, J., & Korson, R. (1992). Social and economic factors in the choice of lung cancer treatment: A population-based study in two rural states. *New England Journal of Medicine, 318,* 612–617.

Greenley, J. R., Mechanic, D., & Cleary, P. D. (1987). Seeking help for psychologic problems: Replication and extension. *Medical Care, 25,* 1113–1128.

Gregorio, D., Cummings, K., & Michalek, A. (1983). Delay, stage of disease and survival among White and Black women with breast cancer. *American Journal of Public Health, 73,* 590–593.

Guarnaccia, P. J., & Parra, P. (1996). Ethnicity, social status, and families' experiences of caring for a mentally ill family member. *Community Mental Health Journal, 32,* 243–260.

Guarnaccia, P. J., Canino, G. J., Rubio-Stipec, M., & Bravo, M. (1993). The prevalence of *ataques de nervios* in the Puerto Rico disaster study: The role of culture in psychiatric epidemiology. *Journal of Nervous and Mental Disorders, 181,* 159–167.

Guendelman, S., English, P., & Chavez, G. (1995). The effects of maternal health behaviors and other risk factors on immunization status among Mexican-American infants. *Pediatrics, 95,* 823–828.

Guerra, L., Mesa, A., Ho, H., Casner, P., & Moldes, O. (1994). Medical residents practices in cancer screening in a Hispanic population. *South Medical Journal, 87,* 631–633.

Harmon, M. P., Castro, F. G., & Coe, K. (1996). Acculturation and cervical cancer: Knowledge, beliefs, and behaviors of Hispanic women. *Women and Health, 24,* 37–57.

Harwood, A. (1977). *Rx: Spiritist as needed: A study of a Puerto Rican community mental health resource.* New York: Wiley.

Harwood, A. (1981a). *Ethnicity and medical care.* Cambridge, MA: Harvard University Press.

Harwood, A. (1981b). Mainland Puerto Ricans. In A. Harwood (Ed.), *Ethnicity and medical care* (pp. 397–481). Cambridge, MA: Harvard University Press.

Haywood, L. J., Ell, K., Sobel, E., deGuzman, M., & Blumfield, D. (1993). Rose questionnaire responses among Black, Latino, and White subjects in two socioeconomic strata. *Ethnicity and Disease, 3,* 303–314.

High, D. M. (1990). Who will make health care decisions when I can't? *Journal of Aging and Health, 2,* 310–325.

Hopkins, R. (1993). Insurance coverage and usage of preventive health services. *Journal of the Florida Medical Association, 80,* 529–532.

Hopkins, R., & Hensley, K. (1993). Breast cancer in Florida women. Incidence and stage at diagnosis. *Journal of the Florida Medical Association, 80,* 468–471.

Hopper, S. V. (1993). The infuence of ethnicity on the health of older women. *Clinics in Geriatric Medicine, 9,* 231–255.

Howard, K. I., Cornille, T. A., Lyons, J. S., Vessey, J. T., Lueger, R. J., & Saunders, S. M. (1996). Patterns of mental health service utilization. *Archives of General Psychiatry, 53,* 696–703.

Hubbell, F. A., Waitzkin, H., Mishra, S. I., Dombrink, J., & Chavez, L. R. (1991). Access to medical care for documented and undocumented Latinos in a southern California county. *Western Journal of Medicine, 154,* 414–417.

Janz, N. K., & Becker, M. H. (1984). The health belief model: A decade later. *Health Education Quarterly, 11,* 1–47.

Javitt, J. C., McBean, A. M., Nicholson, G. A., Babish, J. D., Warren, J. L., & Krakauer, H. (1991). Undertreatment of glaucoma among Black Americans. *New England Journal of Medicine, 325,* 1418–1422.

Jenkins, C. N., Le, T., McPhee, S. J., Stewart, S., & Ha, T. (1996). Health care access and preventive care among Vietnamese immigrants: Do traditional beliefs and practices pose barriers? *Social Science and Medicine, 43*(7), 1049–1056.

Jung, J. H. (1996). Traditional Chinese culture. In N. L. Fisher (Ed.), *Cultural and ethnic diversity: A guide for genetics professionals* (pp. 86–97). Baltimore: Johns Hopkins University Press.

Kang, S. H., Bloom, J. R., & Romano, P. S. (1994). Cancer screening among African-American women: Their use of tests and social support. *American Journal of Public Health, 84,* 101–103.

Kirscht, J. P. (1988). The health belief model and predictions of health actions. In D. S Gochman (Ed.), *Health behavior: Emerging research perspectives* (pp. 27–41). New York: Plenum.

Kleinman, A. (1985). Illness meanings and illness behavior. In S. McHugh & T. M. Vallis (Eds.), *Illness behavior: A multidisciplinary model* (pp. 149–160). New York: Plenum.

Koopman, C., Eisenthal, J., & Stoeckles, J. D. (1984). Ethnicity in the reported pain, emotional distress, and requests of medical outpatients. *Journal of Social Science Medicine, 18,* 487–490.

Lacey, R. N. (1993). Cancer prevention and early detection strategies for reaching underserved urban, low-income Black women. *Cancer, 72* (Suppl.), 1078–1083.

Laguerre, M. S. (1981). Haitian Americans. In A. Harwood (Ed.), *Ethnicity and medical care* (pp.172–210). Cambridge, MA: Harvard University Press.

Landrine, H., & Klonoff, E. A. (1992). Culture and health-related schemas: A review and proposal for interdisciplinary integration. *Health Psychology, 11,* 267–276.

Lannon, C., Brack, V., Stuart, J., Caplow, M., McNeill, A., Bordley, W. C., & Margolis, P. (1995). What mothers say about why poor children fall behind on immunizations: A summary of focus groups in North Carolina. *Archives of Pediatrics and Adolescent Medicine, 149,* 1070–1075.

Lauver, D. (1994). Care-seeking behavior with breast cancer symptoms in Caucasian and African-American women. *Research in Nursing & Health, 17,* 421–431.

Leaf, P. J., Livingston, M. M., Tischler, G. L., Weissman, M. M. , Holzer, C. E., & Myers, J. K. (1985). Contact with health professionals for the treatment of psychiatric and emotional problems. *Medical Care, 23,* 1322–1337.

Leclere, F. B., Jensen, L., & Biddlecom, A. E. (1994). Health care utilization, family context, and adaptation among immigrants to the United States. *Journal of Health and Social Behavior, 35,* 370–384.

Leventhal, H. (1985). Symptom reporting: A focus on process. In S. McHugh & T. M. Vallis (Eds.), *Illness behavior: A multidisciplinary model* (pp. 219–237). New York: Plenum.

Leventhal, H., Zimmerman, R., & Gutmann, M. (1984). Compliance: A self-regulation perspective. In D. Gentry (Ed.), *Handbook of behavioral medicine* (pp. 369–436). New York: Guilford.

Lewis-Fernandez, R., & Kleinman, A. (1995). Cultural psychiatry: Theoretical, clinical, and research issues. *Psychiatric Clinics of North America, 18,* 433–447.

Lipton, J. A., & Marbach, J. J. (1984). Ethnicity and the pain experience. *Social Science Medicine, 19,* 1279–1298.

Loehrer, P. J., Greger, H. A., Weinberger, M., Musick, B., Miller, M., Nichols, C., Bryan, J., Higgs, D., & Brock, D. (1991). Knowledge and beliefs about cancer in a socioeconomically disadvantaged population. *Cancer, 68,* 1665–1671.

Lopez-Rangel, E. (1996). Latino culture. In N. L. Fisher (Ed.), *Cultural and ethnic diversity: A guide for genetics professionals* (pp. 19–35). Baltimore: Johns Hopkins University Press.

Low, S. M. (1985). Culturally interpreted symptoms or culture-bound syndromes: A cross-cultural review of nerves. *Social Science and Medicine, 21,* 187–196.

Mandelblatt, J., Andrews, H., Kerner, J., Zauber, A., & Burnett, W. (1991). Determinants of late stage diagnosis of breast cancer and cervical cancer: The impact of age, social class and hospital type. *American Journal of Public Health, 81,* 646–649.

Manson, A. (1988). Language concordance as a determinant of patient compliance and emergency room use in patients with asthma. *Medical Care, 26,* 1119–1128.

Manson, S. M. (1995). Culture and major depression: Current challenges in the diagnosis of mood disorders. *Psychiatric Clinics of North America, 18,* 487–501.

Marcus, A., Crane, L., Kaplan, C., Reading, A., Savage, E., Gunning, J., Bernstein, G., & Berek, J. S. (1992). Improving adherence to screening follow-up among women with abnormal Pap smears. *Medical Care, 30,* 216–230.

Marin, G., & Marin, B. V. (1991). *Research with Hispanic populations.* Newbury Park, CA: Sage.

Marin, G., Perez-Stable, E. J., & Marin, B. V. (1989). Cigarette smoking among San Francisco Hispanics: The role of acculturation and gender. *American Journal of Public Health, 79,* 196–198.

Marks, G., Solis, J., Richardson, J. L., Collins, L. M., Birba, L., & Hisserich, J. C. (1987). Health behavior of elderly Hispanic women: Does cultural assimilation make a difference? *American Journal Public Health, 77,* 1315–1319.

Marsh, W. W., & Hentges, K. (1988). Mexican folk remedies and conventional medical care. *American Family Physician, 37,* 257–262.

Maynard, C., Fisher, L. D., Passamani, E. R., & Pullum, T. (1986). Blacks in the Coronary Artery Surgery Study (CASS): Race and clinical decision making. *American Journal of Public Health, 76,* 1446–1448.

McCoy, C., Nielson, B., & Chitwood, D. (1991). Increasing the cancer screening of the medically underserved in South Florida. *Cancer, 67,* 1808–1813.

McHugh, S., & Vallis, T. M. (Eds.). (1985). *Illness behavior: A multidisciplinary model.* New York: Plenum.

McKinlay, J. B. (1973). Social networks, lay consultation and help-seeking behavior. *Social Focus, 51,* 275–292.

McManus, M. A., & Newacheck, P. (1993). Health insurance differentials among minority children with chronic conditions and the role of federal agencies and private foundations in improving financial access. *Pediatrics, 91,* 1040–1047.

McMiller, W. P., & Weisz, J. R. (1996). Help-seeking preceding mental health clinic intake among African-American, Latino, and Caucasian youths. *Journal of the Academy of Child and Adolescent Psychiatry, 35,* 1086–1094.

McPhee, S. J., Bird, J. A., Davis, T., Jenkins, C. N., & Le, B. (1997). Barriers to breast and cervical cancer screening among Vietnamese-American women. *American Journal of Preventive Medicine, 13*(3), 205–213.

Mechanic, D. (1982). The epidemiology of illness behavior and its relationship to physical and psychological distress. In D. Mechanic (Ed.), *Symptoms, illness behavior, and help-seeking* (pp. 1–24). New York: Prodist.

Mechanic, D. (1985). Illness behavior: An overview. In S. HcHugh & T. M. Vallis (Eds.), *Illness behavior: A multidisciplinary model* (pp. 101–109). New York: Plenum.

Mechanic, D., Angel, R. J., & Davies, L. (1992). Correlates of using mental health services: Implications of using alternative definitions. *American Journal of Public Health, 82,* 74–78.

Meyerowitz, B., Formenti, S., Ell, K., & Leedom, B. (1996). Latina women with cervical cancer: Psychological distress. Unpublished manuscript. Los Angeles.

Mezzich, J. E., & Raab, E. S. (1980). Depressive symptomatology across the Americas. *Archives of General Psychiatry, 37,* 818–823.

Mirales, M. A. (1989). *A matter of life and death: Health-seeking behavior of Guatemalan refugees in south Florida.* New York: AMS.

Ostrove, N. M., & Baum, A. (1983). Factors influencing medical help-seeking. In A. Nadler & J. Fisher (Eds.), *New directions in helping* (Vol. 3, pp. 107–129). New York: Academic Press.

Pearlman, D. N., Rakowski, W., Clark, M. A., Ehrich, B., Rimer, B. K., Goldstein, M. G., Woolverton, H., & Dube, C. E. (1997). Why do women's attitudes toward mammography change over time? *Cancer Epidemiology Biomarkers and Prevention, 6,* 451–457.

Perez-Stable, E. J., Sabogal, F., Otero-Sabogal, R., Hiatt, R. A., & McPhee, S. J. (1992). Misconceptions about cancer among Latinos and Anglos. *Journal of the American Medical Association, 268,* 3219–3223.

Perez-Stable, E. J., Otero-Sabogal, R., Sabogal, F., McPhee, S. J., & Hiatt, R. A. (1994). Self-reported use of cancer screening tests among Latinos and Anglos in a prepaid health plan. *Archives of Internal Medicine, 154,* 1073–1081.

Richardson, J. L., Marks, G., Solis, J. M., Collins, L. M., Birba, L., & Hisserich, J. C. (1987). Frequency and adequacy of breast cancer screening among elderly Hispanic women. *Preventive Medicine, 16,* 761–774.

Richardson, J. L., Langholz, B., Berstein, L., Burciaga, C., Danley, K., & Ross, R. (1992). Stage and delay in breast cancer diagnosis by race, socioeconomic status, age and year. *British Journal of Cancer, 65,* 922–926.

Ritter, C. (1988). Social supports, social networks, and health behaviors. In D. S. Gochman (Ed.), *Health behavior: Emerging research perspectives* (pp. 149–161). New York: Plenum.

Rogers, C., & Schiff, M. (1996). Early versus late prenatal care in New Mexico: Barriers and motivators. *Birth, 23,* 26–30.

Rogler, L. H., & Cortes, D. E. (1993). Help-seeking pathways: A unifying concept in mental health care. *American Journal of Psychiatry, 150,* 554–561.

Rogler, L. H., Cortes, D. E., & Malgady, R. G. (1991). Acculturation and mental health status among Hispanics: Convergence and new directions for research. *American Psychologist, 46,* 585–597.

Ruiz, M. S., Marks, G., & Richardson, J. L. (1992). Language acculturation and screening practices of elderly Hispanic women: The role of exposure to health-related information from the media. *Journal of Aging and Health, 4,* 268–281.

Schur, C. L., Bernstein, A. B., & Berk, M. L. (1987). The importance of distinguishing Hispanic subpopulations in the use of medical care. *Medical Care, 25,* 627–641.

Seijo, R., Gomez, H., & Freidenberg, J. (1991). Language as a communication barrier in medical care for Hispanic patients. *Hispanic Journal of Behavioral Sciences, 13,* 363–376.

Siddharthan, K., & Ahern, M. (1996). Inpatient utilization by undocumented immigrants without insurance. *Journal of Health Care for the Poor and Underserved, 7*(4), 355–363.

Snow, L. F. (1978). Sorcerers, saints, and charlatans: Black folk-healers in urban America. *Culture, Medicine, and Society, 2,* 60–106.

Snowden, L. R., & Cheung, F. K., (1990). Use of inpatient mental health services by members of ethnic minority groups. *American Psychologist, 45,* 347–355.

Snowden, L. R., Storey, C., & Clancy, T. (1989). Ethnicity and continuation in treatment at a Black comunity mental health center. *Journal of Community Psychology, 17,* 111–118.

Solis, J. M., Marks, G., Garcia, M., & Shelton, D. (1990). Acculturation, access to care, and use of preventive services by Hispanics: Findings from HHANES 1982–84. *American Journal of Public Health, 80* (Suppl.), 11–19.

Spring, M. A., Ross, P. J., Etkin, N. L., & Deinard, A. S. (1995). Sociocultural factors in the use of prenatal care by Hmong women, Minneapolis. *American Journal of Public Health, 85,* 1015–1017.

Starrett, R. A., Bresler, C., Decker, J. T., Walters, G. T., & Rogers, D. (1990). The role of environmental awareness and support networks in Hispanic elderly persons' use of formal social services. *Journal of Community Psychology, 18,* 218–227.

Strogatz, D. S. (1990). Use of medical care for chest pain: Differences between Blacks and Whites. *American Journal of Public Health, 80,* 290–294.

Suarez, L. (1994). Pap smear and mammogram screening in Mexican-American women: The effects of acculturation. *Amerian Journal of Public Health, 84,* 742–746.

Suarez, L., & Pulley, L. (1995). Comparing acculturation scales and their relationship to cancer screening among older Mexican-American women. *Journal of the National Cancer Institute Monograph, 18,* 41–47.

Suarez, L., Lloyd, L., Weiss, N., Rainbolt, T., & Pulley, L. (1994). Effect of social networks on cancer-screening behavior of older Mexican-American women. *Journal of the National Cancer Institute, 86,* 775–779.

Sue, S. (1977). Community mental health services to minority groups: Some optimism, some pessimism. *American Psychologist, 32,* 616–624.

Sue, S., Fujino, D. C., Hu, L., Takeuchi, D. T., & Zane, N. W. S. (1991). Community mental health services for ethnic minority groups: A test of the cultural responsiveness hypothesis. *Journal of Consulting and Clinical Psychology, 59,* 533–540.

Sussman, L. K., Robins, L. M., & Earls, F. (1987). Treatment seeking for depression by black and white Americans. *Social Science and Medicine, 24,* 187–196.

Taylor, S. E. (1990). Health psychology: The science and the field. *American Psychologist, 45,* 40–50.

Thamer, M., Richard, C., Casebeer, A. W., & Ray, N. F. (1997). Health insurance coverage among foreign-born U.S. residents: The impact of race, ethnicity, and length of residence. *American Journal of Public Health, 87*(1), 96–102.

Tortolero-Luna, G., Glober, G. A., Villarreal, R., Palos, G., & Linares, A. (1995). Screening practices and knowledge, attitudes, and beliefs about cancer among Hispanic and non-Hispanic White women 35 years old or older in Nueces County, Texas. *Journal of the National Cancer Institute Monographs, 18,* 49–56.

Tosomeen, A. H., Marquez, M. A.,Panser, L. A., & Kottke, T. E. (1996). Developing preventive health programs for recent immigrants: A case study of cancer screening for Vietnamese women in Olmsted County, Minnesota. *Minnesota Medicine, 79,* 46–48.

Uba, L. (1994). *Asian Americans: Personality patterns, identity, and mental health.* New York: Guilford.

Vega, W. A., Kolody, B., & Valle, R. (1988). Marital strain, coping, and depression among Mexican-American women. *Journal of Marriage and Family, 50,* 391–403.

Vega, W. A., Kolody, B., Valle, R., & Weir, J. (1991). Social networks, social support, and their relationship to depression among immigrant Mexican women. *Human Organization, 50,* 154–162.

Weidman, H. H. (1988). A transcultural perspective on health behavior. In D. S. Gochman (Ed.), *Health behavior: Emerging research perspectives* (pp. 261–280). New York: Plenum.

Weissman, J. S., Stern, R., Fielding, S. L., & Epstein, A. M. (1991). Delayed access to health care: Risk factors, reasons, and consequences. *Annals of Internal Medicine, 114,* 325–331.

Weller, S. C., Pachter, L. M., Trotter, R. T., & Baer, R. D. (1993). Empacho in four Latino groups: A study of intra- and inter-cultural variation in beliefs. *Medical Anthropology, 15,* 109–136.

Wells, K, Golding, J. M., Hough, R. I., & Burnam, M. A. (1989). Acculturation and the probability of use of services by Mexican Americans. *Health Services Research, 24,* 237–257.

Wells, K. B., Golding, J. M., Hough, R. L., Burnam, A., & Karno, M. (1988). Factors affecting the probability of use of general and medical health and social/community services for Mexican Americans and Non-Hispanic Whites. *Medical Care, 26,* 441–452.

Wenneker, M. B., & Epstein, A. M., (1989). Racial inequalities in the use of procedures for the patients with ischemic heart disease in Massachusetts. *Journal of the American Medical Association, 261,* 253–257.

Wilk, R. J. (1986). The Haitian refugee: Concerns for health care providers. *Social Work in Health Care, 11,* 61–74.

Williams, C. A., Beresford, S. A. A., James, S. A., LaCroix, A. Z., Strogatz, D. S., Wagner, E. H., Kleinbaum, D. G., Cutchin, L. M., & Ibrahim,

M. A. (1985). The Edgecombe County High Blood Pressure Control Program III: Social support, social stressors, and treatment dropout. *American Journal of Public Health, 75,* 483–486.

Williams, S. J., Diehr, P., Drucker, W. L., & Richardson, W. C. (1979). Mental health services: Utilization by low income enrollees in a prepaid group practice plan and an independent practitioner plan. *Medical Care, 27,* 139–151.

Woodrow, K. M., Friedman, G. D., Siegelaub, A. B., & Collen, M. F. (1972). Pain tolerance: Differences according to age, sex, and race. *Psychosomatic Medicine, 34,* 548–556.

Yancey, A., & Walden, L. (1994) Stimulating cancer screening among Latinas. *Journal of Cancer Education, 9,* 46–52.

Zambrana, R. E., Ell, K., Dorrington, C., Wachsman, L., & Hodge, D. (1994). The relationship between psychosocial status of immigrant Latino mothers and use of emergency pediatric services. *Health and Social Work, 19,* 93–102.

Zborowski, M. (1952). Cultural components of response to pain. *Journal of Social Sciences, 8,* 16–30.

8

Healing Practices

BONNIE B. O'CONNOR

Introduction

Immigrants to a new country bring with them, as a part of their cultural and experiential heritage, systems of health beliefs and practices that are familiar, are consonant with broader cultural goals and values, and have reputations for efficacy based on many generations of empirical observation and on considerable cultural authority. These healing systems typically remain active and viable in immigrant communities in the new country and often continue to serve as important health care resources over the course of many generations. Acceptance and use of biomedical care does not preclude continued use of indigenous healing practices, nor is use or abandonment of these traditional practices a necessary correlate of acculturation (Castro, Furth, & Karlow, 1984; Gould-Martin & Ngin, 1981; Miller, 1990; Nall & Speilberg, 1978).

There is an immense literature dealing with health beliefs and practices of immigrant and refugee groups in the United States and other countries. Most of this literature is focused on specific ethnic and nationality groups, and the ways in which their particular

systems of health belief and practice interact with use of biomedical health care resources. Because thorough treatment of all indigenous healing systems represented in U.S. immigrant populations is well beyond the scope of a single chapter, and because a substantial literature of population-specific descriptions already exists, my approach to the discussion of healing practices among immigrants departs from this pattern.

This chapter is focused largely on concepts, practices, expectations, and constructions of health, illness, and care that are commonly found across a substantial number of different healing traditions, but that do not comprise a part of the standard medical and public health models of health promotion and disease prevention, and so are likely to be unfamiliar to many American health professionals. My aim is to outline concepts, principles, and data that can be applied broadly to recognize and respond to health-related concerns, beliefs, and behavior in many populations—and so be applicable in novel as well as familiar situations—as opposed to furnishing snapshot summaries of a few.

Culture and Health Care

All healing resources are products of culture and are strongly shaped by the cultures in which they arise (Hufford, 1988). This is as true of modern biomedicine as of the systems that immigrants bring with them to their

BONNIE B. O'CONNOR • Department of Community and Preventive Medicine, MCP♦Hahnemann School of Medicine, Allegheny University of the Health Sciences, Philadelphia, Pennsylvania 19102.

Handbook of Immigrant Health, edited by Loue. Plenum Press, New York, 1998.

adopted homes. It is sometimes difficult for Americans to see anything "cultural" in biomedicine, because of its close congruence with (often tacit) middle-class American macrocultural values. Examples include prizing of individual autonomy, goal orientation, respect for incremental technical training as a source of expertise and authority, the conviction that human beings can and should dominate natural forces and processes, a preference for action in response to challenging situations, a dedication to timeliness and rapid response, a belief that human beings can and should improve themselves and their situations by dint of their own efforts, and a future orientation that includes positive valuation of "planning ahead" and a profound sense that newer technological and theoretical resources are better than older ones (Egeland, 1978; Lock & Gordon, 1988; Stein, 1990; see also Payer, 1988).

Definitions of health, illness, and appropriate care are always culturally derived (Hufford, 1992). Broader values and goals, interwoven in the cultural fabric, undergird attitudes and responses to health and illness: those dealing, for example, with the nature of the universe or of nature and the proper place of humanity within them; with definitions of personhood and appropriate interpersonal relationship; with family and community responsibilities and obligations; with right conduct, a good life, and the means to their achievement; with legitimate sources of knowledge and authority; with the nature and relationships of the human body, mind, and spirit; with moral, ethical, and religious principles; and so forth (O'Connor, 1995).

An example will illustrate. For many cultures, a network of family members is likely to be closely involved in any individual's illness. Family functions can include diagnosis and prescription; preparation and administration of medicaments and foods (not always mutually exclusive categories); close monitoring of bodily functions and signs; treatment decision making; provision of solicitous attentions and diversions; protection of the patient from fearful information and prognostications; constant companionship; protection of the patient's privacy; engagement of traditional specialists when indicated; and, should hospitalization enter the picture, provision of home-prepared foods and attentive monitoring of hospital personnel and interventions to ensure that they are timely, appropriate, and in the patient's best interest (as defined by patient and family).

These actions and expectations reflect definitions and requirements of familial roles, obligations, and interpersonal behavior. In addition they entail (among many other components) cultural values regarding appropriate responses to problems or difficult circumstances (e.g., ignoring, accepting, working through, "fighting"); how persons are defined in relation to self and others (e.g., dependent, interdependent, independent); what constitutes proper and reliable decision making (e.g., individual, collective, elder-controlled); what kinds of exposures (e.g., to natural elements, to specific foods, to information that may provoke strong emotions) are beneficial and harmful; and sources of authoritative judgment and knowledge (e.g., family elder, specialist healer, religious or spiritual functionary, nurse or physician). These broader beliefs and values are not directly "about" health, but they play a defining part in the ways in which people respond to health threats and compromises, and to the maintenance or restoration of desirable states of being.

Healing Systems

Beliefs and practices relating to health are organized into complex and coherent systems of thought and action (Hufford, 1984, 1988) that are articulated, as noted, with larger cultural worldviews. Healing systems include bodies of knowledge and belief, modes of knowledge production, evaluative processes, definitions and categories of health and illness, explanatory models (Kleinman, 1975, 1984) of disease etiology and human function, theories relating cause and nature of illness to preventive and therapeutic choices, specific repertoires of diagnostic and therapeutic actions and *materia medica*, generalist and specialist practitioners and the means to their training and legitimation, self-care modalities, and generative principles for formulating system-consistent responses to new input (O'Connor, 1995). The term "healing system" should be understood to refer to this entire complex of interrelated features (Hufford, 1992). It is of course plausible to focus attention on specific healing beliefs and practices, but it is important when doing so to remain aware of the larger systemic connections that help to maintain their vigor, adaptability to new situations, and resistance to external pressures for change (Hufford, 1992).

Common Concepts

Many of the healing systems used by immigrant populations in the United States share a number of fundamental concepts not found in the conventional medical model (Table 1). For conceptual purposes these can be defined in general terms that cut across systems, bearing in mind that their specific interpretations and nuances vary significantly from system to system.

Health as Harmony and Balance

Central to most nonbiomedical healing systems is a definition of health in terms of harmony or balance. This balance can be among bodily humors or regulatory substances (Assanand, Dias, Richardson, & Waxler-Morrison, 1990; Ramakrishna & Weiss, 1992); innate qualities such as heat and cold (some-

TABLE 1. Common Concepts across Healing Traditions

- Health as harmony or balance
- Integration of body, mind, and spirit
- Vital essence
- Magical and supernatural elements
- Envy and other strong emotions as etiologic factors

times, but not always, related to physical temperatures—see, e.g., Harwood, 1971) or yin and yang; or forces such as expansion and contraction, upward and downward or inward and outward motion. These principles of balance are incorporated into routine health maintenance practices as well as into specific illness treatment protocols. For example, a general awareness of the unhealthful consequences of any form of excess (upsetting the balance too far in one direction) may consciously guide everyday choices of consumption, exposure, social behavior, and other activity (Assanand *et al.,* 1990). Underlying principles of balance enter, in addition, into other aspects of daily life that may not at the moment be associated expressly with health, for example, selection of foods for a meal based on a general sense of what foods do and don't "go together," or what constitutes a wholesome and satisfying meal in particular conditions (e.g., "perfect weather for soup").

Many Latino cultures incorporate a balance between hot and cold properties of bodily functions and states, of symptoms, and of ingested substances into their philosophies of health and healing. Cold conditions are offset with hot foods and medicines, hot conditions with cool ones (because introduction of cold substances would be too abrupt, having a tightening or congealing effect). The goal is to maintain or restore health by moving toward a neutral center, with a preference for remaining slightly on the warm side (Gleave & Manes, 1990; Harwood, 1971, 1981; Schreiber & Homiak, 1981). Hot/cold concerns are also central to healing systems of the Indian subcontinent (Assanand *et al.,* 1990; Ramakrishna & Weiss, 1992), to Haitian healing tradition (LaGuerre, 1981), and to a number of Middle Eastern cultures (Behjati-Sabet, 1990). Arab cultural influences, by way of the historical Moorish occupation of southern Spain, are in fact the likely source of the hot/cold concepts of health and healing common in western hemisphere Spanish-speaking cultures.

In traditional Chinese medicine, which has influenced the healing systems of Vietnam and other southeast Asian cultures, cold and heat (along with many other qualities) are associated with the principles of yin and yang, or *am* and *duong* in their Vietnamese variants (Dinh, Ganesan, & Waxler-Morrison, 1990; Jenkins, Le, McPhee, Stewart, & Ngoc, 1996; Marr, 1987). These essential qualities are complements, are mutually interinfluential, give rise to one another, and transform into each other in a continual ebb and flow (Beinfiend & Korngold, 1991; Kaptchuk, 1983). The balance that is health is a moving, fluid, dynamic balance: not a homeostasis, but an equipoise in which these qualities figure prominently. A suitable image for this type of balance might be that of a hanging mobile: it is never absolutely still, and even slight derangements in one part resonate throughout the whole, causing movement, change, and realignment into one of many possible momentarily balanced arrangements (C. Hudson, personal communication, 1994). Balance is its normative state, but it is a dynamic and processual condition.

In addition to internal states of equilibrium, harmony between the individual and external factors such as social, environmental, spiritual, and cosmological elements may be required for optimal health. A number of cultures recognize social discord as an etiologic factor for illness (see, e.g., Okabe, Takahashi, & Richardson, 1990). Behavioral rules for communication and social interaction incorporate this recognition, placing an emphasis on avoidance of topics, emotional expressions, or breaches of deference that could create disharmony. Balanced life routines that regulate interactions with occupational and social stressors and emphasize the need for adequate rest and appropriate diet (commonly seasonally changeable) may form a part of this broader context of harmony between individuals and their social and environmental surroundings (Boyle, 1989; La-Guerre, 1981; Ramakrishna & Weiss, 1992).

In a great number of cultures, environmental factors such as seasonal change and climatological features are understood to affect health. Times of seasonal change are typically regarded as intervals of particular vulnerability to illness, and special protective steps are taken: particular herbs or seasonal "tonics," specific foods featured or avoided, attention to appropriate dress. Concern with protection from exposure to cold, particularly in the form of cold air, drafts, and wind is virtually universal across cultures as a preventive measure against ill health (although several also recognize health-promoting benefits of fresh air [Boyle, 1989; Ragucci, 1981]). This concern accompanies a pervasive conviction that cold can enter the body and accumulate, causing or contributing to a large variety of maladies both in the immediate run and at future times (Duong, 1987; Ragucci, 1981). In most systems that incorporate these concerns, babies and elders are considered more susceptible than others to environmental influences. In addition, menstruating, pregnant, and postpartum (including postabortion, postmiscarriage) women are especially vulnerable, because their bodies are "open" to the outside environment. Special precautions are typically prescribed for these vulnerable groups.

Spiritual harmony may be defined both in terms of the individual's inner state and in terms of relationships between individuals and spiritual entities that interact with the material world and influence health and general well-being. In Haitian immigrant communities where vodou religious belief is active, individuals have both indirect and direct personal connections with the *loas,* or powerful spiritual entities. The *loas* control or strongly influence all events in life, including sickness and health. Breaches of propriety or expectation with repect to one's *loas* can result in ill health or other misfortune, and *loas* govern all healing herbs (La-Guerre, 1981, 1987; Métraux, 1972; A.N., G.W., *vodouisants,* personal communications, 1996). A parallel situation holds between individuals and the *orichas* in Latino communities (largely Cuban, Puerto Rican, and Dominican) where *santería,* a historical relative of vodou, is practiced.

In many southeast Asian cultures, deceased ancestors remain in active contact with surviving generations of family members and are venerated and provided for in their afterlife. Lapses in responsibility to ancestral spirits may result in illness as punishment, reminder, or means of getting the attention of the living; ancestors may also call attention to other needs by causing illness (Bell & Whiteford, 1987; Chindarsi, 1976; Geddes, 1976; Marr, 1987; Stephenson, 1995). Cosmological factors, including astrological cycles and astronomical events such as eclipses or lunar cycles, may also be identified as affecting health and requiring behavioral adjustments to maintain balance, and individuals may be spiritually connected to or otherwise affected by stars (Davis, 1988; Duong, 1987; Jenkins *et al.*, 1996; Stephenson, 1995).

Integration of Body, Mind, and Spirit

Most nonbiomedical healing systems assume an integration of body, mind, and spirit. The balance and harmony that define health incorporate all of these aspects of persons. Difficulties or imbalances in any of the aspects can produce sickness and symptoms in any of the others. Similarly, treatment interventions may in various circumstances address any aspect and ameliorate the others. Physical injury or disease may bring about mental, emotional, or spiritual unwellness through disturbances of balance. Likewise, emotions (classified variably as mental states or spiritual states, or both) and mental unrest or worry are etiologic factors that may promote mental, emotional, or physical manifestations of illness.

Strong negative emotions tend to be most implicated. In a great many cultures from all around the globe, envy is recognized as a dangerous emotion that can cause illness in the envious person as well as in those who are the objects of envy. Physical manifestations (in either party) include headache, loss of appetite, lassitude, sleep disturbance, and gastric distress. A Korean illness category called *hwabyung* ("fire illness" or "anger illness," *hwa* connoting both fire and anger) is

attributed to "lasting anger, disappointments, sadness, miseries, hostility, grudges, and unfulfilled dreams and expectations" (Pang, 1990, p. 496). Physical manifestations include gastric, cardiac, respiratory, musculoskeletal, and circulatory symptoms, together with "feelings of hotness" and nightmares (Pang, 1990). In traditional Chinese medicine and its related systems positive emotions also have the potential to lead to unhealthful consequences, because excess of any type adversely affects healthful harmony. Excesses of excitement or joy are as disruptive as excesses of anger or sorrow; moderation and balance are the keys.

Parts of these descriptions sound much like psychosomatic theory, but the nature of the interconnections and the mechanisms by which the various aspects are understood to be linked in health and illness are quite different in these healing systems than in the psychosomatic model. Simply to assimilate these explanations to psychosomatic theory would be to make a mistranslation with a resulting loss in sense and meaning, and would surely lead to incomprehension of the view cultural insiders would most likely hold that psychotherapeutic approaches to their illnesses are probably inadequate, if not altogether inapplicable.

In keeping with this integrated sense of the various aspects of persons and their health, many systems do not draw sharp categorical distinctions between mental and physical illness (Duong, 1987; Harwood, 1981; Moon & Tashima, 1982; Novack, 1987; Ramakrishna & Weiss, 1992). Although there typically are distinct concepts of body, mind, and spirit, disturbances in any of these aspects of persons are considered almost invariably interrelated. Specific mental/emotional and spiritual classes of illness may be recognized to exist (though typically considered less commonly occurring than mental and emotional disturbances are in the biomedical view), and may call for the services of a particular specialist in their treatment. In other respects, however, the same sorts of derangements of balance are implicated in all types of disease and illness, and many aspects of treatment are thus quite similar no matter what the problem.

Vital Essence

The human body (as well as other living things in the world) is in a majority of systems conceived as being animated and sustained by a special type of force, energy, or essence whose presence and proper activity are essential to life and health. In several Spanish-speaking cultures, this essence is spiritual, a person's soul. Separation of the soul from the body in life (discussed later) is a serious occurrence which if not remedied can lead to severe or chronic illness, and in time to death. In the Haitian vodou tradition the animating and life-sustaining principle is the *gros bon ange* ("big good angel"), which "enters the individual at conception and functions only to keep the body alive. At clinical death, it returns immediately to God and once again becomes part of the great reservoir of energy that supports all life" (Davis, 1988, p. 186).

In the traditional Chinese healing system the animating principle is a metaphysical force called *qi* (sometimes anglicized as *chi*). It is a unique force likened (in terms comprehensible in the American macro-cultural framework) to "matter on the verge of becoming energy, or energy at the point of materializing" (Kaptchuk, 1983, p. 35). *Qi* is transformative, warming, sustaining, protective, regulating. It is itself always in motion, and is the source of all movement in the body at every level of functioning. There are diagnostic methods for ascertaining the strength and the quality of motion of *qi*, and "specific treatments for supplementing its deficiency, draining its excess, and regulating its flow" (p. 37). *Qi* is derived from food and from air, but there is a part of each individual's *qi*, received from his or her parents, whose source is the primordial *qi* of the universe, thus linking persons and their health to the cosmos.

Magical and Supernatural Elements

Quite a number of healing systems recognize a role for magical and supernatural elements in disease etiology. These may include interventions by deities or spirits in retribution for dereliction of religious or family duty (categories which sometimes overlap, as in ancestor veneration) or for unintentional slights and aggravations (Bliatout, 1982; Chindarsi, 1976); states of possession, physical invasion, or harrassment by demonic, evil, or otherwise undesirable entities (Bell & Whiteford, 1987; Brainard & Zaharlick, 1989; Duong, 1987); spiritual causes such as soul loss or capture (Davis, 1988; Dinh *et al.*, 1990; Harwood, 1981; Rubel, O'Nell, & Collado-Ardón, 1984; Stephenson, 1995); and malign human agency such as cursing, hexing, and sorcery (Bell & Whiteford, 1987; Davis, 1988; Harwood, 1981; LaGuerre, 1981; Ragucci, 1981).

Some illness categories are specific to supernatural causation. In addition, many cultures recognize the possibility of variable causation for *any* type of disease or illness (e.g., mental illnesses, infectious diseases, cancers). Particular aspects or details of a given illness episode may indicate that supernatural etiological factors are involved. Within the Haitian folk healing tradition, a supernatural origin for disease may be suggested by sudden and severe onset or by a very protracted course (LaGuerre, 1981); for many Latino cultures, by lengthy duration and failure to respond to usual standard treatment (Harwood, 1981; Schreiber & Homiak, 1981; Trotter & Chavira, 1981); for medically plural cultures, by inability of a medical doctor to arrive at a diagnosis or identify a cause for troubling symptoms (Bell & Whiteford, 1987; Glasgow & Adaskin, 1990). For traditional Hmong, although many natural causal factors are recognized in ill health, supernatural selection of the victim is almost always implied, explaining in part why this person, at this time, should be injured or fall ill (Geddes, 1976). Whenever magical or supernatural causes are involved, they must also be properly addressed in the healing effort or else illness can be expected to recur, even if symptoms abate for the near term. Some of these types of healing measures can be carried out on one's own or in the context of the family (e.g., through prayer, offerings, observances to spiritual entities or ancestors, ritual baths and cleansings), while others require the interventions of a specialist practitioner (*curandera*, shaman, sorcerer, religious authority, spiritual healer).

Envy

As mentioned previously, the emotion of envy can cause ill health. In the envious person him or herself this happens through disruption of internal balance and harmony. In the object of envy, ill effects are brought about through an implicit curse or, more commonly, through a strong or covetous gaze or evil eye. The glance of the evil eye may be cast both intentionally and unintentionally (Assanand *et al.* 1990; Harwood, 1981; Ragucci, 1981). In several Latino cultures, for example, the simple fact that a possession or a family member may attract admiration and compliments suggests the possibility of underlying envy of which the admirer may even consciously be unaware (e.g., "What a beautiful shawl!" [implied: "I wish I had one . . ."]).

Measures to counteract the possible ill effects include spitting (sometimes between the first two fingers, sometimes thrice) (Kraut, 1994), belittling rejoinders (e.g., "she's just an ordinary kid, really," or "it's old, but still serviceable"), utterance of formulaic phrases, and use of protective amulets or power objects. When the object of envy is a person, especially a child, a countermanding gesture such as a small symbolic pinch or tap (to the cheek or arm, for instance) can provide a little offsetting "insult" to neutralize the admiring compliment. In the case of objects, if one can bear or afford to part with them, giving the admired item as a gift to the admirer dispels envy. Evil-eye beliefs and practices are found in all circum-Mediterranean cultures, in Islamic cultures, Anglo-Celtic cultures, and many African and Asian cultures.

For some southeast Asian cultures, envy creates hazards through supernatural channels. Direct expressions of compliments and admiration to people are considered dangerous in Hmong culture, for example, because they may attract the attention and possessive envy of spirits, who may then try to come and take away the object of desire (X.C., author interview, 1985). Though its mode of action is variable across cultures, envy poses a genuine threat, and is not taken lightly. (During a 1989 fieldwork visit to Philadelphia's Puerto Rican community, I found myself driving behind a car bearing the artfully painted slogan *"La envidia mata"* [envy kills]. Warnings of this type are not metaphorical.) Together with protective objects or amulets and specific preventive actions, behavioral and conversational norms help defend against this type of health risk.

"Folk" Illnesses

General

Immigrants' indigenous healing traditions include illness taxonomies, and these typically contain some illnesses not recognized in biomedical diagnostic categories as "actual" diseases or medical syndromes. These illnesses are generally referred to by academics and Western health professionals as "folk" illnesses (or sometimes as "culture-bound syndromes"). The notion of "folk" illness is an academic construct that takes the nosological and etiological categories of biomedicine as its point of departure. The implication of the label is usually that an illness so referenced is not "real," or at best is not "really" what people who accept it as real believe it to be. This is an etic, or cultural outsiders', viewpoint that is of course not shared by cultural insiders.

As a linguistic convenience I also use the term *folk illness,* but specify that in my usage the term is intended to convey only the limited meaning, "categories of illness well recognized in various cultural settings, but not known in biomedical nosology." Cultural insiders refer to each such illness by its own culturally supplied name. Folk illnesses, like other illnesses, have recognized etiologies, particular constellations of symptoms, identified sequelae, and specified preventive and therapeutic measures. *Hwabyung,* briefly described earlier, is an example of such an illness (see also Duong, 1987; Harwood, 1981; Rubel, 1964; Rubel *et al.,* 1984; Schreiber & Homiak, 1981; Trotter, 1985; Trotter & Chavira, 1981).

By this definition, it could be said that in traditional Chinese medicine *all* illness/imbalance classifications (or "heteropathies"—changes that "violate [the] normal order" [Sivin, 1987, p. 49]) are folk illnesses. Because the understanding of human physiology and organ system function in this system are almost wholly incongruent with those found in modern biomedicine, the classification of illness states, their causal factors, and their configurations of signs and symptoms does not "map" readily onto biomedical nosology. Biomedical diagnostic entities are susceptible of numerous traditional Chinese interpretations, while the Chinese names for particular heteropathic constellations have no referents at all in biomedicine. Even the meanings attached to terms held in common, such as "blood," "breath," or the names of organs, differ enormously between the two systems (Zhang & Hsu, 1990).

Some folk illnesses may represent local names and differing symptom patterns of currently recognized medical disorders (Hufford, 1988, 1992; Rubel, 1964; Rubel *et al.,* 1984), while others do not seem to have medical correlates (although they do tend to be reinterpreted in psychiatric terms by American health professionals, often inappropriately). In either case, aspects of the etiologic explanatory model of folk illnesses will definitely depart from the conventional medical model, as previous discussion demonstrates,

and treatment will follow the system-congruent reasoning: cooling excess heat, restoring proper motion of *qi,* dispelling wind, extirpating evil influences, and so on. (These causal and therapeutic considerations are, of course, not confined to folk illnesses. They also apply to medically recognized diseases, thus providing one of the important reasons why indigenous healing traditions continue to be used by immigrant populations even when they accept and use biomedicine.)

Soul Loss

Each cultural repertoire is likely to contain some folk illness categories of its own. In addition, there are some illnesses widely recognized across cultures (but not in biomedicine). Of these, perhaps the most ubiquitous is soul loss, sometimes academically referred to as "magical fright" (see Simons & Hughes, 1985). Recognition that human beings have (one or more) souls is a cultural commonplace. Souls are usually thought to depart the body at or immediately after death, under proper conditions (but see O'Connor, 1995, chapter 4). In addition, in many cultures it is understood that souls may leave the body during life; the reasons for this separation vary across cultures.

In many Latino cultures, soul separation during life happens under circumstances of shock or severe hardship. In some cultural settings, souls leave the body during sleep, and their experiences on their wanderings produce dreams and the information dreams convey (Chindarsi, 1976). In traditional Hmong culture, souls may be attracted to beautiful surroundings and simply linger there (Bliatout, 1982). Both Hmong and Vietnamese cultural systems recognize that wandering souls also may become lost or ensnared, or enter into another living (animal or human) being (Chindarsi, 1976; Geddes, 1976; Stephenson, 1995; Thao, 1986). Both Haitian vodou and Hmong spiritual systems recognize the possibility of soul capture—in the former by human sorcerers, in the latter typically by wicked or spiteful spirits (Davis,

1988; Geddes, 1976). Across these and other cultures, soul loss can be caused by a sudden severe fright, trauma, or emotional shock brought on by such varying events as witnessing or suffering a frightening accident or brutality, receiving bad news for which one is unprepared, experiencing extended extreme hardship, or being caught up in terrifying natural events such as earthquakes.

Like many recognized medical conditions, soul loss is both a sickness in itself and a contributing factor in other illnesses. It is always serious, and if not properly treated can lead to death. It is important for health professionals who work with immigrant individuals and communities not to dismiss or trivialize soul loss and other folk illnesses since, at least for some of these illnesses, there is evidence that their sufferers are at increased risk for general morbidity and mortality (Rubel *et al.*, 1984). Indications are that treatment outcomes for some folk illnesses are best when the appropriate traditional remedies or practitioners provide the treatment (Rubel *et al.*, 1984), and in some cases traditional treatments may be of clinical consequence (Trotter, 1985).

Common Therapeutic Practices

Use of medicinal herbs and other natural substances, prayers and other religious and spiritual actions, and physically applied therapies are common preventive and therapeutic actions across cultural traditions. Specific theories of the modes of action of these therapies, and of the relationship between the therapeutic modality and the specific health condition for which it is applied, vary across traditions in keeping with system-specific explanatory models of health and illness.

Although it has been customary in the past for scholars of folk medical traditions to classify therapeutic modalities as being *either* material *or* magicoreligious, this is a misleading dualism that reflects the taxonomic categories of the scholars, not of the healing systems and their larger cultural frameworks.

Just as most of these healing systems conceptually integrate body, mind, and spirit in health and illness, so too do they integrate in actual practice material and spiritual/magical/metaphysical healing modalities and goals.

Natural Substances

Every culture of which we have knowledge has developed a *materia medica* of locally available natural substances—botanical, animal, and mineral. These natural medicines are used according to a variety of theoretical models of their modes of action; the pharmacological-biochemical model does not always apply. Herbs and other natural medicaments are used for their physical actions and effects and for their metaphysical properties such as hot/cold or *yin/yang* qualities and effects; for spiritual qualities associated with them, such as purity, patience, inner strength, or calm; for effects they will have on the vital essence; or for their capacity to absorb and carry away negative influences.

Natural medicaments may be taken internally as teas or soups, or along with foods, both specifically as medicines and as culinary spices intended to promote both flavor and beneficial effect. They are used as inhalants and as components of baths and steamings, in ointments and salves, ear and eye drops, douches and enemas, poultices, wet or dry packs, massage compounds, and in moxibustion (the burning on or very near the skin surface of tiny amounts of dried, compressed herbs, usually Chinese mugwort leaves). Specific substances may be used to "sweep" the body in ritual cleansings, drawing out disease-causing malignancies. Eggs or small live animals are also used for this purpose in many settings, because their life force may successfully substitute for the vital essence of the patient as a target for malign forces, possessing spirits, and other agents of disease that may be able to be transferred out of the patient. In several Latino cultures rue (the herb of sorrow and regret) is commonly used for this purpose.

Any natural substances, and any of their various modes of use, may be intended to bring about physical, mental, emotional, or spiritual effects. An herb taken internally is as likely to be intended to bring about changes in the state or motion of vital essence, or to promote courage or sexual vigor, as it is to alleviate a physical symptom of illness. An herbal rubdown or sweeping may be used to draw out a fever or put an end to respiratory symptoms, as well as to deal with spiritual or metaphysical aspects of illness.

Religious and Spiritual Actions

Religious and spiritual actions commonly used to promote health and healing include prayer, meditation, reading or recitation of sacred texts, recitation of verbal charms and brief formulaic utterances to ward off evil influences, laying on of hands, offerings of food and other goods to ancestors and other spiritual entities, visits to holy sites and healing shrines, temporary internment in places of worship or spiritual contemplation, spiritual cleansings, soul callings and restorations, use of amulets and other protective items, and a huge array of additional actions too numerous and varied to list completely. Physical practices such as *tai chi* or *qi gong* (exercises that entail voluntary control of the movement of *qi* in the body) are undertaken to promote spiritual as well as physical well-being. Prescription or administration of botanical medicaments may occur in a religious healing setting, such as a *santería* "reading" (spiritual diagnostic encounter) or celebratory service. Specific herbs or other material substances may also be taken internally or applied externally to achieve spiritual health ends, and any therapeutic action taken to promote balance (e.g., needling of particular acupuncture points, dietary changes, behavioral recommendations) may be intended to promote spiritual health and harmony.

Physical Therapies

Massage and rubbing are physical therapies found in a majority of immigrant healing traditions. Differing styles of massage follow a variety of underlying explanatory models. For example, abdominal massage is used in Mexican and Mexican American healing traditions to bring about specifically physical ends: alleviation of intestinal gas or of muscle pain and cramping, or release of stuck digestive products that are thought to adhere to the stomach lining, causing the folk illness *empacho* (Harwood, 1981; Schreiber & Homiak, 1981; Trotter, 1985). The southeast Asian massage style usually rendered in English as "acupressure" uses digital or manual pressure on energy meridians and points to remove blockages in the flow and make alterations in the behavior of *qi*.

Cupping is a treatment technique found in many cultural traditions. Small cups, tubes, or jars made of metal, wood, bamboo, or glass are heated and placed on the skin—most often on the back and upper shoulders. The heating process creates a vacuum, and the cups adhere to the skin by suction, drawing the skin underneath them up into a rise. When the cups cool sufficiently for the suction to be broken, they self-detach. This treatment usually leaves round, red marks or ecchymoses on the treated area. Depending on the cultural tradition, the treatment is intended to draw impurities, "bad blood," or "wind" (southeast Asian traditions) out of the body through the skin (Duong, 1987). If blood is specifically to be released, small cuts may be made in the skin before placement of the cups, and may be visible afterwards in the center of the residual marks.

Dermabrasion with the edge of a lubricated spoon or other implement, or with a lubricated coin (and for this reason called "coining" in English) is another physical therapy found in southeast Asian healing systems. Its purpose is typically to remove "wind" in the body—a serious health risk that can cause such a variety of diseases as "dizziness, stroke, spasm, vertigo, urticaria, pruritis, cold cough [*sic*], sore throat, arthritis, allergies, and neurologic problems" (Duong, 1987, p. 239). As with cupping, dermabrasive techniques usually leave reddened marks or bruises, again a sign of the "wind" rising to the surface of the body to be dissipated. The marks made by coining are typically striations. The marks of cupping and coining, together with small burns or blisters that may result from moxibustion, have been mistaken in the United States for signs of abuse, especially when seen on children (Yeatman & Dang, 1980; Yeatman, Shaw, Barlow, & Bennett, 1976).

Practitioners

Self-care or family care and home-based first aid account for a great proportion of all healing actions, in both immigrant and native-born populations. In most immigrant healing traditions, common household items such as eggs, lemons, or garlic and other foodstuffs are used medicinally and their proper preparation and applications tend to be matters of general knowledge. Many U.S. immigrant households maintain an herb or medicine garden, even in fairly challenging urban environments and cold climates. Although there are nearly always some changes in the garden inventory in the new homeland, medicinal plants and their seeds come with immigrants as important possessions and prized resources (U.S. Agricultural Service regulations to the contrary notwithstanding). Plants that will grow here, indoors or out, are carefully tended; new arrivals to established immigrant communities help to replenish supplies of medicinals that cannot readily be grown or acquired here.

Specialist practitioners are found in most systems. These commonly include midwives, massagers, bonesetters, blood-stoppers, healers of burns and other skin conditions, spiritual specialists, and herbalists or "leaf doctors" (see LaGuerre, 1981, 1987). The knowledge and practice of herbalists typically extends to animal and mineral natural substances in addition to botanicals. Chinese "herbalism," for example, includes such nonbotanical substances as deer antler, bear gall bladder, rhinoceros horn, and dried insects and reptiles of various kinds. The *curandero/a* ("healer"), well known in most Spanish-speak-

ing cultures, is often a general practitioner, using both material and spiritual modalities to treat an array of ills. Some *curanderos* specialize in spiritual problems, or the spiritual aspects of common illnesses (Trotter & Chavira, 1981). Spiritualist healers and mediums (found in many Latino traditions) carry out their diagnostic and healing activities with the aid of spirit guides who come to them with information (see Harwood, 1977; Trotter & Chavira, 1981), while shamanic healers enter trance states or make ecstatic journeys into the spirit realm to receive diagnostic and etiologic information and to negotiate with supernaturals for the well-being of their patients (Brainard & Zaharlick, 1989; Mottin, 1984).

Pluralism of Health Care Resources

The typical pattern of use of available health care resources for immigrant populations in the United States is pluralistic, incorporating a variety of traditional healing resources as well as biomedical ones. For some groups, this was the normative pattern in their home countries and it represents nothing new in their resettlement; for others, the addition of biomedicine or the augmentation of its role provides a new alternative. (It should be noted in this connection that referring to indigenous healing practices as "alternative" assumes biomedicine to be the norm and other practices to be departures from that norm. From the perspective of those immigrants who have not had previous extensive experience with the biomedical system, it is biomedicine that is "alternative," and it may be regarded with much caution and skepticism.) The extent to which specific groups have made use of traditional healing systems in their countries of origin and their extent of familiarity with biomedicine prior to immigration appear to vary by social class for many populations.

Education and Health Care Pluralism

Pre-immigration variation in familiarity with and acceptance of biomedine is attributable largely to the correlation of social class with patterns of rural or urban residence and the concentration of biomedical resources in urban middle- and upper-class areas in many countries. Preferential use of biomedicine or of traditional resources does not correlate reliably with formal educational attainment, since in many countries health care is pluralistic at all social class levels and (at least some major aspects of) traditional systems are well accepted and influential across the board (Assanand *et al.,* 1990; Behjati-Sabet, 1990; Brainard & Zaharlick, 1989; Dinh *et al.,* 1990; Gould-Martin & Ngin, 1981; Jenkins *et al.,* 1996; Lai & Yue, 1990; Miller, 1990; Ramakrishna & Weiss, 1992; Stephenson, 1995). In these circumstances, biomedicine is but one of many available resources for health care. This is an important point for American health professionals to bear in mind, in view of the pervasive belief in the United States that higher education correlates positively with preferential acceptance of biomedicine.

Acculturation and Health Care Pluralism

It has long been assumed that the traditional healing systems of immigrants coming to the United States and other developed nations would (and should) in due course be replaced by biomedicine, as part of the process of acculturation. As a corollary, the degree of rejection or abandonment of traditional health beliefs and practices, accompanied by acceptance of biomedicine, has been presumed to be a measure of acculturation—what Stephenson (1995, p. 1636) has called the "compliance model of assimilation." Such a replacement has not come about, as the continued vigor of healing traditions closely associated with specific cultural heritage groups clearly demonstrates (Hufford, 1984; O'Connor, 1995). These health care resources continue to be much used even when immigrants have access to health insurances, as in the United States, or free biomedical health care, as in Canada, but must defray

the costs of their traditional care completely out of pocket (O'Connor, 1995; Stephenson, 1995).

Degree of acculturation or assimilation cannot reliably be correlated with continued use of traditional healing methods (Castro *et al.,* 1984; Jenkins *et al.,* 1996; Miller, 1990; Nall & Speilberg, 1978; Tripp-Reimer, 1983). Indeed, Miller (1990) reported that among her study population of Korean immigrants the most assimilated and most highly educated were more likely than others to seek the services of acupuncturists and traditional herbalists. Recent discoveries regarding use of complementary and alternative medicine (CAM) by "mainstream," and thoroughly acculturated, American populations similarly reveal substantial use of nonbiomedical health care options; indeed CAM resources are most used, and used in the greatest variety, by the well-educated middle class (Astin, 1998; Eisenberg *et al.,* 1993). These findings suggest that, across populations, "the conflict between modern knowledge and alternative practice has been overstated" (Hufford, 1995, p. 57).

Patterns of Resort

The pursuit of relief from troublesome health conditions prompts people of any ethnicity or national origin to pursue combinations or sequences of remedial actions, and to continue—and diversify—their efforts until the desired result is attained. Unless the initial presenting symptoms are very alarming, it is likely that first recourse is to home-based first aid measures, such as herbs, teas, and soups, special foods, rest, over-the-counter preparations (which, depending on the community, may be manufactured or natural products, or both), and so forth. If these measures are not sufficiently effective, others may be added or substituted. For instance, the local herbalist may be consulted to verify, augment, or replace one's home herbal efforts; another general or specialist traditional practitioner may be consulted; or the medical doctor may be paid a visit. Any of these resources may be used either sequentially or simultaneously, and addition of new resources does not necessarily replace use of prior ones.

The order in which various resources are brought to bear on a particular health problem may vary along several dimensions: by cultural pattern, by ethnicity, by generation, by gender, by illness type, by particular illness episode, by availability and access, and, of course, by individual preference. Immigrant groups in the United States retain use of their indigenous healing resources even as they add or increase their use of conventional biomedicine, and individuals apply the same forms of reasoning to their decisions about when to use both biomedical and indigenous modalities.

If an illness is acute or the symptoms severe, members of several Asian groups may turn to biomedicine early on, as it is felt to be especially well suited to these circumstances (Ramakrishna & Weiss, 1992; Stephenson, 1995). Participants in the Haitian folk healing system may be inclined to start with simultaneous use of medical help for symptom control and other avenues for spiritual or supernatural intervention, since the sudden and acute onset of an illness may indicate supernatural elements in its etiology (LaGuerre, 1981). The etiologic explanation of the illness is crucial to the healing strategy. Illnesses with etiologic factors not addressed by biomedicine (spiritual causes, sorcery, imbalances of humors, innate qualities, and so forth) will be treated with modalities that properly address these issues, quite often together with medical therapy. Similarly, if biomedicine is thought to address symptoms but not root causes, systems will be combined for most complete benefit. Each system provides a part of what is needed for optimal recovery.

Studies in the literature record some patterns of resort that suggest underlying rules of thumb applicable across groups. For several Asian populations, for example, traditional healing methods seem to be preferred for chronic and degenerative illnesses, and biomedicine for acute ones (Assanand et al.,

1990; Okabe et al., 1990; Ramakrishna & Weiss, 1992; Stephenson, 1995). In a population of Vietnamese refugees in Canada, biomedicine tended to be preferred for treating infectious diseases and traditional methods for functional disorders, colds, and influenza (Stephenson, 1995). It must be stressed in this connection, however, that population-based data are not reliable predictors for the behavior of particular individual members.

Ethnic and religious diversity in immigrant populations contribute to the formation of differing patterns of resort. Among southeast Asian groups, for example, Brainard and Zaharlick (1989) found that ethnic Lao refugees in Franklin county, Ohio, tended to show the greatest use of the biomedical system and the lowest reliance on traditional healers, while Hmong refugees (also from Laos) showed the reverse pattern. Cambodian refugees in the study had relatively high rates of use of the biomedical system and did not appear to demonstrate any overall preference for either their traditional system or biomedicine, and Vietnamese refugees tended to begin with indigenous resources and move to biomedicine only when these failed (Brainard & Zaharlick, 1989). Religious and philosophical convictions, such as the Buddhist expectation that a certain amount of discomfort and even suffering are normative and to be expected in life, the Islamic acceptance that illness and other events of serious consequence are in the hands of God (Behjati-Sabet, 1990), or the Taoist view that "when things are permitted to take their natural course, they move toward perfection and harmony" (Nguyen, 1985, p. 410) help to shape health interventions and responses to illness.

Traditional Explanatory Models and Conventional Biomedicine

One important aspect of the conjoint use of biomedical and traditional healing resources is the application of culturally specific explanatory models of health and illness to both systems, often with the result that biomedical therapies are mitigated and sometimes modified by traditional resources and reasoning. For example, in hot/cold conceptual systems, prescription and over-the-counter pharmaceuticals are commonly assimilated to the hot/cold categories. Hot prescription medications may not be taken if the illness is itself a hot condition, or they may be discontinued if they produce side effects suggesting that they have brought about an over-hot state (Dinh *et al.,* 1990; Harwood, 1981; Ramakrishna & Weiss, 1992; Trotter, 1985).

If pharmaceuticals are felt to be producing an imbalance, they may be continued but counteracted by other actions or substances (Ramakrishna & Weiss, 1992; Stephenson, 1995) as long as their adverse unbalancing effect does not go too far. In several southeast Asian cultures Western pharmaceuticals are felt in general to be very strong—perhaps too strong for the Asian constitution or body type and size, or to be hot by nature and hard on the body. To mediate these potantially harmful qualities, dosages may be reduced or the duration of medication time shortened (or both), or a course of prescription medication may be followed or accompanied by one or more traditional remedies to counteract the hot properties of the drug and help revitalize the constitution (Dinh *et al.,* 1990; Nguyen, 1985; Stephenson, 1995).

Traditional Healing Systems and the Barrier Theory

It is a common concern among health professionals, and a frequently expressed speculation in the literature, that existence and persistence of traditional health beliefs and practices among immigrant and refugee populations may act as barriers to use of biomedical services. Education about the benefits of biomedical preventive and therapeutic measures is proposed as an important countermeasure to reduce "underutilization" of services. (Appropriate and adequate service utilization are calculated from the biomedical perspective.) To date, however, only one empirical study of this contention has been pub-

lished, and its findings do not support "the hypothesis that traditional beliefs and practices act as barriers to access to Western medical care or to utilization of preventive services" (Jenkins *et al.,* 1996, p. 1054; see also DeSantis & Thomas, 1990).

In an interview study of 215 Vietnamese immigrants in San Francisco and Alameda counties, California, Jenkins and colleagues (1996) found that traditional health beliefs and practices were common, but were not correlated with any health care access variables but one: "[t]hose who reported more traditional health beliefs were slightly more likely to have a regular doctor" (p. 1052). Having a regular doctor, in turn, was the most consistent predictor of use of conventional preventive health care services. Overall, there was no evidence that interviewees reporting more traditional health beliefs and practices were less likely to use conventional preventive health services as a result of their continued acceptance of traditional healing methods. This discovery suggests, in turn, that there is no reason to suppose that the traditional Vietnamese explanatory model of illness is harmful or that attempts should be made to change it (Jenkins *et al.,* 1996), a finding with potent implications for health professionals, health educators, and health services researchers.

Definition, Meaning, and Cultural Authority

Cultural values provide the foundations for definitions of and meanings attached to health, illness, and care. In some cultures, for example, even slight symptoms are considered adequate justification for initiating treatment or seeking medical or other professional health care advice (Okabe *et al.,* 1990), while in others a person is hardly to be defined as truly ill or in need of remedial intervention unless incapacitated or unable to carry out usual duties and activities (DeSantis, 1993; Duong, 1987; Thao, 1986). Attention and concern may focus more intensely on some body systems or sets of symptoms than on others. For example, blood and its condition and functions are a focal point in Haitian culture (LaGuerre, 1981); gastrointestinal symptoms in Mexican culture (Schreiber & Homiak, 1981); *qi* and its states of flow in traditional Chinese medicine (Kaptchuk, 1983); humoral equilibrium in the Ayurvedic tradition of the Indian subcontinent (Ramakrishna & Weiss, 1992); respiratory symptoms in Puerto Rican culture (Harwood, 1981); and symptoms produced by "wind" in the body in Vietnamese tradition (Duong, 1987).

Matters of value and meaning are always matters of cultural authority. This has implications for health services design for immigrant populations, inasmuch as American determinations of what constitutes proper and appropriate care may not be shared by patients with other cultural values, both in terms of addressing etiological concerns, as we have seen, and in terms of meeting expectations for care (see, e.g., Arruda, Larson, & Meleis, 1992). A good illustration comes from a fieldwork interview of mine with a young Hmong woman in Philadelphia, who expressed confusion as to the motives of American physicians and nurses who seemed to her to put unwarranted pressures on Hmong women (herself included) to come to medical offices for prenatal care, and who assumed, apparently, that women who did not come to medical offices frequently during their pregnancies were not receiving prenatal care.

She wondered if these health professionals were unaware (and if so, why they were) that older Hmong women assiduously see to the special health requirements of young pregnant women: monitoring their diets, dress, and activities; administering herbs and other medicaments; tracking physical and emotional changes; and giving instruction and advice, to protect against risks and promote optimal health for both mother and baby (M.C., author interview, 1993). In the traditional Hmong view, prenatal care is also considered important, but it is administered by older female relatives and community members, and is not considered a medical matter.

The ministrations, wisdom, and direct personal experience of these women are likely to be more highly valued by traditional Hmong women as sources of prenatal care and advice than are those of doctors (particularly male doctors). In the American health professional view, prenatal care is by definition a medical matter, and the technical training and expertise of health professionals is more highly valued than the advice and attentions of even very experienced laypersons. This mismatch in values and definitions can lead to an unwitting standoff, in which the health professional is urging prenatal care on a woman who is, in her view, already receiving it. Even when the differences are articulated, the difference in values and attribution of cultural authority may lead the prospective patient to decline the recommended medical service.

Variation, Change, and Diversity

Descriptions of culturally specific systems of values, beliefs, and practices must be understood to be descriptions of cultural *repertoires* of possibilities (O'Connor, 1995) and not of "what [name of group] believe or do." Just as there are tremendous differences among groups, there is substantial variability within any cultural group, with different individuals drawing in varied ways from the available cultural repertoire. The term "cultural diversity," nowadays so prominent in both professional and popular parlance, should be understood to have a dual meaning, referring as much to diversity *within* cultures as among them.

As acculturative processes exert their influences, it is likely that intragroup variability will increase. Changes will occur in the healing systems themselves, by virtue of inaccessibility of certain herbs or substances in the country of resettlement, changes in illness patterns in new locations and circumstances, unavailability of some traditional specialists in resettlement communities, interaction with biomedicine and other cultural influences, and so on. Healing traditions, always dynamic in their indigenous settings, continue to be so in diaspora. Individual responses, both to acculturation and to the changed healing systems, are variable: some will continue wholeheartedly to embrace traditional ways; some will accept certain changes, but not others; some will reject practice but retain philosophical underpinnings (and others vice versa); some will at varying paces leave the indigenous healing tradition behind.

Generational succession again increases variability. Some third- and fourth-generation offspring (and beyond) will no longer have any familiarity with the indigenous tradition; some will retain parts of it; others may seek, embrace, and reinvigorate it as part of an affirmation or reestablishment of cultural or ethnic identity. Enough participation in indigenous healing systems typically persists to assure their perpetuation in the cultural repertoire through many successive generations, as individual identity-group members selectively continue to use the systems as active health care options.

Conclusion

Among the many cultural resources that immigrants bring with them to their countries of resettlement are systems of health promotion and healing that are interwoven with their broader cultural worldview. These systems have longstanding reputations for efficacy rooted in generations of experience and observation. They carry substantial cultural authority, and provide articulated theories of health, illness, and care that are quite often incongruent with the biomedical model. Recent research suggests that there is no necessary or predictable correlation between continued acceptance of indigenous healing systems and level of acculturation to the host culture, and that, contrary to prior presumption, persistence of traditional health beliefs and practices does not necessarily act as a barrier to use of biomedical services. This finding calls into question the common supposition that traditional systems' explanatory models are potentially harmful and should be changed through health education.

The adaptive process of acculturation is "a cultural negotiation that [involves] all aspects of life, including that dealing with health" (Kraut, 1994, p. 281). Multiple studies indicate that the typical pattern of use of health care resources for immigrants is plural, integrating both traditional and biomedical resources in a system of self-triage based on articulable explanatory models and etiological and therapeutic principles. For some groups this continues a pattern followed in their countries of origin; for others it is novel. Health professionals can gain much through understanding the cultural repertoires of their immigrant patient populations, while bearing in mind that the knowledge of the repertoire is not predictive of the belief or behavior of individual members of the culture. Immigrants' healing systems are important cultural and community resources, and are best recognized as such by health professionals. Additional services believed important or essential by American providers are likely to meet with the greatest success in immigrant patient populations when offered in culturally responsive and culturally appropriate ways that make an effort to supplement, rather than to supplant, valued healing traditions.

References

Arruda, E. N., Larson, P. J., & Meleis, A. I. (1992). Comfort: Immigrant hispanic cancer patients' views. *Cancer Nursing, 15*(6), 387–394.

Assanand, S., Dias, M., Richardson, E., & Waxler-Morrison, N. (1990). The South Asians. In N. Waxler-Morrison, J. M. Anderson, & E. Richardson (Eds.), *Cross-cultural caring: A handbook for health professionals in Western Canada* (pp. 141–180). Vancouver, British Columbia, Canada: University of British Columbia Press.

Astin, J. A. (1998). Why patients use alternative medicines. *Journal of the American Medical Association, 279,* 1548–1553.

Behjati-Sabet, A. (1990). The Iranians. In N. Waxler-Morrison, J. M. Anderson, & E. Richardson (Eds.),

Cross-cultural caring: A handbook for health professionals in Western Canada (pp. 91–115). Vancouver, British Columbia, Canada: University of British Columbia Press.

Beinfiend, H., & Korngold, E. (1991). *Between heaven and earth: A guide to Chinese medicine.* New York: Ballantine.

Bell, S. E., & Whiteford, M. (1987). Tai Dam health care practices: Asian refugee women in Iowa. *Social Science and Medicine, 24*(4), 317–325.

Bliatout, B. T. (1982). *Hmong sudden unexpected nocturnal death syndrome: A cultural study.* Portland, OR: Sparkle.

Boyle, J. S. (1989). Constructs of health promotion and wellness in a Salvadoran population. *Public Health Nursing, 6*(3), 129–134.

Brainard, J., & Zaharlick, A. (1989). Changing health beliefs and behaviors of resettled Laotian refugees: Ethnic variation in adaptation. *Social Science and Medicine, 29*(7), 845–852.

Castro, F. G., Furth, P., & Karlow, H. (1984). The health beliefs of Mexican, Mexican American and Anglo American women. *Hispanic Journal of Behavioral Sciences, 6*(4), 365–383.

Chindarsi, N. (1976). *The religion of the Hmong Njua.* Bangkok, Thailand: Siam Society.

DeSantis, L. (1993). Haitian immigrant concepts of health. *Health Values: Achieving High Level Wellness, 17*(6), 3–16.

DeSantis, L., & Thomas, J. T. (1990). The immigrant Haitian mother: Transcultural nursing perspective on preventive health care for children. *Journal of Transcultural Nursing,* 2(1), 2–15.

Davis, E. W. (1988). *Passage of darkness: The ethnobiology of the Haitian zombie.* Chapel Hill: University of North Carolina Press.

Dinh, D.-K., Ganesan, S., & Waxler-Morrison, N. (1990). The Vietnamese. In N. Waxler-Morrison, J. M. Anderson, & E. Richardson (Eds.), *Cross-cultural caring: A handbook for health professionals in Western Canada* (pp. 181–213). Vancouver, British Columbia, Canada: University of British Columbia Press.

Duong, V. H. (1987). The Indochinese patient. In R. B. Birrer (Ed.), *Urban family medicine* (pp. 238–242). New York: Springer-Verlag.

Egeland, J. A. (1978). Ethnic value orientation analysis. In *Miami Health Ecology Project report* (Vol. 2). Miami, FL: University of Miami.

Eisenberg, D. M., Kessler, R. C., Foster, C., Norlock, F. E., Calkins, D. R., & Delbanco, T. L. (1993). Unconventional medicine in the United States. *New England Journal of Medicine, 328*(Jan. 28), 246–252.

Geddes, W. R. (1976). *Migrants of the mountains: The cultural ecology of the Blue Miao (Hmong Njua) of Thailand.* Oxford, England: Clarendon/Oxford University Press.

Glasgow, J. H., & Adaskin, E. (1990). The West Indians. In N. Waxler-Morrison, J. M. Anderson, & E. Rich-

ardson (Eds.), *Cross-cultural caring: A handbook for health professionals in Western Canada* (pp. 214–244). Vancouver, British Columbia, Canada: University of British Columbia Press.

Gleave, D., & Manes, A. S. (1990). The Central Americans. In N. Waxler-Morrison, J. M. Anderson, & E. Richardson (Eds.), *Cross-cultural caring: A handbook for health professionals in Western Canada* (pp. 36–67). Vancouver, British Columbia, Canada: University of British Columbia Press.

Gould-Martin, K., & Ngin, C. (1981). Chinese Americans. In A. Harwood (Ed.), *Ethnicity and medical care* (pp. 130–171). Cambridge, MA: Harvard University Press.

Harwood, A. (1971). The hot/cold theory of disease: Implications for the treatment of Puerto Rican patients. *Journal of the American Medical Association, 216,* 1153–1158.

Harwood, A. (1977). *Rx: Spiritist as needed: A study of a Puerto Rican community mental health resource.* Ithaca, NY: Cornell University Press.

Harwood, A. (1981). Mainland Puerto Ricans. In A. Harwood (Ed.), *Ethnicity and medical care* (pp. 397–481). Cambridge, MA: Harvard University Press.

Hufford, D. J. (1984). *American healing systems: An introduction and exploration.* Hershey: Pennsylvania State University School of Medicine.

Hufford, D. J. (1988). Contemporary folk medicine. In N. Gevitz (Ed.), *Other healers: Unorthodox medicine in America* (pp. 228–264). Baltimore: Johns Hopkins University Press.

Hufford, D. J. (1992). Folk medicine in contemporary America. In J. Kirkland, H. Mathews, C. W. Sullivan, III, & K. Baldwin (Eds.), *Herbal and magical medicine: Traditional healing today* (pp. 14–31). Durham, NC: Duke University Press.

Hufford, D. J. (1995). Cultural and social perspectives on alternative medicine: Background and assumptions. *Alternative Therapies in Health and Medicine, 1*(1), 53–61.

Jenkins, C. N. H., Le, T., McPhee, S., Stewart, S., & Ngoc, T. H. (1996). Health care access and preventive care among Vietnamese immigrants: Do traditional beliefs and practices pose barriers? *Social Science and Medicine, 43*(7), 1049–1056.

Kaptchuk, T. (1983). *The web that has no weaver: Understanding Chinese medicine.* New York: Congdon and Weed.

Kleinman, A. (1975). Explanatory models in health care relationships. In National Council for International Health, *Health of the family* (pp. 159–172). Washington, DC: National Council for International Health.

Kleinman, A. (1984). Indigenous systems of healing: Questions for professional, popular, and folk care. In J. W. Salmon (Ed.), *Alternative medicines—popular and policy perspectives* (pp. 251–258). New York: Tavistock.

Kraut, A. M. (1990). Immigrant attitudes toward physicians in America. *Journal of the American Medical Association, 263*(April 4), 1807–1811.

Kraut, A. M. (1994). *Silent travelers: Germs, genes and the "immigrant menace."* Baltimore: Johns Hopkins University Press.

LaGuerre, M. S. (1981). Haitian Americans. In A. Harwood (Ed.), *Ethnicity and medical care* (pp. 172–210). Cambridge, MA: Harvard University Press.

LaGuerre, M. S. (1987). *Afro-Caribbean folk medicine.* South Hadley, MA: Bergin & Garvey.

Lai, M. C., & Yue, K.-M. K. (1990). The Chinese. In N. Waxler-Morrison, J. M. Anderson, & E. Richardson (Eds.), *Cross-cultural caring: A handbook for health professionals in Western Canada* (pp. 68–90). Vancouver, British Columbia, Canada: University of British Columbia Press.

Lock, M., & Gordon, D. (Eds.). (1988). *Biomedicine examined.* Dordrecht, The Netherlands: Kluwer Academic.

Marr, D. G. (1987). Vietnamese attitudes regarding illness and healing. In N. G. Owen (Ed.), *Death and disease in Southeast Asia* (pp. 162–186). Oxford, England: Oxford University Press, 1987.

Métraux, A. J. (1972). *Voodoo in Haiti.* New York: Schocken.

Miller, J. K. (1990). Use of traditional Korean health care by Korean immigrants to the United States. *Sociology and Social Research, 75*(1), 38–48.

Moon, A., & Tashima, N. (1982). Help seeking behavior and attitudes of southeast Asian refugees [Report typescript]. San Francisco: Pacific Asian Mental Health Research Project.

Mottin, J. (1984). A Hmong shaman's séance. *Asian Folklore Studies, 43,* 99–108.

Nall, F., & Spielberg, J. (1978). Social and cultural factors in the responses of Mexican-Americans to medical treatment. In R. A. Martinez (Ed.), *Hispanic culture and health care: Fact, fiction, folklore* (pp. 000–000). St. Louis, MO: Mosby.

Nguyen, M. D. (1985). Culture shock—A review of Vietnamese culture and its concepts of health and disease. *Western Journal of Medicine, 142,* 409–412.

Novack, G. (1987). Medical practice among Haitians. In R. B. Birrer (Ed.), *Urban family medicine* (pp. 235–237). New York: Springer-Verlag.

O'Connor, B. B. (1995). *Healing traditions: Alternative medicine and the health professions.* Philadelphia: University of Pennsylvania Press.

Okabe, T., Takahashi, K., & Richardson, E. (1990). The Japanese. In N. Waxler-Morrison, J. M. Anderson, & E. Richardson (Eds.), *Cross-cultural caring: A handbook for health professionals in Western Canada* (pp. 116–140). Vancouver, British Columbia, Canada: University of British Columbia Press.

Pang, K. Y. C. (1990). *Hwabyung:* The construction of a Korean popular illness among Korean elderly immigrant women in the United States. *Culture, Medicine and Psychiatry, 14,* 495–512.

Payer, L. (1988). *Medicine and culture: Varieties of treatment in the United States, England, West Germany, and France.* New York: Penguin Books.

Ragucci, A. J. (1981). Italian Americans. In A. Harwood (Ed.), *Ethnicity and medical care* (pp. 211–263). Cambridge, MA: Harvard University Press.

Ramakrishna, J., & Weiss, M. G. (1992). Health, illness, and immigration. East Indians in the United States. *Western Journal of Medicine, 157*(3), 265–270.

Rubel, A. J. (1964). The epidemiology of a folk illness: *Susto* in Hispanic America. *Ethnology, 3*(3), 268–283.

Rubel, A. J., O'Nell, C., & Collado-Ardón, R. (1984). *Susto: A folk illness.* Berkeley: University of California Press.

Schreiber, J. M., & Homiak, J. P. (1981). Mexican Americans. In A. Harwood (Ed.), *Ethnicity and medical care* (pp. 264–336). Cambridge, MA: Harvard University Press.

Simons, R. C., & Hughes, C. C. (1985). *The culture-bound syndromes: Folk illnesses of psychiatric and anthropological interest.* Dordrecht, The Netherlands: Reidel.

Sivin, N. (1987). *Traditional medicine in contemporary China.* Ann Arbor: University of Michigan, Center for Chinese Studies.

Stein, H. F. (1990). *American medicine as culture.* Boulder, CO: Westview.

Stephenson, P. H. (1995). Vietnamese refugees in Victoria, B. C.: An overview of immigrant and refugee health care in a medium-sized Canadian urban centre. *Social Science and Medicine, 40*(12), 1631–1642.

Thao, X. (1986). Hmong perception of illness and traditional ways of healing. In G. L. Hendricks, B. T. Downing, & A. Deinard (Eds.), *The Hmong in transition* (pp. 365–378). New York: Center for Migration Studies of New York and Southeast Asian Refugee Studies Project of the University of Minnesota.

Tripp-Reimer, T. (1983). Retention of a folk-healing practice (matiasma) among four generations of urban Greek immigrants. *Nursing Research, 32*(2), 97–101.

Trotter, R. T., III. (1985). Folk medicine in the Southwest: Myths and medical facts. *Postgraduate Medicine, 78*(8), 167–179.

Trotter, T. R., III, & Chavira, J. A. (1981). *Curanderismo: Mexican American folk healing.* Athens: University of Georgia Press.

Yeatman, G. W., & Dang, V. V. (1980). Cao gio (coin rubbing): Vietnamese attitudes towards health care. *Journal of the American Medical Association, 244,* 2748–2749.

Yeatman, G. W., Shaw, C., Barlow, M. J., & Bartlett, G. (1976). Pseudobattering in Vietnamese children. *Pediatrics, 58*(4), 616–618.

Zhang, Q., & Hsu, H.-Y. (1990). *AIDS and Chinese medicine: Applications of the oldest medicine to the newest disease.* Long Beach, CA: OHAI.

9

The Role of the Family and the Community in the Clinical Setting

CAROL R. HOROWITZ

Introduction

When providers care for immigrant patients or clients, we are usually working with human beings whose backgrounds, values, health seeking behaviors, and coping strategies strongly differ from our own. In order to accomplish our goals of reducing suffering, improving quality of life, and helping them gain or develop control over their health, we clearly need biomedical information. This must be supplemented by information about patients' social and economic situations and their beliefs and values, as these are strongly related to their mental and physical health and our ability to provide effective care.

Health workers, however, often know little about where and with whom their patients live, or their life stories. As health care becomes more technical and cost motivated, we have less time and opportunity to get to know patients and to focus on nontechnical aspects of care. We are often taught to reduce patients' subjective experiences of illness into

objective terms, which can be counted, weighed, imaged, and compared with a "normal" standard. We are taught to focus on smaller and smaller pieces of the human puzzle in order to learn the truth about human illness.

Unfortunately, we may be left with an unsettling feeling, as we focus on a patient's electrolyte imbalances, aching backs, legal and insurance problems, but do not truly understand why our patient is suffering. If we pull our lens back and view patients not merely as autonomous physical beings, but as members of families and communities, we can begin to uncover root causes of problems and develop appropriate, practical approaches to their needs.

There are several reasons we should focus on getting to know our patients' families and communities. First, such knowledge can help us improve our ability to directly meet the biomedical and psychosocial needs of our patients. This may be through helping us understand symptoms and health behaviors or through learning about common conditions from their country of origin. Second, we can learn effective and respectful ways to communicate with members of our patients' culture, which can both enhance our ability to deliver quality care and help us avoid a feeling of

CAROL R. HOROWITZ • Departments of Health Policy and Medicine, Mount Sinai Medical Center, New York, New York 10029.

Handbook of Immigrant Health, edited by Loue. Plenum Press, New York, 1998.

"getting nowhere." Third, such knowledge can enlighten us about problems that involve our patients' families and community, such as violence and unemployment. These are inseparable from health problems and it is impossible to improve certain individual conditions without addressing them. Finally, patients, families, and communities have problems that they can begin to solve if they are given some power and control over their situations.

Patients come from cultures with histories and traditions as resilient as our personal and medical cultures. Just as we cannot view an organ in isolation from the rest of the human body (e.g., we cannot treat heart disease without examining a person's diet, stress, and exercise levels), we should not work with an individual without recognizing and understanding the person's family and community. In developing ties with communities so that we can understand their unique concerns and experiences, and working with families to learn about patients' situations and cultures, we will be building some of the most important, informative, and rewarding partnerships of our careers. More important, we will have family and community members who share our goal of improving the lives of our patients, and who have knowledge, experience, and unique capabilities to effect meaningful improvements in culturally appropriate, effective delivery of health care.

The Importance of Immigrants' Families and Communities in the Clinical Setting

Cultural beliefs give meaning to health and illness experiences by providing the individual with culturally acceptable causes for illness, recognizing that something is wrong, interpreting what it might be, organizing a plan of action and a help seeking strategy, and determining desired outcomes (A. Kleinman, 1978). Most of these junctures occur in people's families and communities, not in a medical center. What is an ominous dream? A burning in the belly? Just as providers learn

differential diagnoses, patients have their own strategies for symptom recognition, diagnosis, and treatment. An individual in crisis or sickness will first make personal attempts to alleviate distress or illness. If this is unsuccessful, the person will enlist the support of family, social network, or community. If this fails, the individual will seek more formal channels. Patients use culturally defined explanatory models, in this context, to explore their health problems and decide among treatment alternatives.

All provider–patient encounters are cross-cultural experiences. With the triumph of scientific medicine, doctors and patients ceased sharing a similar view of the body and of the determinants of health and disease (Rosenberg, 1979). The biomedical model (the physician's folk model; Engel, 1981) commonly conflicts with the model for causation held by most laypersons. This is especially true when patients are from wholly different backgrounds or countries than their providers.

When patients leave their families and communities to visit heath workers, it is in a setting that is culturally different from that of the provider and that of the patient, with its own set of rules. In this environment, both the provider and the client aim to elucidate the reason for illness or the best way to maximize health, and to leave the encounter with a care plan that is acceptable in all three cultures (the patient's, the provider's, and the medical establishment's).

Health care providers to immigrants are commonly faced with interactions in which values, beliefs, and ways of communicating conflict with those of patients. Why does a Bengali man smile and nod that he understands and will do what we suggest, and then not appear to do anything? Why does an Eritrean woman insist on having someone else's permission before having a procedure when she is an autonomous adult? Why do Hmong parents refuse to consent to a lifesaving treatment for their child? Why is a Vietnamese man telling us about his dreams? We may react to such instances by distancing ourselves from patients or blaming the patient for being ignorant, noncompliant, unmotivated, difficult, or for wasting our time with insignificant problems.

As providers, we cannot simply use our personal understanding of the importance of family and community to gauge their importance for someone of a different background than ours. In health and illness, an ethnic group's shared beliefs, symbols, and customs serve as common reference points that members use to judge the appropriateness of their decisions and actions.

However, patients are not wholly products of their culture, just as they are not merely products of their biomedical composition. It is important not to exoticize and stereotype patients, their families, and their communities. There are idiosyncratic individualities that transcend cultural norms. There are variations both within and between cultures, and within and between generations that are due to extracultural factors, such as economic status, education, and experience. It is not necessary to generalize beliefs and practices to every member of a culture. "Although ethnicity captures the larger cultural component of human experiences, we must not permit our awareness of a culture to erode its member's individual identities and dignity" (Anderson, 1988).

The Role of Family

Family solidarity is an asset in coping with illness and health maintenance (Hott, 1977). As Whittaker said, "I don't believe in people any more, only in families—people are just bits of families" (Christie-Seely, 1984, p. 13). Family members can facilitate and provide care, report symptoms, assist in decision making, and help patients adopt healthy lifestyles and cope with illness. Alternatively, family issues may foster the development of stress-related illnesses and distract patients from obtaining needed care. It is important to assess an immigrant family's supports and the influence family members have on a patient's diagnosis and treatment. Providers can

learn to both solicit families' help and advice, and understand how family problems contribute to illness. "Whether the clinician likes it or not, what happens in the office with the individual patient will automatically affect the family. . . . The question, therefore, is not *whether* the clinician will intervene at the family level, but of *how* he or she will intervene" (p. 21; emphasis in original).

Definition of Family

A family is a group of two or more persons, joined by ties of blood, marriage, or adoption (formal or informal), that create and maintain a common culture. Family may include "relatives" who have helped or been part of important matters and events in the past. If a still wider view of family is adopted, one could include "natural support systems" (Delgado & Humm-Delgado, 1982) or "social networks" (Unger & Powell, 1980). These individuals and groups (relatives, friends, neighbors) band together to help each other. This may be a germane definition in refugee and immigrant communities where family friends or neighbors adopt a close kin role in lieu of dispersed family members.

Changes in Family with Immigration

The family is continually shaping and being shaped by the social forces surrounding it (Reinhardt & Quinn, 1977). Through immigration, resettlement, and acculturation, families fragment, schisms develop between generations, and there is a shift to focus on nuclear family. As families become more mobile, smaller isolated nuclear groups with fewer natural supports become responsible for larger shares of the economic and social burden. Nonetheless, support networks may be particularly important during times of stress, such as immigration or illness (Canino & Canino, 1982). Strong kinship bonds may also be necessary for survival in new and potentially hostile environments of immigrants.

Immigrant families may have different family structures and rely on family for functions we handle without family in our own cultures. They may have been raised in extended families and socialized for a life with close interdependency with several family members. Their family bonds may be different from those of many Americans. For example, in Asian families, vertical relationships (e.g., parent–child) often take precedence over horizontal relationships (e.g., husband–wife) and in other cultures women may rely most heavily on sisters or close female friends.

Intergenerational relationships will be affected by immigration. Family values are often less strongly held by second- and third-generation immigrants. These shifts may particularly affect older immigrants. Attitudes toward aging may change and intergenerational assistance may decline (Cox & Gelfand, 1987). Family "back home" was a center of power. With a breakdown of extended family structure and an emphasis on individualism, children may feel less obliged to take care of their aged parents and intolerant of an older family member's attempts to influence family decisions. However, immigrants may retain a traditional family value that children should take care of their older parents. Furthermore, professional and institutional assistance may be an alien concept for elderly persons who do not want to rely on others, do not know how to ask for help, or are hesitant to accept it from outsiders. A strong sense of family responsibilities can arouse shameful feelings in persons asking for external help (Cheung, 1989).

Social services for immigrant families often focus on assimilation, assuming that all newcomers want to assimilate. Immigrants may not want to give up their cultural values and assimilate. They may fear losing their cultural identity. These factors exaggerate the problems common to all elderly persons, including illiteracy, isolation, immobility, and a lack of service connections and may make them a particularly vulnerable immigrant population.

Families who do not have, or who lose family supports may also be among the most vulnerable. When minority patients lost informal (family) supports, they increased their use of formal services, suggesting that formal services may be a substitute for the help given by family members (Cox & Gelfand, 1987). Such families also may have language problems, fear of losing their cultural identity, and fear of or unfamiliarity with nonethnic environments. Studies of these problems stress that patient services should be provided in a simulated family setting, include peer support groups, be in a familiar and accessible place, not place too much emphasis on assimilation, and allow patient input (Lin *et al.*, 1991).

Even family members who remain devoted to one another may not be able to help in times of illness or crisis. They can become overwhelmed by their own responsibilities and not be able to assist in care, or be unable to help because of their own financial, time, intellectual, or emotional limitations. Others may encourage the patient to reject health care and prevention. In fact, they can inadvertently contribute to deterioration in care through misunderstandings or misconceptions.

Family's Response to and Role in Illness

Family structure, function, and the role of the family during illness differ considerably across cultures (Lock, 1984). This may affect the way illnesses are perceived, labeled, and handled. When ill, individuals will rely on different family members to different degrees depending on their culture and upbringing. Clinicians may inadvertently leave nontraditional but key "relatives" out of discussions, decision making, and informed consent.

Patients may need to cope with their illness in a new, foreign way and be expected to do so without their usual allies. For example, a person who needs to be hospitalized may be both unfamiliar with Western-style hospitals and separated from the family support system (who usually tend to sick relatives). In this environment, it is understandable that family members want to visit patients freely (not just during visiting hours), bring certain foods, and perform certain rituals (such as burning incense). If families are not allowed to do such things, and if clinicians allow only spouses to participate actively in care, tension and animosity may develop between patients, relatives, and the hospital staff.

Family's Role in Illness Prevention and Health Promotion

Most health prevention occurs outside of medical settings. Clinicians may recommend certain screening tests and dietary and lifestyle modifications, but the decision to comply with these recommendations and the likelihood they will be adhered to depend on patients and their families. Do they trust you? Do they understand the purpose of tests and other suggestions and think they are worthwhile and important? Do they have the knowledge, resources, and time to come for testing, alter their diet, or begin exercising?

Providers cannot learn the answers to these questions without having a rapport, not only with the patients, but also with the people with whom they live, eat, and make decisions. For example, foods can represent home and cultural solidarity to families. If clinicians want patients to lower caloric, fat, salt, or sugar intake, or to increase fluid and vegetable intake, they need to understand potential barriers. Families may adhere to traditional diets to maintain their cultural identity. They may have a different concept of being overweight (there is, to many, such a thing as "too thin"). They may be resistant to drinking water, either because it was a source of disease in their country of origin (as were fresh vegetables), or because they feel it will make them gain weight. They may not be able to afford fish, or certain vegetables, and they may not know how to cook the foods you consider nutritionally important. Although they think they are avoiding salt, they may be eating foods laden with salt (such as fish sauce) without being aware of the salt content.

In these cases, it important to first understand the family's current habits and beliefs. Who cooks, who shops, what is commonly eaten? With this information in hand, you can then suggest dietary alterations that are compatible with their traditional diet. Similarly, you can elicit their understanding of prevention and disease, and teach them why a screening test is important, how and where it will be done, who will do it (e.g., that a woman technician can perform a mammogram if modesty is a concern), and how the results will be used. Some East African patients believe blood drawing takes from them a large proportion of their blood, which may not be replaced; blood drawing therefore may contribute to illness. If you have this understanding in advance, you can preempt their concern with an explanation of why the test is important, and the facts that only a small amount of blood will be taken, the blood will be replaced in days, and the test results will be used in an important way.

Immigrant Families Have Problems Just as Nonimmigrant Families Do

In the family therapy literature, there is ample information about how individual problems affect families and how family problems affect individuals' health. Many health workers are not familiar with the relationship between families and health. Furthermore, family problems may appear different if they are manifested in a family with a different structure and culture. Therefore, these problems may be more difficult to identify and address in immigrant families. Diagnosis, treatment, and compliance may be improved by understanding how individual symptoms or illnesses support the disturbed functioning of the family.

A family member needs to be understood as part of a whole. Family problems result from the way family members relate to one another, not just from the behavior of a single person (Christie-Seely, 1984). Each person's actions affect others and a chain reaction can be set off. Family members then collaborate to keep conflicts going. Triangles tend to form in families so that if there is an unsettled conflict, another member (such as a child) is brought into the relationship to compensate.

The "typical" family problems commonly seen by family therapists may be exaggerated in immigrant families. As they adapt to their new environment, they may lose the external support and comfort they had, unmasking or exaggerating conflicts. Children, who often are more literate and the only English-speaking members of the family, may be pressured to take on parentlike roles of interacting with agencies and other groups. They may become involved in activities their parents do not understand or sanction, but which are accepted and expected in the new culture (e.g., dating, staying out late). They may lose the ability to communicate with their older relatives if they lose fluency in their native tongue as they become fluent in English. Older generations may feel abandoned, lost, and frustrated by their younger family members. Families who lose the ability to communicate and understand each member's interests and priorities are more vulnerable to developing problems.

Patients may have family issues that are not spurred by conflicts (such as those just outlined) and are not recognized as serious (such as abuse), but which are important and affect our ability to deliver health care. Patients may, for example, have family members who are missing, or who remained in their country of origin; this may result in reactive depression, tension, and financial hardship. The patient may have witnessed or heard about family members who died or were tortured, causing Posttraumatic Stress Disorder or other stress-related disorders. Immigrant families also have stress due to economic hardship, social isolation, and difficulty acculturating. Arab immigrants surveyed stated that family stress was one of the top five most prevalent health or illness problems that affected them or their families in the past year (Laffery *et al.*, 1989). In fact, much of the time the ability to stay healthy, given the hostile environments immigrants often come from, may be more remarkable than the fact that many immigrants have some symptom or other (Antanovsky, 1979).

Providers and patients may not think these family problems are in the medical purview, so they may not be shared. However, they will affect care seeking (i.e., by distracting a patient from complying with visits or therapies) and may cause somatic symptoms that are pursued unnecessarily with potentially harmful diagnostic tests and therapies. These somatic symptoms may often lead to unnecessary medical interventions because, while many American clinicians recognize culture-bound symptoms of stress common in the United States (e.g., tension headaches), we may be unaware of stress-related symptoms common in other countries and cultures, for example, urinary or abdominal burning.

Christie-Seeley (1984) suggested some simple guidelines for working with families in general, and these apply to immigrant families. Clinicians should (1) be nonjudgmental, not taking sides with one family member, (2) not compound family labeling by medical labels or diagnoses where these are unnecessary, (3) not collaborate to maintain triangulation or blame, (4) encourage communication among family members, (5) understand how illness and dysfunction repeat over generations, (6) be a therapeutic optimist, emphasizing family strengths and the ability to change.

Family as Decision Maker and Partner

While there is an individualistic tradition of self-reliance and independence prevalent in the United States, many cultures stress mutual dependency and family loyalty, insisting that the needs of the family should take precedence over any individual's need. Immigrant families may rely on family for functions we handle without family in our own cultures. Patients may be more closely dependent on family input in their health care. Illness is often considered a family rather than an individual problem. In fact, patient autonomy may be redefined as family autonomy for some immigrant groups (e.g., needing the family's permission or input to decide on or agree to a treatment). The Ethiopian family has been described as working as a unit to help patients obtain health care (Beyene, 1992).

Patients may even try to reach family members in remote villages, or refugee camps, before making decisions we consider urgent. Families influence patients' choices of type of care, provider, and treatments, both before and after we see them. This may explain why a patient does not comply with our recommendations, or why his or her decisions "mysteriously" change from one visit to the next.

Family's importance may dominate over individual members. Therefore, any information, including diagnostic facts is seen as belonging to the family. Family members often break bad news to the patient at an appropriate time and place. Leaving the family out of the loop in the care of such patients may be time efficient in the short run, but cause problems for the provider and the patient in the long run.

Furthermore, patients often hope or plan to return to their country of origin in the future, to rejoin their family. Decisions they make may reflect the place they hope to live, not the place they currently live. For example, a Somali woman may want her daughter to be circumcised because that practice is expected in Somalia (where she hopes her daughter will return), despite the fact that it is illegal in the United States.

Family as Support System

Families may be support systems to cope with stress and maintain health. Some social service groups consider such families at high risk for mental health problems precisely because they lack extended family supports. Elderly Hispanic immigrants revealed that family orientation was one of the six themes in their concept of good health. For them, this included having family to help and understand them and fulfilling a need to understand how their own illness would affect their family (Ailinger & Causey, 1995). Vietnamese refugees interviewed in the United States overwhelmingly stated that social support, fear of interacting with Americans, and marital status had significant direct effects on the their sense of well-being (Van Tran & Wright, 1986). A study assessing social aspects of refugee adjustment among Vietnamese in the United States (Haines, Rutherford, & Thomas, 1981) found that families had an unwavering dedication to extended family, providing unconditional assistance and even taking on jobs to be able to send packages back home. Individuals, in this group, were defined in terms of specific relations with other family members.

In a study of family involvement of Asians and Caucasians in the treatment of schizophrenic patients (Cheung, 1989), 69% of Asian patients had at least one family member and 46% had multiple family members accompany patient to sessions, versus 12% and 8% respectively for Caucasians. Cheung concluded that noncultural factors such as language difficulties and problems with transportation are not likely the main reasons for this difference. The involvement of immigrant family members represented a substantial effort and sacrifice. Asian families often are able to provide more constant and persistent emotional and material support to their sick members. Cheung also concluded that it is important to include family in the clinical evaluation, treatment planning, and continuing care of Asian psychiatric patients. Unfortunately, many clinicians do not involve or welcome family participation on a routine basis. In this population, neglect or rejection of the family will add to disruption of the therapeutic relationship. This may be one of the major reasons for the poor performance of many community mental health clinics in providing services to Asian patients.

Providers and Families

Immigrant families may close their boundaries to their new environment as a way of protecting their identity or integrity (Christie-Seeley, 1984). They may refuse to learn the language or customs of the new environment, prohibit children from associating with outsiders, or avoid health care settings. This may be the case especially in cultures where there is already a tendency to have closed boundaries. Patients may seek care only for emergencies, such as a traumatic injury, but retreat in lieu of follow-up. Boundaries may then diminish as families slowly acculturate. This may be facilitated if their early encounters are with "outsiders," such as health workers, who are respectful of their culture and sensitive to their concerns.

It is challenging for clinicians to become accustomed to working with families. Interviews of providers of refugee care in Minnesota found that they had reservations about making major changes in their practices to accommodate members of immigrant patients' extended families. However, some acknowledge that providers do not recognize that the head of the household's permission is necessary to allow certain things to occur (Ohmans, Garrett, & Traichel, 1996). We can all learn from families how to better care for patients and how to identify family problems specific to or worsened by cultural and immigration issues.

The Role of Community

The role of immigrant communities in care of patients has much in common with the role of the family. Communities can be our partners, teachers, and barometers. Community problems can manifest as epidemics, such as violence, but their input and leadership solve health problems. Community groups may be invisible to many clinicians. However, it is easy to find groups: In New York City, for example, there were more than 7,000 volunteer neighborhood groups organized in minority communities as far back as two decades ago (Citizens Committee for New York City, 1976). By working with communities, health workers may contribute to prevention and early recognition of illness, influence adaptation to it, better educate patients, and develop an appreciation for eco-

nomic and personal needs for improving the health care system (Reynolds & Cluff, 1976).

Communities can assist patients and providers with functions such as communication, crisis intervention, providing emotional support, care of the ill, and housing. Community organizations have credibility with their constituents, knowledge of relevant channels of communication, and familiarity with cultural values. Clinicians can learn the nature of the community and what communities need and want from health centers. They can also learn traditional mechanisms for participation, which may be different from our Western forms (Oakley, 1989). Furthermore, clinicians can obtain valuable feedback. How can we can find out why an ethnic group of patients stops coming to our health center unless we have good communication with one of their community leaders who can inform us that we inadvertently offended one of the group's members during a past encounter?

Providers usually have little contact with patients' natural support systems or their community. However, we can draw on information about communities to understand a person's values, beliefs, coping mechanisms, and self-concepts. Program planners should understand the natural support systems in relation to needs assessment, outreach, information and referral, staff development, and resource development. Social welfare policy makers should strengthen the natural support system of immigrant communities by making affirmative action guidelines strong and explicit regarding funding, staffing, and target groups, providing technical assistance to implement culture-specific components of these policies. These all should take advantage of the inherent strengths of these support systems and avoid undermining them, while not using their existence as an excuse not to provide services (Canino & Canino, 1982).

Definition of Community

Higgs and Gustafson (1985) define a community as a group of individuals with a common perspective or identity which differentiate them from other groups. They function through a social system to meet their members' needs in a larger social environment. Their identity can be based on culture, beliefs, or mores. Population aggregates defined by demographic features (e.g., elderly persons, an occupational group, or persons with a specific illness or serviced by a particular hospital) are sometimes considered a community, especially for needs assessments (Reinhardt & Quinn, 1977). These aggregates may form into a type of community, for example, an advocacy group.

Geographic communities are usually called neighborhoods. While geographically delineated communities may be easy to identify, communities defined by common characteristics, such as culture, beliefs, or customs, are more difficult to delineate. One cannot, for example, assume that all Eastern Orthodox Russian immigrants live or worship in the same area, or belong to the same organization. Communities exist in a larger environment, so that interaction takes place among members of the community and between them and the surrounding communities and the environment. Individuals often identify with more than one community at a time, such as being Hispanic and Catholic, or Irish and handicapped.

Evolution of Communities

Communities change and evolve over time, with varying degrees of activity and inactivity. Crises, celebrations, and religious occasions may spark cohesiveness or disparity. Traditional communities bound by geography and culture have diminished. The growth of industrialization, transportation, urbanization, racial and ethnic integration, and specialized agencies that can subdivide communities all contribute to isolation of former community members from one another. Communities are less cohesive and less capable of and likely to work together to solve a wide array of problems. Instead, different members may go to different places to solve different needs.

Resurgence of Community–Hospital Partnerships

Robert Kane (1974) noted,

It is ironic that a profession [health care] which began in the community should suddenly need to discover it. Yet, several centuries of gradually institutionalized medicine, followed by a technological revolution, progressively moved medical science farther from the people to be served and closer to the artificial life support system of the medical center. Medical care providers formed communities of their own where they spoke with a special language and became dependent on a complicated network of machinery. The ill entered this world of medical science for intermittent encounters—therapeutic or otherwise—without disturbing the medical milieu. (p. 3)

We are now rediscovering the community at large as we become aware of the vast gap that exists between the knowledge we have acquired and the implementation of that knowledge. We are developing social and preventive roles to treat chronic diseases with multifactorial determinants. We are rediscovering community clinics and community-based training of health workers.

Types of Community Participation in Heath Care

Oakley (1989) described two major forms of community participation in health care: participation as a means and participation as an end. Participation can first be a means to achieve a goal set by an agency or organization that has the power to control necessary resources. With this form, community members tend to be passive participants cooperating (or being co-opted) in a delivery system in which they have some influence (such as commentary or advice) but no control. Their participation may end once a project is completed. This top-down approach may be used when conducting needs assessments, developing community education materials, or soliciting information about the beliefs and practices of a cultural group.

The second form of participation, participation as an end, is more substantive and structural. In this dynamic, bottom-up approach, the goal is to build the confidence and solidarity of a community and create a permanent structure that lasts beyond a project and enables a community to remain involved in members' health care. Such participation may originate from a health system or a community perspective and may involve forming a new community health organization or use of an existing community-level organization. This approach may be used when trying to enable an immigrant community to advocate for the meeting of members' health needs, and to tackle some of the other problems underlying human illness, such as lack of insurance, poverty, poor sanitation, or unsafe working conditions.

Many of us did not receive adequate training to understand the complexities of the system we are trained for and work within. "While most health professionals doubtless want to help their patients, the micro-politics of medical encounters limit providers' capacities to respond to their patients' contextual difficulties" (Waitzkin, 1991, p. 6). We may, for example, misunderstand and therefore ignore or even condone the social conditions influencing their illness. Bottom-up approaches allow us to learn about and address these problems.

Community involvement should be local and indigenous (based on the existing community structure), be created,if possible, as a result of local initiatives, be representative of interests of groups in the community whose involvement is being sought, and be able to develop as a legitimate formal representative body. Therefore, it is important to develop a means for supporting the communities and their organizations. This means that a health organization should include a political commitment to the community and the process of participation, a reorientation of the bureaucracy to be flexible and have a bottom-up approach to community involvement, and a commitment to helping the group develop a capacity for self-management.

Community as a Source of Risk Factors for Stress or Illness

Clinicians can find explanations for tensions and crises that burden the community and increase office visits by observing the activities and interrelations of community subsystems such as law enforcement, health care and religion (Jerome-Forget & Paradis, 1984). By observing, reading about, and asking questions about community histories and current events, clinicians can also learn what health hazards exist in the community. Are members likely to be employed? Poor? Elderly? Part of intact families? Safely and securely housed? As explained earlier, these can all be risk factors for stress or stress-related illness that effect how patients are diagnosed and treated. Related problems are difficult to solve without an understanding of these risk factors and without community partners to help address them.

Community as Partners in Making Care Plans

Immigrant communities may have cultural or religious beliefs that we need to acknowledge in order to make heath care plans with our patients. When patients hear that you as a clinician understand and respect their community's values and practices, this may vastly increase their trust and allow you to introduce them to ideas and practices you think are important. For example, if you want an Indian to cut down on fat, it may be more "impressive" if you discussed cutting down on cooking oil than beef (which they are less likely to eat). This requires that you first ask a community member about typical foods and how they are cooked and then use this knowledge when beginning conversations with similar patients.

Health programs have erred in the past, as Deinard and Dunnigan (1987) explained, by failing to recognize that good health care requires compromises between the different cultural perspectives of the clinician and the patient. In their maternal and child clinic which cared for Southeast Asian refugees, serious problems occurred because clinicians did not have adequate background information about patients before recommending care plans. Physicians wrote prescriptions that were not filled and patients refused to be treated for asymptomatic cases of parasitic diseases and tuberculosis and tried to find alternative providers. Physicians learned from these problems that patients did not understand the reasoning behind many recommendations, and the advice given did not seem to fit the problems they were worried about. They realized that indigenous caregivers, if incorporated into the medical staff could have helped to avoid many problems.

There may be long-standing beliefs that interfere with diagnoses and treatments unless we work with communities to understand them. For example, many adult Muslims are required to abstain from food and drink from sunrise to sunset during the entire month of Ramadan, usually in March or April (Rashed, 1992). While dispensation from fasting is allowed during illness and pregnancy, people may still choose to fast during these times. First, they may not know about the exemptions. Second, they may not consider themselves ill and providers may be unaware that they plan to fast and may not explain the importance of eating or changing medication use. For example, if a diabetic believes that this chronic condition is not really an illness (as it is asymptomatic), he may take his medication before sunrise and fast all day, not knowing he is at risk of life-threatening hypoglycemic episodes. Third, some Muslims, such as pregnant women, may choose to fast because they do not want to have to make up the time later, when they would be the only member of the family fasting (Hoskins, 1992). While this may be safe for some women, it may be a danger for others, such as those who have severe emesis (vomiting) due to morning sickness.

We can work with the community to increase provider and patient awareness and to devise practical solutions. Some diabetic patients may be able to decrease their medication doses and still safely fast. Patients who need certain medications may be able to take them once or twice (rather than three or four times) daily, so that they are taken during the night hours. Health workers can postpone nonemergency diagnostic tests until after Ramadan, if patients prefer. (This, of course, means the provider has already recognized that the patient's hesitancy to undergo the test is because they do not want to have it during the holiday.) Patients who need to eat or take medications during the day may receive special dispensations from local Muslim leaders. As an example, health workers in England worked with a local Muslim leader who provided a written statement outlining the current teaching on fasting for Ramadan during pregnancy, which midwives copied and used when seeing women who were fasting (Reeves, 1992).

All these rather simple but very effective solutions require that providers recognize this religious practice common to a community they serve, work with community leaders to understand the practice, and develop practical, mutually acceptable solutions to medical challenges. Just as a surgeon determines the best approach to remove a tumor without damaging an adjacent organ, providers must determine the best way to allow patients to protect both their health and their personal values and beliefs. We cannot maximize health-related quality of life without securing both.

We can learn what community norms are and how these will affect our ability to work with patients. For instance, many Indochinese people rely on family and community elders to make decisions about medical care (Hoang & Erikson, 1988). If there is a particular practice we find objectionable, but which is widely accepted and expected in a community, we are likely to have difficulty changing this behavior by speaking with just one patient and may simply alienate that patient if we try. We could work with elders and leaders to understand the rationale and importance of the practice and determine whether it is safe to condone it. For example, many Vietnamese practice *cao gio,* or coining, to treat physical symptoms and they have a negative view of physicians who do not condone it (Yeatman & Dang, 1980). Clinicians may decide that this is not an unsafe practice. They may ask about it when taking a history (e.g., "have you tried *cao gio,* was it helpful"). This may lend credibility to a provider and a feeling of being understood on the part of patients. It may also open a dialogue by which to learn about other practices in the community.

On the other hand, we may identify practices we consider unsafe or dangerous. We may be able to explain this to community members, who if they agree, may be able to help us communicate this and put forth an acceptable alternative behavior. The practice of female circumcision, or traditional female genital surgery, is such an example. If we blanketly condemn the practice and display our revulsion to circumcised women and their communities, we may inadvertently drive them away from the health care they need and from an opportunity we have to teach them about the harms of the practice. We cannot simply medicalize this ancient practice and eradicate it as if it were a disease. However, through collaborative educational efforts that partner health workers and immigrant communities (including efforts to raise the social and economic status of women), we can impact the practice (Horowitz & Jackson, 1997).

Community as Patient Advocate

At times, health workers may feel as if their goals of improving health conflict with community goals of preserving cultural integrity. However, in most instances, health workers and communities want similar things for patients. These partnerships can yield impressive gains for patients. Health workers, for instance, are often frustrated by the fact that they do not have trained interpreters for their patients. They may need to rely on inappropriate surrogates such as family members, other patients, or gestures to communicate. In this case, neither immigrant communities nor providers are receiving what they need to promote health. Providers could complain to

their health organizations and community members could complain to each other or to other advocacy groups. Alternatively, they could work together, combining skills and political clout, and lobby for change.

First they may be able to organize volunteer interpreters (such as unemployed or retired community members) who would be trained by hospital staff to interpret. The duo could write grants to foundations to pay for interpreters, or a hospital–community fundraiser could generate some capital to pay for this needed function. Meanwhile, the partners could lobby hospitals to provide a longer term solution by paying for interpreter services and local governments to mandate that hospitals provide interpreter services.

Learning about Subpopulations

There is a burgeoning literature about immigrant and refugee health and cultural beliefs and practices. Some clinicians could consider merely reading about their patient populations in books and articles. However, they would be missing the "fine points" about the patients they care for. While published information about Hispanics, Asians, or other groups may be helpful in initially understanding a group or culture that is foreign to us, to treat a group such as Hispanics as a homogeneous population may be doing us and our patients a disservice. Communities differ because there are subpopulations within these ethnic and cultural groups. They also differ based on their past experiences and their current economic and health situations.

For example, there is much research comparing attributes such as health utilization, attitudes, income, and education of Hispanics with that of White Americans and African Americans. However, there is dramatic variation within the Hispanic population. Hispanics, by virtue of their common language or Spanish surnames may present a blurred picture of the health care needs and uses of each group. The aggregation of culturally distinct subgroups into a more inclusive Hispanic category assumes that citizens of Mexican,

Cuban, and Puerto Rican extraction have similar needs and experience similar barriers in using health services. However, persons of Puerto Rican origin use health care services very differently from persons of Cuban or Mexican extraction. For instance, they are almost twice as likely to use a hospital outpatient department or emergency department as their usual source of care instead of a doctor's office. They are less likely to have private insurance (Schur, Bernstein, & Berk, 1987).

And even within a Hispanic immigrant subpopulation (e.g., Cubans), there will be differences. Is the population from a rural or urban area? Are they political or economic refugees? Are they educated and do they have job skills? Have they previously been exposed to Western medicine? Providers can answer these questions by finding out what local community groups work with Cuban patients and asking them about the population in their area, rather than assuming that all Cuban immigrants to the United States are alike.

Even well-meaning articles introducing a population to Westerners have the potential of creating stereotypes that may interfere with patient care. Written materials can also quickly become outdated, as cultures are not static. It is helpful to know that a cultural or immigrant group may tend to act or think in a certain way at a certain time, but overgeneralization may lead to losing the ability to tailor care to individuals. For example an article about Arab immigrants explains that they do not expect personal care from health professionals; they expect an effective cure. They have great respect for authority figures and technological medicine, and discomfort with revealing detailed personal information to strangers. Therefore, the more intrusive the procedure, the better the potential for recovery (Meleis, 1981). This last description may be true of many Arab Americans, but to assume that all prefer such technical, intrusive, and nonpersonal attention may cause providers to alienate as many patients as they satisfy.

It is important, therefore, learn about local subpopulations through local community groups. Even with this information, it should be understood that all people are different, and that one should make sure their own patients fit the "stereotype" of their culture, without assuming that this is the case. For example, clinicians may discover that an immigrant group does not usually shake hands when first meeting someone. The clinician may then decide not to offer their hand to such patients. However, if the community is acculturated, they may expect their clinician to offer this greeting and feel insulted if he or she does not. Therefore, it may be best to say to a person of this group, when first meeting them; "I often shake hands with a person when I first meet them; what do you do?"

Alternative or Complementary Medical Providers and Traditional Healers

Traditional healers are often important in immigrant communities. Their use increases in populations which have recently migrated to urban areas and their availability appears to facilitate acculturation (Press, 1978). Even if allopathic providers cannot cite bodies of empirical evidence proving the benefits of these therapies, they may be very effective for certain conditions. Moreover, immigrant groups have relied on them for centuries, and will not stop doing so merely because they immigrate. Traditional medicine may be an important part of a patient's support system. Rather than discouraging or belittling such healers, it would be beneficial to understand the types of problems our patients use them for, ensure that they are not using unsafe products, and help them negotiate the difference between problems which may and may not be addressed by alternative practices (Eisenberg, 1997). For example, muscular pain may be treatable by acupuncture, but serious trauma should be treated in a hospital setting.

The Community as Partners in Needs Assessment and in Research

All steps of investigations, such as needs assessments, surveys, and health services research can benefit from community input. In developing a research question or identifying the needs to be assessed, it is helpful to obtain a community perspective. Aday, Chiu, and Andersen (1980) described four issues in cross-cultural research where such collaborations could be fruitful. First, communities can assist in defining the population to be studied, including identifying and efficiently sampling groups that comprise only a small proportion of the total population in an area. Second, they can help the investigator understand and minimize issues of lack of cooperation and nonresponse due to cultural or language barriers. Third, they can assist with technical issues, such as preparation of field materials and recruitment and training of staff, or conducting interviews with non-English-speaking respondents. Fourth, they can help identify biases in the data that might result from issues such as the sensitivity of subject matter relative to certain cultural groups.

Finally, through this process, you can develop relationships with community members, giving them employment or volunteer opportunities, a say in how they are being looked at, a chance to develop skills, and inspiration to advocate for their own interests. If a new immigrant community has not yet organized, your process of identifying leaders and members who are interested in furthering their group's interests and bringing these individuals together may be the spark that ignites the formation of a new community group.

By including the community in research projects, you can increase the likelihood that the work will be germane to the people you are trying to understand or help, and you can increase the quality of the work by avoiding or understanding potential biases and problems. You will also have members of the community who can help you ensure that both your question and the way you answer it make sense to the people you are describing. For example, when we prepared guidelines for the care of circumcised women, we solicited circumcised women's perspectives to prepare the guidelines and showed the guidelines to a diverse group of women in our

community to determine their appropriateness and relevance.

McPhee has been a pioneer in improving cancer screening and prevention for minority communities (especially the Vietnamese) in the San Francisco area (Pham & McPhee, 1992). He and his colleagues have exemplified the idea of community involvement in research and programmatic innovations. They have investigated smoking habits of Vietnamese in their country of origin and in the United States, analyzed their knowledge, attitudes, and beliefs about cancer screening and cancer and worked with communities to identify barriers to care. Using such information, they have partnered with community leaders to pilot programs (such as for smoking cessation) on Vietnamese radio and television programs.

Steps to Improving Understanding of and Working with Immigrant Families and Communities

There are six steps clinicians can take to improve patient care through working with immigrant families and communities.

1. Get to Know Yourself

Patients enter their providers' offices with culture-bound definitions of health and illness. Similarly, providers enter the health professions with culture-bound conceptions. Patients' and providers' ideas change as they are socialized into the health system. This can cause a schism between the provider and patients, but it can be narrowed if providers become more aware of their own backgrounds and beliefs about health and illness and more sensitive to the issues surrounding health care and to the beliefs of the patient.

Spector (1991), for example, asks providers to look at themselves, their families, and their communities to understand their own definitions of health and illness and their own patterns of health behavior. Health workers can, for example, question themselves (as they should their patients), using Kleinman's (1978) explanatory models of illness, or the Kune-Karrera and Taylor questions (1995; explained later). By becoming aware of their own attitudes toward illness and its treatments, providers avoid imposing ethnocentric limits on medical encounters that would insist that our way of providing health care is the best or only way (Reinhardt & Quinn, 1977). Patients may choose to seek care elsewhere if we cannot compromise and solicit and respect their perspective.

2. Get to Know the Families of Your Patients and Their Health Seeking Behavior Patterns

Kune-Karrera and Taylor (1995) reviewed ways to elicit immigrants' health care perceptions and to learn about immigrants' cultures, experiences, and current situations. While their lengthy suggestions were written for pediatricians, they can be adapted easily for use with all immigrant groups and shortened for use in busy clinical settings. It may be useful to take a simple genogram, describing the family members, where they live, and who is missing or dead. One can place a circle around all people who live with the patient, and note whom the patient may particularly rely on or whom they have problems with. This simple diagram can serve as a reference (which can be updated) to facilitate working with the family. Another simple way to learn about families is to ask about holidays and other important occasions (who is there, who will be missed, what is done). This is a good way to build rapport and find out who and what is important to your patients. The suggestions listed in the following section are also useful in getting to know families.

3. Get to Know the Communities Common to Your Setting

Clinicians can establish a knowledge base of diseases common to certain immigrant groups (e.g., tropical diseases) and the history, culture, and psychosocial environment of im-

migrants' homelands. This information can be obtained through discussions with local community members and leaders and reading.

A. Read about Communities of Interest

There are many articles that teach about immigrant groups and cultures (e.g., Campbell & Chang, 1973; Ruiz, 1985). There are also sources of information being compiled by groups who work with immigrants and multicultural populations. The Community House Calls Program (described in "Model Programs" later) and the Cross-Cultural Health Care Project of the Pacific Medical Center have information about communities in the Seattle area on their websites. One can order "Voices of the Community" profiles from the latter group by calling 206-326-4161, or writing to them at 1200-12th Avenue South, Seattle, WA 98144. The New York Task Force on Immigrant Health in New York City has a bibliography of immigrant health articles and information sheets about practices and beliefs of ethnic groups around maternal and child health (New York University, 550 First Avenue, New York, NY 10016).

Clinicians can also read and learn about other health workers' experiences of learning how to serve an immigrant community. For example, Ellis (1982) described a county hospital obstetric and nurse-midwifery service for Southeast Asian refugees. This program incorporates outreach to bring women into care, ways to introduce them to the hospital, preferences for birthing rooms, learning to share traumatic refugee experiences, dietary tips (such as culturally acceptable ways to increase calcium in their diets), and understanding of cultural stoicism.

B. Take a Course

Providers can take a course to learn more about working with communities or about cross-cultural communication. The Cross-Cultural Health Care Project serves as a bridge between communities and health care institutions to ensure full access to quality health care that is culturally and linguistically appropriate. It maintains a center of cultural competence to make educational materials available, provide innovative and professional training for medical interpreters, and provide cultural competency training for health care providers. Information about their excellent educational programs and other functions can be obtained at the address listed earlier.

C. Enhance Community Relations

Clinicians can develop relationships between health centers and the community. This may include volunteering to give lectures about health topics of community interest. In exchange, community members can come to your health center and lecture your group about their community. Let community members work with you. High school students and others can volunteer to work in clinics, and clinics can hire community members, when appropriate, to become part of their health care team. Medical students and residents from your center can work with communities and return to the center to present a community profile, in conjunction with a community member, to health workers.

D. Have a Forum for the Community

A community forum is useful for understanding problems as they occur. Open lines of communication can allow you to learn of community challenges, such as an outbreak of violence or a new wave of immigrants, to learn of times when you may have inadvertently alienated a population, and to gauge the effects of a program or intervention on a community. It is important for providers to simply listen to the members of the community. Providers will become more effective and patient communities more satisfied.

E. Get to Know the Formal and Informal Resources

Use community resources to help enhance your ability to improve patients' health. Re-

sources may include community centers, school groups, and personnel and charitable organizations. Help patients who do not understand how to take advantage of community services learn what is available and how to access it. Social workers may be particularly instrumental in this regard.

4. Get to Know Some of the Traditional Practices and Remedies Used by Families and Communities and Work with Them, Not against Them

A. M. Kleinman (1980) has developed a widely used explanatory model of illness to elicit signs and symptoms by which an illness is recognized and the illness's presumed causes, recommended therapies, and prognosis. These types of questions can be used to determine, in a nonjudgmental way, how patients think about their health. Accept practices and remedies deemed safe, as this may improve patients' perceived health, and their trust and confidence in you.

5. Get to Know How a Community Deals with Common Illnesses or Events, and Keep This in Mind as You Proceed

Learn about traditional definitions of health and illness and traditional names and symptoms of common diseases. Harwood (1981) has written helpful guidelines for culturally appropriate health care, including recognizing intra-ethnic variations in clinical care, eliciting concepts of disease and expectations for care, and treating culture-specific syndromes.

6. Think of Things from the Patients', Their Families', and the Community's Perspective

Patients may not prefer to live in the United States, they may not have a choice of providers, and they may not be familiar with Western medical care. They are often of different ethnicity, race, and class. An empathic imagination will help you more clearly understand help seeking, help rejecting, and other health behaviors.

Model Programs for Working with Families and Communities

These examples of model programs exemplify different perspectives on how to improve patient care through working with families and communities. There is little empiric evidence analyzing the effects of such programs on health utilization, outcomes, or patient satisfaction. However, such programs appear to be innovative, sustainable, and practical. There is a great need for more formal and rigorous evaluation in this area.

Ethnic Obstetric Liaison Program in Australia (Ganguly, 1995) aims to promote the health of women of non-English-speaking backgrounds. The program recruited bicultural, bilingual liaison officers who were midwives or midwifery students to provide information and support to pregnant women and new mothers from emerging immigrant and refugee communities. Officers provided services to the patients and in-services to hospital staff on cultural beliefs and practices relating to pregnancy and childbirth. While hospital staff commonly cited problems dealing with communication, teaching their patients, understanding their cultural practices, and coping with relatives and visitors, 78% reported significant improvements since initiation of the program. They also succeeded in educating women about services available to them, educated them about tests and procedures, and improved attendance at prenatal classes.

In another Australian project, bilingual health educators were recruited form several immigrant groups to conduct group sessions on breast and cervical cancer screening. As a result of the meetings, health workers learned why cervical smears were not taken regularly, such as lack of information and embarrassment about using a male physician. The pro-

ject helped raise the self-esteem of the workers, who, like many other immigrants, had suffered because their overseas qualifications had not been recognized. Participating women had raised awareness and confidence levels and the staff were sensitized to the problems experienced by women in their attempts to gain access to the health services

The authors of these program evaluations concluded that the programs were fulfilling a need to provide learning and culturally appropriate information to women. This included recruiting and training workers with whom the women could relate. To be most effective, programs must target clients and health service providers and focus health promotion not only on health issues, but also on related issues of access, child care, and understanding the system.

Community House Calls Program, Harborview Medical Center, Seattle, Washington. This program aims to decrease sociocultural barriers to care for non-English-speaking ethnic populations and enhance communication between patients and providers. The program employs Interpreter Cultural Mediators, trained interpreters (who are refugees themselves) chosen from each racial or ethnic community to interpret during clinic visits, help patients get other services (such as housing), and explain the Western system of medicine to immigrants. They also work with community advisers, respected members of refugee communities, who help educate the hospital and providers about refugees' cultures, daily lives, and problems, and help interpreters reach out to people who need help. Their website (http://www.hslib.washington.edu/clinical/ethnomed) has valuable information on the program, how to set up a similar program, ethnic communities they serve, and cross-cultural communication.

Boriken Neighborhood Health Center, East Harlem, New York, has been in operation since 1968 (Deuschle, 1983). It was founded when the East Harlem Tenants Council became interested in health services delivery. They requested technical assistance from Mount Sinai Medical Center in the development of a primary care program. The Boriken center has remained a community-governed and -managed health center, and has since obtained strong financial support from federal, state, and city sources. This demonstrates how existing health organizations can work with community organizations to develop a strong and sustainable health center to fulfill unmet needs of the community. In this way, the health organization did not need to change their existing structure or service aims to offer the services to the Boriken community, but could be very instrumental in helping others meet this aim.

Conclusion

Many health providers have not been taught how to work with immigrant populations. By learning about immigrant health care, providers can transform experiences where they are frustrated and confused by patients of different cultures into some of the most rewarding and productive relationships of their practices. One way to foster understanding and communication is to acknowledge and work with the families and communities of our immigrant patients.

Most providers have been trained to work with patients on a one-to-one basis. As with all aspects of health education, it is often most informative to combine individual patient information with that learned from a larger group of individuals who are in a similar situation. For example, when a provider sees a patient with kidney failure, he or she will read about the course and treatment of the disease as studied in a larger population, and explore psychological adjustments made by other such patients. This chapter encouraged providers to similarly explore the world of their immigrant patients.

Immigrants' families and communities can be our partners and our teachers. They can help us understand our patients' attitudes, values and behaviors, and help us communicate more effectively. They can work with us to tackle issues, ranging from compliance with medications to smoking and domestic violence, in mutually acceptable ways. As a result, patients and their familes can become healthier and more satisfied, providers can increase their effectiveness, and communities can develop new ways to lead efforts to assess and improve the health of their members.

References

Aday, L. A., Chiu, G. Y., & Andersen, R. (1980). Methodological issues in health care surveys of the Spanish heritage population. *American Journal of Public Health, 70,* 367–374.

Ailinger, R. L., & Causey, M. E. (1995). Health concept of older Hispanic immigrants. *Western Journal of Nursing Research, 17,* 605–613.

Anderson, E. T., & McFarlane, J. (1988). *Community as partner: Theory and practice in nursing.* Philadelphia: Lippincott-Raven.

Antanovsky, A. (1979). *Health, stress and coping.* San Francisco: Jossey-Bass.

Beyene, Y. (1992). Medical disclosure and refugees: Telling bad news to Ethiopian patients. *Western Journal of Medicine, 157,* 328–32.

Campbell, T., & Chang, B. (1973). Health care of the Chinese in America. *Nursing Outlook, 21,* 245–249.

Canino, G., & Canino, I. A. (1982). Culturally syntonic family therapy for migrant Puerto Ricans. *Hospital and Community Psychiatry, 33,* 299–303.

Cheung, M. (1989). Elderly Chinese living in the United States: Assimilation or adjustment? *Social Work, 34,* 457–461.

Christie-Seely, J. (1984). *Working with the family in primary care: A systems approach to health and illness.* New York: Praeger.

Citizens Committee for New York City. (1976). State of the Neighborhoods report. New York: Author.

Cox, C., & Gelfand, D. (1987). Familial assistance, exchange and satisfaction among Hispanic, Portuguese, and Vietnamese ethnic elderly. *Journal of Cross-Cultural Gerontology, 2,* 241–255.

Cox, C., & Monk, A. (1990). Minority caregivers of dementia victims: A comparison of Black and Hispanic families. *Journal of Applied Gerontology, 9,* 340–354.

Deinard, A. S., & Dunnigan, T. (1987). Hmong health care: Reflections of a six-year experience. *International Migration Review, 21,* 857–865.

Delgado, M., & Humm-Delgado, D. (1982). Natural support systems: Source of strength in Hispanic communities. *Social Work, 27,* 83–89.

Deuschle, K. W. (1983). Community oriented primary care: Lessons learned in three decades. In E. Connor & F. Mullan (Eds.), *Community oriented primary* care: New directions for health services delivery (pp. 6–20). Washington, DC: National Academy Press.

Eisenberg, D. M. (1997). Advising patients who seek alternative medical therapies. Annals of Internal Medicine, 127, 61–69.

Ellis, J. (1982). Southeast Asian refugees and maternity care: The Oakland experience. Birth, 9, 191–194.

Engel, G. (1981). The need for a new medical model: A challenge for biomedicine. In A. L. Caplan, H. T. Englehardt, & J. McCartney (Eds.), Concepts of health and disease: Interdisciplinary perspectives (pp. 589–607). Reading, MA: Addison-Welsley.

Ganguly, I. (1995). Promoting the health of women of non-English-speaking backgrounds in Australia. World Health Forum, 16, 157–163.

Haines, D., Rutherford, D., & Thomas, P. (1981). Family and community among Vietnamese refugees. International Migration Review, 15, 310–319.

Harwood, A. (1981). Guidelines for culturally appropriate care. In A. Harwood (Ed.), Ethnicity and medical care (pp. 482–507). Cambridge, MA: Harvard University Press.

Higgs, Z. R., & Gustafson, D. G. (1985). Community as client: Assessment and diagnosis. Philadelphia: Davis.

Hoang, G. N., & Erikson, R. V. (1988). Cultural barriers to effective medical care among Indochinese patients. Annual Review of Medicine, 36, 229–239.

Horowitz, C. R., & Jackson, J. C. (1997). Female "circumcision": African women confront American medicine. Journal of General Internal Medicine, 12, 491–499.

Hoskins, A. (1992). Pregnancy and fasting during Ramadan [Letter]. British Medical Journal, 304, 1247.

Hott, J. R. (1977). Mobilizing family strengths in health maintenance and coping with illness. In A. M. Reinhart & M. D. Quinn (Eds.), Current practice in family-centered community nursing. St. Louis, MO: Mosby.

Jerome-Forget, M., & Paradis, G. (1984). The Community. In J. Christie-Seely (Ed.), Working with the family in primary care: A systems approach to health and illness (pp. 62–72). New York: Praeger.

Kane, R. L. (1974). Community medicine: What's in a name? In R. L. Kane (Ed.), The challenges of community medicine (pp. 3–18). New York: Springer.

Kleinman, A. (1978). Clinical relevance of anthropological and cross-cultural research: Concepts and strategies. American Journal of Psychiatry, 135, 427–431.

Kleinman, A. M. (1980). Patients and healers in the context of culture. Berkeley: University of California Press.

Kune-Karrera, B. M., & Taylor, E. H. (1995). Toward multiculturality: Implications for the pediatrician. Pediatric Clinics of North America, 42, 21–30.

Laffery, S. C., Meleis, A. I., Lipson, J. G., Solomon, M., & Omidian, P. A. (1989). Assessing Arab-American health care needs. Social Science and Medicine, 29, 877–883.

Lin, K., Miller, M. H., Poland, R. E., Nuccion, I., & Yamaguchi, M. (1991). Ethnicity and family involvement in the treatment of schizophrenic patients. Journal of Nervous and Mental Disease, 179, 631–633.

Lock, M. (1984). The relationship between culture and health or illness. In J. Christie-Seely (Ed.), Working with the family in primary care: A systems approach to health and illness (pp. 73–92). New York: Praeger.

Meleis, A. I. (1981). The Arab American in the health care system. American Journal of Nursing, 81, 1180–1183.

Oakley, P. (1989). Community involvement in health development. Geneva, Switzerland: World Health Organization.

Ohmans, P., Garrett, C., & Traichel, C. (1996). Cultural barriers to health care for refugees and immigrants: Providers' perceptions. Minnesota Medicine, 79, 26–28.

Pham, C. T., & McPhee, S. J. (1992). Knowledge, attitudes and practices of breast and cervical cancer screening among Vietnamese women. Journal of Cancer Education, 7, 305–310.

Press, I. (1978). Urban folk medicine. American Anthropologist, 80, 71.

Rashed, A. H. (1992). The fast of Ramadan—No problems for the well: The sick should avoid fasting. British Medical Journal, 304, 521–522.

Reeves, J. (1992). Pregnancy and fasting during Ramadan [Letter]. British Medical Journal, 304, 843–844.

Reinhardt, A. M., & Quinn, M. D. (1977). Current practice in family-centered community nursing. St. Louis: Mosby.

Reynolds, R., & Cluff, L. (1976). The medical school and the health of the community: Programs developing at the University of Florida. American Journal of Public Health, 61, 1196–1207.

Rosenberg, C. E. (1979). The therapeutic revolution: Medicine, meaning and social change in nineteenth century America. In M. J. Vogel & C. E. Rosenberg (Eds.), The therapeutic revolution: Essays on the social history of American medicine (pp. 3–25). Philadelphia: University of Pennsylvania Press.

Ruiz, P. (1985). Cultural barriers to effective medical care among Hispanic-American patients. Annual Review of Medicine, 36, 63–71.

Schur, C. L., Bernstein, A. B., & Berk, M. L. (1987). The importance of distinguishing Hispanic subpopulations in the use of medical care. Medical Care, 25, 627–641.

Spector, R. E.. (1991). Cultural diversity in health and illness. Norwalk, CT: Appleton and Lange.

Unger, D. G., & Powell, D. R. (1980). Supporting families under stress: The role of social networks. Family Relations, 29, 566–574.

Van Tran, T., & Wright, R. (1986). Social support and subjective well being among Vietnamese refugees. *Social Service Review, 60,* 449–459.

Waitzkin, H. (1991). *The politics of medical encounters.* New Haven, CT: Yale University Press.

Yeatman, G. W., & Dang, V. V. (1980). Cao gio (coin rubbing): Vietnamese attitudes towards health care. *Journal of the American Medical Association, 244,* 2748.

10

Folk Illnesses

ROBERTA D. BAER, LAUREN CLARK, AND CAROLINE PETERSON

Introduction

Folk illnesses are one aspect of the culture of immigrants that can interfere with their ability to use the formal health care system, because of the lack of understanding among many health care professionals of the nature of these illnesses. This chapter addresses a number of issues related to beliefs in folk illnesses among immigrants to the United States, including (1) the contrast between folk and biomedical illnesses, (2) theoretical issues associated with the term *folk illness* and the related term *culture-bound syndromes,* (3) differences in understanding of disease causality in folk medicine and biomedicine, (4) examples of folk illnesses in mainstream American populations and in more recent immigrants, (5) recommendations for clinicians in dealing with patients presenting with folk illnesses, and (6) recommendations for further research on these topics.

Folk Illnesses Contrasted with Biomedical Illnesses

Culture can be defined as the beliefs and behaviors shared by a cultural group. Just as any cultural group has beliefs and behaviors related to marriage, religion, and other areas of life, every cultural group has beliefs and behaviors on issues of health and illness. Particular approaches to staying healthy and treating illness develop in each culture, as do specialists in these areas. These systems can be referred to as folk medical systems (Lieban, 1977). Folk medical systems have systems of disease classifications; use a variety of therapies, including magico-religious, mechanical, and chemical procedures; incorporate prophylactic practices; and use various types of health care specialists, including herbalists, diviners, shamans, midwives, and masseurs (Lieban, 1977).

Folk medical systems, often referred to as ethnomedical systems (Lieban, 1977) can be contrasted with biomedicine (also often referred to as allopathic medicine). The latter term refers to the medicine of the twentieth century Western world, which has come to have worldwide influence (Hahn, 1985). In the industrialized countries, biomedicine is the dominant medical system and philosophy, although increasing dissatisfaction with this medical system has led to an increase in use

ROBERTA D. BAER AND CAROLINE PETERSON • Department of Anthropology, University of South Florida, Tampa, Florida 33620-9951. LAUREN CLARK • School of Nursing, University of Colorado Health Sciences Center, Denver, Colorado 80262.

Handbook of Immigrant Health, edited by Loue. Plenum Press, New York, 1998.

of alternative therapies, even among mainstream Americans (Eisenberg *et al.,* 1993). Biomedicine is concerned with the treatment of diseases, not of persons. A recognized disease is considered to be the same wherever it occurs, regardless of the culture of the individual in whose body it is found (Lieban, 1977). Allopathic or biomedical cures usually focus on manipulation of some aspect of the body and the organs within it through administration of pharmaceuticals or application of surgery.

While most users of folk medical systems usually combine ethnomedical services with those of biomedically trained practitioners (Lieban, 1977), there are a number of important differences between the two types of health care systems. Folk medicine tends to be concerned with a wider range of phenomena that can be termed "illnesses." These include diseases, but also encompass the importance of the patient's experience of the problem and the social and other implications of the disease. Therefore, folk medical cures often include actions directed at social and spiritual universes of the patient. In addition to this broader perspective on some of the conditions addressed by biomedicine, folk medicine also identifies and treats illnesses not within the biomedical realm, that is, folk illnesses.

Theoretical Issues Related to the Terms *Folk Illness* and *Culture-Bound Syndrome*

Whether a patient's problem is a disease to be treated within the realm of the biomedical system or a folk illness within the purview of a folk health system, patients who have symptoms with social meanings are not only diseased or ill, they are sick. The concept of sickness differs from disease and illness in that it recognizes the social milieu in which the sufferer lives. The social acknowledgment that one is, indeed, ill and the ensuing social response to that illness constitute the condition of sickness (Young, 1982). What symptoms count as sickness in one situation

may not be considered sickness at all in another, and it is this area of cross-cultural difference in the construction of socially recognized sickness that continues to fascinate health care practitioners and anthropologists alike.

Historically, symptoms or symptom clusters not recognized in biomedical classification systems as legitimate illnesses have been referred to as folk illnesses. Anthropologists characteristically study illnesses in foreign places or among ethnic groups at home, and those symptom clusters that strike observers as odd, dramatic, exotic, or deviant have been labeled folk illnesses or culture-bound syndromes. The general and inclusive term *folk illness* designates any indigenously perceived illness entity (R. C. Simons & Hughes, 1985). Differences between the definition of folk illness and culture-bound syndrome are fuzzy, but one distinction is the emphasis on biocultural or social explanations for folk illnesses and the importance of universal psychogenic symptomatology in the study of culture-bound syndromes (Low, 1985).

Culture-bound syndromes form a subset of folk illnesses, and are composed of only those folk illnesses that include alterations of behavior and of experience prominently among their symptomatology (R. C. Simons & Hughes, 1985) and where the behavioral alteration is restricted in distribution to discrete areas of the globe (R. Simons, 1980). Furthermore, culture-bound syndromes can be viewed in two ways: as *eccentricities* in the cultural systems of societies in which they are endemic, or *psychopathologies* in Western psychological medicine (p. 195; emphasis added).

The ethnocentricity of a bifurcated classification system, with legitimate biomedical illnesses on the one hand and questionable folk illnesses on the other, has not been lost on anthropologists, who contend that folk illnesses can be found even within the biomedically hegemonic U.S. culture. Scrutinizing the culture-bound label, Hahn (1985) contended that it is solipsistic, reductionistic, and contributes to the fragmentation of human experience into disciplines of study. In a humorous vein, Hahn provided instructions for finding a culture-bound syndrome, illustrating the egotistical and ethnocentric possibilities:

1. An observer with some training in Western medicine visits a foreign setting.
2. The observer notices a behavior that seems strange by his own standards of normality, yet he does not know how to label the behavior in his own classification scheme.
3. Local people provide a label for the behavior.
4. The observer returns home with a wonderful prize: a new culture-bound syndrome with a colorful local label!
5. The observer, having established the new condition, cross-culturally exports it by finding similar conditions in other settings to which he can apply the label.

R. Simons (1980) noted that without a local label, one has not found a culture-bound syndrome. For example, people who are easily startled in the United States do not share a label for their hyperstartling. But in Malaysia, hyperstartlers are named in a diagnostic group as suffering from *latah* and their symptoms are codified. The human experience may be similar, with similar physiologic or psychologic processes, but until the symptoms are labeled, a culture-bound syndrome does not exist.

One small corner of the theoretical debate surrounding culture-bound syndromes is occupied by good-natured criticism of the process of finding such syndromes. More ardent discussion revolves around the most explanatory factors or frameworks contributing to the production of culture-bound syndromes. Various theoretical frameworks employed in the study of culture-bound syndromes are described later.

Latah was one of the first culture-bound syndromes to enflame the debate of culture or nature in the etiology and expression of symptoms. *Latah* is a folk illness reported in Java, Malaysia, and Indonesia. It is associated with hyperstartling, and is characterized by the "involuntary blurting of obscene words or phrases, compulsive imitation of the words or actions of others, and compulsive, unquestioning obedience when ordered to perform actions which may be ridiculous" (Geertz, 1968, p. 93). These symptoms are often brought on by a loud noise initiated (often deliberately) by another person that startles the afflicted person. In support of a universal biological explanation of *latah,* R. Simons (1980) concluded that the syndrome is a culture-specific exploitation of a neurophysiologically determined behavioral potential shared by all humans. Which facets of the behavioral biology of startle are exploited and which ignored, what cultural themes startle phenomena illustrate and exemplify, and who may tease whom within what limits, are all culture specific (R. Simons, 1980). Furthermore, the range of *latah* symptoms, from the mild to the most severe cases, can be observed cross-culturally. The cross-cultural difference, argued R. Simons, is in the vocabulary for identifying and naming the symptoms as a discrete illness. Countering arguments that he dismissed the symbolic aspects of *latah,* R. Simons (1983b) argued that the uncontestably symbolic aspect of *latah* does not negate its biological basis.

Kenny (1978, 1983) disagreed with Simons's biological explanation. Whereas R. Simons (1980) "wished to derive *latah* from a culture-specific exploitation of a neurophysiological potential, I see *latah* as a culture-specific exploitation of a meaning potential implicit in a limited human repertoire of concepts pertaining to order" (Kenny, 1983, p. 161). More simply stated, *latah* is a cultural performance, or even a theatrical production, with symptomology chosen for its meaning within a specific cultural context. By looking at those afflicted—the marginalized, socially disadvantaged, or postmenopausal women—Kenny (1978) insists that *latah* is a symbolic protest. Instead of a biological symptom indicating mental illness, *latah* is a cultural marker of marginality. The best explanation from this symbolic viewpoint is that culture-bound syndromes arise from group mythology and ideology about the nature of the self. In refuting this argument, R. Simons (1983a) countered that there is no epidemiologic indication that *latah* is over-represented among marginalized people. Even if such data existed, the correlational and causal components would likely never be unraveled. R. Simons (1980) conceded that the body is, indeed, a symbol, then quickly insisted, "But the body is also a body" (p. 173).

The famous *latah* debate on the influence of nature and culture has continued to shape ideas about culture-bound syndromes. Using a different set of culturally mediated psychological symptoms, Kleinman (1986a, 1986b) examined neurasthenia in China and depression in North America to understand cultural differences in the salience of psychiatric diagnoses. Neurasthenia is as common a diagnosis in China as depression is in North America, and Kleinman links both to the theoretical construct of somatization. Somatization indicates the processes of communication and exchange through which a bodily idiom of distress signifies and negotiates social and personal problems (Kleinman, 1986b). Somatization is a unifying construct, in that it occurs worldwide. Kleinman proposed that somatic expressions of distress and despair illustrate the embodiment and manipulation of core cultural systems of meanings, norms, and power. Extending the position that the body is a cultural symbol, Kleinman used case studies to illustrate how the most powerless members of a cultural group may experience a progression from work and family problems to hopelessness and demoralization, leading to undermined self-esteem, blocked behavioral alternatives, depression, and somatic preoccupation, amplification, and chronicity. Far from being only a symbolic marker of social despair, however, somatization has not only social causes but social uses as well (Kleinman, 1986b). Although not malingering, a person afflicted with a culture-bound syndrome may derive benefits from the sick role in family

and work situations. Using the somatization construct, the tension between culture or nature explanations is tempered. "Pain, psychic or somatized, is an expression of the universal constant—human misery and distress—that is differentially molded by culture" (Finkler, 1986, p. 505). The new theoretical core becomes the cultural elaboration of the universal common pathway through which human misery is expressed. The body–mind dualism, assumed in prior theoretical explanations, was eliminated in Kleinman's formulation of culture-bound syndromes.

In summarizing various theoretical viewpoints, Hahn (1985) identified three ontological positions. The first, considered the Exclusionist interpretation of culture-bound syndromes, posits that there are culture-free symptoms and culture-bound ones. The culture-free might be illustrated by measles or smallpox, which have an identifiable causative agent to which human beings react more or less uniformly. The culture-bound syndromes, in contrast, involve socially learned responses to distress. In this formulation, there are two sets of illnesses, the biological and the culturally expressed psychological ones. A second theoretical possibility is called the Inclusionist Nature–Culture Continuum, positing that all conditions are some combination of natural, cultural, cognitive, and psychodynamic factors. There is, then, no culture-bound or culture-free illness, because all illnesses are a mixture of elements. For example, measles could be placed at the more natural end of the continuum, and *latah* at the more cultural end, with perhaps alcoholism and depression somewhere near the midpoint. The third interpretation of culture-bound syndromes is the Inclusionist Egalitarian position. From this viewpoint, all conditions are considered equally culture-bound, rendering the concept of a set of culture-bound syndromes useless. What is gained by considering culture-bound syndromes in this tripartite theoretical categorization? First, the limitations of the Exclusionist model become obvious. The Inclusionist models remind us that our own forms of suffering do not cover the spectrum of the possible. Finally, possibilities for future research are clarified when the philosophical underpinnings of each position are described.

Research that could be considered an example of the Inclusionist Egalitarian position explored the utility of the culture-bound syndrome concept and suggested a more useful concept: culturally interpreted symptoms. Low's (1985) examination of the symptom of *nerves* cross-culturally began with her fieldwork in Costa Rica, where *nervios* was an established mode of communicating psychosocial distress. Low learned, however, that nerves was an illness label used cross-culturally, from Kentucky to Newfoundland, but in each culture with specific networks of meaning. The label of culture-bound syndrome seemed useless and conceptually misleading as a descriptor of a syndrome not bound by culture, but shared across cultures. A better concept, Low proposed (pp. 187–188), was culturally interpreted symptoms. A set of psychosomatic symptoms usually considered within the culture-bound category can alternatively be considered culturally interpreted symptoms on three levels: (1) symptoms are culturally expressed through the body as a symbol system, (2) symptoms are culturally received, sorted, and identified in theories of disease and cultural rules, (3) symptoms are given sociocultural meanings based on values and social systems. Although symptoms may be shared cross-culturally, the three-level analysis makes clear the distinct cultural pattern in the translation of biophysiological diseases into socioculturally understood sicknesses.

In summary, a theoretical review of folk illnesses and culture-bound syndromes reveals the ongoing dialogue about the links between the human body as a biophysiological entity and the body as a symbol in a cultural system. Each debate and addition to the theoretical literature on culture-bound syndromes has enriched the dialogue. In particular, Low's (1985) ideas about culturally interpreted symptoms and Kleinman's

(1986a, 1986b) emphasis on somatization as a means of expressing misery and despair have shifted the focus away from contests over the boundaries of nature and culture and toward a reconsideration of the human experience—both mind and body—within sociocultural environments where sickness is experienced and enacted.

For the entire range of folk illnesses (including culture-bound syndromes), there is no one discipline with the theoretical or practical answers to questions about physiologic pathways explaining the symptoms, the cultural meaning of those symptoms, or appropriate and maximally effective treatment. Although some anthropologists or biomedical practitioners may claim explanations or expertise in the area, others believe carving up folk illnesses to fit into academic disciplines is a "polarization [that] is both unfortunate and unnecessary. It is possible to consider factors [related to folk illnesses] in many disciplines simultaneously" (R. C. Simons & Hughes, 1985, p. 26). Exploring the frontier of what is known about folk illnesses challenges health care practitioners, patients, anthropologists, and health care systems to reconsider the range of human experience and suffering.

Differences in Understanding Disease Causality in Folk Medicine and Biomedicine

One of the greatest barriers to understanding folk illnesses and culture-bound syndromes is created by the complexity of the beliefs associated with illness causality in these systems. Folk medical systems can be divided into two categories: naturalistic and personalistic. In naturalistic medical systems, illness is believed to be caused by an active, purposeful agent. This agent may be a human being (such as a sorcerer or witch), a supernatural being (a god), or a nonhuman entity (such as an evil spirit, ghost, or ancestor). The person has become ill as a result of punishment or aggression against him and the reasons for his illness concern him alone (Foster & Anderson, 1978).

In a personalistic medical system, there is no concept of accident, and the same causality is believed to be behind all types of personal misfortune, of which illness is only one example. Usually, two types of curers are required for healing. The first and most important is a shaman or diviner to determine the immediate cause of the problem, and, particularly, who is responsible. The key question to be answered is not "what," but rather "who." Once that has been determined, another type of healer is used to address the symptoms of the illness. At times, even a biomedically trained practitioner is used to address symptoms once the cause has been determined. The often supernatural or nonhuman nature of the causal agents in personalistic systems means that magic and religion are often important parts of such systems and the treatments they espouse (Foster & Anderson, 1978).

Naturalistic medical systems explain illness in more impersonal terms and do not address life's other problems. Health exists when an equilibrium is maintained among elements in the body; illness is the result of a disturbance in the balance. Examples of forces that can disturb the balance of the body are heat, cold, or strong emotions. The role of the curer is to determine what type of medicine, herbs, or other treatments are necessary to restore the disturbed balance. The lack of superhuman beings or entities in illness causality means that most treatments usually do not include religious or magical elements. There is very little focus on diagnosis; often the cause is determined by the patient or family of the patient. The main role of the healer in naturalistic systems is to provide relief from symptoms (Foster & Anderson, 1978).

These two etiological systems are not mutually exclusive, and many folk medical systems use elements of both in the explanation of illness causality. Believers in folk medicine also may use biomedical practitioners to address the symptoms of illnesses of both types of causality.

Examples of Folk Illnesses among Immigrants and Mainstream American Populations

Folk medical healers treat a wide range of illnesses, from those also treated by biomedical practitioners, to those that it is believed that they, alone, can address, that is, folk illnesses. While folk illnesses are often considered to be found only in small minority populations, recent research suggests that belief in folk medical systems and folk illnesses is also common among mainstream populations in the United States. Even among biomedical practitioners, common folk health beliefs and practices have been identified, raising questions about the possibility that anyone can be completely insulated from the permeating cultural influences of folk health systems (Roberson, 1987). While all cultural beliefs will vary in any population due to intracultural diversity, related to levels of education, social class, language spoken, level of acculturation, and so on, some of these folk illness beliefs and their associated folk treatments are extremely widespread, even among the contemporary middle class (Brown & Marcy, 1991; Eisenberg *et al.,* 1993).

The following section briefly reviews some of the folk illnesses seen in various populations. (If more information is needed on particular groups, several cultural assessment guides for practitioners are available; see "Additional Resources" at the end of this chapter.) While some of the same illness terms are seen in more than one culture (as discussed in the case of *nervios* [Low, 1985], as well as by Davis and Low [1989] and Davis and Guarnaccia [1989]), each illness is discussed as the ethnic group under consideration defines it. As Kay (1979) noted, lexemic change and semantic shift render illness labels indefinite cross-culturally and even intraculturally over time. "Just because a common folk term is still used, it does not mean that the word still encodes the same features for all users" (Kay, 1977a, p. 163). Currently, cross-cultural research is under way to begin to determine the extent to which an illness, such as "empacho," is really the same thing across the range of Latino populations who identify this illness (Weller, Pachter, Trotter, & Baer, 1993). In this case, some beliefs about causes, symptoms, and treatments of this illness do cross cultures; others do not. A similar pattern appears to exist for several other common folk illnesses, including *nervios* (Baer, 1997), *susto* (Weller, 1996), *caida de mollera* (Weller, 1997), and *mal de ojo*. For example, in a study of *nervios* among Mexicans, Mexican Americans, Puerto Ricans in Hartford, Connecticut, and Guatemalans, Baer (1997) found that *nervios* covers a broad range of mental health conditions. Symptoms include headache, feeling of choking, cold sweats, swollen or bloated stomach, bad temper, crying, agitation, insomnia, depression, feeling hopeless about one's life, and shaking and trembling.

Anglo Americans

One folk illness that has been noted among Anglo Americans (Baer *et al.,* in review), African Americans (L. Pachter, Niego, & Pelto, 1996), and English-speaking Puerto Ricans (L. Pachter *et al.,* 1996), is "folk flu." This illness was first identified by McCombie (1987) in the southwestern United States. She found no overlap between the biomedically defined respiratory illness named influenza (caused by *Hemophilus influenza*) and the folk category of "flu." Folk flu is characterized as a gastrointestinal illness with vomiting and diarrhea, among other symptoms. Using a folk diagnosis of flu may serve important social functions; the label can be applied to almost any illness. With a culturally recognized, legitimate diagnosis in hand, the anxiety of the patient is relieved, as the condition is understood to be a temporary interruption of role responsibilities with anticipated complete restoration to full health in a short time. Since everyone is susceptible to folk flu, the individual is not ill as the result of a social transgression (as in the case of a venereal disease or a smoking-related pulmonary condition). Social functions of a diagnosis of "flu" include the legitimization of a patient's abrogation of social or professional obligations without creating concern or embarrassment (McCombie, 1987).

Ritenbaugh (1982) has suggested that other health problems, including some recognized by the biomedical community, may indeed be culture-bound syndromes. These syndromes, Ritenbaugh stresses, can be recognized by the problematic therapeutic relationships typical of them. She points specifically to obesity, a "disease" classification that has become increasingly problematic. Until the present century, mild to moderate obesity was considered a sign of health, beauty, or both in the United States; this continues to be the situation in many contemporary societies. A major factor in the changing view of mild obesity in the United States has been the classification system used by insurance companies for deciding who should be charged higher rates. By the late 1950s, the decision had been made to accept the weight of individuals of 25 years of age as ideal; the fact that most individuals increase their weight up to about 50 years of age was ignored. On the basis of a weak link found by the Framingham study between cardiovascular disease and being extremely overweight, "obesity, as a disease, was born" (p. 355). However, regardless of the fact that this association was found exclusively in a male population, weight standards for women have exhibited a steady downward trend. The tremendous cultural emphasis on thinness in women is an important factor in the other current epidemic among Anglo American females, eating disorders (Parker *et al.,* 1995).

African Americans

African Americans may also hold various folk medical beliefs and experience a range of folk illnesses the etiologies of which frequently are divided into the realms of natural and unnatural (or personalistic). Some researchers have suggested that due to the personalistic belief system the sick person is thought to be a victim and therefore is not wholly responsible for his or her health status (Lassiter, 1995). Other researchers have contended that African Americans view illness as disharmony with one's soul and therefore maintaining good health is a personal responsibility (Jackson, 1981). A natural illness is provoked when the dictums of good health are broken by not eating well, not maintaining a regular schedule of rest, recreation, and worship, and not leading a moral lifestyle (Jackson, 1981; Lassiter, 1995). Agents of naturalistic illnesses include microbes, inadequate rest, poor nutrition, accidents, environmental pollutants, hot and cold imbalances, positive and negative imbalances, or alterations in the blood. An unnatural illness is caused by the intervention of evil influences, or more innocuously may be due to stress or worry. Unnatural agents include ghosts, souls, deities, devils, witches, shamen, or priests (Lassiter, 1995).

Many African American folk illnesses are due to altered states of the blood. Blood is considered to be in continual flux, responding to internal and external stimuli as varied as food, seasons, temperature, emotions, and hygiene (Snow, 1974). These conditions include bruised blood, high blood, low blood, bad blood, blood clots, thick blood, thin blood, and unclean blood (Jackson, 1981; Snow, 1974). Bruised blood is the blood left after tissue is injured; it is darker because it is not moving. High blood can cause one to feel dizzy and lead to falling-out (to be described later). High blood is caused by blood collecting high up in the body or due to an increase in blood volume; it may be treated with Epsom salts and vinegar. Low blood, contrarily, is considered to be a lack of blood or inadequate iron. Bad blood is contaminated blood and may be provoked by natural causes or supernatural causes, or may be hereditary. Usually there is an insinuated sanction for inappropriate social behavior if this label is applied; for example, syphilis is sometimes referred to as bad blood. Blood clots are described as blood that stops moving and is associated with abdominal cramps or leg cramps especially during menses. This condition may be accompanied by thick blood or colds. Thick blood moves more slowly and may cause circulatory problems; it may also be laden with more impurities than is ideal. Hot foods, for instance, are thought to thicken the blood. Thin blood makes one more susceptible to respiratory problems and becoming chilled; it may also be related to low blood or low iron. Finally, unclean blood is a natural accumulation of impurities in the blood over time. Due to the tendency for these impurities to accumulate, regular sexual activity, bowel elimination, sweating, bleeding, and purges are thought to assist the body in maintaining clean blood.

Other types of African American folk illness include tedder, gas, falling-out, ear noises, and cold (Jackson, 1981; Snow, 1974). Tedder is a scalp condition that manifests whitish, dry, scaly patches with hair loss in the area. This condition is most common in children and is highly communicable. Gas is thought to be located in the stomach, but has the capacity to produce pain in other parts of the body including the shoulders and the chest. It is caused by consuming heavy foods. Falling-out, also known as indisposition, occurs when someone collapses suddenly. Their eyes may be open but unfocused and they are unable to hear. Falling-out is preceded by weakness and dizziness and is caused by high blood (Hughes, 1985). Ear noises may prognosticate impending death since ringing or buzzing in the ears are interpreted to be the spirits calling. Finally, cold is embodied in air, winds, water, dew, and food. Menstruating women are especially susceptible to getting cold and the condition can be very dangerous and could even kill a person.

The African American folk health belief system may identify supernatural involvement with accidents, paralyzing stroke, the birth of children with congenital problems, or sudden death (Snow, 1974). No supernatural illness responds to biomedical intervention as they are believed to be caused by rootwork, or witchcraft. Most of the African Americans who believe in supernatural illness hold that rootwork is only viable if all involved parties believe in its potency (Rosereto, 1973). Root-work may induce symptomology distinct from that recognized as illness by biomedicine and may require a positive rootworker to reverse the hex (Rosereto, 1973; Snow, 1993).

Haitian Americans

Folk illnesses are also common among populations of recent immigrants to the United States. Among Haitian Americans, illness is thought to be caused by a disequilibrium between internal and external qualities such as hot and cold air or food, and gas, or by angry spirits; germs are not widely recognized etiological agents. Health is produced by proper eating, exercising, sleeping, and hygiene (Lassiter, 1995). There is an external locus of control for falling ill and individuals may not consider their own actions to be related to their health problems. Disease for Haitian Americans can also be divided into two types, natural and supernatural. Natural diseases are characterized by having familiar symptoms of short duration (Laguerre, 1981). The most dangerous types of natural disease are those caused by blood problems such as an alteration in the volume, quality, and color of the blood or changes in the movement of the blood. The blood may be hot, cold, thin, thick, weak, yellow, spoiled, turned to water, or dark (Laguerre, 1981; Lassiter, 1995). Hot blood causes a high fever and is provoked by being overly nervous, exerting oneself intellectually or physically, giving birth, or sleeping. Cold blood may be caused by malaria or may naturally cool while sitting. Thin blood causes one to appear pale and may be caused by fright or by hypertension. Thick blood produces itching. Weak blood causes physical or mental weakness. Yellow blood occurs when there is bile in the blood. Spoiled blood may be caused by fright and is associated with venereal disease; it may also be associated with emotions, sexual exposure to bad people, magic, or consumption of inappropriate foods. Blood turns to water when one has been drinking too much alcohol and may result in pleurisy or tuberculosis. Dark blood is indicative of a terminal illness.

Other types of natural illnesses include gas, milk complications, the wandering womb, fright, perdition, alterations in the body's hot/cold balance, bone displacement, and the movement of disease (Laguerre, 1981; Lassiter, 1995). Gas problems are associated with the location and movement of gas in the body. Gas entering the ears causes headaches, gas entering the body via the mouth causes stomachaches, and gas traveling from the stomach to the legs causes rheumatism. Gas may also produce pain and anemia. Complications with mother's milk occur if a woman becomes angry or frightened. Haitian Americans hold that anger induces the milk to travel to the woman's head which brings headaches, depression, and psychoses. This condition is not only dangerous for the mother but also for the baby as the milk could mix with blood and poison the baby. Another danger is that the milk may become too thick and cause impetigo. Wandering womb occurs postpartum in some Haitian Americans with symptoms of dizziness, weakness, and confusion. The womb is believed to wander because it misses the baby it held for 9 months, and is in search of its friend. Fright is characterized by partial blindness and headache. It may occur when a person becomes upset due to bad news or some threat to the person's well-being. When those things occur, blood rushes to the head producing the typical symptoms. Another type of natural illness is know as perdition. Perdition is when a baby is trapped in the womb for extended periods of time, up to many years. This illness is caused by a woman walking barefoot on wet surfaces, lifting heavy objects, or experiencing excessive stress. These conditions reverse the baby's growth until the baby resumes its original microscopic status. It will maintain that state until the conditions that provoked perdition are ameliorated; at that point the normal 9-month pregnancy will resume. Hot and cold disequilibrium occur if one consumes foods, or exposes oneself to conditions, that are too hot or too cold in a humoral (not temperature) sense.

Supernatural illnesses occur suddenly and are thought to be caused by angry spirits (Lassiter, 1995). To honor the spirits and keep them content, ceremonies must be performed regularly; voodoo may play a role in this. Thus, there is a dependency created between people and spirits; the spirits need the people to maintain their own position in the spiritual hierarchy, and the people need the spirits to protect them and offer them health (Laguerre, 1981). The cure for supernatural illness is realized only when the breach in the relationship between the person and the spirits is remediated.

Haitian American patients will generally present with vague descriptions of their symptoms since they believe that when the person is ill the entire body is ill (Laguerre, 1981). Health is considered to be a personal responsibility and the patient may be reluctant to recount specific symptoms to the physician but instead relate what condition they believe they have and wait for the doctor to confirm the diagnosis.

Vietnamese Americans

Vietnamese Americans have a holistic concept of health wherein health is dependent on family, religion, food, morality, and metaphysical forces. Illness may be caused by natural forces, disequilibrium, supernatural forces, or germs (Lassiter, 1995). Natural illnesses occur when the individual is no longer in balance with nature. These conditions are treated by interventions such as massage and avoidance of any excesses in an attempt to promote the body's natural recuperative powers. Supernatural illnesses are caused by gods, demons, and spirits. Illnesses of disequilibrium are caused by loss of balance of hot and cold or yin and yang. Causality is a major theme in Vietnamese cosmology, and horoscopy and individual destiny, based on the star under which the person was born, are large influences in health (Stephenson, 1995).

In Vietnamese cosmology, the body has three souls and nine vital spirits. The primary soul maintains the life force, the secondary soul is the seat of intelligence, and the tertiary soul is for the senses. If any of the souls or spirits leave, illness will shortly follow. For this reason when many Vietnamese persons leave an area they will make noise or talk loudly to alert the souls and spirits that it is time to go. Because the souls are so important, they must be honored after their vessel persons die. If the souls are not honored they may return as evil spirits. Evil spirits may also come from dogs, pigs, cats, water, and fire; it is those evil spirits that bring disease (Grossinger, 1987). If a person does experience soul loss she or he will be thin, tired, and pale. Because of the possibility of soul loss, many Vietnamese would rather avoid surgery, thus eliminating the risk of soul loss during anesthesia-induced unconsciousness.

Some Vietnamese view Western medicine in opposition to traditional medicine. However, this opposition is not an anathema; rather traditional and Western medicine are viewed as yin–yang influences: both are important, but should never be used simultaneously. Western medicine is thought to be hot, while traditional medicine is cool. Within Vietnamese traditional medicine, familial and social responses to illness are emphasized rather than the techniques of Western health care traditions (Moore, Van Arsdale, Glittenberg, & Aldrich, 1980). One popular form of Vietnamese treatment intervention for myalgias, dengue, fevers, influenza, headaches, the common cold, and other conditions is *cao gio* (Stephenson, 1995). *Cao gio* consists of dermabrasion by coining, cupping, moxibustion, or pinching. With coining, a mentholated coin is rubbed all over the chest or the back. Cupping consists of placing a heated glass on the area of complaint or on an associated area and creating a vacuum. This vacuum is believed to draw out the infection. With moxibustion, a burning plant (or piece of a plant) or cigarette is briefly placed on the skin. Finally, pinching may be performed with the fingers or with tweezers.

All of these forms of intervention break the superficial capillaries, resulting in ecchymosis (L. M. Pachter, 1994). Coin rubbing may look like abuse in children; therefore, health care professionals must take a careful history and make observations of parent–child interaction to determine the etiology of bruising (Golden & Duster, 1977).

Preventative care is also practiced by Vietnamese. One example is that postpartum Vietnamese women are encouraged to follow strict sanctions including avoidance of raw vegetables, sunshine, limited bathing, and enforced bed rest of 1 month or more. If these practices are not followed, death could result since the delivery caused her body to become overly heated (Moore *et al.,* 1980).

Cuban Americans

For Cuban Americans, good health is a balance of humans with their environment, natural with supernatural, mind with body, and hot with cold (Lassiter, 1995). Illness can be separated into two types: physical and metaphysical. Physical illnesses may be due to a hot–cold imbalance, a deficiency of a body substance, or an obstruction. A subset of physical illnesses for Cuban Americans are many common folk illnesses, including *empacho* and *mal aire. Empacho* is believed to be caused by consuming starchy, heavy foods and is most common among children. *Mal aire* is believed to be caused by an excess of heat (from exercise or a fever) or too much cold (from water or wind) leading to the chief complaints of back pain and muscle spasms that may cause paralysis and respiratory disorders. Metaphysical illnesses, unlike physical illnesses, are believed to be caused by God's will, magical forces, evil spirits, or human forces. *Susto* and *mal de ojo* are two types of metaphysical illnesses. *Susto* is thought to be caused by a traumatic event causing the spirit to flee and demonstrating the symptoms of anorexia, ensuing weight loss, listlessness, and pallor. *Mal de ojo* is caused by a strong person whose envy or admiration deleteriously affects the health of susceptible persons. Children and women are thought to be the most susceptible and therefore should protect themselves by wearing gold or jet beads or amulets in the shape of a hand. The protective amulets are representative of the influences of *santeria* and *brujeria* (witchcraft) on Cuban folk medicine. Both *santeria* and *brujeria* are derived from West African religious and healing traditions (Ruiz, 1985); *santeria* is most often used as a mental health care system (Sandoval, 1979).

Mexican Americans

Mexican American folk illnesses fall into two categories: those with natural causes and those caused by witchcraft (Schreiber & Homiak, 1981). Health, in general, is thought to be produced when social and spiritual realms are harmonious. There is no real differentiation between psychic and somatic disorders. A wide repertoire of herbal and other types of home remedies are used by this ethnic group (Kay, 1996).

The three dominant concepts in Mexican American folk illnesses (soul loss, humoral theory, and blood loss) attest to the concurrent psychic and somatic elements of illness. Soul loss is caused by fright, spirit intrusion, object intrusion, breach of taboo associated with shame, fear, disillusion, anger, or envy. The humoral theory posits that health is a balance of hot and cold; conversely illness is caused when there is internal or external exposure to excessive hot or cold. Finally, any type of blood loss can cause weakness and illness. Natural illnesses include *mollera caida, empacho, mal ojo, susto, bilis, latido, tripa ida, mal aire, chipil,* and *pasmo* (Kay, 1977a; A. Rubel, 1960; Schreiber & Homiak, 1981; Trotter, 1985; Trotter, Montellano, & Logan, 1989). *Mollera caida* usually occurs in infants, though recent research has established that there is an adult form as well (Weller, 1996); symptoms include sunken anterior fontanelle, the inability to suckle, diarrhea, crying, and fever. *Empacho* is characterized by abdominal pain, fever in the stomach, thirst, and a swollen abdomen. It is caused by food becoming stuck in the digestive tract and is frequently due to social norms requiring people to eat food to be polite even if the food is not desired. If the condition is not treated expeditiously it may result in death (Schreiber & Homiak, 1981). *Mal ojo* is accompanied by headaches, nervousness, a rash, weeping, diarrhea, vomiting, crying, fever, and disturbed sleep. It is caused by an adult staring at a less powerful person, usually a child. *Susto* also has symptoms of stomachache and diarrhea and may result in death. It is characterized by anxiety, anorexia, insomnia, irritability, trembling, diarrhea, and depression. For the older person, *susto* may be fatal or cause tuberculosis. Researchers have traditionally associated this condition with role conflicts and social inadequacies. However, recent studies have suggested that *susto* is associated with increased morbidity and mortality (Baer & Penzell, 1993; A. Rubel *et al.,* 1984), and that the element of soul loss is of less importance than that of fright in contemporary understandings of causality of the illness (Weller, 1997).

There are relatively few nonnatural types of disease in Mexican American cosmology. These are believed to be caused by witchcraft and may be illustrated by *mal puesto. Mal puesto* has psychological and somatic symptoms that are not easily classified (Hughes, 1985). It is usually caused by a disruption of social relationships and may lead to infertility or insanity.

Puerto Rican Americans

For Puerto Ricans, good health is a gift from God and allows one to participate in the workforce and to be a good provider (Brosnan, 1976). Ill health, conversely, is a punishment for wrongdoing, though not necessarily exclusively since life is full of suffering. Illness may be due to combining hot and cold food inappropriately or chilling oneself by walking in the rain. When one is suffering from too much heat, the appropriate treatment is an attempt to balance that state with something cold. There are also physiological

and spiritual causes of illness, as mental and physical functioning of the body are believed to be inseparable (Delgado, 1979). Therefore, spiritualists are often used, particularly in the case of emotional or mental health–related complaints (Harwood, 1977). Witchcraft may also play a role if an individual falls ill for no cause. *Mal de ojo* is one type of illness caused by envy. To cure this illness the cause of the ailment must be found. Puerto Ricans also share with Mexicans and Cubans a belief in the folk illness *empacho* (L. Pachter *et al.,* 1992), discussed earlier, as well as in the illness *nervios*. Guarnaccia, De La Cancela, and Carrillo (1989) have suggested that the related problem, *ataques de nervios,* is an expression of grief and anger, related to the process of migration; causality is the disruption of family systems and concerns about family members at home.

Summary

In summary, these folk illness systems of African Americans, Haitian Americans, Vietnamese Americans, Cuban Americans, Mexican Americans, and Puerto Rican Americans are distinct from biomedicine in that they see the body in a more holistic fashion where social, physical, and psychological elements are interdependent. These systems also have a tendency to dichotomize illness into the etiologies of natural and supernatural. Because of the complex beliefs and conditions recognized in these systems specialized ethnomedical health care providers exist in these communities to meet the needs of these populations.

Recommendations for Clinicians in Dealing with Patients Presenting with Folk Illnesses

One of the most useful results flowing from the literature on folk illnesses has been the critical reappraisal of biomedical nosologies. The diagnostic categorical schema used in *DSM-IV* (American Psychiatric Association, 1994) or *ICD-9*, for example, are based on implicit values and assumptions, to which practitioners must be attuned and skeptical. A culturally informed use of diagnostic categories means not only knowing the culture of the person being evaluated in sufficient detail to make a valid behavioral assessment, "[but also] resisting taking the values and meanings of one's own culture (and social class) for granted when dealing with a patient" (Hughes, 1985, p. 21). Practitioners sensitized to folk illnesses improve their practice through including a cultural assessment in the conduct of patient history, focusing on symptoms as opposed to rushing to a diagnostic conclusion, and remaining open to the possibilities for concurrent use of folk remedies and biomedical treatments.

There are a number of issues of critical importance to the clinician in dealing with folk illnesses and folk medical systems in general. Patients who believe in these systems will use them for biomedical as well as folk illnesses. In biomedical illnesses, folk remedies may be used in combination with those of biomedicine. A patient being treated by a physician for a biomedically defined "disease" may be complementing such treatments with more traditional ones. The danger is that folk treatments may interfere with biomedical treatments, through interaction of aspects of the two types of remedies or drugs. It is therefore important that the clinician win the trust of the patient and learn whether folk remedies are being used. If so, and if they pose a problem for the biomedical treatment, efforts should be made to find a way that both types of treatments can be used without negative interactions. If necessary, the biomedical treatment should be changed; it is unlikely that a patient who believes in the power of folk remedies will abandon these merely on the advice of a clinician.

In the case of folk illnesses, it is generally believed that biomedical health care workers are unable to effectively treat such problems. Folk treatments will be used, and only if they are not effective will biomedical health care resources be pursued. In addition, many be-

lievers in folk medical systems report negative interactions with health care providers if the former suggest that their problem is a folk illness (Baer *et al.*, 1989). For this reason, they may use treatments that are potentially dangerous (such as lead oxides to treat *empacho* among Mexicans and Mexican Americans) (Trotter, 1985), or delay biomedical consultation until the problem is extremely serious.

However, recent research has shown that regardless of differences in understanding the causality of many folk illnesses between the biomedical and folk sectors, many folk illnesses are accompanied by physiological symptoms that are amenable to biomedical attention (Baer & Bustillo, 1993; Baer & Bustillo, n.d.). The best approach for the clinician is to avoid discussions of causality, or even labeling of the condition, but rather, to focus on the symptoms for which biomedicine can offer relief. A sympathetic practitioner who takes this approach and encourages the patient to seek a folk healer for other aspects of the problem, will find that patients will be willing to use biomedicine for some aspects of the treatment of folk illnesses.

Recommendations for Further Research on These Topics

In an epidemiologic sense, the incidence and prevalence of folk illnesses are difficult to determine. "How many cases of *susto* occurred in Texas last year?" or "What percentage of babies will be affected with *mal de ojo* at some point in their first 2 years of life?" are fascinating questions to consider, but difficult to answer. Some well-done studies have provided answers to epidemiologic questions about folk illnesses (e.g., Baer & Bustillo, 1993; Chiu, Tong, & Schmidt, 1972; Higginbotham, Trevino, & Ray, 1990; Pachter *et al.*, 1996) and demonstrate effective and innovative methods for studying folk illnesses. Research related to folk illnesses involves challenges of definition and measurement, appreciation for strengths and weaknesses in large-scale surveys, and inclusive consideration of biomedical, folk, and lay domains of care for the identification and treatment of folk illnesses.

Challenges to the effective definition and measurement of folk illnesses arise from the nature of folk illnesses as culturally located and incompatible with the biomedical paradigm. Determining an operational definition for the identification of the folk illness to be studied is one obstacle, and accurately measuring incidence or prevalence is another. Researchers will certainly uncover more challenges in the conduct of an investigation of folk illnesses. However, some of the key issues at this point are described in the following sections.

Definitional Issues

Clear definitions of folk illnesses exist (see the "Glossary of Culture-Bound or Psychiatric Syndromes" in R. C. Simons & Hughes, 1985; see also Kay, 1977b; Rubel, O'Nell, & Collado-Ardon, 1984), but the defining symptoms vary among subcultural groups (see Low, 1985) and may change over time (see Crandon-Malamud, 1991; Finerman, 1989; Kleinman, 1986a). Although there is consensus at some level among members of a culture group about what symptoms constitute any specific folk illness, there is seldom an authoritative definition against which to compare clusters of reported symptoms. The *DSM-IV* (the canon of mental illnesses in Western biomedical culture) provides authoritative lists of criteria for the differentiation and diagnosis of mental disorders such as schizophrenia and depression, but there is no corollary to the *DSM-IV* to aid in the differential diagnosis of *mal aire* and *susto.* It is difficult to measure what is not clearly defined.

Despite the relative lack of official diagnostic categories for folk illnesses, there is no lack of informal criteria for the diagnosis of folk illnesses. One promising area of research has been the systematic definition and differentiation of folk illnesses, both intraculturally and cross-culturally (Garro, 1986; Weller & Dungy, 1986). A study in this vein may select a folk illness, identify the main attributes of the illness, rank order those attributes in order of importance, and then examine a population to determine the level of consensus among members of the group regarding the characteristics of the illness. Curers and laypeople may have different models of the illness, for example, or men and women may demonstrate different levels of knowledge about the illness, or older and younger generations may disagree about illness causation. Research addressing definitional and consensus issues assists clinicians in listening more sensitively for core attributes of folk illnesses in patient encounters.

Measurement Issues

Challenges to the valid and reliable measurement of folk illness incidence include lack of written records about folk illness cases, lack of objective laboratory data confirming the diagnosis, and the weaknesses of self-reported data. First, in retrospective studies of disease categories acknowledged in biomedical nosologies, a fundamental research tool is medical chart review for tabulation of cases or risk factors within a specified population. Unlike standard biomedical diagnostic categories, the diagnosis of a folk illness would rarely, if ever, show up in a medical record. Even if a patient is seeking help with symptoms related to a folk illness, the suspected folk illness may not have been reported to the practitioner, detected by the practitioner, or committed to writing in the chart. Consequently, measurement of folk illness incidence would be fruitless using medical record data. Second, unlike illnesses with a laboratory indicator, folk illnesses are undetectable using standard laboratory analyses of urine, feces, blood, or tissue samples. The application of a folk illness label to symptoms is a matter of symptom interpretation far more than symptom quantification in terms of deviations from normal chemistry or histology. Screening populations for folk illnesses using laboratory indicators is therefore pointless.

Finally, studies of folk illness incidence and prevalence must rely on self-reported symptoms and diagnoses. Asking someone if he or she has suffered from a particular illness is the most direct way of ascertaining lifetime incidence. Complicating this seemingly direct approach is the fact that many childhood folk illnesses would not be recalled by an individual, since the experience occurred when he or she was too young to recall it. In these instances, researchers have asked mothers as surrogate informants about the incidence of folk illnesses among their children (e.g., Baer & Bustillo, 1993; Baer *et al.,* 1989). Another confounding variable in self-reports of folk illnesses is the tendency for informants to respond with socially desirable answers to questions posed by researchers. Especially when the research setting is a clinic or hospital and the investigator is a nurse or physician, patients feel uncomfortable answering honestly that their problem is not the biomedical diagnosis listed on the chart, but a problem with a hex or folk illness. Selecting interviewers with linguistic and cultural backgrounds similar to those interviewed is hypothesized to facilitate more accurate self-reporting (Higginbotham *et al.,* 1990).

One large-scale survey with both strengths and limitations deserves special mention as an example of epidemiologic research on folk illnesses and folk practitioners (Higginbotham *et al.,* 1990). Using data collected as part of the Hispanic Health and Nutrition Examination Survey (HHANES), investigators conducted a secondary analysis of data from 3,623 Mexican Americans (ages 18 to 74 years) residing in the southwestern United States. Each of these informants was asked, "There are some providers of health care that we sometimes go to, such as *curanderos, sobadores,* herbalists, spiritualists, and others. Have you seen or talked to any of these persons for health care during the past 12 months?" Only 4.2% (148 of the sample of

3,623) responded affirmatively as to use of such practitioners. Users of *curanderos* were more likely to be male, have lower levels of education, be foreign born, report their health as fair or poor, and speak Spanish during the interview. No effect of acculturation was detected. The strengths of this study included the stratified random sample of Hispanics selected from the Southwest and the comprehensive list of folk healers included in the question. The finding that 4.2% of Mexican Americans interviewed used folk healers in the previous year corresponds with earlier research showing that relatively few Mexican-origin residents in the United States consulted folk healers (Snow, 1974).

Skaer, Robinson, Sclar, and Harding (1996) attempted to compensate for the general overrepresentation of more highly educated higher income individuals, and those with telephone access in population samples such as HHANES in a study conducted in rural eastern Washington state in six rural health clinics. Clinics such as these serve low-income migrant populations. Included in this study were woman of less than 20 years of age, who were interviewed by bilingual female medical assistants and nurses. More than 21% of the women reported using curanderos in the past 5 years (vs. a 12-month reporting period for the HHANES study). This is comparable to the 20% rate of curandero treatment reported by Risser and Mazur (1995) in Houston at a pediatric primary care clinic, and to the 17% of mothers in a California study reporting that they used or would use a *curandera* as the initial source of care for the children's illnesses (Mikhail, 1994). These studies suggest that research methods in the study of folk illnesses and utilization of the folk health care sector vary and may account for differences in results. There is also reason to believe that large-scale telephone interviews with government sponsorship using population samples may produce different results from studies with interview components using convenience samples from low income and migrant populations. Studies quantifying the effect of folk illnesses and folk healers in immigrant populations must be carefully scrutinized, since methodological decisions so closely affect results.

A common limitation in studies seeking to examine and quantify folk illnesses and use of folk health care systems is the minimization of lay diagnosis and treatment. Lay providers of care, such as friends and family, are not considered curanderos, but may possess expertise and skill in treating folk illnesses and routine acute illnesses (Chrisman & Kleinman, 1983). One informant in an Arizona study of Mexican Americans (Clark, 1992) reported the following: "There's a medicine [in a local Mexican pharmacy] for *empacho*. I can't remember the name, I just know what it looks like." This mother treated *empacho* at home on her own, most likely using *pamita*, or tansy mustard seed. The mother then continued, illustrating another level of lay care: "Sometimes my daughter gets *empacho* when she swallows her gum. And my mom will rub her back and pop it. If it pops three times, that means they're really *empachado*." In this family, when children were afflicted with *empacho* they were treated at home by their own mother or by their grandmother, but in neither instance were these treatments considered to be care by a *curandero*. In another study, 53% of a sample of Mexican and Mexican American farmworker women in Florida admitted to treating folk illnesses in their own children (Baer & Bustillo, 1993). Although the 4.2% estimate of *curandero* use often cited from the HHANES study suggests low utilization of folk healers, it provides unreliable information about the incidence of folk illnesses and the entire realm of treatment options for Hispanics in the Southwest. Low utilization rates of healers in both biomedical and folk settings suggests a major emphasis on household strategies to ameliorate minor symptoms, with symptom severity the major determinant of physician utilization when household strategies fail (Markides, Levin, & Ray, 1985).

For many immigrant families, management of illness symptoms at home is paramount given biomedical health care may be unavailable, inaccessible, unaffordable, or culturally unappealing (Chesney, Chavira, Hall, & Gary, 1982; Estrada, Trevino, & Ray, 1990; Higginbotham *et al.*, 1990; Lewin-Epstein, 1991; A. J. Rubel & Garro, 1992). Considering these deterrents to use of the biomedical health care system, sufferers and their families turn to the arsenal of home treatments at their disposal, including over-the-counter medications; prescription medications saved from prior illnesses or obtained illegally, home remedies, or medications transported to this country from other parts of the world (Clark, 1992; Logan, 1988). Practitioners and researchers alike are most effective in studying folk illnesses and folk health systems when the rigid conceptual boundaries between health care systems are removed to acknowledge the fluid entry and exit of curers from different health systems in the sufferer's experience of illness.

To truly understand and measure prevalence and treatment of folk illnesses will necessitate departures from the types of research instruments we have used to date. *We need to understand what to ask;* for example, Baer and Bustillo (1998) suggested that our research methods may have obscured our current understanding of the treatment of folk illnesses. Most research asks interviewees how they treat particular folk illness (see, e.g., Weller *et al.*, 1993). However, since the cause of many folk illnesses is in the spiritual or social sphere, the treatments for the cause of the illness may be nonphysiological. Baer and Bustillo (1998) suggested that those who believe in folk illnesses may separate treatments for causes and treatments for symptoms, and that the latter may be of a more biological-physiological nature. However, our research has asked only about treatments for causes, so we lack a complete understanding of how these illnesses are handled. As discussed earlier, we also need to ask about informal and lay treatments for folk illnesses to appreciate the full picture of the interplay between self-care, lay care, folk care, and biomedical care.

We also need to understand what not to ask: Surveys must be constructed to use terms that are meaningful to the populations being studied (see, e.g., Baer, 1996), and must acknowledge the reality that in many folk medical systems, curers are a heterogeneous group in which formal curers such as *curandaras* overlap with laypersons (e.g., knowledgeable grandmothers). Folk medical systems are not biomedicine, and the types of health surveys and question content used in biomedical surveys will not produce meaningful data. But folk medical systems and the folk illnesses and culture-bound syndromes they address are an important aspect of the health culture of many mainstream and immigrant populations, and it is our responsibility to learn how to understand and evaluate the contributions of these other approaches to health care.

Conclusions

Folk illnesses continue to influence the health care needs and overall health of many mainstream as well as immigrant populations. Ethnomedical systems parallel biomedical systems to provide health care, and at times the two systems respond simultaneously or serially to the same constellation of patient symptoms. Decades of theoretical debate over the nature of folk illnesses have produced the conclusion that folk illnesses are not neatly categorized as either strictly cultural illnesses or merely pathophysiologic variation. Models for considering folk illnesses and the subset of culture-bound syndromes have also been discussed.

Examples of folk illnesses among Anglo Americans, African Americans, Haitian Americans, Vietnamese Americans, Cuban Americans, Mexican Americans, and Puerto Ricans suggest wide variability in the range and interpretation of folk illnesses among these ethnic groups. Clinicians who reflectively practice will become aware of cultural influences in biomedical classification systems and will acknowledge the plurality in

the way patients assemble medical systems to treat symptoms. Clinicians are also encouraged to offer treatment for symptoms within the area of their expertise to ease suffering, while suggesting consultation outside the biomedical system for those folk illness symptoms and causes that biomedicine cannot treat.

While there has been a great deal of research on the topic of folk illnesses and culture-bound syndromes, a number of issues are still to be clarified, including how some of these illnesses are defined, both intra- and interculturally, and how incidence and prevalence of these illnesses can better be measured. Research on treatment must be broadened to include self- and lay care, and attention is needed to the issues of treatment of causes and treatment of symptoms.

References

American Psychiatric Association. (1994). *Diagnostic and statistical manual of mental disorders* (4th ed.). Washington, DC: Author.

Baer, R. (1996). Health and mental health among Mexican-American migrant workers: Implications for survey research. *Human Organization, 55,* 58–66.

Baer, R. (1997, March 4–9). "Nervios" in four Cultures. Paper presented at the meetings of the Society for Applied Anthropology, Seattle, WA.

Baer, R., & Bustillo, M. (1993). Susto and mal de ojo among Florida farmworkers: Emic and etic perspectives. *Medical Anthropology Quarterly, 15,* 90–100.

Baer, R., & Bustillo, M. (1998). Caida de Mollera among children of Mexican migrant workers: Implications for the study of folk illnesses. *Medical Antrhopology Quarterly, 12*(2), 241–249.

Baer, R, & Penzell, D. (1993). Susto and pesticide poisoning among Florida farmworkers. *Culture, Medicine and Psychiatry, 17,* 321–327.

Baer, R., Garcia de Alba, J., Cueto, L., Ackerman, A., & Davison, S. (1989). Lead-based remedies for empacho: Patterns and consequences. *Social Science and Medicine, 29*(12), 1373–1379.

Baer, R., Weller, S., *et al.,* (submitted). Cross-cultural perspectives on the common cold. *Human Organiz.*

Brosnan, J. (1976). A proposed diabetic educational program for Puerto Ricans in New York City. In P. Brink (Ed.), *Transcultural nursing* (pp. 263–275). Englewood Cliffs, NJ: Prentice-Hall.

Brown, J.S., & Marcy, S. A. (1991). The use of botanical for health purposes by members of a prepaid health plan. *Research in Nursing and Health, 14,* 330–350.

Chesney, A. P., Chavira, J. A., Hall, R. P., & Gary, H. E., Jr. (1982). Barriers to medical care of Mexican-Americans: The role of social class, acculturation, and social isolation. *Medical Care, 20*(9), 883–891.

Chiu, T. L., Tong, J. E., & Schmidt, K. E. (1972). A clinical and survey study of latah in Sarawak, Malaysia. *Psychological Medicine, 2,* 155–165.

Chrisman, N. J., & Kleinman, A. (1983). Popular health care, social networks, and cultural meanings: The orientation of medical anthropology. In D. Mechanic (Ed.), *Handbook of health, health care, and health professions* (pp. 569–590). New York: Free Press.

Clark, L. (1992). Women's domestic health work in poverty: A comparison of Mexican American and Anglo households. Doctoral dissertation, University of Arizona, Tucson.

Crandon-Malamud, L. (1991). *From the fat of our souls: Social change, political process, and medical pluralism in Bolivia.* Berkeley: University of California Press.

Davis, D., & Guarnaccia, P. (1989). Health culture and the nature of nerves. *Medical Anthropology, 11*(1), 1–13.

Davis, D., & Low, S. (1989). *Gender, health and illness.* New York: Hemisphere.

Delgado, M. (1979). Herbal medicine in the Puerto Rican community. *Health and Social Work, 4*(2), 24–40.

Eisenberg, D., Kessler, R., Foster, C., Norlock, F., Calkins, D., & Delbanco, T. (1993). Unconventional medicine in the United States: Prevalence, costs, and patterns of use. *New England Journal of Medicine, 328*(4), 246–252.

Estrada, A. L., Trevino, F. M., & Ray, L. A. (1990). Health care utilization barriers among Mexican-Americans: Evidence from HHANES 1982–84. *American Journal of Public Health, 80* (Suppl.), 27–31.

Finerman, R. (1989). Tracing home-based health care change in an Andean Indian community. *Medical Anthropology Quarterly, 3*(2), 162–174.

Finkler, K. (1986). Review of Social origins of distress and disease: Depression, neurasthenia, and pain in modern China (by Arthur Kleinman). *Current Anthropology, 27*(5), 505–506.

Foster, G., & Anderson, B. (1978). *Medical Anthropology.* New York: Wiley.

Garro, L. C. (1986). Intracultural variation in folk medical knowledge: A comparison between curers and noncurers. *American Anthropologist, 88,* 351–370.

Geertz, H. (1968). Latah in Java: A theoretical paradox. *Indonesia, 5,* 93–104.

Golden, S. M., & Duster, M. C. (1977). Hazards of misdiagnosis due to Vietnamese folk medicine. *Clinical Pediatrics, 16*(10), 949–950.

Grossinger, R. (1987). *Planet Medicine: From stone age shamanism to post-industrial healing.* Berkeley, CA: North Atlantic.

Guarnaccia, P., De La Cancela, V., & Carrillo, E. (1989). The multiple meanings of ataques de nervios in the Latino community. *Medical Anthropology, 11*(1), 47–62.

Hahn, R. A. (1985). Culture-bound syndromes unbound. *Social Science and Medicine, 21*(2), 165–171.

Harwood, A. (1977). *RX: Spiritist as needed.* New York: Wiley.

Higginbotham, J. C., Trevino, F. M., & Ray, L. A. (1990). Utilization of curanderos by Mexican Americans: Prevalence and predictors findings from HHANES 1982–84. *American Journal of Public Health, 80* (Suppl.), 32–35.

Hughes, C. G. (1985). Glossary of "Culture-bound" or folk psychiatric syndromes. In R. C. Simons & C. C. Hughes (Eds.), *The Culture-Bound Syndromes: Folk illnesses of psychiatric and anthropological interest* (pp. 475–497). Boston: Reidel.

Jackson, J. J. (1981). Urban Black Americans. In A. Harwood (Ed.), *Ethnicity and medical care* (pp. 37–129). Cambridge, MA: Harvard University Press.

Kay, M. (1977a). Health and illness in a Mexican-American barrio. In E. G. Spicer (Ed.), *Ethnic medicine in the Southwest* (pp. 99–166). Tucson: University of Arizona Press.

Kay, M. (1977b). *Southwestern medical dictionary: Spanish/English, English/Spanish.* Tucson: University of Arizona Press.

Kay, M. (1979). Lexemic change and semantic shift in disease names. *Culture Medicine and Psychiatry, 3,* 73–94.

Kay, M. (1996). *Healing with plants in the American and Mexican West.* Tucson: University of Arizona Press.

Kenny, M. (1978). Latah: The symbolism of a putative mental disorder. *Culture, medicine and psychiatry, 2*(3), 209–231.

Kenny, M. (1983). The Latah problem revisited. *Journal of Nervous and Mental Disorders, 171*(3), 159–167.

Kleinman, A. (1986a). *Social origins of distress and disease: Depression, neurasthenia, and pain in modern China.* New Haven, CT: Yale University Press.

Kleinman, A. (1986b). Social origins of distress and disease: Depression, neurasthenia, and pain in modern China [Book review]. *Current Anthropology, 27*(5), 499–504.

Laguerre, M. (1981). Haitian Americans. In A. Harwood (Ed.), *Ethnicity and medical care* (pp. 172–210). Cambridge, MA: Harvard University Press.

Lassiter, S. M. (1995). *Multicultural clients: A professional handbook for health care providers and social workers.* Westport, CT: Greenwood.

Lewin-Epstein, N. (1991). Determinants of regular source of health care in black, Mexican, Puerto Rican, and non-Hispanic white populations. *Medical Care, 29*(6), 543–557.

Lieban, R. W. (1977). The field of medical anthropology. In D. Landy (Ed.), *Culture, disease, and healing* (pp. 13–31). New York: Macmillian.

Logan, K. (1988). "Casi como doctor": Pharmacists and their clients in a Mexican urban context. In S. van der Geest & S. R. Whyte (Eds.), *The context of medicines in developing countries* (pp. 107–129). Dordrecht, The Netherlands: Kluwer Academic.

Low, S. M. (1985). Culturally interpreted symptoms or culture-bound syndromes: A cross-cultural review of nerves. *Social Science and Medicine, 21*(2), 187–196.

Markides, K. S., Levin, J. S., & Ray, L. A. (1985). Determinants of physician utilization among Mexican-Americans. *Medical Care, 23*(3), 236–246.

McCombie, S. (1987). Folk flu and viral syndrome: An epidemiological perspective. *Social Science and Medicine, 25*(9), 987–993.

Mikhail, B. I. (1994). Hispanic mothers' beliefs and practices regarding selected children's health problems. *Western Journal of Nursing Research, 16*(6), 623–638.

Moore, L. G., Van Arsdale, P. W., Glittenberg, J. E., & Aldrich, R. A. (1980). *The biocultural basis of health*. St. Louis, MO: Mosby.

Pachter, L., Bernstein, B., & Osorio, A. (1992). Empacho in a mainland Puerto Rican clinic population. *Medical Anthropology, 13*(4), 285–299.

Pachter, L., Niego, S., & Pelto, P. (1996). Differences and similarities between health care providers and parents regarding symptom lists for childhood respiratory illnesses. *Ambulatory Child Health, 1,* 196–204.

Pachter, L. M. (1994). Culture and clinical care. *Journal of the American Medical Association, 271*(9), 690–694.

Parker, S., Nichter, M., Nichter, M., Vuckovic, N., Sims, C., & Ritenbaugh, C. (1995). Body image and weight concerns among African Americans and White adolescent females. *Human Organization, 54*(2), 103–114.

Risser, A. L., & Mazur, L. J. (1995). Use of folk remedies in a Hispanic population. *Archives of Pediatric and Adolescent Medicine, 149*(9), 978–981.

Ritenbaugh, C. (1982). Obesity as a culture bound syndrome. *Culture, Medicine and Psychiatry, 6,* 347–361.

Roberson, M. H. B. (1987). Folk health beliefs of health professionals. *Western Journal of Nursing Research, 9*(2), 251–263.

Rosereto, L. R. (1973). Root work and the root doctor. *Nursing Forum, 12*(4), 414–426.

Rubel, A. (1960). Concepts of disease in Mexican-American culture. *American Anthropologist, 62,* 795–814.

Rubel, A., O'Nell, C., & Collado-Ardon, R. (1984). *Susto: A folk illness*. Berkeley: University of California Press.

Rubel, A. J., & Garro, L. C. (1992). Social and cultural factors in the successful control of tuberculosis. *Public Health Reports, 107*(6), 626–636.

Ruiz, P. (1985). Cultural barriers to effective medical care among Hispanic-American patients. *Annual Review of Medicine, 36,* 63–71.

Sandoval, M. (1979). Santeria as a mental health care system. *Social Science and Medicine, 13B,* 137–151.

Schreiber, J. M., & Homiak, J. P. (1981). Mexican Americans. In A. Harwood (Ed.), *Ethnicity and medical care* (pp. 264–336). Cambridge, MA: Harvard University Press.

Simons, R. (1980). The resolution of the latah paradox. *Journal of Nervous and Mental Disorders, 168*(4), 195–205.

Simons, R. (1983a). Latah II: Problems with a purely symbolic interpretation. *Journal of Nervous and Mental Disorders, 171,* 168–175.

Simons, R. (1983b). Problems with a purely symbolic interpretation. *Journal of Nervous and Mental Disorders, 171,* 168–175.

Simons, R. C., & Hughes, C. C. (Eds.). (1985). *The Culture-bound syndromes: Folk illnesses of psychiatric and anthropological interest*. Boston: Reidel.

Skaer, T. L., Robinson, L. M., Sclar, D. A., & Harding, G. H. (1996). Utilization of curanderos among foreign born Mexican-American women attending migrant health clinics. *Journal of Cultural Diversity, 3*(2), 29–34.

Snow, L. F. (1974). Folk medical beliefs and their implications for care of patients. *Annals of Internal Medicine, 81,* 82–96.

Snow, L. F. (1993). *Walkin' over medicine*. Boulder, CO: Westview.

Stephenson, P. H. (1995). Vietnamese refugees in Victoria, BC: An overview of immigrant and refugee health care in a medium-sized Canadian urban centre. *Social Science and Medicine, 40*(12), 1631–1642.

Trotter, R. (1985). Greta and Azarcon. *Human Organization, 44*(1), 64–72.

Trotter, R., Montellano, B., Logan, M. (1989). Fallen fontanelle in the American Southwest: Its origin, epidemiology, and possible organic causes. *Medical Anthropology, 10*(4), 211–221.

Weller, S. (1996, November 20–24). Latino folk illness beliefs. Paper presented at the 95th annual meeting of the American Anthropological Association, San Francisco, CA.

Weller, S. (1997, March 4–9). Latino beliefs about mollera caida. Paper presented at the meetings of the Society for Applied Anthropology, City, State.

Weller, S., & Dungy, C.I. (1986). Personal preferences and ethnic variations among Anglo and Hispanic breast and bottle feeders. *Social Science and Medicine, 23*(6), 539–548.

Weller, S., Pachter, L., Trotter, R., & Baer, R. (1993). Study of intra- and inter-cultural variation in beliefs about empacho. *Medical Anthropology, 15,* 109–136.

Young, A. (1982). The anthropologies of illness and sickness. *Annual Review of Anthropology, 11,* 257–285.

Additional Resources

Cultural assessment guidebooks for practitioners often provide a summary of cultural beliefs related to health, illness, and treatment for various ethnic groups. The following list provides practitioners with further reading materials.

Geissler, E. M. (1994). *Pocket guide to cultural assessment.* St. Louis, MO: Mosby.

Lipson, J. G., Dibble, S. L., & Minarik, P. A. (1996). *Culture and nursing care: A pocket guide.* San Francisco: University of California, School of Nursing.

Schrefer, S. (1994). *Quick reference to cultural assessment.* St. Louis, MO: Mosby.

Spector, R. E. (1996). *Guide to heritage assessment and health traditions.* Stamford, CT: Appleton and Lange.

11

Ethical Issues in Immigrant Health Care and Clinical Research

PATRICIA A. MARSHALL, BARBARA A. KOENIG,
PAUL GRIFHORST, AND MIRJAM VAN EWIJK

Introduction

In the past decade, the number of immigrants and refugees has increased dramatically in various nations throughout the world. Ethnic conflict in Africa, Eastern Europe, and elsewhere has resulted in large numbers of individuals living in diaspora. Those in search of better economic conditions or political asylum emigrate to countries where opportunities for safety and security are thought to exist. Thus, in the context of health care delivery, particularly in urban centers, cultural pluralism is the norm rather than the exception. In pluralistic societies, where the influx of immigrant and refugee populations has grown, interactions between patients and health professionals from different ethnic backgrounds are becoming routine.

Attention to ethical issues associated with health care delivery and clinical research in culturally diverse settings has been notably absent from scholarly and public debates. In recent years, however, interest has grown (Connor & Fuenzalida-Puelma, 1990; Pellegrino & Flack, 1992; Pellegrino, Corsi, & Mazzarella, 1992; Veatch, 1989). Scholars have begun to explore a number of issues, including the international application of research ethics (Angell, 1988; Brody, 1998; Christakis, 1988, 1992; Christakis & Panner, 1991; Lane, 1993; Loue, Okello, & Kawuma, 1996; Marshall, 1992a; Schoepf 1991), the application of informed consent (Ijsselmuiden & Faden, 1992; Kaufert & O'Neil, 1990; Levine, 1993), disclosure of medical information (Beyene, 1992; Carrese & Rhodes, 1995; Pellegrino, 1992b; Surbone, 1992), the role of the family (Muller & Desmond, 1992), withdrawing or withholding medical interventions (Blackhall, Murphy, Frank, Michel, & Azen, 1995; Caralis, Davis, Wright, & Marcial, 1993; Klessig, 1992), and child abuse and neglect (Baylis & Downie, 1997).

In this chapter, our primary objective is to examine ethical problems that occur in the provision of health care to immigrant and refugee populations. A full treatment of the

PATRICIA A. MARSHALL • Medical Humanities Program, Loyola University Chicago, Maywood, Illinois 60153.   BARBARA A. KOENIG • Center for Biomedical Ethics, Stanford University, Palo Alto, California 94304.   PAUL GRIFHORST AND MIRJAM VAN EWIJK • European Research Center on Migration and Ethnic Relations, Utrecht University, Utrecht 3584CS, The Netherlands.

Handbook of Immigrant Health, edited by Loue. Plenum Press, New York, 1998.

myriad and complex moral dilemmas surrounding health care for this population is beyond the scope of this paper. Instead, we focus on a limited number of significant issues using case examples to illustrate the problems addressed. We begin with a brief exploration of the ethical foundations of clinical practice and medical research. Four important areas of ethical concern for refugee and immigrant health care are then highlighted. First, we examine the relevance of cultural beliefs and values for ethical problems that arise in patient care, focusing specifically on respect for persons and the articulation of individual autonomy. Second, we address problems associated with communication, with special attention to ethical issues surrounding the use of interpreters. Third, we explore ethical dimensions of access to care, concentrating on problems associated with discrimination and political repression. Fourth, we examine ethical problems associated with clinical research; in this section we are particularly concerned about the application of informed consent and the protection of confidentiality.

Finally, we offer practical guidelines for clinicians facing ethical dilemmas in cross-cultural interactions with patients. We argue that three elements are essential in successfully resolving moral problems in cross-cultural patient care and clinical research: an ability to communicate effectively with patients and their families; sufficient understanding of the patient's cultural background; and identification of culturally relevant value conflicts.

Ethical Foundations of Medical Practice and Clinical Research

Bioethics is the term generally used to refer to moral dilemmas associated with the development and application of Western biomedical technology. As Fox and Swazey (1984) have noted, bioethics emerged in the 1960s as an interdisciplinary field of inquiry concerned with the moral, social, and religious issues surrounding the rise of new scientific technologies and their medical applications. Thus, the interests of bioethicists have paralleled advances in basic biomedical science and clinical research. Early experiments with human organ transplantation focused attention on the meaning of personhood, the definition of death, and the allocation of scarce medical resources (Rothman, 1991). These problems remain important areas of inquiry for bioethicists. Similarly, there has been an ongoing concern with scientific investigations and the potential risks for human subjects involved in research (Beecher, 1966; Levine, 1986; National Commission for the Protection of Human Subjects of Biomedical and Behavior Research, 1978; Veatch, 1991). Currently, there is an extensive literature addressing a range of problems such as medical interventions and end-of-life decision making (Schneiderman & Jecker, 1995; Teno, Hill, & O'Connor, 1994), reproductive technologies (Lauritzen, 1993), physician-assisted suicide (Wier, 1996), and applications of genetic research (Frankel & Teich, 1994). The scope of the problems addressed in bioethics is expansive and will evolve with scientific and technological developments.

Theoretical Orientations in Bioethics

Bioethics is decidedly interdisciplinary in its intellectual foundations. Historically, the fields of moral and political philosophy, theological ethics, law, and medicine have all played a role in its development. However, the discipline of moral philosophy has dominated the theoretical orientation and practical applications of bioethics. Analytic philosophy emphasizes an Enlightenment concern with the *rational* man and is characterized by a strong focus on individual rights. Indeed, Fox (1990) and others (Hoffmaster, 1990; Marshall & Koenig, 1996) have argued that the orientation of bioethics reflects the strong emphasis on individualism and autonomy in the United States.

Because of its grounding in analytical philosophy, bioethics has relied primarily on the language of principles and rights (Beauchamp & Childress, 1993; Englehardt, 1986; Pellegrino & Thomasma, 1989; Veatch, 1981). Ethical problems have traditionally been analyzed based on the Western philosophical principles of respect for autonomy, beneficence, nonmaleficence, and distributive justice. The principle of respect for autonomy, sometimes called respect for persons, refers to the obligation to honor the wishes of a competent individual regarding health care or participation in scientific research. A belief that individuals have the capacity to exercise free will, to act with self-determination, is vitally important to the principle of autonomy: "The autonomous person is one who not only deliberates about and chooses such plans, but who is capable of acting on the basis of such deliberations" (Beauchamp & Childress, 1979, p. 56). Requirements for informed consent and confidentiality in the provision of health care and the implementation of research appeal to and are justified by the principle of autonomy and respect for persons.

The principle of beneficence refers to the obligation of health providers to act in a way that benefits the health and well-being of patients; conversely, the principle of nonmaleficence concerns the obligation to do no harm. Taken together, the principles of beneficence and nonmaleficence emphasize the importance of maximizing benefits and minimizing potential harms (Beauchamp & Childress, 1993; Frankena, 1973). The principle of justice is closely linked to issues of equality and fairness in determining who receives the benefits and who bears the burdens of health care and clinical research. Certain populations—racial minorities, refugees, immigrants, the poor—are particularly vulnerable to discrimination and injustices in the implementation of health care delivery and scientific investigations.

In recent years, the "principles approach" to ethical dilemmas in health care has come under heavy criticism. Dissatisfaction with the weaknesses of the positivist orientation of Western, "Anglo-American" philosophy has led to the development of alternative paradigms for analyzing medical morality. The conceptual frameworks and methodologies of casuistry (Jonsen & Toulmin, 1988), virtue ethics (MacIntyre, 1984; Pellegrino & Thomasma, 1993), narrative ethics (Hunter, 1991), feminist ethics (Tong, 1996; Wolf, 1996), and relational and communitarian ethics (Benner, 1991; Loewy, 1991) reflect the diverse range of ethical approaches now being developed. While these approaches vary in their underlying theoretical foundations, they share a fundamental recognition of the importance of human relationships and contextual features in defining moral dilemmas and bioethical practices. The result is a growing acknowledgment among bioethicists that ethical reasoning must include attention to social practices rather than only abstract moral propositions (Weisz, 1990).

Cultural Diversity and Bioethics

In their recent analysis of ethical issues in biomedicine, Marshall and Koenig (1996) explored the application of bioethics in culturally diverse environments. They suggested that medical ethics *across* cultures includes "the lived experience of human suffering in the context of disease, the moral discourse of healers and patients, the development and use of healing modalities, the professional organization of practitioners, and the social and economic regulation of medical environments" (p. 350). They argued that cultural difference has been virtually transparent in bioethics, despite the fact that biomedicine is an international enterprise and cross-cultural encounters between patients and providers in Western and non-Western nations are routine experiences.

Philosophers and theologians have begun to address the relevance of cultural difference to bioethics. Although several volumes have examined religious and cultural perspectives regarding medical ethics (Pellegrino *et al.,* 1992; Veatch, 1989), a number of scholars have questioned whether an "ethnic perspective" on bioethics can be philosophically justified (Dula, 1994; Dula & Goering, 1994;

Garcia, 1992). Only recently have the challenges to bioethics practices in multicultural societies been examined systematically. In his discussion of the possibility of a transnational bioethics, Pellegrino (1992a) suggested that the science, technology, and morality of biomedical ethics are deeply ingrained with distinctly Western values that are "often alien, and even antipathetic, to many non-Western world views" (p. 191). The existence of cultural pluralism and the inevitable presence of very different social values among diverse populations led Engelhardt (1991) to argue that secular bioethics may be the only solution.

In their discussion of intercultural moral reasoning, Marshall, Thomasma, and Bergsma (1994) explored several examples of ethical problems associated with scientific technologies in cross-cultural context. The Remmelink Report on the status of euthanasia in the Netherlands and the ethics of abortion for sexual preference in India are two cases used to illustrate their point that misunderstandings may occur on many different levels: intercultural, intracultural, and contextual. They concluded that while consensus on specific issues may not be achieved, communication may be enhanced if there is at least minimal agreement on the meaning and value of ethical concepts and a genuine commitment to discerning cultural context. Jecker, Carrese, and Pearlman (1995) also emphasized the importance of respecting cultural difference in their discussion of resolving ethical dilemmas in clinical cases involving Native American Navajo individuals. These investigators called attention to cultural differences between Anglo and Navajo worlds; moreover, they acknowledged that fundamental differences exist among people who share the same traditions and "world view." Their analysis demonstrates that the Navajos are no more unidimensional in their beliefs and values than are people of any ethnic or cultural heritage.

Koenig and Gates-Williams (1995) highlighted important issues surrounding bioethics practices in cross-cultural context in their exploration of cultural diversity and care of the dying. They outlined an approach to understanding cultural difference in patient care that takes into account a range of factors, including the language and style of communication used by the patient and family to talk about the diagnosis and prognosis, determination of decisional authority, consideration of religious beliefs, gender, and age, and consideration of the political and historical context, particularly problems associated with poverty, refugee status, or lack of access to care. A similar approach for addressing cultural dimensions in medical care was suggested by Orr, Marshall, and Osborn (1995) in their analysis of cross-cultural issues in clinical ethics consultations.

In his critique of the theoretical foundations and applications of bioethics, Kleinman (1995) proposed that the process of "cultural engagement" is vital to ethical deliberation. He argued strongly that dismissing the relevance of culture in this process denies the fact that the deliberative process is itself both cultural and contextualized. Kleinman suggested that bioethics shares the limitations of biomedicine in its refusal to engage with the major non-Western moral traditions and to question the "orthodox sources of the self within the western philosophical tradition" (p. 1669). Moreover, just as the biomedical model of disease silences and constrains the patient's experience with illness, bioethics too often reconstructs the moral problem into philosophical abstractions removed from the suffering of the individual. Marshall and Koenig (1996) concurred with Kleinman and argued that moral dimensions of health care beliefs and practices are culturally constituted, embedded in religious and political ideologies that influence individuals and communities at particular biographical and historical moments.

In his discussion of ethical relativism and morality, Shweder (1990) argued for a version of qualified ethical relativism based on his assertions that there are genuine and significant differences between the moral codes of different people and that more than one rationally defensible moral code exists. According to Shweder, a universalistic approach to moral reasoning is unrealistic. The cultural constructs of ethics, morality, and health and illness are negotiable and dynamic entities. Therefore, a single worldview, a unidimensional perspective that represents cultural beliefs about medical morality is impossible to achieve. The alternative is an ethical framework that takes into account diverse cultural practices that may be repugnant in light of idealized "universal" standards of morality.

Respect for Persons and the Expression of Autonomy in Immigrant Health

Central to the principle of respect for persons is the belief in the ability of individuals to act as autonomous agents. However, the capacity for autonomous action may be hindered because of immaturity, illness, or incarceration; cultural beliefs and practices that emphasize community or family decision making as opposed to individual choice also influence the expression of autonomy. Immigrants and refugees often come from cultural environments where decisions are made traditionally by authority figures in the family or community. Cultural elements are embedded in the pattern of meanings that form the basis of medical practices, knowledge of disease, and expectations about what constitutes a healing relationship (B. J. Good, 1994; Kleinman, 1980). Thus, in the context of health care, an individual's cultural heritage provides an interpretive framework not only for beliefs about the cause and symptomology of illness, but also for the negotiation of treatment decisions.

Although Western-trained physicians are encouraged to be sensitive to the ethnic backgrounds of patients, the realization of this ideal in medical practice may be difficult. Too often, there is a tendency to stereotype patients based on their ethnicity, language, or appearance. When this occurs, assumptions are made by health providers about what the patient understands, knows, or wants in regard to medical care. Moreover, the tendency

to categorize patients on the basis of their ethnic or cultural background obscures the importance of other influential factors such as age, class, gender, and religion. However, differences between patients and providers representing diverse cultural worlds are more pronounced because of the substantive content of beliefs about healing and the modes of expressing these beliefs (Ware & Kleinman, 1992). For example, beliefs concerning the use of traditional healers or alternative therapies such as prayers, herbal remedies, or ritual practices may be in direct conflict with the views of Western-trained physicians. As Lock (1993) pointed out, deeply embedded cultural beliefs are often misunderstood or viewed as obstacles to the provision of "good" scientific medical care.

Current biomedical practices emphasize strongly the importance of self-determination and autonomy in decisions about medical care. Yet, the centrality of patient autonomy and a patient's right to decide represents a decidedly Western philosophical orientation. For example, the application of informed consent for medical treatment, disclosure of medical information, and the implementation of advance directives, which emphasize a patient's "right" to limit or withdraw unwanted therapy, presuppose a particular kind of patient. Koenig (1993) suggested that this "ideal" patient possesses a clear understanding of the illness, prognosis, and treatment; a belief that it is possible to control the future; the perception of freedom of choice; and a willingness to discuss topics of sickness and death openly. This idealized view of the patient reinforces and sustains the underlying belief that individuals actually have the capacity for self-determination and autonomous decision making.

Immigrants or refugees from non-Western cultures may not share the proclivity for autonomous informed consent, advance care planning, or the disclosure of distressing medical news. In his discussion of the application of informed consent in international settings, Levine (1991) recognizes the problem of incommensurability between particular Western and non-Western cultural beliefs. Christakis (1992) supported Levine's (1991) rejection of "universal" standards regarding informed consent because of different perspectives on the nature of the "person" in diverse cultures (e.g., DeCraemer, 1983; Shweder, 1990). Levine (1991, 1993) and Christakis (1992) acknowledged both the necessity and the importance of accommodating the informed consent process to the particular constraints of interactions involving patients from non-Western cultural backgrounds.

In the United States, and to varying degrees in other Western nations, a patient's right to confidentiality and the truth about a diagnosis and prognosis is thought to facilitate patients' participation in the process of making treatment decisions. For example, M. D. Good, Good, Schaffer, and Lind's (1990) analysis of the treatment of cancer in the United States suggested that oncologists view frank and open discussions as essential in forging partnerships with their patients. However, divergent beliefs and practices about truth telling and confidentiality may inhibit interactions between health providers, patients, and their families. This was precisely the issue in a case reported by Orr and colleagues (1995) involving a Mexican American patient. The patient, a 76-year-old man, was diagnosed with lymphoma. His family did not want him to know the seriousness of his condition. The dilemma was solved when his physician agreed to a compromise: he would not tell the patient anything the patient did not want to know. In this way, the physician applied what Freedman (1993) has called "offering the truth" to patients. Freedman suggested asking patients if they would like to discuss any concerns they might have about their illness, and if they want to know any information about their diagnosis or prognosis. In this way, providers honor their own belief in respecting a patient's "right to know" and a family's desire to protect a loved one from information that is thought to be emotionally upsetting.

A recent comprehensive study on ethnic diversity and beliefs about patient autonomy found significant differences among African Americans, European Americans, Korean Americans, and Mexican Americans (Blackhall et al., 1995). Findings revealed that the great majority of the African Americans (88%) and the European American (87%) believed that a patient should be told the truth about a diagnosis of metastatic cancer, compared with only 65% of the Mexican Americans and 47% of the Korean Americans. Similar results occurred when respondents were asked if they believed that a patient should be told of a terminal prognosis. In addition, the investigators found that African Americans and European Americans were more inclined to believe in a model of decision making based on individual autonomy, while Korean Americans and Mexican Americans favored a family-centered model of decision making. Similarly, Orona, Koenig, and Davis (1994), in their report on nondisclosure among ethnically diverse patients, found that Chinese Americans and Mexican American patients with cancer were inclined to hold a family-centered model of decision making.

In their discussion of several cases from an ongoing study of end-of-life care for immigrant patients terminally ill with cancer, Hern, Koenig, Moore, and Marshall (1998) illustrated the challenge of negotiating Western notions of respect for individual autonomy when they are in conflict with traditional non-Western views on how to properly care for a dying family member. They described the difficulties faced by the patient, family members, and staff when decisions must be made concerning medical interventions. For example, a 42-year-old Vietnamese immigrant living in California was diagnosed with metastatic cancer. Miss Tai, who spoke only Cantonese, lived with her aging parents and younger brother and sister. In interviews with Miss Tai, she suggested that her brother was the primary decision maker concerning her medical care. Her brother not only provided considerable support for his sister, he often acted as the interpreter for his sister. Referring to his desire to protect his sister from emotional pain, he said in an interview,

"At the beginning when the doctor told me that she had the cancer, I told my family not to tell my sister because I was worried that she could not face the fact, that she would be too sad. . . . But later on, the doctor told her so she knew." His position regarding disclosure was directly opposed to the view of the oncologist. Indeed, the oncologist, who insisted on the use of an interpreter to communicate with the patient, said, "I could not withhold information from her. I am so against that, that if it came to that I would have insisted that they get another physician." Moreover, the physician described the family as "abnormal" in the way they withheld information from Miss Tai. The physician expressed frustration and anger because the patient did not seem able to make decisions on her own.

Another case described by Hern and colleagues (1998) documented the confusion that sometimes occurs in interactions between immigrant patients and their providers when they have different opinions about the effectiveness of therapeutic remedies and diagnostic tests. In contrast to Miss Tai, Mrs. Laing, a 43-year-old immigrant from southern China, was diagnosed with adenocarcinoma metastatic to her brain. She was described by herself, her family, and the physician as the primary decision maker regarding her medical care. In this way, she conformed to the accepted Western pattern in which patients want to be informed about their medical condition and actively participate in decisions about treatment. Mrs. Laing indicated during an interview that if she was unhappy with her treatment, she would request that it be discontinued. At one point during her therapy, she refused radiation treatment to shrink the tumor in her brain. However, one of the research team observed an interaction in which Mrs. Laing asked for a CT scan. Unknown to the physician, she had been using traditional Chinese medicines and she wanted to determine whether they were working. The physician had trouble understanding why she would request a CT scan when she had refused radiation therapy.

As long as the physician or other health provider defines what information is relevant and "understandable" to patients, patients' autonomy, their right to be informed, is subject to limitations beyond their control. Immigrants and refugees are especially vulnerable to being poorly informed about their medical treatment. In the Netherlands, for example, pregnant women and foreign-born patients with tuberculosis are tested routinely for HIV when they are hospitalized because they are thought to be at risk for AIDS. An HIV test requires the permission of the patient, but informed consent is often avoided for various reasons. Some health practitioners argue that they are not trained in communicating about such a difficult topic; others believe it is too complicated to explain the procedure and the possible consequences of the test to people who are unable to speak Dutch. Grifhorst and van Ewijk, two of the authors of this chapter, are currently conducting research on treatment for tuberculosis among immigrants and refugees to the Netherlands. They describe a case involving a woman named Soleani, an Afro Caribbean immigrant from the Dominican Republic. She was 31 years old and employed as a social worker. She had recently divorced and moved with her two children from a small village to a larger town. After caring for her sick mother in the Dominican Republic for several weeks, she returned to the Netherlands with complaints of fatigue, loss of appetite, and continual coughing at night. She sought help from a general practitioner who referred her immediately to the clinic for further tests. That same day, Soleani was transferred to a specialized hospital because of a progressive contagious tuberculosis.

Soleani was embarrassed about her diagnosis and afraid that others would learn about her disease. Since her resettlement in the Netherlands, she often experienced the negative stereotypes associated with her immigrant status, including the suggestion that she must be a prostitute. She had worked hard to overcome this stigma. Yet, she was threatened by another stigma because of her diagnosis of tuberculosis—a disease that she associated with the poor and marginalized. Subsequently, in the hospital, she was stunned when she learned that she had been tested for HIV—yet another stigmatizing illness. A nurse told her that her HIV test was negative, expecting Soleani to be relieved. Instead of being happy at this news, Soleani was shocked by the total lack of information concerning the test. Her permission for HIV testing was never obtained.

Elsewhere, Marshall (1992a) has argued that "[t]he key to understanding moral dilemmas surrounding disclosure of medical information rests on two factors: first, beliefs on the part of both patients and practitioners about what is appropriate to say regarding the diagnosis and prognosis of illness; and second, beliefs about the character and disposition of the patient-practitioner relationship" (p. 59). She suggested that when patients expect to be told the truth, withholding information may be viewed as a betrayal of trust. Conversely, if patients expect health providers and family members to be guarded, telling the truth about an illness might be experienced as indifference to the healing relationship between patient and providers, and abandonment of the protective relationship between family members.

Ethical Problems in Communication

General Issues

Communication between patients and providers may be difficult to achieve when the clinical relationship extends across cultural boundaries. In addition, misunderstandings and miscommunication about medical interventions and decision making are more likely to occur when patients and practitioners speak different languages. In this section, three problems influencing the ethical treatment of immigrants and refugees are addressed: (a) language barriers in medical interactions; (b) cultural norms governing the substance and context of medical conversa-

tions, with attention to problems surrounding disclosure of information and confidentiality; and (c) beliefs about decisional authority in regard to medical interventions.

Language barriers represent perhaps the most profound obstacle to communication in medical encounters with immigrants and refugees. A case involving a refugee in the Netherlands illustrates the problems that arise when patients and practitioners are incapable of communicating because of language differences. This case documents the diminished capacity for providers to be morally responsible in their interactions with patients when language barriers exist. Dragan, a 38-year-old man from Yugoslavia had arrived 6 months previously in the Netherlands with his young daughter and pregnant wife. The family asked for asylum and was accommodated in a very small room in one of the emergency shelters for asylum seekers; formerly, the shelter had been a youth hostel. Dragan spoke Croatian and some German and English. When he complained about "sleeping problems," the visiting nurse at the shelter decided he was having difficulties with "adjustment" and referred him to a mental health center. A psychiatrist there assumed that Dragan was suffering from a war trauma. The psychiatrist provided him with a psychotropic drug and, in addition, a letter for the physician who occasionally visited the shelter. In this letter, which was written in Dutch, the psychiatrist defended his prescription of the psychotropic medication, saying that "the patient was talking excitedly and moving his arms a lot." Furthermore, the visiting physician at the refugee shelter was warned to be aware of the possible serious side effects of the medication he prescribed, including symptoms such as "a painful permanent erection."

The psychiatrist did not know about (because he did not ask) the dramatic events that had overwhelmed the young family since their arrival in the Netherlands. Not only had his baby been born 2 moths previously, but also Dragan had recently learned that his parents had been killed in Yugoslavia; in addition, he was diagnosed with a contagious tuberculosis. Two points concerning language are relevant here. First, although the psychiatrist could not communicate effectively with Dragan, he made an assumption concerning Dragan's history. Second, the letter contained information not available to Dragan because he could not read Dutch. The possibility for effective treatment is seriously jeopardized when patient and provider lack the rudimentary skills of communication. In this case, a translator might have been able to shed light on the complex situation surrounding Dragan's adjustment to a new environment.

Language barriers represent only one dimension of effective communication with immigrant or refugee patients. Cultural norms governing the structure and content of discourse in medical encounters are also vitally important. Beliefs and expectations concerning "appropriate" discourse in medical interactions—what is discussed, the timing of the conversation, who is present at the conversation, and who participates in the discussion—influence deliberation over ethical issues such as disclosure of medical information and confidentiality.

Some of the moral and practical complexities of decisions regarding the disclosure of a patient's medical history with family or friends is illustrated in the following story of Hayat, a 30-year-old woman from Somalia, who arrived in the Netherlands in 1993 seeking political asylum. She spent the first 3 years in several refugee camps and just recently received a residence permit that enabled her to move into a small apartment in a large city. Because she was on her own in the Netherlands, she joined a local Somalian community organization, where she had the opportunity to meet other people from Somalia. However, after a fall from an escalator in a shopping mall, Hayat was sent to an acute care teaching hospital where it was discovered that she had tuberculosis. Hayat, ill with pulmonary tuberculosis and TB of the peritoneum, was transferred to be treated in a specialized clinic remote from her place of residence.

At the clinic, she was informed that she might not be able to have children because the TB infection had also damaged her fallopian tubes. Hayat was very upset about the prognosis and did not want anyone to know about her condition. Neither was she willing to reveal the route of infection, because of concerns about her vulnerable social status in the Somalian community since she was a young single woman. On the clinic ward she avoided other patients from Somalia. She also hid herself when Somalian people came to visit their relatives. Horrified by the idea that she would be cast out of her newly established social network, Hayat told her circle of acquaintances by telephone that she was in Paris for a long holiday, staying with her relatives.

Nevertheless, the staff discussed the possibility of contacting friends in her social network to arrange for proper care when she was released from the hospital. A conflict was imminent because the staff believed that her friends should be informed; they believed that the benefits of this course of action definitely outweighed Hayat's concerns about confidentiality. An anthropologist with expertise in Somalian culture was consulted. Referring to recent research findings, she pointed out that for many Somalian people, tuberculosis was still considered to be a highly contagious, incurable, and inheritable disease with serious social and economic consequences. Finally, a consensus was reached. Hayat would remain in the hospital until she was able to take care of herself again. A social worker was asked to take care of her apartment and mail until she was ready to return home.

In addition to language barriers and different beliefs concerning the nature of medical interactions and the appropriateness of disclosing information, effective communication may also be thwarted when patients and practitioners have diverse opinions about who has the authority to decide whether or not a medical intervention should be implemented. In the United States, patients are expected to make decisions for themselves or through designated surrogates. However, many immigrants and refugees come from areas in which decisions are made by family members or community representatives. Beliefs about personhood, individual autonomy, and decisional capacity are embedded in the sociocentric patterns of family ties and community obligations. In certain contexts, religious or tribal leaders, or a patient's extended family may play a significant role in major decisions. Orr and colleagues (1995) described an ethics consultation involving a gypsy woman seriously ill following surgery; in this case, the woman's family brought in their tribal chief to negotiate communication and decision making with the physicians and other members of the health care team.

Problems Associated with the Use of Interpreters

Medical translators are often thought to act as straightforward interpreters of information exchanged between health providers and patients. This perspective minimizes the complexities of the process of interpretation, in which the translator must negotiate not only language, but also cultural and contextual factors. Some of the problems associated with medical interpretation include the inability to easily translate equivalent expressions across languages; paraphrasing that results in omissions or erroneous substitutions of terms; varying levels of comprehension among participants in the interaction; and the influence of conflicting cultural beliefs and values among participants. Drawing on their research with Native Canadian medical interpreters in Winnipeg hospitals, Kaufert and O'Neil (1990) argued that interpreters have a significant impact on medical interactions and their outcomes. They suggest that, in addition to mediating the explanatory models of illness held by clinicians and patients, Native interpreters often introduce their own beliefs and personal agendas into the interaction. Kaufert and O'Neil emphasized the dynamic nature of the interaction. They described the triad that exists between

patient, interpreter, and clinician, in which the process of feeding information back and forth results in a restructuring of both the patient's and the provider's understanding of the medical problem.

It is inevitable that interpreters exercise some degree of control over the communication between health care providers and patients. The influence on communication is articulated through the role of gatekeeping; interpreters make crucial decisions about the selection of information to communicate, the terminology used to express medical concerns, and the simplification of information to suit particular interactions. The modification of the message that the health providers wish to give to patients, and conversely, the response of patients to questions, has ramifications for ethical practices such as informed consent or advance care planning regarding medical interventions.

Wasongarz, Carter, Barnes, and Koenig (1995), as part of an ongoing ethnographic study of end-of-life decision making among culturally diverse patients terminally ill with cancer, explored the way in which medical interpreters influenced decisions such as resuscitation, the limitation of treatments, and the completion of a Durable Power of Attorney for Health Care. These investigators challenge the assumption that interpreters are simply conduits of information between patients and providers. Results of their analysis suggest that interpreters modified language in order to make patients feel more comfortable about their diagnosis and prognosis. Translators were also found to influence the communication process by acting as culture brokers, patient advocates, and counselors. For example, referring to her practice of modifying the words of the provider, one interpreter stated, "When I translated 'death,' I usually would avoid using the word 'death.' For Chinese patients, I would use 'letting go,' 'sleeping,' 'stop eating rice,' and other words to substitute the word 'death'" (p. 13). The investigators suggested that perhaps the interpreter changed the word "death" not only to ease the emotional burden of the patient, but also to ease the discomfort the interpreter felt when telling the patient that he or she is dying.

Wasongarz and associates (1995) called attention to another process of modification in which translators expand on what the physician says in order to communicate a technical medical procedure in culturally appropriate terms. They reported that a Cantonese interpreter spent 15 minutes explaining a lumbar puncture to a patient; the oncologist had communicated this in one sentence.

The existence and effectiveness of translation services in hospitals or clinics varies considerably depending on financial resources and the availability of professional interpreters. In the Netherlands, for example, since the 1970s, well-organized interpreter services have been available for health care providers. However, there is a general compliant that these services are underutilized. This has ramifications for the quality of health care provided to patients who are immigrants and unable to speak Dutch. Laila, for example, was a 24-year-old woman from Morocco; her husband had joined her in the Netherlands 4 years earlier. They lived in a ramshackle two-room apartment in a small industry town. Laila spoke only Arabic and her husband's ability to speak Dutch was very limited. Both had been unemployed for more than a year. Laila was several months pregnant with her second child when she began coughing and having intermittent fevers. She consulted her physician several times, complaining that she did not feel well. But, even in the last 2 months of her pregnancy, when her medical records indicated problems with her blood pressure and weight loss, no special action was taken by the physician or the midwife. On the contrary, despite her worsening condition, and the fact that almost every woman in the Netherlands is advised to have "24-hour hospital delivery," the midwife decided that it would be better for Laila to deliver in an environment familiar to her. However, during labor, Laila developed toxemia. Laila and her newborn son were immediately sent to the hospital. At the hospital, Laila was diagnosed with tuberculosis. Although she had already contaminated her son, the medical staff decided to separate her from her baby. Laila spent 6 weeks in isolation, a period she still remembers as being the most traumatic of the entire event. Throughout the duration of her pregnancy and hospitalization, none of the health providers called for the assistance of an Arabic interpreter.

In contrast to the Netherlands, in the United States there is a scarcity of professional interpreters in health care facilities. However, the need for translation services is overwhelming, particularly in areas where immigrant populations are increasing. For example, at Stanford's university medical center, hospital interpreters have an average of 3,000 patient encounters per month. This dramatic figure calls attention to the need for competent interpreters and effective translation services. Some professionals are calling for the development of standards of practice for medical interpreters; in the states of Washington and Massachusetts, standards have been implemented, along with requirements for continuing education.

When professional interpreters are unavailable, many hospitals and clinics rely on family, friends, and bilingual employees to translate for monolingual patients. Studies have shown, however, that there is a tendency for family members to camouflage, exaggerate, or minimize information (Putsch, 1985). For example, Marshall (1989) described a situation in which a young girl dying of bone cancer was fluent in both English and Spanish. The girl's family spoke only Spanish. The child would sometimes translate for the physicians, nurses, and other staff caring for her. When the girl died, the family was confused and surprised because they claimed they did not understand the gravity of her condition. In an attempt to shield the family, the girl had been providing reassurances that eventually she might be able to go home.

Discussions about death and dying can be especially problematic when family members act as interpreters. Decisions about end-of-life care may be compromised if family members avoid or misconstrue the information because they desire to protect a loved one from disconcerting information. For example, Wasongarz and associates (1995) described a case involving a 71-year-old Columbian man with metastatic lung cancer. He lived with his three daughters, all of whom participated in caring for him at home. One of the daughters had accompanied her father to the clinic and acted as the translator for the providers since he had begun treatment. Early in his therapy, she had requested that the physician not use the word "cancer" around her father because she was afraid it would upset him. After six months of treatment, the physician asked for the assistance of a hospital interpreter to translate for her. Aggressive therapy was no longer an option and she wanted to know how the patient felt about palliative care. In an interview, the physician said:

> Actually, up until yesterday, it wasn't clear to me that he knew what he had, what his prognosis was, why we were doing the radiation treatments. For the longest time they [the daughters] were just telling him that he was sick, that he had something in his lung; that he needed this, that, and the other treatment to get better. So, yesterday, for the first time, I got another interpreter than the daughter to talk to him because I wanted to get a better feel for what he knew he had and why he had been going through this treatment. (p. 17)

In this case, the physician relied on the professional interpreter to investigate the patient's understanding of the seriousness of his illness and to ensure an informed consent. If the physician had relied on the daughter for translation, it is unlikely that this discussion would have occurred.

Access to Health Care

General

Immigrant and refugee populations face a number of challenges regarding access to medical care. Language barriers, poverty, so-cial or geographical isolation, lack of familiarity with the location of services, inability to navigate the complexities of bureaucratic medical systems, and cultural beliefs about illness and healing that may conflict with biomedical treatments represent serious obstacles to accessing health services. The passage of legislation that discriminates against immigrants, along with personal prejudices that make some clinicians reluctant to treat immigrant patients, also undermines access to care for this population.

For example, in the United States, recent federal and state legislation that would block treatment of illegal residents and prevent certain types of medical treatment for legal residents has serious public health implications in addition to reinforcing prejudice toward foreign-born individuals. Studies (Berk, Albers, & Schur, 1996; Thamer, Richard, Casebeer, & Ray, 1997; de la Torre, Friis, Hunter, & Garcia, 1996) have shown that foreign-born individuals are extremely vulnerable to not having health insurance, which limits their access to medical services. Moreover, administrative criteria for utilization of services often prevents these individuals from adequate protection when they seek treatment. The issue of payment for health services, for example, can be an important obstacle to care for practitioners constrained by organizational rules and procedures regarding uncompensated treatment, particularly for undocumented immigrants (Siddharthan & Alalasundaram, 1993).

Differing views about the etiology and treatment of illness significantly influence the utilization of Western medical services. Studies (see, e.g., Bell & Whiteford, 1987; Uba, 1992) point to the hesitation of immigrants to seek help because of unfamiliarity with Western diagnostic techniques, fears related to the potential for misunderstandings about symptoms, or the perception that biomedical treatments may be irrelevant for the specific problem. In addition to cultural beliefs about illness, other factors such as the lack of financial resources to pay for treatments or the living arrangements of immigrants are very important factors in determining access to care. In a study of health care access among Vietnamese immigrants living in the San Francisco area, investigators (Jenkins, Le, Mcphee, Steward, & Ha, 1996) found that poverty and marital status were more likely to predict access to care and utilization of preventive services than traditional health beliefs and practices. Language barriers constitute a major challenge to effective access for immigrant and refugee patients; D'Avanzo (1992) found that Vietnamese refugees in the United States were more willing to seek treatment if translators were available.

Investigations have also called attention to the way in which immigrants combine traditional healing practices with biomedical treatments or selectively use different types of traditional and Western health resources. For example, Gilman, Justice, Saepharn, and Charles (1992) examined the influence of refugee traditions on the use of Western medical services among the Mien from Laos living in Richmond, California; they found that the Mien refugees integrated their traditional practices with the use of biomedical services.

The next section explores problems associated with access to care for immigrants and refugees in the Netherlands, drawing on cases from Grifhorst and van Ewijk's ongoing study of tuberculosis treatment for this population.

Immigrants and Refugees in The Netherlands

In theory, in the Netherlands, everyone has the right to health care. However, barriers exist for those who are not insured. About 65% of the population participates in a mandatory health insurance program because they have some form of legal income through employment or welfare benefits. The premium for health insurance is relative to one's income. Like the health care system, the mandatory health insurance program, although considered to be nonprofit, is privately organized. Extensive public regulation characterizes both,

however. If they have a legal income, immigrants have the same entitlement to health insurance as the native population.

Illegal migrants who do not have opportunities to earn money legally have only limited access to medical services. Some of these individuals, or a family member or employer, pay in cash for the services received; others may use the medical insurance card of a friend, but overall, illegal migrants have been solely dependent on the provision of health care by benevolent practitioners, specialists, midwifes, municipal public health services, and a few free health centers run by volunteers.

Until recently, the use of health care facilities by illegal immigrants has always been considered a problem to be solved mainly by the health care practitioners themselves. The challenges faced by health care providers treating immigrants or refugees have not been a high priority. Generally, practitioners and hospitals have been very inventive in organizing public funding to cover the costs for their free services in cooperation with the local welfare or health insurance agency.

However, in the 1990s, the dominant voice in national political debates has emphasized an exclusionary posture. In 1996, for example, a proposition was approved by the Dutch Parliament that seeks to exclude inhabitants without legal residential status from the job market and the use of social arrangements such as welfare, education, and subsidized housing; in addition, this proposition restricts their access to health care. This proposition (de Koppelingswet) should be understood as part of a whole range of measures, including the tightening of border control and an employer sanction program, intended to regulate immigration.

Parliament has decided that emergency care should remain available and "free" for illegal residents. Moreover, a condition threatening public health, such as tuberculosis, gives illegal migrants the right to a temporary residence permit that entitles them to health insurance. This incentive was initiated to motivate medical compliance among illegal migrants being treated for tuberculosis in order to prevent the development of drug-resistant strains of tuberculosis.

However, the provision of free emergency care is not unconditional. Medical care is provided only under strict conditions: the provider must present evidence that his or her patient is really unable to pay and that the patient's condition is life threatening. Otherwise, like the costs for free nonemergency care, the practitioner (or hospital) will be deemed responsible for the costs. These restrictive measures are concurrent with considerable cuts in the national health budget. Anticipated consequences are that an increasing number of illegal immigrants will be denied access to hospitals and other medical facilities and health care providers will be pressured to become more restrictive in their treatment of uninsured patients. Health care practitioners face considerable conflicts of interest: Should they remain loyal employees and respect the governmental mandates or should they carry out their responsibilities as physicians and nurses to provide care irrespective of institutional rules?

The following cases illustrate the problems surrounding access to medical services for immigrants in the Netherlands. The first example demonstrates the difficulties associated with being an illegal resident. Said was a 27-year-old man from Morocco. He was an undocumented migrant (since 1986), earning a living in the Netherlands by doing a number of jobs. One day, Said was arrested during a police raid in the restaurant where he worked; he was put in prison. There he was diagnosed with tuberculosis and treated with medication for almost 4 months. After Said was discharged he still had to complete his tuberculosis treatment for a period of 5 months; a total of 9 months is required for effective treatment. Therefore, the prison physician ordered him to contact the nearest treatment center for tuberculosis. At the treatment center, however, he was told to check in with the TB service in the town where the police had arrested him.

At this point, Said came across a TB nurse who was concerned with his health and social situation. They agreed that Said would visit the TB clinic once a week to collect his medication. Subsequently, the nurse helped Said to find a place to sleep and helped arrange a temporary visa for the duration of his treatment; the visa entitled him to welfare benefits, including health insurance. The situation was complicated because, technically, the medical service was obliged to report this to the immigration police. However, after the nurse notified the police, Said refused to cooperate any further, even though the police repeatedly requested his treatment status and resident status. As long as Said was being treated for tuberculosis, he enjoyed some legal protection from being deported. When Said neared the end of his therapy, the nurse provided him with enough medicines to bridge the last month. It was no longer necessary for Said to come to the tuberculosis clinic to collect; it is believed that he resumed his life working as an illegal immigrant. The nurse encountered very negative reactions from his colleagues about his approach to Said's problems; some accused him of being "overly involved with an illegal person's fate."

The next case involves a refugee seeking political asylum and illustrates the way in which systemic labeling of an individual as a "difficult patient" by health providers diminishes access to care. Andreo was a 30-year-old school teacher from Tiblishi in Georgia who requested asylum in the Netherlands in December of 1995. While residing in a refugee camp, Andreo began to have fevers and night sweats. Because he feared that Dutch authorities would turn down his application for asylum because of his medical history, he did not seek help nor did he appear for mandatory screening for tuberculosis. Since 1990, he had suffered from tuberculosis, nephrosis, and hepatitis B. All of his problems had been treated poorly because of a dysfunctional health care system due to the political and economic situation in Georgia.

One morning, a roommate alerted a camp nurse when Andreo did not want to leave his bed. Once hospitalized, he was diagnosed with pulmonary TB. After 3 weeks of treatment he was sent back to the camp, where he had to reside pending his asylum procedure, to complete his tuberculosis therapy. From the start, Andreo was convinced that his diagnosis was a medical error. He did not experience any pain in his lungs; instead he felt pain in his liver. Repeatedly, he told the health care practitioners that he was afraid to end up like his father, who had died of liver cancer. However, Andreo's complaint was not taken seriously. When he finally decided to quit his TB treatment, which he believed was extremely harmful for his liver, a note in his medical chart indicated that he was a "difficult man, who did not comply with doctor's orders." Consequently, he was pressured to take his medicines under direct observation of the camp nurse.

Although it is against public health advice to transfer asylum seekers who are under treatment for tuberculosis, Andreo was sent to another refugee camp. There again, he was reluctant to take his TB medication. In addition, he had an argument with the physician about the fact that he had to share a small room with five other men, even though he was sick. In his medical record, Andreo was characterized as a manipulative patient who used his medicines to pressure the staff in order to get privileged treatment. His complaints about his liver were described as "vague," without any empirical grounds.

After Andreo's application for asylum was turned down by the court, his lawyer advised him strongly to get a medical test from his physician, suggesting that he might have a better chance for a residence permit based on humanitarian reasons—in his case, his tuberculosis. Although Andreo had gradually lost his trust in the medical staff of the camp, he felt he did not have much choice except to request further medical tests. The physician, however, was enraged at his request, accusing Andreo of misusing expensive medical care on behalf of his own agenda. The physician refused to cooperate, and denied Andreo further treatment.

These two cases illustrate the profound difficulties associated with access to care for immigrant or refugee patients. The illegal resident status of Said severely compromised his ability to receive effective treatment for his tuberculosis. His desire to be compliant with his medication formally required cooperation with the legal authorities; yet, his reluctance to cooperate is understandable. This case placed both Said and his caretakers in a double bind. If Said or the health providers told the authorities of Said's whereabouts at the end of treatment, Said risked incarceration or deportation. The alternative—not complying with treatment—was equally undesirable. A slightly different issue emerged in Andreo's case. The labeling of Andreo as a "manipulative" and "difficult" patient diminished the capacity of the health providers to treat him effectively. As gatekeepers to the health services provided for immigrants, the physicians had significant power to keep Andreo from receiving adequate care. Their response to Andreo appears punitive. Andreo was being disciplined for obstructionist behavior; he was not treated as a sick patient in need of help.

Participation in Scientific Research

The Nuremberg Trials following World War II established a major initiative concerning the ethical treatment of human subjects in scientific research (Katz, 1972). An important aspect of the Nuremberg Code was its commitment to informed consent in research involving human subjects. Subsequently, other codes of research ethics were developed, including the Draft Code of Ethics on Experimentation prepared by the World Medical Association in Geneva in 1961 and the Helsinki Declaration of 1964. More recently, the World Health Organization and the Council for International Organizations of Medical Sciences (1993) proposed international ethical guidelines for research involving human subjects (Brody, 1998; Levine, 1993).

In the United States, a report on the Tuskegee syphilis study in 1972 gave considerable impetus to the movement toward mandatory review of scientific research protocols. The Tuskegee study, implemented in 1932 in Macon County, Alabama, was designed to examine the natural course of untreated syphilis; the subjects were poor Black men who were not informed about the nature of the study (Jones, 1981). Treatment was not provided for the subjects until 1972, following public disclosure of the investigation. A panel appointed by the Department of Health, Education, and Welfare reviewed the Tuskegee syphilis experiment and in 1974 the National Research Act was passed; this act established the National Commission for the Protection of Human Subjects of Biomedical and Behavioral Research (Faden & Beauchamp, 1986). A number of reports were published by the National Commission concerning human experimentation on human fetuses (1975), prisoners (1976), children (1977), and the institutionalized mentally infirm (1978). Perhaps the most significant document produced by the Commission (1978) was the *Belmont Report,* a document describing basic ethical principles regarding research with human subjects.

Currently, throughout the world, research ethics committees have been established to provide oversight and approval for proposals to conduct studies involving human subjects. In the United States, in 1966, the Public Health Service (USPHS) required the establishment of ethics committees at research institutions. Final regulations concerning policies governing research on human subjects were issued in 1981 by the Department of Health and Human Services (USDHHS, 1981). The federal mandates were clear: any research involving human subjects that is funded by a Department agency, with certain exemptions, must be evaluated by an Institutional Review Board (IRB). Criteria for IRB approval include (1) a sound research design; (2) protection of privacy and confidentiality; (3) equality in treatment of subjects; (4) consideration of risks and benefits; (5) monitoring of data collection; (6) informed consent; (7) documentation of informed consent; and (8) a statement indicating that participation in the research is voluntary and that withdraw-

ing from the study will not result in harm or penalty.

IRBs have had a profound impact on the regulation of research with human subjects (Levine, 1986; Veatch, 1987). While there is consensus about the general purpose of IRBs, significant problems remain in the application of the review process. For example, one problem concerns the selection of committee members (Veatch, 1987). Committees are required to include representatives from non-scientific fields and from the community, but most are dominated by scientists who are responsible for reviewing the research protocols of colleagues and friends. Two issues become apparent. First, questions regarding professional competence arise in determining who is qualified to judge the professional merit of protocols. Second, professional bias may be an obstacle to objectivity regarding determination of harm to research subjects. The strong value placed on promoting scientific research among most IRB representatives may outweigh the concerns of a community representative. Moreover, lay members may experience psychological pressure to reach consensus and therefore they may be inclined to accept the arguments of a "professional." Additional problems center around which studies fall under the guidelines set by IRBs. Research that is perceived to involve minimal risk to subjects is exempt from review. The problem, of course, is one of interpretation regarding the judgment of "minimal risk" (pp. 109–123).

Social scientists have expressed serious reservations about the applicability of IRB regulations for basic and applied social research (e.g., Cassell, 1978; Gray, 1979; Marshall, 1992a; Seiler & Muirtha, 1980; Wax & Cassell, 1979). Critics suggest that many ethical problems encountered in social science research, particularly ethnographic or phenomenological studies, are not addressed by the federal regulations.

Internationally, the numerous codes of ethics governing scientific research with human subjects have been grounded in the same four ethical principles that have dominated health care in general: the principle of autonomy (respect for persons), the principles of beneficence and nonmaleficence, and the principle of justice (U.S. National Commission, 1978; Veatch, 1987). In non-Western and developing countries, investigators (Christakis, 1988, 1992; Christakis & Panner, 1991; Goodgame, 1990; Lane, 1994; Levine, 1991; Loue *et al.,* 1996) have called attention to the problematic development of appropriate standards for ethical conduct in scientific research. Lane (1994) described the development of a code of research ethics in Egypt; she argued that the "social and cultural contexts of the production of biomedical research in Egypt will influence the interpretation and application" (p. 885) of the generally accepted principles of research. Similarly, Loue and colleagues (1996), in their discussion of strategies for developing a Ugandan code of research ethics, suggested that, "although these principles are relevant to research in Uganda, their adoption and implementation must reflect the circumstances and cultural context that are unique to Uganda" (p. 47).

In the next two sections, we address difficulties encountered by health researchers working with immigrant and refugee populations focusing specifically on informed consent and confidentiality.

Informed Consent

Requirements for informed consent in research appeal to and are justified by the principle of autonomy and respect for persons. Informed consent in human subjects research consists of three key elements: the provision of information, comprehension of information, and voluntariness in regard to participation. Each of these dimensions may pose serious challenges to investigators conducting health-related research with immigrant or refugee populations.

Adequate information for potential subjects includes a description of research purposes and a clear delineation of risks and benefits. Relevant information must be com-municated in a manner that is understandable and linguistically appropriate. Potential subjects must be able to comprehend the information being communicated in order to make a decision. As Agich (1988) pointed out, "Ideally, comprehension of the information disclosed should allow the individual's personal beliefs and values to be reflected in any decision" (p. 133). However, immigrants or refugees may not be able to understand adequately because they speak a language different from that of the investigator, or their ability to speak the language of the researcher is limited. Linguistic barriers may be reduced through the use of an interpreter, but potential problems remain, as indicated in the section on the use of interpreters in health care delivery for immigrant and refugee populations. An investigation requiring a translator creates a dual problem for health researchers (Marshall, 1991). First, the investigator depends on the translator to communicate the research objectives correctly and effectively; second, the investigator depends on the translator to actually follow through with the consent which means relaying the information and requesting participation in the study. In situations where a translator is used, consent can be assumed only if the respondent agrees to participate.

Voluntary participation in research depends on the respondent's ability to understand not just the meaning of the research, but the impact it may have on his or her life. Most important, voluntariness implies that an individual participates in research without unnecessary coercion or social pressure. The offer of excessive financial compensation, bribes, or unrealistic promises may constitute coercion, especially if the subject is vulnerable because of social factors such as their ethnicity, poverty, or immigrant status. The voluntary nature of participation in research is influenced significantly by the implicit or explicit power of investigators and the institutions they represent. Thus, as Marshall (1992b) observed, social status and social class differences between investigators and immigrants or refugees, particularly if immigrants are poor or uneducated, may inhibit voluntariness in informed consent.

Scientific research conducted in non-Western settings presents the investigator with additional problems in regard to obtaining informed consent. For example, a number of scholars (Angell, 1988; Newton, 1990) have suggested that the application of Western ethical standards to scientific research conducted in developing countries with divergent cultural norms may be construed as a form of *ethical imperialism*. Yet, as Angell and others (e.g., Barry, 1988; Christakis, 1992; Ekunwe & Kessel, 1984; Levine, 1991) have pointed out, while ethical relativism demands cultural sensitivity to local customs, investigators are never authorized to conduct research without regard to potential harm and without attempts to be informative throughout a project's implementation. In particular, scholars (Angell, 1988) have cautioned against an ethical relativism that would permit the exploitation of populations in non-Western settings in research that would not be allowed in the investigator's home country.

A key issue surrounding informed consent in non-Western settings involves identification of the appropriate person to provide consent (Levine, 1991; Loue *et al.,* 1996). Barry (1988), in his discussion of AIDS research in Africa, described the challenge of translating the concepts of autonomy and personhood: "Personhood is defined by one's tribe, village, or social group" p. 1083; see also DeCraemer, 1983; Ijsselmuiden & Faden, 1992). Tribal elders, community leaders, religious authorities, or family members of the research subject may need to be approached before obtaining consent from individuals. For example, in their discussion of research ethics in Uganda, Loue and colleagues (1996) noted: "Ugandan civil law states that an eighteen-year-old male living at home has the legal right to make his own decisions. Customary law, however, dictates that the son obtain his father's consent prior to entering any obligation. Women . . . often refuse to make a decision regarding their own participation or their child's participa-

tion absent the consent of their partner" (p. 49). Negotiating informed consent with the designated authorities in health research with non-Western populations requires investigators to move beyond narrow definitions of personhood, autonomy and self-determination.

Right to Privacy and Confidentiality

The right to privacy, like informed consent, is justified by the principle of respect for autonomy. The obligation to maintain confidentiality implies that individuals have control over when and how communication about themselves is given to others. Specifically, in the context of scientific research with human subjects, confidentiality suggests that an agreement has been made that limits access to private information.

Investigators conducting health research with immigrant or refugee populations often engage in research involving the collection of sensitive information on the personal lives of study participants, including, for example, detailed descriptions of physical or mental problems, sexual and drug histories, and social networks. Disclosure of personal information, whether it is inadvertent or intentional, could threaten the economic or physical well-being of individual participants, particularly if the individual is an illegal immigrant or a refugee. If research documents are appropriated by governmental or institutional authorities, a participants' welfare is always jeopardized.

Although the assurance of anonymity for subjects is normally extended to participants in health research, it is sometimes difficult to sustain as information about the study becomes public knowledge. This may be especially problematic when research is conducted in small communities where the behavior of individuals is closely monitored, such as refugee camps, or in institutional settings in which information may be shared with professional colleagues or staff. In addition, La Rossa, Bennet, and Gelles (1981) emphasized the need for stringent standards of confidentiality when multiple members of one family are interviewed. In this situation, anonymity is vitally important because of the potential for punitive sanctions against family members if information about certain behavior is revealed. Studies of illegal behavior such as drug abuse, or highly sensitized issues such as sexual abuse, domestic violence, or HIV status, present other problems for health researchers working with immigrant and refugee populations (Leonard, 1990; Stepick and Stepick, 1990).

Conclusions and Recommendations

Ethical problems associated with the provision of health care and the implementation of clinical research for immigrant and refugee populations will continue to challenge health providers. In this chapter, we explored the relationship between cultural beliefs and values and expressions of autonomy in medical interactions, with particular attention to moral dilemmas associated with disclosure of information, protection of confidentiality, and informed consent. We also addressed ethical dimensions surrounding access to care, noting the relevance of poverty, discrimination, and political repression. We believe that three elements are essential to effectively resolving moral problems in cross-cultural patient care and scientific research with immigrants and refugees: an ability to communicate effectively with patients and their families; sufficient understanding of the patient's cultural background; and identification of culturally relevant value conflicts.

Successful communication in medical encounters depends on the ability of providers to understand the language and style of conversation used by the patient and family members to discuss diagnosis, prognosis, and medical treatments. Language barriers can be powerful obstacles to a thoughtful exploration of moral issues that arise in patient care. Even if the patient and provider share the same language, particular words may be unique to certain dialects, inhibiting communication. Family members, who often act as interpreters for patients, may camouflage the information to protect patients from news that is perceived to be emotionally upsetting. Professional interpreters also influence the information being conveyed, modifying the message in order to accommodate linguistic difference or personality style. Two concerns should be addressed in medical interactions with immigrant and refugee patients. First, whenever possible, additional time for discussion with patients should be scheduled in order to allow for longer conversations necessitated by the use of an interpreter. Second, the use of interpreters requires careful attention to the message being conveyed, whether the interpretation is done by a professional translator or a family member; professional interpreters should be used instead of family members when they are available in hospital or clinic settings.

Understanding a patient's cultural background and its impact on ethical dilemmas that arise in patient care requires attention to a range of factors, including consideration of religious beliefs, developmental age, gender, educational background, financial circumstances, social network, and length of time since emigrating or seeking political asylum. Equally important are patients' and families' beliefs about their illnesses and treatments, their beliefs about what actually constitutes a "moral problem" in health care, their comprehension of what providers have discussed with them, and their opinions on what actions—on their part and the provider's part—would resolve the problem.

In the context of health care decision making with patients who are immigrants or refugees, determination of decision-making authority is vital. In the United States, patients or their designated surrogates are expected to make decisions about medical treatments. Cultural traditions that locate decisional authority in tribal elders, religious figures, family heads, or community leaders differ significantly from the Western focus on the individual. Where there is a stronger communitarian perspective, beliefs about the self and individual autonomy are embedded in the sociocentric patterns of family ties and community obligations. Patients and their families should be asked to identify individuals whom it may be important to involve in the decision-making process, and every effort should be made to include them. Both patient and provider lose the opportunity for a more productive and compassionate interaction when the provider avoids negotiation and instead, assumes a "morally" righteous posture in applying the Western principle of respect for personal autonomy.

Ethnic stereotyping is a significant problem in cross-cultural medical interactions. Too often, health practitioners make assumptions about patients' cultural backgrounds and their health care beliefs. For example, Spanish is spoken by immigrants from many different countries; yet, immigrants or refugees from Mexico, Central America, or South America have diverse ethnic identities and cultural traditions. It is impossible to categorically define one "Latino" culture; nor is it possible to define one "African" or "Anglo" culture. Moreover, class, gender, and other social differences blur the distinctiveness of cultural traditions. Expecting patients of similar ethnic groups to act in predictable ways is unrealistic and disrespectful. Asking patients and their families questions about beliefs and practices that may influence the resolution of ethical dilemmas in their particular cases is key to bridging cultural misunderstandings.

Health care practitioners working with immigrant populations cannot become familiar with the language and customs of the myriad cultures represented by patients. Members of the patient's family or community, particularly individuals who are sufficiently bilingual and bicultural, may provide important background information for patients when ethical dilemmas occur. It may also be beneficial to consult with professionals in academic centers or community organizations who are knowledgeable in the language or cultural traditions of immigrant patients. Collaboration with others—professionals and community representatives—enhances the potential for achieving successful outcomes in morally complicated medical encounters.

A key component of resolving medical ethical dilemmas is the identification of value conflicts; this process can be especially troubling for practitioners and patients when the conflicts are based on strong differences in beliefs concerning what represents morally and culturally "appropriate" behavior. In these situations, it is vitally important for the provider to be self-reflective in examining his or her own cultural and professional values regarding the problem being confronted. Unrecognized biases and prejudices inhibit a sensitive and robust treatment of the moral issues that arise. In addition, it is important for health care providers to recognize the vulnerability of patients and to be aware of the power the providers have to influence decision-making processes. The professional status of physicians, nurses, and other members of the health care team can be overwhelming to immigrant and refugee patients who may feel they must comply with treatment recommendations.

Compromise and intellectual flexibility on the part of the provider are necessary when moral conflicts involving cultural differences arise in the course of medical treatment. Identifying the central concerns of patients and their families and being open to various solutions facilitates the process of negotiating a course of action. Rigidity and intractability stalemates interactions and may further alienate a patient or family already experiencing isolation and powerlessness. Engaging in power struggles over Western biomedical customs diminishes opportunities for recognizing a workable solution.

In conclusion, we believe that it is irresponsible to disregard the importance and validity of alternative belief systems held by immigrant and refugee patients. Claims of moral superiority on the basis of membership in the dominant biomedical culture fall short of an ethical response to a medical dilemma. Future research that explores systematically the cultural underpinnings of the resolution of moral problems in health care delivery is needed.

The complexity of the issues involved requires attention to a range of problems concerning the definition of medical ethical dilemmas on the part of patients and providers, the process of negotiating moral disputes in cross-cultural contexts, and the impact of asymmetrical social power among patients and providers in the decision-making process.

Acknowledgments

The work on multiculturalism and bioethics by Barbara Koenig and Patricia Marshall has been supported by the Greenwall Foundation. We want to thank William C. Stubing, president of the Greenwall Foundation, for his belief in the importance of an anthropological perspective on bioethics. The cases reported on cultural diversity and end-of-life care among cancer patients are from a study supported by the National Institutes of Health, RO1NR02906. The cases involving immigrants and refugees come from an ongoing investigation by Paul Grifhorst and Mirjam van Ewijk; the study is supported by the Dutch Praeventiefonds, #002826950.

References

Agich, G. (1988). Human experimentation and clinical consent. In J. Monagle & D. C. Thomasma (Eds.), *A guide for health professionals* (pp. 127–139). Rockville, MD: Aspen.

Angell, M. (1988). Ethical imperialism? Ethics in international collaborative clinical research. *New England Journal of Medicine, 319,* 1081–1083.

Barry, M. (1988). Ethical considerations of human investigation in developing countries: The AIDS dilemma. *New England Journal of Medicine, 319,* 1083–1086.

Baylis, F., & Downie, J. (1997). Child abuse and neglect: Cross-cultural considerations. In H. Nelson (Ed.), *Feminism and families* (pp. 173–187). New York: Routledge.

Beauchamp, T. L., & Childress, J. (1993). *Principles of biomedical ethics* (4th ed.). New York: Oxford University Press.

Beecher, H. K. (1966). Ethics and clinical research. *New England Journal of Medicine, 274,* 1354–1360.

Bell, S. E., & Whiteford, M. B. (1987). Tai Dam health care practices: Asian refugee women in Iowa. *Social Science and Medicine, 24,* 317–325.

Benner, P. (1991). The role of experience, narrative, and community in skilled ethical comportment. *Advances in Nursing Science, 14,* 1–21.

Berk, M. L., Albers, L. A., & Schur, C. L. (1996). The growth in the US uninsured population: Trends in Hispanic subgroups, 1977 to 1992. *American Journal of Public Health, 86,* 572–576.

Beyene, Y. (1992). Medical disclosure and refugees— Telling bad news to Ethiopian patients. In Crosscultural medicine—A decade later [Special issue]. *Western Journal of Medicine, 157,* 328–332.

Blackhall, L. J., Murphy, S. T., Frank, G., Michel, V., & Azen, S. (1995). Ethnicity and attitudes toward patient autonomy. *Journal of the American Medical Association, 274,* 820–825.

Brody, B. A. (1998). *The ethics of biomedical research: An international perspective.* New York: Oxford University Press.

Caralis, P. V., Davis, B., Wright, K., & Marcial, E. (1993). The influence of ethnicity and race on attitudes toward advance directives, life-prolonging directives, life-prolonging treatments and euthanasia. *Journal of Clinical Ethics, 4,* 155–165.

Carrese, J. A., & Rhodes, L. A. (1995). Western bioethics on the Navajo reservation. *Journal of the American Medical Association, 274,* 826–829.

Cassell, J. (1978). Risk and benefit to subjects of fieldwork. *American Sociologist, 13,* 134–143.

Christakis, N. A. (1988). The ethical design of an AIDS vaccine trial in Africa. *Hastings Center Report, 18,* 31–37

Christakis, N.A. (1992). Ethics are local: Engaging crosscultural variation in the ethics for clinical research. *Social Science and Medicine, 35,* 1079–1091.

Christakis, N. A., & Panner, M. J. (1991). Existing international ethical guidelines for human subjects research: Some open questions. *Law, Medicine and Health Care, 19,* 214–221.

Connor, S. S., & Fuenzalida-Puelma H. (Eds.). (1990). *Bioethics: Issues and perspectives.* Washington, DC: Pan American Health Organization.

D'Avanzo, C. (1992). Barriers to health care for Vietnamese refugees. *Journal of Professional Nursing, 8,* 245–253.

DeCraemer, W. A. (1983) Cross-cultural perspective on personhood. *Milbank Memorial Fund Quarterly, 6,* 19–34.

de la Torre, A., Friis, R., Hunter, H. R., & Garcia, L. (1996). The health insurance status of US Latino women: A profile from the 1982–1984 HHANES. *American Journal of Public Health, 86,* 533–537.

Dula, A. (1994). African American suspicion of the healthcare system is justified: What do we do about it? *Cambridge Quarterly of Healthcare Ethics, 3,* 347–358.

Dula, A., & Goering, S. (1994). *"It just ain't fair": The ethics of health care for African Americans.* Westport, CT: Praeger.

Ekunwe, E. O., & Kessel, R. (1984). Informed consent in the developing world. *Hastings Center Report, 14,* 22–24.

Engelhardt, T. H., Jr. (1986). *The foundations of medical ethics.* New York: Oxford University Press.

Engelhardt, T. H., Jr. (1991). *Bioethics and secular humanism: The search for a common morality.* Philadelphia: Trinity.

Faden, R. R., & Beauchamp, T. L. (1986). *A history and theory of informed consent.* New York: Oxford University Press.

Fox, R. C. (1990). The evolution of American bioethics: A sociological perspective. In G. Weisz (Ed.), *Social science perspectives on medical ethics* (pp. 201–220). Philadelphia: University of Pennsylvania Press.

Fox, R. C., & Swazey, J. P. (1984). Medical morality is not bioethics: Medical ethics in China and the United States. *Perspectives in Biology and Medicine, 27,* 336–360.

Frankel, M. S., & Teich, A. H. (Eds.). (1994). *The genetic frontier: Ethics, law, and policy.* Washington, DC: American Association for the Advancement of Science.

Frankena, W. (1973). *Ethics* (2nd ed.). Englewood Cliffs, NJ: Prentice-Hall.

Freedman, B. (1993). Offering truth: One ethical approach to the uninformed cancer patient. *Archives of Internal Medicine, 153,* 572–576.

Garcia, J. L. A. (1992). African-American perspectives, cultural relativism and normative issues: Some conceptual problems. In H. Flack & E. D. Pellegrino (Eds.), *African-American perspectives on biomedical ethics* (pp. 11–65). Washington, DC: Georgetown University Press.

Gilman, S. C., Justice, J., Saepharn, K., Charles, G. (1992). Use of traditional and modern health services by Laotian refugees. *Western Journal of Medicine, 157,* 310–315.

Good, B. J. (1994). Medicine, rationality, and experience: An anthropological perspective. Boston: Cambridge University Press.

Good, M. D., Good, B. J., Schaffer, C., & Lind, S. E. (1990). American oncology and the discourse on hope. *Culture Medicine and Psychiatry, 14,* 59–79.

Goodgame, R. W. (1990). AIDS in Uganda: Clinical and social features. *New England Journal of Medicine, 323,* 383–389.

Gray, B. H. (1979). The regulatory context of social research: The work of the national commission for the protection of human subjects. In C. B. Klockars & F. W. O'Connor (Eds.), *Deviance and decency: The ethics of research with human subjects* (pp. 197–224). Beverly Hills, CA: Sage.

Hern, H. E., Jr., Koenig, B. A., Moore, L. J., & Marshall, P. A. (1998). The difference that culture can make in end-of-life decision making. *Cambridge Quarterly of Healthcare Ethics, 7.*

Hoffmaster, B. (1990). Morality and the social sciences. In G. Weisz (Ed.), *Social science perspectives on medical ethics* (pp. 241–260). Philadelphia: University of Pennsylvania Press.

Hunter, K. M. (1991). *Doctors' stories: The narrative structure of medical knowledge.* Princeton, NJ: Princeton University Press.

Ijsselmuiden, C. B., & Faden, R. R. (1992). Research and informed consent in Africa—Another look. *New England Journal of Medicine, 326,* 830–833.

Jecker, N. S., Carrese, J. A., & Pearlman, R. (1995). Caring for patients in cross-cultural settings. *Hastings center report, 25,* 6–14.

Jenkins, C. N. H., Le, T., Mcphee, S. J., Stewart, S., & Ha, N. T. (1996). Health care access and preventive care among Vietnamese immigrants: Do traditional beliefs and practices pose barriers? *Social Science and Medicine, 43,* 1049–1056.

Jones, J. H. (1981). *Bad blood.* New York: Free Press.

Jonsen, A., & Toulmin, S. (1988). *The abuse of casuistry.* Berkeley: University of California Press.

Katz, J. (1972). *Experimentation with human beings.* New York: Russell Sage Foundation.

Kaufert, J. M., & O'Neil, J. D. (1990). Biomedical rituals and informed consent: Native Canadians and the negotiation of clinical trust. In G. Weisz (Ed.), *Social science perspectives on medical ethics* (pp. 41–64). Philadelphia: University of Pennsylvania Press.

Kleinman, A. M. (1980). *Patients and healers in the context of culture.* Berkeley: University of California Press.

Kleinman, A. (1995). Anthropology of bioethics. In W. Reich (Ed.), *Encyclopedia of Bioethics* (pp. 1667–1674). New York: Macmillan.

Klessig, J. (1992). The effect of values and culture on life-support decisions. In Cross-cultural medicine—A decade later [Special issue]. *Western Journal of Medicine, 157,* 316–322.

Koenig, B. A. (1993). Diversity in decision-making about care at the end-of-life. In *Dying, decision-making, and appropriate care.* Washington, DC: Institute of Medicine/National Academy of Sciences.

Koenig, B. A., & Gates-Williams, J. (1995). Understanding cultural difference in caring for dying patients. *Western Journal of Medcine, 163,* 244–249.

Lane, S. D. (1993). Research bioethics in Egypt. In R. Gillon (Ed.), *Principles of health care ethics* (pp. 885–894). New York: Wiley.

La Rossa, R., Bennet, L. A., & Grelles, R.. (1981). Ethical dilemmas in qualitative family research. *Journal of Marriage and Family, 43,* 303–313.

Lauritzen, P. (1993). *Pursing parenthood: Ethical issues in assisted reproduction.* Indianapolis: Indiana University Press.

Leonard, T. L. (1990). Male clients of female street prostitutes: Unseen partners in sexual disease transmission. *Medical Anthropology Quarterly, 4,* 41–55.

Levine, R. J. (1986). *Ethics and regulation of clinical research* (2nd ed.). Baltimore: Urban and Schwarzenberg.

Levine, R. J. (1991). Informed consent: Some challenges to the universal validity of the western model. *Law, Medicine, and Health Care, 19*, 3–4.

Lock, M. (1993). Education and self reflection: Teaching about culture, health and illness. In R. Masi, L. L. Mensah, & K. McLeod (Eds.), *Health and cultures: Exploring the relationships* (pp. 137–156). Oakville, Ontario, Canada: Mosaic.

Loewy, E. (1991). *Suffering and the beneficent community: Beyond libertarianism.* Albany: State University of New York Press.

Loue, S., Okello, D., & Kawuma, M. (1996). Research bioethics in the Ugandan context: A program summary. *Journal of Law, Medicine & Ethics, 24*, 47–53.

MacIntyre, A. (1984). *After virtue.* Notre Dame, IN: Notre Dame University Press.

Marshall, P. A. (1989). Children in medical settings. In J. Garbarino, F. M. Stott, & the Faculty of the Erikson Institute (Eds.), *What children can tell us* (pp. 266–290). San Francisco: Jossey-Bass.

Marshall, P. A. (1991). Research ethics in applied anthropology. In C. E. Hill (Ed.), *Training manual in medical anthropology* (pp. 213–235). Washington, DC: American Anthropological Association and Society for Applied Anthropology.

Marshall, P. A. (1992a). Anthropology and bioethics. *Medical Anthropology Quarterly, 6*, 47–71.

Marshall, P. A. (1992b). Research ethics in applied anthropology. *IRB: A Review of Human Subjects Research, 14*, 1–5.

Marshall, P. A., & Koenig, B. A. (1996). Anthropology and bioethics: Perspectives on culture, medicine and morality. In C. Sargent & T. Johnson (Eds.), *Medical anthropology: Contemporary theory and method* (2nd ed., pp. 349–373). Westport, CT: Praeger.

Marshall, P. A., Thomasma, D. C., & Bergsma, J. (1994). Intercultural reasoning: The challenge for international bioethics. *Cambridge Quarterly of Healthcare Ethics, 3*, 321–328.

Marshall, P. A., Koenig, B. A., Barnes, D. M., & Davis, A. J. (1998). Multiculturalism, bioethics and end-of-life care: Case narratives of Latino cancer patients. In D. C. Thomasma & J. Monagle (Eds.), *Health care ethics: Issues for the 21st century* (pp. 421–431). Rockville, MD: Aspen.

Muller, J. H., & Desmond, B. (1992). Ethical dilemmas in a cross-cultural context—A Chinese example. In Cross-cultural medicine—A decade later [Special issue]. *Western Journal of Medicine, 157*, 323–327.

National Commission for the Protection of Human Subjects of Biomedical and Behavioral Research. (1978). *The Belmont report: Ethical principles and guidelines for the protection of human subjects of research.* Washington, DC: U.S. Government Printing Office.

Newton, L. H. (1990). Ethical imperialism and informed consent. *IRB: A Review of Human Subjects Research, 12*, 10–11.

Orona, C. J., Koenig, B. A., & Davis, A. J. (1994). Cultural aspects of nondisclosure. *Cambridge Quarterly Healthcare Ethics, 3*, 338–346.

Orr, R. D., Marshall, P. A., & Osborn, J. (1995). Cross-cultural considerations in clinical ethics consultations. *Archives of Family Medicine, 4*, 159–164.

Pellegrino, E. D. (1992a). Intersections of Western biomedical ethics and world culture: Problematic and possibility. *Cambridge Quarterly of Healthcare Ethics, 1*, 191–196 (quotation, p. 191).

Pellegrino, E. D. (1992b). Is truth telling to the patient a cultural artifact? [Editorial]. *Journal of the American Medical Association, 268*, 1734–1735.

Pellegrino, E. D., & Flack, H. E. (1992). *African-American perspectives on biomedical ethics.* Washington, DC: Georgetown University Press.

Pellegrino, E. D., & Thomasma, D. C. (1989). *For the patient's good: The restoration of beneficence in health care.* New York: Oxford University Press.

Pellegrino, E. D., & Thomasma, D. C. (1993). *The virtues in medical practice.* New York: Oxford University Press.

Pellegrino, E. D., Corsi, P., & Mazzarella, P. (Eds.). (1992). *Transcultural dimensions in medical ethics.* Frederick, MD: University Publishing.

Putsch, R. W., III. (1985). Cross-cultural communication: The special case of interpreters in health care. *Journal of the American Medical Association, 254*, 3344–3348.

Rothman, D. (1991). *Strangers at the bedside: A history of how law and bioethics transformed medical decision-making.* New York: Basic Books.

Schneiderman, L. J., & Jecker, N. S. (1995). *Wrong medicine: Doctors, patients, and futile treatment.* Baltimore, MD: Johns Hopkins University Press.

Schoepf, B. G. (1991). Ethical, methodological and political issues of AIDS research in central Africa. *Social Science Medicine, 33*, 749–763.

Seiler, L. H., & Muirtha, J. M. (1980). Federal regulation of social research using "human subjects": A critical assessment. *American Sociologist, 15*, 146–157.

Shweder, R. (1990). Ethical relativism: Is there a defensible version? *Ethos, 18*, 219–223.

Siddharthan, K., & Alalasundaram, S. (1993). Undocumented aliens and uncompensated care: whose responsibility? *American Journal of Public Health, 83*, 410–412.

Stepick, A., & Stepick, C. D. (1990). People in the shadows: Survey research among Haitians in Miami. *Human Organization, 49*, 64–77.

Surbone, A. (1992). Truth telling to the patient [Letter]. *Journal of the American Medical Association, 268*, 1661–1662.

Teno, J., Hill, T. P., & O'Connor, M. A. (1994). Advance care planning: Priorities for ethical and empirical research. *Hastings Center Report, 24* (Suppl.), 1.

Thamer, M., Richard, C., Casebeer, A. W., & Ray, N. F. (1997). Health insurance coverage among foreign-born US residents: The impact of race, ethnicity, and length of residence. *American Journal of Public Health, 87,* 96–102.

Tong, R. (1996). *Feminist approaches to bioethics.* Boulder, CO: Westview.

Uba, L. (1992) Cultural barriers to health care for southeast Asian refugees. *Public Health Reports, 107,* 544–548.

U.S. Department of Health and Human Services (USDHHS). (1981). *Final Regulations Amending Basic HHS Policy for the Protection of Human Research Subjects: Final Rule: 5 CFR 46. Federal Register: Rules and Regulations 46 (16, January 26),* 8366–8392.

U.S. National Commission for the Protection of Human Subjects of Biomedical and Behavior Research. (1978). *Report and recommendations: Research involving those institutionalized as mentally infirm.* Bethesda, MD: U.S. Department of Health, Education and Welfare.

Veatch, R. M. (1981). *A theory of medical ethics.* New York: Basic Books.

Veatch, R. M. (1987). *The patient as partner: A theory of human-experimentation ethics.* Bloomington: Indiana University Press.

Veatch, R. M. (1989). *Cross cultural perspectives in medical ethics: Readings.* Boston: Jones and Bartlett.

Veatch, R. M. (1991). *The physician–patient relationship: The patient as partner: Part 2.* Bloomington: Indiana University Press.

Ware, N. C., & Kleinman, A. R. (1992). Culture and somatic experience. *Psychosomatic Medicine, 54,* 546–560.

Wasongarz, D., Carter, J., Barnes, D. M., & Koenig, B. A. (1995). Bioethics and the intermediary role of interpreters: Negotiating language and emotion. Unpublished manuscript, Stanford University Center for Biomedical Ethics. First presented as a paper at the 1994 annual meeting of the American Anthropological Association, Atlanta, GA.

Wax, M. L., & Cassell, J. (Eds.). (1979). Fieldwork, ethics and politics: The wider context. In M. L. Wax & J. Cassell (Eds.) *Federal regulations: Ethical issues and social research* (pp. 85–101). Boulder, CO: Westview.

Weisz, G. (Ed.). (1990). *Social science perspectives on medical ethics.* Philadelphia: University of Pennsylvania Press.

Wolf, S. (1996). *Feminism and bioethics: Beyond reproduction.* New York: Oxford University Press.

World Health Organization and Council for International Organizations of Medical Sciences (WHO-CIOMS). (1993). *International ethical guidelines for biomedical research involving human subjects.* Geneva, Switzerland: Author.

12

Refugee Health

KAREN N. OLNESS

Overview—Refugee Problems

During the 20th century more than 15 million refugees have relocated to the United States. During the decade from 1986 to 1996 there have been 25 to 30 million displaced persons in the world during any given month. Some of these have become immigrants to the United States, some have returned to their homes, and many are still waiting for permanent relocation. Throughout the 1990s there have been large refugee camps in Asia, Europe, and Africa. Each area has its own unique problems.

The majority of refugee groups throughout the world have evolved from political upheavals and ethnic struggles within their countries of origin. As a result, the refugees suffer not only from physical but also mental trauma. Being a refugee often has lifelong consequences for refugee families even when relocation is rapid, safe, and provides generously for material needs. In fact, most relocations are slow, involve a great deal of chaos, and are accompanied by poverty. In general, refugee settings lack adequate attention and programs for the most vulnerable—pregnant and nursing mothers, children, and the elderly. Although they should provide safety and a haven, refugee settings often contribute to

continuing physical and mental risks for the most vulnerable. These have negative impacts for productivity, economics, and political stability that adversely affect the whole world.

Examples of Refugee Camps

Refugee camps are grim places, in general. Housing is extremely crowded, sanitation is poor, there is a frequent risk of fire, and the noise level is high. In spite of this, refugee men often develop small businesses and are busy (Torjesen, Olness, & Torjesen, 1981). Women are usually very busy with the complexities of carrying food and water from distribution points, cooking, washing, and child care in refugee camps. There seems to be little doubt that women in many refugee settings have large numbers of children (Wulf, 1994). Centers for Disease Control researchers in a refugee camp in Thailand documented that the crude birth rate in 1980 was 55 per 1,000, a high rate (Toole & Waldman, 1988). Unfortunately, the high rates of pregnancy are at the expense of refugee women's already fragile health status. The World Health Organization (WHO) definition of high-risk criteria among pregnant women includes ages under 19 or over 40, women with no accompanying family, illiterate women, women with less than 2 years between births, women suffering acute chronic or medical conditions or infection, women with poor immunization status, or women being served by health providers who

KAREN N. OLNESS • Rainbow Babies and Children's Hospital, Cleveland, Ohio 44106.

Handbook of Immigrant Health, edited by Loue. Plenum Press, New York, 1998.

do not speak their language (United Nations High Commission for Refugees, 1993). Unfortunately, many refugee women fit this definition and the repercussions from high-risk pregnancies for both the women and their infants are negative. For example, the fetus may be at risk from maternal infections with tuberculosis, hepatitis, malaria, gonorrhea, chlamydia, HIV virus, syphilis, or several of these diseases.

Food rations in refugee camps are based mainly on total calorie intake rather than on a population's specific nutritional needs. In many societies women serve the male members of the family and their children before they eat themselves. It is likely that the majority of refugee women suffer from malnutrition, especially iron and calcium deficiencies.

Existing health services in most refugee settings overlook specific needs of women. This ranges from provision of sanitary supplies for menstruating women to provision of birth spacing services. When birth spacing services do exist, they are often insensitive to refugee beliefs, fears, and educational level. Health education regarding sexually transmitted diseases is usually inadequate for both men and women and nonexistent for adolescents. In both Asian and African countries there are beliefs that a man can cure AIDS by having sex with a virgin. This belief has jeopardized the lives of many young females, as young as 4 or 5 years, and caused transmission of HIV infection to them.

Labor and delivery is hazardous in refugee settings. Properly equipped facilities for complicated deliveries are not often available. Many women do not have supportive family members to help them during labor and delivery. Most refugee women will choose to give birth at home, often because they do not like being treated by health professionals who are not of their own gender or ethnic group.

Somali Refugees in Kenya (Wulf, 1994)

Overall conditions of the camps were described as relatively good in 1993. However, the heat, dust, flies, and refuse piles rein-

forced an unrelenting impression of hardship. Camps were divided into sections with leaders, and each section chose a male community health worker. They provided information about hygiene, sanitation, and malaria prevention. Community development workers, some of them female, were also trained to carry out community clean-ups, cooking demonstrations, or protection of the elderly. Every camp had market areas including availability of a kind of pink bubble gum used to sweeten the sharp flavor of khat, the dried green leaf chewed all day by older members. In spite of these relatively well-organized circumstances and reduction of serious malnutrition, there were still many infectious diseases in these camps. Tuberculosis remained common, for example. The birth rate was high and facilities for women at high risk during pregnancy were very limited. Women leaving the camps to gather firewood were frequently raped by roving bandits, young men from the camps, or members of the Kenyan army and police force assigned to protect the camps. Somali women who were raped were then abandoned by their husbands and husbands' families if they became pregnant.

Afghan Refugee Camp Near Hangu, Pakistan (1996)

These camps had existed for about 15 years and were well organized in terms of housing, activities of daily life, and health programs. General food distribution from United Nations agencies was no longer available. Families without an employed male had problems getting adequate food. Each camp had a Basic Health Unit (BHU), open several days of the week and staffed with both Afghan and Pakistani physicians and nurses. Each camp also had volunteer Community Health Workers (CHW) and Community Health Supervisors (CHS). In recent years Volunteer Female Health Workers (FHWs) have also been trained to provide prenatal monitoring and advice to pregnant women and to assist during home deliveries. Although purdah (the requirement that women remain in their family compound) is practiced, exceptions are made to allow women to come to the BHUs where male and female clinics are separated. The BHUs charge refugees, except widows and orphans, for health services.

In general the CHW and FHW teaching, often done while patients wait to be seen, is excellent. For example, they provide discussions on control of mosquitos, flies, and preparation of oral rehydration solution made with wheat and sugar. FHWs have been able to change some traditional practices such as smearing cow dung on umbilical cords shortly after birth. As a female, I was allowed into Afghan homes to meet with women. I was not allowed to photograph women but I could photograph the cows tethered in the home compound. I observed training in preparation for delivery and actual delivery; training uses a box cut to simulate the birth canal. Women laughed when they told me how stupid they used to be about many things, such as smearing cow dung on the umbilical cord.

A major continuing problem in these camps was malnutrition of children. This seemed related to both lack of food and to chronic diarrhea that often affected toddlers. There were many children with evidence of developmental delays, genetic disorders, and cerebral palsy. Some of this may relate to frequent marriages among cousins. Birth rates were high in these camps and most couples were not interested in birth spacing, although there were a few new users of birth control each month. Most girls were not allowed to attend the refugee camp schools, and those who did attend might do so for only 2 or 3 years. Husbands did all family shopping and it was clear that the problem of malnutrition was more likely to be resolved by education of men than of women.

Refugee Camps in Zaire

In 1994 many Rwandans fled from Rwanda into Zaire and Tanzania in the largest mass movement of refugees ever recorded. As a result the refugee camps were incredibly crowded and infectious diseases were rampant during the initial months. Within a few weeks there were 10,000 unaccompanied minors identified, most of them infants or toddlers. Although most Rwandan children were in a normal state of nutrition at the time their families fled, a majority of preschoolers were malnourished within a month of arriving in the refugee camps. Women were also malnourished and many of the lactating women complained about their shortage of breast milk. Women also appeared anxious, depressed, and overwhelmed. In general, Rwandans prefer the privacy of the nuclear family and their usual huts are spread out over hills. Undoubtedly, the proximity of shelters (mostly branches and plastic sheeting from the United Nations) in the refugee camps was stressful for Rwandan women. Most of the women in the camps preferred to give birth in their hut rather than in the camp hospitals because they prefer the squatting position for delivery. This was not allowed in the hospitals.

Rwandan women leave school much earlier than men in order to take on domestic duties. In general, women do most of the work. The insistence on privacy and independence of individual households means that women are unlikely to share new skills or information with neighbors. This reduced the transfer of knowledge about birth spacing, sexually transmitted diseases, and other health matters. At the time of the large refugee exodus, studies indicated that 30% of pregnant women in Kigali were infected with HIV. It is likely that rampant transmission of HIV has continued in the refugee camps.

In November and December 1996 the majority of Rwandan refugees returned to Rwanda. It became apparent that many of the refugees, especially the women, children, and elderly, had been held hostage by Hutu militia who were well organized in the refugee camps and used them for staging their military plans. The return to Rwanda was rapid with little concern for children. Once again, many young children were separated from parents and identified as unaccompanied minors.

What Can We Learn from the Refugee Camp Examples?

Refugees from each of the camps described became immigrants to the United States. It is unlikely that most American health providers would recognize the physical and mental hazards that these immigrants had endured. For example, a 5-year-old child who had become an orphan in one of these settings may have had normal weight on arrival in the United States. Medical records for him may be scanty or nonexistent. But if he suffered severe malnutrition in his first 2 years in the refugee setting, he is likely to have permanent brain injury with learning disabilities that will manifest by age 9 or 10 (Galler, Shumsky, & Morgane, 1996). Former refugee women may continue to have depression. They may be suspicious of Western health providers. They may have chronic ongoing infections or problems resulting from their long period of malnutrition in the refugee camps. It is noteworthy that former refugees often do not discuss the circumstances of their flight or their experiences in the refugee camps. They may be afraid that the information will jeopardize their status in the United States or may simply wish to repress the experience. It is possible for American health care providers to get specific information about various refugee settings from U.N. agencies, from the International Rescue Committee on Refugee Women and Children, or from other nongovernmental agencies (International Federation of Red Cross and Red Crescent Societies, 1996).

Traumatization of Refugees

Traumatization of refugees is often an enduring, cumulative process that continues from the native country and into the country of exile (Kleber, Figley, & Gersons, 1995). The trauma includes political repression, detention, torture, terror, battlefield experiences, disappearance of relatives and friends, separation and loss of families and friends, and hardships during the flight or in the refugee camps. Health programs for refugees must take into account such traumatization.

Uprooting, being forced to leave one's familiar surroundings, involves three forms of loss (Van der Veer, 1995):

1. The loss of love and respect experiencd in the relationship with family and friends.
2. The loss of social status in the country of exile. Most refugees have to start at the bottom of society.
3. The loss of a familiar social environment that gave meaning to life.

Adults

Van der Veer (1995) has described the experiences of refugees in three phases including (1) increasing political repression, (2) major traumatic experiences associated with a variety of emotional reactions, and (3) the phase of exile. The last includes ongoing problems in cultural adjustment, language problems, social isolation, problems in finding work, and receiving bad news from the country of origin.

All health professionals who work with adult refugees need to be sensitive to the prior traumatization and how it is likely to cause both biologic and behavioral problems. It is also important to recognize that mental health interventions appropriate for Americans may not be appropriate for refugees from very different cultures. Americans value individualism and self-analysis. This is not true for many cultures (e.g., Lao or Vietnamese). The idea that symptoms will respond to talking with a stranger over time may make no sense to a refugee. The idea of expressing anger openly is abhorrent to Southeast Asian refugees. Health providers should have some knowledge about the adult refugee's beliefs concerning causes of illness. For example Mollica and Lavelle (1988) reported that Cambodian refugees who had been tortured believed this was done to them because of their karma. They felt responsible for their own suffering.

The need to communicate through interpreters may cause problems for health professionals and for the newly arrived refugee. The choice of an interpreter must take culture into account. Issues such as gender, social status, or prior relationships may make therapy difficult. Westermeyer (1989) noted that some interpreters may have experienced traumas similar to those of the patient. In order to avoid thinking about his or her own issues, the interpreter may evade certain topics, change the subject, or inform the therapist that the interview is too stressful for the refugee.

Because of prior experiences, refugees often have a feeling of being humiliated or powerless. They are likely to be easily offended by anything in the manner of a health professional or his coworkers that resembles indifference, humiliation, or abuse of power. A traumatized refugee requires time, patience, interest, and respect. The health professional should do his or her best to give the refugee a sense of control. It is very important to help adult refugees with ongoing problems related to their traumas, because doing so improves the mental health outlook for the entire family (Gany & DeBocanegra, 1996).

In spite of the liklihood that traumatized refugees often somatize their symptoms, it is important that American health professionals also recognize they may have serious biologic diseases that can cause vague symptoms or psychological problems. For example, vague intestinal complaints may be due to parasites. Intracerebral cysts from parasites may take years to manifest and symptoms may include seizures, headaches, or vague neurologic complaints. Flukes may cause hepatic disease with resultant nausea, anorexia, and weakness. Neuropsychological symptoms may be early signs of AIDS. It is recommended that the newly arrived immigrant from Africa or Asia have stool examinations, hepatitis assays, HIV testing, blood smears, and ultrasound or MRI examinations, depending on symptoms.

Delayed disorders associated with refugee trauma have been reported by Krell (1988).

Psychiatric disorders have manifested decades later in adults who were Holocaust survivors or Japanese concentration camp internees as children.

Children

A defining characteristic of refugee status is loss. Children may lose their toys, clothing, homes, friends, siblings, parents, and grandparents. The loss of a parent is a major disaster for children, and outcomes depend on the developmental stage of the child at the time of the parent's death. The most vulnerable times are in the preschool years and in early adolesence. The risk for psychological morbidity is greater if the death is unanticipated or caused by violence as is the usual situation for a refugee child. Children exposed to war have many psychosocial problems (McCloskey & Southwick, 1996).

Refugee children also suffer long-term problems as a result of severe deprivation of food or medical care. Many refugee children are malnourished. When this occurs prior to age 3 years, there is a strong liklihood of permanent brain injury with cognitive and behavioral impairments that may not be manifest until the school years (Galler *et al.,* 1996).

About a third of children exposed to political violence and trauma have subsequent severe psychological problems. Many children seem to maintain resilience in the face of political violence. It is possible that this relates to habituation, intrinsic temperament, developmental stage when violence occurred, or quality and quantity of family support. However, good studies on long-term outcomes for children exposed to violence do not yet exist (Cairns & Dawes, 1996)

Much research has been done on coping ability. Children who cope well in adversity have been termed "stress resistant" or "resilient" (Garmezy, 1987; Rutter, 1985). Rutter noted that exposure to multiple stressors decreases a child'd ability to cope successfully. Garmezy identified protective factors as personality disposition of the child, a supportive milieu, and an external support system in the community. Werner (1989) also noted that the ability to find emotional support in the community is an important characteristic of children who cope well. It is important to note that refugee children may have parents but that the parents may not be very available because of their own anxiety, grief, and insecurity. The strength of the community is very important for such children, and reestablishment of community in the new country may be problematic. Refugees may themselves be wary about establishing bonds in the community. Refugees tend to reinstitute preexisting ethnic, religious, and political divisions from the society of origin in their groupings in the new country. Racism may be a problem in the new community. Refugee families sometimes move several times within the first years in the United States and this further reduces the liklihood of establishing meaningful community bonds.

Developmental issues separate the refugee child from the refugee adult. Developmental changes may make children more vulnerable in some areas but more adjustable and flexible in others. They have the advantage over their parents in that they ensocialize and acculturate into American society in a way that their parents cannot. Sometimes a role reversal occurs due to more rapid acculturation among refugee children who then assume adult-type roles (e.g., translating for the parent, answering the phone). Parents may have problems adapting to American adolescent culture. Many refugee families may not be headed by a father. This was true for 23% of 37,844 Vietnamese households in the United States in 1976 (Kelly, 1977). Conflicts developed when adolescent sons believed they should dominate their solo-parent mothers.

A study of Cambodian refugee children took place after teachers in Portland, Oregon, observed that Cambodian students demonstrated sudden fear reactions. Psychiatric interviews were then conducted with 46 of the 52 Cambodian students (Kinzie *et al.,* 1986;

Sack, Clarke, & Seeley, 1996). Six children had left Cambodia before Pol Pot and had no major traumas or symptoms. The remaining children had major trauma, including forced labor starvation and loss of family members. Seven saw their own family members killed. Half suffered PTSD by *DSM-III* (American Psychiatric Association, 1980) standards, and 53% had depressive disorders, most of them mild. There was no relationship between the symptoms and age, sex, or type of trauma. There was no evidence of social impairment in school or of antisocial behavior. Authors concluded that school provided a critical culture element in supporting these students during their adjustment to a new country. A follow-up of 27 of the 40 original subjects (Sack *et al.,* 1996) found that 13 had PTSD and 11 had more severe depressive disorders; 15 were still in school and 15 were supporting themselves. Again, no antisocial behavior was reported. The patients' suffering was subjective and private. It is likely that their symptoms will continue indefinitely.

Westermeyer (1991) has noted that refugee children are at increased risk for developing mental health problems include those without their families, children with brain damage from trauma or malnutrition, those in partial families, and those whose parents are psychiatrically or socially disabled (Westermeyer, 1991). Other areas of psychopathology among refugee children include identity conflicts, learning disabilities, mental retardation, major depressions, mania, eating disorders (usually obesity), conduct disorders, posttraumatic stress disorder (PTSD), substance abuse, and parental somatization of refugee children. With respect to the last diagnosis, refugee parents may displace their own anxiety onto normal children. Psychiatric assessment of the parent is indicated in this situation.

The resilience program for children developed by Grotberg (1995) and tested in many countries involves strategies for parents and children to facilitate coping. It is a practical program that may help refugee children while in refugee camps and after resettlement.

Health Problems of Child Refugees

The health problems of child refugees are biologic, psychological, and psychophysiological. Unfortunately, even in the best of refugee management circumstances, children are ill served. While in a refugee setting, a child may receive sufficient food, water, and housing but psychological issues related to the stress of being a child refugee are seldom addressed. Although the manner in which a child reacts acutely or over the long term depends on inherent temperament, available family support, and prior experiences, it is unlikely that any refugee child will escape fear, anxiety, or depression altogether.

In a refugee setting, children are especially vulnerable because of their small size, frequent malnutrition, lack of immunity to new infectious disease agents, and poor health care. Lack of sanitation, crowding, and stress contribute to frequent infectious illnesses among children. Sexual abuse occurs often in refugee camp settings and affects both girls and boys. If parents are present, they are likely to be depressed or preoccupied with problems of daily survival and not as comforting as they might be to their children in normal circumstances. Many refugee children have observed terrible events such as murders of family members, friends, or neighbors. They have lost their familiar and treasured homes, often abruptly. Preschoolers cannot comprehend the disruption, chaos, and agony of their elders.

All of the terrible refugee events are compounded by cross-cultural and language differences when these children arrive in the United States. They may have moved multiple times as refugees and they are likely to move several times after first arrival in the United States. The perception of instability and unpredictability of life continues. They lack language skills to explain their past experiences to relatives or sponsors; in any event, the new friends may themselves be disinterested or unable to relate to the past experiences of refugees.

Evaluation of a Refugee Child

Ideally, a medical evaluation should occur soon after the arrival of the child in the United States. While specific components of laboratory examinations may be eliminated, depending on the location of the refugee camp, all evaluations should assess development, behavior, and learning. Evaluation of learning may not be possible until the child has acquired English language skills but should not be forgotten. Special efforts should be made to help the child feel comfortable during the examination. The examiner should provide toys, allow the parent or a trusted adult to hold the child, and take time for an interpreter to explain each part of the examination to the child.

History

The initial evaluation should include a careful history, including the following:

1. Reason for refugee status, location of original family home, location of refugee camps, duration as a refugee, and stressors as a refugee. Describe a typical day as a refugee child.
2. Family status including list of those who perished in the disaster leading to movement of refugees, current family members available to the child, and health of remaining family members.
3. Nutrition prior to becoming a refugee and while in the refugee camp environment. What type of food was provided to the refugee child? How many meals per day?
4. Illnesses experienced in the refugee camp, history of any epidemics experienced by many in the refugee camp, and type of medical care received.
5. Immunization history.
6. Education history if relevant.
7. Birth history, early child development history, significant illnesses prior to becoming a refugee, family medical history.
8. History of recurrent fevers, worms, loose stools, jaundice, skin rashes,

seizures, wheezing, loss of hearing, visual problems, weight loss.

9. History of sleep problems, eating problems, fears, angry behavior, or other behavior problems that might reflect the refugee experience.

10. What medications is the child currently receiving? What indigenous herbs or medications have been given to the child recently?

Physical Examination

The examination should be thorough with sensitivity to the child's culture and perceptions. For example, if the child is from a Southeast Asian culture, it is not appropriate to touch the child on the head without requesting permission. Permission must also be requested before examining the ears with an otoscope. Special attention should be paid to height, weight, head circumference, and stigmata reflecting malnutrition or child abuse. A careful neuromotor assessment is important, especially for infants and toddlers. If the child is coming from an area endemic for malaria or hepatitis, it is important to palpate the liver and spleen. Skin must also be examined closely to rule out scabies and other parasites as well as to note evidence of indigenous treatment such as coining or cupping.

Laboratory Examinations

Depending on the history and part of world from which the child came, it is appropriate to request hepatitis B screening, HIV screening, VDRL or RPR, liver function tests, hemoglobin/hematocrit, sedimentation rate, urinalysis, stool for ova and parasites, blood lead level, and skin testing for tuberculosis.

Many of these children may not have had immunizations such as rubella, mumps, hemophilus influenza, or hepatitis B. It is important to review immunization history and develop a plan to immunize the child according to U.S. standards. If no immunization history exists, the physician must embark on an accelerated immunization strategy after taking care to be certain the family understands and accepts the plan.

Treatment, Prevention, and Follow-up

It is clearly important to treat existing infectious diseases and to provide family members and sponsors information about how they can avoid contracting the diseases (Franks et al., 1989). Immunizations should be brought up to date. Information should be given about appropriate diet.

Much more difficult is the treatment and follow-up with respect to psychological and developmental issues. Ideally, the refugee child should have access to a child health professional with expertise in these issues as soon as possible after arrival in the United States. If the professional is uncertain about culturally appropriate approaches, it is essential that he or she request this information from someone who is from the same culture and who has lived in the United States for some time.

The Committee on Community Health Services of the American Academy of Pediatrics ([AAP], 1997) recently published a statement to inform practitioners about the special health care needs and vulnerabilities of immigrant children and their families. This article reviews the risk factors of access to health care services, infectious diseases, psychosocial issues, dental disease, and nutritional problems. The committee recommends that pediatricians should oppose denying needed services to any child who resides within the borders of the United States, and that child health providers should educate themselves about the special cultural and medical issues of immigrant children. They should tolerate and respect differences in attitudes and approaches to child rearing and also support the extended immigrant family in health care activities. The committee also recommended that chapters of the American Academy of Pediatrics should define the health care needs of immigrant children in their areas and work with state legislatures and agencies to assure unimpeded access to all medically necessary services for all children.

Special Issues of Internationally Adopted Children

Many internationally adopted children have been refugees in a formal sense, or their past experiences have been analogous to those of refugee children. They have suffered the worst kind of loss, the loss of their parents, and they have often been moved from place to place over relatively long periods of time. The concept of adoption is not one that is known or acceptable in many countries such as Japan, Laos, Uganda, and Pakistan. In these and other countries children without parents may be raised by relatives without formal adoptions or they are often institutionalized. The disruption of early, vital attachment relationships between children and their caretakers is one of the major hidden tragedies of war. With the lack of attachment and lack of cultural stability and restraints, these children are likely to manifest antisocial behavior as adolescents and adults.

Thus, internationally adopted children may be regarded as at risk for all the physical and mental problems of refugee children. In addition, if they are beyond a year of age when adopted, they are likely to have serious problems of attachment. This has been a particular problem for children adopted from Eastern Europe over the past decade (Keck & Kupecky, 1995). Attachment problems are complicated by concurrent cognitive problems that may exist often in those orphans who have been born to alcohol abusing mothers or who experienced early malnutrition.

Such children are often indiscriminately friendly. They do not develop a true preference for their parents. As a result they do not perceive the parents as in charge. Because they may not have experienced loving caretakers who responded quickly to their early needs, they do not trust people, are often too independent, do not recognize risks, and do not develop qualities of empathy and love. Unfortunately, this may often occur in spite of their being placed in responsive, loving families. Such children are often manipulative because that has become a useful survival skill. The adoptive parents may suffer a great deal emotionally, feeling responsible, guilty, and angry. Experienced therapists may facilitate improved bonding, but many of these children do not truly bond and behave in sociopathic ways as they become older. In recent years adoptive parents in the United States formed a Parent Network for Post Institutionalized Children. This group provides resources for families whose adopted children are having attachment difficulties (Address: P.O. Box 613, Meadowlands, PA 15347).

A study of 643 Vietnamese refugee children (Sokoloff, Carlin, & Pham, 1984) found that 72% were adopted and 20% were foster children. Both adoptive and foster parents often said that the first year after placement "drained them emotionally" due to the excessive physical and emotional needs of the children. The children had many adjustment problems. Williams and Westermeyer (1993) reported family problems in four of six unaccompanied refugee adolescents. The strife engendered by the disturbed adolescents reached such an extent in two of the families that the parents eventually divorced. Older refugee children may feel rejected by both their original culture and the resettlement culture and fail to identify with or accept either society. The perception of alienation leads to antisocial behaviors.

There are five clinics in the United States that specialize in internationally adopted children. They are able to provide guidance and resources with respect to both the physical and psychological needs of these children. They are in the Department of Pediatrics, University of Minnesota, Minneapolis, MN, phone 612-626-6777; Department of Pediatrics, Tufts University, Boston, phone 617-636-5071; and in Rainbow Babies and Children's Hospital, Cleveland, Ohio, phone 216-844-3230.

Health Problems of Adult Refugees

General Issues

The health problems of adults include both physical and mental problems. Women are likely to have more problems than men related to discrimination against females in refugee camps. In general, the problems require multidisciplinary interventions from physicians, nurses, social workers, interpreters, and community leaders working together. Health care providers must consider cross-cultural issues such as whether a male physician can examine an adult female refugee. Regarding decisions about medical procedures, it is sometimes difficult to identify the family member who has the authority to make the decision. It may be necessary to involve a grandfather or a grandmother to approve a decision for an adult refugee. There were many problems related to medical procedures when Hmong refugees first arrived in the United States, because health care providers did not understand who were decision makers in the Hmong system.

Health care providers should consider the possibility of the following health problems of adult refugees:

- Posttraumatic stress syndrome
- Depression
- Sexually transmitted diseases, including HIV
- Parasitic diseases
- Infectious diseases such as melioidosis, brucellosis, rickettsial infections, leishmaniasis, and typhoid
- Nutritional deficiencies including iron deficiency, vitamin deficiencies, and micronutrient deficiencies
- Dental problems
- Tuberculosis
- Use of indigenous herbs and drugs that the family may have brought from overseas
- Genetic diseases peculiar to the ethnic group

Adult refugees who are parents have skills in child rearing that are relevant in the society of origin. Most can benefit from education and training in child nutrition, growth and development, management of behavior problems, immunizations, accident hazards, and social resources for parents. For example, Minnesota Early Learning Design (MELD), an agency that provides long-term support groups for parents, included special support groups for Hmong parents. Sometimes the refugee parenting skills may be better than those of parents in the resettlement country. A study comparing Hmong parents and American parents of comparable socioeconomic level in Minnesota found that Hmong children had significantly fewer accidents than the children born in the United States. However, a major problem for Hmong children was obesity, especially in boys. Parents overfed them in the new society.

Refugee parents often perceive themselves losing control as their children outpace them in acquisition of the English language and in cultural adaptation. A Russian father brought his son in for counseling because the 7-year-old boy made fun of his father's poor English. The father, an engineer in Russia, was sad and frustrated. These problems are all too common, and they increase as the children move into adolescence. Most refugee parents can benefit by group sessions for parents like themselves who are immigrants with adolescent children.

Informed Consent and Refugee Patients

Unfortunately, there are examples of researchers taking advantage of refugee patients in research endeavors without adequate consent. This has happened both overseas and in the United States. This also happens with respect to consent for treatment. Consent issues are complicated by the fact that belief systems in some cultures do not hold that the patient should be informed truthfully about diagnosis and prognosis, and that family decision making is preferable to individual decision making.

American informed consent requirements are the most rigid in the world. Full information must be presented to the person about the benefits, adverse effects, and risks of either treatment or a research protocol. The person must be legally competent and understand the information, and then make a voluntary choice free from outside influence or coercion. Each of these elements may pose a problem for refugee patients from different cultures.

Gostin (1995) has recommended that physicians seek an independent ethical review when the patient has different cultural expectations of the therapeutic relationship. Those involved in the review should have experience and understanding of the patient's culture, customs, and language. There can be deviation from usual formal standards of informed consent if the change focuses on patient-centered values. At all times genuine respect for human dignity, including different culture and values, must prevail.

Cross-Cultural Issues

Appraising a patient or parent's cultural beliefs, values, and customs should be an essential part of a health assessment regardless of whether the patient is a refugee (Olness, 1997). Cultural assessments are helpful in understanding patient behaviors that could otherwise be interpreted as negative or noncompliant. Cultural norms are usually unwritten but, nonetheless, are understood as the rules and values by which a culture functions. People are expected to abide by these unwritten rules or norms. When they violate them, they may be criticized or ostracized by others within the culture. Cultural norms include unwritten definitions about what is health and what is sickness.

Americans, although criticized for their lack of awareness about world events, actually are more experienced in relating to multiple cultures than most people in most countries. Because of the hundreds of different cultures and ethnic groups represented in the United States, television, the mobility of the citizens, and universal education, it is rare to find an American who does not know someone of a different racial or ethnic background. American children do not run after strangers of a different skin color yelling "foreigner," as they do in countries such as Laos or Uganda. American health care providers represent a wide spectrum of racial and ethnic backgrounds, but, of course, no individual provider can be knowledgeable about the cultural backgrounds of all patients.

In doing a cultural assessment it is important to consider the following:

1. Are there specific genetic diseases associated with the refugee's racial or ethnic group?
2. What is the refugee patient's interpretation of his or her symptoms?
3. What alternative treatment might he or she already have received?
4. What are the meanings of body language such as head nods? Am I insulting the patient by some of my body language? (e.g., pointing the sole of my foot toward the patient)
5. What are the dietary practices of the patient?
6. Who in the family or tribal constellation makes the decisions about whether or not to accept treatment?
7. Is the interpreter relating well to the patient?

Prevention of Health Problems for Immigrants: Recommendations for Refugee Camps

Those who are decision makers in refugee settings outside the United States are often and understandably preoccupied with issues of water, housing, food, and security. However, recognizing that many refugees will eventually be relocated to new countries and cultures, there is much that can be done to prepare refugees, ensure better health, and reduce problems for the refugees as they become immigrants. Special attention to the most vulnerable (i.e., pregnant or nursing mothers, children, and the elderly) is crucial.

Once the acute settlement needs are over (usually a matter of a few weeks) those in charge of refugee settings should focus on the following:

1. Conducting anthropometric assessments of children under 5 years of age.
2. If malnutrition is found, urgent refeeding programs should be implemented. Also, efforts should be made to define the causes of malnutrition, that is, diversion of available food, improper preparation of food, improper weaning practices, high incidence of infectious diseases, or a combination of factors. Programs should then be implemented to prevent further malnutrition.
3. Facilitation of breast feeding for mothers.
4. Establishment of reproductive health care for women. This is something that occurs rarely in refugee settings (Wulf, 1994).
5. Immunization programs for adults and children.
6. Provision of consistent surrogate mothers to unaccompanied minors.
7. Organized school and recreation programs for children.
8. Literacy programs for refugees who cannot read and write.
9. Surveillance programs not only for infectious diseases and malnutrition but also for child abuse, including sexual abuse of young males and females.
10. Orientation programs for refugees related to new languages, cultures, and occupations.
11. Vocational training programs.

These interventions can do much to reduce physical and psychological problems for new immigrants. Often, there are many well-educated refugees who can work to implement programs such as school, recreation, literacy, and orientation programs.

Training of Refugee Camp Workers

Because of the increasing number of complex humanitarian emergencies in the world, there is now a major effort to develop excellent training for persons who are employed by humanitarian agencies and for the thousands who volunteer to help in refugee situations (Burkle, 1995; Olness, in press). The training is helpful not only for work overseas but also for work in domestic disasters and for work with refugees who are relocated to the United States. In recent years, several training programs have become available in the United States. They include the following:

1. Center for Excellence in Disaster Management and Humanitarian Assistance, University of Hawaii. This center sponsors a 3-week intensive course on Disaster Management in April each year. The director of the course is Frederick Burkle, Jr., M.D., phone 808-973-8387, fax 808-949-4232.
2. HELP program sponsored by the School of Hygiene and Public Health of Johns Hopkins University. This is a 3-week course held in Baltimore each July. The director is Dr. Gilbert Burnham.
3. Management of Complex Humanitarian Emergencies; focus is on children and families. This 1-week course is sponsored by Rainbow Babies and Children's Hospital in Cleveland, Ohio and endorsed by the American Academy of Pediatrics and the International Pediatric Association. The director is Karen Olness, M.D., phone 216-844-3122, fax 216-844-7601, e-mail kno@po.cwru.edu.
4. Interaction program. Interaction, a consortium of 120 nongovernment humanitarian agencies, has received a grant from USAID to develop a de-

tailed curriculum in Management of Complex Humanitarian Emergencies. This course will be a 12-day course, given over 2 weeks and was piloted in 1997. Phone 202-667-8227, fax 202-667-8236.

Recommendations for U.S. Sponsors of Immigrants

These recommendations are based on the author's personal experience with refugees, as well as conclusions from the follow-up study, and recommendations from the American Academy of Pediatrics' Committee on Community Health Services.

Sponsors also benefit from orientation programs. Their misconceptions are often similar to those of the new arrivals. They may be unprepared for cross-cultural differences and unrealistic expectations among the immigrants. They fail to recognize the inherent inner strength and resolve that is part of many new immigrants (Torjesen *et al.*, 1981). They also may not appreciate the long-term effects of cruelty and abuse suffered by refugees and the malnutrition experienced by many of the small child refugees. Sponsors sometimes do too much for immigrants initially and not enough later on in terms of social support.

There are many reports of problems between sponsors and new immigrants. In Buddhist cultures, for example, after an individual has provided assistance such as money or house appliances, it is assumed that he or she has made a commitment to provide in similar fashion forever. The Southeast Asian refugee would consider it appropriate to demand a new house, car, and so on as his or her due. Recently arrived Hmong in Minnesota were told by their sponsor that he was not wealthy and they would need to work together to provide necessities of life. Imagine the surprise of the sponsor to return home to find the proud refugees presenting him with a bag of live squirrels they had captured. They said that this would provide the family meat for the next week! A frequent problem among refugees who are well educated is that they cannot immediately gain employment in their area of expertise and must take more menial tasks, a concept not acceptable to educated people from many Asian or African cultures. This may lead to depression in the new immigrant. Sponsors can do much to guide the new immigrants into an understanding that they do well to gain job experience and a job record in menial work. Two Vietnamese physicians who arrived in Minnesota at the same time demonstrated opposite approaches to this issue. One immediately accepted employment in a nursing home, and used the opportunity to practice his English with the elderly who were only too happy to help him. He also studied for examinations given to foreign medical graduates. He passed the language examinations easily in a year, passed the medical examinations, and obtained an internship within 2 years. His colleague refused to take menial work and 3 years later had still not passed the language examinations.

Sponsors (foster or adoptive parents) of unaccompanied minors may be unprepared for the problems of attachment that are usual. Children may seem initially charming, pleasant, and courteous to anyone but fail to develop a true parent–child relationship with the sponsor or adoptive parent. Such children may also manifest behaviors reflecting their earlier deprivation such as binge eating, hoarding food, and demanding many clothes and toys.

If possible, prospective sponsors should do the following:

1. Learn as much as possible about the culture and language from which the immigrants have come.
2. If unaccompanied minors are involved, meet with persons who have long experience in working with such children and anticipate that therapy will be required by the children.
3. Whenever an immigrant family is involved, share the sponsorship with a small group, for example, several members of the same church or service club.

4. Make arrangements for training in language for adults prior to arrival.
5. Make medical appointments for all members of a new family as soon as possible.
6. Facilitate meals that are familiar to the new family.
7. Find families of the same ethnic group who have been in the community for some time and who are willing to help with orientation.
8. Get children into school as soon as possible. If the school does not have ESL classes, arrange for ESL training for the children.
9. Facilitate self-sufficiency for the family in every way possible.
10. Support new immigrants in taking jobs that may be more menial than their previous profession and explain that this is the American way.

These interventions will increase the likelihood of good mental and physical health among the new immigrants and, therefore, the likelihood that they will be productive citizens.

Summary

Immigrants who arrive as refugees have many more problems than those who arrive directly from their countries of origin. Most refugees have suffered physical and mental traumatization. These experiences may lead to lifelong problems and affect adjustment to life in the United States. Refugees have often spent substantial time living in squalor and are at great risk for health problems, including many infectious diseases and malnutrition. Refugee children have often witnessed atrocities and may arrive as orphans or unaccompanied minors. This may lead to attachment problems in their new families and to PTSD symptoms. On the other hand, many refugees are people of enormous inner strength. The same energy that facilitated their escapes leads them to overcome the trauma and to adjust very well in their new country. American sponsors and health care professionals benefit by orientation to the cultural issues of refugees from specific areas. They then become key figures in facilitating a healthy adjustment for the refugee immigrants.

References

Ahearn, F. L., & Athey, J. L. (1991). *Refugee children: Theory, research, and services.* Baltimore: Johns Hopkins University Press.

American Psychiatric Association. (1980). *Diagnostic and statistical manual of mental disorders* (3rd ed.). Washington, DC: Author.

Burkle, F. M. (1995). Complex humanitarian emergencies: Concept and participants. *Prehospital and Disaster Medicine, 10,* 43–47.

Cairns, E., & Dawes, A. (1996). Children: Ethnic and political violence—A commentary. *Child Development, 67,* 129–139.

Committee on Community Health Services, American Academy of Pediatrics. (1997). Health care for children of immigrant families. *Pediatrics, 100,* 153–156.

Franks, A. L., Berg, C. J., Kane, M. A., Browne, B. B., Sikes, K., Elsea, W. R., & Burton, A. H. (1989). Hepatitis B infection among children born in the United States to Southeast Asian refugees. *New England Journal of Medicine, 321,* 1310–1315.

Galler, J. R., Shumsky, J. S., & Morgane, P. J. (1996). Malnutrition and brain development. In W. A. Walker & J. B. Watkins (Eds.), *Nutrition in pediatrics: Basic science and clinical application* (2nd ed., pp. 194–210). Neuilly-sur-Seine, France: Decker Europe.

Gany, F., & DeBocanegra, H. T. (1996). Overcoming barriers to improving the health of immigrant women. *Journal of the American Women's Medical Association, 5,* 155–160.

Garmezy, N. (1987). Stress, competence, and development: Continuities in the study of schizophrenic adults, children vulnerable to psychopathology, and the search for stress-resistant children. *American Journal of Orthopsychiatry, 57,* 159–174.

Gostin, L. O. (1995). Informed consent, cultural sensitivity and respect for persons. *Journal of the American Medical Association, 274,* 844–845.

Grotberg, E. (1995). *A guide to promoting resilience in children: Strengthening the human spirit.* The Hague, Netherlands: BernardVan lees Foundation.

International Federation of Red Cross and Red Crescent Societies. (1996). *World disasters report.* New York: Oxford University Press.

Keck, G., & Kupecky, R. (1995). *Adopting the hurt child: Hope for families with special needs kids: A guide for parents and professionals.* Colorado Springs, CO: Pinon.

Kelly, G. P. (1977). *From Vietnam to America.* Boulder, CO: Westview.

Kinzie, D., Sack, H. W., Angell, H. R., Manson, S., & Roth, B. (1986). The psychiatric effects of massive trauma on Cambodian children. *Journal of the American Academy of Child and Adolescent Psychiatry, 25,* 370–376.

Kleber, R. J., Figley, C. R., & Gersons, B. P. R. (1995). *Beyond Trauma: Cultural and societal dynamics.* New York: Plenum.

Krell, R. (1988). Survivors of childhood experiences in Japanese concentration camps. *Americal Journal of Psychiatry, 145,* 383–384.

McCloskey, L. L., & Southwick, K. (1996). Psychosocial problems in refugee children exposed to war. *Pediatrics, 97,* 394–397.

Miller, K. E. (1996). The effects of state terrorism and exile on indigenous Guatemalan refugee children: A mental health assessment and an analysis of children's narratives. *Child Development, 67,* 89–106.

Mollica, R. F., & Lavelle, J. P. (1988). Southeast Asian refugees. In L. Comas-Diaz & E. E. H. Griffith, *Clinical guidelines in cross-cultural mental health* (pp. 262–302). New York: Wiley.

Olness, K. (1997). Cross cultural issues in primary pediatric care. In *Primary pediatric care* (3rd ed., pp. 128–135). New York: C. V. Mosby.

Olness, K. (in press). Complex humanitarian emergencies and children: Training programs for those who help. *International Child Health.*

Riley, C., & Smith, D. (1990). The prevalence of post traumatic stress disorder and its clinical significance among Southeast Asian refugees. *American Journal of Psychiatry, 147,* 913–917.

Rousseau, C., Drapeau, A., & Corin, E. (1996). School performance and emotional problems in refugee children. *American Journal of Orthopsychiatry, 66,* 239–251.

Rutter, M. (1985). Resilience in the face of adversity: Protective factors and resistance to psychiatric disorder. *British Journal of Psychiatry, 147,* 598–611.

Sack, W. H., Clarke, G. N., & Seeley, J. (1996). Multiple forms of stress in Cambodian adolescent refugees. *Child Development, 67,* 107–116.

Sokdoff, B., Carlin, J., & Pham, H., (1984). Five-year follow-up of Vietnamese refugee children in the United States. *Clinical Pediatrics, 23,* 565–570.

Toole, M. J., & Waldman, R. J. (1988). An analysis of mortality trends among refugee populations in Somalia, Sudan, and Thailand. *Bulletin of the World Health Organization, 66,* 237–247.

Torjesen, H., Olness, K., & Torjesen, E. (1981). *The gift of the refugees.* Eden Praire, MN: Garden.

United Nations High Commission for Refugees. (1993). *The state of the world's refugees: The challenge of protection.* New York: Penguin.

Van der Veer, G. (1995). Psychotherapeutic work with refugees. In R. J. Kleber, C. R. Figley & B. P. R. Gersons (Eds), *Beyond trauma* (pp. 151–170). New York: Plenum.

Werner, E. E. (1989). High risk children in young adulthood: A longitudinal study from birth to 32 years. *American Journal of Orthopsychiatry, 59,* 72–81.

Westermeyer, J. (1993). Psychiatric services for refugee children: An overview. In F. L. Ahearn & J. L. Athey (Eds) *Refugee children* (pp. 127–162). Baltimore: Johns Hopkins University Press.

Williams, C., & Westermeyer, J. (1993). Psychiatric problems among adolescent Southeast Asian refugees: A descriptive study. *Journal of Nervous and Mental Disease, 171,* 79–85.

Wulf, D. (1994). *Refugee women and reproductive health care: Reassessing priorities.* New York: Women's Commission for Refugee Women and Children.

13

Border Health

LINDA S. LLOYD

Introduction to the United States–Mexico Border

It is frequently said that viruses, pollution, and natural disasters do not recognize international borders. This chapter examines the critical health issues only along the United States–Mexico border. Although there is a limited body of research on border health issues, and much still needs to be done, innovative programs addressing some of the issues facing U.S. and Mexican border communities have been implemented.

The United States–Mexico border region was defined in the 1983 Border Environmental Agreement (El Paso Community Foundation, 1996) as the area within 62 miles (or 100 kilometers) on either side of the almost 2,000-mile-long border between the United States and Mexico. There are an estimated 10 million people living in this area, with most of the population living in or around the 14 pairs of sister cities along the border. Four of the five poorest cities with a population greater than 100,000 in the United States are found along the Texas–Mexico border, with an estimated one out of every three residents living below the federal poverty level (Albrecht, 1993b; Skolnick, 1995). El Paso is the nation's 22nd largest city and has the

fourth lowest per capita income in the United States.

According to the Border Research Institute at New Mexico State University, Hispanics account for 41% of the population in the border area (El Paso Community Foundation, 1996). While the number of newcomers to the area continues to grow rapidly, many of the Hispanic residents have family ties to the area which predate the U.S.–Mexico war of the mid 1800s. In El Paso, 69% of the population is Hispanic (Skolnick, 1995).

An estimated 614 million people crossed between the United States and Mexico in 1994 (El Paso Community Foundation, 1996). The San Diego–Tijuana border crossing is the busiest in the world; an estimated 71.1 million individuals crossed the border in 1995 (San Diego Association of Governments [SANDAG], 1996b). In San Diego County, an average of 67,000 vehicles cross the border every day, with 40,000 alone crossing into San Diego at the San Ysidro crossing point (SANDAG, 1996a). In El Paso, there are approximately 40 million border crossings annually (Skolnick, 1995), with an estimated 52.4 million in 1995.

Rapid population growth has made it difficult for either the U.S. or Mexican government to provide an adequate infrastructure of services such as potable water, sewage disposal, or health care, creating large urbanized areas on both sides of the border with substandard living conditions. In addition, the growth of the *maquiladora* industry and the

LINDA S. LLOYD • Alliance Healthcare Foundation, San Diego, California 92123.

Handbook of Immigrant Health, edited by Loue. Plenum Press, New York, 1998.

North American Free Trade Agreement (NAFTA) have brought increased attention to the border, and the border region is now one of the fastest growing areas in North America. Espinosa-Torres, Hernández-Avila, and López-Carillo (1994) reported that between 1984 and 1994 the population in the border region grew by 60%. *Maquiladoras* or "twin plants" are assembly plants set up in Mexico by foreign companies. All materials are imported into Mexico and assembled at the plants, with the products then being exported to foreign markets. Almost 40% of the plants assemble electronic equipment, materials, and supplies. There are a total of 2,206 *maquiladora* plants in Mexico, with almost 70% located in the border region and close to half a million border residents employed by them (El Paso Community Foundation, 1996; Guendelman & Jasis-Silberg, 1993).

Most of the research published to date has focused on issues such as environmental health, occupational health, communicable disease control, and the utilization of health care services. This chapter examines each of those areas.

Environmental Health

Environmental health is a critical issue for the border region given its rapid industrial growth, uncontrolled housing developments along both sides of the border, and traditional agricultural base. Mexico and the United States share ecosystems, sources of water (rivers and subterranean aquifers), and air; whatever happens on one side of the border has a direct impact on the opposite side of the border.

Housing

The presence of *colonias*—formal, organized neighborhoods characterized by substandard housing, inadequate sewage disposal, and limited to no access to potable water—is seen throughout the Mexican border region. However, Texas and New Mexico are the only states in which *colonias* are encountered in their border areas; neither Arizona nor California have such developments. In the latter two states, small illegal, informal encampments on private property are found. In the United States, the *colonias* are located in unincorporated areas, where state zoning regulations do not apply. It has therefore been difficult to enforce building codes and the provision of adequate sewage and clean water services. Along the U.S. side of the border, houses may be built of wood and brick while others are constructed from cardboard (Albrecht, 1993b). Some families dig shallow wells near the house, but the water is not fit for human consumption due to contamination from the Rio Grande and surface contamination from inadequate human and animal waste disposal (Albrecht, 1993b; Hatcher *et al.,* 1995).

It is estimated that there are at least 11,000 homeless, migrant workers in north San Diego County alone (Regional Taskforce on the Homeless, 1994). These workers are principally employed in the agricultural and construction businesses. Although called "migrant," the majority live and work in north San Diego County; in fact, many have lived in the area for years. These workers live in illegal encampments generally found in proximity to work sites but not on the farmer's or builder's property site; many are hidden in canyons to minimize complaints. Shelters at the encampments reflect the length of time the camp has been in existence, and range from holes dug into the ground and covered by brush to small shacks constructed from scrap cardboard, wood, and plastic sheeting (Chávez, 1992). Sanitation consists of open-air defecation and dumping of trash into nearby bushes or gullies. Water is rarely from a safe source due to the camps' isolation (Muñoz & Adamo, 1994). The encampments are periodically bulldozed by county authorities when they grow too large or following complaints by property owners and neighbors.

Water Pollution

Pollution of water sources creates health hazards such as the transmission of viral, bacterial, and protozoal pathogens, skin diseases, birth defects, and cancers. These health problems may result from drinking contaminated water, eating fish caught in contaminated rivers, and using contaminated water for bathing and playing. In the early 1990s, health care workers and researchers in the Brownsville–Matamoros area documented a sharp increase in birth defects in the area, with anencephaly rates being particularly high (Kelly, 1992). Rates for anencephaly in Brownsville are three times the national average, and in an 18-month period researchers in Matamoros documented at least 42 cases. While the causes of many cases of neural tube defects (anencephaly and spina bifida) are not known, evidence suggests that environmental and occupational exposures to organic solvents, chemicals used in agriculture, and heavy metals may have a possible role (Sever, 1995). While the toxicity of arsenic to humans has been recognized for hundreds of years, its role as a human carcinogen associated with lung and skin cancers has been recognized only fairly recently (Axelson, 1980; Leonard & Lauwerys, 1980; Shalat, Walker, & Finnell, 1996). More recent studies suggest that arsenic be treated as a probable human reproductive toxin, and identify a possible role in spontaneous abortion, cardiovascular defects, and neural tube defects (Shalat *et al.*, 1996). Most exposure of the general population to arsenic (used in pesticides and a number of agricultural and industrial processes) occurs through the ingestion of foodstuffs, including contaminated water, containing both inorganic and organic arsenic (Leonard & Lauwerys, 1980).

The rivers that mark the border, the Rio Grande–Rio Bravo, New, and Tijuana rivers, are all heavily polluted with raw sewage, agricultural runoff contaminated with fertilizers and pesticides, and industrial waste. In a report to the U.S. Congress from the Council on Scientific Affairs of the American Medical Association, it was estimated that 206 million liters of raw sewage are dumped into the rivers each day (Council on Scientific Affairs, 1990). According to the El Paso

Community Foundation (1996), the New River, which crosses the border near Calexico, California, has been called the most polluted river in the United States; 15 human pathogens including the causative agents of hepatitis, polio, cholera, and typhoid fever have been isolated from its waters. A study in a small border community in Texas demonstrated that 35% of children were infected with hepatitis A by 8 years of age; by age 35 almost 90% of the population had been infected (Nickey, 1989). The Texas Department of Health closed a private water system serving the residents of a *colonia* because of high levels of arsenic. Cech and Essman (1992) cited data indicating that only 12% of 128 community water systems in border communities were in compliance with Texas Department of Health regulations, with as many as 34% failing water testing requirements.

Water quality studies have been supported over time by both the U.S. and Mexican governments. Results of a study conducted in the El Paso–Ciudad Juárez sister cities area indicate that both the Rio Grande and groundwater supplies were heavily contaminated with fecal coliforms; this was the result of direct discharge of wastewater into the Rio Grande and the placement of drinking water wells next to open canals carrying untreated domestic and industrial wastewater in Ciudad Juárez (Cech & Essman, 1992). Of 12 samples of well water, 11 (91%) were positive for fecal coliforms and 18 of 30 tap water samples (60%) were positive. Direct discharge of untreated wastewater in the river is due to the fact that Ciudad Juárez, a city of more than 800,000 inhabitants, does not have a wastewater treatment plant. Domestic and industrial wastewater is transported through the city in a large, 16-mile-long, open, unlined canal, known as the Aguas Negras canal, where it is then dumped onto agricultural fields for irrigation purposes or directly into the Rio Grande.

In Matamoros, Mexico, water in a canal behind a *maquiladora* plant contained xylene levels more than 50,000 times the U.S. standard for drinking water. Water from a canal behind a nearby *maquiladora* contained xylene at levels 6,000 times the standard (Kelly, 1992). Alkylbenzenes, including xylene, benzene, and toluene, are chemicals commonly used as solvents or as the starting materials in the chemical synthesis of other chemicals or drugs. Benzene has a demonstrated role in causing leukemias, in particular acute myelogenous leukemia (McMichael, 1988). Exposure to high concentrations of xylene can result in neurophysiological dysfunction and respiratory tract symptoms. Chronic exposure to xylene has been associated with anemia, leukopenia, chest pain, ECG abnormalities, and central nervous system symptoms (Langman, 1994). Many of the *maquiladora* plants use toxic solvents, acids, metal-plating solutions, and other hazardous chemicals. However, there are only two hazardous waste landfills in Mexico, neither one near the border region. Although a 1988 Mexican environmental law requires U.S.-owned *maquiladoras* to return toxic waste to the United States, few have done so and the law is rarely enforced. The clandestine dumping of drums filled with toxic waste has been observed in isolated areas of the Mexican desert (Kelly, 1992; Moure-Eraso, Wilcox, Punnett, Copeland, & Levenstein, 1994).

In San Diego County, water used for irrigation comes from the municipal water system. Other areas of Southern California use reclaimed, treated sewage for irrigation. In one of the first large-scale health surveillance studies conducted in migrant worker encampments in San Diego County (Swerdlow *et al.,* 1992), samples were taken from the 29 water sources identified for the 33 encampments with a water source. Nineteen of the 29 water sources (66%) were farm irrigation systems that camp residents tapped into through hoses or pipes; 9 sources were the municipal water system; and at one camp residents reported buying bottled water. No fecal coliforms were isolated from any of the water samples, although other coliforms were isolated in 11% of the samples from the irrigation systems. Total chlorine was measured as an indication of the potential for contamination of drinking water sources. Of the samples taken from irrigation systems, 38% did not contain total chlorine, while 17% of the samples taken from the municipal water supply were lacking total chlorine. At four camps, residents stated that there were times when water from a nearby river was used for drinking purposes; all three samples from the river were positive for coliforms, including fecal coliforms.

Air Pollution

Air quality in the major sister city areas has been a continuing problem. El Paso and San Diego, the two largest border cities on the U.S. side, routinely violate U.S. National Ambient Air Quality Standards (NAAQS) (El Paso Community Foundation, 1996; Espinosa-Torres *et al.,* 1994). In fact, El Paso complied with NAAQS for carbon monoxide for the first time in 1994, while continuing to violate the standards for ozone, carbon monoxide, and PM10 (particulate material less than 10 microns). San Diego violates NAAQS in ozone and carbon monoxide levels. Other border areas that do not meet air quality standards for PM10 are Imperial County, California, and four border counties in Arizona.

High blood lead levels in residents of El Paso and Ciudad Juárez have been attributed to a smelter on the El Paso side of the border. Petroleum emissions, burning tires, and open burning at dumps in Ciudad Juárez, and smelters and unpaved roads on both sides of the border have been implicated in elevated particle matter in the air. Both Ciudad Juárez and El Paso suffer from very poor air quality (Shields, 1991). Because of this, an innovative program to address air pollution has been developed between El Paso and Ciudad Juárez (Paso del Norte Air Quality Task Force, 1994; Ruth Riedel, Alliance Healthcare Foundation, San Diego, 1996, personal communication). This program included the business sector as an integral part of the planning process, and has had positive results in compliance with reduced emissions of contaminants into the air and a measurable improvement in air quality. The program is novel in that it took a binational approach to develop appropriate control strategies, and involved U.S. and Mexican businesses and governmental agencies in the program.

Each city identified its priority areas for air pollution reduction. For example, in Ciudad Juárez an innovative program to develop and implement environmentally sound methods for the manufacture of bricks has brought together researchers from Ciudad Juárez and El Paso, government agencies, and the owners of brickmaking facilities (Grigsby, 1996). This program promotes the use of low pressure gas as an alternative fuel, and redesigned brick ovens. In El Paso, reductions in vehicular emissions have been targeted by the program. El Paso requires that gasoline be oxygenated with ethanol during the winter months; this reduces carbon monoxide emissions by one third.

Ciudad Juárez and El Paso have developed binational programs for vehicle inspections and body and paint shops (Paso del Norte Air Quality Task Force, 1994). In Ciudad Juárez, inspections of the certified vehicle emissions testing centers were started to ensure that these centers are in compliance with federal and local standards. Many of the chemicals used in body and paint shops have high levels of volatile organic compounds, which contribute to ground level ozone. In Ciudad Juárez, where there are an estimated 300 body and paint shops, it is now required that painting booths be enclosed as a means to control emissions. In El Paso, shops are required to use paints that have lower contents of volatile organic compounds.

Higher carbon monoxide and ozone levels in the United States have been attributed to the use of older vehicles, the lack of emissions controls, and poor quality gasoline in Mexico. Espinosa-Torres and colleagues (1994) have attributed the atmospheric contamination in San Diego and Tijuana to both mobile (cars, cargo and passenger vehicles, and airplanes) and fixed (manufacturing plants and service industries) sources. Given the shared atmospheric conditions in the San Diego–Tijuana area, the diffusion and transport of contaminants negatively affects both sides of the border, regardless of the origin. In contrast, the primary source of contaminants in the Calexico, California–Mexicali area is dust; PM10 sample readings frequently exceed both the 24-hour and annual standards (El Paso Community Foundation, 1996). At least part of the dust problem is a result of the vast agricultural industry found in this area.

Furthermore, the role of water and air pollution is suspected in the high incidence of bone cancer and lupus in an Arizona border community. In Santa Cruz County, Arizona, the rate of multiple myeloma, a type of bone marrow cancer, was found to be 2.4 times higher in the county than the expected rate, and cases of lupus were almost twice as high ("Burning Border Health Issues," 1995a). Residents of Nogales, Santa Cruz County, believe that air pollution caused by burning in a landfill across the border and exposure to sewage and toxic chemicals released into a wash that runs through the city are the principal sources of their health problems. After a meeting to discuss the study results between health officials from Mexico and Arizona, the landfill was closed and a new one, where waste is not burned, was opened farther away.

Occupational Health

Occupational hazards for border region residents include exposure to hazardous chemicals (both industrial and agricultural), long working hours, extended exposure to the elements (e.g., farmworkers), repetitive tasks, and limited work breaks. There are few studies of occupational hazards that focus specifically on the border, and some researchers feel that insufficient attention has been given to studying specific working conditions in the *maquiladora* plants (Espinosa-Torres *et al.,* 1994; Guendelman & Jasis-Silberg, 1993). The results of the few health studies conducted in *maquiladora* plants are inconclusive because of limitations in the study design, problems with recruiting study participants, and reluctance of *maquiladora* management to provide access to workers (Guendelman & Jasis-Silberg, 1993). Research specifically on occupational conditions in the *maquiladoras* is needed given that these plants employ more than 500,000 people, are the fastest growing industry in the border area, have a very high proportion of female workers (approximately 60% of employees in *maquiladoras* are female, compared to 28% in the general workforce), and have a very high employee turnover rate (Guendelman & Jasis-Silberg, 1993; Moure-Eraso *et al.,* 1994). High employee turnover in the *maquiladoras* may be related to greater movement of employees from one job to another, high competition for jobs given the large numbers of migrants to the border cities, pregnancy in female employees, and ill or injured individuals unable to remain in their positions because of work requirements and long commutes to work (Guendelman & Jasis-Silberg, 1993). Reported occupational hazards in the plants include inadequate lighting and ventilation, high noise levels, lack of hygiene, lack of worker insurance, lack of adequate break times, prolonged periods spent on detailed tasks, and exposure to toxic substances (Espinosa-Torres *et al.,* 1994; Guendelman & Jasis-Silberg, 1993).

A study conducted in Tijuana, Mexico, by Guendelman and Jasis-Silberg (1993), compared women working in electronic and garment *maquiladoras*, women working in the service sector, and women who had never entered the labor force. Women in all four groups reported that they considered their health to be fairly good although all four groups had high stress scores. The authors used Cohen's Perceived Stress Scale to measure the sense of control an individual felt over her life. The high stress scores in all four groups indicate that most women had a low sense of control over their lives. The researchers found that although women working in the *maquiladoras* earned less money, worked longer hours, and had less decision-making power in their jobs than women employed in the service industry, they reported equivalent levels of job satisfaction. In addition, *maquiladora* workers did not suffer more functional impairments, depression, or nervousness than service workers. In fact, women in the electronics industry suffered from less nervousness and fewer functional impairments than women in service industries. The authors concluded that the women's positive feelings toward their jobs may be due to the fact that their employment provides them with options other than marriage and childbearing, and better employment possibilities. *Maquiladora* plants tend to be more attractive workplaces and provide more opportunities for social interaction than the poor *colonias* most of the workers live in. Additional research is needed to examine the chronic and potential effects of exposure to hazardous substances on reproduction.

Other authors reported more difficult work conditions, with women reporting sexual harassment, required pregnancy monitoring, pressure on pregnant women to quit, and the required use of company physicians so that occupational accidents or health problems will not be reported to government agencies ("Border Health Hazards," 1995b). Eskenazi and Guendelman (1993) also examined the birthweight of the most recent child of the women in the *maquiladora* study. While rates for fetal loss and time to conception were consistent across the groups studied, occupation was consistently found to be a better predictor for birthweight than parity, age, education, and smoking. Women who worked in either garment or electronic *maquiladoras* had lower birthweight babies than women working in the service sector. The researchers were unable to determine the reasons for lower birthweight of infants of *maquiladora* workers, but suggested that chemical exposures, ergonomic factors, workplace characteristics, and sociodemographic variables may play a role.

Occupational hazards for farmworkers have been documented as being related to exposure to chemicals used in agricultural activities, such as pesticides, fungicides, and fertilizers (Swerdlow *et al.,* 1992), and unsafe work conditions, such as lack of appropriate protective equipment for use while spraying fields and long work hours with few breaks. However, little has been published about the concerns of migrant farmworkers themselves. In a project at a unique shelter for homeless working men in north San Diego County, the residents identified topics for discussion at the weekly health sessions (Catholic Charities, 1995). Shelter staff then coordinated the session with an appropriate speaker and educational materials. In several instances, shelter residents prepared and presented information to new arrivals at the shelter. Examples of topics requested have been care and prevention of back injuries; first aid; alcoholism; sexually transmitted diseases; food preparation; care of upper respiratory infections; and disaster preparadeness, including earthquakes and floods. Given that the majority of the residents worked in agriculture or construction, topics related to occupational hazards were frequently requested, such as the prevention and care of lower back injuries and first aid. Men with work-related injuries were seen in the shelter; their injuries included eye problems, fractures from falls, and wounds that had not healed properly. In one instance, a paraplegic victim of a work-related accident was dropped off at the shelter after discharge from the hospital, although the shelter was not equipped to deal with problems associated with his care.

Communicable Diseases

Communicable disease control is of great concern to both sides of the border, given the large numbers of individuals who cross the border each day. Many of the diseases that affect the border populations are associated with poverty: overcrowding, substandard housing, and inadequate water and sanitation infrastructures. An additional challenge to disease control in the border region is the cross-border health care seeking behavior of individuals who are ill. This practice may lead to interrupted treatment schedules, a lack of communication between Mexican and American medical personnel due to language barriers, and differences in standards of diagnosis and practice (HIV/STD Subcommittee of the California/Baja California Binational Health Council, 1995; Warner & Reed, 1993). For communicable disease control to be effective in the border region, the health departments on each side of the border need to better articulate ways in which the two very different health systems can interact.

Suárez y Toriello and Chávez (1996), in their profile of the U.S.–Mexico border region, compared disease patterns of the border region with that seen in both the United States and Mexico as a whole. The infant mortality rate in Mexico is three times higher than that of the United States, and the rate for the north Mexican border states is two to three times higher than the rate seen in the neighboring U.S. states. Seventy-two percent of the deaths in the Mexican border region were due to four causes: problems arising during the perinatal period, pneumonia, congenital defects, and intestinal infections. While infant mortality due to infections represented 39% of all deaths in the Mexican border states, only 2.7% of all infant deaths in the U.S. border states were due to infections. When one examines causes of infant mortality within specific populations in the U.S. border states, patterns similar to those seen in Mexico emerge.

In Webb County, Texas, the combined incidence rate for hepatitis A and hepatitis of unspecified form was 103 per 100,000, as compared to 13 per 100,000 for the state of Texas (Council on Scientific Affairs, 1990); unspecified strains of hepatitis were reported at almost seven times the national rate (Jones, 1989). In a 1989 study conducted in a small border community in Texas, very high rates of hepatitis A were found, even though the majority of the population was born in the United States (54%) (Hatcher *et al.,* 1995; Nickey, 1989). Of the remaining study participants, 26% were born in Ciudad Juárez and 21% were born in other parts of Mexico or Latin America. Hatcher and colleagues reported that Texas, Arizona, and all of the Mexican border states reported higher rates of hepatitis A along their border areas. The authors attributed these high levels to the poor sanitary conditions that exist along the border.

Incidence rates for shigellosis and salmonellosis were 39 and 52 per 100,000, respectively, compared with state rates of 11 and 15 per 100,000 (Council on Scientific Affairs, 1990). The border rate for amebiasis is more than three times the national rate (Jones, 1989). Although much of the burden of gastrointestinal infections is due to lack of a clean and safe water supply, resolution of the water problems along the border continues to be a significant challenge.

Rabies has become a serious problem in Texas counties along the U.S.–Mexico border (Council on Scientific Affairs, 1990). Rabies had been confined to sporadic cases in coyotes. However, in the late 1980s, an epizootic of canine rabies was detected in Starr County, Texas (Clark *et al.,* 1994). While the outbreak initially involved primarily coyotes, cases of rabid domestic dogs have continued to increase since it began. Furthermore, it had spread to at least 12 counties by 1992. The lack of rabies vaccination on the Mexican side of the border and easy movement across the border by animals appears to have contributed to the spread of rabies to domestic dogs on the U.S. side of the border (Warner, 1991). Serological and genetic analyses support this notion (Clark *et al.,* 1994).

Mosquito-borne diseases, tuberculosis, and HIV/AIDS serve as specific examples of the unique health challenges present along the border.

Mosquito-Borne Diseases

Neither malaria nor dengue fever are considered to be problems in the United States, although Mexico does have outbreaks of both these mosquito-borne febrile diseases. Health

officials in the United States maintain mosquito spraying programs in order to control the mosquito vectors of diseases. However, in 1986 there was an outbreak of locally transmitted malaria in San Diego County (Maldonado *et al.,* 1990). There were a total of 28 cases, with 2 local residents and 26 Mexican migrant workers affected. An epidemiological study of the outbreak ruled out importation of the cases, and determined that local transmission had occurred because the men slept in the open in close proximity to a marshy area where *Anopheles hermsi* was known to be breeding. This outbreak is believed to have been the largest of its kind in the United States since 1952.

Dengue fever and dengue hemorrhagic fever have become endemic in Mexico (Centers for Disease Control and Prevention [CDC], 1996b). In 1980, after 2 years of intense dengue transmission in Mexico, Texas documented the first cases of indigenously transmitted dengue fever in the United States since 1945 (CDC, 1996b, Warner, 1991). Mexico experienced its most recent outbreak in mid 1995 through early 1996 (CDC, 1996b). Health officials in Mexico notified Texas state health authorities of the outbreak because the mosquito vector is present year-round in the southern area of Texas, and because of the frequent movement of people across the border. A total of 29 laboratory-diagnosed cases of dengue fever were detected in Texas residents; it was determined that 7 of these cases were acquired through local transmission.

In an interview with Skolnick (1995), Dr. Laurance Nickey, Director of the El Paso City–County Health and Environmental District, reported the practice of health workers from El Paso joining Mexican health workers to spray the Aguas Negras sewage canal in Ciudad Juárez to prevent mosquito breeding in the stagnant waters. Ciudad Juárez does not have sufficient funds for adequate mosquito control, which increases the possibility of viral encephalitis transmission in both Ciudad Juárez and El Paso given the proximity of the two cities.

Tuberculosis

Tuberculosis (TB) rates along the border are twice as high as the national rates, and single-drug-resistant tuberculosis rates are higher in Hispanic than non-Hispanic border populations. The CDC (1996a) reported that between 1985 and 1995, cases of TB in foreign-born persons living in the United States increased 61%; these cases account for 22% of all TB cases in the United States. Of foreign-born individuals with TB, 22% were born in Mexico (8% of the national total), and the states of California, Texas, New Mexico, and Arizona accounted for 81% of Mexican-born TB patients.

In 1995, an epidemiologic study to characterize patterns of immigration and migration and health-seeking behaviors of foreign-born Hispanic TB patients was initiated between the CDC and local health departments of the four U.S. border states (CDC, 1996a). Single-drug-resistant TB was found to differ significantly between foreign-born Hispanic patients (1.7 to 5.0 times higher) and U.S.–born Hispanic patients (1.7 to 3.2 times higher) when compared with U.S.–born non-Hispanic patients (CDC, 1996a). Multidrug-resistant TB was found to be 6.8 times higher among foreign-born Hispanic TB patients than among U.S.–born non-Hispanic patients, while rates of foreign-born and U.S.–born Hispanic patients were similar. In Tijuana, Mexico, drug resistance has been seen in up to 50% of the TB cases, while drug resistance was seen in 43% of cases in Project Juntos in Ciudad Juárez (Skolnick, 1995). Because the level of resistance to isoniazid (INH) is close to 4% for U.S.–born Hispanic patients, and higher than that for foreign-born Hispanic patients, the CDC recommends an initial four-drug regimen for treating TB in patients who live in the border region (CDC, 1996a).

Gellert and Pyle (1994) report that antibiotic-resistant tuberculosis may be increasing due to the practice of self-medication through the purchase of drugs without a prescription in Mexico. A volunteer visited 17 pharmacies in the Mexican city of Nogales and requested information on how to treat a bad cough in her child. In response to this question, all the pharmacists recommended an antibiotic, with 35% suggesting amoxicillin. In response to the next question as to what the pharmacist would recommend if the cough was tuberculosis, 82% (14) told the woman to seek medical attention. However, 92% offered to sell her a rifampin suspension when she requested it, even though the product is labeled as one for which a prescription is required. The authors concluded that improved coordination and regulation of these drugs, along with an education program for pharmacists on their appropriate dispensation, should be made to avoid even more drug-resistant forms of tuberculosis.

Project Juntos is an example of a binational tuberculosis control program between El Paso and Ciudad Juárez (Skolnick, 1995). Started in the early 1990s, this project helped to establish a TB control division in the health department in Ciudad Juárez. The El Paso health department assists with laboratory testing and the two health departments work together in binational control activities. In the San Diego–Tijuana area, a subcommittee of the California/Baja California Binational Health Council was formed in 1992 to address binational TB control. The Tuberculosis Subcommittee was successful in raising funds to implement a binational laboratory coordination program, standardize diagnosis and treatment protocols, and develop a binational transportation system and educational programs for professionals and the community from both sides of the border.

The CDC currently supports five binational TB control projects in sister city areas along the border. This innovative collaboration between the CDC, local U.S. health departments, and the Ministry of Health in Mexico focuses on training personnel and develops binational TB prevention and control programs (CDC, 1996a). Binational programs are particularly important for TB control since the treatment regimen is at least 6 months long; movement across the border increases the number of individuals who are lost to follow-up; and the possibility that family members may reside on both sides of the border, which may limit control of contacts (Albrecht, 1993a). In some active TB patients, tracking family members and other individuals who might have been exposed, such as work colleagues and school classmates, has required a significant binational effort between the local health departments (CDC, 1991).

HIV/AIDS

Of all the Mexican border states, Baja California Norte has the highest AIDS case rate (59 per 100,000 inhabitants), and it is estimated that one out of every 1,669 inhabitants either has AIDS or has died of AIDS (Secretaria de Salud, 1996). In addition, the northern border states account for 12% of all AIDS cases in Mexico. If one compares the number of AIDS cases diagnosed in San Diego County through 1994 (6,300) with that of Baja California (614), one can see that there is a tenfold difference between the two sister cities. However, in San Diego County there were more than 300 Mexican-born AIDS cases, supporting the belief that AIDS cases are significantly underreported in Mexico. Reasons given for underreporting are limited resources for epidemiological activities, incomplete diagnosis and follow-up of AIDS cases, and reluctance of physicians to report cases because of fear of discrimination for the patient (HIV/STD Subcommittee of the CA/Baja CA Binational Health Council, 1995).

Tijuana continues to account for the majority of AIDS cases in Baja California (67% in 1994). Transmission modes reported for cases in Baja California were 48% in homosexual or bisexual men; 7% injecting drug users; 17% through heterosexual contact; 2% perinatal; and 21% unknown (Secretaria de Salud, 1996). However, the Secretary of Health of Mexico reports that the large unknown category is due to the fact that in Mexico many AIDS cases are identified through death certificates and transmission routes are not investigated. The states of Baja California and Sonora report the highest number of AIDS cases associated with injection drug use in men, 4.5% and 5.5%, and women, 2.8% and 3.7%, respectively. As presented by González-Block and Hayes-Bautista (1991), HIV in Mexico is principally transmitted sexually, with male bisexual practices more common in Mexico than in the United States. However, the number of AIDS cases associated with injection drug use is very low in Mexico when compared with injection drug use among Latino populations in the United States (González-Block & Hayes-Bautista, 1991).

Cross-Border Utilization of Health Care Services

Several cases of well-off Mexican nationals entering the United States to receive health care services paid through the public sector have been reported in the news media (Eisenstadt & Thorup, 1994). These cases have perpetuated the public's feeling that the U.S. health care system is being abused by poor Mexican immigrants, regardless of the fact that the individuals caught defrauding the medical system were well-to-do Mexicans. There is also evidence that Mexican Americans have lower health care use rates than the overall population (Estrada & Hughes, 1990; Guendelman & Jasis, 1990). Hayes-Bautista (1996) reported that Latinos in general have much lower utilization of health care services rates, fewer days in the hospital, and lower hospital costs than the general population. While much attention has been given to the use of medical services in the United States by Mexican nationals, little attention has focused on the use of Mexican health care services by U.S. residents. Studies have documented cross-border health service seeking behaviors (Guendelman & Jasis, 1990), in which poorer U.S. residents tended to go to Mexico for more affordable care while more affluent Mexicans came to the United States for health services (Homedes *et al.,* 1994; Thompson, 1994).

Arizona–Sonora

In a survey of physicians and dentists living in border towns of Arizona and Sonora, 20% of the patients seen in practices located in Mexico were U.S. residents, while only 7% of the patients seen in practices located on the U.S. side of the border were Mexican nationals (Homedes *et al.,* 1994). In addition, Mexican health providers reported higher proportions of patients visiting them two to three times a year than U.S. physicians reported for their Mexican patients (median 50% vs. 25%).

U.S. physicians and dentists reported that Mexican nationals came to the United States for health care because of superior services, referrals by other providers or friends, dissatisfaction with Mexican services, and bilingual providers. Health problems seen by U.S. providers were related primarily to cardiovascular disease, accidents, and endocrine and respiratory problems. Mexican physicians and dentists reported that U.S. residents sought health care services in Mexico because of cheaper services, better quality of care, and more culturally appropriate care. These providers reported seeing U.S. patients for respiratory problems, infectious diseases, and perinatal services. However, in terms of the number of Mexican practitioners who saw patients with specific health problems, more than 50% of the providers saw individuals with respiratory problems and at least 25% treated infectious diseases, cardiovascular disease, and digestive problems, or provided prenatal care.

Language has long been identified as a barrier to accessing services, especially by monolingual populations. Given the large proportion of U.S. residents in the Arizona border area who speak both Spanish and English, it was not surprising to see that 86% of providers in Arizona employ bilingual personnel, although only 17% reported being bilingual themselves (Homedes *et al.,* 1994; Nichols, LaBrec, Homedes, & Geller, 1994). In Sonora, only 13% of the providers reported employing bilingual personnel, although 25% were bilingual. In addition, 26% of the Mexican health care professionals reported receiving at least some of their medical training in the United States, while only 9% of U.S. providers received any part of their training in Mexico.

Homedes and colleagues (1994) reported that the cross-border use of health services was identified as a problem by 62% of the U.S. providers and by 42% of the Mexican providers. Reasons given included financing and quality of care issues due to a lack of continuity with the patient, and the absence of medical records. Eight percent of Mexican providers also mentioned that seeing U.S. patients raised legal and ethical concerns because patients requested treatments not yet approved by the U.S. Food and Drug Agency. Although reimbursement for care was reported as a problem when seeing patients from across the border, 89% of Arizona providers reported that their Mexican patients paid in cash and that 9% had insurance. Only 4% of U.S. residents seeking services in Sonora had insurance, and 96% paid for services in cash.

Another component of the survey of health care providers in the Arizona–Sonora border area was a survey of health care providers in the city of Tucson, Arizona (Nichols *et al.,* 1994). Seventy-nine percent indicated that they saw at least one Mexican resident a week, although the authors state that this may be an overestimate given difficulties in distinguishing between residents of Mexico and U.S. residents of Mexican descent. Tucson providers indicated that they were most frequently consulted for problems of the circulatory and digestive systems. While border area providers characterized 64% of their cases as acute care and 23% as chronic diseases, Tucson providers saw fewer acute care cases (45%) and more chronic diseases (38%), and twice as many rehabilitation cases (6% vs. 3%). These differences demonstrate the need to examine the types of medical services being utilized in different border areas. Patients from Mexico seeking services just over the U.S. side of the border tended to be poorer, presented more acute cases in serious condition, and more cases related to injuries or poisonings. Patients from Mexico seen in Tucson provider offices tended to be wealthier, in better health, and sought more care for chronic diseases or specialized health care (Nichols *et al.,* 1994).

San Diego–Tijuana

Guendelman and Jasis (1990) conducted a study in Tijuana, Baja California, to determine whether the Mexican border populations who temporarily cross over the border burden the public health services in the United States. Tijuana was selected as the study site since it is the largest Mexican border city (more than 788,000 inhabitants in 1990) and the border crossing between Tijuana and San Diego is the busiest in the United States. A total of 660 households were randomly selected and interviewed. Findings demonstrated that use of health services in the United States was low, with only 2.5% of households reporting use of services in the United States in the previous 6 months. In contrast, more than 40% used services only in Tijuana. Of the 2.5% of the respondents who used services in the United States, 47% were U.S. residents or citizens entitled to those services. Another 42% held a border passport that allowed them to legally enter the United States for short visits, and only 11% illegally crossed the border for health care purposes.

Contrary to the popular belief that Mexicans cross the border to obtain free services, 39% of the individuals reporting use of U.S. health care services stated they paid cash for those services, 20% were covered by third-party insurance, and 32% were covered by public funds (including Medicare, Medicaid, and free services). Of those using the U.S. health system, 84% of the visits were to private-sector physicians and only 15% were in the public sector. Reasons given for use of the U.S. health system were treatment for an illness, reproductive health care, and physical examinations. Respondents (64%) also reported high out-of-pocket costs for medical care in Mexico (Guendelman & Jasis, 1990).

Guendelman and Jasis (1990) also reported that of the study population with insurance coverage in the United States, 65% exclusively sought services in the United States; 4% used services in both countries; and 31% used only Mexican health services. Of the respondents with insurance coverage in Mexico, 98% used only Mexican services. The authors concluded that the Mexican border population does not represent a large burden on U.S. public health care.

In further analyses of the data generated through the project just mentioned, Guendelman (1991) examined reasons that Mexicans crossed the border for health care services. She found that in this study population, the majority of Mexicans using U.S. health services were upper middle class, and more than 50% were U.S. residents or citizens entitled to receive the benefits through their participation in the U.S. labor force. Results indicated that the strongest predictor for utilization of health services in the United States by Mexicans was insurance coverage. Other factors identified as significant contributors to access to U.S. health care services were transportation and socioeconomic status. Not surprisingly, individuals with more resources were not only better able to access those services but accessed them more consistently over time.

In response to concern voiced by public officials of increasing use of U.S. maternity services by Mexican women, Guendelman and Jasis (1992) examined the factors associated with childbirth and the utilization of maternity services in California and Mexico by women who were living in Tijuana and had had a child in the previous 5-year period. Women were asked to participate in focus group sessions, during which attitudes and values that influenced the decision of the woman to give birth in a U.S. or Mexican facility were examined. The authors found that of the 184 women who had been living in Tijuana and had had a child within the previous 5 years, 89.6% gave birth in Mexico and 10.4% gave birth in the United States. Examination of sociodemographic characteristics indicated that upper- and middle-income women were more likely to give birth in the United States, and that 73.8% of all U.S. deliveries were in the private sector. A full 89.5% of women who gave birth in the United States reported paying for at least part of the delivery costs, with 82.3% fully paid in cash and 17.7% paid in installments. The remainder of the U.S. deliveries were paid through private insurance (10.5%). None of the women reported obtaining public benefits for the U.S. delivery, although some reported attempts to obtain such coverage.

Reasons given for choosing to deliver in the United States as opposed to Mexico included citizenship opportunities (47%) and better attention and technology (45%); only 8% mentioned special services (such as WIC or food coupons) or a more comfortable hospital stay. Among women giving birth in Tijuana, the majority (74.6%) reported greater familiarity with maternity services or the right to free services or insurance coverage in Mexico (13.9%). Only 11.5% felt that quality of care was better in Mexico than in the United States. The authors concluded that Mexican women crossing the border to give birth in the United States represent a very low public health burden since most births taking place in the United States were in the private sector, were paid for in cash, and were to women of middle and upper socioeconomic status. The prime motivators for giving birth in the United States were potential U.S. citizenship and the quality of hospital care, rather than attempts to obtain free care (Guendelman & Jasis, 1992).

In interviews with undocumented workers living in migrant encampments in north San Diego County, Eisenstadt and Thorup (1994) examined the issue of access to U.S. health care services and actual utilization of those services by poor Mexican migrant workers. Individuals indicated that fear of the authorities and lack of knowledge about how to access services were major barriers to seeking health care in the case of immigrant workers. Another barrier identified was the lack of transportation. This is consistent with the

Guendelman (1991) study, where the availability of transportation was a significant predictor for utilization of U.S. health services. One individual living in an encampment stated that neither he nor anyone else in his family had used any health or social service since their arrival 3 years earlier, with the exception of public education for the children (Eisenstadt & Thorup, 1994). These workers also found it difficult to cross the border to access health care in Mexico given their undocumented status and potential problems crossing back into the San Diego.

Arredondo-Vega (1996) examined the use of Mexican medical services by U.S. nationals in the San Diego–Tijuana region. He found that the low cost of medical services, the low cost of pharmaceuticals, and differences in controls and restrictions over prescription medicines all contributed to the use of Mexican health care services by U.S. nationals. In a survey of 10 Tijuana clinics and hospitals in 1994–95, 8 reported that they had American clients. Services utilized by U.S. resident patients were outpatient care and gynecology-obstetrics. Other services were general surgery, plastic surgery, and dentistry. When ranked by order of importance, outpatient care and hospitalization were services ranked as those with greatest demand, and alternative treatments for cancer, traumatology, and orthopedics ranked second. This study also revealed that purchasing medications is also commonplace due to the fact that drugs are often cheaper and easier to obtain in Mexico than in the United States. Many of the clinics catering to Americans are located near the border crossing, thereby reducing the length of time spent traveling to the clinic once the border has been crossed.

Mexican Health Care Utilization by Retired U.S. Citizens and Residents Living in Mexico

There are a large number of U.S. citizens who live in Mexico. According to estimates from the United States State Department (Warner & Reed, 1993), in 1988 there were an estimated 396,000 Americans living in Mexico. An additional 203,000 were in Mexico as tourists; this figure includes retired Americans living in Mexico for part of the year. Many of the U.S. nationals resident in Mexico are individuals who have retired to Mexico because of a more appealing climate and the lower cost of living (Warner & Reed, 1993). In Baja California alone, Arredondo-Vega (1996) reports an estimated 60,000 Americans; approximately 50% (30,000) live in the city of Tijuana.

A policy research project was undertaken to examine health services in Mexico for U.S. citizens and residents and the use of U.S. services by Americans resident in Mexico (Warner & Reed, 1993). Interviews were conducted with individuals living in Mexico, with service providers, and with health insurance companies. In interviews with retired individuals living in different parts of Mexico, retirees reported problems with reimbursement from Medicare and Blue Cross for medical costs incurred in Mexico. Since Medicare and Veteran's Administration benefits are not applicable in Mexico, a number of individuals reported that the main reason they used health services in the United States was this restriction in coverage. In general, interview respondents expressed a high degree of confidence in the Mexican medical system, and felt that dollars could be saved if Medicare would allow for reimbursement to Mexican providers. While there are private Mexican insurance plans, many of the interviewees indicated that they could not afford the premiums and expressed concern with some companies' practice of cutting off individuals at a certain age. However, a large number of Americans reported purchasing coverage on an annual basis through the Mexican Institute of Social Security (IMSS) (Warner & Reed, 1993).

Border Health Services

Health services on the border were surveyed to determine what percentage of the patients seen in these facilities are U.S. resi-dents and how they pay for health care (Warner & Reed, 1993). Two physicians in private practices (one in Reynosa and the second in Matamoros) serving a substantial number of U.S. residents were interviewed. Both served between 150 and 250 clients from the United States on a monthly basis, and both reported that 95% of their U.S. patients are Hispanic. Both physicians indicated that it is very difficult for them to collect from U.S. insurance companies, and that 90% of their patients paid cash.

Private hospitals were also included in the study. In Matamoros, the Hospital y Centro de Especialidades Médico Quirúrgicas has a special arrangement directly with the Eagle Bus Manufacturing Company and H.E.B. grocery stores. The Hospital y Centro directly bills Eagle Bus Manufacturing for services provided to employees. Most of the Eagle Bus Manufacturing employees using the services at the Hospital y Centro are Hispanics. In Reynosa, the Plaza Internacional Hospital has established special arrangements with companies located along the border. About 50% of the patients seen at the hospital are from the United States, and 95% of these are Hispanic. About 90% of all Plaza Internacional's clients pay directly for services with insurance. A number of hospitals near the border that treat U.S. residents are found in Ciudad Juárez and Nuevo Laredo; some U.S. insurance companies will reimburse these hospitals.

Cross-Border Purchase of Pharmaceuticals

Anecdotal information from interviews with migrant workers in San Diego indicate that a number of individuals cross the border in order to purchase prescription medications (Swerdlow *et al.*, 1992). Not only are the pharmaceuticals less expensive but some prescription drugs, antibiotics in particular, are available over-the-counter and the individual does not need to see a doctor in order to obtain a prescription. However, as discussed earlier, problems due to self-medication are being increasingly seen, such as the emergence of drug-resistant TB strains (Gellert & Pyle, 1994).

A survey of 79 patients from a university medical clinic to determine use of pharmacies located across the border in Ciudad Juárez was conducted by Casner and Guerra (1992). Of the individuals interviewed, 81% reported having purchased medication in Ciudad Juárez and 55% reported purchasing medications in Mexico several times a year. A total of 69% had purchased medications in Ciudad Juárez the previous month, and 28% in the previous week. The most common types of medications purchased were high blood pressure medication and antibiotics. Of those who had purchased medications in Mexico, 75% did so without a prescription. Reasons given by the respondents for purchasing medications in Mexico were that it was less expensive (49%) and that they did not require a prescription (20%).

Seventy-two percent of the interviewees reported that the medication they purchased was recommended by someone other than a physician, such as a friend, a relative, a pharmacist, or themselves (Casner & Guerra, 1992). This high level of self-medication is of great concern to health care providers given the potential for serious side effects when multiple drugs are taken at the same time or are not taken in appropriate doses.

In the study by Warner and Reed (1993), a survey of prices in pharmacies along the border revealed that prices for medications in the United States were anywhere from 35% to 1000% greater than the same name brand medication across the border in Mexico. While U.S. nationals purchased pharmaceuticals in Mexico because of lower costs, Mexican nationals reported purchasing drugs they were unable to obtain in Mexico in U.S. pharmacies. A 1987 change in Texas prescription laws allows Texas pharmacies to fill prescriptions from health providers anywhere in the United States, Canada, and Mexico. This law has greatly increased the ability of Mexican nationals to access U.S. pharmaceutical products.

Americans are increasingly seeking alternative care clinics that have sprung up along the border (Warner & Reed, 1993). These clinics offer treatments that may be considered illegal or are not readily available in the United States. According to the Office of Technology Assessment (OTA) in Washington, D.C. (Warner & Reed, 1993), most of the patients who seek these services tend to be well-educated, middle- to upper-middle-class individuals. While the clinics will work with the client to obtain reimbursement from insurance companies, most require cash payments for treatments received.

Summary and Conclusions

Many of the diseases that affect border populations are associated with poverty, overcrowding, substandard housing, pollution, and inadequate health and social services infrastructures. The United States–Mexico border region is unlike any other region in either country. The border has experienced very high growth rates in the past 15 years, and continues to be a magnet for individuals seeking employment both in Mexico and the United States. The creation of the "twin plant" or *maquiladora* system along the Mexican side of the border has fueled an industrial boom. However, these *maquiladoras* also bring their own challenges, especially in the areas of disposal of toxic wastes and working conditions. The environmental situation of the border area is considered by many public health officials, researchers, and communities to be a "disaster," with long-term consequences for the health of the population.

The United States and Mexico share ecosystems, water supplies, and air. Some of the health problems that have been identified are increased levels of cancers, birth defects such as anencephaly, certain autoimmune disorders, and a number of other communicable diseases (e.g., salmonellosis, shigellosis, TB, hepatitis A). Both the United States and Mexico have laws that prohibit or control much of the environmental degradation which is taking place along both sides of the border, but lack of funding to enforce legislation cripples U.S. and Mexican environmental agencies. "Politics," according to some health officials and researchers, prevents truly collaborative projects from being implemented. Examples are the lack of U.S. financial support for a cross-border wastewater treatment plant in El Paso–Ciudad Juárez, and significant resistance by San Diego County residents for a San Diego–Tijuana plant. The impact of human and agricultural wastewater dumped into border rivers (such as the Rio Grande and the Tijuana River) is seen daily in water samples that are positive for fecal coliforms; viruses are found in some areas, as well as arsenic and other contaminants. In San Diego County, popular beach areas are frequently closed due to contamination. In El Paso, ground water contamination is a serious problem in the *colonias* that have sprung up around the city. Similarly, air quality in the major sister cities is unacceptably poor.

The border region is characterized by a dynamic economy, which the North American Free Trade Agreement has helped to promote. Yet, the region is one of the poorest in the United States, with rates of tuberculosis, hepatitis A infection, and salmonellosis-shigellosis two to three times higher than national rates. The southern border areas of the four U.S. border states also have higher rates than those seen statewide. Given the rapid industrial development the region has undergone, difficult working conditions and occupation-associated health problems are an emerging concern.

There are few occupational health studies of industries along the border. Such studies have been difficult to conduct because companies refuse to allow employees at their *maquiladora* plants to participate. Guendelman and Jasis-Silberg (1993) have discussed the possibility of a "healthy worker" effect on the results of their study of women working in *maquiladora* plants. They noted that electronics *maquiladoras*, in particular, tend to be more selective in their hiring, and target young, single women without children for employment. Another factor contributing to difficulties in long-term studies is the high employee turnover rate in the *maquiladora* plants.

Guendelman and Jasis-Silberg (1993) suggested that future studies examine the long-term reproductive outcomes and other sequelae and diseases that may result from occupational exposure to chemicals or other toxins. These authors also stated that future occupational studies should take into account not only conventional indicators of health, such as physical examinations and laboratory tests, but also workers' perceptions, feelings, and health beliefs. These data would shed more light on the patterns of disease within the *maquiladora* population.

The use of health services on the U.S. side of the border by Mexican nationals appears to be less than what the American public popularly believes. In fact, recent research revealed a pattern of U.S. health services utilization by wealthier Mexicans, with poorer Americans using Mexican health care services. Numerous individuals cross the border into Mexico regularly to purchase prescription medications. As discussed earlier, self-medication without a physician's supervision can lead to increased drug resistance and the risk of reactions among medications.

For the health of border residents to improve, significant efforts at creating binational programs are urgently needed. A good example is the El Paso–Ciudad Juárez air pollution control program, in which appropriate strategies were identified for each city with the collaboration of public agencies, businesses, and researchers.

References

Albrecht, L. (1993a). International effort battles TB along border. *Texas Medicine, 89*(12), 28.

Albrecht, L. (1993b). Troubling waters: sister cities struggle with health conditions on the U.S.–Mexico border. *Texas Medicine, 89*(10), 24–25.

Arredondo-Vega, J. A. (1996, October 30). *The use of Mexican medical services by American nationals.*

Paper presented at the Border Health Working Group meeting, San Diego, CA.

Axelson, O. (1980). Arsenic compounds and cancer. *Journal of Toxicology and Environmental Health, 6*(5–6), 1229–1235.

Border health hazards. (1995b). [Editorial]. *Multinational Monitor, 16*(4), 22–23.

Burning border health issues. (1995a). [Editorial]. *Environmental Health Perspectives, 103*(6), 542–543.

Casner, P.R., & Guerra, L. G. (1992). Purchasing prescription medication in Mexico without a prescription. *Western Journal of Medicine, 156*(5), 512–516.

Catholic Charities. (1995). *Comprehensive preventive health project at La Posada de Guadalupe.* Final report submitted to the Alliance Healthcare Foundation, San Diego, CA.

Cech, I., & Essman, A. (1992). Water sanitation practices on the Texas–Mexico border: Implications for physicians on both sides. *Southern Medical Journal, 85*(11), 1053–1064.

Centers for Disease Control and Prevention. (1991). Tuberculosis transmission along the U.S.–Mexico border—1990. *Morbidity and Mortality Weekly Report, 40*(22), 373–375.

Centers for Disease Control and Prevention. (1996a). Characteristics of foreign-born Hispanic patients with tuberculosis—Eight U.S. counties bordering Mexico, 1995. *Morbidity and Mortality Weekly Report, 45*(47), 1032–1036.

Centers for Disease Control and Prevention. (1996b). Dengue fever at the U.S.–Mexico border, 1995–1996. *Morbidity and Mortality Weekly Report, 45*(39), 841–844.

Chávez, L. R. (1992). *Shadowed lives: Undocumented immigrants in American society* (Case Studies in Cultural Anthropology). Fort Worth, TX: Harcourt Brace Jovanovich College Publishers.

Clark, K. A., Neill, S. U., Smith, J. S., Wilson. P. J., Whadford, V. W., & McKirahan, G. W. (1994). Epizootic canine rabies transmitted by coyotes in south Texas. *Journal of the American Veterinary Medical Association, 204*(4), 536–540.

Council on Scientific Affairs. (1990). A permanent U.S.–Mexico Border Environmental Health Commission. *Journal of the American Medical Association, 263*(24), 3319–3321.

Eisenstadt, T. A., & Thorup, C. L. (1994). *Caring capacity versus carrying capacity: Community responses to Mexican immigration in San Diego's North County* (Monograph Series 39). San Diego, CA: Center for U.S.–Mexican Studies, University of California.

El Paso Community Foundation. (1996). *The border. The United States/Mexico international boundary.* El Paso, TX: El Paso Community Foundation.

Eskenazi, B., & Guendelman, S. (1993). A preliminary study of reproductive outcomes of female maquiladora workers in Tijuana, Mexico. *American Journal of Industrial Medicine, 24,* 667–676.

Espinosa-Torres, F., Hernández-Avila, M., & López-Carillo, L. (1994). NAFTA: A challenge and an opportunity for environmental health. The case of the maquiladoras. *Salud Pública de México, 36*(6), 597–616 (in Spanish).

Estrada, A. L., & Hughes, A. (1990). *Hispanic health care needs along the United States/Mexico border and the training needs of health providers.* Southwest Border Rural Health Research Center, College of Medicine, University of Arizona, Tucson, AZ.

Gellert, G. A., & Pyle, N. G. (1994). Pharmacy practice and antibiotic-resistant tuberculosis along the U.S.–Mexico border [Letter to the editor]. *Journal of the American Medical Association, 271*(20), 1577–1578.

González-Block, M. A., & Hayes-Bautista, D. E. (1991). AIDS: The silent threat to binational security. *Salud Pública de México, 33*(4), 360–370 (in Spanish).

Grigsby, C. O. (1996, May 15–17). *Air pollution reduction in the Mexican brickmaking industry.* Paper presented at the Philanthropy on the Border Binational conference, El Paso, TX/Ciudad Juárez, Chihuahua, Mexico.

Guendelman, S. (1991). Health care users resident on the Mexican border: What factors determine choice of the U.S. or Mexican health system? *Medical Care, 29*(5), 419–429.

Guendelman, S., & Jasis, M. (1990). Measuring Tijuana residents' choice of Mexican or U.S. health care services. *Public Health Reports, 105*(6), 575–583.

Guendelman, S., & Jasis, M. (1992). Giving birth across the border: The San Diego–Tijuana connection. *Social Science and Medicine, 34*(4), 419–425.

Guendelman, S., & Jasis-Silberg, M. (1993). The health consequences of maquiladora work: Women on the U.S.–Mexican border. *American Journal of Public Health, 83*(1), 37–44.

Hatcher, J., Hopewell, J., Guardiola, A., Jacquart, K., Moreau, W., Stys, J., DeNino, L., & Warner, D. (1995). *The border health authority: Issues and design* (U.S.–Mexican Occasional Paper No. 6). Austin: Lyndon B. Johnson School of Public Affairs, University of Texas.

Hayes-Bautista, D. E. (1996, October 30). *Work force issues and options in the border states.* Paper presented at the Border Health Working Group meeting, San Diego, CA.

HIV/STD Subcommittee of the California/Baja California Binational Health Council. (1995). *STD/HIV/AIDS Prevention and Education Project.* Proposal submitted to the Border Health Office, Pan American Health Organization, El Paso, TX.

Homedes, N., Chacón-Sosa, F., Nichols, A., Otálora-Soler, M., LaBrec, P., & Alonso-Vázquez, L. (1994). Utilization of health services along the Arizona–Sonora border: The providers' perspective. *Salud Pública de México, 36*(6), 633–645.

Jones, D. B. (1989). Trouble on the border: International health problems merge at the Rio Grande. *Texas Medicine, 85*(8), 28–33.

Kelly, M. E. (1992). Free trade: The politics of toxic waste. *Report on the Americas, 26*(2), 4–7.

Langman, J. M. (1994). Xylene: Its toxicity, measurement, of exposure levels, absorption, metabolism, and clearance. *Pathology, 26*(3), 301–309.

Leonard, A., & Lauwerys, R. R. (1980). Carcinogenicity, teratogenicity, and mutagenicity of arsenic. *Mutation Research, 75*(1), 49–62.

Maldonado, Y. A., Nahlen, B. L., Roberto, R. R., Ginsberg, M., Orellana, E., Mizrahi, M., McBarron, K., Lobel, H. O., & Campbell, C. C. (1990). Transmission of *Plasmodium vivax* malaria in San Diego County, 1986. *American Journal of Tropical Medicine and Hygiene, 42*(1), 3–9.

McMichael, A. J. (1988). Carcinogenicity of benzene, toluene, and xylene: Epidemiological and experimental evidence. *IARC Scientific Publications, 85*, 3–18.

Moure-Eraso, R., Wilcox, M., Punnett, L., Copeland, L., & Levenstein, C. (1994). Back to the future: Sweatshop conditions on the Mexico–U.S. border: I. Community health impact of maquiladora industrial activity. *American Journal of Industrial Medicine, 25*, 311–324.

Muñoz, G., & Adamo, L. C. (1994). *Safe water and sanitation for homeless migrant farm and day workers in North San Diego County.* Final report submitted to the Alliance Healthcare Foundation, San Diego, CA.

Nichols, A. W., LaBrec, P. A., Homedes, N., & Geller, S. E. (1994). Utilization of medical services in Arizona by residents of Mexico. *Salud Pública de México, 36*(2), 129–139 (in Spanish).

Nickey, L. N. (1989). Economics, disease burden U.S.-Mexico border [Editorial]. *Texas Medicine, 85*(8), 8.

Paso del Norte Air Quality Task Force. (1994). *Sharing a common airshed.* El Paso, TX: El Paso City-County Health and Environmental District.

Regional Taskforce on the Homeless. (1994). *Homeless farmworkers and day laborers: Their conditions and their impact on the San Diego Region.* San Diego, CA: Author. (Population estimates were updated in July, 1994.)

San Diego Association of Governments. (1996a, November). Border area transportation. *SANDAG Special Report,* San Diego, CA.

San Diego Association of Governments. (1996b). *Economic bulletin.* San Diego, CA: Author.

Secretaria de Salud y CONASIDA. (1996). Epidemiological data on AIDS, epidemiological data on STDs: Data through the fourth trimester, 1995. *SIDA–ETS, 1*(3), i–xxi (in Spanish).

Sever, L. E. (1995). Looking for causes of neural tube defects: Where does the environment fit in? *Environmental Health Perspectives, 103* (Suppl. 6), 165–171.

Shalat, S. L., Walker, D. B., & Finnell, R. H. (1996). Role of arsenic as a reproductive toxin with particular attention to neural tube defects. *Journal of Toxicology and Environmental Health, 48*(3), 253–272.

Shields, J. (1991). Ambient air arsenic levels along the Texas–Mexico border. *Journal of the Air and Waste Management Association, 41,* 827–831.

Skolnick, A. A. (1995). Along the U.S. southern border, pollution, poverty, ignorance, and greed threaten nation's health. *Journal of the American Medical Association, 273*(19), 1478–1482.

Suárez y Toriello, E., & Chávez, O. E. (1996). *Profile of the United States–Mexico border.* Mexico City, Mexico: Federación Mexicana de Asociaciones Privados de Planificación Familiar.

Swerdlow, D. L., Muñoz, G., Lobel, H., Waterman, S., Agraz, A., Ginsberg, M., Peter, C., & Ramras, D. (1992). *Health surveillance in migrant camps, San Diego County: July 1991–June 1992.* Final report submitted to the Alliance Healthcare Foundation, San Diego, CA.

Thompson, W. W. (1994). Cross-border health care utilization and practices of Mexican-Americans in the lower Rio Grande valley. *Border Health Journal, 10*(2), 1–9.

Warner, D. (1991). Health issues at the U.S.–Mexican border. *Journal of the American Medical Association, 265*(2), 242–247.

Warner, D. C., & Reed, K. (1993). *Health care across the border: The experience of U.S. citizens in Mexico* (U.S.–Mexican Policy Report No. 4). Austin: Lyndon B. Johnson School of Public Affairs, University of Texas.

14

Migrant Health

MARIE NAPOLITANO AND BRUCE W. GOLDBERG

Introduction

The migrant labor force in the United States is composed predominately of agricultural workers. Although some of the workforce in the entertainment, tourism, and other employment sectors is seasonal or migratory, these numbers are inconsequential when compared with the numbers of migrant and seasonal agricultural workers. Migrant farmworkers perform physically demanding and hazardous work, experience poor living conditions, and have inadequate access to medical and social services. The majority of migrant farmworkers are immigrants and they endure racial discrimination, disruption of cultural traditions and practices, language barriers, and an often unpredictable and stressful lifestyle. Consequently, migrant farmworkers and their families have different and more complex health problems than those of the general population. Although we recognize the significance of the health problems among migrant families and their children, this chapter focuses primarily on the migrant and seasonal farmworker.

Estimates of the numbers of migrant and seasonal farmworkers in the United States vary from one to five million. This disparity is due to differences in definitions, divergent methodologies for estimating the numbers of migrant workers, and whether dependents are included. There is no uniform definition of migrant and seasonal farmworkers. The Office of Migrant Health defines a migrant farmworker as an individual "whose principal employment is in agriculture on a seasonal basis, who has been so employed within the last 24 months and who establishes for the purpose of such employment a temporary abode" (U.S. Department of Health and Human Services [USDHHS], 1980). Seasonal farmworkers are those who work cyclically but do not migrate.

Comprehensive and accurate data regarding migrant and seasonal farmworkers are lacking. Although migrant and seasonal farmworkers are two distinct populations, there are many demographic and occupational similarities between the two groups. Therefore, much of the available data regarding these two groups are often obtained and reported as an aggregate. When reliable distinctions between the two groups can be made we do so; otherwise, the term *migrant farmworker* can be assumed to refer to both migrant and seasonal farmworkers in the aggregate.

MARIE NAPOLITANO • Department of Primary Care, School of Nursing, Oregon Health Sciences University, Portland, Oregon 97201. BRUCE W. GOLDBERG • School of Medicine, Oregon Health Sciences University, Portland, Oregon 97201.

Handbook of Immigrant Health, edited by Loue. Plenum Press, New York, 1998.

Demographics

The Office of Migrant Health estimates there are three million migrant and seasonal farmworkers and their dependents in the United States (Wilk, 1988). California, with 23%, has the largest share of migrant farmworkers and Texas is second with 12%. Sixty-eight percent of migrant farmworkers are employed in eight states (in descending order: California, Texas, Florida, Washington, Michigan, Oregon, North Carolina, and Georgia) (Larson & Plascencia, 1993).

Migrant farmworkers have generally confined themselves to three "streams" or geographic areas of employment. The home state is usually in the south and is referred to as downstream, while the work states are upstream. The east coast stream originates from a home base in Florida and extends up the east coast of the United States to the northern Atlantic states. The midwestern stream originates in Texas and extends throughout the plains states, middle western states, and parts of the Rocky Mountain states. The western stream originates in California and Arizona and extends northward to Washington through the agricultural areas west of the Rockies (Meister, 1991). However, as workers increasingly travel throughout the country seeking employment, these streams are becoming less distinct. Migrants in the northwest, southwest, and northeast generally work with fruit and nut crops and those in the middle west and western plains states work field crops. The southeast is predominated by vegetable crops and has the highest percentage of hand harvesting work in the country.

The demographics of migrant farmworkers in the United States has changed dramatically in the past 50 years. In the 1930s and 1940s the majority of migrant farmworkers were White and born in the United States. Today, the migrant farm labor force in the United States is generally composed of immigrants from Latin American countries, particularly young Mexican men (Mines, Gabbard, & Samradick, 1993). Seventy-three percent of all migrant farmworkers are male and 55% were born in Mexico. This is a relatively young population, with a median age of 31 years. Seventy percent of the total migrant work force is Hispanic. Foreign-born workers comprise 60% of the migrant workforce and this group is almost exclusively (96%) from Latin American countries.

Most foreign-born workers are legally authorized to work in the United States; however, a significant number of migrant farmworkers (20%) are unauthorized (Mines, Scabbard, & Boccalandro, 1991). Legal issues surrounding work status and immigration are extremely sensitive to many migrant workers. Many workers, both authorized and unauthorized, live in fear of immigration and legal authorities. Therefore, the validity of data surrounding numbers of unauthorized workers remains questionable. Of the 40% of the workforce born in the United States, 60% are White, non-Hispanic, 31% are Hispanic, and 6% African American.

Poverty and low education are significant issues among migrant farmworkers. Nearly one half (46%) of all farmworkers and more than three quarters (77%) of undocumented farmworkers live below the poverty threshold (Mines et al., 1993). Yet, despite the high poverty levels, only 20% get need-based social services such as food stamps. Fifty-three percent of migrant workers have less than 8 years of formal, school-based education. Spanish is the primary language for nearly two thirds of all migrant farmworkers and only 40% speak or read English well. Most migrants are married and 57% reside with their families at their work site.

True migratory farmworkers comprise approximately 40% of the farm labor workforce. These migratory workers are primarily employed as harvesters and are predominantly newer immigrants. About two thirds of these migratory workers come to the United States from a home base in Mexico, follow crops for a period of time, and then return home. The other one third remain in the United States, following crops from one location to another (Mines et al., 1993).

There is increasing evidence that over time the immigrant farm labor work forces move away from migratory patterns and tend to settle permanently. This process begins with predominantly immigrant, migrant workers performing the most difficult and least skilled tasks such as harvesting. As these unskilled laborers repeatedly work in areas, some eventually become rooted and begin to settle down. Concomitant with this is a tendency for these workers to graduate into more desirable and higher paying semiskilled jobs such as irrigating, pruning, and spraying. While this pattern is more widespread in the western United States, evidence suggests that it is occurring in increasing numbers in the east (Mines *et al.*, 1993).

Life as a Migrant Farmworker

The majority of migrant farmworkers work in three major areas of agriculture: field crops and orchards, nurseries, and canneries. Their lives consist of following crops, nursery, or cannery work on a seasonal basis and returning to a homebase for part of a year, usually in California, Texas, Florida, or Mexico. Some follow employment opportunities continuously throughout the year. Life in the migrant stream involves decision making regarding traveling for work without certainty of employment or housing and moving without feeling a sense of having arrived and being settled. It involves working many hours in difficult physical conditions.

Employment for migrant farmworkers is unpredictable due to the uncertainty of the health of crops and the availability of work on arrival. Timing of crops may vary each year due to weather conditions often making the availability of work not coincide with arrival dates. Many migrant farmworkers risk arriving early at a job site simply to ensure themselves employment.

Decision making regarding travel for work is often based on little or no information about the availability of employment at the arrival site. When information regarding work is obtainable, the sources can be word of mouth from other workers, employer notices in local newspapers, calling growers, and recruitment by crew bosses. Information about housing is even more difficult to obtain.

Availability of housing for migrant farmworkers is less than adequate. During migration, migrant farmworkers may live in employer-provided housing, private camps, state camps (California), rental apartments, or rental hotel rooms. Data from California, Oregon, and Washington show that the total amount of housing available for migrant farmworkers, including private camps, employer-provided housing, and California's state-run camps, provides less than 30% of the needed capacity in those three states (U.S. General Accounting Office [USGAO], 1992). Employer-provided housing is decreasing as many aging camps are being demolished and not being replaced and growers are closing camps rather than paying fines for violations. A survey done by CASA of Oregon in 1990 indicated that the vast majority of farmworkers and their families do not live in labor camps but are living in rental housing under crowded and substandard conditions (Pallack, 1991). When attempting to rent housing, migrant farmworkers face considerable obstacles such as excessive rent, substantial deposit amounts, long-term leases, lack of credit, discrimination, and a sparse rural renting market (Lopez, 1995). When housing is not available or the obstacles become too great, migrant farmworkers and their families may end up living in their cars.

Inadequate funds are available for construction of sufficient farmworker housing (Lopez, 1995). A national effort to solve this problem is the Rural Housing and Community Development Service Section 514/516 programs that provide loans to growers and loans and grants to nonprofit sponsors of farmworker housing. However, federal funds for farmworker housing have been cut (USGAO, 1992). Most states and local governments have not addressed this problem. A few exceptions, however, do exist. The state of Oregon grants growers a tax credit to provide housing for farmworkers and California operates state housing centers. California, Florida, Ohio, Oregon, and Virginia have migrant farmworker housing programs which offer assistance to groups that construct or rehabilitate hired migrant farmworkers' housing (USGAO, 1992). Nonprofit organizations have attempted to fill the void in farmworker housing. For example, the Delmarva Rural Program has developed more than 30 units of housing in Delaware and Maryland (Lopez, 1995). In Oregon, the Housing Development Corporation has been building quality migrant farmworkers' housing (approximately 91 units) for over 13 years in Washington County.

To a large extent, the condition of farmworker housing is inadequate. Migrant farmworkers may be living in substandard housing such as shacks and barns or in overcrowded bungalows, trailers, dormitories, apartments, or hotel rooms (USGAO, 1992). Their living quarters may lack electricity, plumbing, heating or cooling, adequate ventilation, more than one exit, screens over windows, laundry facilities, and recreational facilities. Reports, however, cite that farmworker housing has improved to some extent (National Advisory Council on Migrant Health [NACMH], 1995; Pallack, 1991). A survey done by CASA of Oregon in 1990 found that the majority of employer-provided housing was in good physical condition (Pallack, 1991).

The Health of Migrant Farmworkers

Just as uncertainty pervades the lives of migrant farmworkers, uncertainty pervades our picture of their health. The literature cites the poor health of this population and their special health concerns (Dever, 1991; Goldsmith, 1989; NACMH, 1995). However, the available epidemiologic data needed to build a clear picture of their health status are less than adequate. First, precise migrant population data are missing and inaccuracies (e.g., the use of different definitions for migrant farmworkers) exist in the data that are available (Rust, 1990). Lack of accurate population data results in inaccurate numbers being used as denominators in morbidity and mortality calculations (indicators of health sta-

tus). Second, comprehensive health data are missing. A national farmworker health data reporting system does not exist nor do population health surveys identify migrant farmworkers in most cases (D. Slesinger, 1992). Other health data sources are useless or limited for this population (e.g., lack of a category on death certificates for migrant agricultural worker). Third, the interaction of migration with income, educational level, physical-cultural-social factors, genetic makeup, and past life history and the resultant impact on the health of migrant farmworkers have not been examined. The very nature of the migrant lifestyle for this population contributes to the difficulties in filling these gaps resulting in an uncertain picture of the health status of the migrant population.

The few insights from the literature as to the health status of migrant farmworkers come from studies based on migrant health clinic records or convenience samples of small segments of the migrant population. There is uncertainty as to just how representative of the entire migrant population these data are. Records from migrant health clinics reveal dermatitis, injuries, respiratory problems, musculoskeletal problems, eye problems, gastrointestinal problems, and diabetes as the most frequently reported health problems (Slesinger, 1992). The majority of clinic encounters tend to be for acute illness rather than chronic illness or preventive care (Wilk, 1986). One larger study by the Migrant Clinicians Network (Dever, 1991) sampled utilization data from four migrant health centers in Texas, Michigan, and Indiana, and from community health data collected from two control group counties. This study concluded that migrant farmworkers have more multiple and complex health problems; they suffer more frequently from infectious diseases; they have more clinic visits for otitis media, pregnancy, hypertension, contact dermatitis, eczema, and medical supervision of children. Diabetes and hypertension increasingly accounted for more visits as age increased.

Insights into specific health problems for this population result from studies using convenience samples of migrant farmworkers. However, studies are minimal and therefore may not present an accurate picture of these problems. The majority of studies have focused on occupational health problems.

Occupational and Environmental Health Problems

The work of migrant farmworkers exposes these individuals to numerous occupational and environmental hazards many of which have been poorly quantified for this population (Rust, 1990). Occupational and environmental risks are virtually inseparable for the majority of migrant farmworkers. Although hazards may be job-specific (field worker, farm machinery handler, nursery worker, cannery worker), overall this population faces many occupational and environmental risk categories such as injuries, crowded living conditions, pesticide exposure, lack of field sanitation, and unfavorable climate conditions.

Occupational health risks can and do result in numerous physical and health problems. In order to understand the actual and potential occupational health problems for migrant farmworkers, the National Institute for Occupational Safety and Health's (NIOSH) list of Leading Work-Related Diseases and Injuries (Millar, 1991) for all agricultural workers serves as a worthwhile starting point. Documentation (examples in parentheses) exists for migrant farmworkers in each of these categories; however, studies are sparse and do not present a clear picture of the scope of health problems encountered by this population within each category. The list includes:

1. Occupational lung diseases such as reduced lung functioning (Gamsky, Schenker, McCurdy, & Samuels, 1992), asthma, and pneumonia.
2. Musculoskeletal injuries such as tendenitis, repetitive motion trauma, falls from ladders, neck-shoulder-back pain (Mines & Kearney, 1982; D. P. Slesinger & Cautley, 1981; Wilk, 1986).

3. Occupational cancers such as skin and bladder cancers and leukemia (Moses, 1989; Zham & Blair, 1993).
4. Severe occupational traumatic injuries such as machine-related fatalities (S. D. Ciesielski, Hall, & Sweeney, 1991), electrocutions, suffocations, amputations, and eye injuries.
5. Occupational cardiovascular disease such as heat stroke (Brown, 1991).
6. Disorders of reproduction such as miscarriages (De la Torre & Rush, 1989), infertility (Whorton, Milby, Krauss, & Stubbs, 1979), limb reduction birth defects (Schwartz & LoGerfo, 1988), premature births, and pregnancy complications (Wilk, 1986).
7. Neurotoxic disorders such as neurologic dysfunction (Hays & Laws, 1991; Sharp, Eskenazi, Harrison, Callas, & Smith, 1986).
8. Noise-induced hearing loss (Bernhardt & Langley, 1993; Crutchfield & Sparks, 1991).
9. Dermatological conditions such as dermatitis (Gamsky *et al.*, 1992; O'Malley, Smith, Krieger, & Margetich, 1990; Schuman & Dobson, 1985), burns, and lacerations.
10. Psychological disorders such as stress and depression (De Leon Siantz, 1990; Vega, Warheit, & Palacio, 1985).
11. Infectious diseases such as acute gastroenteritis and zoonosis (S. D. Ciesielski, Seed, Ortiz, & Metts, 1992; Kligman, Peate, & Cordes, 1991; Ungar, Iscoe, Cutler, & Bartlett, 1986).

Other health problems secondary to environmental risks for the migrant farmworker include allergic reactions, drowning in ditches, respiratory problems due to exposure to cold and wet weather conditions (NACMH, 1995), urinary tract infections due to lack of sanitation facilities (Bechtel, Shepherd, & Rogers, 1995; Wilk, 1986), and lower extremity infections and cellulitis due to inadequate foot protection. Although all occupational and environmental hazards can pose major health threats for the migrant farmworker, the seriousness and presumed prevalence of injuries and pesticide exposures warrant particular attention to these health risks.

Injuries

Agriculture is consistently rated as one of three most hazardous occupations (Rust, 1990). Injuries are reported as the leading cause of mortality and morbidity among agricultural workers (U.S. Department of Labor [USDL], 1988; Wilk, 1986). The National Safety Council's 1988 survey of 127,169 farm family members (Hosken, Miller, & Hanford, 1988) and the CDC/NIOSH publication *Epidemiology of Farm-Related Injuries: Bibliography with Abstracts* (USD-HHS, 1992a) serve as good references on the diversity of agricultural injuries. However, a comprehensive surveillance system for injuries does not exist and many of the data sources used to compile statistics for agricultural injuries have limitations (Gerberich *et al.,* 1992). For example, workmen's compensation data which are used for compiling injury statistics are inconsistent or lacking for agriculture due to exemptions, exclusions, and loopholes in state laws (Mobed, Gold, & Schenker, 1992). Data are also lacking on the nature and consequences of agricultural injuries (Mobed *et al.,* 1992). Therefore, an accurate understanding of the scope and features of injuries for all agricultural workers is currently not possible.

Insights into this problem specifically for migrant farmworkers are further hampered by reporting inadequacies. For example, federal law exempts farms with fewer than 10 workers, which accounts for many of the farms hiring migrant farmworkers, from reporting injuries. Also, no category exists for migrant farmworkers on farm injury reports; therefore, injury data tend to combine farmers and all types of farmworkers. However, a broad range of injuries have been identified as significant for migrant farmworkers. These include fractures or sprains from falls

from ladders or equipment; sprains or strains from prolonged stooping, heavy lifting, and carrying; amputations, deaths, crush injuries from tractors, trucks, or other machinery; pesticide poisoning, electrical injuries; carbon monoxide poisoning from running equipment in enclosed areas, and drowning in irrigation ditches (S. D. Ciesielski, Hall, & Sweeney, 1991; Mines & Kearney, 1982). The few studies that exist on injuries of migrant farmworkers support this broad range of injury types. One study in California reported injuries from machinery, falling stacks of containers, heavy loads, and falling from ladders (Mines & Kearney, 1982). Another study in North Carolina also reported numerous injuries from machinery (S. D. Ciesielski, Hall, & Sweeney, 1991).

Pesticides

Pesticides are used extensively in agriculture. The Environmental Protection Agency (EPA) estimated that 817 million pounds of pesticides were used for agricultural purposes in 1991 (EPA, 1992). Pesticides are known to be harmful to the environment and in particular to ecosystems. Although toxicity data are not complete on all pesticides, many pesticides are known to be toxic to humans causing a wide range of adverse health effects.

The number of migrant farmworkers affected by pesticides and other chemicals, the levels of exposure, and the health consequences for this population are not known. The EPA has estimated that 300,000 migrant farmworkers suffer acute illnesses annually as a result of pesticide exposure (Wilk, 1986). Our lack of understanding regarding this problem with migrant farmworkers results from multiple deficiencies. For example, states may lack mandatory reporting; local, state, and federal agencies may not have sufficient resources for identifying violations of required reporting; migrant farmworkers may not seek medical care for known exposures; health professionals may not recognize signs and symptoms of exposures; and health problems secondary to pesticide exposure may not present for an extended period of time.

The work and living environment of the migrant farmworker presents numerous sources of pesticide exposure. Mobed, Gold, and Schenker (1992) categorized these sources of exposure as avoidable (e.g., diluting and mixing pesticides, applying pesticides, being sprayed), unavoidable (e.g., drifts, contact with residues) and unknown (contaminated water, contaminated fruits and vegetables). Pesticides are readily absorbed through the skin and respiratory and gastrointestinal tracts. The main route for occupational exposures is the skin (Spear, 1991) and there may be greater absorption by migrant farmworkers due to lack of washing facilities (D. P. Slesinger & Ofstead, 1989; Zham & Blair, 1993).

The migrant farmworker's dwelling can be a major source of contamination for the worker and his family. Migrant farmworker housing may be located adjacent to fields that have been contaminated with pesticides (Soliman, Derosa, Mielke, & Bota, 1993) and may be exposed to drifts of pesticides during and following application of pesticides. Housing may be located where posted signs regarding pesticide applications cannot be seen by the migrant farmworker and his family. Field-adjacent housing and other housing used by migrant farmworkers may have been sprayed with pesticides to control for rodents and roaches. Migrant farmworker housing can be contaminated by the farmworkers themselves inadvertently carrying pesticides home from work on their clothes, skin, hair, tools, and vehicles. One study found organophosphate compounds in 62% of household dust samples tested in homes of farmers and migrant farmworker families living within 200 feet of an orchard (Simcox, Fenoke, Wolz, Lee, & Halma, 1995). According to McCauley (1996), pesticides may persist in dwellings longer than in outdoor environments due to the lack of degradative environmental processes such as sun, rain, and microbial activity.

Organophosphate anticholinesterase pesticides comprise the largest group of pesticides in current use (Kaloyanova & Batawi, 1991; Lotti, 1992). Acute neurological illness can be caused by overexposure to these pesticides and other organophosphates and carbamates (Hays & Laws, 1991; Sharp et al., 1986). Organophosphates and carbamates work by inhibiting the activity of cholinesterase, an enzyme essential for normal neuromuscular functioning. As exposure to these pesticides increases, cholinesterase activity as measured by blood cholinesterase level decreases (McCauley, 1996). Migrant farmworkers and their children who were exposed to pesticides have been found to have lower levels of cholinesterase (S. Ciesielski, Loomis, Mims, & Auer, 1994; Richter, 1992).

Mild psychological and behavioral deficits such as changes in the speed and precision of answering questions, impaired judgment, poor comprehension, and decreased ability to communicate reportedly occur after exposure to anticholinesterase pesticides and can persist for weeks and months (Sidell, 1992). Other acute health manifestations of pesticide exposure include abdominal pain, ataxia, nausea, diarrhea, dizziness, vomiting, headache, malaise, skin rashes, and eye irritation (Moses, 1989; Wilk, 1986) . Acute severe pesticide poisoning can result in death (Moses, 1989).

The long-term health effects due to acute and low-dose, long-term pesticide exposures are unclear in general. Because of the exposure risks migrant farmworkers confront, long-term and chronic health problems due to pesticides are major concerns for this population (Mobed et al., 1992; Schenker & McCurdy, 1988; Sharp et al., 1986). However, studying long-term effects in the migrant population poses numerous methodological challenges such as long-term follow-up and controlling for confounding factors.

Associations have been made between long-term exposures and several types of cancer, neurotoxic effects, and reproductive problems (Blair & Zahm, 1991; Moses, 1989; Sharp et al., 1986). Most epidemiologic studies on carcinogenicity and pesticides have focused on farm owners or farm machinery operators. Studies with farmers consistently have shown increases in risks for cancers including leukemia, non-Hodgkin's lymphoma, Hodgkin's disease, multiple myeloma, and cancer of the stomach, prostate, and testes (Zham & Blair, 1993). The few studies and case reports that exist for migrant farmworkers have findings similar to those with farmers; however, these findings also have shown excesses for cancers of the buccal cavity, pharynx, lung, and liver (Moses, 1989; Zham & Blair, 1993).

Polyneuropathy and neurobehavioral effects are two additional chronic or delayed effects from acute high-dose or chronic low-dose pesticide exposure (Sharp et al., 1986). Findings of the long-term effects from exposure to pesticides on human reproduction are inconsistent except for the relationship between male infertility and dibromochloropropane which is banned in the United States (Sharp et al., 1986; Whorton et al., 1979). Spontaneous abortions, premature births, pregnancy complications, fetal malformation or growth retardation, cancer among offspring, and abnormal development of infants exposed to chemicals in breast milk were cited by Wilk (1986) as potential problems.

Other health problems attributed to chronic pesticide exposure include limb reduction birth defects (Schwartz & LoGerfo, 1988), and chronic dermatitis, fatigue, headache, sleep disturbances, anxiety, blood disorders, and abnormal liver and kidney function (Moses, 1989; Wilk, 1986).

Other Significant Health Problems for the Migrant Population

The number of migrant farmworkers who are HIV seropositive is higher than in the general population and appears to be increasing (Centers for Disease Control [CDC], 1992; Jones, 1992; Lyons, 1992). Included in these numbers are women farmworkers who have been infected from heterosexual contact (Skjerdal, Misha, & Benavides-Vaello, 1996). The vulnerability of this population stems from a high number of risk factors such as substance abuse (National Migrant Resource Program, 1993; Skjerdal et al., 1996), a lack of health education opportunities, and physical and social isolation. Certain cultural factors also can contribute to the HIV disease picture for migrant farmworkers. These include the infrequent use of condoms (Ryan, Foulk, Lafferty, & Robertson, 1988), the multiple-person use of syringes for medications to treat different illnesses ("Be Aware! Common Cultural Practices and AIDS," 1987; Lafferty, 1991), and the use of folk medicine which can delay diagnosis of AIDS ("Be Aware!" 1987). Studies have found a lack of knowledge among migrant farmworkers regarding HIV and its transmission (Bletzer, 1995; Ryan et al., 1988; Skjerdal et al., 1996; Vasilion, 1992).

Migrant farmworkers have higher rates of tuberculosis infection than the general population (CDC, 1992) especially those who have immigrated from regions with known high rates such as Latin America, Southeast Asia, and Haiti. The prevalence rates reported from studies done in the late 1980s in Delaware, Virginia, and North Carolina have all been very similar: 37%–44% (S. D. Ciesielski, Seed, Esposito, & Hunter, 1991; Jackson, Mercer, Miller, & Simpson, 1987; Wingo et al., 1986). Migratory lifestyle complicates the treatment of active tuberculosis because it interferes with or prevents long-term follow-up, contact screening, and access to care; the cost of medication and fear of the INS are also factors.

Dental decay, including baby bottle tooth decay, is a prevalent problem in migrant children (Call, Entwistle, & Swanson, 1987; Koday, Rosenstein, & Lopez, 1990; Weinstein, Domoto, Wohlers, & Koday, 1992; Woolfolk, Hamard, Bagramian, & Sgan-Cohen, 1984). In addition, adult migrant farmworkers endure high rates of dental disease. A study in Colorado found adult migrant farmworkers to have a higher rate of periodontal disease than Hispanic groups in the Southwest (Weinstein *et al.,* 1992). Lack of dental insurance and the high cost of dental care are mainly responsible for the low incidence of dental care among migrant farmworkers and their children. The Migrant Head Start program screens all enrolled migrant children for dental decay but the program is unable to find sufficient dentists to treat the children (Marco Beltran, Oregon Migrant Head Start Program, personal communication, 1996). Koday found a high rate of treatment and sealant use in migrant children in central Washington probably due to that migrant clinic's priority for dental care (Koday *et al.,* 1990).

Although diabetes and hypertension are cited as prevalent reasons for clinic encounters, there is a dearth of information about these conditions for this population. Nutritional status, domestic violence, substance abuse, and mental health are also cited as significant health concerns for the migrant farmworker population but little information is available. In addition, the health needs of migrant farmworkers from their perspective have not been identified. With regard to their perceived health status, D. P. Slesinger and Ofstead (1993) reported that one third (33.6%) of migrant farmworkers surveyed in Wisconsin felt that their health was fair or poor compared with 9.4% of the U.S. population. Only 13.3 % of these migrant workers rated their health as excellent as compared with 40.2 % of the U.S. population.

Access to Health Care

As previously documented, measures of the health status of migrant farmworkers lag behind those of the rest of the population. While some of this can be attributed to underlying social and occupational conditions, it is also evident that migrant farmworkers experience limited access to medical care. The Migrant Health Act, signed into law in 1962, was established to improve the delivery of primary and supplemental health care services to migrant and seasonal farmworkers in the United States. Funded under Section 329

of the Public Health Service and administered by the Bureau of Primary Health Care, the program currently funds more than 100 organizations in 41 states and provides services at more than 400 clinic sites. Yet, the program is able to serve less than 20% of the migrant farmworker and dependent population (NACMH, 1995).

Inability to afford care is among the leading impediments to access to health care. Over half of migrant farmworkers' medical bills are paid by federal migrant health funds, 17% by Medicaid, and approximately 14% by out-of-pocket expenditures (D. P. Slesinger & Ofstead, 1993). The Medicaid program was established to assist the poorest Americans gain financial access to medical care and indeed most migrant farmworkers fit the profile of the population Medicaid was designed to help. Yet, migrant farmworkers appear to have more difficulty accessing Medicaid benefits than any other population in the country (NACMH, 1995). Although the reasons for this are complex, a great deal is related to a disparity between the organizational structure of the Medicaid program and the farmworker lifestyle.

Although Medicaid is a federal mandate, it is administered by individual states. Farmworkers must apply within the state where they reside and there is no transfer of benefits between states. States are allowed up to 45 days to process applications and once an individual is approved, depending on the state, eligibility must be revalidated every 1 to 6 months. Migrant farmworkers have often moved on to the next state before eligibility can be established. In addition, the seasonal nature of farm work brings about widely fluctuating monthly incomes such that during some of the productive months workers and their families may not be eligible for benefits. Finally, even if farmworkers have Medicaid coverage, they often have difficulty finding providers who will treat them.

Overcoming financial barriers to medical care has been a central issue in U.S. health care policy over the past 30 years. However, there is a growing understanding that even if financial access to care is guaranteed, there are a number of nonfinancial barriers that impede access to primary health care. Unfortunately, few studies have developed models that predict the extent to which these nonfinancial barriers affect access to primary health care (Cary *et al.*, 1995).

Among the most frequently cited nonfinancial barriers to care are language, transportation, culture, mobility, and occupational factors. Farmworkers often labor far longer than the traditional 8-hour workday, leaving no time at the end of the workday to get medical care. In addition, the seasonal nature of agricultural work means that farmworkers make every effort to maximize their income earning work hours whenever work is available. Farmworkers are thus reluctant to take time off from work to obtain medical care as any interruption to the workday results in decreased income and spawns the fear of being viewed as lazy by employers or crew chiefs.

Transportation and geographic factors affect farmworkers' ability to access health care. Given the rural locations of worksites, great distances must often be traveled to clinics or hospitals. Transportation is unreliable and expensive and most migrant farmworkers do not own a vehicle (Mines *et al.*, 1991). Furthermore, the mobility of farmworkers results in great difficulty obtaining continuity of care.

The farmworker population is composed of people from a mixture of ethnicities and culture. Language and cultural differences may leave farmworkers unaware that the services they need are available. Migrant health centers make every effort to minimize the barriers of language and culture yet often are unable to provide sufficient numbers of bilingual staff. Recent changes in local migrant stream demographics add to these difficulties. For example, over the past 10 years indigenous Guatemalans have been the most rapidly increasing population among the east coast migrant stream. Of these individuals, roughly 40% speak only a local dialect. In addition, most of these individuals have never heard about, nor know

how to protect themselves from communicable diseases such as tuberculosis, HIV, and STDs (East Coast Migrant Health Project, 1996).

Although bilingual and bicultural clinic staff help improve access to care, farmworkers by the nature of their work and lifestyle are an extremely hard to reach population. Thus, many migrant health clinics have been expanding their community outreach services. The federal Migrant Health Program defines outreach as making services known to the population and ensuring that they can access all the available services. Such programs should be accessible, acceptable, improve effectiveness of health services, provide comprehensive health services, and be appropriate to the population being served (National Migrant Resource Program, 1993).

Outreach programs take a variety of forms. They may provide home or work site health education, social services, transportation, or "mobile" clinics that provide agricultural field-based or "satellite" medical care. An increasing number of outreach programs utilize lay or peer workers recruited from the indigenous cultures of communities that they serve. The lay health worker model is commonly used in developing countries where access to professionals is extremely difficult. In the United States they have been used increasingly to provide services to poor and medically underserved populations. Lay health worker programs in migrant farmworker communities have been successful in bridging the sociocultural gap between professional providers and their families and in providing health education and support (Meister, Warrick, Zapien, & Wood, 1992; Warrick, Wood, Meister, & Zapien, 1992).

Finally, access to dental and mental health care is even more problematic than primary medical care. Over 25% of migrant health clinics provide no dental services (National Migrant Resource Program, 1995). Furthermore, many state Medicaid programs provide limited or nonexistent dental benefits making access to community dental providers even more difficult.

The stresses associated with a poor, migrant lifestyle often with limited social support and cultural isolation greatly increase the risk for mental illness (Laughlin, 1977). Local mental health services for migrant farmworkers are often insufficient to meet the needs of this unique population. Understanding a farmworker's primary language and culture are or critical importance in providing effective mental health care. Furthermore, mobility greatly complicates the provision of mental health care.

Legislative Protection for Migrant Farmworkers

Loopholes in laws and deficiencies in enforcement result in farmworkers' not being adequately protected by state and federal laws (NACMH, 1995). The General Accounting Office (GAO) of the Human Resources Division analyzed the extent to which selected federal laws, regulations, and programs protect the health and well-being of migrant farmworkers. The conclusions stated that this population is not adequately protected; therefore, their health and well-being are at risk (GAO/HRD-92-46 Hired Farmworkers' Health at Risk). The GAO found: (1) lack of adequate protection form pesticides due to insufficient information and lack of enforcement of regulations; (2) inadequate field sanitation; (3) inadequate protection for children on farms; (4) lack of health care due to inadequate program; and (5) lack of social security benefits due to employer underreporting and lack of information given to migrant farmworkers.

Lack of Adequate Protection from Pesticides

The Environmental Protection Agency (EPA) regulates pesticides and their uses and maintains specific standards for protecting farmworkers exposed to agricultural pesticides. The EPA modified its standards in 1992 in order to increase protection for migrant farmworkers. These standards include prevention of exposure to pesticides, mitigation of exposures, and information to migrant farmworkers about the hazards of the pesticides. The standards require that employers inform workers about the specific pesticides being used and the dangers from exposure in writing. Employers must also provide training on the prevention of exposure and the treatment of poisonings. Timely warnings must be given to workers who will be in fields treated with pesticides. A lack of enforcement and the absence of a reporting mechanism for violations contribute to a large extent to the lack of protection from pesticide exposure for migrant farmworkers. In addition, exemptions from the standards have been granted for such reasons as economic hardship for the employer (NACMH, 1995).

OHSA's responsibility is to adopt and enforce specific standards to help ensure a safe and healthy workplace for all employees. With respect to pesticides at the work site, OHSA has deferred to EPA standards. However, OHSA can approve state plans for worker protection (such as pesticide protection) that are more stringent than federal regulations. State plans can be more effective; however, states may cite the lack of resources to effectively enforce their plans to protect farmworkers (USGAO, 1992).

Inadequate Field Sanitation

OHSA regulations require that basic field sanitation be provided to farmworkers. Farms with fewer than 10 workers are exempted from these regulations except for the states of Washington, Oregon, Arizona, and Alaska, which have more stringent state laws. Violations of the law are numerous. A Department of Labor 1990 national survey of farmworkers revealed that 31% worked in fields without drinking water, handwashing facilities, or toilets (USGAO, 1992). Other studies have found even less access (Sweeney & Ciesielski, 1990). Limited federal resources prevent effective enforcement of the regulations (USGAO, 1992).

Less Protection for Children on Farms

Federal legislation allows children to work in agriculture at a younger age than other industries. For example, a 16-year-old adolescent is allowed to operate such machines as tractors, hay bailers, or grain combines. Children ages 12–13 years can work in agriculture outside school hours with parental consent.

Enforcement of child labor laws by the Department of Labor may be ineffective (USGAO, 1992). The National Child Labor Committee (a child labor advocacy group) estimated that 100,000 children of farmers and farmworkers work illegally on farms and one million child labor violations occur due to lack of enforcement and low penalties (USGAO, 1992). Children of migrant farmworkers usually work in the fields to contribute to low family income and for lack of available child care facilities (USGAO, 1992).

Lack of Health Care due to Inadequate Program Assistance

The Medicaid and Migrant Health Programs should serve as safety nets for the health care for migrant farmworkers. However, for a variety of reasons, these programs may not be serving this population adequately. Medicaid benefits may not be available to migrant farmworkers because they are undocumented; they leave the state for work before their applications are processed; or they receive benefits from one state that are not honored by medical providers in another state (USGAO, 1992).

The Migrant Health Program serves fewer than 20% of migrant farmworkers (NACMH, 1995). As discussed under access to health care, budget constraints due to inadequate funding do not allow migrant health clinics to serve all migrant farmworkers in their dispersed locations.

Lack of Social Security Benefits

Migrant farmworkers may receive fewer Social Security (SSI) benefits than other workers which means less financial support when they retire or become disabled. This results from employers' not reporting the total income of all their hired farmworkers. Migrant farmworkers may also be unaware of the SSI program for age, blindness, or disability.

Other federal laws specifically do not cover migrant farmworkers. For example, the National Labor Relations Act protects the rights of employees to organize and bargain collectively; however, it specifically excludes migrant and seasonal migrant farmworkers. Some states such as California do allow employees this right. The Federal Unemployment Tax Act provides income to workers during periods of unemployment; however, migrant and seasonal migrant farmworkers are excluded. The Workers Compensation Law provides assistance to workers injured on the job, but only 27 states provide coverage to migrant farmworkers and only 14 of these provide migrant farmworkers coverage equal to that of other workers (McCauley, 1996).

Future Changes and Directions

As evidenced by the information presented previously in this chapter, the health of migrant workers is as much related to housing, working conditions, and social factors as it is to the structure of the health care delivery system. To adequately address the health care needs of the migrant worker will require more than simply providing medical services. It will necessitate coordination and integration of the vast array of social, legal, medical, and employment-related services and delivery of these services in a manner that minimizes barriers and promotes accessibility.

Indeed, it is the concepts of coordination, integration, and portability around which the future health delivery system for migrant workers should be constructed. The lifestyle of the migrant worker and the demands of their jobs call for a system in which workers and their families can receive the services they need and interact with the providing agencies and programs in one location. Such a location should serve as a centralized source of information for the worker and for service agencies. Reliable and consistent information would be available and a centralized database would minimize duplicative paper work, documentation, registration, and other data collection. Funding sources could thus be consolidated and used more efficiently.

In addition to being geographically centralized, services and benefits must be "portable." The ability for migrant workers and their families to transfer eligibility for state-administered programs such as Medicaid and cash assistance from one state to another is essential. Such a system would ideally allow migrant workers to receive those benefits for which they qualify seamlessly and without interruption or reapplication, regardless of where they were living or working.

Reducing the barriers to effective service brought about by differences in language, culture, and literacy requires that all services be delivered in a culturally and linguistically appropriate manner. Ideally, staff persons should be multilingual and multicultural. Hours of operation would be designed to meet the needs of the population being served and reliable transportation would be made available to those in need.

Within the confines of health delivery systems, services will also need to be coordinated and consolidated. Mental, dental, and direct medical care should be provided in a centralized location and with a coordinated information and medical record system. The medical record should be accessible to all those providing health care services to migrant workers and their families. The facilitation of outreach and work site or camp–based health delivery and education requires a complete medical record that can easily be transferred from a health center to another local. In addition, such records should be accessible at migrant health delivery sites in other states. The existing technology surrounding computerized medical records is sufficient to allow for such a system. However, the infrastructure and financial support for such a system must be established.

References

Be aware! Common cultural practices and AIDS. (1987). *Migrant Health Newsline, 4,* 1.

Bechtel, G. A., Shepherd, M. A., & Rogers, P. W. (1995). Family, culture, and health practices among migrant farmworkers. *Journal of Community Health Nursing, 12,* 15–22.

Bernhardt, J., & Langley, L. (1993). Agricultural hazards in North Carolina. *North Carolina Medical Journal, 54,* 512–515.

Blair, A., & Zahm, S. (1991). Cancer among farmers. *Occupational Medicine State of the Art Reviews, 6,* 335–354.

Bletzer, K. V. (1995). Use of ethnography in the evaluation and targeting of HIV/AIDS education among Latino farm workers. *AIDS Education and Prevention, 7,* 178–191.

Brown, D. W. (1991). Heat and cold in farmworkers. *State Art Review of Occupational Medicine, 6,* 371–389.

Call, R., Entwistle, B., & Swanson, T. (1987). Dental caries in permanent teeth in children of migrant farm workers. *American Journal of Public Health, 77,* 1002–1003.

Cary, A. H., Goldberg, B. W., Jobe, A. C., McCann, T., Skupien, M. B., Troxel, T. M., & Williams, D. R. (1995). If we fund it, will they come? Researching nonfinancial barriers to primary health care. *Family & Community Health, 18,* 69–74.

Centers for Disease Control. (1992). *Prevention and control of tuberculosis in migrant farm workers* (HHS Publication No. [CDC] 92-8017). Washington, DC: U.S. Government Printing Office.

Ciesielski, S., Esposito, D., Protiva, J., & Pielhl, M. (1994). The incidence of tuberculosis among North Carolina migrant farmworkers, 1991. *American Journal of Public Health, 84,* 1836–1838.

Ciesielski, S., Loomis, D., Mims, S., & Auer, A. (1994). Pesticide exposure, cholinesterase depression, and symptoms among North Carolina migrant farmworkers. *American Journal of Public Health, 84,* 446–451.

Ciesielski, S. D., Hall, S. P., & Sweeney, M. (1991). Occupational injuries among North Carolina migrant farmworkers. *American Journal of Public Health, 81,* 926–927.

Ciesielski, S. D., Seed, J. R., Esposito, D. H., & Hunter, N. (1991). The epidemiology of Tuberculosis among North Carolina migrant farm workers. *Journal of the American Medical Association, 265,* 1715–1719.

Ciesielski, S. D., Seed, J. R., Ortiz, J. C., & Metts, J. (1992). Intestinal parasites among North Carolina migrant farmworkers. *American Journal of Public Health, 82,* 1258–1262.

Crutchfield, C., & Sparks, S. (1991). Effects of noise and vibration on farm workers. *Occupational Medicine: State of the Art Reviews, 6,* 355–369.

De la Torre, A., & Rush, L. (1989). The effects of health care access on maternal and migrant seasonal farmworker women infant health of California. *Migrant health Newsline, Clinical Supplement*, 1–3.

De Leon Siantz, M. L. (1990). Correlates of maternal depression among Mexican-American migrant farmworker mothers. *Journal of Community Psychology, 3*, 9–13.

Dever, A. (1991). *Profile of a population with complex health problems*. Austin, TX: Migrant Clinicians Network.

Diaz, J. O., Trotter, R. T., & Rivera, V. A., Jr. (1989). *The effects of migration on children: An ethnographic study*. State College, PA: Centro de Estudios Sobre la Migracion.

East Coast Migrant Health Project. (1996). *Changes in the east coast migrant stream*. Washington, DC: Author.

Gamsky, T. E., McCurdy, S. A., Wiggins, P., Samuels, S. J., Berman, B., & Shenker, M. B. (1992). Epidemiology of dermatitis among California farm workers. *Journal of Occupational Medicine, 34*, 304–310.

Gamsky, T. E., Schenker, M. B., McCurdy, S. A., & Samuels, S. J. (1992). Smoking, respiratory systems and pulmonary function among a population of Hispanic farmworkers. *Chest, 101*, 1361–1368.

Gerberich, S., Gibson, R., Gunderson, P., Melton, L., French, L., Renier, C., True, J., & Carr, W. (1992). Surveillance of injuries in agriculture. In U.S. Department of Health and Human Services, *Papers and Proceedings of the Surgeon General's Conference on Agricultural Safety and Health* (pp. 161–178). Washington, DC: USDHHS.

Goldsmith, M. (1989). As farmworkers help keep America healthy, illness my be their harvest. *Journal of the American Medical Association, 261*, 3207–3213.

Hays, W., & Laws, E. (1991). *Handbook of chemical toxicology*. London: Academic Press.

Hosken, A. F., Miller, T. A., & Hanford, W. D. (1988). *Occupational Injuries in Agriculture—A 35 State Summary* (Report No. DSR-87-0942). Morgantown, WV: National Institute for Occupational Safety and Health.

Jacobson, M. L., Mercer, M. A., Miller, L. K., & Simpson, T. W. (1987). Tuberculosis risk among migrant farmworkers on the Delmarva penninsula. *American Journal of Public Health, 77*, 29–32.

Jones, J. (1992) HIV-related characteristics of migrant workers in rural South Carolina. *Migrant Health Newsline* (Clinical suppl., March/April), 4.

Kaloyanova, F., & Batawi, M. (1991). *Human toxicology of pesticides*. Boca Raton, FL: CRC.

Kligman, E. W., Peate, W. F., & Cordes, D. H. (1991). Occupational infections in farmworkers. *State Art Review of Occupational Medicine, 6*, 429–446.

Koday, M., Rosenstein, D. I., & Lopez, G. M. (1990). Dental decay rates among children of migrant workers in Yakima, WA. *Public health Reports, 105*, 530–533.

Lafferty, J. (1991). Self-injection and needle sharing among migrant farmworkers [Letter to the editor]. *American Journal of Public Health, 81*, 221.

Lambert, M. I. (1995). Migrant and seasonal farmworker women. *Journal of Obstetric, Gynecologic, and Neonatal Nursing, 24*, 265–268.

Larson, A. L., & Plascencia, L. (1993). *Migrant Enumeration Project 1993*. Rockville, MD: Bureau of Primary Health Care.

Laughlin, J. A. (1977). *Foreigners in their own land: The migrant and mental health*. Chicago: Illinois Migrant Council.

Lopez, N. C. (1995, Fall). Meeting the challenge: Providing migrant farmworker housing. *Rural Voices*, 3–7.

Lotti, M. (1992). The pathogenesis of organophosphate polyneuropathy. In *Critical reviews in toxicology* (pp. 465–487) Boca Raton, FL: CRC.

Lowengart, R., & Peters, J. (1987). Childhood leukemia and parents' occupational and home exposures. *Journal of the National Cancer Institute, 79*, 39–46.

Lyons, M. (1992). Study yields HIV prevalence for New Jersey farmworkers. *Migrant Health Newsline* (Clinical suppl., March/April), 1–2.

McCauley, L. (1996). Reducing pesticide exposure in minority families (USDHNS-PHS. Grant No. ES-96-005). Portland, OR: CRUET–Oregon Health Sciences University.

Meister, J. L. (1991). The health of migrant farm workers. In *Occupational medicine: State of the art reviews* (Vol. 6, pp. 503–510). Philadelphia: Hanley & Balfus.

Meister, J. S., Warrick, L. H., Zapien, J. G., & Wood, A. H.. (1992). Using lay health workers: Case study of a community-based prenatal intervention. *Journal of Community Health, 17*, 37–51.

Mentzer, M., & Villalaba, B. (1988). *Pesticide exposure and health: A study of Washington farmworkers*. Granger, WA: Evergreen Legal Services, Farmworker Division.

Millar, J. D. (1991). Papers and proceedings of the Surgeon General's Conference on Agricultural Safety and Health. NIOSH Publication (pp. 92–105). Cincinnatti, OH: National Institute for Occupational Safety and Health.

Mines, R., & Kearney, M. (1982, April). *The health of Tulare County farmworkers: A report of 1981 survey and ethnographic research*. Visalia, CA: Tulare County Department of Health.

Mines, R., Gabbard, S., & Boccalandro, B. (1991). *Findings from the National Agricultural Worker's Survey. (NAWS) 1990: A demographic and employment profile of perishable crop farm workers* (U.S. Department of Labor, Office of Program Economics Research Report No. 1). Washington, DC: U.S. Government Printing Office.

Mines, R., Gabbard, S., & Samadrick, R. (1993). *U.S. farmworkers in the post-IRCA period*. Washington, DC: U.S. Department of Labor.

Mobed, K., Gold, E., & Schenker, M. (1992). Occupational health problems among migrant and seasonal farm workers. *Western Journal of Medicine, 157*, 367–373.

Moses, M. (1989). Pesticide-related health problems and farmworkers. *American Association of Occupational Health Nurses Journal, 37*, 115–130.

National Advisory Council on Migrant Health. (1995). *Losing ground: The condition of farmworkers in America*. Bethesda, MD: Department of Health and Human Services/Health Resources and Services Administration, Bureau of Primary Health Care, Migrant Health Branch.

National Migrant Resource Program. (1993). *1993 recommendations of the National Advisory Council on Migrant Health*. Austin, TX.

National Migrant Resource Program. (1995). *Dental survey*. Austin, TX.

O'Malley, M., Smith, C., Krieger, R., & Margetich, S. (1990). Dermatitis among stone fruit harvesters in Tulare County. *American Journal of Contact Dermatology, 1*, 100–111.

Pallack, K. (1991). *Oregon farm labor housing survey*. Newberg, OR: CASA of Oregon.

Richter, E. (1992). Aerial application and spray draft of anticholinesterases: Protective Measures. In B. Ballatyne & T. Aldridge (Eds.), *Clinical and experimental toxicology of organophosphates and carbamates* (pp. 623–631). Oxford, England: Butterworth-Hunenian.

Rust, G. S. (1990). Health status of migrant farmworkers: A literature review and commentary. *American Journal of Public Health, 80*, 1213–1217.

Ryan, R., Foulk, D., Lafferty, J., & Robertson, A. (1988). *Health knowledge and practices of Georgia's migrant and seasonal workers relative to AIDS: A comparison of two groups*. Georgia Southern College, Center for Rural Health (p. 1), as cited in National Resource Program Fact Sheet (1992).

Sasao, T., & Sue, S. (1993). Toward a culturally anchored ecological framework of research in ethnic-cultural communities. *American Journal of Community Psychology, 21*, 705–727.

Schenker, M. B., & McCurdy, S. A. (1988). Pesticides, viruses, and sunlight in the etiology of cancer among agricultural workers. In C. Becker (Ed), *Cancer prevention strategies in the workplace* (pp. 29–37). New York: Hemisphere.

Schuman, S., & Dobson, R. (1985). An outbreak of contact dermatitis in farmworkers. *Journal of the American Academy of Dermatology, 13*, 220–223.

Schwartz, D. A., & LoGerfo, J. P. (1988). Congenital limb reduction defects in the agricultural setting. *American Journal of Public Health, 78*, 654–657.

Sharp, D. S., Eskenazi, B., Harrison, R., Callas, P., & Smith, A. H. (1986). Delayed health hazards of pesticide exposure. *Annual Review of Public Health, 7*, 441–471.

Sidell, F. (1992). Clinical considerations in nerve agent intoxication. In S. Somani (Ed.), *Chemical warfare agents*. New York: Academic Press.

Simcox, N. J., Fenoke, R. A., Wolz, S. A., Lee, I., & Halma, D. A. (1995). Pesticides in household dust and soil: Exposure pathways for children of agricultural families. *Environmental Health Perspectives, 103*, 1126–1134.

Skjerdal, K., Misha, S., & Benavides-Vaello, S. (1996). A growing HIV/AIDS crisis among migrant and seasonal farmworker families. *Migrant Clinicians Network Streamline, 2*, 1–3.

Slesinger, D. (1992). Health status and needs of migrant farm workers in the United States: A literature review. *Journal of Rural Health, 8*, 227–234.

Slesinger, D. P., & Cautley, E. (1981). Medical utilization patterns of Hispanic migrant farmworkers in Wisconsin. *Public Health Reports, 96*, 255–263.

Slesinger, D. P., & Ofstead, C. (1990). *Migrant agricultural workers in Wisconsin*. 1989: Social, economic, and health characteristics. Madison: University of Wisconsin, Department of Rural Sociology.

Slesinger, D. P., & Ofstead, C. (1993). Economic and health care needs of Wisconsin migrant farmworkers. *Journal of Rural Health, 9*, 138–148.

Soliman, M. R., Derosa, C. T., Mielke, H. W., & Bota, K. (1993). Hazardous waste, hazardous materials and environmental health equality [Review]. *Toxicology and Industrial Health, 9*, 901–912.

Spear, R. (1991). Recognized and possible exposure to pesticides. In W. J. Hayes & E. Laws (Eds.), *Handbook of pesticide toxicology: Vol I. General principles* (pp. 245–274). San Diego, CA: Academic Press.

Sweeney, M., & Ciesielski, S. (1990, April). *Where work is hazardous to your health*. Raleigh, NC: Farmworkers Legal Services of North Carolina.

Ungar, B. L., Iscoe, E., Cutler, J., & Bartlett, J. G. (1986). Intestinal parasites in a migrant farmworker population. *Archives of Internal Medicine, 146*, 513–515.

U.S. Department of Labor. (1988). Occupational injury and illness incidence rates by industry. *Monthly Labor Review*, 118–119.

U.S. Department of Labor. (1989). *Occupational Injury & Illnesses, 1989*. Washington, DC: National Bureau of Labor Statistics.

U.S. Department of Health and Human Services. (1980). *Migrant health program target population estimates*. Rockville, MD: Author.

U.S. Department of Health and Human Services. (1992). *Papers and proceedings from the Surgeon General's Conference on Agricultural Safety and Health* (Vol. 15). Washington, DC: U.S. Government Printing Office.

U.S. Environmental Protection Agency. (1992). *Pesticide industry sales and usage. 1990 and 1991 market estimates*. Washington, DC: Author.

U.S. General Accounting Office. (1992). *Hired farmworkers: Health and well-being at risk* (Publication No. GAO/HRD-92-46). Washington, DC: Author.

Vasilion, T. M. (1992). Knowledge of AIDS among female Hispanic migrant farmworkers in Virginia. *Migrant Health Newsline* (Clinical suppl., March/April), 2–4.

Vega, W., Warheit, G., & Palacio, R. (1985). Psychiatric symptomatology among Mexican American farmworkers. *Social Science Medicine, 20,* 39–45.

Warrick, L. H., Wood, A. H., Meister, J. S., & Zapien, J. G. (1992). Evaluation of a peer health worker prenatal outreach and education program for Hispanic farmworker families. *Journal of Community Health, 17,* 13–26.

Weinstein, P., Domoto, P., Wohlers, K., & Koday, M. (1992). Mexican-American parents with children at risk for baby bottle tooth decay: Pilot study at a migrant farmworkers' clinic. *Journal of Dentistry for Children, 59,* 376–383.

Whorton, D., Milby, T., Krauss, R., & Stubbs, H. (1979). Testicular function in DBCP exposed pesticide workers. *Journal of Occupational Medicine, 21,* 161–166.

Wilk, V. A. (1986). *Occupational health of migrant and seasonal farmworkers in the United States.* (2nd ed.). Washington, DC: Farmworker Justice Fund.

Wilk, V. A. (1988). *Occupational health of migrant and seasonal workers in the U.S.: Progress report.* Washington, DC: Farmworker Justice Fund.

Wingo, C., Borgstrom, B., & Miller, G. (1986). Tuberculosis among migrant farm workers—Virginia. *Journal of the American Medical Association, 256,* 977, 981.

Woolfolk, M., Hamard, M., Bagramian, R., & Sgan-Cohen, H. (1984). Oral health of children of migrant farm workers in northwest Michigan. *Journal of Public Health Dentistry, 44,* 101–105.

Zham, S. H., & Blair, A. (1993). Cancer among seasonal farmworkers: An epidemiologic review and research agenda. *American Journal of Industrial Medicine, 24,* 753–766.

15

Health and Disease among Hispanics

SYLVIA GUENDELMAN

Introduction

The racial and ethnic composition of the United States is markedly influenced by a rapidly growing Hispanic population. From 1900 to 1996, the Hispanic population increased from less than 1% of the total U.S. population to almost 9% (U.S. Bureau of the Census, 1993). Estimated at 22.8 million, Hispanics are projected to be the largest ethnic group by the year 2000 (U.S. Bureau of the Census, 1993).

The health profile of Hispanics reflects the young age, high immigration flow, and low socioeconomic levels of this population (U.S. General Accounting Office, 1992). Proportionally, more Hispanics than non-Hispanic Whites (hereafter referred to as Whites) die from homicide and accidents during their adolescence and young adulthood. Hispanic morbidity is also higher for infectious diseases such as tuberculosis, septicemia, viral hepatitis, meningitis, pneumonia, and AIDS (Furino, 1992). In addition, Hispanics have a higher morbidity rate than Whites for a number of chronic illnesses including diabetes,

hypertension, cardiopulmonary problems, allergies, liver disease, and stroke ("Prevalence and Impact of Arthritis by Race and Ethnicity," 1995). Ethnic differences in morbidities such as tuberculosis and cervical cancer partly reflect barriers to access to health insurance and health services among Hispanics ("Prevalence and Impact of Arthritis," 1995; U.S. General Accounting Office, 1992). Yet, prevalence of the two main causes of death in the nation, namely, heart disease and cancer, are lower among Hispanic than White adults (W. Vega, 1994).

Indeed, a paradox exists with regard to Hispanic health status. The health profile of immigrant adults, including women of reproductive age, is better than expected in light of the disadvantaged conditions and barriers to access to care that they face (Furino, 1992; Guendelman, 1995b; W. Vega, 1994). Immigrant Hispanics constitute a young population with a strong work ethic and family orientation. These factors may protect them against adverse health outcomes.

The purpose of this review is to examine the patterns of health and disease of the Hispanic population taking a life cycle perspective. Biological and social factors are known to affect health throughout life and have cumulative effects (World Bank, 1994). In this review, the health status of pregnant women and infants, children between the ages of 1

SYLVIA GUENDELMAN • School of Public Health, University of California, Berkeley, California 94720-7360.

Handbook of Immigrant Health, edited by Loue. Plenum Press, New York, 1998.

and 12, adolescents, adults, and the elderly is described, following a brief demographic profile. Given that children, youth, and women of reproductive age comprise a large segment of the population, particular emphasis is placed on a health assessment of these target groups. Due to space limitations only outcome indicators of physical health are presented. Considering the heterogeneity in the Hispanic population, variations in health by country of origin and acculturation are highlighted whenever information is available. Finally, some implications of this health assessment for health promotion and disease prevention interventions are discussed.

The information presented in this chapter is useful to clinicians working with Hispanic immigrants because it identifies risks and protective factors that characterize the health profile of this population. The epidemiologic evidence also sensitizes the clinician to important differences among the Hispanic subpopulations and the underlying social and cultural conditions that influence the health status of immigrants. By gaining understanding of these issues, clinicians will be in a better position to make accurate assessments and prescribe culturally sensitive interventions that promote, restore, or maintain the health of immigrants. Researchers will also find the epidemiological evidence summarized in this chapter helpful insofar as it points out areas of vulnerability and strengths for Hispanics and identifies gaps in knowledge where future research can make significant contributions.

The Demographic Profile

High fertility and immigration account for the rapid growth of the Hispanic population. With a median age 9 years younger than Whites, the majority of Hispanics are of childbearing age. Culturally, Hispanics place strong values on family and child rearing which leads to a high fertility rate (Molina, 1994). In 1990, 14% of all births in the United States were to Hispanic women; the majority were births to Mexican women.

This decade marks the highest peak in U.S. immigration (legal and undocumented), with a high proportion of immigrants coming from Latin America (Fix & Passe, 1994). While accurate estimates of the number of undocumented immigrants are not available, it is estimated that more than 60% of the 3.2 million undocumented immigrants in the United States are from Mexico and other parts of Central America, and the Caribbean (Molina, 1994).

Historically, Hispanics are an extremely diverse population with a rich mosaic of differing ethnic heritage. Mexicans, the largest ethnic group in this country, make up 64.3% of all Hispanics. Puerto Ricans (10.6%), Cubans (4.7%), Central and South Americans (13.4%), and other Hispanics (7%) comprise the rest. More than 90% of Hispanics live in 10 states including California, Texas, Arizona, New Mexico, New York, and Florida. Hispanics are also well represented in Illinois and Colorado (Furino, 1992).

Proximity, occupational opportunities, and family ties encourage Hispanics to settle in metropolitan areas, with Puerto Ricans living predominantly in New York, Cubans in Florida, and Mexicans and Central Americans in Texas and California. The agricultural industry, especially in the southwest, is supported primarily by Mexican seasonal or permanent laborers, many of whom are undocumented. Both geography and legal status are important determinants of access to health services and of health status for Hispanics.

On average, Hispanic families are larger than White families. More than one half of Hispanic families consist of at least four members compared to three members among White families. Mexican, Central American, and South American families have the largest household size with almost one fifth of these being composed of more than six persons (U.S. Bureau of the Census, 1993). While the majority of Hispanic families are headed by a married couple, almost a fourth are headed by single women. Mexican and Cuban families are more likely to have households headed by a parental dyad while Puerto Ricans show a striking rate of female-headed households. More than 60% of children of parents of Puerto Rican descent live in single-parent families, a condition strongly associated with poverty (The Commonwealth Fund, 1995).

Poverty, low education, ineligibility for government funded health and social services, and lack of insurance coverage are paramount challenges facing Hispanics today. In 1993, one third of Hispanic families lived in poverty (U. S. Bureau of the Census, 1993). The median income of Hispanic households was nearly 70% lower than for White households. Statistics are even grimmer for children: almost 40% are living in poverty (The World Bank, 1994). Many live in poor or near-poor working families earning incomes below 200% of the federal poverty level. Undocumented status, low education, and lack of proficient English ability channel people into secondary labor markets which provide low salaries and no fringe benefits including health insurance. Almost 40% of Hispanic adults lacked health insurance in 1994 (Landale & Oropesa, 1995).

Although educational attainment has improved for Hispanics since 1980, the levels remain much lower than for non-Hispanics. A significant number of immigrants have less than a fifth-grade education. Only one half of young Hispanic adults report earning a high school diploma and less than 10% report earning a bachelor's degree. According to the last census, Cubans were more likely to have a bachelor's degree (25.1%), while Mexicans and Puerto Ricans were the least likely to attain a college education.

Partly as a result of low education, there continues to be a vast disparity between employment opportunities and income earnings capacity for Hispanics and Whites. While Hispanic representation in managerial and professional positions has increased in the past decade, the majority of Hispanics, both men and women, are employed in the service or manufacturing industry, agriculture, or construction (U.S. Bureau of the Census, 1993).

There is disagreement about whether Hispanics are climbing the economic ladder

across generations, the way earlier waves of European immigrants did. A recent study from southern California, where 21% of the nation's Hispanics are concentrated, indicates the presence of a flourishing Hispanic middle class. The middle class is progressing due to household income pooling rather than educational advancement (G. Rodriguez, 1996).

These varied demographic and historical characteristics influence the health of Hispanics of all age groups.

Maternal and Child Health

Previous studies on the reproductive health of Hispanic women consistently highlight three important findings. First, Hispanic women, who are younger, poorer, less educated and generally tend to initiate prenatal care later than White women, have birth outcomes that are comparable to those of White women (Cohen, Friedman, Hahan, Lederman, & Munoz, 1993; Guendelman & Abrams, 1994; Guendelman, Gould, Hudes, & Eskenazi, 1990; Ventura, 1988). Birth outcomes are usually measured by indicators such as birthweight, preterm birth, neonatal, postneonatal, and infant mortality. Except for preterm births and neonatal mortality, the birth outcomes of Hispanic women are not significantly different from those of Whites (Table 1) (Balcazar & Aoyama, 1991; J. E. Becerra, Hogue, Atrash, & Perez, 1991; *Monthly Vital Statistics Report,* 1996; Williams, Binkin, & Clingman, 1986).

Second, important ethnic variations exist in the maternal risk profiles and the birth outcomes of Hispanic subpopulations. National and local data indicate that Puerto Ricans, who have higher percentages of unmarried mothers, teenage mothers, and smokers during pregnancy (Kleinman, 1990; Ventura, 1988) also show the poorest birth outcomes. In contrast, Cuban Americans, who have the highest educational attainment, show the best outcomes (Cohen *et al.,* 1993; Ventura, 1988). Mexican Americans, despite their lower socioeconomic status, have significantly better outcomes than Puerto Ricans

TABLE 1. Birth Outcomes among Hispanic Subgroups and Non-Hispanic Whites

Indicators	Puerto Ricans	Mexican Americans	Cuban Americans	All Hispanics	Non-Hispanic Whites	Reference
% Low birth weight	9.3	5.7	5.9	6.2	5.6	Mendoza *et al.*
<2500 grams	7.9	4.9	4.8	5.5	4.7	(1991); Becerra *et al.* (1991)
% Very low birth weight	1.6	1.0	1.0	1.1	0.9	Mendoza *et al.*
<1500 grams	1.3	0.8	0.8	0.9	0.7	(1991); Becerra *et al.* (1991)
Teen preterm births (prior to 37 week gestation)	14.6	13.5	12.6	13.7	11.4	Mendoza *et al.* (1991)
Neonatal mortality (birth–28 days) (per 1,000 live births)	4.7	4.2	3.3	4.1	4.3	*Monthly Vital Statistics Report* (1996)
Post neonatal mortality (28 days –364 days) (per 1,000 neonatal survivors)	3.0	2.6	2.1	2.6	2.5	*Monthly Vital Statistics Report* (1996)
Infant mortality (per 1,000 live births)	7.6	6.8	5.4	6.7	6.8	*Monthly Vital Statistics Report* (1996)

(Table 1) (J. E. Becerra *et al.*, 1991; Cohen *et al.*, 1993; Guendelman *et al.*, 1990; *Monthly Vital Statistics Report*, 1996).

Finally, foreign-born women have more favorable birth outcomes than U.S.-born women of Hispanic descent (J. E. Becerra *et al.*, 1991; J. Collins & Shay, 1994; J. C. Collins & David, 1990; Guendelman *et al.*, 1990; Scribner & Dwyer, 1989; Williams *et al.*, 1986). In one recent study in Chicago, U.S.–born Mexican and other Hispanic mothers in very low-income census tracts had rates of infants with low birth weight of 14% and 15%, respectively, while foreign–born Hispanic mothers residing in similar areas had rates of 3% and 7% (Scribner & Dwyer, 1989). The low birth weight rate of foreign–born mothers was 40% lower than that of low-income White mothers (Camilli, McElroy, & Reed, 1994). Similarly, data from the Hispanic Health and Nutrition Examination Survey (HHANES), which is the largest health survey available on Hispanics, reveal that first-generation Mexican Americans have lower rates of low birth weight (3.9%) than the second generation (6.1%) (Guendelman *et al.*, 1990). Other investigations reveal that Puerto Rican–born Hispanics have lower rates of low-weight births than women born in the continental United States (J. E. Becerra *et al.*, 1991; Cohen *et al.*, 1993).

The Epidemiological Paradox

It is intriguing to note that while Hispanic women have risk profiles similar to African American women showing impoverished, poorly educated, and medically underserved conditions, they have birth outcomes far superior, and closer to those of White women (California Department of Health Services, 1994; J. Collins & Shay, 1994; Guendelman, 1995c; Institute of Medicine, 1985; Shiono & Behrman, 1995). The favorable birth outcomes of Hispanic women despite the high prevalence of risk factors that have traditionally been associated with poor birth outcomes is often referred to as an epidemiological paradox.

Attempts to unravel this paradox have primarily focused on Mexican Americans. This population tends to experience delayed entry into prenatal care, have larger families with shorter birth-spacing intervals, and higher rates of teen pregnancy than Whites, yet enjoys positive birth outcomes at an equivalent rate (Guendelman, 1995c). It is especially puzzling that Mexican-born women, who tend to be even poorer, less educated, and face more difficulties in access to care than native-born Mexican Americans, have more favorable pregnancy outcomes (Guendelman, 1995c).

Research indicates that there are no straightfoward explanations for the epidemiological paradox of positive pregnancy outcomes in the at-risk Mexican American population. Several hypotheses have surfaced that point to deficits among immigrants, such as an underreporting of infant deaths and ethnic misclassification in birth or death certificates. The possibility that excess fetal deaths might eliminate weaker fetuses before birth is another proposed explanation (Powell-Griner & Streck, 1982). However, a California study of low-income women found that fetal death rates among Hispanics was somewhat lower than the rate among Whites (Guendelman, Chavez, & Christianson, 1994).

Other hypotheses focus on the positive or "protective" factors that may contribute to healthy outcomes. Selective migration may favor healthy mothers and healthy babies insofar as individuals with economic resources, skills, and good health are more likely to migrate from Mexico (Guendelman, 1995c). In addition, immigrant mothers may bring with them certain attitudes, values, and behaviors that protect them against stresses and other harmful conditions associated with poverty and resettlement in a new society. A compelling explanation from the "prevention" perspective is that immigrants may be profiting from sociocultural and behavioral factors whose benefits outweigh the risks stacked against them. Healthy habits such as refraining from the use of tobacco, alcohol, and illicit drugs during pregnancy, and good nutrition are associated with good pregnancy outcomes. Kinship networks and family stability are other potential explanations of healthy outcomes for Hispanic newborns.

Healthy Habits of Women of Reproductive Age

Studies show that Hispanic women consistently report lower rates of tobacco use than White women. Guendelman and Abrams (1994) compared 664 Mexican American women in the Hispanic HANES and 1,156 White women in the second national HANES (NHANES) across stages of the reproductive cycle and found that whereas 23% of Mexican American women smoked in the interconceptional period, only 8.1% smoked during pregnancy. In contrast, among White women there were nearly twice as many interconceptional smokers (43%). This level remained high during pregnancy at 37.3%.

Evidence from a recent study at a prenatal clinic in Tucson, Arizona, showed that Mexican American smokers are more likely to abstain from smoking during pregnancy than White smokers (Camilli et al., 1994). Of the 200 Mexican American women participating in the study, 24% smoked in the year prior to their pregnancy compared with 51% of the 131 non-Hispanic White women participants. While only 19% of the Mexican American women had smoked during any part of their pregnancy, 48% of their White counterparts had done so. In addition, Mexican Americans smoked almost 5 fewer cigarettes per day than non-Hispanic Whites (6.9 vs. 11.8). After controlling for age and amount of smoking, the odds of abstaining from cigarettes during pregnancy were 4.7 times higher for Mexican American than non-Hispanic White women (Guendelman et al., 1994).

In a study exploring perinatal substance use among almost 30,000 women attending 202 hospitals in California in 1992, W. A. Vega, Kolody, Hwang, and Noble (1993) found that Hispanic women, primarily of Mexican descent, were far less likely than White women to have reported that they smoked during pregnancy (3.3% vs. 14.8%). Foreign-born Hispanic women were 3.6 times less likely to smoke than native-born Hispanics (1.8% vs. 6.6%) (W. A. Vega et al., 1993). Since evidence shows a clear and consistent association between low birth weight, infant mortality, and smoking during pregnancy, the low rate of smoking for Hispanic women is clearly advantageous (Guendelman, 1995c).

Alcohol use during pregnancy has been associated with both short- and long-term negative health effects for infants, including congenital malformations, mental retardation, and low birth weight (Chomitz, Cheung, & Leiberman, 1995). While evidence is mixed, alcohol use during pregnancy appears to be low among Mexican American women. In W. A. Vega and colleagues' (1993) study, positive alcohol screens were more likely among Hispanic (both U.S.– and foreign-born) than White women (6.9% vs. 6.1%). Yet in Guendelman and Abrams' (1994) study using Hispanic HANES data, pregnant Mexican American women on average consumed .02 daily servings of alcohol compared to .08 servings among pregnant White women.

Prenatal use of controlled substances has been correlated with fetal growth retardation, perinatal death, and pregnancy and delivery complications (Fricker & Segal, 1978; Lifschitz, Wilson, & Smith, 1983; Oleske, 1977; Robins, Mills, Krulewitch, & Herman, 1993; Zelson, Rubio, & Wasserman, 1971). In the drug exposure study by W. A. Vega and colleagues (1993), significantly fewer Hispanics tested positive for any drug at the time of delivery than did White women (2.8% vs. 6.8%). Foreign-born Hispanic women had even lower prevalence rates of drug abuse (W. A. Vega et al., 1993). Recent studies conducted in San Diego supported the findings of much lower rates of illicit drug usage for Hispanic women compared with White women (Rumbaut & Weeks, 1994).

The intake of specific minerals, vitamins, and proteins have been related to pregnancy outcomes for all ethnic groups (Abrams & Berman, 1993; Institute of Medicine, 1990). Guendelman and Abrams (1994) compared the intake of eight nutrients between Mexican American women and non-Hispanic White women of reproductive age. Immigrant women born in Mexico had a higher average intake of protein, vitamins (A, C, folic acid), and calcium relative to the recommended dietary allowance standards than White women or U.S.–born Mexican Americans (Guendelman, 1995c). Although this study did not follow women through their pregnancies, the results suggest that nutrition may help to explain the much lower rate of low birth weight among foreign-born Mexican American women than

among U.S.–born women of Mexican descent (California Department of Health, 1987; Guendelman et al., 1990).

Kinship Networks and Family Stability

Social factors related to family and social networks seem to provide clues to better reproductive health. Research on Hispanics describe the centrality of the family and the closeness of kinship ties (Bean, Russell, & Marcum, 1977; Keefe, Padilla, & Carlos, 1979; Swicegood, Bean, Stephen, & Opitz, 1988; Triandis, Sashima, Hui, Losanshy, & Marin, 1982). Hispanic kinship networks and support may translate into more knowledge about healthy pregnancies, encourage positive behaviors, and lessen stress during pregnancy, all of which promote healthy birth outcomes. They may also alter hormonal and immunological responses associated with pregnancy complications (McClean, Hatfield-Timajchy, Wingo, & Floyd, 1993).

Compared with non-Hispanic Whites, Mexican Americans have a higher proportion of husband–wife families and lower rates of divorce and separation. Family stability among Mexican Americans appears to be highest among ever-married women who have the lowest educational level and the highest use of Spanish exclusively (Frisbie & Bean, 1995). Family stability may play a role in the case of teenage pregnancies as well. Teen pregnancy appears to be more common and more culturally accepted among Hispanics than Whites and infants of Hispanic teen mothers are often cared for by extended family (R. Becerra & de Anda, 1984).

Prolonged Protection into Early Childhood

A question remains whether the protective factors available during pregnancy continue to sustain the health of Hispanic children after they are born. A study by Guendelman, English, and Chavez (1995) assessed more than 700 infants in San Diego County to determine whether health advantages at birth are retained at 8 to 16 months of age or if instead, socioeconomic conditions deplete healthy status at birth.

According to this study, among the infants born without serious medical problems, almost three fourths (74%) remained healthy; that is, they had no history of serious infectious disease. For 26% of the infants, health status was eroded by social conditions. The prevalence of serious infectious diseases such as bronchitis or pneumonia among these infants was comparable with that of non-Hispanic infants raised in central Harlem and other disadvantaged communities. Factors associated with illness were large households, barriers to care, and maternal characteristics. In households with more than 10 members, the odds of an ill child were approximately 4.5 times larger than homes with only 2 to 4 members. Mothers who experienced barriers to pediatric care were twice as likely to have an ill child. Moreover, maternal characteristics including smoking, pregnancy complications, and employed status were found to positively correlate with child illness. In addition, those mothers that were newcomers to the United States and spoke Spanish exclusively were more likely than non-newcomers to have ill children. These findings suggest that while a protective sociocultural orientation may buffer the infant from environmental insults and detrimental effects of poverty *in utero,* it may not be strong enough to counteract these effects after the infant is born.

The Effects of Acculturation

As women become more acculturated their risk profile changes. They tend to smoke, drink, and use illicit drugs at a higher rate and their diet deteriorates. Changes in the risk profile are accompanied by changes in birth outcomes (Guendelman & Abrams, 1994; W. A. Vega *et al.,* 1993). Although the Hispanic HANES study by Guendelman and colleagues (1990) found that second-generation Mexican American women had worse health outcomes than first-generation women, a more recent study by Guendelman and English (1995) reveals that it might take only 5 years after moving to the United States for Mexican immigrant women to begin to show changes in risk profiles and birth outcomes.

In their study of more than 1,000 immigrants in two California counties, Guendelman and English (1995) found that long-term residents living in the United States for 5 years or more were more likely to smoke, have unplanned pregnancies, suffer pregnancy complications, and to deliver preterm and low–birth weight infants than newcomers living in the United States less than 5 years. These findings suggest that birth outcomes may be highly sensitive to acculturative effects. Foreign-born women seem to enjoy the advantages of a protective sociocultural orientation which becomes eroded with acculturation and time spent in the United States.

Health Status among Children 1–12 Years of Age

Children's health has improved steadily in recent years due to immunization and nutrition programs, safety regulations, advances in medical technology, and public assistance programs that promote access to health services (Coiro, Zill, & Bloom, 1994). Despite progress, ethnic disparities in maternal perceptions of children's health and in health status indicators continue to exist. Two to three times as many Hispanic mothers (11.4% Mexican American, 15.2% Puerto Rican, and 16.5% Cuban American) as White mothers (5%) rate their children in poor health (Mendoza *et al.,* 1991). Evidence suggests an association between health perceptions and actual health status (Mendoza *et al.,* 1991). On a number of health status indicators Hispanic children are at increased risk in comparison with Whites: immunization coverage is lower while the risk for infectious diseases, chronic diseases such as asthma and lead poisoning, oral health, and unintentional injuries is higher (Table 2) (Arfaa, 1981; Bass, Mehta, & Eppes, 1992; Bates, 1995; "Blood Lead

Levels Among Children," 1995; California Department of Health Services, 1996; Carter-Pokras & Gergern, 1993; Casey Foundation, 1996; "Children at Risk from Ozone Air Pollution," 1995; "Firearm-Related Deaths," 1992; Fischbach, Lee, Englehart, & Wheeler, 1993; Guendelman, 1995a; Ismail & Szpunar, 1990; Ismail, Burt, Brunelle, & Szpunar, 1988; "Leads from the MMWR," 1988; Lee, Gomez-Marin, & Lee, 1996; Looker, Johnson, McDowell, & Yetley, 1989; Markland & Durand, 1976; Marks, Halpin, Irvin, Johnson, & Keller, 1979; Matteucci, Holbrook, Hoyt, & Molgaard, 1995; Mayer & Le Clere, 1994; McCormick, Zee, & Heiden, 1982; National Institute of Dental Research, 1989; Salas, Heifetz, & Barrett-Connor, 1990; San Francisco Department of Public Health, 1995; Sargent *et al.*, 1995; Sargent, Stukel, Dalton, Freeman, & Brown, 1996; Snyder, Mohle-Boetani, Palla, & Fenstersheib, 1995; U.S. Department of Health and Human Services, 1993; "Vaccination Coverage of 2-Year-Old Children," 1994; Waldman, 1996; P. Wood, Humberto, Hidalgo, Prihoda, & Kromer, 1993); D. Wood *et al.*, 1995.

Infectious Disease

Vaccine Preventable Disease

The Centers for Disease Control estimate that while 75% of the nation's children entering kindergarten are immunized (Casey Foundation, 1996), only 65% complete the basic immunization series by their second birthday. This coverage is far below the year 2000 national objective to vaccinate 90% of children in this age group. Although school-age Hispanic children seem to have coverage comparable to White children ("Vaccination Coverage," 1994), Hispanic 2-year-olds trail behind. For instance, the 1996 California Kindergarten Retrospective Survey examined the proportion of California kindergarten children who were up to date for immunizations at 24 months. According to this survey, 51.5% Hispanic children were up to date with their immunizations compared with 65.7% White children (California Department of Health Services, 1996).

Because of poverty, urban living, and multiple barriers to access to care, Hispanic chil-

TABLE 2. Health Status among Hispanic Subgroups and Non-Hispanic White Children

Health indicators or profile	All Hispanics	Mexican American	Puerto Rican	Cuban American	Non-Hispanic Whites	Reference
Immunization	51.5	—	—	—	65.7	California Dept. of Health Services (1996)
Prevalence of chronic medical conditions	—	3.9	6.2	2.5	3.8	Mendoza *et al.*, (1991)
Asthma % active (per 1,000)	—	4.5	8.8	20.1	6.4	Carter-Pokras & Gergern (1993)
Lead exposure 6 months to 5 years	1.3	—	—	—	1.2	Sargent *et al.* (1995)
Iron deficiency	18	—	—	—	11.6[a]	Sargent *et al.* (1996)
Bilateral hearing loss (per 1,000)	—	27.6	68.3	67.7	15.5	Lee *et al.* (1996)
% with 1 or more diagnosis of ocular disorder	22.3	—	—	—	25.2	Fischbach *et al.* (1993)
Rate of decayed, missing, or filled teeth (DMF)	—	2.13	2.07	2.96	1.97	Ismail & Szpunar (1990); National Inst. Dental Research (1989)
Motor vehicle accidents	36.2	—	—	—	34.0	Waldman (1996)

dren are at an increased risk for sporadic out-breaks of communicable diseases such as measles. In Los Angeles County during the 1980s measles epidemic, Hispanic children had a risk that was 12.6 times greater for contracting measles than non-Hispanic Whites and 3.6 times greater risk than African Americans ("Leads From the MMWR," 1988; D. Wood et al., 1995).

Other risk factors found to inhibit full immunization coverage include demographic characteristics such as single-parent status, lack of English proficiency, and increased parity, as well as life stressors and maternal health risk behaviors (Guendelman, 1995a; Markland & Durand, 1976; Marks et al., 1979; San Francisco Department of Health, 1995). In a recent California study, incomplete immunization status among infants under 16 months of age was strongly associated with maternal risk behaviors (Guendelman, 1995a). Smoking, alcohol consumption, and failure to use car seatbelts increased the likelihood of inadequate immunization coverage. When these behaviors were grouped into a maternal risk index, which also included the failure to safeproof electrical outlets and a poor organization of the home environment, a dose–response effect was found. Specifically, the odds of a delay in the immunization schedule increased 38% with each increase in the maternal risk score (Guendelman, 1995a). Evidence further suggests that while prenatal care and family size are strongly associated with underimmunization coverage at 3 months, as age increases beyond infancy, maternal and child characteristics appear to be less significant while insurance coverage and access to a regular source of care gain importance as determinants of immunization (D. Wood et al., 1995).

Parasites

Because parasitic diseases are endemic in many Latin American countries, screening for parasites has become a more prevalent health care practice in the United States. Soil-transmitted parasites such as round-worm, hookworm, and whipworm, and protozoa parasites such as giardia are prevalent in migrant farmworker communities, as well as among recent immigrants from Central America and border populations. Cystercercosis, a helminthic infection of the central nervous system known to cause seizures is a relatively common parasitic disease in the Southwest particularly among immigrant children (Arfaa, 1981; McCormick et al., 1982).

Crowded living conditions and exposure to other children may exacerbate the problem. In a study at a Massachusetts community clinic, 35% of 124 children screened were carriers of pathogenic parasites; Brazilian and Central American children demonstrated the highest rates (Bass et al., 1992). A similar study in a Los Angeles clinic found parasitic prevalence among half of a sampled group of 125 foreign-born Central Americans. In contrast, a parasite prevalence rate of only 14% was reported for U.S.–born Central American children (Salas et al., 1990).

Chronic Medical Conditions

Asthma

Childhood asthma, affecting 5 million children, is the most common pediatric chronic illness. It is the leading cause of school absenteeism and childhood hospitalization, disability, and childhood morbidity. According to Hispanic HANES data, the highest prevalence of active childhood asthma in the United States occurs in the Puerto Rican community (11.2%) (Carter-Pokras & Gergern, 1993). Secondhand smoke, along with poverty, urban living, and poor housing, has been associated with increasing rates of asthma among Puerto Ricans. Prevalence rates are also elevated among Cuban Americans (8.8%) compared with White non-Hispanic children (6.4%). Although rates among Mexican Americans are lower (4.5%), they may be deflated due to underreporting (P. Wood et al., 1993).

Poverty-related conditions such as exposure to environmental toxins in urban areas, respiratory infections that spread in overcrowded housing arrangements, and antigens such as cockroaches and mites exacerbate asthmatic symptoms. Almost 70% of Hispanic children reside in high ozone areas which place them at risk for asthma. In addition, studies show that asthma is more debilitating to poor children without access to regular medical care than non-poor children (Bates, 1995; "Children at Risk," 1995; P. Wood *et al.*, 1993).

Lead Exposure

While the rate of lead poisoning nationwide appears to be declining because of elimination of lead in gasoline, Hispanic and African American children remain at high risk for lead exposure ("Blood Lead Levels," 1995; Sargent *et al.*, 1995).

Living in old rented homes in poor urban areas increases the likelihood of lead exposure for Hispanic children. For instance, in a 1993 screening in Rhode Island, Hispanic children, while comprising less than 5% of the population, accounted for 35% of the elevated blood lead levels. Children under the age of 2 living in old, deteriorating houses appeared to be particularly at risk ("Blood Lead Levels," 1995).

Another study conducted in California found that Mexican-born children's high rate of lead was due to the following exposures while they were living in Mexico: leaded gasoline emissions, lead-glazed ceramics, lead-based paints, and lead in canned food and beverages (Snyder *et al.*, 1995).

Iron-Deficiency Anemia

The past 20 years have shown a decline in the prevalence of iron deficiency in U.S. children, probably as a result of fortification of infant foods with iron and nutritional programs. Despite this decline, children of minority status who live in poverty and are ineligible for assistance programs remain at risk for iron deficiency (Sargent *et al.*, 1996).

Data on iron deficiency in Hispanic children is limited, especially for those under 5

years of age. Yet, one study conducted in Massachusetts with almost 12,000 children between the ages of 6 months and 5 years found that 18% of Hispanic children were iron deficient compared with 11.6% of the rest of the population (Sargent *et al.*, 1996). However, lead levels among children 9 months to 5 years of age were not higher among Hispanics compared with Whites in a recent study conducted in San Francisco (San Francisco Department of Public Health, 1995). A comparison between NHANES and Hispanic HANES data on iron status showed no differences between Hispanic and White children over 5 years of age (Looker *et al.*, 1989).

Eye and Ear Disorders

There has been little research on the prevalence of eye and ear disorders in Hispanic children. Ethnic comparisons for eye disorders show similar prevalences for Hispanic and White children (Fischbach *et al.*, 1993). In contrast, data collected by the Hispanic HANES and NHANES surveys show a higher prevalence of hearing problems at or above the 30db hearing threshold level among Hispanics, with strikingly high numbers for Cuban American (11.7%) and Puerto Rican (9.6%) children compared with White children (3.7%). Although findings are inconsistent, higher rates of otitis media at an early age in Hispanics versus non-Hispanics may partly account for the higher rates of hearing loss (Lee *et al.*, 1996).

Oral Health

Oral health is an extremely good indicator of socioeconomic status. One measurement of oral health status refers to the score of decayed, missing, and filled teeth (DMFT) and the prevalence of gum disease or gingivitis. Hispanic HANES data for 1982 to 1984 revealed that almost half of the children ages 5 to 17 years were free from cavities with DMFT scores similar to other groups (Ismail & Szpunar, 1990; National Institute of Dental

Research, 1989). However, low-income families reported children to be twice as likely to have cavities (National Institute of Dental Research, 1989). Furthermore, gingivitis was prevalent in more than two thirds of Mexican Americans (Ismail *et al.*, 1988). Similarly, a screening of 6- and 7-year-old immigrant and refugee children in San Francisco showed a DMFT score double the average as compared with same-age native-born children of all ethnicities ("Leads from the MMWR," 1988). One third of the immigrant or refugee children were reported to have serious dental conditions in comparison with only one tenth of nonimmigrant children (D. Wood *et al.*, 1995).

Unintentional Injuries

Unintentional injuries, the leading cause of child death, has claimed more children's lives annually than the next six causes of childhood deaths combined (U.S. Department of Health and Human Services, 1993). Motor vehicle accidents were the leading cause of injury-related deaths in 1990, resulting in one third of accidental deaths of children under 5 years of age and almost one half of accidental deaths of children under the age of 10 (Waldman, 1996).

Ethnic minority children are disproportionately affected by injuries (Mayer & Le Clere, 1994). For example, a study of injured children in a San Diego trauma center found that compared with White children, Hispanic children had significantly longer stays in intensive care units; this speaks to the severity of injuries. While Hispanic children were more likely to be struck by a vehicle as a pedestrian, they were less likely than White children to be injured from falls (Matteucci *et al.*, 1995). In addition, Hispanic children were significantly less likely to have been restrained in motor vehicle accidents and to have worn a helmet in motorcycle and bicycle accidents (Matteucci *et al.*, 1995).

The use of preventive devices such as smoke detectors, car seats, and seat belts decreases the risk for childhood unintentional injuries. National data indicate that Hispanics utilize injury preventive measures less than Whites. A 1990 survey showed that while 68.2% of Whites had functional smoke detectors in their homes, only 54.7% of Hispanics were protected by such devices. Furthermore, the frequency of car seat and seat belt usage among Whites (60%) was higher than among Hispanics (45%) (Mayer & Le Clere, 1994).

Firearm-related deaths have recently surpassed motor vehicle accidents to become the leading cause of injury-related mortality for children over 10 years of age in some southwestern states. In 1990, Hispanic and White youngsters had similar firearm-related death rates at 17.4 per 100,000 and 16.8 per 100,000, respectively, rates far below those for African Americans at 32.3 per 100,000 ("Firearm-Related Deaths," 1992).

The Health Status of Adolescents

Hispanic adolescents, whose numbers are expected to more than double between 1980 and 2030 from 4.7 million to 9.6 million, account for the fastest growing group of minority youths in the United States (Children's Defense Fund, 1990). A variety of socioeconomic factors including living in poor, female-headed households, dropping out of school, and lack of health insurance coverage place these youngsters at risk for negative health outcomes (Children's Defense Fund, 1990; Lieu, Newacheck, & McManus, 1993; P. Smith, McGill, & Watt, 1987). A survey conducted in 1988 of more than 7,000 youths ages 10–17 showed that compared to 11% of Whites and 16% of African Americans, 28% of Hispanics lacked health insurance (Lieu *et al.*, 1993).

From a health standpoint, Hispanic youth have high rates of risk-taking behaviors, teenage pregnancy, and sexually transmitted diseases (STDs) including HIV (Brindis, 1992; "Preliminary Data on Births and Deaths," 1995). Further, the prevalence rates of obesity, violence-related injuries, and substance abuse are more elevated than the rates for White youth (Table 3) (Adams, Schoenborn, Moss,

Warren, & Kann, 1995; Must, Gortmaker, & Dietz, 1994; Rodriguez & Brindis, 1995; Schinke, Orlandi, & Vaccaro, 1992).

These adverse health outcomes not withstanding, progress in some health-related behaviors should be noted. The birth rate for Hispanic teens mirrored the nation's in 1995 and declined up to 3% from 1994. Further, the rate of births to unmarried adolescents declined by 5% for this time period ("Preliminary Data," 1995).

Risk-taking Behaviors

Evidence suggests that Hispanic adolescents engage in more risk-taking behaviors than White youth of comparable age groups (Brindis, Wolfe, & McCarter, 1995). Ethnic differentials in smoking, drinking, and consumption of illegal drugs have been particularly noted. Hispanic youth, of which 14% smoke, have the highest smoking prevalence rate, followed by 12% of Whites, 11% of African Americans, and 9% of Asians (Moreno et al., 1991). In 1993, almost 46% of Hispanics ages 12 to 21 had smoked at least one entire cigarette in their lifetime (Adams et al., 1995). This puts Hispanics at a higher risk for developing a smoking habit than other ethnic groups. While the level of smoking is higher for older adolescents and for males, it is the younger adolescents and

TABLE 3. Health Status for Hispanic and Non-Hispanic White Adolescents

Health indicators	All Hispanics	Non-Hispanic Whites	Reference
Smoking	51.3%	48.5%	Schinke et al. (1992)
Alcohol consumption	72.5%	76.1%	Schinke et al. (1992);
males	29.9%	33.4%	Adams et al. (1995)
females	25.5%	33.5%	
Illegal drugs: Marijuana	37.1%	26.4%	Schinke et al. (1992)
Cocaine	9.6%	6.7%	
Smoking	51.30%	48.50%	
STDs:			
gonorrhea rate: males	439.2/100,000	151/100,000	Brindis (1992)
females	389.1/100,000	359/100,000	
syphilis rate: males	30.4/100,000	1.4/100,000	
females	21.7/100,000	4.2/100,000	
HIV	15%	42%	
Childbearing 15–19 years	106.2/1,000	50.3/1,000	"Prelim. Data" (1995)
Pregnancy desired	37%	42%	Smith et al. (1987)
Ever had intercourse	49%	52%	Brindis (1992)
Obesity prevalence: males	23.2%	15.8%	Must et al. (1994)
females	21.9%	15%	
Homicide-related injuries			Rodriguez &
(age 15–24): males	26.2/100,000	9.1/100,000	Brindis (1995)
females	5.6/100,000	3.9/100,000	
Nonfatal intentional			Rodriguez &
injuries: males	48.3/1,000	39.7/1,000[a]	Brindis (1995)
females	23.9/1,000	22.6/1,000[a]	
Weapon carrying: gun	17.2%	21.9%	Adams et al. (1995)
knife	59.3%	59.3%	
other	23.5%	18.9%	
Suicide attempts (see also Guendelman, 1995c)			Vega et al. (1993)
males	9.0%	6.9%	
females	17.5%	19.3%	

[a] Includes all non-Hispanic races

the females who attempt to give up this habit. For example, in 1992, 69% of all smokers ages 12 and 13, as well as 62% of females and 52% of males ages 14 to 17, had attempted to quit smoking at least once during the previous 6 months.

Although it is illegal in the United States for a minor to purchase tobacco products, the percentage of smokers ages 12 to 17 who regularly purchase their own cigarettes has been climbing since 1989. For Hispanic adolescents, this rate has climbed 17% from 1989 to 1993 compared to 3.4% for Whites. Further, Hispanics seem less likely than non-Hispanics to have ever been asked for proof of age when purchasing cigarettes ("Accessibility of Tobacco Products to Youths Aged 12–17 Years," 1996).

Cultural norms may indirectly contribute to adolescent smoking behaviors. For instance, while Mexican American parents are no more likely than non-Hispanics to be accepting of their children's smoking, they may unknowingly contribute to this problem by prompting their children to engage in smoking-related behaviors. These prompts, which include asking the adolescent to help the parent light the cigarette or to purchase cigarettes for the parent, in turn increase the adolescent's risk for cigarette smoking (Moreno et al., 1991).

Smoking is associated with the consumption of other addictive substances such as alcohol and illegal drugs (Marcell, 1994). In 1990, of 1,500 San Francisco high school students surveyed, at least 26% of Hispanic adolescents drank some type of alcohol once a week or more; at least 13% drank daily to the point of intoxication (Morales, 1990). While Hispanic women are cited in the literature as more likely to abstain from alcohol, this study found no significant gender differences. Drinking was significantly higher for Central American adolescents. High rates of alcohol consumption may account for Hispanics being overrepresented in arrests due to driving while intoxicated (Felix-Ortiz & Newcomb, 1992). In a recent study Schinke and colleagues (1992) found no correlation

between ethnicity and substance use among Hispanic and White adolescents. Nonetheless, adolescents with average and lower than average grades appeared to be at higher risk for substance abuse.

Thirty-one percent of the nation's youth 12 to 21 years of age have ever used an illegal substance, in the form of either street drugs or medication without a doctor's prescription, with marijuana use being most commonly reported (Adams et al., 1995). Among Hispanic adolescent males, history of drug use (29.9%) is not statistically different from that of White adolescent males (33.4%) and both these rates are slightly higher than for African Americans (27.5%). In contrast, the percentage of Hispanic adolescent females ever having used drugs is lower than that of White females (25.5% vs. 33.5%) but slightly higher than the rate for African Americans (23.1%) (Adams et al., 1995).

Gender differences in risk-taking behavior may be partially explained by cultural norms that allow for young Hispanic girls to receive more protection from their parents than males (Marcell, 1994; Sokol-Katz & Ubrich, 1992). Furthermore, cultural double standards allow males more freedom for experimentation (Baird, 1993). These norms may account for less female engagement and delay in initiating risky behaviors such as sexual intercourse, involvement with alcohol and drugs, and violent behavior.

It has been shown that Hispanic adolescents, excluding Cuban Americans, tend to engage in more risk-taking behavior if they come from female-headed households (Marcell, 1994; Sokol-Katz & Ulbrich, 1992). Further, the risk of violent crime as well as other types of victimization is three times greater for Hispanic families living in poverty (M. Rodriguez & Brindis, 1995). Nevertheless, native-born Hispanics are more likely to use alcohol and marijuana compared with foreign-born Hispanics, who are generally poorer (Brindis et al., 1995). Such evidence suggests that in addition to socioeconomic factors, acculturation poses a risk for unhealthy habits among teenagers.

Sexually Transmitted Diseases

Hispanic adolescents regardless of gender report having less open communication with their parents or other adults regarding issues of sexuality (Brindis, 1992; Marchi & Guendelman, 1994–1995). Women in particular feel less able to initiate such discussion for fear of being perceived as disrespectful (Flores-Ortiz, 1994). Family communication patterns combined with low access to formal information about reproductive issues and to health care puts this population at risk for transmission of STDs, HIV, and pregnancy (Brindis *et al.,* 1995). Living in communities with high prevalence of STDs and a low use of condoms adds to the risk of these adverse outcomes.

In 1994, 372 teens between 13 and 19 years of age had AIDS (Centers for Disease Control, 1997). Hispanic adolescents have twice the rate of AIDS as compared with White adolescents (K. Smith, McGraw, Crawford, Costa, & McKinley, 1993). This rate is attributed to an abundance of high-risk practices, such as unprotected sex and intravenous drug use, in this population (Flores-Ortiz, 1994). HIV risk is elevated for females because the risk for HIV is higher among Hispanic male partners (K. Smith *et al.,* 1993).

Overall, the rates of most STDs are highest among sexually active teenagers because they are more likely than adults to engage in unprotected sex and have multiple partners who often have STDs (Centers for Disease Control, 1995). The prevalence of STDs such as gonorrhea, chlamydia, and syphilis continue to be disproportionately higher for Hispanic youth than they are for Whites (Centers for Disease Control, 1995). The most current estimates indicate that 21.3 and 266.2 per 100,000 of 10- to 14-year-old and of 15- to 19-year-old Hispanics, respectively, were treated for gonorrhea in 1994. That same year, only 11 per 100,000 of Whites ages 10 to 14 and 156.1 of those ages 15 to 19 were treated for this condition (Centers for Disease Control, 1995). Unfortunately, while rates of gonorrhea have been declining for all adoles-

cents ages 10 to 19, they have been climbing steadily for Hispanics ages 10 to 14 since 1991.

Childbearing

Hispanics overall begin childbearing relatively early compared with Whites. Mexican Americans have the highest fertility rates and Cuban Americans the lowest (Aneshensel, Fielder, & Becerra, 1989; Brindis, 1992; Children's Defense Fund, 1990). Although 45% of single Hispanic adolescents ages 15 to 19 report having had sexual intercourse, a rate lower than that of African Americans at 61% or Whites at 52%, their rates of giving birth to a live infant (15%) are over twice as high as that of Whites of the same age group (7%) (Aneshensel *et al.,* 1989). Further, Hispanic females make up only 9% of the adolescent population of the United States, yet they account for 14% of all births to adolescent mothers, and they are more likely than Whites or African American teens to give birth again within 3 years of their first birth (Children's Defense Fund, 1990).

There are several reasons for Hispanic adolescents' high rates of parity. First, they tend to have a smaller knowledge base of reproductive and contraceptive issues than White adolescents. For example, only 20% of Hispanic adolescent immigrants report always using birth control compared with 33% of U.S.–born Hispanics and 35% of White adolescents (Brindis *et al.,* 1995). Second, among pregnant teens, Hispanics tend to be less likely to terminate the pregnancy (Aneshensel *et al.,* 1989). Further, young Hispanics appear to consider their pregnancy a *happy time* (R. Becerra & de Anda, 1984) regardless of the timing and do not expect their families or peers to react negatively to the news of the pregnancy (R. Becerra & de Anda, 1984; P. Smith *et al.,* 1987; Sokol-Katz & Ulbrich, 1992).

Compared to more than 50% and 60%, respectively, of their White and African American counterparts, only 27% of Hispanics in 1987 who had a child during their teen years had completed high school by their mid-twenties (Brindis, 1992; Children's Defense Fund, 1990). Further, twice as many Hispanics are out of school right before or immediately following a delivery. These ethnic or racial differentials may be partially rooted in cultural expectations that prescribe that motherhood become the primary responsibility for the pregnant Hispanic mother (Brindis, 1992).

Obesity

While it has been difficult to track trends of obesity in adolescents, it appears that the prevalence in Hispanic teens has been increasing in recent years (Malina, 1993). Especially Hispanic adolescent males have a higher prevalence of obesity compared with other racial or ethnic groups. The prevalence of obesity among Hispanic adolescent girls is second only to African Americans and is three times more prevalent for females living in poverty (Must et al., 1994). Not only has adolescent obesity been linked to increased obesity-related morbidity in adulthood, but the adverse social and psychological consequences of obesity in youth may be as detrimental as long-term physical health problems (Must et al., 1994). Obesity in adolescence has been associated with less acceptance by peers, discrimination by significant adults, poor body image, poor self-concept, depression, problems in family relations, and poor school performance.

Violence and Unintentional Injuries

Hispanic communities bear a disproportionate share of violence-related death and injury compared with the general population. Homicide has been labeled as the second leading cause of death among Hispanic teens and young adults (M. Rodriguez & Brindis, 1995). In 1991, the rate for Hispanic adolescent males was four times the rate for White teens ages 15–24 (M. Rodriguez & Brindis, 1995). Hispanic women experience violence at five times lower levels than males. Based on 1991 statistics, the rate for females was 5.6 per 100,000 compared to 26.2 per 100,000 for males (M. Rodriguez & Brindis, 1995).

In 1990, guns accounted for one in every four deaths among persons between the ages of 15 and 24 and for 77% of homicides among adolescents ages 15 to 19 (M. Rodriguez & Brindis, 1995). Forty-one percent of male Hispanic high school students reported carrying a gun; this rate was much higher than that of White male adolescents at 28.6%. Also Hispanic adolescent females reported carrying a gun over twice as often as White females ("Physical Fighting Among High School Students," 1992; M. Rodriguez & Brindis, 1995).

Violent crimes, including rape, robbery, and assault, occur at much higher rates for Hispanic adolescents than for youth of other ethnicities. For example, the rate of victimization for Hispanic males is approximately 48 per 1,000 compared to 40 per 1,000 for non-Hispanic males. The risk of engaging in fights at school is also higher for Hispanics than Whites perhaps because Hispanic adolescents face more learning difficulties particularly if English is their second language. Educational attainment is inversely associated with violence (M. Rodriguez & Brindis, 1995). Sixteen percent of adolescent males and 4.4% of adolescent females reported having had a recent fight in school that required medical treatment compared to 10% of White males and 2.4% of White females ("Physical Fighting," 1992). In addition, household burglary and larceny is 65% higher for Hispanics at 240 per 1,000 than for non-Hispanics (M. Rodriguez & Brindis, 1995).

The consumption of alcohol or illegal drugs is also associated with serious youth crime and with injuries due to driving under the influence. Hispanic teens who consume alcohol, drugs, or both tend to do so in higher quantities than adolescents from other ethnicities. Poverty plays an important role in the rates of consumption since there exists a higher concentration of alcohol outlets in low-income and ethnic minority neighborhoods ("Physical Fighting," 1992; M. Rodriguez & Brindis, 1995).

Suicide

Suicide is the third leading cause of death among teenagers between the ages of 15 and 19 years (Burge, Felts, Chenier, & Parrillo, 1995) and is becoming a serious problem among males ages 15 to 24 years (Adams *et al.*, 1995). Hispanics show low rates of suicide yet have high levels of suicidal attempts. Risks for suicidal ideation behaviors include acute stress; depression and low self-esteem, or mental health problems; family dysfunction; substance abuse; limited social opportunities; and poor academic performance. Multiple risk factors have been shown to increase the prevalence of suicide ideation and attempts among all adolescents (Burge *et al.*, 1995).

Drug use and immigrant status are consistently related to high levels of suicide ideation among Hispanic adolescents. While in one study conducted in multiethnic Miami, 12- to 14-year-old Cuban Americans had the lowest suicidal ideation, Nicaraguans had the highest lifetime prevalence of suicide attempts. High alcohol use was a frequently reported risk factor among Cubans whereas family substance abuse was more commonly reported among Nicaraguans and other Hispanics. Youngsters suffering from stresses due to acculturation show heightened vulnerability for suicide attempts, but the extent to which posttraumatic stress disorders or other experiences of migration influence suicidal attempts or ideation is not known (W. Vega *et al.*, 1993).

Acculturation

Acculturation, defined as the level of immigrants' adaptation to the mainstream culture, has diverse implications for the health of Hispanic adolescents. Low acculturation, for example, can serve to buffer the teenager from multiple risk factors associated with the lifestyle of mainstream adolescents. For instance, adherence to traditional cultural val-

ues among Mexican American adolescents, such as protecting virginity and abstinence from addictive substances in girls and valuing the family among males, can be salutogenic insofar as it has been linked to lower rates of delinquent behavior in males (Marcell, 1994), and to later onset of first intercourse among females (Marcell, 1994; Reynoso, Felice, & Shragg, 1993). Conversely, low acculturated individuals are more likely to be of low socioeconomic status and experience barriers to care. Consequently they tend to suffer from poorer health outcomes such as oral health (Marcell, 1994).

Adult Health Status

Another Epidemiological Paradox

The health of Hispanic adults tends to be much better than is expected given their socioeconomic status and is comparable to or often better than that of Whites of similar poverty levels (Table 4) (Council on Scientific Affairs, 1991; Nickens, 1991; Perez-Stable, Marin, & Marin, 1994; Sorlie, Backlund, Johnson, & Rogot, 1993; W. Vega, 1994). For example, Hispanics have lower rates of cardiovascular disease and lung cancer (W. Vega, 1994), and lower mortality rates for these diseases across income groups compared with Whites (Sorlie *et al.*, 1993; Winkleby, Fortmann, & Rockhill, 1993). Rates of breast, prostrate, and colorectal cancer are also better than or similar to the rates for Whites (Bassford, 1995). Furthermore, the overall mortality rate for Hispanics over 65 years of age is significantly lower than that of Whites (3,482/100,000 and 5,106/100,000, respectively) (W. Vega, 1994). This epidemiological paradox found among adults is similar to that found among women of reproductive age with respect to birth outcomes.

Cultural aspects such as an extended family and community system, combined with diets reflective of their country of origin, have been cited as positively influencing the health of Hispanics (Winkleby *et al.*, 1993).

TABLE 4. Health Status among Hispanic Subgroups and Non-Hispanic White Adults

Health indicators	Puerto Rican	Cuban American	Mexican American	All Hispanics	Non-Hispanic Whites	Reference
Diabetes (ages 45–74)	26.1%	15.8%	23.9%			Council on Scientific Affairs (1991)
Overweight						Vega (1994); Council Scientific Affairs (1991)
males	25%	29%	30%			
females	37%	34%	39%		27%	
Hypertension			18%		19.2%	Centers for Disease Control (1995); Caralis (1992)
males				15%		
females				10.1%		
Tuberculosis				18.3/100,000	9.1/100,000	Vega (1994)
Syphilis						Vega (1994)
males				22.8/100,000	2.9/100,000	
females				10.7/100,000	1.8/100,000	
HIV/AIDS				14%		Council on Scientific Affairs (1991)
HIV				20%		Vega (1994)
females						
Smoking	41.3%	42.8%	43.6%	23%	25.6%	Council on Scientific Affairs (1991); Perez-Stable et al. (1994)
Arthritis				11.2%	15.2%	"Prelim. Data" (1995)

Chronic Diseases

These favorable outcomes not withstanding, low-income Hispanics who tend to be uninsured and lack access to care remain at risk for cardiovascular disease and certain cancers. Hypertension often goes unrecognized and untreated among low-income Hispanics who have a high prevalence of hypertension (Caralis, 1992; Council on Scientific Affairs, 1991). Furthermore, issues of compliance with treatment prevail, and almost half of those who know they are hypertensive do not take medications to regulate their condition; of those who do take blood pressure–regulating medicines, less than one quarter actually have the disease under control (Caralis, 1992). These factors may explain why despite having lower heart disease mortality rates than other ethnic groups, Hispanics have not been as successful as Whites or African Americans in lowering their rates of cardiovascular diseases (Caralis, 1992). In addition, when data is analyzed by gender, Hispanic women may have more risks and a higher prevalence for cardiovascular disease than White women (Chipella & Feldman, 1995).

Low-income Hispanics may lack the necessary knowledge to be able to detect cancer's early warning signs and may be less likely or able to seek health care (Villar & Menck, 1994). This may impact the prevalence of cancer of the stomach, esophagus, pancreas, and cervix which are significantly higher in this population (Council on Scientific Affairs, 1991). Mexican Americans tend to begin treatment for cancer later than other Hispanic groups; they consequently tend to have worse outcomes than Puerto Ricans or Cuban Americans (Villar & Menck, 1994).

Hispanic adults are also at risk for other chronic diseases such as diabetes and arthritis. Of Hispanics ages 45 to 74, 26.2% of Puerto Ricans, 23.9% of Mexican Americans, and 15.8% of Cuban Americans suffer from type II, non-insulin-dependent diabetes mellitus (Council on Scientific Affairs, 1991).

While diabetes affects Cuban Americans at rates similar to those of non-Hispanic Whites, Puerto Ricans and Mexican Americans have rates of diabetes that are two to three times higher than Whites (Burge *et al.,* 1995; W. Vega, 1994). Of Hispanics with diabetes, Mexican Americans tend to have six times more complications, including end-stage renal disease and retinopathy, than Whites (W. Vega, 1994).

A correlation has been found between diabetes in Hispanics and obesity and diet (Council on Scientific Affairs, 1991). This finding is of special concern in light of the fact that close to one third of Hispanics are overweight, that Mexican Americans tend to have higher levels of cholesterol and triglycerides than Whites, and that the prevalence of a sedentary lifestyle is higher among Hispanics than among Whites (Perez-Stable *et al.,* 1994).

Self-reported, age-adjusted rates of arthritis are significantly lower for Hispanics (11.2%) than they are for Whites (15.5%). Nevertheless, the proportion of Hispanics (22.2%) who report having a physical limitation attributed to this condition is higher than that reported by Whites (17.5%) ("Prevalence and Impact of Arthritis by Race and Ethnicity," 1995). A higher prevalence of functional impediments may be associated with obesity and low socioeconomic status ("Prevalence and Impact," 1995).

Communicable Diseases

Communicable diseases such as tuberculosis, STDs, and AIDS continue to be of primary concern for adult Hispanics in the United States (W. Vega, 1994).

While the rate of tuberculosis for the native-born population is continuously decreasing ("Tuberculosis Morbidity," 1996) the rates of diagnosis are rising in the foreign-born population (Cantell, Snider, Cauthen, & Onorato, 1995). This is particularly evident among Mexicans who comprise a large percentage of new immigrants (J. Collins & Shay, 1994). Furthermore, tuberculosis is significantly more prevalent among Hispanics than among

Whites, 22.4/100,000 vs. 4/100,000, respectively (Cantell *et al.,* 1995). Although the number of reported cases dropped slightly among Hispanics from 1994 to 1995 (Bassford, 1995), a comparison of the tuberculosis rates from 1985 through 1992 shows that Hispanics made up 33% of the excess cases compared to 18% for Whites.

Among sexually transmitted diseases, the rates of syphilis are exponentially larger in Hispanics, 10.7/100,000 in women and 22.8/100,000 in men, than in Whites, 1.8/100,000 in women and 2.9/100,000 in men (W. Vega, 1994). Further, chancroid, chlamydia, and gonococcus all affect Hispanics disproportionately (W. Vega, 1994). With respect to AIDS, Hispanics account for 14% of all reported cases (Council on Scientific Affairs, 1991). Among Hispanics, Puerto Ricans are at highest risk for contracting HIV with rates up to seven times higher than those of Whites (Diaz, Buehler, Castro, & Ward, 1993). More than 65% of reported cases of AIDS among men born in Central and South America, Cuba, and Mexico were associated with male to male sex and less than 10% of transmission in this group was linked to injection drug use (Diaz *et al.,* 1993). By contrast, 61% of AIDS cases among Puerto Rican men were attributed to injection drug use and only 22% were associated with male to male sex (Diaz *et al.,* 1993). Among U.S.–born Hispanics, 51% of the AIDS cases were associated with male to male sex and 35% with injection drug use (Diaz *et al.,* 1993).

Hispanic women have one of the most rapid growths of infection and account for 20% of all HIV in women (W. Vega, 1994). Both foreign- and native-born women have higher rates of transmission through sexual contact with an injection drug user than non-Hispanic White women (Diaz *et al.,* 1993). Similar to the situation of adolescents, limited knowledge of the disease and its prevention, as well as cultural norms limiting condom use, help aggravate this problem among adult Hispanic women (Council on Scientific Affairs, 1991).

Risk-Taking Behaviors

Hispanic adults, not unlike teenagers, tend to engage in risky behaviors that have been linked to negative health outcomes (W. Vega, 1994). The rate for heavy alcohol use, for example, is slightly higher for Hispanics (7.3%) than for Whites (6.4%) or Blacks (4.8%) (U.S. Department of Health and Human Services, 1997). This may account for Hispanics, in particular Mexican Americans and Puerto Ricans, being at very high risk for alcoholism and cirrhosis of the liver (Burge et al., 1995). The pattern of drinking for Latino males often includes a period of abstention followed by binge-type drinking which is more likely to be excessive than non-Hispanics' drinking (Perez-Stable et al., 1994).

Hispanics also have a disproportionate number of deaths related to narcotic addictions (Burge et al., 1995). Marijuana and cocaine use varies by Hispanic origin group but tends to be more prevalent among Puerto Ricans (W. Vega, 1994). In 1994, 1.1% of all Hispanics identified themselves as current cocaine users compared to only .5% of Whites. Nonetheless, Hispanics have the lowest rates of overall substance abuse, 5.4%, when compared with Whites, 6%, or Blacks, 7.3% (Department of Health and Human Services, 1997). This lower rate is remarkable in that Hispanics report higher levels of exposure to drugs when compared with Whites. In a 1994 survey, 9.7% reported having been approached by a drug seller and 18% of them reported having witnessed a drug deal in their neighborhood; Whites reported approximately 5% for each instance (www.health.org, 1997).

Although some studies have found that Hispanic smokers are at higher risk for being heavy smokers (20+ cigarettes daily), adult Hispanics have smoking rates that are slightly lower than that of Whites or African Americans, 23%, 25.6%, and 26.2%, respectively (Perez-Stable et al., 1994). Similar to the situation of adolescents, female adults' smoking rates tend to be significantly lower than those of their male counterparts. In 1990, for example, 16.3% of Hispanic women smoked compared with 30.9% of males (Perez-Stable et al., 1994). It must be noted that this discrepancy in gender-specific smoking patterns has helped to lower the rates of smoking prevalence for this population. Among all Hispanics, those who are less acculturated smoke significantly less and are more likely to make an attempt to quit smoking than those more acculturated (Palinkas, Pierce, Rosbrook, Pickwell, & Bal, 1993). In addition, Hispanic men and women are more likely to be occasional smokers than other groups, and although they are aware of the harmful effects of cigarettes, they are less likely to believe that smoking is addictive (Palinkas et al., 1993).

Oral Health

The oral health of Hispanics follows their socioeconomic profile: those living in poverty have a significantly higher number of decayed or missing teeth (Watson & Brown, 1995). The fact that Hispanics are less likely than Whites or African Americans to have dental insurance, and that 7% of Hispanic adults have never visited a dentist, leads to their being twice as likely as Whites to have an untreated oral disease (Watson & Brown, 1995). Furthermore, Hispanics receive emergency dental work more often than Whites or African Americans (Watson & Brown, 1995). Among Hispanics, Puerto Ricans tend to have the highest rates of gingivitis and periodontal disease and Mexican Americans have the highest rates of untreated tooth decay (Watson & Brown, 1995). In addition to difficulties of access to dental care, a lack of adherence to regular oral hygiene and knowledge of the importance of oral hygiene may also be associated with adverse dental health for Hispanics.

Elderly Adults

Across ethnic subgroups, Puerto Ricans tend to have more limitation of activities and more acute conditions than Mexican Americans, but Cuban Americans usually have the best health status (Council on Scientific Affairs, 1991; W. Vega, 1994). Studies show that despite elderly Hispanics being in better health than their White counterparts, they perceive their health status to be worse than that reported by Whites (Villa, Cueliar, Gamel, & Yeo, 1993). While rates of cardiovascular disease and cancer are not significantly different from those of White seniors, older Hispanics experience a higher prevalence of non-insulin-dependent diabetes mellitus morbidity and mortality than do other populations (Bassford, 1995; Villa *et al.,* 1993). In addition, older Hispanics are at higher risk for obesity, hypertension, and cancers of the liver, pancreas, stomach, and cervix. Possibly due to high rates of smoking by Hispanic elderly males when young, this population suffers from a higher prevalence of chronic obstructive pulmonary disease and lung cancer than younger Hispanics (Bassford, 1995).

Similar to the situation of their younger counterparts, barriers to health care such as lack of health insurance and language difficulties negatively affect the level of care that older Hispanics receive. Poor access contributes to the low rates of preventive health screenings in this population (Bassford, 1995). Consequently, although elderly Hispanics experience hearing loss at rates up to 48%, less than 10% report using a hearing aid (Bassford, 1995). Their oral health also tends to suffer: 24% of elderly Hispanics have never seen a dentist compared to 0.5% of Whites (Watson & Brown, 1995). And, possibly due to an underdiagnosing of depression, suicide rates for Puerto Rican and Cuban American males which peak between 25 and 35 years of age, rise again in the later years (Bassford, 1995). Despite these vulnerabilities, the lower mortality rates of Hispanic seniors compared with Whites attests to the remarkable sturdiness of Hispanic elderly persons.

Conclusion and Implications for Health Promotion and Disease Prevention

This review summarized the available epidemiologic literature on Hispanics across the life cycle. Several limitations in the studies that were reviewed require that the epidemiologic findings be interpreted with caution. A large body of evidence is based on secondary data which have some shortcomings. For instance, while the Hispanic HANES has generated important population-based estimates of health outcomes and risk and protective factors, it is already quite dated. Data for this one-time cross-sectional survey were collected in 1982–1984. Surveys conducted more recently do not sample sufficiently large numbers of Hispanics to allow for reliable calculation of estimates. In addition, public data sets such as birth and death certificates and registries on reportable diseases such as STDs or cancer often classify ethnic groups in different ways. Moreover, the registries may be incomplete. Furthermore, the census undercount of minority groups, and particularly of undocumented groups, may lead to inflated estimates of disease incidences and mortality rates among Hispanics and within subpopulations of Hispanics. Some of the studies that were reviewed used primary data collected with purposive samples in local communities. These data, although current, cannot yield population-based rates.

Although data limitations leave many gaps in information, the accumulated evidence attests to the wide heterogeneity among Hispanic subpopulations by socioeconomic status, country of origin, length of stay in the United States, acculturation, and migration background. From a lifestyle perspective the health profile of Hispanics is mixed. On the one hand, Hispanic adults, including women of reproductive age, do not seem to conform to the traditional "minority health profile." Despite facing socioeconomic disadvantages and barriers to care, Hispanics compared with Whites fare comparably if not better than Whites on major outcomes such as birth outcomes, cardiovascular diseases, and certain types of cancer. On the other hand, beyond favorable outcomes at birth, children and youth stand a high risk of unintentional injuries, chronic illness, and infectious diseases. And, regardless of age, Hispanics have elevated prevalences of high-risk behaviors and oral health problems. These vulnerabilities appear to be largely associated with living in poverty, disadvantaged neighborhoods, and stresses related to acculturation.

The most effective ways to improve health status among Hispanics may be through a combination of health promotion and disease prevention strategies and through improvements in access to care and health insurance coverage. Health promotion strategies must address the underlying causes of health problems by providing information and skills to individuals to reduce risk behaviors and increase or reinforce protective behaviors. In addition, addressing health problems in the Hispanic community will require strong local community leadership and the development of collaborative efforts among health organizations, non-health sectors, the media, and community residents. These collaborative efforts must address the social and environmental conditions that contribute to risk factors in Hispanic communities, including issues of poverty, violence, poor housing, anti-immigrant feelings, a deteriorating educational system, and lack of health insurance coverage for the working poor and near poor.

Acknowledgments

I would like to thank Veronica Angulo and Jana Oxenreider, two graduate students in the School of Public Health, who helped in the preparation of this manuscript, devoting many hours of their time, and Lora Santiago for clerical support.

References

Accessibility of tobacco products to youths aged 12–17 years—United States, 1989 and 1993. (1996). *Morbidity and Mortality Weekly Report, 45,* 125–129.

Abrams, A., & Berman, C. (1993). Women, nutrition and health. *Current Problems in Obstetrics, Gynecology and Fertility, 1,* 3–61.

Adams P., Schoenborn, C., Moss, A., Warren, C., & Kann, L. (1995) Health-risk behaviors among our nation's youth: United States, 1992. *Vital and Health Statistics Series 10: Data from the National Health Interview Survey, 192,* 1–51.

Aneshensel C., Fielder, E., & Becerra, R. (1989). Fertility and fertility-related behavior among Mexican-American and non-Hispanic white female adolescents. *Journal of Health and Social Behavior, 30,* 56–76.

Arfaa, F. (1981). Intestinal parasites among Indochinese refugees and Mexican immigrants resettled in Contra Costa County, California. *Journal of Family Practice, 12,* 223–226.

Baird, T. (1993). Mexican adolescent sexuality: Attitudes, knowledge, and sources of information. *Hispanic Journal of Behavioral Sciences, 15,* 402–417.

Balcazar, H., & Aoyama, C. (1991). Interpretative views on Hispanics' perinatal problems of low birth weight and prenatal care. *Public Health Reports, 106*(4), 420–425.

Bass, J., Mehta, K., & Eppes, B. (1992). Parasitology screening of Latin American children in a primary care clinic. *Pediatrics, 89*(2), 279–283.

Bassford, T. (1995). Health status of Hispanic elders. *Ethnogeriatrics, 11,* 25–37.

Bates, D. (1995). Observation on asthma. *Environmental Health Perspectives, 103,* 243–246.

Bean, F., Russell, L., & Marcum, J. (1977). Familism and marital satisfaction among Mexican-Americans: The effects of family size, wife's labor force participation, and conjugal power. *Journal of Marriage and Family, 39,* 759–776.

Becerra, J. E., Hogue, C. J., Atrash, H. K., & Perez, N. (1991). Infant mortality among Hispanics: A portrait of heterogeneity. *Journal of the American Medical Association, 265,* 217–221.

Becerra, R., & de Anda, D. (1984). Pregnancy and motherhood among Mexican-American adolescents. *Health and Social Work, 2,* 106–123.

Blood lead levels among children—Rhode Island, 1993–1995. (1995). *Morbidity and Mortality Weekly Report, 44*(42), 788–791.

Brindis, C. (1992). Adolescent pregnancy prevention for Hispanic youth: The role of schools, families, and communities. *Journal of School Health, 62*(7), 345–351.

Brindis C., Wolfe, A., & McCarter, V. (1995). The associations between immigrant status and risk-behavior patterns in Latino adolescents. *Journal of Adolescent Health, 17,* 99–105.

Burge, V., Felts, M., Chenier, T., & Parrillo, A. (1995). Drug use, sexual activity, and suicidal behavior in U.S. high school students. *Journal of School Health, 65,* 222–227.

California Department of Health Services, Center for Health Statistics. (1987). *California birth cohort file.* Sacramento, CA: Center for Health Statistics.

California Department of Health Services. (1994). *Analysis of health indicators for California's minority populations.* Sacramento, CA: Center for Health Statistics.

California Department of Health Services. (1996). *Immunization Branch 1996 Kindergarten Retrospective Survey*. Sacramento, CA: Author.

Camilli, A., McElroy, L., & Reed, K. (1994). Smoking and pregnancy: A comparison of Mexican-American and non-Hispanic white women. *Obstetrics and Gynecology, 84,* 1033–1037.

Cantell, M., Snider, D., Cauthen, G., & Onorato, I. (1995). Epidemiology of tuberculosis in the United States, 1985 through 1992. *Journal of the American Medical Association, 272,* 535–539.

Caralis, P. (1992). Coronary artery disease in Hispanic Americans. *Postgraduate Medicine, 91,* 179–188.

Carter-Pokras, O., & Gergern, P. (1993). Reported asthma among Puerto Rican, Mexican-American, and Cuban children, 1982 through 1984. *American Journal of Public Health, 83*(4), 580–582.

Casey Foundation. (1996). *Kids Count data book* (State profile of child wellness). Baltimore: Author.

Centers for Disease Control. (1995, September 1). "Hypertension Among Mexican-Americans—United States, 1982–1984 and 1988 to 1991 [http://wonder.cdc.gov/WONDER/anon/ANON1128/MMRW1.00.ex].

Centers for Disease Control. (1997, January 15). Count of AIDS cases as of December 1994; by age: Ages 0–54; Hispanics (N = 76), 323.

Centers for Disease Control, Division of STD Prevention. (1995). *Sexually transmitted disease surveillance, 1994.* (U.S. Department of Health and Human Services, Public Health Service). Atlanta, GA: Author.

Children at risk from ozone air pollution—United States, 1991–1993. (1995) *Morbidity and Mortality Weekly Report, 44*(16), 309–312.

Children's Defense Fund. (1990). *Latino youths at a crossroads.* Washington, DC: Author.

Chipella, N., & Feldman, H. (1995). Renal failure among male Hispanics in the United States. *American Journal of Public Health, 85,* 1001–1004.

Chomitz, V. R., Cheung, L., & Leiberman, E. (1995). The role of lifestyle in preventing low-birthweight. *Future of Children, 1,* 121–138.

Cohen, B., Friedman, D., Hahan, C., Lederman, L., & Munoz, D. (1993). Ethnicity, maternal risk, and birth weight among Hispanics in Massachusetts, 1987–89. *Public Health Reports, 108*(3), 363–371.

Coiro, M., Zill, N., & Bloom, B. (1994). Health of our nation's children. *Vital and health statistics, Series 10, data from the National Health Interview Survey, No. 191* (DHHS Publication No. [PHS] 95–1519). Washington, DC: U.S. Department of Health and Human Services.

Collins, J., & Shay, D. (1994). Prevalence of low birth weight among Hispanic infants with United States–born and foreign–born mothers: The effect of urban poverty. *American Journal of Epidemiology, 139*(2), 184–191.

Collins, J. C., & David, R. J. (1990). The differential effect of traditional risk factors on infant birthweight among blacks and whites in Chicago. *American Journal of Public Health, 80,* 679–681.

The Commonwealth Fund. (1995). *National comparative survey of minority health care.* Unpublished manuscript, The Commonwealth Fund.

Council on Scientific Affairs. (1991). Hispanic health in the United States. *Journal of the American Medical Association, 265,* 248–252.

Diaz, T., Buehler, J., Castro, K., & Ward, J. (1993). AIDS trends among Hispanics in the United States. *American Journal of Public Health, 83,* 504–509.

Felix-Ortiz, M., & Newcomb, M. (1992). Risk and protective factors for drug use among Latino and white adolescents. *Hispanic Journal of Behavioral Sciences, 14,* 291–919.

Firearm-related deaths—Louisiana and Texas, 1970–1990. (1992). *Morbidity and Mortality Weekly Report, 41*(13), 213–221.

Fischbach, L., Lee, D., Englehardt, R., & Wheeler, N. (1993). The prevalence of ocular disorders among Hispanic and Caucasian children screened by the UCLA mobile clinic. *Journal of Community Health, 18*(4), 201–211.

Fix, M., & Passe, J. (1994). *Immigration and immigrants setting the record straight.* Washington, DC: Urban Institute.

Flores-Ortiz, Y. (1994). The role of cultural and gender values in alcohol use patterns among Chicana/Latina high school and university students: Implications for AIDS prevention. *International Journal of the Addictions, 29,* 1149–1171.

Fricker, H., & Segal, S. (1978). Narcotic addiction, pregnancy, and the newborn. *American Journal of Diseases of Children, 132,* 360–366.

Frisbie, W., & Bean, F. (1995). The Latino family in comparative perspective: Trends and current conditions. In C. Jacobson (Ed), *Racial and ethnic families in the United States* (pp. 29–71). New York: Garland.

Furino, A. (Ed.). (1992). *Health and policy and the Hispanic.* Boulder, CO: Westview.

Guendelman, S. (1995a). The effects of maternal health behaviors and other risk factors on immunization status among Mexican-American infants. *Pediatrics, 95*(6), 823–827.

Guendelman, S. (1995b). *Immigrants may hold clues to protecting health during pregnancy: Exploring a paradox.* Paper presented at the 1995 Wellness Talk, University of California, Berkeley.

Guendelman, S. (1995c). Immigrants may hold the clues to protection of health during pregnancy: Exploring a paradox. *Wellness Series, 47*–75.

Guendelman, S., & Abrams, B. (1994). Dietary, alcohol, and tobacco intake among Mexican-American women of childbearing age: Results from the HHANES data. *American Journal of Health Promotion, 8*(5), 363–372.

Guendelman, S., English, P., & Chavez, G. (1995). Infants of Mexican immigrants: Health status of an emerging population. *Medical Care, 33*(1), 41–52.

Guendelman, S., & English, P. (1995). The effect of United States residence on birth outcomes among Mexican immigrants: An exploratory study. *American Journal of Epidemiology, 142*(9), 530–538.

Guendelman, S., Gould, J. B., Hudes, M., & Eskenazi, B. (1990). Generational differences in perinatal health among the Mexican American population: Findings from HHANES 1982–84. *American Journal of Public Health, 80* (Suppl.), 61–65.

Guendelman, S., Chavez, G., & Christianson, R. (1994). Fetal deaths in Mexican American, black, and white non-Hispanic women seeking government-funded prenatal care. *Journal of Community Health, 19*(5), 319–330.

Institute of Medicine, Committee to Study the Prevention of Low Birthweight. (1985). *Preventing low birthweight.* Washington, DC: National Academy Press.

Institute of Medicine. (1990). *Nutrition during pregnancy.* Washington, DC: National Academy Press.

Ismail, A., & Szpunar, S. (1990). The prevalence of tooth loss, dental caries, and periodontal disease among Mexican-Americans, Cuban-Americans, and Puerto Ricans: Findings from HHANES 1982–1984. *American Journal of Public Health, 80,* 66–70.

Ismail, A., Burt, B., Brunelle, J., & Szpunar, S. (1988). Dental caries and periodontal disease among Mexican-American children from five southwestern states, 1982–1983. *Morbidity and Mortality Weekly Report, CDC Surveillance Summaries, 37*(SS3), 33–45.

Keefe, S., Padilla, A., & Carlos, M. (1979). The Mexican American extended family as an emotional support system. *Human Organization, 38,* 144–152.

Kleinman, J. C. (1990). Infant mortality among racial/ethnic minority groups, 1983–1984. *Morbidity and Mortality Weekly Report, 39* (SS-3), 31–39.

Landale, N., & Oropesa, R. (1995) *Immigrant children and the children of immigrants: Inter- and intra-ethnic group differences in the United States.* (Research Paper 95-02). East Lansing: Michigan State University, Population Research Group.

Leads from the MMWR. Measles—Los Angeles County, California, 1988. (1988). *Journal of the American Medical Association, 261*(8), 1111–1115.

Lee, D., Gomez-Marin, O., & Lee, H. (1996). Prevalence of childhood hearing loss. *American Journal of Epidemiology, 144*(5), 442–448.

Lieu, T., Newacheck, P., & McManus, M. (1993). Race, ethnicity, and access to ambulatory care among U.S. adolescents. *American Journal of Public Health, 83*(7), 960–965.

Lifschitz, M., Wilson, G., Smith, E., & Desmond, M. (1983). Fetal and postnatal growth of children born to narcotic dependent women. *Journal of Pediatrics, 102,* 686–691.

Looker, A., Johnson, C., McDowell, M., & Yetley, E. (1989). Iron status: Prevalence of impairment in three Hispanic groups in the United States. *American Journal of Clinical Nutrition, 49,* 553–558.

Malina, R. (1993). Ethnic variation in the prevalence of obesity in North American children and youth. *Critical Reviews in Food Science and Nutrition, 33,* 389–396.

Marcell, A. (1994). Understanding ethnicity, identity formation, and risk behavior among adolescents of Mexican descent. *Journal of School Health, 64,* 323–327.

Marchi, K., & Guendelman, S. (1994–1995). Gender differences in the sexual behavior of Latino adolescents: An exploratory study in a public high school in the San Francisco Bay area. *International Quarterly of Community Health Education, 15,* 209–226.

Markland R., & Durand, D. (1976). An investigation of sociopsychological factors affecting infant immunization. *American Journal of Public Health, 66,* 168–170.

Marks, J., Halpin, T., Irvin, J., Johnson, D., & Keller, J. (1979). Risk factors associated with failure to receive vaccinations. *Pediatrics, 64,* 304–309.

Matteucci, R., Holbrook, T., Hoyt, D., & Molgaard, C. (1995). Trauma among Hispanic children: A population-based study in a regionalized system of trauma care. *American Journal of Public Health, 85*(7), 1005–1007.

Mayer, M., & Le Clere, F. (1994). Injury prevention measures in households with children in the United States. 1990. In *Advance data from vital and health statistics* (Vol. 250, pp. 1–16). Hyattsville, MD: National Center for Health Statistics.

McClean, D., Hatfield-Timajchy, K., Wingo, P., & Floyd, R. (1993). Psychosocial measurement: Implication for the study of preterm delivery in black women. *American Journal of Preventive Medicine, 9* (Suppl. 6), 39–81.

McCormick, G., Zee, C., & Heiden, J. (1982). Cysticercosis cerebri—Review of 172 cases. *Archives of Neurology, 39,* 534–539.

Mendoza, F., Ventura, S., Valdez, R., Castillo, R., Saldivar, L., Baisden, K., & Martorelli, R. (1991). Selected measures of health status for Mexican-American, mainland Puerto-Rican, and Cuban American children. *Journal of the American Medical Association, 265*(2), 231.

Molina, M. (1994). *Latino health in the U.S.: A growing challenge.* Chicago: American Public Health Association.

Morales, E. (1990). *Cadre evaluation report: (Year three) Demonstration project funded by the Office of Substance Abuse Prevention, U.S. Department of Health* (Technical report, Community Substance Abuse Services). San Francisco: Department of Public Health.

Moreno, C., Laniado-Laborin, R., Sallis, J., Elder, J., De Moon, C., Castro, F., & Devsaransingh, T. (1991). Parental influences to smoke in Latino youth. *Preventive Medicine, 23,* 48–53.

Must, A., Gortmaker, S., & Dietz, W. (1994). Risk factors for obesity in young adults: Hispanics, African-

Americans, and whites in the transition years, age 16–28 years. *Biomedicine and Pharmacotherapy, 48,* 143–156.

National Institute of Dental Research. (1989). Oral health of United States children: 1986–87 (NIH Pub. No. 89-2247). Bethesda, MD: National Institute of Health.

Nickens, H. (1991). The health status of minority populations in the United States. *Western Journal of Medicine, 155,* 27–32.

Oleske, J. (1977). Experiences with 118 infants born to narcotic-using mothers. *Clinic Pediatrics, 16,* 418–423.

Palinkas, L., Pierce, J., Rosbrook, B., Pickwell, S., & Bal, D. (1993). Cigarette smoking behavior and beliefs of Hispanics in California. *American Journal of Preventive Medicine, 9,* 331–337.

Perez-Stable, E., Marin, G., & Marin, B. (1994). Behavioral risk factors: A comparison of Latinos and non-Latino whites in San Francisco. *American Journal of Public Health, 84,* 971–976.

Physical fighting among high school students—United States, 1990. (1992). *Morbidity and Mortality Weekly Report, 41,* 91–94.

Powell-Griner, E., & Streck, D. (1982). A closer examination of neonatal mortality rates among the Texas Spanish surname population. *American Journal of Public Health, 72*(9), 993–999.

Preliminary data on births and deaths—United States, 1995. (1995). *Morbidity and Mortality Weekly Report, 45,* 914–919.

Prevalence and impact of arthritis by race and ethnicity—United States, 1989–1991. (1995). *Morbidity and Mortality Weekly Report, 45,* 373–378.

Reynoso, T., Felice, M., & Shragg, G. (1993). Does American acculturation affect outcome of Mexican-American teenage pregnancy? *Journal of Adolescent Health, 14,* 257–261.

Robins, L., Mills, J., Krulewitch, D., & Herman, A. (1993). Effects of in utero exposure to street drugs. *American Journal of Public Health, 83,* 12.

Rodriguez, G. (1996). *The emerging Latino middle class.* Malibu, CA: Pepperdine University Press.

Rodriguez, M., & Brindis, C. (1995). Violence and Latino youth: Prevention and methodological issues. *Public Health Reports, 110,* 260–267.

Rumbaut, R., & Weeks, J. (1994, November 1). *Unraveling a public health enigma: Why do immigrants experience superior perinatal health outcomes?* Paper presented at the 122nd annual meeting of the American Public Health Association, Washington, DC.

Salas, S., Heifetz, E., & Barrett-Connor, E. (1990). Intestinal parasites in Central American immigrants in the United States. *Archives of Internal Medicine, 150,* 1514–1516.

San Francisco Department of Public Health. (1995). *Newcomer children in San Francisco: Their health and well-being.* A report by the Child Health Initiative for Immigrant/Refugee Newcomers Project, 18–27.

Sargent, J., Brown, M., Freeman, J., Bailey, A., Goodman, D., & Freeman, D. (1995). Childrens lead poisoning in Massachusetts communities: Its association with sociodemographic and housing characteristics. *American Journal of Public Health, 85*(4), 528–534.

Sargent, J., Stukel, T., Dalton, M., Freeman, J., & Brown, M. (1996). Iron deficiency in Massachusetts communities: Socioeconomic and demographic risk factors among children. *American Journal of Public Health, 86*(4), 643–648.

Schinke, S., Orlandi, M., & Vaccaro, D. (1992). Substance use among Hispanic and non-Hispanic adolescents. *Addictive Behaviors, 17,* 117–124.

Scribner, R. S., & Dwyer, J. H. (1989). Acculturation and low birthweight among Latinos in the Hispanic HANES. *American Journal of Public Health, 79,* 1263–1267.

Shiono, P. H., & Behrman, R. E. (1995). Low birthweight: Analysis and recommendations. *Future of Children, 5*(1), 4–18.

Smith, K., McGraw, S., Crawford, S., Costa, L., & McKinley, J. (1993). HIV risk among Latino adolescents in two New England cities. *American Journal of Public Health, 83,* 1395–1399.

Smith, P., McGill, L., & Watt, R. (1987). Hispanic adolescent conception and contraception profiles. *Journal of Adolescent Health Care, 8,* 352–355.

Snyder, D., Mohle-Boetani, J., Palla, B., & Fenstersheib, M. (1995). Development of a population-specific risk assessment to predict elevated blood lead levels in Santa Clara County, California. *Pediatrics, 96*(4), 643–648.

Sokol-Katz, J., & Ulbrich, P. (1992). Family structure and adolescent risk-taking behavior: A comparison of Mexican, Cuban, and Puerto Rican Americans. *International Journal of the Addictions, 110,* 260–267.

Sorlie, P., Backlund, E., Johnson, N., & Rogot, E. (1993). Mortality by Hispanic status in the United States. *Journal of the American Medical Association, 270,* 2464–2468.

Swicegood, G., Bean, F., Stephen, E., & Opitz, W. (1988). Language usage and fertility in the Mexican-origin population of the United States. *Demography, 25*(1), 17–33.

Triandis, H., Sashima, Y., Hui, H., Losanshy, J., & Marin, G. (1982). Acculturation and biculturalism indices among relatively acculturated Hispanic young adults. *Interamerican Journal of Psychology, 16,* 140–149.

Tuberculosis morbidity—United States, 1995. (1996), *Morbidity and Mortality Weekly Report, 45,* 365–370.

U.S. Bureau of the Census. (1993). The Hispanic population in the United States: March 1993. In *Current population reports population characteristics* (pp. 000–000). Montgomery, AL: U.S. Department of

Commerce Economics and Statistics Administration, Bureau of the Census.

U.S. Department of Health and Human Services. (1997, January 8). Patterns: Patterns of Drug Use in 1994. [www.health.org/pubs/94hhs/patterns.htm].

U.S. Department of Health and Human Services, Public Health Service. (1993). Advance report of final mortality statistics. 1991. *Monthly Vital Statistics Report, 40*(2), Hyattville, MD: National Center for Health Statistics.

U.S. General Accounting Office. (1992). Hispanic access to health care: Significant gaps exist. In *United States General Accounting Office report to Congressional requesters*. Washington, DC: Author.

Vaccination coverage of 2-year-old children—United States, 1992–1993. (1994). *Morbidity and Mortality Weekly Report. 43,* 282–283.

Vega, W. (1994) Latino outlook: Good health, uncertain prognosis. *Annual Review of Public Health, 15,* 39–67.

Vega, W., Gil, A., Warhelt, G., Apospori, E., & Zimmerman, R. (1993). The relationship of drug use to suicide ideation and attempts among African-American, Hispanic, and white non-Hispanic male adolescents. *Suicide and Life Threatening Behavior, 23,* 110–119.

Vega, W. A., Kolody, B., Hwang, J., & Noble, A. (1993). Prevalence and magnitude of perinatal substance exposures in California. *New England Journal of Medicine, 329,* 850–854.

Ventura, S. J. (1988). Birth of Hispanic parentage, 1985. *Monthly Vital Statistics Reports, National Center for Health Statistics, Hyattsville, MD, 36*(11), 88–112.

Villa, M., Cueliar, J., Gamel, N., & Yeo, G. (1993). *Aging and health: Hispanic American elders*. Stanford, CA: Stanford Geriatric Education Center.

Villar, H., & Menck, H. (1994). The National Cancer Data Base report on cancer in Hispanics. *Cancer, 74,* 2386–2395.

Waldman, B. (1996). Demographics almost 19 million childhood injuries result in 11 thousand deaths. *Journal of Dentistry for Children,* 54–59.

Watson, M., & Brown, L. (1995). The oral health of U.S. Hispanics: Evaluating their needs and their use of dental services. *Journal of the American Dental Association, 126,* 789–795.

Williams, R. L., Binkin, N. J., & Clingman, R. J. (1986). Pregnancy outcomes among Spanish surname women in California. *American Journal of Public Health, 76,* 387.

Winkleby, M., Fortmann, S., & Rockhill, B. (1993). Health-related risk factors in a sample of Hispanics and whites matched on sociodemographic characteristics. *American Journal of Epidemiology, 137,* 1365–1373.

Wood, D., Donald-Sherbourne, C., Halfon, N., Tucker, B., Ortiz, V., Hamlin, J., Duan, N., Mazel, R., Grabowsky, M., Brunell, P., & Freeman, H. (1995). Factors related to immunization status among inner-city Latino and African-American preschoolers. *Pediatrics, 96*(2), 295–301.

Wood, P., Humberto, A., Hidalgo, M., Prihoda, T., & Kromer, M. (1993). Hispanic children with asthma: Morbidity. *Pediatrics, 91*(1), 62–69.

The World Bank. (1994). *A new agenda for women's health and nutrition*. Washington, DC: Author.

Zelson, C., Rubio, E., & Wasserman, E. (1971). Neonatal narcotic addiction: 10-year observation. *Pediatrics, 48*(2), 178–189.

16

Asian Pacific Islander Health

ERIKA TAKADA, JUDY M. FORD, AND LINDA S. LLOYD

Introduction

Asian Pacific Islander Americans (A/PI), one of the United States' smallest subpopulations at 3% of the total U.S. population (1990 U.S. Census, in Lum, 1995), is also the fastest growing minority group in the United States. Three factors contribute to its rapid increase in size. The Immigration Act of 1965, which did away with country quotas and promoted the reunification of immigrant families, the steady influx of Southeast Asian refugees since 1975, and the contemporary stream of Asian immigrants into the United States swelled the A/PI population 141% between 1970 and 1980. Between 1980 and 1990, the population continued to grow and doubled in size from 3.5 million to more than 7 million (Burr & Mutchler, 1993; Lin-Fu, 1988). With this continued rate of growth, the U.S. Asian Pacific Islander population is estimated to reach 10 million by the year 2000 (Lin-Fu, 1988).

Asian Pacific Islander Americans are often grouped together and considered as one homogeneous group, resulting in generalizations about the population as a whole. Asian Pacific Islanders are, in fact, highly diverse. They consist not only of Asian immigrants

(i.e., those from China, Japan, Korea, Vietnam, Philippines, Thailand, India, Cambodia, Laos, etc.) which account for 93% of all A/PIs, but also of Pacific Islander immigrants (i.e., those from Hawaii, Samoa, Guam, Fiji, etc.) which constitute the remaining 7% (Browne & Broderick, 1994; Lin-Fu, 1988). In addition to the numerous nationalities represented among A/PIs, this population is composed of more than 30 distinct cultures, each with its own language, religion, or life philosophy governing individual, family, and group interactions (Browne & Broderick, 1994). According to 1990 U.S. Census data, there are 29 different Asian groups and 20 Pacific Islander groups which collectively speak more than 100 languages (Loue, Lloyd, & Loh, 1996). Therefore, to effectively study and understand the Asian American population, we must take into account the diversity of the group.

One of the generalizations that continues to be made about Asian Pacific Islander populations is that they are a "model minority," that is, that they are uniquely successful without many problems or needs (Lin-Fu, 1988). Another is that A/PIs are a population of higher socioeconomic status (SES) (Takeuchi & Young, 1994). The A/PI population is, in fact, highly diverse and bipolar in socioeconomic status. For example, the bipolar nature of SES among A/PIs can be seen in comparing the more acculturated and higher SES of Japanese Americans, whose migration history dates back to 1885, with

ERIKA TAKADA • Division of Health Promotion, Graduate School of Public Health, San Diego State University, San Diego, California 92182. **JUDY M. FORD** AND **LINDA S. LLOYD** • Alliance Healthcare Foundation, San Diego, California 92123.

Handbook of Immigrant Health, edited by Loue. Plenum Press, New York, 1998.

the less acculturated and lower SES of Southeast Asian Americans, a more recent refugee group to the United States. Such stereotypes as "the model minority" have led to a lack of understanding of the specific health problems and health care needs for the population as a whole, as well as within the population. Some A/PI ethnic groups may be more at risk for health problems than others (e.g., diabetes in Japanese Americans, cancer in Pacific Islanders); other groups may have more severe barriers to health services, such as language proficiency. The generalizations also mask the need for collecting national health data in a stratified fashion. Health care providers, researchers, and policy makers are unable to recognize the differences that exist, or even the distinct groups that make up the population, due to a lack of group-specific information.

Migration patterns between the subgroups also influence the diversity of health issues among the A/PI population. For example, although the Chinese, Japanese, and Koreans have a long history of immigration to the United States, for both Chinese and Korean Americans the majority of the population are still foreign-born (Barringer, Gardner, & Levin, 1993). Filipinos have been considered U.S. nationals due to U.S. occupation of the country, and therefore may not have suffered as much discrimination under earlier immigration laws. Recent studies have shown that Filipinos account for the second highest number of immigrants annually, after Mexicans (Agbayani-Siewert, 1994). The most recent group of Asian immigrants is predominantly from Southeast Asia. This migration resulted primarily from the war in Southeast Asia and the genocidal regime of Pol Pot in Cambodia between 1975 and 1979. Southeast Asians have generally had higher levels of stress and trauma related to their migration experience, and tend to be less educated than other subgroups.

The purpose of this chapter is to identify and discuss the health status of Asian Pacific Islander Americans by focusing on the heterogeneity of the population and by identifying the most prevalent health issues affecting the different groups making up the A/PI populations. Given that there is no "typical" Asian Pacific Islander community, generalizations from one A/PI subgroup to other A/PI subgroups with respect to health-seeking behaviors and use of Western or traditional healing practices, are problematic. The diverse health needs and illnesses suffered by the A/PI communities are made apparent, as are the gaps in knowledge that exist due to a lack of group-specific information. The barriers in access to care, infectious disease, mental health issues, chronic disease, health risk factors, and relevant migration patterns, are highlighted. In addition, recommendations are provided on how to improve our knowledge base in these health areas and how to effectively address those health care needs for the subgroups identified.

Access to Care

Socioeconomic Barriers

Studies that show low rates of health services utilization and low numbers of uninsured among A/PIs give the impression that this group has few health problems and is relatively well insured (Mayeno & Hirota, 1994; Smith & Ryan, 1987). However, further analysis of the data shows that low rates of health services use are due not to low need, but to lack of access to the mainstream health care system. Likewise, data which show low numbers of uninsured are typically gained from national studies. Such studies suffer from low numbers of Asian Americans surveyed, relative to other groups, and the tendency not to break down Asian American groups but to collapse their data with that of Whites (Mayeno & Hirota, 1994). Such practices mask the true level of uninsured among Asian Americans and fail to show that, like other groups in the United States, Asian Pacific Islander Americans are subject to the same socioeconomic barriers that limit access to the health care system.

Despite the stereotype of the "successful" or "model" minority (i.e., an upwardly mobile, well-established group with few problems and few health needs), poverty and lack of health insurance are significant barriers to care for Asian Americans. According to the 1980 U.S. Census, while 7.5% of all Asian Americans had an annual family income above $50,000, there were significant concentrations in the lower income brackets (Mayeno & Hirota, 1994). In fact, Asian American families with incomes below the federal poverty level were found to be poorer than any other group. In addition, of all racial or ethnic groups, Asian Americans had the highest proportion (24.2%) of unrelated persons (individuals not living in the same household) with annual incomes below $2,000 (Mayeno & Hirota, 1994). Local surveys provide not only more detail through identification of specific ethnic groups within the Asian Pacific Islander populations, but they also reveal a better picture of the impact poverty has on local populations of Asian Americans. For example, a San Diego survey of Asian Americans (including Hmong, Khmer, Chinese, and Vietnamese) found that 75.8% lived below the poverty level, while a San Francisco Bay area survey of Vietnamese found that 53% reported incomes below the federal poverty level (Mayeno & Hirota, 1994).

Lack of health insurance is another barrier to access to health care for many Asian Americans. Like national income data, the national data on health insurance coverage of Asian Americans gives the impression that, as a group, they are well insured (Mayeno & Hirota, 1994). Again, relatively small numbers of Asian Americans are included in national surveys, and oftentimes those surveyed are more highly educated and have higher incomes (with a greater potential to afford health insurance or to get it through their employer) than the general population of Asian Americans. For example, Japanese Americans overall have achieved a relatively high level of socioeconomic status with good access to health care largely because their immigration pattern and history is quite different from that of more recent migrant groups. Given that greater than 70% of the current Japanese American population was born in the United States, acculturation levels and familiarity with the health care system are significantly different from those of the less well-established Asian Americans (Takeuchi & Young, 1994). Generalizing the Japanese American experience to all A/PI groups creates the image, nationally, that Asian Americans are relatively well insured, while state and local data document a different picture of the state of health insurance coverage among Asian Americans.

Although the unemployment rate among Asian Americans is relatively low, many work in low-wage jobs, such as in factories and the service industry. Such jobs typically do not offer employer-based health insurance and do not pay sufficiently to allow workers to purchase their own health insurance. For example, a study conducted in Boston's Chinatown found that 61% of those who were uninsured were employed; and two thirds of the employed uninsured had annual incomes below $10,000 (Mayeno & Hirota, 1994). A study conducted in California in 1989 found that Asian Americans were the racial–ethnic group least likely to have access to employer-based health insurance, with 20% of nonelderly Asian Americans surveyed uninsured. Local surveys in Chicago found that 30.5% of Chinese and 40.9% of Koreans surveyed in 1990 and 1989, respectively, were uninsured (Mayeno & Hirota, 1994).

Therefore, data on Asian American poverty and health insurance rates, especially national studies, should be cautiously considered as only partially reflecting the true status of these indicators. Until we can do a better job at the national level of providing group-specific data on Asian Americans, local data must be used to gain a more comprehensive understanding of the financial need among Asian Americans and how this need impacts their access to, and utilization of, the health care system.

Systemic and Cultural Barriers

Cultural issues serve as barriers to the health care system for Asian Americans in addition to, and oftentimes over and above, socioeconomic issues. Cultural issues specific to Asian Pacific Islanders such as language, health and illness conceptualization, and values governing interpersonal relationships, can serve as barriers to access to the U.S. health care system. These issues often clash with the structure and process of the health system. In addition, inherent in the structure of the health care system are systemic barriers, such as lack of Asian American professionals and lack of understanding of the differences in health and illness conceptualization among practitioners, which impede A/PI use of the health care system.

The groups that make up the Asian Pacific Islander population have certain similarities with respect to the systemic and cultural issues that are barriers to the U.S. health care system, and are similarly impacted by those barriers. For many, language is a major barrier to access to care. This is particularly true for the A/PI elderly who have lower levels of literacy in English, as well as in their native language (Browne & Broderick, 1994; Douglas & Fujimoto, 1995; Lew, 1991). Limited reading skills in one's native language and in English has a negative impact on accessing care because of the need to read and understand health facilities signs, paperwork, informational materials, and to comprehend health practitioner instructions (Mayeno & Hirota, 1994). In a 1988 study of Southeast Asians in San Diego, 60% of those surveyed cited language as a major problem in obtaining health care, with 58.8% of Chinese surveyed reporting that they could not read English (Mayeno & Hirota, 1994). In response to low levels of English literacy, bilingual written materials have often been used to reach Asian American populations. However, given that native language literacy can be low as well, bilingual written materials have limited value for helping Asian Americans, especially elderly Asian Americans, overcome the language barriers. For example, the Oakland Chinese Community Survey (Mayeno & Hirota, 1994) found that 38% of those surveyed could not read Chinese. A similar study conducted in Chicago's Chinatown found that 23% of respondents could read Chinese "a little" or "none."

Acculturation also influences the degree to which traditional versus Western medicine is used among Asian Americans. Those who are more acculturated to U.S. society tend to rely more on Western medical practices. Therefore, the young are less likely than the elderly to rely solely on traditional and herbal medical practices, which elderly Asian Americans may use even to the exclusion of Western medicine. As a result, it can often be difficult to convince some groups of the utility of Western practices (Browne & Broderick, 1994; Douglas & Fujimoto, 1995). Health professionals need to be aware of these preferences as some herbal medicines are quite potent on their own, and may have harmful effects if used in conjunction with prescribed Western medicines. One example is a case report of strychnine poisoning in a Cambodian woman using a traditional remedy to alleviate a gastrointestinal disorder (Katz, Prescott, & Woolf, 1996). The authors pointed out that although there are other toxins that can cause seizures, the use of traditional medicines containing strychnine should be investigated in Southeast Asian patients with severe abdominal distress and seizures.

The systemic barriers that compound the difficulties presented by other barriers to care include the scarcity of professionals who can speak the patient's native language; the limited number of professionals who will take the time to make sure that the patient and his or her family understand how the system works; the absence of professionals who understand the cultural context of the patient and who can manage their care within that context; the lack of bilingual staff trained in medical terminology; and reliance on interpreters who use literal medical translations that patients cannot understand.

Explanatory Models for Health and Illness Conceptualization

It can be said that, as a group, Asian Pacific Islanders conceptualize health and illness differently from the Western concept of health and illness; however, it is the Western medical perspective that drives the U.S. health care system. Culturally specific explanatory models for health and illness explain how an individual interprets and then addresses an episode of illness. For example, Filipinos consider health to depend on maintaining equilibrium in the body and a harmonious balance between the individual and his or her environment (Flaskerud & Soldevilla, 1986). Thus, illness is the result of imbalance, potentially caused not only by pathogens, poisons, and heredity, but also by inappropriate behavior, shame, social irresponsibility, divine retribution, or some combination. Koreans and Chinese have similar beliefs about health and illness (Anonymous, 1991; Chin, 1992; Kim & Rew, 1994; Zane, Sue, Hu, & Kwon, 1991). These groups tend to use a combination of traditional and Western medicine to treat their ills, depending on the health problem. Traditional medicine is used to reestablish internal or external balance that has been disrupted, the root cause of the illness, and Western medicine is used to alleviate symptoms such as pain.

As seen with Chinese, Koreans, and Filipinos, Southeast Asians also view health as a state of equilibrium. For example, the Vietnamese believe that disease and illness is caused by an imbalance of *am* and *duong* (yin and yang) (Jenkins *et al.,* 1996), and use herbal medicines restore balance. Cambodians, Hmong, and Lao believe that internal disequilibrium can be caused by changes in diet, climate, or familial discord (Miller, 1995; Shimada, Jackson, Goldstein, & Buchwald, 1995; Uba, 1992). Illness can also result from one's karma, which is believed to be the result of past actions during previous incarnations. A fatalistic attitude in which illness and suffering are an inevitable part of life is also a common belief (Uba, 1992), and,

as a result, value is placed on the denial or tolerance of physical pain (Jenkins *et al.,* 1996). Traditional remedies include herbal medicine, coin rubbing, cupping, therapeutic burning, and acupuncture (Jenkins *et al.,* 1996; Miller, 1995; Uba, 1992).

In an effort to determine whether traditional health beliefs impeded access to the U.S. health care system, Jenkins and colleagues (1996) examined and analyzed the relationship between traditional beliefs and practices and access to care in a sample of Vietnamese in the San Francisco Bay area. Interestingly, their findings did not support the hypothesis that traditional beliefs and practices were barriers to accessing or utilizing U.S. health care services. Rather, demographic and access variables such as socioeconomic status, marital status, employment, age, and language proficiency were found to be stronger predictors of access to medical care and utilization of preventive services. In addition, some differences in the greater use of traditional remedies by more recent Vietnamese immigrants may be a result of official Vietnamese government sanction of traditional remedies, since Western medicine was often scarce and expensive in Vietnam (Jenkins *et al,* 1996).

There is little published information on access issues for the Pacific Islander population. It is known, however, that before seeking and utilizing Western health services, many Pacific Islander patients will use prayer and *fofo,* traditional remedies such as herbal potions, massage, dietary restrictions, and therapeutic incantation (Barker, 1991). They, too, often continue the traditional treatments in addition to Western medical practices.

Accessing the U.S. health care system is dependent on the type of illness for all A/PI groups. For psychosomatic complaints, such as chronic headache, muscle aches, and body pain, many will use Western medicines and practices (Chin, 1992; Flaskerud & Soldevilla, 1986). However, the Asian Pacific Islander's concept of mental illness prevents appropriate use of the U.S. mental health system. This is discussed in further detail later in this chapter.

Treatment Compliance

Attitudes toward medication and treatment compliance are directly related to culturally specific explanatory models for health and illness; some authors have called for health care professionals to develop an understanding of health concepts held by the groups seen frequently in their health system (Lew, 1991; Miller, 1995; Rairdan & Higgs, 1992; Shimada *et al.,* 1995). For example, fears of "soul loss" as a result of surgery, and fear of reincarnation without the missing organ or limb have been reported as barriers to acceptance of surgical interventions for Cambodians and Hmong (Lew, 1991; Rice, Ly, & Lumley, 1994; Shimada *et al.,* 1995). Health professionals without sufficient understanding of the language and the culture, including cultural interpretations of health and illness, are significant barriers to health care utilization for Asian Americans.

Western medicine is also often viewed by Asian Americans as "strong," and therefore capable of throwing off one's internal balance. While the U.S. health care system views patients who do not follow therapeutic instructions as noncompliant, this failure may be more related to a culturally defined compliance, in which patients do not view themselves as noncompliant but rather as managing their illness appropriately. In a study of Cambodian patients seen in a clinic in Seattle, Washington, the principal reasons for noncompliance with medications were misunderstandings about what the medication was for, its side effects, concerns about the effects of Western medicine on "internal strength," and local concepts about pharmacokinetics (Shimada *et al.,* 1995). Patients explained their decisions to discontinue or to selectively reduce the dosage of medications according to the Cambodian view of the body and understanding of how pharmaceuticals react with or affect the body (e.g., belief that low "inner strength" would be aggravated by taking "strong" medicines, concern that there would be a reaction in the stomach if more than one medication was taken at the same time). In addition, the authors found that patients were, in some cases, intentionally noncompliant by not taking the medication or by changing the treatment regimen. In other cases, compliance was compromised unintentionally when they modified the dose thinking the drug was being used to treat another health condition or waited significant periods of time between doses to reduce side effects. The authors stated that these pharmacokinetic concepts are found in other Asian cultures in areas with greater reliance on milder herbal treatments and low exposure to Western medicine.

Role of the Family and Interpersonal Values in Illness Management

In serving the health care needs of A/PIs, health professionals must come to understand and respect the important role of the family, as well as the values governing interpersonal conduct. In Asian cultures, the needs and wants of the family take priority over the individual and, therefore, planning and following a treatment regimen may require family decision making. Kinship relationships are highly valued and relatives depend on one another for emotional, financial, and psychological support (Abrantes, 1994; Browne & Broderick, 1994; Chin, 1992). The family assumes the responsibility for communication between the health practitioner and the patient to ensure accurate transfer of information. This is especially important for elderly patients, who are more likely to comply with treatment regimens when the family is involved in the decision making (Browne & Broderick, 1994; Douglas & Fujimoto, 1995). Miller (1995) recommended that the health care provider speak to the oldest male member of the family about diagnoses and treatment regimens first and, for female patients, that the husband be allowed into the examining room to provide comfort and support. This family decision-making approach may conflict with Western concepts of autonomy and an individual's right to self-determination, with patients alone expected to provide informed consent regarding their medical care. Although it is recognized that family members may be involved in discussions around medical care, the U.S. health care system requires that the patient be responsible for the final decision. For further discussion on this issue, please refer to Chapter 11 (this volume).

Thus, to effectively serve the health care needs of the individual patient, health practitioners must include the family in planning a treatment regimen. This is a difficult task, as the U.S. health care system treats the individual, not the family. In addition, practitioners in managed care systems are rewarded for efficiency, which may mean less time with patients and their families and may not be conducive to meeting the needs of individuals unfamiliar with the U.S. health care system.

There is a tendency among Asian groups not to complain, to be modest and accepting of life situations, and to be indirect and avoid confrontations and unpleasantries in their interpersonal interactions. For example, interpersonal interactions for Filipinos are governed by the concepts of reciprocal obligation (*utang ng loob*), shame (*hiya*), self-esteem (*amor proprio*), and getting along with others (*pakikisama*) (Abrantes, 1994; Browne & Broderick, 1994). As a result, Asian Americans tend not to question authority (Abrantes, 1994; Chin, 1992; Zane *et al.,* 1991). Noncompliance may result because Asian patients may not wish to contradict or question a physician, and may not mention that a prescribed medication is ineffective or that they are experiencing side effects. Deference to providers may also inhibit questions about the therapeutic regimen because questions may be viewed as a lack of respect (Miller, 1995).

Reaching Asian Americans and adequately serving their health needs requires much more than a translator. A system of care that requires Asian Americans, and especially recent immigrants, to disclose problems, to question authority figures, and to expose themselves physically or emotionally to strangers cannot be effective in meeting their

needs. Cultural values that govern health beliefs and interpersonal behavior must be considered in the organization and delivery of health and mental health services in order to effectively serve this population.

Infant Health Outcomes

The impact of limited access to the U.S. health care system by Asian Americans can be seen in a variety of health issues. We use infant health outcomes as an example of the impact of limited access to health care. Infant health outcomes among Asian American subgroups indicate that there are differences between them with respect to access to prenatal care. While as a group Asian Americans have the lowest infant mortality rate compared with other U.S. ethnic minority groups, recent studies have found that there are Asian American subgroup differences with respect to infant mortality, as well as prenatal care and birth weight outcomes (Fuentes-Afflick & Hessol, 1997; Mayeno & Hirota, 1994). For example, Hawaiian data from a 1989 study found that while 30.1% of all mothers with live births had no prenatal care in the first trimester, 32.7% of Filipinas and 62.6% of Samoans had no prenatal care in the first trimester (Zane, Takeuchi, & Young, 1994). In a 1997 study of the impact of Asian ethnicity on prenatal care and birth weight outcomes, 12.6% of Filipina, 6.9% of Chinese, and 11.0% of Korean women reported inadequate prenatal care (Fuentes-Afflick & Hessol, 1997). Although inadequate prenatal care was, in general, significantly associated with low birth weight, it was not consistently predictive of the birth outcome. For example, prenatal care utilization was more predictive for low birth weight for Cambodian and Laotian women than for Filipino women.

Barriers to accessing prenatal care services by Hmong women were identified in two studies (Jambunathan & Stewart, 1995; Spring, Ross, Etkin, & Deinard, 1995). Jambunathan and Stewart report the following reasons for delaying prenatal care: attending school, lack of someone to take care of other children, transportation problems, and not wanting to be touched by doctors and nurses because "touching the baby too much" could cause a miscarriage. A study by Spring and colleagues (1995) reported that the pelvic exam was considered to be "unacceptable" to 61% of the women interviewed because of embarrassment and shame, and that this feeling significantly limited prenatal visits. Other barriers reported were discontinuity in physician care, language barriers, and clinic hours. While the rates of infant mortality, low birth weight and inadequate prenatal care for these subgroups are relatively low, differences among the subgroups do exist. Further studies must be conducted to understand why some subgroups do not access the system to the extent other Asian Americans do for their prenatal care.

Elderly Health

It is projected that by the year 2050, 20% of the nation's elderly persons will be from minority communities. This projected growth in the minority elderly population is based on two factors: the steadily growing proportion of ethnic minorities in the population, with Asian Americans representing the fastest growing minority group, and the growth of the minority elderly population, which is exceeding that of the White elderly population (Browne & Broderick, 1994). It is well known that many Asian Americans, particularly Chinese and Japanese, have longer life expectancies than White Americans. This fact is often used, along with low health care utilization rates, to demonstrate that Asian American elderly people have few health needs. In fact, Asian American elderly individuals show a greater prevalence of certain conditions such as hypertension, osteoporosis, and dementia, than the general population (Browne & Broderick, 1994). For example, Chinese and Korean women are more susceptible to osteoporosis because they consume too little calcium and protein (Douglas & Fujimoto, 1995).

Group-specific data reveal that health issues that affect A/PI elderly persons are

masked by low utilization rates and the generalization of longer life expectancies to all A/PIs. Further inquiry is needed to identify effective means by which elderly Asian Americans can be engaged in order to increase their access to the mainstream health care system and to effectively diagnose and treat their illnesses. This understanding should be used not to find ways to subvert those beliefs with mainstream ideologies, but to find out where Western medicine can fit into their conceptualizations so that medical practices will be seen as a familiar help and not a foreign hindrance to their health.

Infectious Diseases

Acquired Immune Deficiency Syndrome

Prevention education for HIV and AIDS has ignored, to some extent, Asian Pacific Islander subpopulations due to the low number of AIDS cases among A/PI communities. In 1990, the Centers for Disease Control and Prevention reported that Asian Americans represented 0.6% of all AIDS cases in the United States, with the lowest rate of AIDS cases, 3.8 per 100,000, as compared with other racial or ethnic groups (Gock, 1994). Although the numbers themselves may be small when compared with other ethnic groups, an examination of trends in the number of AIDS cases highlights some disturbing statistics. The annual rate of increase in reported AIDS cases for Asian Pacific Islanders between 1987 and 1990 is similar to that seen for *all* other racial and ethnic minorities combined: In 1987 the annual rate for A/PIs was 66% while it was 65% for other ethnic minorities; in 1988 it was 47% and 43%, respectively; and for 1990 it was 39% and 39%, respectively (Gock, 1994). Gock also cited a study conducted by the National AIDS Network in 1989 in which the incidence of AIDS in Asian Pacific Islander communities was found to be doubling about every 10 months. In addition, in cities with large concentrations of Asian Americans, this group had the highest rate of increase in reported AIDS cases compared with other ethnic groups (Brown, 1992; Gock, 1994).

As with other health issues, local or statewide studies provide a more detailed picture of the impact of AIDS on Asian Americans. National surveillance data tend not to provide a breakdown of AIDS cases among Asian Americans by ethnic group or country of origin. For example, a study conducted in Los Angeles County in 1989 found that, of all the reported AIDS cases among Asian Americans ($N = 150$), Filipinos accounted for 29.3% of the cases, followed by Japanese (17.3%) and Chinese (14.0%). Koreans accounted for only 2.7% of the cases (Gock, 1994).

Despite the growing numbers of AIDS cases among Asian Americans, many still consider AIDS not to be a problem for Asian Americans (Brown, 1992). This lack of concern, coupled with widely held stereotypes about Asian American "immunity" to the disease as well as AIDS being a disease of gay White men and drug users, has led to complacency regarding the AIDS issue (Brown, 1992; Gock, 1994). Studies on AIDS-related knowledge, attitudes, beliefs, and behaviors among various A/PI subgroups indicate low levels of knowledge about HIV transmission (Gock, 1994; Loue et al., 1996). In a San Diego County survey of 282 individuals representing 11 different A/PI communities, only 48% identified either unprotected anal or vaginal intercourse as a means of HIV transmission, with the majority being unable to correctly identify even one medically accepted cause of HIV transmission. Other reasons for HIV infection given included casual contact with an HIV-infected person and karmic destiny (Loue et al., 1996). Sexually active young adult Asian Americans engage in the same sexual behaviors, putting them at high risk for HIV infection, as young White, Hispanic, and African Americans. In the San Diego study and in three studies cited by Gock, even respondents with an understanding of HIV transmission engaged in high-risk behaviors such as unprotected sex with multiple partners or unprotected sex with prostitutes.

Thus, HIV prevention and AIDS education targeting A/PI communities are needed to impact risky sexual behavior and to dispel myths regarding the disease as well as perceived personal susceptibility. Prevention and education programs have been shown to be effective among high-risk A/PI populations. For example, a 1995 San Francisco study of 329 homosexual A/PI men found that short-term, culturally relevant sessions reduced HIV risk among the participants (Choi, Lew, Vittinghoff, 1996). Participants in a three-hour group counseling and skills building training session reported increased knowledge about AIDS, more concern about HIV infection, and fewer sexual partners at the 3-month follow-up. This study shows how even relatively brief counseling sessions can have a positive impact on the knowledge and behavior of high-risk A/PI populations. More work is necessary in this area to find out what types of prevention and education programs would be effective for other high-risk A/PI populations, such as injection drug users and their partners, and those engaged in high-risk heterosexual behaviors.

Challenges for HIV prevention programs are the diversity of Asian Pacific Islander communities and the myths that A/PIs are not affected by this disease. There are features common to A/PI cultures that can be used as the basis for developing communication strategies; A/PI cultures are generally "collectivist," valuing the community as opposed to the individualistic cultures of the Western world (Brown, 1992; Catolico, 1997). They emphasize modesty and privacy and not the explicit discussion of risk behaviors. These common features cannot, however, ignore the need to develop specific strategies for high-risk subgroups within the broader A/PI community, such as gay and bisexual A/PIs, limited-English-language individuals, and heterosexual men and women with multiple partners. Education and prevention efforts need to specifically target Asian Americans not only with information about HIV transmission and safe sex practices, but also with information to dispel the myth that Asian Americans need not be concerned about this disease. Without a culture-specific focus, the effectiveness of education and prevention efforts will be limited and the number of AIDS cases will continue to grow.

Hepatitis B

More than 200 million people around the world are chronically infected with the hepatitis B virus (HBV); 75% of these live in Asia (Hann, 1994). Therefore, it is not surprising that hepatitis B is more common among Asian Americans than any other racial or ethnic group in the United States. With proper screening and immunization the risk of transmission of HBV can be almost eliminated. Left unscreened, HBV can lead to cancer (hepatocellular carcinoma), chronic active hepatitis, and chronic liver disease (Mayeno & Hirota, 1994). In the United States, an estimated 10% to 15% of Southeast Asian refugees (approximately 100,000 people) are chronic carriers of the virus (Jackson, Rhodes, Inui, & Buchwald, 1997). A study assessing the incidence of HBV infection among Korean Americans in New York, New Jersey, Philadelphia, Washington, D.C., and Baltimore found that 42% of asymptomatic HBV carriers tested positive for chronic hepatitis and 11% tested positive for cirrhosis of the liver (Hann, 1994).

Perinatal transmission is the most common form of HBV transmission among Asian Pacific Islander Americans in the United States (Mayeno & Hirota, 1994). This is made clear in the disproportionate representation of Asian American women among those who give birth to HBV carrier infants. In 1991, while 3.2% of total U.S. births were to Asian American women, a staggering 54% of those infants tested positive for HBV (Mayeno & Hirota, 1994). These data show that the risk of perinatal transmission of HBV for Asian American women is 16 times greater than it is for the entire U.S. population. In 1984, the U.S. Public Health Service's Immunization Advisory Committee recommended that pregnant women of Asian Pacific Islander origin be screened for HbsAg positivity so that the infants of carrier mothers can be immunized (Lin-Fu, 1988). Given that certain groups of Asian Americans do not adequately use prenatal care and health care providers who see these women may not know about HBV, many Asian American women remain at risk for transferring the virus to their babies. Even programs identifying high-risk pregnant women may not be successful in obtaining compliance from the mother for the series of HBV immunizations for the infant. In a 1988 study, the CDC reported that only 2% of the Southeast Asian refugees in the United States have been immunized (Jenkins et al., 1990).

Knowledge of hepatitis B is low in some Asian populations. An important barrier to vaccine acceptance relates to how the various A/PI communities interpret liver disease and its causal factors; not all groups recognize the relationship between liver disease and the virus (Jackson et al., 1997; Sworts & Riccitelli, 1997). Of 215 Vietnamese respondents in the San Francisco Bay area, 48% had never heard of hepatitis B (Jenkins et al., 1990). Jackson and colleagues (1997) conducted semistructured, open interviews with 34 adult Cambodian refugees, including chronic carriers and persons with symptoms of active liver disease. They found that although Cambodian translators explained that the Khmer words commonly used to describe hepatitis B reflected the organ damage that results from hepatitis B infection (i.e., "liver disease"—*rauk tlaam* or "swollen liver disease"—*rauk hoem tlaam*), 82% of the respondents did not understand the phrases. Of the 6 respondents with active liver disease, only 2 recognized the term "liver disease," while 4 other respondents (3 non-HBV carriers and 1 carrier) were familiar with it. Three of the remaining 28 respondents reported hearing the term and associated it with heavy alcohol use but not hepatitis.

All respondents associated a self-limiting rash with a "weak" liver, but were unable to identify other illnesses associated with the liver (Jackson *et al.,* 1997). This study demonstrates the importance of selecting words that identify recognizable concepts of culturally specific explanatory models and that reflect the community's experience and social context of the illness when translating medical terminology into other languages. Given the high incidence of this disease, its asymptomatic stages, the high perinatal transmission rate and the variety of disorders that can result when left undetected, it is important to specifically target Asian Americans with HBV education, prevention, screening, and treatment services that address local explanatory models for liver disease.

Tuberculosis

Asian Americans are also disproportionately infected with tuberculosis (TB). In 1989, while the Asian American population was 2.9% of the total U.S. population, Asian Americans accounted for 17.6% of all reported tuberculosis cases in the United States (Mayeno & Hirota, 1994). With a tuberculosis incidence rate more than six times higher than the U.S. population as a whole, efforts at screening for TB among Asian Americans must be improved. The high incidence of TB among Asian Americans is largely due to its high endemicity in Asian countries or refugee camps where many of the Southeast Asian immigrants to the United States lived while awaiting entry. While testing positive for TB is grounds for exclusion from entry into the United States, many may be asymptomatic at the time of screening, and therefore can serve to infect other people when their TB becomes active (Mayeno & Hirota, 1994). Thus, not only are targeted TB education, screening, and treatment services needed, but the screening also needs to be conducted repeatedly to pick up asymptomatic cases.

Mental Health

While many Asian Pacific Islander Americans are familiar with mainstream medical care for physical ailments, fewer are familiar with the mental health system. Even Filipinos, who as a group have been exposed to U.S. medical care longer than others, are not as familiar with or accepting of U.S. mental health services (Flaskerud & Soldevilla, 1986). Lack of acceptance of U.S. mental health care springs from the differences between A/PI and Western concepts of mental health and mental illness. Many A/PIs express depression and anxiety somatically. Some believe that the tendency to somatize mental health problems occurs because of the stigma and shame associated with mental illness (Flaskerud & Soldevilla, 1986; Kim & Rew, 1994; Ying, 1990). When Asian Americans do access health facilities for mental or emotional problems, they tend to present with more severe psychiatric disorders that emerge after a period of denial. Families attempt to care for mentally ill individuals in an effort to prevent the shame that results when outsiders to the family know that there is a problem. Thus, individuals with mental illness are presented to mental health facilities only after the family can no longer tolerate aberrant behaviors, at which time the disorder tends to be more severe.

Micro and macro perspectives of psychological well-being reflect individual versus community approaches to mental health. Catolico (1997) proposed that the macro perspective may more closely fit the family decision-making process seen across A/PI communities. In her study of Cambodian refugee women and mental health services, Catolico called for mental health providers to reframe their approach to psychological well-being. The micro perspective of psychological well-being focuses on the individual and deemphasizes reliance on an extended social support system, thereby potentially separating the individual from his or her own cultural values. The macro perspective, on the other hand, views psychological well-being as a socially defined and socially constructed notion. The use of concepts that are closer to Cambodian explanatory models and that are relevant to Cambodian perspectives of health and illness, such as harmony and balance, may reduce marginalization of Cambodian women in the health care system.

Use of Mental Health Services

A number of Asian and Pacific Islander populations share perceptions on mental health issues. Koreans refer to the state of somatizing emotional problems as *hwa byung*. Typical complaints include body aches, anxiety, dizziness, fatigue, irritability, and loss of appetite (Flaskerud & Soldevilla, 1986; Kim & Rew, 1994). Asian Americans may attribute symptoms of mental illness to karma, the result of offending ancestral spirits (Ong, 1995), possession by supernatural, evil spirits (Flaskerud & Soldevilla, 1986), impropriety, character weakness, and misdeeds or a failure to be fair (Flaskerud & Soldevilla, 1986; Kim & Rew, 1994; Ying, 1990). Means to address the mental disorder may include utilizing traditional practitioners to restore balance in the body and the environment, praying to ancestors, keeping busy so one "does not think so much," and using one's will power and "strength of mind" (Flaskerud & Soldevilla, 1986; Frye & D'Avanzo, 1994; Handelman & Yeo, 1996; Kim & Rew, 1994; Ong, 1995). Western medicine may also be used to relieve physical symptoms of the emotional disorder. Because of the preference for the use of traditional healers and family assistance, very little is known regarding the specific mental health needs of Asian Americans unless they are very ill (Flaskerud & Soldevilla, 1986; Kim & Rew, 1994; Kuo, 1984; Ying, 1990).

It is difficult to bring A/PIs into the mental health system and to effectively diagnose emotional disorders. Carlson and Rosser-Hogan (1993) pointed out that the majority of services targeting Southeast Asian refugees, aimed at making them self-sufficient in as short a time as possible, are job training and English language classes. Psychological counseling for recent immigrants is severely limited by a lack of funding and a lack of mental health professionals familiar with the culture of the refugees. Ong (1995) stated that

diagnostic categories used in the U.S. mental health system may not accurately describe or reflect the mental status of Southeast Asian immigrants, and may inadvertently invalidate the patient's own understanding of his or her life and culture. The type of facility used by Asian Pacific Islanders has also been shown to have a significant impact on the diagnosis of mental illness. Flaskerud and Akutsu (1993) found that Asian Americans in Los Angeles County seen at ethnic-specific clinics by Asian therapists were less likely to be classified as psychotic than were Asian American clients seen by Asian and White therapists at mainstream clinics. These differences in diagnoses may be due to different practices or it may be that ethnic-specific centers and therapists elicit more comprehensive information and utilize cultural understanding of presenting symptoms to obtain a more accurate diagnosis. On the other hand, ethnic-specific centers may be more acceptable to A/PI clients, allowing them to present at earlier, less severe, stages of an illness (Flaskerud & Akutsu, 1993).

The Asian Pacific Islander populations are divided into non–Southeast Asian and Southeast Asian for the following sections due to the substantial literature on mental health issues affecting the Southeast Asian populations. This division is made given the quantity of published studies on the mental health status of Cambodians, Laotians, Hmong, and Vietnamese.

Non-Southeast Asian Populations

To date, the most common mental health problems seen among non–Southeast Asian populations such as Filipino, Korean, and Chinese Americans include depression, marital and family discord, schizophrenia, and problems associated with loss of self-esteem, loss of social status, and shame (Agbayani-Siewert, 1994; Flaskerud & Soldevilla, 1986; Kim & Rew, 1994; Kuo, 1984; Lum, 1995; Ying, 1990). Much of the social and emotional stress experienced is related to immigration, underemployment, and the cultural dissonance that occurs with attempts to adjust to life in the United States. Employment for many Asian Americans, especially Filipinos and Koreans, often does not reflect the education or social status they attained in their native country.

Mental health problems manifest themselves in a variety of ways. For example, there is a higher suicide rate among elderly Japanese and Chinese Americans, with Japanese American women 75 years and older and *issei* (first-generation) men over 85 exhibiting higher rates than the non-Asian population (Lum, 1995). Other studies have found that the suicide rate among Chinese American elderly women is as high as 10 times that for White women (Browne & Broderick, 1994). Not surprisingly, depression is widespread in the elderly. Japanese American elders demonstrate their depression through exaggerated anxiety over minor changes in physical or mental functions (Douglas & Fujimoto, 1995). The authors attributed the frequency of depression in this population to tension in intergenerational relationships and changes in functional status. Lum (1995) identified trauma related to migration and immigration, isolation from peers, poverty, and alienation from younger family members as risk factors for mental health problems.

When considering mental health problems of Pacific Islanders, and Samoans in particular, it is important to understand the concept of the *'aiga,* or the extended family. Samoans take pride in the ability of the *'aiga* to look after their own family members (Barker, 1991). They turn to help outside the *'aiga* only after the resources of the family are exhausted. Family members and the *'aiga* have a high tolerance for absorbing deviant behavior and physical or mental differences within the family. Western psychiatric care is used only as a last resort or at the behest of formal agencies (Barker, 1991). However, the *'aiga* can also be a source of much stress for an individual striving to meet the demands and expectations of an extended family. This is true whether the family unit is in the United

States or in the home country. Family expectations include a stable marriage, a large family, employment, remittances sent back to the extended family in the home country, and community leadership. Samoans must deal with these issues in addition to the stresses of migration and acculturation.

Southeast Asian Populations

For some Southeast Asian groups, most of the published health literature focuses on mental health issues, with limited reports on physical health problems. By focusing on mental health to the exclusion of other health problems, important epidemiological information may be missed, such as increases in cardiovascular diseases, cancer, and drug use. One reason for the strong mental health focus may be that in some groups, notably Cambodian refugee families, very high levels of stress have been identified (Carlson & Rosser-Hogan, 1993; Frye & D'Avanzo, 1994; Handelman & Yeo, 1996; Sack *et al.,* 1993). Refugee status for Vietnamese immigrants has been identified as one of the strongest predictors of mental health problems (Flaskerud & Soldevilla, 1986; Lum, 1995).

Adolescents

Few studies examine the mental health of Asian Pacific Islander children and adolescents. However, a longitudinal study of Cambodian adolescents who lived through the genocidal Pol Pot regime from 1975 to 1979 and are now living in the United States with their families, showed high levels of posttraumatic stress disorder (PTSD), depression, and anxiety disorder when first interviewed in 1984 (Clarke, Sack, & Goff, 1993; Sack *et al.,* 1993). This group of adolescents was reinterviewed in 1987 and 1990 to determine how the rates of PTSD and depressive and anxiety disorders would vary years after the traumatic event. Also, researchers wished to determine the functional status of the now young adults using their own War Trauma

Scale and Resettlement Stressor Scale (Sack *et al.,* 1993). The authors found in the 1984 interview that PTSD, diagnosed in 50% of the study population, and depressive disorders, also found in 50%, were closely linked. However, in the 1990 follow-up interview, the two diagnoses were no longer linked. Clinical depression had almost disappeared and was seen in only 6% of the group, although signs of PTSD were still present in 38% of the youth. These young people were functioning well, and the persistence of PTSD did not appear to significantly impact their performance in school or on the job.

Adults and the Elderly

Chronic physical complaints of Southeast Asian Americans have been described by a number of authors as somatizations of depression, anxiety, or posttraumatic stress disorder (Carlson & Rosser-Hogan, 1993; D'Avanzo, Frye, & Froman, 1994; Flaskerud & Soldevilla, 1986; Handelman & Yeo, 1996; Kroll *et al.,* 1989; Lum, 1995). Southeast Asian individuals with mental health problems are cared for by the family at home until the behavior becomes unmanageable. When they do present to health facilities, they exhibit symptoms such as heart palpitations, chest pain, shortness of breath, headache, fatigue, loss of appetite, and body pains, which the patient would not attribute to a mental or emotional disorder (Flaskerud & Soldevilla, 1986; Handelman & Yeo, 1996; Kroll *et al.,* 1989).

Lum (1995) cited a study of Southeast Asian refugees seen in a psychiatric clinic where 70% met the criteria for PTSD. According to Palinkas and Pickwell (1995), Cambodian refugees living in the United States have higher levels of both physical and psychological illness than other Southeast Asian groups. This higher incidence of health problems is a result of the genocide and other trauma experienced during the Pol Pot regime, the war in Southeast Asia, and from migration and resettlement experiences, which generally included time in a refugee camp before resettlement in the United States.

Tran (1993) reported that depression is commonly found among Vietnamese patients diagnosed with a mental disorder, and is often related to loss of status, role changes, generational conflicts, unfulfilled expectations of social and economic attainment, and the dependency of young and old family members. This depression is compounded by delayed response to the premigration and escape experiences of many Vietnamese immigrants (Lin-Fu, 1988; Tran, 1993). The trauma of the Vietnam war was enhanced by severe hardship during migration either overland through Cambodia or on overcrowded boats and years in refugee camps. The added stress of resettling in the United States and adjusting to a new language, culture, and values has left Vietnamese refugees at high risk for emotional disorders (Flaskerud & Soldevilla, 1986). In a 1995 report by Lum, a 20% prevalence rate for depression was found in Vietnamese patients seen in public health clinics.

For some refugees, time may eventually ease the pain but for many others such psychological trauma is often suppressed. When Asians with PTSD are admitted to mental health facilities, manifestations are often more severe than in other ethnic groups (Flaskerud & Soldevilla, 1986). Carlson and Rosser-Hogan (1993) interviewed a nonclinical random sample of 50 Cambodian adult refugees living in Greensboro, North Carolina (mean age: 42 years; range: 21–65 years) and found a PTSD rate of 86%, which is similar to that found in a comparable group of Cambodian refugees living in California. Other studies have reported rates of PTSD ranging from 22% to 92%. The authors stated that rates of depression (80%) and anxiety (78%) were also high in their sample. Despite the frequency of these problems, only one of the study participants sought and received mental health care services.

A lack of understanding of culturally specific explanatory models may affect diagnosis of presenting symptoms by the doctor, as well as patient compliance with Western treatment regimens. Handelman and Yeo (1996) found that examining culturally specific concepts led to a better understanding of chronic somatic complaints among Cambodian refugees. In a study to elucidate causal factors underlying chronic symptoms seen in Cambodian refugee patients, Handelman and Yeo compared a group of adult Cambodians receiving psychiatric care with a nonclinical sample of adult Cambodians. Headache was the most frequent chronic symptom reported by respondents in both groups, and equal numbers reported cardiovascular and pulmonary symptoms (chest pain, shortness of breath, chronic cough, wheezing, and palpitations). Nonclinical participants also reported musculoskeletal symptoms (muscular pain, joint pain). Although chronic headache was reported by both groups, it was the only symptom significantly associated with being under psychiatric care and having depression. Although all participants identified multiple causes for their chronic complaints, "extreme sadness" (*pruiy chiit*) and "thinking too much" (*kiit chraen*) were the most commonly given reasons by both groups. These have been reported to be culture-bound syndromes associated with PTSD by other authors (Frye & D'Avanzo, 1994; Moore & Boehnlein, 1991). Other explanations given were physical stress, aging, "imbalance" (*tiet akrak*), and karma (*tweu lam*). The authors recommended that complaints of chronic headache in Cambodian patients should serve as a reminder to physicians to evaluate the patient for depression.

One published study (Moore & Boehnlein, 1991) examining psychiatric disorders in Mien refugees from highland Laos identified issues similar to those faced by the Cambodian population. Trauma related to war, geographic dislocations, and forced migration from Laos to the United States caused high levels of PTSD and major depression generally expressed through somatic symptoms. Moore and Boehnlein suggested that a central role of therapy should be to help patients reestablish their equilibrium with their environment, and that clinicians should expect long-term therapeutic relationships with their Mien patients because of the chronicity of their symptoms. The authors also demonstrated through case studies that traditional Mien and Western healing practices can co-exist in the provision of care and are more effective in the long run.

Family Stress

Frye and D'Avanzo (1994) examined family stress, violence, and emotional distress among Cambodian refugee women living in inner city environments in Long Beach, California, and Lowell, Massachusetts. Headache was identified as the most prevalent symptom of the culture-bound syndrome "thinking too much," followed by chest pain, palpitations, shortness of breath, excess sleeping, and withdrawal, all classic symptoms of anxiety. Differences were noted between the two groups when asked about the causes of "thinking too much." The Long Beach cohort indicated that memories of the Pol Pot regime were the leading cause. The Lowell group stated that financial difficulties were the main cause. The Lowell cohort was generally poorer, less educated, younger, and had more young dependents than the Long Beach group. When asked how they coped with "thinking too much," the majority of women from both sites stated that they would avoid sad thoughts and being alone; however, some women also mentioned suicide as an alternative. Similar strategies, with the exception of suicide, were identified for helping a family member cope with "thinking too much." When asked how they would deal with a family member who became physically or emotionally violent while suffering from "thinking too much," more women from Long Beach stated they would "talk softly" to the individual and would deal with the situation within the family. However, half of the Lowell cohort indicated that they would call the police if necessary.

Although Asian Americans have some of the lowest levels of alcohol use, some authors have reported an increase in use as Asians acculturate (D'Avanzo et al., 1994). The use of alcohol and drugs to relieve stress resulting from "thinking too much" was reported by some women in a study conducted by Frye and D'Avanzo (1994). Frye and D'Avanzo's Lowell cohort reported more use of alcohol, while the Long Beach cohort reported greater use of prescription drugs, primarily sleeping pills, for self-treatment. The authors concluded that withdrawal and avoidance of conflict in response to stress leave Cambodian women more vulnerable to victimization in the urban environments they live in, and at greater risk for possible alcohol and drug abuse (D'Avanzo et al., 1994; Frye & D'Avanzo, 1994).

Chronic Diseases

The two most important chronic diseases studied among the ethnic subgroups of Asian Pacific Islander Americans have been cancer and heart disease. The groups most studied have been Chinese and Japanese, most likely because of their larger numbers in the Asian American population and the longer length of time they have been in the United States, as compared with other Asian American subgroups. Very little data on chronic diseases are available on South and Southeast Asian immigrant populations. Data on Pacific Islander subgroups are particularly limited since these groups were not counted separately until the 1980 U.S. census. The only Pacific Islander ethnic group identified separately prior to that time was the Hawaiians.

Studies have shown a gradient in mortality for certain chronic diseases (Imazu et al., 1996; Nichaman et al., 1975; Syme et al., 1975; Zane et al., 1994). First-generation immigrants tend to reflect patterns of risk and mortality that more closely resemble those in their country of origin, while generations farther removed tend to reflect patterns that more closely resemble that of the general U.S. population (Lum, 1995). Significant changes in health-related behaviors as individuals move from one country to another, as well as changes observed across succeeding generations, may all contribute to the observed gradients in chronic disease prevalence in Asian Pacific Islander immigrant populations (Barringer et al., 1993).

Cardiovascular Disease

Hypertension

Although hypertension is fairly common among some Asian American groups, Asians generally have lower rates of hypertension than Whites. This statistic does not reflect, however, the significantly lower levels of information Asians have about hypertension, and their lower rates of blood pressure screening and medication treatment (Chen et al., 1994; Mayeno & Hirota, 1994). For Asian Americans, hypertension is influenced by stress related to immigration and acculturation, body weight, country of origin, and demographic factors such as age and gender (Zane et al., 1994). In a study of Boston Chinese immigrants, blood pressure levels were correlated with age and gender among Chinese elderly. While the prevalence of hypertension was significantly less than that of elderly White Americans, and closely resembled the patterns of the elderly population in mainland China, hypertension prevalence increased by age and was significantly higher among elderly Chinese women than Chinese men (Zane et al., 1994). Other researchers have noted changes to higher fat diets after immigration, and Bates (1989) reported moderate to high total cholesterol levels in 24% of Southeast Asians seen in a clinic setting.

A 1996 study by Imazu and colleagues compared the prevalence and risk factors of high blood pressure among Japanese living in Hiroshima, Japan; Honolulu, Hawaii; and Los Angeles, California. The prevalence rates of hypertension in Honolulu, Los Angeles, and Hiroshima were 42.6%, 37.2%, and 29.7%, respectively. Even more interesting is that the majority of the Japanese studied in Hawaii and California were first-generation immigrants. In examining interpopulation differences among the genetically similar population of Japanese living in different areas, the differences can be attributed primarily to culture and environment (Imazu et al., 1996; Nichaman et al., 1975; Syme et al., 1975).

Studies of hypertension among Korean Americans have also found lower rates as compared with the general U.S. population, with differences by gender (Korean American men have a much higher prevalence rate, 22.4%, than Korean women, 3.2%) (Zane et al., 1994). While no correlation has been reported between dietary factors and hypertension for this group, family history has been found to be a major risk factor for Korean American men. The prevalence of hypertension among Filipinos in the United States is the highest compared with any other Asian American subgroup. In a 1984 study by Stavig et al., Filipinos had higher rates of uncontrolled hypertension than did the Chinese and Japanese Americans surveyed. While elevated blood pressure among Asian Americans was 18.3%, 24.5% of Filipinos had elevated blood pressure (Zane et al., 1994). Further study is required to understand the root causes of the high rates of hypertension among Filipino Americans and Korean American men.

In a "Heart Health" intervention targeting Southeast Asians conducted by Chen and colleagues (1994), only 3.6% of Cambodian, 1.8% of Lao, and 4.3% of Vietnamese study participants were able to define what blood pressure was prior to the intervention. Similarly low levels of knowledge with respect to ways to prevent heart disease were seen among the three groups. Using indigenous outreach workers, multiple communication strategies were developed to inform the target population in their own languages about the importance of monitoring blood pressure and ways to prevent heart disease. Postintervention, significant gains ($p < 0.01$) were seen in all three groups with respect to correctly defining blood pressure (Cambodian = 59%, Lao = 51%, and Vietnamese = 62%) and prevention of heart disease (Cambodian = 86%, Lao = 76%, and Vietnamese = 77%). This study demonstrates that culturally and linguistically appropriate health education interventions are effective in increasing knowledge on specific health issues, although the authors recommended further study to examine whether actual behavior changes occurred.

Coronary Heart Disease

With regard to heart disease, Asian Americans show lower levels of mortality than U.S. Whites but their mortality rates exceed those in their country of origin. For example, in a 1987 study by King and Locke of ischemic heart disease (IHD) among Chinese immigrants, mortality due to IHD was significantly lower than that of U.S. Whites, but far exceeded that of their country of origin (King & Locke, 1987). Similar results were found in a smaller study of coronary heart disease mortality among Filipinos in Hawaii (Barringer et al., 1993).

The well-known Ni-Hon-San study published in the 1970s explored the gradient in the incidence of coronary heart disease (CHD) among Japanese in Japan, Hawaii, and California. The study showed the significance of the variety of CHD risk factors for one Asian ethnic group living in very different environmental and cultural conditions, with the gradient in CHD risk factors increasing from Japan to California (Syme et al., 1975). Among the biochemical risk factors measured—cholesterol, glucose, and uric acid—the levels were significantly lower for men in Japan than in California or Hawaii in every age group (Nichaman et al., 1975). Mortality attributed to CHD in the three geographic locations also corresponded to the gradient pattern found in the biochemical variables. The diet consumed by Japanese Americans is generally higher in animal fat, dairy, and simple carbohydrates; when combined with a more sedentary lifestyle as seen in the United States, these conditions lead to an increase in the risk factors for cardiovascular disease.

Smoking

Cigarette Smoking

Smoking is a major cause of coronary heart disease. In the United States, smoking rates have been found to be higher among recently immigrated Asians, due to the fact that smoking in Asian countries is more prevalent than in the United States. With increased acculturation, smoking prevalence rates decline among Asian Americans in a manner that resembles the pattern of decline in smoking that has occurred in the general U.S. population over the past 30 years (Zane et al., 1994). However, studies have consistently found high rates of smoking among Asian American subpopulations, with significantly higher rates among Asian American men than women and rates of 55% and higher among immigrants from Southeast Asia (Moeschberger et al., 1997; Zane et al., 1994).

Cigarette smoking rates among Cambodian and Lao men are among the highest reported in the United States. Moeschberger and colleagues (1997) reported smoking prevalence rates of between 33% and 55% for Cambodian, 72% for Lao, and 56% for Vietnamese males, compared to 32% of non-Asian U.S. men (Imazu et al., 1996), with no indication of a decline such as that seen in smoking prevalence rates for White and African American males (0.57% and 0.67% per year, respectively). Given these high rates, it is expected that increasing morbidity and mortality due to cardiovascular disease and lung cancer will be seen in this group. Moeschberger and colleagues developed profiles of current smokers, former smokers, and nonsmokers for Cambodian, Lao, and Vietnamese men to identify smoking cessation strategies appropriate for each group. They found that those who quit smoking tended to be older, employed, more assimilated in U.S. culture, and of Cambodian ethnicity. In contrast, current smokers tended to be older than nonsmokers, not in the labor force, traditionally oriented to their native culture, less educated, and of Vietnamese or Lao ethnicity. Currently, few smoking cessation programs specifically target Southeast Asian men.

Betel Quid Chewing

While Asian women do not traditionally smoke cigarettes, in some areas of South and Southeast Asia chewing of the betel nut is common among older women. Although a decline in this practice has been noted in some countries, it continues among older women (Reichart, Schmidtberg, & Scheifele, 1996). The betel quid, a combination of areca nut (the betel nut), betel leaf, lime paste, and leaf tobacco, is placed between the gum and the cheek and then chewed for long periods of time; sometimes the tobacco is placed on the opposite side of the mouth and chewed simultaneously (Pickwell, Schimelpfening, & Palinkas, 1994; Reichart et al., 1996). The ingredients are easy to find in Asian markets in the United States, and come in prepackaged sets. The betel mixture permanently stains the teeth and mouth of the individual a dark color. Health risks associated with betel chewing are oral cancer, oral leukoplakia, and mucosal lesions known as "betel chewer's mucosa," which have been suggested to represent an early form of submucous fibrosis (Reichart et al., 1996). In a study of Cambodian women refugees participating in the Cambodian Home Health Care Project in San Diego, California, Pickwell and colleagues (1994) noted that betel quid chewers were generally over 50 years of age and started using betel after the birth of their first child. Betel chewing was found to be an important social activity for adult women. Most of the women did not identify any physical effects from chewing betel, although most acknowledged that the practice was highly addictive. None of the women viewed chewing betel as a health risk even though many indicated that smoking tobacco could cause lung cancer. However, they did not see an association between tobacco that is chewed and tobacco that is smoked.

Both Pickwell and colleagues (1994) and Reichart and colleagues (1996) found that young Cambodian women are not continuing the practice of chewing betel as they move into the adult social world. While this might be expected for Cambodian women living in the United States, Reichart's findings were from a study conducted in three small villages in Cambodia. This finding reflects other studies which indicate that the prevalence of betel chewing is slowly declining in most South and Southeast Asian countries, while remaining stable in others (e.g., Taiwan) (Reichart *et al.,* 1996). The authors suggested that betel chewing may be less appealing to younger women due to the staining around the mouth by the betel juice.

Cancer

Early studies of cancer among Chinese Americans found that Chinese were at relatively high risk for cancer of the nasopharynx, liver, and esophagus, and at relatively low risk for breast and prostate cancer (Barringer *et al.,* 1993; Lum, 1995). These risk patterns followed closely those for Chinese in Asia. However, investigators have found that the longer immigrants lived in the United States, the more like the U.S. population their risk patterns became for certain cancers. For example, a 1990 study of colorectal cancer among Chinese Americans found that colorectal cancer was significantly associated with saturated fat intake and a sedentary lifestyle, and that the risk of colorectal cancer for Chinese immigrants increased with the number of years lived in the United States (Barringer *et al.,* 1993). Japanese Americans have also been found to have a high frequency of certain cancers. Stomach cancer occurs at a rate almost three times that of the White population (Barringer *et al.,* 1993). There has also been a steady rise in the incidence of colorectal cancer, as well as an upward trend in breast cancer among Japanese American women (Lin-Fu, 1988; Lum, 1995).

Of the minority groups examined by the 1985 U.S. Department of Health and Human Services Secretary's Task Force on Black and Minority Health, Hawaiians had the highest rate of breast cancer at 33.6/100,000, compared with 26.6/100,000 in non-Hispanic Whites and 26.3/100,000 in African Americans. The average annual age-adjusted cancer mortality rate was 200.5 for Hawaiians compared to 163.6 for Whites. A 1996 report showed some of the first data on the incidence and relative risk of cancer among American Samoans, the second largest Pacific Islander group in the United States after Hawaiians (17% of all Pacific Islanders) (Mishra, Luce-Aoelua, Wilkins, & Bernstein, 1996). Using data from the Los Angeles County/University of Southern California Cancer Surveillance Program and the Hawaii Tumor Registry, Mishra and colleagues found that American Samoans had higher relative risks for cancer of the nasopharynx, stomach, liver, gallbladder, lung, thyroid, and corpus uteri, as well as leukemia. They had lower relative risks for cancers of the colon, bladder, and cervix. However, because census information on the different Pacific Islander groups was not collected until 1980, data reported to the Cancer Surveillance Program and the Tumor Registry may be incomplete and unreliable primarily due to underestimations. These preliminary data suggest a need for preventive attention to American Samoans, as well as a closer examination into the lifestyle and culture of this population in order to better understand the site-specific high incidences of cancer. This study also shows a need for more adequate data collection in order to better address the cancer-related health issues of the Pacific Islander populations.

A study comparing local data on cancer screening among Asian Americans with data from the National Health Interview Survey found that levels of cancer screening for Asian Americans were significantly lower than for the U.S. population as a whole (Mayeno & Hirota, 1994). While 9% of the U.S. population reported never having had a Pap smear, 32% of Vietnamese in San Francisco and 45% of Chinese in Oakland reported never having had a Pap smear. Sixty-two percent of the U.S. population reported never having had a mammogram, while 82% of San Francisco Vietnamese and 74% of Oakland Chinese reported never having had a mammogram (Mayeno & Hirota, 1994).

According to three recently published studies on cancer screening in Cambodian and Lao women, little has been available in the literature on cancer rates for these two

Southeast Asian populations (Bailey *et al.,* 1996; Kelly *et al.,* 1996; Yi & Prows, 1996). All three studies identified significant cultural barriers to breast and uterine cervical cancer screening. These include embarrassment over the physical exam; cultural constraints around being touched by a stranger, especially a male doctor; belief that cancer cannot be treated; and fear of large medical facilities and the equipment used. Two of the studies developed and evaluated interventions to increase screening rates (Bailey *et al.,* 1996; Kelly *et al.,* 1996).

Common themes between the interventions developed for Cambodian (Bailey *et al.,* 1996; Kelly *et al.,* 1996) and Lao (Bailey *et al.,* 1996) women were the need to dedicate significant individual time to explain why screenings are necessary, explain the purpose of the equipment, provide an opportunity for women to socialize with each other as well as the program organizers before starting sessions, ensure that female doctors carried out the exams, and explain results once they were received. Southeast Asian immigrant women have some of the lowest literacy and socioeconomic levels among Asian and Pacific Islander immigrant groups, and therefore tend to access preventive services at much lower rates than other groups (Bailey *et al.,* 1996). Although Kelly and colleagues (1996) reported that their multidimensional approach to cancer screening for Cambodian women was labor intensive and expensive, they conclude that the approach was critical in order to persuade women to undergo screening for both breast and uterine cervical cancer (74% were screened). They also suggested that this approach can be used to address other health issues for other immigrant groups with low acculturation levels.

While Asian women in Asia have lower rates of breast and uterine cervical cancers, and these rates increase after immigration, they are often still lower than the rates in other U.S. populations. However, the risks to health and well-being caused by a lack of screening for cervical and breast cancer are significant enough to call for further study in this area. It is important to understand the barriers to screening for these cancers and to determine what services or programs are necessary to effectively reach this population with regular screening services.

Diabetes

Obesity has been found to be a significant problem for some Asian American populations, placing them at risk for related disorders such as heart disease and diabetes. While for some obesity is related to family history, lifestyle, and dietary habits, for others, such as Korean Americans, the risk for obesity increases with length of residence in the United States. The increase in obesity observed with length of residence in the United States is more marked among Korean men than women (Zane *et al.,* 1994). Obesity has been found to be related to economic and gender factors as well. Affluent Korean men tend to be more obese than those who are less affluent, whereas the converse is true for Korean women. For other Asian subgroups, obesity was also significantly more prevalent among the men than the women. Gender differences in obesity are further illustrated in data that indicate that of the Asian American subgroups studied, only Samoan women were found to have higher percentages of obesity than men.

The high rate of obesity found in certain subgroups of Asian Pacific Islanders has implications for related illnesses such as diabetes. However, since precise data on the incidence and prevalence of diabetes among A/PIs are not available, only prevalence estimates can be used to estimate the degree to which Asian Pacific Islander Americans suffer from this disorder (Zane *et al.,* 1994). National prevalence estimates of diabetes range from 2% to 18%, based on data for these populations in overseas settings. However, state-level data on diabetes mortality among Asian Pacific Islanders give a more precise picture of the impact of this disease. Data compiled in California in 1988 and 1989 showed that Samoans had the highest age-adjusted diabetes mortality rates of all Asian Pacific Islanders, exceeding that of White Americans by 47% (Zane *et al.,* 1994). Chinese and Korean Americans showed diabetes mortality rates (6.0–7.5/100,000 and 4.5/100,000, respectively) that were significantly lower than that of White Americans (10.7/100,000). In Hawaii, Filipino, Chinese, and Korean Americans showed diabetes mortality rates exceeding that of White Americans by two- to threefold (Zane *et al.,* 1994). According to Lum (1995), there is a higher prevalence of diabetes and glucose intolerance among Japanese Americans than among non-Hispanic Whites. This higher rate is attributed to a genetic predisposition of Japanese to diabetes that is triggered through acculturation to the Western lifestyle, namely the American diet.

Conclusions and Recommendations

Asian Pacific Islanders are a very diverse group with respect to health status. Examining this population as one homogeneous group is not an effective way of assessing their needs since their diversity is rooted in the customs and traditions of their countries of origin. This diversity extends through their patterns of migration to their lifestyles in the United States. Although the availability of national data on specific subgroups in the Asian Pacific Islander population is inadequate, significant work has been done at the state and local levels on the mental health needs of Asian Pacific Islanders and the impact of cultural differences on their access to the mainstream U.S. mental health care system. The results of those studies show that significant differences in premigration experiences, expectancies of and preparation for life in the United States, language proficiency, economic attainment, and employment status can have negative effects on the mental health of Asian immigrants. Studies analyzing cultural differences have found that conceptualizations of health and illness and

the values that govern interpersonal interaction differ significantly between Asian immigrants and U.S. society. All of these differences hinder access to the mainstream U.S. health care system, especially for those who utilize traditional health practices (i.e., the elderly and those who have most recently migrated).

Other significant health issues for Asian Pacific Islander Americans that need to be studied and monitored are infectious diseases (e.g., hepatitis B, tuberculosis, AIDS), chronic disease (e.g., cancer, hypertension, diabetes) and infant outcomes (e.g., infant mortality, prenatal care, low birth weight). Recent results have shown that while Asian Americans account for small proportions of cases in these disease areas overall, there are significant differences among the subgroups that make up the Asian Pacific Islander population, some of which are disproportionately affected by certain diseases. These differences show that certain groups of Asian Americans lack access to screening and treatment services, increasing their susceptibility to poor health outcomes. These differences also show the ineffectiveness of some programs aimed at lowering the rates of morbidity, for example, screening pregnant A/PI women for HBV to reduce perinatal transmission of the virus. Although the recommendation to screen pregnant A/PI women was made in 1984, in 1988, there was only a 2% HBV immunization rate. Such results show that screening and treatment efforts need to be targeted and accompanied by knowledgeable health providers who can recognize these specific health issues. In addition, there is a need for more education, prevention, and intervention outreach to groups of Asian Pacific Islanders in order to improve their health outcomes.

This chapter and other research have shown that there are significant gaps in knowledge regarding the health issues and health care needs of Asian Pacific Islanders. While there has been a significant amount of research in the area of mental health, other health areas have not received the same attention. The following are recommendations concerning how to effectively identify and address the health care needs of Asian Pacific Islander Americans and recommendations for future research that will broaden our knowledge base for this target population.

General Recommendations

1. *Increase efforts to explore and study the specific subgroups that make up the Asian Pacific Islander population.* Data that are group specific will be more useful in understanding group-related health behaviors, health needs, and occurrences of disease and illness. Stratified data will help develop appropriate services and programs that are more effective in meeting those needs.

2. *Develop health services and programs using state and local data, which can provide more specific information on the groups in an area, until national data are group-specific for Asian Pacific Islander Americans.* Relying on broad national data that may not adequately represent some subgroups may result in health problems being missed or underestimated.

3. *Conduct more research in areas other than mental health for Asian Pacific Islander Americans.* While mental health is an important issue, the longer Asian immigrants are in the United States, the more they will resemble the general U.S. population in the incidence and prevalence of disease and illness related to the U.S. lifestyle, such as hypertension, heart disease, and obesity. It is necessary to understand the causal factors (i.e., hereditary, biological, behavioral, and psychosocial) of these disorders among A/PIs in order to develop appropriate services and programs to meet their long-term needs.

4. *Explore various means of communication in order to effectively provide Asian Pacific Islander Americans with health education and screening and treatment information.* This information, whether orally or visually communicated, should be provided in a culturally appropriate manner that increases understanding of the health issue in the cultural context of the specific subgroup. Identification of communication channels should take into account low literacy levels in both English and native languages as well as preferred methods for receiving information and discussing health problems (including the source of the information and the setting in which it is delivered).

5. *Provide culturally appropriate services through mainstream facilities.* Rather than dismiss underutilization of health services as merely a cultural barrier for the patient to overcome, changes must be made in the system to facilitate access to services. Trained translators and interpreters are needed to address language barriers, but cannot replace providers who understand the culture and the conceptualizations of health and illness that Asian Pacific Islanders have. Such providers are key to incorporating the U.S. medical system and its practices in a framework that the patient will understand and be able to manage within his or her cultural framework. Mainstream health facilities should collaborate with ethnic-specific clinics in predominantly Asian immigrant communities to develop a process of diagnosis and treatment that effectively meets the needs of Asian Pacific Islander Americans.

Issue-Specific Recommendations

1. Use local data on poverty and health insurance rates for Asian Pacific Islander Americans to more accurately assess the impact of these factors on access to and utilization of health services.

2. Include specific HIV/AIDS education and prevention strategies for high-risk

subgroups within the broader A/PI community, such as gay or bisexual and limited-English-language individuals, and heterosexual men and women with multiple partners.

3. Develop hepatitis B education, prevention, screening, and treatment services that reflect culturally specific explanatory models of the disease, including translations of medical terminology and means of transmission.

4. Reduce tuberculosis (TB) transmission by conducting TB education, prevention, and treatment services in various stages over time in order to promptly identify individuals who may originally have screened negative, but have subsequently developed active TB.

5. Develop frameworks for mental health which reflect the role of the extended family in decision making and the local concepts of health and illness.

6. Determine barriers to screening for cancer, in particular breast and uterine and cervical cancers, and develop effective outreach strategies to increase cancer screening rates in the A/PI communities.

References

Abrantes, P. (1994). The impact of race and culture on adolescent girls: Four perspectives. *Women's Health Issues, 4*(2), 85–91.

Agbayani-Siewert, P. (1994, September). Filipino American culture and family: Guidelines for practitioners. *Journal of Contemporary Human Services,* 429–438.

Anonymous. (1991, Summer). [Editorial]. *Journal of Christian Nursing,* 5–6.

Bailey S., Bennett, P., Hicks, J., Kemp, C., & Warren, S. H. (1996). Cancer detection activities coordinated by nursing students in community health. *Cancer Nursing, 19*(5), 348–352.

Barker, J. C. (1991). Pacific Island migrants in the United States: Some implications for aging services. *Journal of Cross-Cultural Gerontology, 6,* 173–192.

Barringer, H. R., Gardner, R. W., & Levin, M. J. (1993). *Asians and Pacific Islanders in the United States.* New York: Russell Sage Foundation.

Brown, W. J. (1992, August). Culture and AIDS education: Reaching high-risk heterosexuals in Asian-American communities. *Journal of Applied Communication Research,* 275–291.

Browne, C., & Broderick, A. (1994). Asian and Pacific Island elders: Issues for social work practice and education. *Social Work, 39*(3), 252–259.

Burr, J. A., & Mutchler, J. E. (1993). Nativity, acculturation, and economic status: Explanations of Asian American living arrangements in later life. *Journal of Gerontology, 48*(2), S55–S63.

Carlson, E. B., & Rosser-Hogan, R. (1993). Mental health status of Cambodian refugees ten years after leaving their homes. *American Journal of Orthopsychiatry, 63*(2), 223–231.

Catolico, O. (1997). Psychological well-being of Cambodian women in resettlement. *Advances in Nursing Science, 19*(4), 75–84.

Chen, M. S., Anderson, J., Moeschberger, M., Guthrie, R., Kuun, P., & Zaharlick, A. (1994). An evaluation of heart health education for Southeast Asians. *American Journal of Preventive Medicine, 10*(4), 205–208.

Chin, S. Y. (1992). Cross-cultural medicine a decade later: This, that and the other: Managing illness in a first-generation Korean-American family. *Western Journal of Medicine, 157*(3), 305–309.

Choi, K. H., Lew, S., Vittinghoff, E., Catania, J. A., Barrett, D. C., & Coates, T. J. (1996). The efficacy of brief group counseling in HIV risk reduction among homosexual Asian and Pacific Islander men. *AIDS, 10,* 81–87.

Clarke, G., Sack, W. H., & Goff, B. (1993). Three forms of stress in Cambodian adolescent refugees. *Journal of Abnormal Child Psychology, 21*(1), 65–77.

D'Avanzo, C. E., Frye, B., & Froman, R. (1994). Culture, stress and substance use in Cambodian refugee women. *Journal of Studies on Alcohol, 55*(4), 420–426.

Douglas, K. C., & Fujimoto, D. (1995). Asian Pacific elders: Implications for health care providers. *Clinics in Geriatric Medicine, 11*(1), 69–82.

Flaskerud, J. H., & Akutsu, P. D. (1993). Significant influence of participation in ethnic-specific programs on clinical diagnosis for Asian-Americans. *Psychological Reports, 72,* 1228–1230.

Flaskerud, J. H., & Soldevilla, E. Q. (1986). Pilipino and Vietnamese clients: Utilizing an Asian mental health center. *Journal of Psychosocial Nursing, 24*(8), 32–36.

Frye, B. A., & D'Avanzo, C. D. (1994). Cultural themes in family stress and violence among Cambodian refugee women in the inner city. *Advances in Nursing Science, 16*(3), 64–77.

Fuentes-Afflick, E., & Hessol, N. A. (1997). Impact of Asian ethnicity and national origin in infant birth weight. *American Journal of Epidemiology, 145*(2), 148–155.

Gock, T. S. (1994). Acquired Immunodeficiency Syndrome. In N. W. S. Zane, D. T. Takeuchi, & K. N. J. Young (Eds.), *Confronting critical health issues of Asian and Pacific Islander Americans* (pp. 247–265). Thousand Oaks, CA: Sage.

Handelman, L., & Yeo, G. (1996). Using explanatory models to understand chronic symptoms of Cambodian refugees. *Clinical Research and Methods, 28*(4), 271–276.

Hann, H. W. L. (1994). Hepatitis B. In N. W. S. Zane, D. T. Takeuchi, & K. N. J. Young (Eds.), *Confronting critical health issues of Asian and Pacific Islander Americans* (pp. 148–173). Thousand Oaks, CA: Sage.

Imazu, M., Sumida, K., Yamabe, T., Yamamoto, H., Ueda, H., Hattori, Y., Miyauchi, A., Hara, H., & Yamakido, M. (1996). A comparison of the prevalence and risk factors of high blood pressure among Japanese living in Japan, Hawaii, and Los Angeles. *Public Health Reports, 3* (Suppl. 2), 59–61.

Jackson, J. C., Rhodes, L. A., Inui, T. S., & Buchwald, D. (1997). Hepatitis B among the Khmer: Issues of translation and concepts of illness. *Journal of General Internal Medicine, 12*(5), 292–298.

Jambunathan, J., & Stewart, S. (1995). Hmong women in Wisconsin: What are their concerns in pregnancy and childbirth? *Birth, 22*(4), 204–210.

Jenkins, C. N. H., McPhee, S. J., Bird, J. A., & Bonilla, N. T. H. (1990, July). Cancer risks and prevention practices among Vietnamese refugees. *Western Journal of Medicine, 153,* 34–39.

Jenkins, C. N. H., Le, T., McPhee, S. J., Stewart, S., & Ha, N. T. (1996). Health care access and preventive care among Vietnamese immigrants: Do traditional beliefs and practices pose barriers? *Social Science and Medicine, 43*(7), 1049–1056.

Katz, J., Prescott, K., & Woolf, A. D. (1996). Strychnine poisoning from a Cambodian traditional remedy. *American Journal of Emergency Medicine, 14*(5), 475–477.

Kelly, A. W., Chacori, M. D. M. F., Wollan, P. C., Trapp, M. H., Weaver, A. L., Barrier, P. A., Franz III, W. B., & Kottke, T. E. (1996). A program to increase breast and cervical cancer screening for Cambodian women in a midwestern community. *Mayo Clinic Proceedings, 71*(5), 437–444.

Kim, S., & Rew, L. (1994). Ethnic identity, role integration, quality of life, and depression in Korean-American women. *Archives of Psychiatric Nursing, 8*(6), 348–356.

King, H., & Locke, F. B. (1987). Health effects of migration: U.S. Chinese in and outside the Chinatown. *International Migration Review, 21,* 555–575.

Kroll, J., Habenicht, M., Mackenzie, T., Yang, M., Chan, S., Vang, T., Nguyen, T., Ly, M., Phommasourvanh, B., Nguven, H., Vang, Y., Souvannasoth,

L., & Cabugao, R. (1989). Depression and post-traumatic stress disorder in Southeast Asian refugees. *American Journal of Psychiatry, 146*(12), 1592–1597.

Kuo, W. H. (1984). Prevalence of depression among Asian Americans. *Journal of Nervous and Mental Disease, 172*(8), 449–457.

Lew, L. S. (1991). Elderly Cambodians in Long Beach: Creating cultural access to health care. *Journal of Cross-Cultural Gerontology, 6,* 199–203.

Lin-Fu, J. S. (1988). Population characteristics and health care needs of Asian Pacific Americans. *Public Health Reports, 103*(1), 18–27.

Loue, S., Lloyd, L., & Loh, L. (1996). HIV prevention in U.S. Asian Pacific Islander communities: An innovative approach. *Journal of Health Care for the Poor and Underserved, 7*(4), 364–376.

Lum, O. (1995). Health status of Asians and Pacific Islanders. *Clinics in Geriatric Medicine, 11*(1), 53–67.

Mayeno, L., & Hirota, S. M. (1994). Access to health care. In N. W. S. Zane, D. T. Takeuchi, & K. N. J. Young (Eds.), *Confronting critical health issues of Asian and Pacific Islander Americans* (pp. 347–375). Thousand Oaks, CA: Sage.

Miller, J. A. (1995). Caring for Cambodian refugees in the emergency department. *Journal of Emergency Nursing, 21*(6), 498–502.

Mishra, S. I., Luce-Aoelua, P., Wilkens, L. R., & Bernstein, L. (1996). Cancer among American-Samoans: Site-specific incidence in California and Hawaii. *International Journal of Epidemiology, 25*(4), 713–721.

Moeschberger, M. L., Anderson, M. A. S., Kuo, Y-F., Chen, M. S., Wewers, M. E., & Guthrie, R. (1997). Multivariate profile of smoking in Southeast Asian men: A biochemically verified analysis. *Preventive Medicine, 26*(1), 53–58.

Moore, L. J., & Boehnlein, J. K. (1991). Treating psychiatric disorders among Mien refugees from highland Laos. *Social Science and Medicine, 32*(9), 1029–1036.

Nichaman, M. Z., Hamilton, E. B., Kagan, A., Grier, T., Sacks, S. T., & Syme, S. L. (1975). Epidemiologic studies of CHD and stroke in Japanese men living in Japan, Hawaii, and California: Distribution of biochemical risk factors. *American Journal of Epidemiology, 102,* 491–501.

Ong, A. (1995). Making the biopolitical subject: Cambodian immigrants, refugee medicine and cultural citizenship in California. *Social Science and Medicine, 40*(9), 1243–1257.

Palinkas, L. A., & Pickwell, S. M. (1995). Acculturation as a risk factor for chronic disease among Cambodian refugees in the United States. *Social Science and Medicine, 40*(12), 1643–1653.

Pickwell, S. M., Schimelpfening, S., & Palinkas, L. A. (1994). "Betelmania": Betel quid chewing by Cambodian women in the United States and its potential health effects. *Western Journal of Medicine, 160*(4), 326–330.

Rairdan, B., & Higgs, Z. R. (1992, March). When your patient is a Hmong refugee. *American Journal Nursing,* 52–55.

Reichart, P. A., Schmidtberg, W., & Scheifele, C. (1996). Betel chewer's mucosa in elderly Cambodian women. *Journal of Oral Pathology & Medicine, 25*(7), 367–370.

Rice, P. L., Ly, B., & Lumley, J. (1994). Childbirth and soul loss: The case of a Hmong woman. *Medical Journal of Australia, 160*(9), 577–578.

Sack, W. H., Clarke, G., Him, C., *et al.* (1993). A 6-year follow-up study of Cambodian refugee adolescents traumatized as children. *Journal of the American Academy of Child and Adolescent Psychiatry, 32*(2), 431–437.

Shimada, J., Jackson, J. C., Goldstein, E., & Buchwald, D. (1995). "Strong medicine": Cambodian views of medicine and medical compliance. *Journal of General and Internal Medicine, 10*(7), 369–374.

Smith, M. J., & Ryan, A. S. (1987). Chinese-American families of children with developmental disabilities: An exploratory study of reactions to service providers. *Mental Retardation, 25*(6), 345–350.

Spring, M. A., Ross, P. J., Etkin, N. L., & Deinard, A. S. (1995). Sociocultural factors in the use of prenatal care by Hmong women, Minneapolis. *American Journal of Public Health, 85*(7), 1015–1017.

Stavig, G. R., Igra, A., & Leonard, A. R. (1984). Hypertension among Asians and Pacific Islanders in California. *American Journal of Epidemiology, 119*(5), 677–691.

Sworts, V. D., & Riccitelli, C. N. (1997). Health education lessons learned: the H.A.P.I. Kids Program. *Journal of School Health, 67*(7), 283–285.

Syme, S. L., Marmot, M. G., Kagan, A., Kato, H., & Rhoads, G. (1975). Epidemiologic studies of CHD and stroke in Japanese men living in Japan, Hawaii, and California: Introduction. *American Journal of Epidemiology, 102,* 477–480.

Takeuchi, D. T., & Young, K. N. J. (1994). Overview of Asian Pacific Islander Americans. In N. W. S. Zane, D. T. Takeuchi, & K. N. J. Young (Eds.), *Confronting critical health issues of Asian and Pacific Islander Americans* (pp. 3–21). Thousand Oaks, CA: Sage.

Tran, T. V. (1993). Psychological traumas and depression in a sample of Vietnamese people in the United States. *Health and Social Work, 18*(3), 184–194.

Uba, L. (1992). Cultural barriers to health care for Southeast Asian refugees. *Public Health Reports, 107*(5), 544–548.

Yi, J. K., & Prows, S. L. (1996). Breast cancer screening practices among Cambodian women in Houston, Texas. *Journal of Cancer Education, 11*(4), 221–225.

Ying, Y. W. (1990). Explanatory models of major depression and implications for help-seeking among immigrant Chinese-American women. *Culture, Medicine and Psychiatry, 14,* 393–408.

Zane, N. W. S., Sue, S., Hu, L., & Kwon, J. H. (1991). Asian-American assertion: A social learning analysis of cultural differences. *Journal of Counseling Psychology, 38*(1), 63–70.

Zane, N. W. S., Takeuchi, D. T., & Young, K. N. J. (1994). *Confronting critical health issues of Asian and Pacific Islander Americans.* Thousand Oaks, CA: Sage.

17

African Health

MARLENE FAUST, JAMES C. SPILSBURY, and SANA LOUE

Background

The number of African immigrants admitted to the United States has risen dramatically since the 1970s. The United States admitted 80,779 immigrants during the 1970s. During the following decade, the number of immigrants more than doubled to 176,893. This upward trend in migration is apparently continuing into the 1990s, with 83,781 African immigrants admitted from 1991 to 1993 alone (U.S. Department of Justice, 1993).

Many of these individuals have been admitted into the United States as refugees. From 1971 to 1980, a total of 2,991 African refugees were admitted into the United States. Many of these individuals (1,307 or 43%) came from Ethiopia. The number of refugees admitted from Africa increased 10-fold to 22,149 in the 1980s. In 1991–1992 alone, almost 10,000 African refugees were admitted as permanent residents, with the majority of these individuals (6,850 or 74%) from Ethiopia (U.S. Department of Justice, 1995). This surge of African immigrants to

the United States underscores the importance of educating health care workers about the special medical needs of this group.

In general, several factors have prompted immigration. Individuals may be seeking economic opportunities or fleeing the hardships of war, famine, or political unrest. Others may immigrate for social reasons (Takougang, 1995). These are the same motivations that have contributed to recent African migration to the United States. A brief review of the factors underlying recent waves of immigration from Nigeria, Sudan, and Ethiopia illustrates these motivations.

Nigeria, with a population of approximately 100 million, is not only the most populous African country, but is also one of the most potentially wealthy (Ekwe-Ekwe, 1990). However, the high hopes that many Nigerians had for their country were destroyed by continuing conflict within its borders. From 1967 to 1970, the Biafran civil war initially drove Nigerians from their homeland. Following the war, the country's gross national product (GNP) steadily rose, due mainly to the oil industry. Government corruption and poor investments eventually resulted in a huge government deficit, estimated to be 10% of the country's GNP (Pedder, 1993a) and a soaring inflation rate that has reached 100% (Adams, 1994). Consequently, Nigeria is now considered one of Africa's poorest countries. The educational system is understaffed due to low wages and campuses are often shut down. This eco-

MARLENE FAUST • School of Medicine, Case Western Reserve University, Cleveland, Ohio 44106-4945. JAMES C. SPILSBURY • Department of Anthropology, Case Western Reserve University, Cleveland, Ohio 44106. SANA LOUE • Department of Epidemiology and Biostatistics, School of Medicine, Case Western Reserve University, Cleveland, Ohio 44106-4945.

Handbook of Immigrant Health, edited by Loue. Plenum Press, New York, 1998.

nomic situation has prompted the migration of many of Nigeria's skilled and professional individuals to other countries (Pedder, 1993a).

In the early 1990s, Sudan suffered from increased fighting and shortages of food (Toole & Waldman, 1993). The number of individuals admitted to the United States doubled during 1990 and 1991 and continued to remain high through 1993 (U.S. Department of Justice, 1993).

Recent changes in the patterns of immigration from Ethiopia to the United States further illustrate the impact of these various motivating factors on immigration patterns. Prior to the 1980s, the majority of Ethiopians who entered the United States were from Ethiopia's educated class or came in search of education in the United States. Many were also fleeing political persecution (McCaw & DeLay, 1985). The state of higher education is poorly managed in Ethiopia, with universities understaffed and professors underpaid (Pedder, 1993b). Originally, many of the students who came to the United States planned to return to their homeland after completing their education. One study reported that prior to 1974, 95% of Ethiopian residents in the United States were students who intended to return to Ethiopia after finishing their education (Beyene, 1992). However, this situation began to change in the 1970s and students began to settle in the United States instead of returning home (Takougang, 1995).

There are several possible explanations for this shift. A Marxist regime was in power in Ethiopia in the earlier period and there was little political or individual freedom. Consequently, students who became familiar with Western democratic governments may have had little desire to return to such an oppressive political situation. During this same time, civil wars raged not only in Eritrea and Tigray, but throughout Africa. The Ethiopian civil war, begun in 1961, has been Africa's longest war. It has caused the death of more than a quarter million people and the displacement of three quarters of a million people (Kaplan, 1988). Several African countries, which would have potentially provided refuge for the

Ethiopian immigrants, also faced depressed economies, as well as high unemployment rates and low wages (Takougang, 1995).

Events in other African countries have also caused new waves of migrants to seek refuge in the United States. The recent war and genocide in Rwanda, involving the murder of as many as 1 million people, has sent the nation reeling. Some reports state that since the massacres began, 1.2 million individuals have fled the country, causing a refugee crisis unparalleled in world history (Watson, 1994). Other crises causing population displacement have occurred across Africa in countries such as Somalia, Liberia, Angola, and Mozambique (Toole, 1995).

Within the past decade, there has been a shift in the African populations that migrate to the United States. While previously, the immigrants from Africa were educated or professional people, recently the majority of individuals who migrate are from rural populations (McCaw & DeLay, 1985). Rural immigrants tend to be less assimilated to Western ways and medicine than are immigrants from the educated classes. They are also less likely to speak English and more likely to be in poorer health. One study estimated that 84% of the Ethiopian refugees examined by the participating health providers could not speak English (McCaw & DeLay, 1985). This has serious ramifications in the delivery of proper health care to these individuals (Chester & Holtan, 1992; Rafuse, 1993).

Additional factors also impact the volume and nature of immigration from Africa to the United States. The U.S. Congress is responsible for setting annual ceilings on the number of immigrants allowed entry through the usual immigration process. The number of individuals permitted entry as refugees, rather than through the more cumbersome immigration process, is set yearly by both Congress and the State Department (Freeman, 1994). Other democratic governments have set up different policies concerning the control of migration. In Europe, countries do not accept equal responsibility in welcoming refugees. For example, Germany has taken in half of all asylum seekers across Europe, totaling 438,000 admissions in 1992 (Wihtol De Wenden, 1994). France has recently adopted stricter policies on the number of individuals granted asylum due to an increasing number of applicants. While only 4% of asylum seekers were refused entry in 1976, 85% were refused admission in 1990. Presently, one third of applicants to France derive from African nations (Wihtol De Wenden, 1994). Great Britain takes a very conservative approach to immigration, still selecting individuals based on ethnicity or national origin (Freeman, 1994).

Since 1987, the United States has used HIV status as a criterion for screening individuals seeking to enter the country (Fairchild & Tynan, 1994). While this decision was made in an attempt to protect the public health of the country, it has resulted in immigration barriers to individuals thought to be from "high-risk" areas, such as the Caribbean and Africa. The "blood ban" on immigrants that originated in 1984 was extended to include not only Haitians but central Africans in 1986 and sub-Saharan Africans in 1990 (Fairchild & Tynan, 1994).

Newly arrived immigrants tend to settle where they have family ties, such as friends and relatives; where there are large concentrations of individuals with their ethnic background; and where there are opportunities for employment (Takougang, 1995). The greatest concentrations of Ethiopian immigrants are currently located in large metropolitan areas, such as Washington, D.C., Los Angeles, Boston, New York City, San Francisco, and Chicago (Beyene, 1992). This distribution can probably be attributed to greater opportunities for employment and the more tolerant racial climate of larger cities (Takougang, 1995).

Despite the large numbers of African immigrants resident in the United States and the increasing numbers being admitted to this country, little data are currently available concerning the health status of African immigrants to the United States. Pertinent information is available regarding African immigrants to other industrialized Western countries.

However, three considerations might limit the applicability of these data to the United States. First, much of the health data relating to immigrants to other Western countries address the concerns of refugee populations, which may differ significantly from nonrefugee immigrants in socioeconomic status and health status before and after immigration. Second, exclusion criteria and mandatory screening procedures vary by country, so the range of diseases with which immigrants enter their new country will differ across countries. Those individuals with specified diseases will be a priori inadmissible to countries excluding them on the basis of those diseases. Immigrants infected with HIV, for instance, are routinely excluded from the United States. Consequently, one would expect to see a relatively low prevalence of HIV in the immigrant community, unless the infection is contracted after arrival in the United States. Third, compared to countries with national health care systems, the "for pay" nature of the U.S. system may lead to delayed utilization of health services, resulting in increasing severity of presenting conditions among immigrants who do seek treatment.

In spite of these concerns, the experience of other industrialized countries with African immigrants may still be relevant to an American clinician, and the following discussion supplements information dealing with immigrants to the United States with that from other Western countries. This section is not intended as an exhaustive description of every possible disease that an African immigrant may present to an American clinician, but rather as illustrative of the types of diseases that may be observed and concerns that should be noted.

Maternal and Child Health

A longitudinal study of 238 immigrant women in Ottawa, Canada, found that Somali women had the lowest prenatal class attendance rates, compared with those of Lebanese, Polish, and Vietnamese immigrant women.

Somali women were among the most recent of the immigrants and a large proportion of them (60.7%) had entered as refugees. Of the four immigrant groups, they were more likely to report only fair or poor language ability in both French and English. This lack of language ability in either of the official languages was determined to be an important barrier to attendance at prenatal care classes. The researchers suggested the use of alternative models of care among non-English-, non-French-speaking immigrant groups, such as a "train the trainer" model, reliance on home visits by a paraprofessional from that immigrant community, and reliance on cultural brokers. (Edwards, 1994).

A study of birth outcomes of three cohorts of women with live singleton births in Washington state during the years 1980 through 1991 indicated that Ethiopian-born women were more likely to be older and married than U.S.–born women, and less likely to smoke. The Ethiopian women were significantly more likely to have high birth weight in babies than were the U.S.–born mothers (RR = 4.0). The authors of the study postulated that the favorable pregnancy outcomes among the Ethiopian women were attributable to greater emotional and psychological support as compared with that provided to U.S.–born Black women, better nutritional status among Ethiopian women, and genetic differences between the Ethiopian women and the U.S.–born Black women.

Breastfeeding appears to be more common among African immigrant women in France than among French-born women. Immigrant women from Africa are less likely than French women to be seropositive for either toxoplasmosis or rubeola (Bourdillon *et al.,* 1991).

A study of 5,508 births selected at random from 1981 national survey data found that occupational activity during pregnancy appears to be less common among immigrant women from North Africa than among French-born women. The occupational activity appeared to increase, though, as the educational level of the women increased. During the first trimester of pregnancy, North African women were more likely to carry heavy loads or stand for extended periods of time in conjunction with their work than were the French women (Stengel, Saurel-Cubizoles, & Kaminski, 1986).

The developmental milestones of some infants may be delayed due to malnutrition and parasitic infections. Assessment of these milestones may be rendered more difficult due to the lack of accurate birth records (Salzer & Nelson, 1983). Some children may have received uvulectomies. Many female children may have undergone clitorectomies prior to their arrival in the United States. Salzer and Nelson have reported the case of a toddler who was treated for tapeworm infestation with "fire therapy," which involved burning the skin on the abdomen with a stick that had been heated in fire. Iron deficiency anemia is not uncommon. (Salzer & Nelson, 1983).

Infectious Disease

Tuberculosis

In general, immigrant groups from African countries with high TB prevalence rates may reflect those high rates (Mortensen, Lang, Storm, & Viskum, 1989; Wartski, 1991). Articles concerning the health of African immigrants to the United States highlight the potential problem of TB in this group. For instance, a study of 239 Ethiopian immigrants to two major American cities found that 72% of these individuals were PPD positive, four (3.4%) had abnormal chest X rays, and one had a case of active pulmonary TB (Parenti, Lucas, Lee, & Hollenkamp, 1987). Moreover, immigrants of any age group may be infected. In a study conducted in Buffalo, New York, 1 of a total of 9 pediatric Somalian and Zairian refugees examined at a local hospital was PPD positive (Meropol, 1995), and almost 25% of TB cases in Ethiopian immigrants to Israel from 1980 to 1988 were 14 years old or younger (Wartski, 1991). An investigation of tuberculosis in two public schools in Scarborough, Ontario, Canada, found 11 children of a Somalian immigrant family with active pulmonary tuberculosis (Rothman & Dubeski, 1993).

Experience with immigrant TB in other Western countries indicates that occurrence of extrapulmonary TB is not rare. From 1989 to 1991, approximately 11% of the 261 cases of TB among Ethiopian immigrants to Israel was extrapulmonary (Wartski, 1993). The frequency by site of all 120 cases of extrapulmonary TB found in Ethiopians migrating to Israel since 1980 follows: lymph, 61%; bone, 13%; abdomen, 13%; skin and subcutaneous tissue, 4%; renal tract, 2%; pericardium, 2%; meninges, 2%; and other sites, 3% (Wartski, 1993). Extrapulmonary TB has also been noted in cases of African immigrants to the United Kingdom (Wells, Northover, & Howard, 1986; Wilkins & Roberts, 1985), Denmark (Mortensen et al., 1989), and Canada (Hanania & Hoffstein, 1993). In Western countries, correct diagnosis of extrapulmonary TB may be challenging because of its relative rarity. For example, Hanania and Hoffstein reported that skeletal TB and tuberculous lymphadenitis may mimic malignant lymphoma. Abdominal TB may also be easy to overlook because patients present with vague symptoms such as weight loss, malaise, pryrexia, and abdominal tenderness (Wells et al., 1986). In dealing with African immigrant populations, clinicians should be highly suspicious of symptoms resembling TB and maintain awareness of the various unusual and misleading manifestations of this infectious disease (Oren, Jamal, London, & Viskoper, 1991).

Malaria

Because malaria is endemic throughout much of Africa, occurrence of malaria in African immigrants should not be surprising. The experience of Ethiopian immigrants to Israel suggests that the likelihood of immigrants arriving infected with this disease is directly related to endemicity levels in their origin and staging points (Slater, Greenberg, & Costin, 1993). As an example, more than 60% of the immigrants to Israel in 1988 who had spent weeks in refugee camps located in malaria-endemic areas of Ethiopia arrived there infected with malaria. In contrast, in 1990 immigrants came from malaria-free regions of Ethiopia and, consequently, showed a very low prevalence rate of malaria parasitemia (0.15%).

In Great Britain, Phillips-Howard, Bradley, Blaze, and Hurn (1988) found that from 1977 to 1986, more than 80% of the 5,015 cases of *P. falciparum* malaria were acquired in sub-Saharan Africa. During this time period, the number of cases from Anglophone West Africa more than doubled from 147 to 409 and represented more than 60% of all the *P. falciparum* infections from Africa. Many of these cases, though, occurred in short-term migrants. Of note, the highest attack rates were observed in settled immigrants returning to their home countries to visit friends and relatives (316 per 100,000 for Africans and 331 per 100,000 for Asians). Clinicians in the United States should, therefore, recognize the potential risk of malarial infection incurred by African immigrants who return home for periodic visits.

Sexually Transmitted Diseases

The experience of American and other industrialized nations indicates that the prevalence of sexually transmitted diseases (STDs) among African immigrants generally reflects the prevalence levels found in the immigrants' home countries. For example, hepatitis B virus (HBV) is common in sub-Saharan Africa, where 5%–15% of the population are believed to be chronic carriers (Chen et al., 1993). Not surprisingly, then, Crysel and colleagues (1991) reported elevated crude HBV prevalence rates among immigrants to the United States from Ethiopia (9.4%) and Angola (7.1%). Similar rates have also been reported among sub-Saharan African immigrants in France (Roudot-Thoraval et al., 1989), and infection rates as high as 76% have been reported among Ethiopian immigrants to Israel (Hornstein et al., 1991). HBV is responsible for considerable morbidity and mortality arising from acute and chronic hepatitis, cirrhosis, and primary hepatocellular carcinoma (Crysel *et al.*, 1991). These data suggest that U.S.–born infants of women emigrating from countries with elevated HBV rates are at substantial risk of HBV infection. Consequently, the Centers for Disease Control (CDC) recommend that all pregnant women immigrants be screened for HB surface antigen to identify infants needing HBV vaccination and other appropriate treatment (Crysel *et al.*, 1991). Moreover, Poland (1995) recommended that HBV negative women immigrants of reproductive age be immunized.

Immigrants' syphilis rates also seem to mirror prevalence in the home country. Parenti and colleagues (1987) found a prevalence rate of 7.5% in a sample of 239 Ethiopian immigrants to the United States, which is somewhat less than the prevalence rate of 12.5% found in P. S. Friedman and Wright's (1977) study of obstetrical patients in Addis Ababa. Parenti and colleagues recommended that screening procedures for immigrants include rapid plasma reagin test confirmed, as needed, with fluorescent *Treponema* antibody absorption test (RPR/FTA).

Infection with a *Treponema* species need not involve the central nervous system (CNS) or cardiovascular system. An Ethiopian immigrant to Israel presenting with painful bilateral periostitis of the tibia was found to have treponemal bone disease, indicating that the diagnosis of this disease should be considered in persons emigrating from endemic areas who present with chronic skin or bone lesions (Sperber, Stemmer, Sobel, & Schlaeffer, 1989).

Because current U.S. law forbids immigration of individuals infected with HIV, it is not expected that large numbers of HIV seropositive Africans are migrating to the United States. The inability of screening tests, however, to reliably detect highly divergent strains of HIV found in central Africa, such as group O, raises the possibility that some West African immigrants to the United States

may be infected with HIV (Schable *et al.*, 1994). Too, once they arrive, immigrants are subject to the same risks of infection as "indigenous" Americans and may also be subjected to elevated risk of infection if they return to their country of origin for visits. If African immigrants become infected with HIV, results of a retrospective cohort study of 96 seropositive sub-Saharan African immigrants living in London indicate that survival experience of African immigrants with HIV is more similar to that of patients born in developed countries than that of patients in the countries of origin (Low, Paine, Clark, Mahalingam, & Pozniak, 1996).

A recent study of HIV knowledge and behavioral risks of foreign-born Boston public school students found that Black students born outside the United States were less knowledgeable about HIV transmission than Black students born in the United States (Hingson *et al.*, 1991). It is unclear from this study, however, what proportion of individuals had immigrated from Africa. The Toronto, Ontario, Canada, community has pursued a rather innovative approach to HIV education in the African community through the formation of Africans United to Control AIDS. The organization provides educational materials and conducts public forums and workshops for members of the African communities; the majority of the members of these communities are from South Africa, Somalia, Ethiopia, Nigeria, Ghana, Uganda, and Cape Verde (Nakyonyi, 1993).

Intestinal Parasites

Available studies indicate that African immigrants to the United States often arrive with intestinal parasites. Parenti and colleagues' (1987) examination of 191 Ethiopian immigrants revealed that 70 (36.7%) had at least one parasite, and 10.5% had two or more. The most common parasite found was the protozoan *Giardia lamblia* (11.5%), followed by the helminths *Trichuris trichuria* (4.2%), *Schistosoma mansoni* (4.2%), hookworm, and *Hymenolepsis nana*. Likewise, 5 of 14 (36%) pediatric Somalian, Ethiopian, and Zairian refugees examined in Buffalo, New York, were found to be infected with pathogenic parasites, and the African immigrant group's infection prevalence of 36% was higher than that of pediatric refugees from either Vietnam (24%) or Eastern Europe (5%) (Meropol, 1995).

Clinicians treating African immigrants should be aware that individuals with intestinal parasites present with extremely variable clinical symptoms, which can often mimic common Western conditions (Hoffman, 1989). For example, an intestinal parasite can cause acute epigastric pain or gastrointestinal bleeding associated in the West with typical gastroenteritis, peptic ulcer disease, or biliary colic. Similarly, acute massive upper gastrointestinal bleeding, commonly caused by peptic ulcer disease, varices, and Mallory-Weiss tears, may result from worm-induced hepatosplenic disease. A large number of parasites may produce an acute obstructive syndrome analogous to biliary colic. Moreover, acute abdominal cases of apparent right upper quadrant origin, usually attributed in the West to trauma, biliary tract or peptic ulcer disease, pneumonia, empyema, or hepatitis, may also result from helminth infections. Both hydatid disease of the liver and amoebic liver abscess are important diseases of the Third World, and may need to be added to the diagnostic considerations when examining African immigrants.

Of the parasitic helminths, *Strongyloides stercoralis* represents a unique danger because of its auto-infection potential. Cases of strongyloidiasis range in severity from asymptomatic to fatal hyperinfection (Chu, Whitlock, & Dietrich, 1990). Adult worm infestations may last over 30 years in the same individual (Hoffman, 1989), and larval forms may persist up to 40 years after acquisition (Chu *et al.,* 1990). Even asymptomatic infection requires appropriate treatment because of the threat of hyperinfection. Cases of *S. stercoralis* infection, one life threatening, have been documented in African immigrants to the United States (Bhatt, Cappell, Smilow,

& Das, 1990; Parenti *et al.,* 1987). Bhatt and colleagues concluded that strongyloidiasis should be included in the differential diagnosis of obscure gastrointestinal bleeding in persons from endemic areas. Of note, chronic strongyloidiasis is gaining importance with immune-compromised patients (Chu *et al.,* 1990). In the case of one Ghanaian immigrant to the United Kingdom, hyperinfection developed because of immunosuppression resulting from chemotherapy for adult T-cell leukemia-lymphoma (Pagliuca, Layton, Allen, & Mufti, 1988). This case underscores the need to test for *S. stercoralis* in immigrants from endemic areas before beginning any immunosuppressive therapy (Pagliuca *et al.,* 1988).

In general, clinicians should acquire the habit of asking immigrants about their geographic history and lifestyle to determine the possibility of exposure to intestinal parasites, for example, freshwater exposure to *Schistosoma spp.,* soil exposure to hookworm (Hoffman, 1989). Moreover, blood work and stool examinations of these patients need to be performed by experienced technicians.

Dermatologic Conditions

A clinician evaluating an immigrant with cutaneous abnormalities should consider the possibility of infection (Kelsall & Pearson, 1992). Such consideration has been problematic for general practitioners because texts and training have focused on the appearance of skin disease in Europeans and North Americans of European descent (Graham-Brown *et al.,* l990). A symposium held at an international dermatology conference in 1988 marked the first real recognition of the problem of dermatologic infections in immigrant populations with darker skin color (Graham-Brown *et al.,* 1990). Graham-Brown and colleagues reported that clear differences exist between immigrant and indigenous populations, most notably in the amount of "imported" infectious disease and pigmentation problems. These authors also recognized the importance of sociocultural factors, such as the use of emollients and oils, the frequency of bathing, and women's acceptance of male dermatologists as health care providers. Moroccan and Cape Verde immigrants to Rotterdam had much greater frequency of vitiligo, dermatophytosis, and alopecia areata than did the indigenous population. African immigrants in South London had a much lower incidence of skin cancer and "suspicious" pigmented lesions, nevi, and other minor skin blemishes than did indigenous Londoners. However, immigrants' curly hair resulted in higher prevalence of ingrown hair and folliculitis of the scalp, resulting in hair loss, abscess formation, and keloid scarring. For unknown reasons, African immigrants also suffer from sarcoidosis, keloid scars, lichen striatus, eczematides, and lupus erythematosus more than do indigenous Londoners. The Leicester population of immigrant Asian Ugandans and immigrant Africans from Uganda's neighbor states suffer from infectious diseases such as tuberculosis, leprosy, and mycetomas that are rare in the indigenous population (Graham-Brown *et al.*, 1990). Finally, Ethiopian immigrants to Israel showed higher rates of leprosy and onchoceriasis than did indigenous Israelis (Nahmias *et al.*, 1993). Both of these diseases are endemic in Ethiopia.

Anthrax

Disease preventive measures may have eliminated certain infectious diseases in the United States but not in endemic areas where an immigrant originates (Paulet, Caussin, Coudray, Selcer, & de Rohan Chabot, 1994). A case report of a 33-year-old West African immigrant in France is illustrative. This individual returned to Senegal and Gambia for a 3-month visit. Three days after his return to France, he was hospitalized for asthenia, dysnopea, mucopurulent expectoration, and moderate diarrhea. Blood cultures revealed the presence of *Bacillus anthracis*. Despite antibiotic therapy initiated the second day of hospitalization, he died. Paulet and colleagues concluded that clinicians should en-tertain the diagnosis of anthrax when treating septic syndromes in patients from endemic areas because the risk of a fatal outcome increases with delayed diagnosis.

Chronic Disease

African immigrants to the United States present to clinicians with a variety of chronic diseases. Not all of these diseases are acquired in the home country before immigrating to the United States. In fact, some chronic diseases occur in very low frequency in sub-Saharan Africa, and increase in frequency in these groups after immigration, as they acquire risk levels equal to that of the indigenous population. The increased risk of acquiring chronic diseases seems to be related to immigrants' exposure to new diets and lifestyle in their host country. For example, prevalence of varicosis is very low in African populations, but children of African immigrants seem to acquire the same risk of developing this condition as does the host-country population (Carpentier & Priollet, 1994). The risk most likely increases because of the immigrants' change to the low-fiber diet common in industrialized countries. Besides varicosis, multiple sclerosis (MS) is rare in both sub-Saharan Africa and in African immigrants to the United Kingdom; however, children of these immigrants also experience an increased risk of MS roughly equal to that of the indigenous population (Elian, Nightingale, & Dean, 1990).

Diabetes also apparently falls into this category. Little published research exists pertaining to diabetes among African immigrants to Western countries. Available data are limited to the case of immigrants to Israel. Medalie, Papier, Goldbourt, and Herman's (1975) 5-year prospective study of diabetes incidence among 10,000 Israeli municipal workers revealed an average annual incidence of 8.4 per 1,000 for those individuals born in North Africa or Israel, compared to 11.2 per 1,000 for those born in Asia, 7 per 1,000 for those born in southeast Europe, and 5.6 per 1,000 for those born in eastern and central Europe. Investigations of diabetes prevalence among newly arrived Ethiopians during the large migrations of 1984–1985 and 1991 revealed prevalence rates of 0.4 percent and 0 percent, respectively (Rubinstein, Graf, Landau, Reisin, & Goldbourt, 1991; Rubinstein, Graf, & Villa, 1993). Upon exposure to a Western diet and lifestyle, though, diabetes prevalence rises: Cohen, Stein, Rusecki, and Zeidler (1988) found a prevalence of 8.9% among a group of 158 young-adult Ethiopians who had lived in Israel for 2.5–4 years, and Rubinstein, Graf, and Villa (1993) expect that diabetes prevalence will rise in the 1991 immigrant "cohort" as exposure to a Western diet increases.

Coronary Vascular Disease (CVD)

A search of the literature revealed no information concerning CVD among African immigrant groups to the United States. Some studies, however, have been implemented concerning CVD among African immigrants to other Western countries. Balarajan (1991) studied mortality from ischemic heart disease and cerebrovascular disease among several immigrant groups to England and Wales for the time periods 1970–1972 and 1979–1983, including those from African commonwealth countries. For both time periods, Balarajan found excess deaths due to ischemic heart disease in African immigrant males ages 20–69 (standardized mortality ratios or SMR of 116 for 1970–1972 and 113 for 1979–1983) compared with the indigenous population (England and Wales rates of 1979–1983 as standard) but no such excess for African immigrant women. From 1979 to 1983, mortality from ischemic heart disease among men ages 20–69 years was highest in Indians (SMR = 136), followed by Irish (SMR = 114), Polish (SMR = 114), Africans (SMR = 113), and Scots (SMR = 111). The lowest rates were experienced by Caribbean men (SMR = 45). Overall, African male immigrants experienced a 3% decline in the ischemic heart disease SMR between 1970 and 1972 and 1979 and 1983. Of note, African men showed a greater excess of death at younger ages. Insufficient number of deaths of young women precluded analysis by age groups.

Examination of mortality rates from cerebrovascular disease showed a high excess of deaths among African immigrant men and women from 1970 to 1972 (SMRs of 264 and 253, respectively). These rates were exceeded only by those among Caribbean immigrants (SMRs of 271 for men and 307 for women). However, between 1970–1972 and 1979–1983, mortality from cerebrovascular disease fell significantly in most immigrant groups. SMRs among African male immigrants for the time period 1979 to 1983 was 163, while that for African immigrant women was 139. These ratios represent a 38% decline in African men and a 45% decline in African women. As in the earlier time period, from 1979 to 1983 the greatest mortality rates for cerebrovascular disease were observed in Caribbean immigrants (SMR = 176 for men and 210 for women). Excess cerebrovascular mortality observed in African men was greatest among those ages 40–69.

Balarajan (1991) raised the possibility that the excess in deaths from ischemic heart disease and cerebrovascular disease in African immigrant men and from cerebrovascular disease in African immigrant women might be linked to diabetes, which also produces excess mortality in Africans. Balarajan called for further research to determine why excess deaths from CVD occur in immigrant groups.

In contrast to Balarajan's (1991) results for England and Wales, Nahmias and colleagues (1993) reported no evidence of CVD in Ethiopian immigrants to Israel. Moreover, other research on Ethiopian immigrants to Israel has revealed that while blood pressure of newly arrived Ethiopians is markedly lower than that of indigenous Israelis, it increases, particularly diastolic pressure, as the time an immigrant spends in Israel increases (Goldbourt, Khoury, Landau, Reisin, & Rubinstein, 1991; Goldbourt, Rosenthal, & Rubinstein, 1991; Rubinstein, Goldbourt, et al., 1993).

Occasionally, African immigrants present with coronary disease rarely observed in

Western clinics. For example, mitral subannular left ventricular aneurysms seem to be confined to Black Africans and have been found in at least one sub-Saharan African immigrant to Canada (Fitchett & Kanji, 1983). Although such conditions are rare, their recognition and management are important because they are responsible for a significant number of cases of cardiac failure, arrhythmia, and systemic embolism in African populations.

Cancer

Before immigration, sub-Saharan Africans are subjected to several pathogens that are believed to be associated with various cancers: *Schistosoma hematobium* and bladder cancer, Hepatitis B virus and liver cancer, human papillovirus and cervical cancer, Epstein-Barr virus and Burkett's lymphoma (Kagawa-Singer, 1995).

Examination of mortality rates reveals cancer patterns different between African immigrants and indigenous populations. Bouchardy, Parkin, Wanner, and Khlatt (1996) found that compared to local-born French, immigrants from Algeria, Morocco, and Tunisia from the time period 1979 to 1985 had a generally lower risk of death from cancer at all sites except the nasopharynx, gallbladder, and bladder (Algerian only). Moreover, Egyptian immigrants experienced higher mortality rates from leukemia and lymphoma than did local-born French, which was not particularly surprising since the world's highest lymphoma mortality rates are found in Northern Africa (Pisani, Parkin, & Ferlay, 1993). Bouchardy's (1996) group suggested that specific cultural and behavioral factors may have contributed to the different cancer patterns observed. For example, a rich vegetable diet and low level of alcohol consumption may be related to decreased rates of aero-digestive and liver cancers; consumption of other dietary items (e.g., cured meats, spices) may be related to the increased rates of nasopharynx cancer; and previous infection with *Schistosoma hematobium* may be related to the elevated rate of bladder cancer in Algerian immigrants.

In a similar study, Grulich, Swerdlow, Head, and Marmot (1992) examined cancer mortality during 1970–1985 among West African (Sierra Leone, Ghana, Nigeria, Gambia) and East African (Kenya, Malawi, Tanzania, Uganda, Zambia) immigrants to England and Wales. They found that compared with the indigenous population, overall cancer mortality was significantly raised in West African males, nonsignificantly raised in West African females, and lower in East African males and females. The increased risk in West African men seemed primarily caused by rates of liver cancer over 30 times that of the local population. Liver cancer is, in fact, a major public health problem in the West African community in England and Wales and is most likely related to the high prevalence of hepatitis B in this group. Rates of prostatic cancer and non-Hodgkins lymphoma were also elevated in West African males. West African immigrants of both sexes showed significantly decreased mortality from lung and brain cancer.

East African immigrants, predominantly Asian in ethnicity, had significantly lower rates of lung cancer and melanoma. In addition, males suffered significantly lower mortality from Hodgkin's disease and from stomach, pancreatic, and testicular cancers, while East African women had significantly lower rates for cervical cancer. On the other hand, East African immigrants had 5 to 10 times the mortality from cancers of the oral cavity and had significantly higher mortality from cancers of the pharynx (males). Compared to English and Welsh populations, rates of testicular cancer, ovarian cancer, lung cancer, melanoma, and Hodgkin's disease among all African immigrants were low, while multiple myeloma rates for African immigrant males were significantly higher.

The Iscovitch, Steinitz, and Andreev (1993) study of more than 8,200 Ethiopian immigrants to Israel shows some similarity with the experience of immigrants to the United Kingdom and France: low overall cancer rates compared to indigenous Israelis; a high prevalence of liver cancer, believed to be associated with hepatitis B virus; and high rates of non-Hodgkins lymphoma in males. In contrast to rates in their country of origin, Ethiopian female immigrants experienced high rates of thyroid cancer.

Peptic Ulcers

African immigrant workers in Europe are reported to be at increased risk for peptic ulcers compared with indigenous populations. This has been attributed to the practice of self-prescribing nonsteroidal anti-inflammatory drugs to relieve muscle discomfort at the end of the workday and an elevated prevalence of *Helicobacter pylori,* a bacterium recently associated with ulcers (Lonardo *et al.,* 1990; Lonardo *et al.,* 1994).

Mental Health and Illness

There has been little research in the area of mental health among African immigrants to the United States. Much of what has been written derives from studies conducted in Europe, Israel, and Canada.

Diagnosis

A number of researchers have reported increased rates of mental illness among African immigrants, compared with native-born individuals. Both Bagley and Rwegellera, relying on psychiatric registers, found an increased prevalence of schizophrenia and affective psychosis among West African immigrants to the United Kingdom (Bagley, 1971; Rwegellera, 1977). Kidd (1965) reported an increase in general psychiatric morbidity among West African students, as compared to U.K.–born controls. Littlewood and Lipsedge (1981) noted an increased rate of schizophrenia in patients from West Africa from their retrospective study of psychotic patients in a London psychiatric unit, although the cause of this increased rate remained unclear. A study of first admission rates for schizophrenia in the Netherlands found high rates of first admissions among young male immi-

grants from Morocco, as compared with the native-born population (Selten & Sijben, 1994). Ndetei (1986) attributed his finding of an increased prevalence of paranoid disorders among African patients in a London hospital to "cultural factors." He specifically noted that more than half of the 34 African patients in the sample attributed their illness to poison, evil spirits, witchcraft, or magic. Majid (1992) has offered an alternative explanation for Africans' apparent vulnerability to certain forms of mental illness, arguing that it may result from the stress of migration, culture change, racial prejudice, and discrimination.

Severe psychopathology has also been documented among Ethiopian immigrants to Israel. Arieli and Ayche (1993) found a high prevalence of nightmares and sleep disturbances as long as 6 years after immigration. Low income and high unemployment were associated with the presence of severe psychopathology. Ratzoni and colleagues (1993) found an increased prevalence of dissociative disorders among Ethiopian adolescents in their study of hospitalized adolescent and adult Ethiopian immigrants in Israel. Researchers in Canada have noted an apparent increased risk of suicide among immigrants from South Africa. (Rich, Kliewer, & Ward, 1988).

A not insignificant proportion of African immigrants to the United States may have come as refugees, who are fleeing their country to escape persecution or who are in fear of being persecuted if they remain there. That flight may have involved arrest, detention, torture, imprisonment, starvation, and disease. (Chester & Holtan, 1992; Kemp, 1993; McCaw & DeLay, 1985). Settlement in the new country may have been accompanied by a loss of status, employment, family, or possessions; an absence of social support; discrimination; and significant cultural differences between the country of origin and the location of resettlement (Orley, 1994). Consequently, immigrants arriving as refugees may be at particularly high risk of mental disorder. It should be noted, however, that these disorders are not specific to refugees alone;

neither are they specific to immigrants from Africa.

The use of torture against political detainees and prisoners of conscience has been documented in more than 90 countries (Roth, Lunde, Boysen, & Genefke, 1987), including Ethiopia, North Africa (Roth *et al.,* 1987), and Uganda (Amnesty International, 1985). Amnesty International reported in the mid 1980s, for example, that female detainees in Uganda were subjected to group rape, and pregnant detainees were kicked in the abdomen to precipitate spontaneous abortion. Male detainees were subjected to the application of electricity, the beating and pulling of the genitals, and the crushing of the testicles with cattle-gelding instruments (Amnesty International, 1985). Other reports have indicated a relatively high prevalence of sexual torture among female detainees in African nations. (Lunde & Ortmann, 1990). Five major political purposes for the use of sexual torture have been identified: to destroy a woman's personal identity, to punish a woman who did not conform to cultural norms, to exact revenge on a segment of the population, to exploit a woman's vulnerability in an unprotected situation, and to gather information about a husband's activities (Dutch Medical Group, 1985). The prevalence of sexual torture in non-Western countries is not known (Mollica & Son, 1989).

Despite the passage of time since the torture, refugee survivors of torture may continue to experience not only physical symptoms but emotional and psychological symptoms as well. (For a discussion of methods of torture and the motivations underlying the practice of torture, see Roth *et al.,* 1987.) Psychological sequelae, not specific to patients from African nations, may include confusion and disorientation, memory disturbances, poor concentration, anxiety, depression, irritability, aggressiveness, emotional lability, self-isolation or social withdrawal, lack of energy, insomnia, nightmares, and sexual dysfunction (Goldfeld, Mollica, Pesavento, & Faraone, 1988; Petersen, Christensen, Kastrup, Thomsen, & Folspang, 1994).

Posttraumatic stress disorder may occur in response to this trauma; that response may be either delayed or protracted. Most commonly, the disorder manifests within 6 months of the traumatic event. Diagnosis requires exposure to a traumatic event and symptoms from each of three clusters: intrusive recollections, avoidant or numbing symptoms, and hyperarousal symptoms (American Psychiatric Association, 1994). Symptoms may include flashbacks, recurring dreams, persistent remembering, or psychogenic amnesia.

Adjustment disorders may occur as the result of a stressful life event such as migration. A diagnosis of adjustment disorder, which refers to a state of subjective distress and emotional disturbance, encompasses culture shock and grief reaction. Symptoms generally abate within 6 months following the cessation of the stress or its consequences.

Unlike posttraumatic stress disorder and adjustment disorders, acute stress reactions are transient and usually abate within several days of the occurrence of exceptional physical or mental stress. Diagnosis requires an immediate clear and temporal connection between the stressor and the onset of the symptoms, which may include withdrawal from expected social interaction, narrowing of attention, disorientation, anger or verbal aggression, despair or hopelessness, inappropriate overactivity, or uncontrollable and excessive grief, evaluated in accordance with local cultural standards (World Health Organization, 1993a, 1993b).

These traumatic experiences may predispose the refugee patient to distrust the health care provider. The provision of care may be rendered even more difficult due to language differences, socioeconomic differences between the patient and the provider, and the provider's lack of experience with cross-cultural situations.

Consequently, it is not surprising that African immigrants' utilization of services is often less than that of the native-born population. Rwegellera (1980) found that African immigrants to the United Kingdom were reluctant to contact their general practitioner for a referral for hospitalization. Rwegellera attributed this to a lack of understanding of the physician's role or potential helpfulness. A study of Moroccan immigrants in Belgium concluded that this immigrant community made less use of psychiatric services than did the native-born population, although there is insufficient evidence to conclude that Moroccan immigrants experience less psychiatric illness (Bastenier & Dassetto, 1980).

Methodological Concerns

Interpretation of this body of research is problematic for a number of reasons. First, many of the data bases and samples used for these studies were themselves problematic due to small sample size and selection bias. A number of studies examining rates of hospitalization for mental illness, some of which relied on preexisting databases, failed to distinguish between voluntary and compulsory admissions. Second, researchers may have misdiagnosed symptoms in patients from a different culture due to lack of familiarity with the norms specific to the patient's culture and misunderstandings due to differences in language. The PTSD model, in particular, has been criticized as narrow, a pathologization of normal psychological process, and ethnocentric in its view of the expression of traumatic stress (M. Friedman & Jaranson, 1994). Third, classification of patients' origins, for example, East Africa, West Africa, are inconsistent between studies, rendering interstudy comparisons difficult. Finally, it is unclear to what extent study findings pertaining to African immigrants to countries outside of the United States are applicable to African immigrants to the United States.

Dental Health

Literature relating to preventive care and health education among African immigrants is sparse. Israeli researchers have found that, compared with Israeli adults and data from the WHO data bank, adult immigrants to Israel from rural Ethiopia have a relatively healthy periodontal status, despite a lack of regular dental visits and the absence of home oral hygiene maintenance (Sgan-Cohen, Steinberg, Zusman, Naor, & Sela, 1993). One Swedish study, which relied on a national data registry, found that immigrants' utilization of dental services was low. Among the 23 Ethiopians in the sample, the average length of time between arrival in Sweden and first visit to the dentist was 4.9 years (Zimmerman, Bornstein, & Martinsson, 1995).

Nutrition

A recent Canadian survey of single male Ethiopian refugees in Ottawa, found that the mean nutrient intakes are generally adequate due to the frequent consumption of nutrient-dense foods. However, body mass index and arm circumference were low in comparison with Canadian and American standards. These lower values were associated with a lack of domestic skill (McIsaac, Tucker, Gray-Donald, & Stafford-Smith, 1991).

Health Care Delivery

It is important for several reasons that health care providers understand the culturally mediated health behaviors of their African patients. First, patients may present to health care providers for treatment of an illness that has no counterpart in Western medicine. Moroccan immigrants, for example, may report *le-riah,* a syndrome characterized by dizziness, rapid heart beating, wandering pains, and weakness, found predominantly in women (Peeters, 1986). Second, patients may self-medicate using remedies that are potentially injurious. Geophagia, which has been noted in Africa (Reid, 1992), can lead to gastrointestinal impaction, decreased iron absorption, and anemia (Roselle, 1970). In addition, the care provider will be better able to communicate with his or her patient if there is a mutual understanding of health terms, illness, and the postulated cause of that illness (Groce & Zola, 1993; Pachter, 1994). Some African patients, for example, may believe that a disability results from divine punishment or witchcraft (Groce & Zola, 1993). A physician's approach to a disabled patient, and the patient's response to his or her physician, will necessarily be tempered by the physician's awareness—or lack of it—of this interpretation.

U.S. physicians emphasize the open disclosure of diagnosis and the accompanying prognosis, often in conjunction with obtaining informed consent for treatment. Beyene (1992) has contrasted this U.S. emphasis on autonomy and self-reliance, leading to full disclosure to the individual patient, with the Ethiopian values of paternalism and protection, which provide for family ownership of all diagnostic facts. Although honesty is also highly valued within Ethiopian culture, "[t]ruth is socially defined," meaning that deception is acceptable in order to avoid offending or hurting another. Beyene has therefore recommended that physicians involve the patient's family members in the patient's care in order to reduce the patient's anxiety.

Innovative approaches may be required to facilitate immigrants' access to needed services. The Texas Department of Health, for instance, developed a screening program in the early 1980s, in order to connect refugees with significant health problems to the public health system for assessment and referral. Sponsoring agencies introduce the immigrants to the screening program, which then provides a complete medical assessment (Anonymous, 1993).

Health-Related Cultural Practices in African Immigrants

Genital Mutilation

Traditional female genital surgery, or female genital mutilation (FGM) as it has become known in industrialized nations, is widespread in Africa, occurring in 26 countries on the continent and affecting millions of women (Lalonde, 1995). In Somalia alone, more than 80,000 procedures are performed annually (Gallo, 1988). As immigration of Africans to the United States increases, it is increasingly likely that health care providers, often without any experience in dealing with FGM, will be faced with providing clinical services to women who have undergone the procedure (Arbesman, Kahler, & Buck, 1993; Baker, Gilson, Vill, & Curet, 1993). Moreover, although FGM is illegal in the West, the experience of other industrialized countries indicates that children of immigrants may be at risk of FGM in their host country: 10,000 girls in the United Kingdom (Trevelyan, 1994; Walder, 1995) and more than 16,000 young women and girls in France (Gallard, 1995). Figures for those at risk in the United States are not available. In Arbesman and collleagues' (1993) survey of a convenience sample of 12 Somali refugee women in Buffalo, New York, 5 women indicated that the practice of FGM was good and 7 said that they would support the procedure being performed on their daughters. However, these results may not accurately represent the views of all African immigrants, especially the children of immigrants (Trevelyan, 1994). In fact, the Board of Immigration Appeals, in ruling that the threat of FGM is a legitimate form of persecution for the purposes of asylum, granted asylum to a young girl from Togo who refused to return home for the procedure (Dugger, 1996b).

Complications from FGM are extensive and depend on the type of operation and hygienic conditions at the site of the procedure. Surgical procedures range from removal of the prepuce of the clitoris to the removal of the clitoris, the labia minora, and the medial part of the labia majora coupled with stitching together of the vaginal wall (Black & Debelle, 1995). Short-term complications, which may arise if the operation was performed unhygienically, include primary or secondary hemorrhage, sepsis, septicemia, and tetanus (Black & Debelle, 1995). Long-term genitourinary complications include dyspareunia, poor urinary stream, hematocolpos, vesicovaginal or rectovaginal fistula, keloid formation, implantation dermoid cysts, dysmenorrhea, chronic pelvic infection, recurrent vaginitis and urinary tract infections, infertility, painful intercourse, and lack of sexual pleasure (Arbesman et al., 1993; Baker et al., 1993; Black & Debelle, 1995). The major obstetrical complications include difficulty in performing vaginal examinations and a prolonged second stage of labor because of the inability of the fibrosed and rigid vulva to expand, which necessitates an anterior episiotomy (Arbesman et al., 1993; Baker et al., 1993). In unattended labor, women often suffer perineal tears, fistulae, hemorrhage, infection, and fetal asphyxia or death (Arbesman et al., 1993; Baker et al., 1993). Moreover, in health care facilities unaccustomed to treating women with FGM, clinicians may react with incomprehension and even hostility if the woman requests resuturing (Black & Debelle, 1995). Finally, because FGM is an emotionally traumatic event, several long-term psychological complications, including chronic irritability, reactive depression, hallucinations, and psychosis, may occur (Arbesman et al., 1993).

Cases of women with FGM receiving obstetrical and gynecological services in the United States have included Somalian refugees in Buffalo, New York (Arbesman et al., 1993), Ethiopians in Chicago (Salzer & Nelson, 1983), and a Sudanese woman in Albuquerque, New Mexico (Baker et al., 1993). Omer-Hashi (1994), a midwife trained in Somalia and member of Ontario, Canada's FGM Prevention Task Force, advises that clinicians providing health care to women who have undergone FGM demonstrate great sensitivity and cultural awareness, particularly because many of these women may be unfamiliar with medical technology or male caregivers. In particular, health care providers should not express shock and should always ask the woman's permission before allowing other clinicians to examine them. The caregiver should provide early prenatal counseling before defibulation to reduce stress and enable the patient to make informed decisions regarding her care and clinicians should learn a variety of methods to open the scar tissue to permit intercourse and vaginal delivery (Baker et al., 1993; Lalonde, 1995; McCleary, 1994; Omer-Hashi, 1994). Further, after defibulation, women will need counseling to increase self-esteem, to learn about normal anatomy and their altered function and appearance, menstruation, urination, and intercourse, and about the use of a water-based lubricant during intercourse to lessen the pain.

Uvulectomy

Salzer and Nelson (1983) reported examining the 20 children of 8 Ethiopian refugee families in Chicago and discovering that all children had undergone an uvulectomy. This procedure is commonly performed on African children in order to treat cough, sore throats, and to "keep a child from talking too much" (Salzer & Nelson, 1983, p. 452). Severe complications from uvulectomies, such as hemorrhage and infection (Einterz, Einterz, & Bates, 1994; Prual, Gamatie, Djakounda, & Huguet, 1994) are usually immediate. Consequently, they are not likely to be seen by U.S. clinicians unless the uvulectomy was performed after immigration. Chronic complications, however, might be observed and include modification of nasal speech, palatal scarring, and recurrent tonsillitis (Hartly & Rowe-Jones, 1994; Prual et al., 1994; Wind, 1984).

Child-Rearing Practices

Child-rearing practices vary widely around the world. Some cultures' child-disciplining practices may be viewed as "extreme" or "abusive" by Western standards but normal and acceptable by those societies practicing them and may even be sanctioned legally. Thus, administering hot pepper to a child's ano-genital region (LeVine & LeVine, 1981) and severe beating for minor offenses such as lying or stealing (Okeahialam, 1984) would most likely constitute abusive behavior in the United States, but not necessarily in the country of origin.

Upon arrival in the United States, immigrants find themselves in a social and legal environment that may differ greatly from that of their country of origin. A recent New York City child abuse case underscored the challenges faced by both immigrant parents in their attempts to raise their children in a new environment and American social services in their efforts to deal with immigrant populations in a culturally sensitive manner that still protects children from maltreatment (Dugger, 1996a). In this case, a Nigerian adult male defended himself against a charge of child abuse by claiming that the corporal punishment he administered to his son, which broke the boy's wrist, was standard child-disciplining behavior in Nigeria. Consultation with other Nigerian immigrants in the United States, however, revealed that this man's behavior transgressed the bounds of acceptable behavior in Nigeria as well, and the adult was charged with assault. The approach used in this case demonstrates a useful method for American health care providers when dealing with instances where child maltreatment is suspected: input from other immigrants of that ethnicity may be indispensable in interpreting the behavior and deciding on the correct course of action.

Conclusion

African immigrants to the United States constitute a diverse group in terms of their immigration experiences, their customs and traditions, and their approaches to health and illness. Research is needed to better understand the impact of these differences on their health status and their ability and willingness to access traditional Western care. Significant health issues that require attention include issues relating to maternal and child health, infectious diseases such as tuberculosis and malaria, and chronic diseases such as cancer and coronary vascular disease.

It is clear that significant gaps exist in our knowledge regarding the health issues and the health needs of African immigrants to the United States. These gaps can only be narrowed through the development of systems designed to collect data relating to specific subgroups. Health care providers should be provided with additional training that will allow them to address their African immigrant patients in a culturally sensitive manner, with an understanding of the many issues and barriers that may hinder their patients' decision making or participation in the medical system.

References

Adams, P. (1994). Reign of the generals. *Africa Report, 36,* 26–29.

American Psychiatric Association. (1994). *Diagnostic and statistical manual of mental disorders* (4th ed.). Washington, DC: Author.

Amnesty International. (1985). *Uganda: Evidence of torture.* London: Author.

Anonymous. (1993). Refugee program sensitive to cultural, medical needs. *Texas Medicine, 89,* 46–47.

Arbesman, M., Kahler, L., & Buck, G. M. (1993). Assessment of the impact of female circumcision on the gynecological, genitourinary and obstetrical health problems of women from Somalia: Literature review and case series. *Women and Health, 20,* 27–42.

Arieli, A., & Ayche, S. (1993). Psychopathological aspects of the Ethiopian immigration to Israel. *Israel Journal of Medical Science, 29,* 411–418.

Bagley, C. (1971). Mental illness in immigrant minorities in London. *Journal of Biosocial Science, 3,* 449–459.

Baker, C. A., Gilson, G. J., Vill, M. D., & Curet, L. B. (1993). Female circumcision: Obstetric issues. *American Journal of Obstetrics and Gynecology, 169,* 1616–1618.

Balarajan, R. (1991). Ethnic differences in mortality from ischaemic heart disease and cerebrovascular disease in England and Wales. *British Medical Journal, 302,* 560–564.

Bastenier, A., & Dassetto, F. (1980). Immigres et sante. Les immigrés et l'hôpital [Immigrants and health. Immigrants and the hospital]. *Consommation des soins et motalités d'utilisation de l'institution hospitalière.* Feres: Louvain-La-Neuve.

Beyene, Y. (1992). Medical disclosure and refugees: Telling bad news to Ethiopian patients. *Western Journal of Medicine, 157,* 328–332.

Bhatt, B. D., Cappell, M. S., Smilow, P. C., & Das, K. M. (1990). Recurrent massive upper gastrointestinal hemorrhage due to *Strongyloides stercolis* infection. *American Journal of Gastroenterology, 85,* 1034–1036.

Black, J. A., & Debelle, G. D. (1995). Female genital mutilation in Britain. *British Medical Journal, 310,* 1590–1592.

Bouchardy, C., Parkin, D. M., Wanner, P., & Khlatt, M. (1996). Cancer mortality among North African migrants in France. *International Journal of Epidemiology, 25,* 5–13.

Bourdillon, F., Lombrail, P., Antoni, M., Benrekassa, J., Bennegadi, R., Leloup, M., Huraux-Rendu, C., & Scotto, J. C. (1991). La sante des populations d'origine etrangere en France [The health of populations of foreign origin in France]. *Social Science and Medicine, 32,* 1219–1227.

Carpentier, P., & Priollet, P. (1994). *Epidémiologie de l'insuffisance veineuse chronique* [Epidemiology of chronic venous insufficiency]. *La Presse Médicale, 23,* 197–201.

Chen, N., Lesavre, P., Noel, L. H., Mattlinger, B., Simon, P., Ramée, M. P., Menault, M., & Lévy, M. (1993). How frequent are hepatitis B virus markers in adult patients with glomerular diseases in a low endemic country. *Nephron, 63,* 400–403.

Chester, B., & Holtan, N. (1992). Working with refugee survivors of torture. *Western Journal of Medicine, 157,* 301–304.

Chu, E., Whitlock, W. L., & Dietrich, R. A. (1990). Pulmonary hyperinfection syndrome with *Strongyloides stercoralis. Chest, 97,* 1475–1477.

Cohen, M. P., Stein, E., Rusecki, Y., & Zeidler, A. (1988). High prevalence of diabetes in young adult Ethiopian immigrants to Israel. *Diabetes, 37,* 824–27.

Crysel, C., Wong, M. P., Broun, B., Cochran, J., & Morales, B. (1991). Screening for hepatitis B virus infection among refugees arriving in the United States 1979–1991. *Morbidity and Mortality Weekly Report, 40,* 784–786.

Dugger, C. W. (1996a, February 28). Immigrant cultures raising issues of child punishment. *New York Times,* pp. A1, A12.

Dugger, C. W. (1996b, June 14). U.S. grants asylum to woman fleeing genital mutilation rite. *New York Times,* p. A1.

Dutch Medical Group. (1985, March 22–24). *Medical treatment of refugees/torture victims.* Paper presented at the international meeting on Amnesty International medical work, London.

Edwards, E. (1994). Factors influencing prenatal class attendance among immigrants in Ottawa-Carleton. *Canadian Journal of Public Health, 85,* 254–258.

Einterz, E. M., Einterz, R. M., & Bates, B. M. (1994). Traditional uvulectomy in northern Cameroon [Letter]. *Lancet, 343,* 1644.

Ekwe-Ekwe, H. (1990). *Conflict and intervention in Africa.* New York: Saint Martin's.

Elian, M., Nightingale, S., & Dean, G. (1990). Multiple sclerosis among United Kingdom–born children of immigrants from the Indian subcontinent, Africa, and the West Indies. *Journal of Neurology, Neurosurgery, and Psychiatry, 53,* 905–911.

Fairchild, A. L., & Tynan, E. A. (1994). Policies of containment: Immigration in the era of AIDS. *American Journal of Public Health, 84,* 2011–2022.

Fitchett, D. H., & Kanji, M. (1983). Mitral subannular left ventricular aneurysm: A case presenting with ventricular tachycardia. *British Heart Journal, 50,* 594–596.

Freeman, G. P. (1994). Can liberal states control unwanted immigration? *Annals of the American Academy of Political and Social Science, 534,* 17–30.

Friedman, M., & Jaranson, J. (1994). The applicability of the posttraumatic stress disorder concept to refugees. In A. J. Marsella, T. Bornemann, S. Ekblad, & J. Orley (Eds.), *Amidst peril and pain: The mental health and well-being of the world's refugees* (pp. 207–227). Washington, DC: American Psychological Association.

Friedman, P. S., & Wright, D. J. (1977). Observations on syphilis in Addis Ababa: 2. Prevalence and natural history. *British Journal of Venereal Diseases, 53,* 276–280.

Gallard, C. (1995). Female genital mutilation in France. *British Medical Journal, 310,* 1592–1593.

Gallo, P. (1988). Female circumcision in Somalia. *Mankind Quarterly, 29,* 165–180.

Goldbourt, U., Khoury, M., Landau, E., Reisin, L. H., & Rubenstein, A. (1991). Blood pressure in Ethiopian immigrants: Relationship to age and anthropologic factors, and changes during their first year in Israel. *Israel Journal of Medical Sciences, 27,* 264–267.

Goldbourt, U., Rosenthal, T., & Rubenstein, A. (1991). Trends in weight and blood pressure in Ethiopian immigrants in their first few years in Israel: Epidemiologic observations and implications for the future. *Israel Journal of Medical Sciences, 27,* 260–263.

Goldfeld, A. E., Mollica, R. F., Pesavento, B. H., & Faraone, S. V. (1988). The physical and psychological sequelae of torture. *Journal of the American Medical Association, 259,* 2725–2729.

Graham-Brown, R. A., Berth-Jones, J., Dure-Smith, B., Naafs, B., Pembroke, A. C., Harth, W., Gollnick, H., Orfanos, C., Kurwa, A., & Bowry, V. (1990). Dermatologic problems for immigrant communities in a western environment. *International Journal of Dermatology, 29,* 94–101.

Groce, N. E., & Zola, I. K. (1993). Multiculturalism, chronic illness, and disability. *Pediatrics, 91,* 1048–1055.

Grulich, A. E., Swerdlow, A. J., Head, J., & Marmot, M. G. (1992). Cancer mortality in African and

Caribbean migrants to England and Wales. *British Journal of Cancer, 66,* 905–911.

Hanania, N., & Hoffstein, V. (1993). Tuberculosis presenting with generalized lymphadenopathy, pulmonary infiltrates, and bone destruction in a young man. *Archives of Internal Medicine, 153,* 1265–1267.

Hartly, B. E., & Rowe-Jones, J. (1994). Uvulectomy to prevent throat infections. *Journal of Laryngology and Otology, 198,* 65–66.

Hingson, R. W., Strunin, L., Grady, M., Strunk, N., Carr, R., Berlin, B., & Craven, D. E. (1991). Knowledge about HIV and behavioral risks of foreign-born Boston public school students. *American Journal of Public Health, 81,* 1638–1641.

Hoffman, S. H. (1989). Tropical medicine and the acute abdomen. *Emergency Medicine Clinics of North America, 7,* 591–609.

Hornstein, L., Ben-Porath, E., Cuzin, A., Baharir, Z., Rimon, N., & Nahmias, J. (1991). Hepatitis B virus infection in Ethiopian immigrants to Israel. *Israel Journal of Medical Sciences, 27,* 268–272.

Iscovitch, J., Steinitz, R., & Andreev, H. (1993). Descriptive epidemiology of malignant tumors in Ethiopian Jews immigrating to Israel, 1984–89. *Israel Journal of Medical Science, 29,* 364–367.

Kagawa-Singer, M. (1995). Socioeconomic and cultural influences on cancer care of women. *Seminars in Oncology Nursing, 11,* 109–119.

Kaplan, R. D. (1988). *The wars behind the famine.* Boulder, CO: Westview.

Kelsall, B. L., & Pearson, R. D. (1992). Evaluation of skin problems. *Infectious Disease Clinics of North America, 6,* 441–471.

Kemp, C. (1993). Health services for refugees in countries of second asylum. *Nursing Review, 40,* 21–24.

Kidd, C. B. (1965). Psychiatric morbidity among students. *British Journal of Preventive and Social Medicine, 19,* 143–150.

Lalonde, A. (1995). Clinical management of female genital mutilation must be handled with understanding and compassion. *Canadian Medical Association Journal, 152,* 949–950.

LeVine, S., & LeVine, R. (1981). Child abuse and neglect in sub-Saharan Africa. In J. Korbin (Ed.), *Child abuse and neglect: Cross-cultural perspectives* (pp. 35–55). Berkeley: University of California Press.

Littlewood, R., & Lipsedge, M. (1981). Some social and phenomenological characteristics of psychotic immigrants. *Psychological Medicine, 11,* 289–302.

Lonardo, A., Grisendi, A., Della Casa, G., Ferrari, A. M., Pulverenti, M., & Melini, L. (1990). Peptic ulcer in migrants: Seven case-reports from Italy. *Recenti Progressi in Medicina, 81,* 502–503.

Lonardo, A., Grisendi, A., Frazzoni, M., Della Casa, G., Pulvirenti, M., & Melini, L. (1994). The immigrant worker's ulcer. *Gastroenterologie Clinique et Biologique, 18,* 90.

Low, N., Paine, K., Clark, R., Mahalingam, M., & Pozniak, A. L. (1996). AIDS survival and progression in black Africans living in south London, 1986–1994. *Genitourinary Medicine, 72,* 12–16.

Lunde, I., & Ortmann, J. (1990). Prevalence and sequelae of sexual torture. *Lancet, 336,* 289–291.

Majid, A. (1992). Mental health of ethnic minorities in Europe [Letter]. *World Health Forum, 13,* 351–352.

McCaw, B. R., & DeLay, P. (1985). Demographics and disease prevalence of two new refugee groups in San Francisco: The Ethiopian and Afghan refugees. *Western Journal of Medicine, 143,* 271–275.

McCleary, P. H. (1994). Female genital mutilation and childbirth: A case report. *Birth, 21,* 221–224.

McIsaac, J. B., Tucker, K. L., Gray-Donald, K., & Stafford-Smith, B. (1991). Nutritional status of single male government-sponsored refugees from Ethiopia. *Canadian Journal of Public Health, 82,* 381–384.

Medalie, J. H., Papier, C. M., Goldbourt, U., & Herman, J. B. (1975). Major factors in the development of diabetes mellitus in 10,000 men. *Archives of Internal Medicine, 135,* 811–817.

Meropol, S. B. (1995). Health status of pediatric refugees in Buffalo, NY. *Archives of Pediatric and Adolescent Medicine, 149,* 887–892.

Mollica, R. F., & Son, L. (1989). Cultural dimensions in the evaluation and treatment of sexual trauma: An overview. *Psychiatric Clinics of North America, 12,* 363–379.

Mortensen, J., Lange, P., Storm, H. K., & Viskum, K. (1989). Childhood tuberculosis in a developed country. *European Respiratory Journal, 2,* 985–987.

Nahmias, J., Greenberg, Z., Berger, S. A., Hornstein, L., Bilgury, B., Abel, B., & Kutner, S. (1993). Health profile of Ethiopian immigrants in Israel: An overview. *Israel Journal of Medical Sciences, 29,* 333–343.

Nakyonyi, M. M. (1993). HIV/AIDS education participation by the African community. *Canadian Journal of Public Health* (Suppl. 1), S19–S23.

Ndetei, D. M. (1986). Paranoid disorder—Environmental, cultural, or constitutional phenomenon? *Acta Psychiatrica Scandinavia, 74,* 50–54.

Okeahialam, T. C. (1984). Child abuse in Nigeria. *Child Abuse and Neglect, 8,* 69–73.

Omer-Hashi, K. H. (1994). Commentary: Female genital mutilation: Perspectives from a Somalian housewife. *Birth, 21,* 224–226.

Oren, S., Jamal, J., London, D., & Viskoper, J. R. (1991). Extrapulmonary tuberculosis: Five case reports. *Israel Journal of Medical Sciences, 27,* 390–393.

Orley, J. (1994). Psychological disorders among refugees: Some clinical and epidemiological considerations. In A. J. Marsella, T. Bornemann, S. Ekblad, & J. Orley (Eds.), *Amidst peril and pain: The mental health and well-being of the world's refugees* (pp. 193–227). Washington, DC: American Psychological Association.

Pachter, L. M. (1994). Culture and clinical care: Folk illness beliefs and behaviors and their implications for health care delivery. *Journal of the American Medical Association, 271,* 690–694.

Pagliuca, A., Layton, D. M., Allen, S., & Mufti, G. J. (1988). Hyperinfection with strongyloides after treatment for adult T cell leukaemia-lymphoma in an African immigrant. *British Medical Journal, 297,* 1456.

Parenti, D. M., Lucas, D., Lee, A., & Hollenkamp, R. H. (1987). Health status of Ethiopian refugees in the United States. *American Journal of Public Health, 77,* 1542–1543.

Paulet, R., Caussin, C., Coudray, J. M., Selcer, D., & de Rohan Chabot, P. (1994). *Forme Viscérale de Charbon Humain Importé d'Afrique* [Visceral anthrax imported from Africa]. *La Presse Médicale, 23,* 477–478.

Pedder, S. (1993a, August 21). Anybody seen a giant? *Economist,* S3–S4.

Pedder, S. (1993b, August 21). Breaking the cycle. *Economist,* S8–S10.

Peeters, R. F. (1986). Health and illness of Moroccan immigrants in the city of Antwerp, Belgium. *Social Science and Medicine, 22,* 679–685.

Petersen, H. D., Christensen, M. E., Kastrup, M., Thomsen, J. L., & Folspang, A. (1994). General health assessment in refugees claiming to have been tortured. *Forensic Science International, 67,* 9–16.

Phillips-Howard, P. A., Bradley, D. J., Blaze, M., & Hurn, M. (1988). Malaria in Britain: 1977–86. *British Medical Journal, 296,* 245–248.

Pisani, P., Parkin, D. M., & Ferlay, J. (1993). Estimates of the worldwide mortality from eighteen major cancers in 1985: Implications for prevention and projections of future burdens. *International Journal of Cancer, 55,* 891–903.

Poland, G. A. (1995). Immunizing the adult immigrant patient: What to do when there are no records. *Minnesota Medicine, 78,* 18–20.

Prual, A., Gamatie, Y., Djakounda, M., & Huguet, D. (1994). Traditional uvulectomy in Niger: A public health problem? *Social Science and Medicine, 39,* 1077–1082.

Rafuse, J. (1993). Multicultural medicine: Dealing with a population you weren't quite prepared. *Canadian Medical Association Journal, 148,* 282–285.

Ratzoni, G., Ben Amo, I., Weizman, T., Weizman, R., Modai, I., & Apter, A. (1993). Psychiatric diagnoses in hospitalized adolescent and adult Ethiopian immigrants in Israel. *Israel Journal of Medical Science, 29,* 419–421.

Reid, R. M. (1992). Cultural and medical perspectives on geophagia. *Medical Anthropology, 13,* 337–351.

Rich, V., Kliewer, R. H., & Ward, R. H. (1988). Convergence of immigrant suicide rates to those of destination country. *American Journal of Epidemiology, 127,* 640–653.

Roselle, H. A. (1970). Association of laundry starch and clay ingestion with anemia in New York City. *Archives of Internal Medicine, 125,* 57–61.

Roth, E. F., Jr., Lunde, I., Boysen, G., & Genefke, I. K. (1987). Torture and its treatment. *American Journal of Public Health, 77,* 1404–1406.

Rothman, L. M., & Dubeski, G. (1993). School contact tracing following a cluster of tuberculosis cases in two Scarborough schools. *Canadian Journal of Public Health, 84,* 297–302.

Roudot-Thoraval, F., Kouadja, F., Wirquin, V., Thiers, V., Avons, P., Brechot, C., & Dhumeaux, D. (1989). *Prévalence du portage de l'antigène Hbs et des marqueurs de réplication virale B dans une population de femmes enceintes, en France* [Prevalence of Hbs antigen carriers and markers of B virus replication in a population of pregnant women in France]. *Gastroenterologie Clinique et Biologique, 13,* 353–356.

Rubinstein, A., Graf, E., Landau, E., Reisin, L. H., & Goldbourt, V. (1991). Prevalence of diabetes mellitus in Ethiopian immigrants. *Israel Journal of Medical Sciences, 27,* 252–254.

Rubinstein, A., Goldbourt, U., Shilbaya, A., Levtov, O., Cohen, G., & Villa, Y. (1993). Blood pressure and body mass index in Ethiopian immigrants: Comparison of Operations Solomon and Moses. *Israel Journal of Medical Science, 29,* 360–363.

Rubinstein, A., Graf, E., & Villa, Y. (1993). Prevalence of diabetes mellitus in Ethiopian immigrants: Comparison of Moses and Solomon Immigrations. *Israel Journal of Medical Science, 29,* 344–346.

Rwegellera, G. G. C. (1977). Psychiatric morbidity among West Africans and West Indians living in London. *Psychological Medicine, 7,* 317–329.

Rwegellera, G. G. C. (1980). Differential use of psychiatric services by West Indians, West Africans and English in London. *British Journal of Psychiatry, 137,* 428–432.

Salzer, J. L., & Nelson, N. A. (1983). Health care of Ethiopian refugees. *Pediatric Nursing, 9,* 449–452.

Schable, C., Zekeng, L., Pau, C. P., Hu, D., Kaptue, L., Gurtler, L., Dondero, T., Tsague, J. M., Schochetman, G., & Jaffe, H. (1994). Sensitivity of United States HIV antibody tests for detection of HIV-1 group O infections. *Lancet, 344,* 1333–1334.

Selten, J. P., & Sijben, N. (1994). First admission rates for schizophrenia in immigrants to the Netherlands: The Dutch National Register. *Social Psychiatry and Psychiatric Epidemiology, 29,* 71–77.

Sgan-Cohen, H. D., Steinberg, D., Zusman, S. P., Naor, R., & Sela, M. N. (1993). Peridontal status among adult immigrants from rural Ethiopia. *Israel Journal of Medical Science, 29,* 407–410.

Slater, P. E., Greenberg, Z., & Costin, C. (1993). Imported malaria from Ethiopia—End of an era? *Israel Journal of Medical Science, 29,* 383–384.

Sperber, A. D., Stemmer, S., Sobel, R. J., & Schlaeffer, F. (1989). Treponemal bone disease in an Ethiopian immigrant. *Israeli Journal of Medical Science, 25,* 459–461.

Stengel, B., Saurel-Cubizoles, M. J., & Kaminski, M. (1986). Pregnant immigrant women: Occupational activity, antenatal care and outcome. *International Journal of Epidemiology, 15,* 533–539.

Takougang, J. (1995). Recent African immigrants to the United States: A historical perspective. *Western Journal of Black Studies, 19,* 50–57.

Toole, M. J. (1995). Mass population displacement: A global challenge. *Infectious Disease Clinics of North America, 9,* 353–366.

Toole, M. J., & Waldman, R. J. (1993). Refugees and displaced persons. *Journal of the American Medical Association, 270,* 600–604.

Trevelyan, J. (1994). A woman's lot. *Nursing Times, 90,* 48–50.

U.S. Department of Justice. (1993). *Statistical yearbook of the Immigration and Naturalization Service.* Washington, DC: Author.

U.S. Department of Justice. (1995). *Statistical yearbook of the Immigration and Naturalization Service.* Washington, DC: Author.

Walder, R. (1995). Why the problem continues in Britain. *British Medical Journal, 310,* 1593–1594.

Wartski, S. A. (1991). Tuberculosis in Ethiopian immigrants. *Israel Journal of Medical Sciences, 27,* 288–92.

Wartski, S. A. (1993). Tuberculosis case finding and treatment in Ethiopian immigrants to Israel, 1989–1991. *Israel Journal of Medical Sciences, 29,* 376–380.

Watson, P. (1994). Purging the evil. *Africa Report, 39,* 13–16.

Wells, A. D., Northover, J. M. A., & Howard, E. R. (1986). Abdominal tuberculosis: Still a problem today. *Journal of the Royal Society of Medicine, 79,* 149–153.

Wihtol De Wenden, C. (1994). The French response to the asylum influx, 1980–93. *Annals of the American Academy of Political and Social Science, 534,* 81–90.

Wilkins, E. G. L., & Roberts, C. (1985). Superficial tuberculous lymphadenitis in Merseyside: 1969–1984. *Journal of Hygiene (Cambridge), 95,* 115–122.

Wind, J. (1984). Cross-cultural and anthropobiological reflections on African uvulectomy. *Lancet, 2,* 1267–1268.

World Health Organization. (1993a). *The ICD-10 classification of mental and behavioral disorders: Diagnostic criteria for research.* Geneva, Switzerland: Author.

World Health Organization. (1993b). *The international statistical classification of diseases and health-related problems: The ICD-10.* Geneva, Switzerland: Author.

Zimmerman, M., Bornstein, R., & Martinsson, T. (1995). Utilization of dental services in refugees in Sweden. *Community Dentistry and Oral Epidemiology, 23,* 95–99.

18

Infectious Diseases

KEITH B. ARMITAGE AND ROBERT A. SALATA

Introduction

Many parasitic infections and other geographically restricted diseases occurring in refugees and immigrants are unfamiliar to health care professionals whose training and clinical experience is limited primarily to the United States. Emerging infections are becoming larger problems, and there are significant challenges with old foes such as tuberculosis and malaria. The appearance of human immunodeficiency virus (HIV) as an endemic sexually transmitted disease in many less developed countries will continue to be an issue in immigrants and refugees. At the same time, HIV has changed the incidence and presentation of many other diseases.

Healthcare workers faced with the challenge of infections in immigrants and refugees must appreciate a number of signs and symptoms and assimilate them into proper geographical context in order to reach a rational plan for diagnosis and management. Some infections of immigrants and refugees, such as falciparum malaria, are acute and life threatening, and require prompt diagnosis and treatment. In other cases, a chronic or subacute problem may re-quire an ongoing, systematic approach to diagnosis.

In this chapter, we outline an approach to infectious diseases in immigrants and refugees, beginning with a discussion of screening issues, geographic health risks, and an overview of common syndromes seen in this population. This is followed by a description of selected infectious agents, detailing the epidemiology, clinical presentation, and approach to diagnosis and treatment.

General Approach

When refugees or immigrants present with signs and symptoms of infection, potential etiologies depend on the geographic origin of the patient, the relative incidence of various diseases and their incubation period, the likelihood of insect or certain other exposures, and specific clinical findings (Table 1). A good history is of paramount importance; assistance with language and an understanding of religion and culture are often vital. Obtaining a precise geographic history is essential as many infectious agents occur more commonly in or are restricted to certain worldwide areas (discussed later). Questions about insect exposures, contaminated food and water consumption, sick contacts, and the possibility of immunosuppression are critical. It is important to inquire about traditional forms of treatment that may mask symptoms or confuse the clinical picture.

KEITH B. ARMITAGE AND ROBERT A. SALATA • Division of Infectious Diseases, University Hospitals of Cleveland, Cleveland, Ohio 44106-5083.

Handbook of Immigrant Health, edited by Loue. Plenum Press, New York, 1998.

TABLE 1. Medical Evaluation of Immigrants and Refugees from Developing Countries

History
Identify where patient has been, and when. Ask about specific exposures to insects, water, food. Inquire about medication, traditional healing methods, immunization history.

Physical examination
General examination with particular attention to adenopathy, hepatosplenomegaly, skin lesions, pulmonary findings.

Laboratory tests
CBC, eosinophil count; if anemia present, iron studies, hemoglobin electrophoresis. Three stools for ova and parasites. Stool culture, especially if food handler. Hepatitis B serology; HIV serology if sexually active or pregnant; syphilis serology. Chest X ray; urinalysis.

Thorough physical examination is essential, but may be hindered by poor facilities, lack of privacy, and the embarrassment of the patient. Areas of particular importance include the skin and mucous membranes, assessment for adenopathy, and careful pulmonary and abdominal examinations. Lymphadenopathy should raise the suspicion for tuberculosis, tularemia, plague, filariasis, scrub typhus, visceral leishmaniasis, toxoplasmosis, trypanosomiasis, HIV infection, and secondary syphilis. Hepatosplenomegaly may indicate typhoid fever, brucellosis, tularemia, leptospirosis, visceral leishmaniasis, and schistosomiasis. Splenomegaly is common in patients with chronic or recurrent malaria. The approach to subjects presenting with rash is discussed later.

Laboratory evaluation should be driven by the differential diagnosis. For several infections, the chance of rapid identification is enhanced by immediate examination of fresh specimens (e.g., stool for amebae, blood smears for malaria, borellia, trypanosomes). Stool examination to detect ova or larva of intestinal helminths remains the mainstay in diagnosing these infections. Examination of stool for polymorphonuclear cells is easily accomplished and is useful in differentiating inflammatory causes of diarrhea (e.g., *Salmonella, Shigella,* invasive *E. coli*) from noninflammatory etiologies (e.g., viruses, *Giardia, Cryptosporidium,* enterotoxigenic *E. coli*). Anemia and peripheral eosinophilia are common and are discussed later. Thrombocytopenia may be seen in malaria and dengue fever, and leukopenia may be seen in malaria, typhoid fever, rickettsial disease, brucellosis, and viral infections. Liver function abnormalities often provide important information for conditions such as hepatitis, malaria, leptospirosis, or rickettsial diseases, and chest X ray findings may be characteristic in patients with pulmonary syndromes or subdiaphragmatic disease (e.g., amebic liver abscess). Current mechanisms exist for screening for infections in immigrants and refugees, including tests for TB, HIV, hepatitis B, and syphilis. Tuberculin skin testing should be done in all subjects, and testing for HIV, hepatitis B, and syphilis done in groups known to be at risk (see later sections). Other screening tests used in refugees and immigrants include a hematocrit and eosinophil count and stool examination (see later sections). Most infections in immigrants and refugees cannot be detected by routine screening, and an evaluation for specific infections should be based on clinical and epidemiological grounds.

Geographic Health Risks

In a broad sense, specific health risks may be encountered more frequently in different areas of the world. It is difficult, however, to accurately assess the degree of risk in each area or in individual patients. The following is a general discussion of the geographic distributions of potential infectious diseases in selected areas.

Africa

Northern Africa, characterized by fertile coastal areas and a desert hinterland with oases, has minimal endemic arthropod-borne disease although cases of dengue fever, filariasis, leishmaniasis, malaria, relapsing fever, Rift Valley fever, sandfly fever, typhus, and West Nile fever do occur. Food and waterborne diarrheal diseases are endemic as well as typhoid fever and hepatitis A. Schistosomiasis is prevalent in the Nile Valley. Intestinal helminthic infections, brucellosis, giardiasis, echinococcosis, polio, and trachoma are also encountered.

Sub-Saharan Africa, dominated by tropical rain forests, wooded steppes, desert, and savanna, lies entirely in the tropics. Arthropodborne infections are a major cause of morbidity. Malaria (especially *P. falciparum*) occurs throughout. In addition, filariasis, onchocerciasis, leishmaniasis, trypanosomiasis, relapsing fever, tick-associated typhus, plague, hemorrhagic fever, and yellow fever occur in these countries. Water and foodborne diseases are highly endemic. In addition to infections listed as seen in Northern Africa, other conditions include hepatitis E, cholera, and paragonimiasis. Hepatitis B is also hyperendemic. Other infections seen in this area of the world include meningococcal meningitis, polio, trachoma, and Lassa fever; Ebola and Marburg hemorrhagic fever are present but reported infrequently.

Southern Africa varies physically from deserts to fertile plateaus and plains to temperate areas of the coast. Special considerations here include Crimean-Congo fever, malaria, typhus, tick-bite fever, and occasional cases of trypanosomiasis in Botswana and Namibia. Hepatitis B is hyperendemic. Hepatitis A, amebiasis (especially in South Africa), and typhoid fever are reported from this area. Schistosomiasis has been reported from Botswana, Namibia, Swaziland, and South Africa.

The Americas

Central America and the Caribbean are areas that include tropical rain forests and deserts with areas of equable tropical climate. Malaria exists in many of these countries. Cutaneous and mucocutaneous leishmaniasis occur in Central America and visceral disease is seen in El Salvador, Guatemala, Honduras, and Mexico. Onchocerciasis is seen in parts of Mexico and Chagas' disease is observed in rural central America. Dengue fever and Venezuelan equine encephalitis are reported. Food and waterborne diseases including amebic and bacterial dysenteries are common. Hepatitis A is reported. Cases of cholera are being reported in Central America but not in the Caribbean. Brucellosis occurs in the northern parts of Central America. Typhoid fever and shigellosis reported from Central America have been associated with drug-resistant organisms. *Fasciola hepatica* is endemic in Cuba. Haiti has a high rate of malaria, filariasis, tularemia, tuberculosis, and HIV infection.

Equatorial South America includes the Amazon basin, savanna zones, and dry tropical forest. Insect-related illnesses abound, including falciparum and vivax malaria, Chagas' disease, leishmaniasis, onchocerciasis, plague, yellow fever, bartonellosis, Orgya fever, louse-borne typhus and sandfly-borne disease. Diarrheal diseases are common and include amebiases, bacterial enteritis, and helminthic infections. Schistosomiasis occurs in Brazil, Suriname, and Venezuela. Hepatitis A occurs frequently. Brucellosis occurs and echinococcus is seen in Peru. Cholera has become endemic in these areas since 1991. Other infections including rodent-borne arenavirus hemorrhagic fever (Bolivia), hepatitis B and D (Amazon), meningococcal meningitis (Brazil), and rabies have been encountered from tropical South America.

Asia

East Asia encompasses the countries of China, Korea, Japan, and Mongolia and is geographically dominated by mountain complexes, desert, forests, and subtropics in the southeast. Malaria now occurs only in China. Cases of filariasis are still encountered in south China. Visceral leishmaniasis is resurging in China. Hemorrhagic fever with renal syndrome, Korean hemorrhagic fever, dengue fever, and Japanese encephalitis are other insect-related infections seen in these countries. Mite-borne or scrub typhus is encountered in southern China, Japan, and Korea. Diarrheal disease and hepatitis A are common in most countries. Hepatitis E is prevalent in western China. Schistosomiasis is endemic in the Yangtze river basin. Clonorchiasis and paragonimiasis are reported in China, Japan, Macoa, and Korea, and fasciolopsiasis in China. Hepatitis B is highly endemic throughout all countries.

Southeast Asia and southern Asia include areas of tropical and monsoon forests, savannas, dry tropical forests, steppes, deserts, and high mountain ranges. Arthropod-borne infections are important causes of morbidity in these countries with malaria, filariasis, plague (Vietnam), Japanese encephalitis, dengue and dengue hemorrhagic fever, typhus, visceral leishmaniasis (Bangladesh, India, and Nepal), cutaneous leishmaniasis (Afghanistan, India, Iran and Pakistan), and Crimean-Congo hemorrhagic fever (western South Asia) seen frequently. Food- and waterborne diseases are common and include cholera, amebic and bacterial dysenteries, typhoid fever, hepatitis A and E, intestinal nematodes, fasciolopsiasis, clonorchiasis, and opisthorchiasis. Melioidosis is encountered in Southeast Asian countries. Brucellosis and echinococcosis are seen in many countries of south Asia. Hepatitis B is highly endemic. Meningococcal meningitis has been reported in India and Nepal. Poliomyelitis continues to be seen in many of these countries. Rabies is seen as a hazard in most countries. Urban areas of these countries are experiencing marked increases in cases of HIV infection: cases are expected to escalate further given the high population densities in these areas, and sexual practices and injection drug abuse in some areas.

Western Asia encompasses the countries of Bahrain, Cyprus, Iraq, Israel, Jordan, Kuwait, Lebanon, Oman, Qatar, Saudi Arabia, Syria, Turkey, United Arab Emirates (UAE), and Yemen. Special health risks in these areas include cutaneous leishmaniasis, murine and tick-borne typhus, relapsing fever, typhoid fever, brucellosis and hepatitis A, and foci of echinococcosis are seen. Outbreaks of cholera and meningococcal meningitis have been reported among pilgrims to Mecca and Medina.

Oceania

Major concerns for insect-associated or food- and waterborne illnesses occur in Melanesia and Micronesia–Polynesia. Malaria is endemic in Papua New Guinea. Filariasis is widespread. Mite-borne typhus is seen in Papua New Guinea. Dengue fever occurs in epidemics in most islands. Diarrheal diseases, typhoid fever, and helminthic infections are frequent. Hepatitis A is also a major concern. Hepatitis B is endemic. Trachoma is seen in Melanesia.

Common Syndromes

Fever

Fever in immigrants and refugees requires prompt evaluation to differentiate falciparum malaria from other causes. It is critical to maintain a high index of suspicion for infection with *P. falciparum* as the presentation can be nonspecific, patients may not have fever at the time they seek medical attention, and other symptoms of malaria are easily confused with viral illnesses. All immigrants and refugees arriving from or living in malarious areas who present with fever should have thick and thin blood smears to evaluate for malaria. Malaria is discussed in greater detail later.

In the approach to immigrants or refugees with fever, a careful history is important, with the focus on geographic exposure, the duration and nature of the fever, insect and water (drinking or wading) or contaminated food exposures, and exposure to soil or sick contacts (Bell, 1985). An evaluation for other symptoms such as headache, cough, gastrointestinal symptoms, rigors, sweats, and rash is critical. Important physical findings that may suggest the etiology of fever include rash, petechiae, conjunctivitis, pharyngeal hyperemia, pulmonary rales or consolidation, lymphadenopathy, hepatosplenomegaly, cardiac murmurs, vaginal or urethral discharge, and neurologic findings.

Once malaria has been excluded, the approach to the differential diagnosis in the refugee or immigrant with fever can be based on the incubation period, the acuity of the illness, and accompanying symptoms. The incubation period can be particularly helpful if the timing of potential exposures can be determined (Table 2). Patterns of fever can sometimes be helpful, although it is hazardous to exclude an infection such as malaria or typhoid fever because the patient does not follow the textbook description. A regular, intermittent fever pattern can be suggestive of malaria. Episodes of fever separated by several days of normal temperatures is suggestive of relapsing fever due to borreliosis, but can be seen in malaria, brucellosis, and African trypanosomiasis. Unremitting fever in which the fever always remains elevated is suggestive of classic typhoid fever. Double quotidian fever (two spikes a day not related to antipyretics) is seen in classic visceral leishmaniasis, but can be seen in early malaria and endocarditis.

The presence of jaundice should raise the possibility of hepatitis, yellow fever, amebic liver abscess, or typhoid fever (Zuckerman, 1996). The presentation of typhoid fever and other enteric fever syndromes can be nonspecific and patients often lack classic findings such as rose spots. Persistent high fever and relative temperature–pulse dissociation are classic; typhoid fever is discussed in more detail later. Other infectious syndromes with a relatively short incubation period include various rickettsial diseases, brucellosis, typhus, Q fever, and relapsing fever. Dengue fever and other arboviruses should be considered in patients with acute febrile illnesses. There has been a marked increase in the reported cases of dengue fever in the first half of the 1990s (Gubler & Clark, 1995), and other arboviral infections are also reported with increasing frequency. The presentation of dengue fever and other arbovirus can be nonspecific with high fever as the only major manifestation, or patients can present with headache, severe myalgias, rash, or hemorrhagic complications.

Brucellosis can present with a relatively long incubation period, as can visceral leishmaniasis, amebiasis, African trypanosomiasis, and several helminthic infections such as schistosomiasis, strongyloides, and filariasis. Malaria can present with a long incubation and relapsing course, particularly in nonfalciparum malaria in which the liver phase is untreated or partially treated. Individuals from endemic areas who are partially immune can

TABLE 2. Approach to Immigrants and Refugees with Fever

Short incubation		Long incubation	
Acute course	Prolonged/relapsing course	Acute course	Prolonged/relapsing course
Malaria	Typhoid fever	Malaria	Tuberculosis
Arbovirus infection	Brucellosis	Amebiasis	Amebiasis
Rickettsiosis	Q fever	Leptospirosis	Brucellosis
Brucellosis	Acute schistosomiasis	African trypanosomiasis	Filariasis
Typhus	Relapsing fever	Actinomyces	Leishmaniasis
Influenza	Tuberculosis	Rabies	Trypanosomiasis
Yersinia pestis		Hepatitis B	Meliodosis
Leptospirosis			Paragonimiasis
Yellow fever			Strongyloidiasis
			Schistosomiasis
			Typhoid fever

present with atypical manifestations of falciparum malaria.

Tuberculosis should be considered in patients with fever and a long incubation period. Pulmonary symptoms should increase the suspicion for tuberculosis (TB), but the absence of respiratory complaints does not rule out TB; extrapulmonary infection should be considered in cases of prolonged occult fever, especially when liver enzyme or hematologic abnormalities exist. Other infections that can present with a long incubation period and pulmonary symptoms include paragonimiasis and melioidosis.

Eosinophilia

Clinically significant eosinophilia that merits further investigation is indicated by an absolute eosinophil count of over 500 cells per cubic millimeter determined on at least two occasions (Mahmoud & Austin, 1980). In immigrants and refugees, eosinophilia is most frequently associated with helminthic infection. Most helminthic infections that are limited to the gastrointestinal tract do not cause eosinophilia, and there is a strong association between tissue invasion (i.e., involvement of tissues outside the gastrointestinal tract) and the presence and magnitude of eosinophilia. In contrast to helminths, protozoan parasites rarely if ever are associated with eosinophilia. Exceptions to this rule include the intestinal protozoa *Dientamoeba fragilis* and *Isospora belli*. Helminths associated with eosinophilia include many tissue nematodes such as *Wuchereria bancrofti, Brugia malayi, Loa loa, Onchocerca volvulus, Dracunculus medinensis, Toxocara canis,* and *T. catis, Trichinella spiralis, Angiostrongylus cantonensis;* migrating larvae of the gut nematodes *Ascaris lumbricoides, Necator americanus, Ancylostoma duodenale,* and *Strongyloides stercoralis;* tissue trematodes such as *Schistosoma spp., Fasciola hepatica, Paragonimus westermani;* and tissue cestodes such as *Echinococcus granulosus.*

Each of the helminths just listed has a specific geographic distribution, and obtaining a detailed geographic history is an essential part of the evaluation. The first laboratory investigation should be an examination of a fresh stool specimen for ova and parasites, which if initially negative should be repeated daily for a total of three examinations. A chest X ray to evaluate for tropical pulmonary eosinophilia should be done, particularly in the presence of any pulmonary symptoms. If stool examinations are unrevealing, day and night blood tests for microfilaria, skin snips for onchocerciasis, and superficial rectal biopsies for *Schistosome* ova may be indicated. Serologic tests are available for diagnosing strongyloides, schistosomiasis, visceral larva migrans, and some filarial diseases. Serologic testing has a limited role in evaluation when other tests are unrevealing, particularly in subjects with limited exposures; these tests may be difficult to interpret in patients who are long-term residents of endemic areas. In one study of Southeast Asian refugees, strongyloidiasis and hookworm were the most common conditions associated with eosinophilia (Nutman *et al.,* 1987).

Despite a full evaluation, as many as 30%–50% of immigrants and refugees with eosinophilia will not have a specific etiology determined; most of these have a helminthic infection that has escaped diagnosis (Spry, 1980). Empiric antihelminthic therapy with thiabendazole, mebendazole, or albendazole may be indicated, and if not successful diethycarbamizine or praziquantel should be considered.

Diarrhea

Diarrhea may be the most common symptom experienced by immigrants and refugees (Table 3). In these patients, diarrhea may be acute or chronic. Diarrhea of less than 2 weeks duration is considered acute. In tropical countries, acute diarrhea is endemic, as well as occurring in epidemics, with substantial morbidity and mortality, particularly among young children. There are a wide variety of enteropathogens that cause diarrhea with a short

TABLE 3. Overview of Differential Diagnosis of Diarrhea in Immigrants and Refugees

Acute	Bloody	Chronic
Salmonella	Shigella	Giardiasis
Malaria	Campylobacter	Cryptosporidium
Cholera	Amebiasis	Isosporiasis
Escherichia coli	Enteroinvasive *E. coli*	Topical sprue
Schistosomiasis	Salmonella	Strongyloidiasis
Food poisoning	Yersinia sp.	Schistosomiasis
Rotavirus	Balantidiasis	AIDS associated diarrhea
Norwalk-like virus	Antibiotic-associated colitis	Trichuriaisis (heavy infection)
Other viral	Aeromonas	Clonorchiasis
	Schistosomiasis	Microsporidium
	Trichuriasis	
	Non-cholera vibratos	

incubation period in immigrants and refugees, including *Salmonella sp., Shigella sp., E. coli, Campylobacter,* rotavirus, and protozoan parasites. These enteric pathogens circulate in the community, and at times are isolated from asymptomatic as well as symptomatic subjects.

The role of antimicrobial therapy in the management of acute diarrhea is limited. For many enteropathogens such as *Salmonella* and *E. coli,* antimicrobial therapy in mild cases has not been proven to have a benefit, and in the case of *Salmonella* may prolong the carrier state. For dysentery due to *Shigella sp.* or *E. histolytica,* antimicrobial therapy is indicated, and for cholera, antimicrobial therapy can decrease the volume of fluid lost. Antimicrobial resistance is a growing problem in some enteropathogens, such as *Shigella* and *Salmonella* (Tauxe, Puhr, & Wells, 1990). Epidemics of acute diarrhea due to enteropathogens are common, particularly in crowded conditions such as those found in refugee camps. In this setting, steps to ensure the safety of the water supply, improve hygienic conditions, and decrease person-to-person spread are critical.

A large number of conditions, both infectious and noninfectious, can lead to chronic diarrhea, or diarrhea present for more than 4 weeks (Gianella, 1986). Patients with chronic diarrhea can be further subdivided based on the presence or absence of malnutrition, blood in the stool, or both. Patients with chronic diarrhea, no malnutrition, but blood present in the stool should be evaluated for colonic neoplasia or parasite-associated conditions such as ameboma, whipworm colitis, chronic campylobacteriosis, and schistosomiasis. Inflammatory bowel disease, which is being recognized with increasing frequency in tropical and developing countries, should also be considered.

Patients without blood in the stool but with signs or symptoms of malnutrition usually have an underlying malabsorption syndrome, which may be due to a variety of conditions. Among the infectious causes are tropical sprue, bacterial overgrowth syndrome, and several parasitic infections including *Giardia lamblia, Strongyloides stercoralis, Capillaria,* and *Cryptosporidium.* Some cases of filariasis can cause lymphatic obstruction that can lead to chronic diarrhea, as can intestinal pseudoobstruction due to Chagas' disease. The term *tropical enteropathy* has been used to describe a syndrome of malabsorption and minor intestinal mucosal abnormalities seen in otherwise healthy subjects from tropical countries. Tropical enteropathy is thought to be an adaptation to frequent enteric infections. There are a wide variety of noninfectious causes of malabsorption that may be encountered in immigrants and refugees that are beyond the scope of this chapter.

Chronic diarrhea, malnutrition, and wasting are common manifestations of HIV infection in tropical countries (Serwadda, Mugerwa, & Sewankambo, 1985). Referred to as "slim disease" in many parts of Africa, this syndrome has not been linked to one specific pathogen. It may be related to multiple enteric pathogens, or to involvement of the bowel mucosa due to HIV infection itself. Many enteric pathogens have more severe and prolonged courses in patients with AIDS (discussed further later).

Rash

Skin lesions can be part of a systemic illness or may represent an isolated dermatosis (Table 4). Subjects presenting with rash and

TABLE 4. Dermatologic Signs and Symptoms of Infections

Sign or symptom	Infection
Analgesia	Leprosy
Pruritis	Enterobiasis
	Onchocerciasis
	Toxocariasis
Rash	Dengue
	Measles
	Meningiococcus
	Enteroviral exanthams
	Rickettsial diseases
	Typhoid
	Syphilis
	Viral hemorrhagic fevers
Localized swelling	Chagas' disease
	Gnathostomiasis
	Loiasis
	Myiasis
	Pinta
Ulcer, eschar, abscesses	Anthrax
	Chagas' disease
	Chancroid
	Cutaneous leishmaniasis
	Lymphogranuloma venereum
	African trypanosomiasis
	Syphilis
	Scrub typhus, other rickettsial diseases
	Yaws

constitutional symptoms such as fever, weight loss, sweats, or other symptoms should be evaluated for systemic illnesses that are associated with rash based on the patient's specific exposures, geographic origin, and syndrome. Diagnostic considerations in subjects presenting with fever and a skin ulcer or sore include tularemia, plague, anthrax, trypanosomiasis, scrub typhus, leishmaniasis, rickettsialpox, nocardiosis, blastomycosis, and pyogenic infections. The differential diagnosis in subjects with fever and a rash should include rickettsial diseases such as scrub typhus and spotted fever, dengue fever and other arthropod-borne hemorrhagic fevers, typhoid fever, leptospirosis, rat bite fever, acute schistosomiasis, measles, rubella, and secondary syphilis.

Several important primarily dermatologic conditions that Western-trained health care workers may not be familiar with deserve special mention. Leprosy (*Mycobacterium leprae*) is prevalent in India, China, Korea, tropical Asia and Africa, areas of Latin America, and some Pacific islands (Binford, Mayers, & Walsh, 1982). Infection, spread by nasopharyngeal secretions of infected patients, is facilitated by crowded conditions. The leprosy bacillus primarily affects skin, peripheral nerves, and mucous membranes. Leprosy is a heterogeneous disorder, with tuberculoid, lepromatous, and intermediate forms. In tuberculoid leprosy, subjects in the early stage present with demarcated, sparse, hypoaesthetic, asymmetric skin lesions. In early lepromatous leprosy, subjects may have erythematous nodules, papules, or macules. Nasal stuffiness, epistaxis, conjunctivitis, and uveitis are also seen. In advanced disease, tropical ulcers, muscle wasting, paralysis, tenderness, and enlargement of the peripheral nerves may be seen. The diagnosis can be made by the demonstration of acid-fast bacilli in skin biopsies. The diagnosis of leprosy often carries a social stigma, and the health care worker should be aware of the social consequences of such a diagnosis. Drug treatment can be complicated and lengthy. Commonly employed agents include dapsone, rifampin-rifabutin, clofazamine, ethionamide, and aminoglycosides.

Cutaneous leishmaniasis, discussed later, presents as painless skin nodules or ulcerating lesions. The nonvenereal spirochetes *Treponema carateum* (yaws) and *Treponema carateum* (pinta) are seen most often in tropical areas where there is crowding and poor hygiene (Antal & Causse, 1985). They occur most often in children and adolescents, and are spread by direct inoculation through broken skin. Yaws presents as a single papilloma that may expand to form multiple papillomatous lesions which may ulcerate. In advanced cases, multiple crops of lesions, gummas, and bone lesions may occur. Pinta presents as a scaly papule which progresses to a maculopapular erythematous rash at the site of the primary lesions. Both yaws and pinta can be diagnosed by the demonstration of spirochetes in early lesions, and can be successfully treated with penicillin.

Anthrax (*Bacillus anthracis*) is endemic in agricultural areas and is most often seen in workers with exposure to animal hides and hair (Longfield, 1984). Cutaneous anthrax presents initially as a painless, itchy papule that becomes vesicular and then forms a black eschar. Untreated lesions can disseminate and lead to sepsis or meningitis. The organism can usually be cultured from the lesion, and the lesions can be infectious. Cutaneous anthrax responds to penicillin, erythromycin, or chloramphenical. Anthrax can also present with inhalation-pulmonary or gastrointestinal forms, due to inhalation or ingestion of the spores, respectively. Both pulmonary and gastrointestinal anthrax usually proceed rapidly to sepsis and have high fatality rates.

Many helminths enter the human host through the skin usually without clinical symptoms or with pruritus at the site of penetration as the most common manifestation. Cutaneous manifestations can be seen in strongyloidiasis, hookworm infection, schistosomiasis, and toxocariasis. Several animal helminths (e.g., *Toxocara sp.*) enter the human host through the skin and migrate in the subcutaneous tissues producing cutaneous larva migrans (Zaiman, 1995). The lesions usually begin as nodules, which, as the larva migrate, become pruritic, serpiginous, and erythematous. Animal helminths cannot successfully complete their life cycle in humans and usually die within a few weeks. Symptomatic cases can be treated with topical or oral thiabendazole.

Refugees or immigrants exposed to crowded conditions or poor sanitation are at risk for scabies and lice. Myiasis, a superficial skin condition caused by the laying of fly eggs and their development into larva in the skin, is not uncommon in tropical countries (Guillozot, 1980). Subjects with myiasis present with one or more nodules, which may be confused with boils due to *Staphylococcus aureus*. Myiasis can be treated with surgical incision; in some cases the larva can be induced to migrate out by application of petroleum jelly and an occlusive dressing that suffocates the larva. Pyogenic infections due to *Staphylococcus* and *Streptococcus* are also common in tropical regions, as are dermatophyte infections such as tinea capitis or tinea pedis. Skin reactions to insect bites are common and should be considered in subjects with pruritic dermatoses.

Pulmonary Syndromes

Many systemic infections have pulmonary manifestations, and there are several bacteria and parasites that should receive strong consideration when refugees and immigrants present with respiratory symptoms (see Table 5). Tuberculosis, discussed later in detail, is endemic throughout most of the world, and is the most common serious and contagious pulmonary infection. Paragonimiasis (discussed later) and melioidosis can mimic tuberculosis. Melioidosis is caused by the gram-negative bacillus *Pseudomonas pseudomallei* that is found in soil in Southeast Asia. Infected patients can present acutely with pneumonia and sepsis, or the infection can be chronic in nature with patients presenting with upper lobe cavitary lesions on

TABLE 5. Parasites Causing Pulmonary Disease

Parasite	Pulmonary syndrome	Distribution	Transmission	Diagnosis
Helminths				
Ascariasis	Tropical pulmonary eosinophilia	Tropics	Fecal–oral	Stool for O & P, sputum for larvae
Capillariasis	Tropical pulmonary eosphiphilia	Thailand, Philippines	Raw fish	Stool for O & P, sputum for larvae
Dirofilariasis	Solitary nodule	Southern U.S.	Mosquito borne	Radiology, tissue
Echinococcosis	Pulmonary cysts	Worldwide;	Canine feces rural livestock	Radiology, serology
Filariasis	Tropical pulmonary eosinophilia	Tropics	Insect borne	Blood smear; serology
Gnathosgomiasis	Tropical pulmonary eosphiphilia	Thailand, Japan	Raw fish, fowl; fresh water	Tissue
Hookworm	Tropical pulmonary eosinophilia	Tropics; subtropics	Soil–skin	Stool for O & P
Paragonomiasis	Parasitic bronchietasis	China, Korea, Latin America, Africa	Raw crabs, crayfish	Sputum, stool for O & P
Schistosomiasis	Cor pulmonale	Asia, Africa, Caribbean	Fresh water, contact	Stool, urine smear for eggs
Strongyloidiasis	Tropical pulmonary eosinophilia	Tropics; subtropics	Soil–skin	Stool or sputum for larvae
Toxocariasis	Pneumonitis with eosinophilia	Worldwide	Dog or cat feces	Serology, tissue biopsy
Protozoa				
Amebiasis	Abscess	India, Mexico, South Africa	Food, water fecal–oral	Serology
Malaria	Pulmonary edema	Africa, Latin America, Asia	Mosquito borne	Blood smear
Toxoplasmosis	Pneumonitis in comprised host	Worldwide	Cat feces, raw meat	Serology, tissue biopsy

chest X ray. Therapy with fluoroquinolones, or tetracycline plus chloramphenicol or sulfonamides is effective.

Pulmonary infiltrates and eosinophilia can occur with several intestinal helminths that have a migratory phase in the lung as part of their life cycle (ascariasis, hookworm infection, or strongyloidiasis) (Ottesen & Nutman, 1992). Fleeting infiltrates, cough, eosinophilia, and wheezing may occur after recent infection, when the parasite migrates from the gastrointestinal tract to the lungs before returning to the gut to complete its life cycle. Examination of stool and sputum is sometimes helpful in establishing an etiologic diagnosis, and repeating stool exam several weeks after presentation is often

useful. Symptomatic treatment with bronchodilators may be necessary; definitive therapy with antihelminthic agents may need to be repeated after the agent has completed the lung migratory phase of the life cycle.

Human infection with dog or cat *Toxocara sp.* results in tissue invasion (visceral larva migrans) (Glickman & Schantz, 1981). Subjects can present with cough, wheezing, pulmonary infiltrates, and eosinophilia. Tropical pulmonary eosinophilia also occurs as part of a syndrome due to the nematodes *Wuchereria bancrofti* and *Brugia malayi*. Nocturnal cough, eosinophilia, and a response to therapy with diethylcarbamazine or ivermectin are typical. Schistosomiasis, discussed later, can present with pulmonary syndromes, either as part of the acute infection syndrome (Katayama fever) or in chronic disease (cor pulmonale).

Because the unique life cycle of *S. stercoralis* produces autoinfection resulting in persistent infection for years, strongyloidiasis deserves special mention in immigrants who present with eosinophilia and pulmonary infiltrates. Autoinfection can produce mild symptoms years after exposure, and immunodeficient patients can present with severe disease. Immunosuppression due to medications such as corticosteroids or underlying disease including HIV infection can lead to the hyperinfection syndrome with dissemination of the parasite into many organs, including the lungs; cough and sputum production are a common feature in this setting (Anydia, Doppl, & Battmane, 1994). Polymicrobial bacteremia and meningitis with adult respiratory distress syndrome can also occur. The diagnosis can be made by identification of *Strongyloides* larva in the sputum or stool. Supportive care and therapy with thiabendazole or ivermectin are indicated, but the syndrome has a high mortality rate. Care should be taken in giving immunosuppressive therapy to subjects who may harbor *Strongyloides stercoralis,* and screening examinations of the stool should be undertaken before such therapy is undertaken.

Echinococcosis, discussed later, should be considered in patients from parts of the world where sheep and cattle are raised who present with complicated cystic lesions on chest X ray. Pulmonary cysts due to echinococcosis are usually asymptomatic, and appear on X ray as well-demarcated, thin-walled cysts. Most often lung cysts coexist with hepatic involvement.

Patients with amebic liver abscess can present with pulmonary symptoms due to pleural or pulmonary reaction in association with adjacent liver abscess or, more rarely, due to rupture of a liver abscess into the pleura or lung parenchyma. An elevated right hemidiaphragm or right lower lobe atelectasis, or both, on chest X ray is common in patients with amebic hepatic abscess (Ravdin, 1995).

Immigrants and refugees with HIV infection and other immunocompromising states are susceptible to pulmonary infections due to a variety of opportunistic pathogens such as *Pneumocystis carinii, M. tuberculosis, Mycobacterium avium-complex* or *M. kansasii, Toxoplasma gondii,* and *Strongyloides stercoralis.*

Anemia

Anemia is very common in refugees and immigrants, occurring in 20%–40% in some groups (Fleming, 1987). Anemia in these patients may be part of a systemic illness or due to an otherwise asymptomatic infection that leads to iron deficiency. Systemic illness such as visceral leishmaniasis, tuberculosis, AIDS, malaria, and typhoid fever often have anemia as part of the clinical presentation. Patients with anemia and symptoms of weight loss, fever, adenopathy, or other symptoms should be evaluated for an underlying systemic illness driven by the specific signs, symptoms, and exposures.

Nutritional deficiency, particularly iron deficiency, is a common manifestation of otherwise asymptomatic helminthic infection (Baker, 1981). Hookworm is frequently associated with iron deficiency, but other helminths have also been implicated, and polyparasitism is common. Women of childbearing age are particularly at risk for severe iron deficiency due to menstrual and gastrointestinal iron loss combined with poor nutrition. Patients with suspected iron deficiency anemia should have stool examined for ova and parasites, and empiric antihelminthic therapy with mebendazole should be considered if stool studies are negative.

Tropical sprue should be considered in individuals with anemia due to folate or vitamin B12 deficiency. Tropical sprue is associated with small bowel malabsorption due to an unidentified infectious agent or agents that occur throughout the world in tropical or subtropical regions (Gianella, 1986). Tropical sprue may follow an acute episode of diarrhea, particularly in short-term visitors to endemic areas, or may present more insidiously. Subjects with tropical sprue present with evidence of small bowel malabsorption with steatorrhea, weight loss, nutritional deficiencies, and crampy abdominal pain. Prolonged therapy with antibiotics such as tetracycline may result in remission, and spontaneous remissions occur. Folate and B12 should also be administered and usually result in resolution of anemia. B12 deficiency can also be seen with fish tapeworm infection due to *Diphyllobothrium latum.*

Noninfectious causes of anemia such as thalassemia or other hemoglobinopathies also need to be considered in immigrants and refugees, and hemoglobin electrophoresis considered in unexplained anemia.

Sexually Transmitted Diseases

Sexually transmitted diseases (STDs) are an increasingly important cause of morbidity and mortality around the world; most notably the last quarter of the 20th century has seen the emergence of HIV as an STD in most parts of the world. The specific causative agents of STDs and their epidemiology vary with geography and culture (Perine, 1994). STDs that infrequently cause infection in the developed world such as chancroid, lymphogranuloma venereum (LGV), and donovanosis are much more common in the developing world, particularly the tropics (Piot & Holmes, 1990). Commonly encountered infections such as gonorrhea and syphilis are seen more often in the developing world, and complications of STDs such as urethral strictures, pelvic inflammatory disease (PID), and infertility are more common. STDs, particularly those associated with genital ulcers such as chancroid, syphilis, and genital herpes are important cofactors in the transmission of HIV (Robinson, Mulder, Auvert, & Hayes, 1997).

Gonorrhea, chlamydia, and syphilis are the most common STDs. Gonorrhea is estimated to have a prevalence of 3% to 18% of women and 4% to 9% of men in developing countries (Daly *et al.,* 1994). The etiologic agent of gonorrhea is *Neisseria gonor-*

rhoeae, a fastidious gram-negative coccus that is found only in humans. Clinical manifestations of gonorrhea include urethritis, epididymitis, proctitis, cervicitis, endometritis, and salpingitis. Complications include infertility and ectopic pregnancy in women and urethral stricture in men. Gonorrhea is also an important cause of neonatal ophthalmologic infection, which leads to blindness in up to 20% of untreated cases, and is an important cause of blindness in Africa. Gonorrhea can be diagnosed by culture of cervical discharge in women or smear of culture of urethral discharge in men. Penicillin, once the mainstay of therapy for gonorrhea, is ineffective in many parts of the world due to the development and spread of resistance. Alternative therapies include ceftriaxone, which is considered the mainstay of therapy for gonorrhea but has the disadvantage of being significantly more expensive than penicillin, and spectinomycin, which is ineffective in some parts of the Far East. Fluoroquinolones have been shown to be effective in uncomplicated urethritis, but increasing resistance to this class of antibiotics is also observed. Neonatal ophthalmologic infection can be treated with topical silver nitrate.

Chlamydia trachomatous, the principal cause of nongonococcal urethritis, is an important cause of PID and infertility in women, and is also the etiologic agent of lymphogranuloma venereum (LGV). *C. trachomatous* is also an important cause of neonatal ophthalmologic infection. In men, LGV presents with a genital papule or ulcer (which is often asymptomatic) followed in weeks to months by acute tender inguinal lymphadenopathy frequently accompanied by systemic symptoms. In women, LGV presents as acute proctocolitis, and can be complicated by peroneal stricture and fistulae. *Chlamydia* can be diagnosed by a variety of antigen staining techniques; culture requires live cell lines and is not commonly used. Tetracyclines or erythromycin are the mainstays of therapy.

Primary syphilis, due to infection with *Treponema pallidum,* presents with a painless genital ulcer that spontaneously heals. Secondary syphilis follows 1 to 6 months later in approximately 25% of patients and has multiple manifestations including rash that typically involves the palms and soles, fever, malaise, and adenopathy. Untreated secondary syphilis may become latent, or tertiary syphilis may develop years later, with destructive lesions known as gummas that can involve a variety of tissues including bone, skin, the central nervous system, and the cardiovascular system. Congenital syphilis occurs when primary or secondary syphilis accompanies pregnancy, and can result in major sequelae for the fetus including hepatosplenomegaly, rash, arthritis, and anemia. In some tropical countries the prevalence of syphilis in pregnant women is 10% to 15%, and congenital syphilis is one of the top five causes of perinatal mortality. A history of genital ulcers or other symptoms suggestive of syphilis should be sought in women seeking prenatal care with the goal of therapeutic intervention to prevent neonatal infection.

The diagnosis of syphilis can be made by demonstration of the organism from samples obtained from primary or secondary lesions, but the diagnosis is most often made serologically. Serologic tests can be divided into treponemal tests (e.g., FTA), which represent specific antibodies directed against treponemal antigens, and nontreponemal tests (e.g., VDRL, RPR) which represent nonspecific antibodies in response to infection. Interpretation of serologic tests requires some caution, with some pitfalls unique to patients from tropical countries. Nonvenereal treponemes may serve as cross-reacting antigens, and patients with yaws or pinta can have positive treponemal antibodies. There are a variety of conditions that can produce false positive nontreponemal tests, such as chronic parasitic or bacterial infection and rheumatic diseases. In addition, nonvenereal syphilis is endemic in western Asia, northern Africa, and Australia. Also known as bejel, nonvenereal syphilis is transmitted by contaminated drinking and eating utensils, and

presents as lesions on the face and oropharynx. Tertiary complications similar to those seen in venereal syphilis can occur. Serologic tests are indistinguishable from those in venereal syphilis.

Therapy of primary and secondary syphilis can be accomplished with a single dose of benzathene penicillin. Latent syphilis, tertiary syphilis, congenital syphilis, and neurosyphilis require longer and more intensive courses of antibiotics, and health care providers should consult a reference text for details.

The interaction of syphilis and HIV deserves mention. Genital ulcers due to syphilis enhance the transmission of HIV. In developed countries syphilis and HIV are epidemiologically linked; this may be true for developing countries, but data are lacking (Bassett et al., 1996; Boyer, Barrett, Peterman, & Bolan, 1997; Klouman et al., 1997; Mbizvo et al., 1996; Musher, 1991; Nunn, Kengeya-Kayondo, Malamba, Seeley, & Mulder, 1994). In addition, HIV affects the natural history of syphilis; HIV infected patients are more likely to have secondary and neurosyphilis, and the time course may be compressed. HIV infected patients are also more likely to fail treatment (Beck et al., 1996).

Chancroid is a genital ulcer disease due to infection with Hemophilus ducreyi, a small gram-negative rod. Chancroid is common in the tropics and in some tropical countries is the most common cause of genital ulcer disease (Ronald & Plummer, 1985). It is seen less often in temperate areas. Contact with a prostitute is an important risk factor in the United States, Thailand, and Kenya (Plummer et al., 1983). Patients present with a papule that enlarges into a tender ulcer that can be distinguishable from a primary syphilitic ulcer by its irregular edge, exquisite pain, and friable granulation tissue in the base. Multiple ulcers may be present, and adenopathy is common. Diagnosis is usually made on clinical grounds as isolation of the organism is difficult and other techniques for diagnosis are not available. Antibiotic therapy with erythromycin, trimethoprim-sulfamethoxazole, ceftriaxone, and fluoroquinolones is effective, although resistance in developing in some areas, and local resistance patterns should be determined.

Donovanosis is a genital ulcer disease due to infection with the bacterium *Calymmatobacterium granulomatosis* which is endemic in southeast Asia, southern India, the Caribbean, and parts of Africa and South America. Donovanosis begins as a papule that progresses to a large ulcer. The lesions are usually painless. Untreated cases can be complicated by scarring and deformation. Diagnosis is based on the demonstration of intracytoplasmic "Donovan bodies" on tissue smears. Trimethoprim-sulfamethoxazole is the mainstay of therapy.

Selected Infectious Agents

Viruses

Dengue Fever

Dengue viruses are responsible for two disease syndromes, classic dengue fever and dengue hemorrhagic fever–dengue shock syndrome (DHF-DSS) (Halstead, 1990). Dengue viruses are small enveloped RNA viruses that are transmitted to humans by *Aedes aegypti* mosquitoes. Dengue occurs in nearly all tropical countries, with recent epidemics documented in Central and South America. Epidemics are most common during the rainy season, and usually occur at altitudes of less than 2,000 feet. Classic dengue fever occurs after an incubation period of 2 to 7 days with the sudden onset of high fever, headache, backache, myalgias, and arthralgias (hence the name "break bone fever"). Therefore, febrile illnesses lasting for more than 10 to 14 days are not likely related to hemorrhagic fever syndrome. Facial flushing and conjunctivitis also commonly occur, and during days 2 to 6 of the illness patients may experience nausea, vomiting, anorexia, hyperesthesia, taste aberrations, and adenopathy. Within a day or two of de-

fervescence, a generalized morbilliform rash may occur, and fever may return with the rash, producing a biphasic fever curve (Trofa *et al.,* 1997).

DHS-DSS occurs in subjects with preexistent nonneutralizing antibody to the virus, and is more common in children. The presence of antibody-antigen complexes leads to the activation of the cytokine and coagulation cascades with resultant increase in capillary permeability and coagulopathy. DHS-DSS usually begins like dengue fever, with the development of severe symptoms during day 2 to 5 of the illness. DHS-DSS is characterized by hypotension, petechiae, and ecchymoses, and in severely affected patients, renal failure and gastrointestinal hemorrhage (Anonymous, 1996; Gubler & Clark, 1995).

Dengue infection can be diagnosed serologically. No specific therapy is available; management is based on supportive care with antipyretics for fever and myalgias, and fluid and electrolyte management in patients with DHS-DSS.

Yellow Fever Virus

Yellow fever is an acute mosquito-borne viral infection that results in fever, jaundice, proteinuria, and hemorrhage. Yellow fever virus is a small RNA virus. There are two epidemiologic forms: a sylvan or jungle type that is predominant in South America and an urban form that exists in Africa. In the sylvan form, monkeys are the primary host and a variety of mosquito vectors spread the virus to humans, who are incidental hosts. In the urban form, humans are the primary host, and the virus is spread by *Aedes aegypti* mosquitoes. In both cases, the disease occurs with increased frequency during the rainy season, and outbreaks occur with a periodicity of 5 to 10 years. In South America, most cases occur in young men with rural occupations, while in Africa cases occur most often in children (Monath, 1987).

The incubation period is 3 to 6 days and is followed by a spectrum of disease that ranges from mild to severe. Milder cases are characterized by fever, headaches, and myalgias lasting a few days. Severe cases are characterized by high fever, chills, severe headache, lumbosacral back pain; myalgias anorexia, nausea, and vomiting occur less frequently. There may be a relative bradycardia despite a high temperature. This initial phase lasting approximately 3 days may be followed by a brief defervescence, which is followed by the reappearance of fever, vomiting, epigastric pain, jaundice, and prostration. Oliguric renal failure and bleeding diathesis may occur including disseminated intravascular coagulation. Case fatality rates of icteric yellow fever are 20% to 50%, with most deaths occurring on days 7 to 10. Definitive diagnosis can be made on the basis of serologic tests. There is no specific therapy; supportive care should be given to patients with severe disease. A safe and effective vaccine exists which after one injection conveys protection in 7 to 10 days that lasts 10 years. The vaccine contains live virus and should not be given to children younger than 6 months, pregnant women, or immunocompromised patients, including those with AIDS.

Undifferentiated Arboviral Viruses

There is a heterogeneous group of viruses that occur in specific geographic locations that have in common transmission by insect bites and the production of a febrile illness. There are at least 80 arthropod-borne viruses that are known to infect humans; most produce a mild, nonspecific febrile illness (Tesh, 1990).

Chikungunya fever occurs throughout most of sub-Saharan Africa, India, Southeast Asia, Indonesia, and the Philippines. The Chikungunya virus is transmitted by *Aedes* mosquitoes, and produces a febrile illness characterized by headache, myalgias, and a maculopapular rash affecting primarily the trunk and extremities. Joint pain can be a severe; lymphadenopathy and leukopenia can occur. The illness can be diagnosed serologically. Treatment is supportive. Ross River virus is antigenically similar to Chikungunya

virus and produces a similar illness. Ross River fever occurs in Australia, New Guinea, and the South Pacific islands.

West Nile fever occurs in rural areas of Africa, southern Europe, and central and south Asia. The West Nile fever virus is transmitted to humans from avian hosts by mosquito vectors. Epidemics occur during the rainy season when there is maximal mosquito activity. The clinical manifestations are usually mild in children, but can resemble a dengue-like illness in adults. Rarely meningoencephalitis occurs, most often in elderly and debilitated patients. The diagnosis of West Nile fever can be made serologically, and the disease is treated symptomatically.

Phlebotomus fever, also known as sandfly fever, is produced by a group of viruses transmitted by the bite of phlebotamine (sand) flies. Phlebotomus fever occurs throughout rural areas of northern Africa, southern Europe, and central Asia. In temperate regions, the illness occurs mostly in the summer months. In children, phlebotomus fever is usually mild. In adults, the illness is characterized by the abrupt onset of fever, headache, photophobia, myalgias, conjunctival injection, nausea, and vomiting. Leukopenia is common. The illness usually lasts 2 to 4 days. Diagnosis is made serologically; therapy is supportive.

Rift Valley fever occurs throughout Africa. The Rift Valley fever virus is transmitted to humans through direct contact or aerosols from tissues of infected animals, particularly sheep and cattle. The disease is most often seen in animal herders, veterinarians, and slaughterhouse workers. The usual clinical presentation is that of a nonspecific febrile illness. Rarer presentations include hemorrhagic fever with hepatic necrosis, encephalitis, and loss of vision due to retinal vasculitis and edema. Serologic diagnosis is available, but is complicated by cross-reactivity with phlebotomus fever viruses, which clinically presents in a very similar manner. Management is supportive. A vaccine exists for persons at high risk.

Oropouche fever occurs in northern South America, particularly the Amazon River basin of Brazil. The Oropouche fever virus is transmitted to humans by the bite of *Culicoides* midges. The disease occurs both in urban and sylvan cycles. The disease is characterized by the sudden onset of high fever, chills, dizziness, headache, myalgias, arthralgias, nausea, and vomiting after an incubation period of 4 to 8 days. The illness usually lasts from 2 to 5 days and complications are not seen. Oropouche fever can be diagnosed serologically; therapy is supportive.

Viral Hemorrhagic Fevers

Viral hemorrhagic fevers have received worldwide public attention in the past decade with the publicity surrounding Ebola virus. Viral hemorrhagic fevers are zoonoses with distinct geographic distributions (LeDuc, 1989). There are a wide variety of hemorrhagic fever syndromes that are discussed briefly. Yellow fever and dengue viruses fall into this category, and were discussed earlier.

Arenaviruses are a group of viruses that cause chronic infections in rodents and humans acquire disease by contact with rodent urine. Cases are largely confined to rural areas where rodent hosts are found. Lassa virus is responsible for Lassa fever, and is found in forest and savanna areas of western Africa. After an incubation period of 7 to 18 days, patients present with fever, arthralgias, headache, and malaise. More severely affected patients present with encephalopathy, seizures, and sensorineural hearing loss. Bleeding occurs in 15% to 20%; the fatality rate is 1% to 3%.

Junin virus causes Argentine hemorrhagic fever, which occurs in humid grasslands in that country. Bolivian hemorrhagic fever caused by the Machupo virus causes a similar illness that occurs in the plains of Bolivia, Paraguay, and western Brazil. Patients infected with these viruses have more hemorrhagic complications than those with Lassa. The initial presentation is similar to Lassa, with fever and malaise, which thereafter may progress to bleeding, hypotension, and neurologic complications.

All three viruses can be diagnosed serologically. Supportive care is often required. Lassa fever can be transmitted from person to person and isolation and barrier precautions should be instituted in suspected cases. The antiviral drug ribavirin has shown efficacy in cases of Lassa, particularly when begun early in the illness. Argentine hemorrhagic fever has been treated with convalescent-phase plasma with success in reducing mortality. There are currently no vaccines available for these viruses.

Ebola and Marburg viruses are found localized to the forest and savanna areas of sub-Saharan Africa (McCormick & Fisher-Hoch, 1990). The animal reservoir is unknown, and most cases are the result of human-to-human transmission most often due to contact with body fluids, blood, blood products, or needle exposure. Airborne transmission has not been confirmed. Both viruses cause a hemorrhagic fever with a high mortality. The incubation is 10 to 20 days for Ebola and 4 to 9 days for Marburg. Initial manifestations include fever, headache, and malaise followed by bleeding in 80% of cases. Adult respiratory distress syndrome and neurologic complications are seen. The mortality rate is estimated to be 30% for Marburg and 50% to 90% for Ebola. These infections can be diagnosed serologically or by electron microscopy. Body fluid precautions are essential.

Hantaviruses are a group of enveloped viruses which worldwide are responsible for two related disease syndromes: hemorrhagic fever with renal syndrome (HFRS) and nephrophagia epidemica (NE) (McCormick & Fisher-Hoch, 1990). A third syndrome, hanta pulmonary syndrome, geographically restricted to the United States, has recently been described. Hantaviruses are present in rodent populations and transmission to humans occurs through contact with rodent feces or urine. The incubation period is 12 to 21 days. HFRS is seen in rural and urban areas of Asia, China, Japan, and Korea where rodent exposure in likely. The HFRS illness usually begins abruptly with chills, fever, lethargy, headache, anorexia, nausea, vomiting, abdominal pain, and diarrhea. In severe cases this is followed by hypotension and bleeding diathesis (Mertz, Hjelle, & Bryan, 1997; Warner, 1996). The mortality of HFRS is 3% to 5%. NE is a milder form seen mostly in Scandinavia in which deaths are rare. Hantavirus infection can be diagnosed serologically. Ribavirin may reduce morbidity and mortality if administered early in the disease; the benefit of such therapy in hanta pulmonary syndrome has not been established (Fisher-Hoch *et al.,* 1995).

Congo-Crimean hemorrhagic fever (CCHF) occurs throughout Africa, Asia, and eastern Europe (McCormick & Fisher-Hoch, 1990). The disease is transmitted to humans through the bite of ixodid ticks or through direct contact with infected animals; a variety of domestic and wild animals serve as reservoirs. The illness should be considered in patients with animal exposure or seasonal exposure to the tick vector. CCHF has an incubation period of 3 to 6 days. The illness is characterized by the acute onset of fever, chills, severe headache, back pain, arthralgias, and abdominal pain. Conjunctivitis, pharyngitis, and palatal petechiae are seen. Manifestations of the bleeding diathesis are seen on day 3 to 5 of the illness. CCHF can be diagnosed serologically. The mortality of severe CCHF is 40% to 90%. Ribavirin may be effective but clinical trials are lacking (Fisher-Hoch *et al.,* 1995; Tignor & Hanham, 1993).

Rabies

Rabies is a common problem in tropical countries, occurring more often in urban settings because of the larger concentration of dogs in these areas. It is estimated that at least 96% of cases are related to canine exposures (Warrell & Shope, 1990). The disease is most common in young males, who have a comparatively high rate of dog bites. Rabies virus causes a fatal meningoencephalitis. The incubation period averages 20 to 90 days but can range from 4 days to years. Vague symptoms of fever and malaise may precede the onset of encephalitis, which in acute cases is followed by the rapid onset of paralysis and death. Reflex spasms of the inspiratory muscles associated with intense fear of water is classic. Less acute cases with slower onset of paralysis occur. There is no specific therapy and the mortality rate approaches 100%. The diagnosis can be made by demonstration of the virus in pathologic specimens or serologically. Rabies can be prevented by vaccination, and postexposure prophylaxis with rabies immune globulin should be given to patients with possible exposure according to published schedules.

Polio

Despite widespread vaccination in many countries, polio remains a devastating disease in many parts of the developing world where access to polio vaccine is limited (World Health Organization Consultation Group in Poliomyelitis, 1985). Most infections are asymptomatic or produce a nonspecific self-limited illness; aseptic meningitis and paralytic poliomyelitis occur less frequently. Aseptic meningitis due to the polio virus is indistinguishable from other causes of viral meningitis. Paralytic polio occurs due to destruction of the anterior horn cells of the spinal cord and presents as flaccid paralysis, most characteristically asymmetrically in the lumbar area. Other areas of the spinal cord may be involved and produce a variety of neurologic syndromes. Children are most susceptible due to the age-dependent acquisition of antibody; older children and adults are more likely to have symptomatic and paralytic forms.

Polio can be diagnosed serologically or by isolation of the virus in stool. Therapy is symptomatically limited to treatment of muscle spasm and physical therapy in paralytic cases. Polio is highly preventable by vaccination.

Measles

Measles continues to be widespread in many parts of the world where less than 50%

of the children are vaccinated. There are an estimated 2 million deaths per year worldwide attributable to measles (Halsey & Job, 1990). The measles virus is highly contagious and is spread from person to person by respiratory droplets. The virus produces an acute febrile illness characterized by cough, coryza, and a maculopapular rash. In the developing world, the vast majority of cases are in children. In some industrialized countries young adults are also susceptible. The illness usually occurs 9 to 10 days after exposure. Small bluish-white papules with an erythematous base (Koplik spots) occur in most patients; they are seen in the first 2 days of the illness with fever but before the onset of the rash. The rash usually begins on the face and then spreads with diffuse maculopapular lesions which may become confluent. Complications of measles include pneumonia due to the virus or from secondary bacterial infection, otitis media, croup, diarrhea, seizures, and encephalitis. In young infants in developing countries, the illness has a case fatality rate that approaches 25%.

Measles can be diagnosed serologically. Therapy is supportive, with fluids and nutritional support as needed. Vitamin A supplementation has been shown to decrease the acute mortality associated with measles, and in populations where vitamin A deficiency is likely, children should receive supplementation (Hussey & Klein, 1990). Measles is preventable with the administration of a live, attenuated vaccine.

Hepatitis A and E

Hepatitis A is endemic throughout the world and infection in childhood is frequent in developing countries (Feinstone, 1996). Infection in children is usually mild and anicteric. Cases in adults produce jaundice approximately half the time but mortality is less than 0.3% and long-term sequelae are rare. Hepatitis A is related to the enteroviruses and is spread by the fecal-oral route. There is only one serotype and infection provides lifelong immunity. It is rare for individuals who grew up in developing countries to be nonimmune and to develop jaundice as an adult. Nonimmune health care workers exposed to food and water in developing countries are at high risk for hepatitis A. They should receive hepatitis A vaccine or immune globulin.

Hepatitis E has epidemiologic and clinical characteristics similar to hepatitis A. Epidemics of hepatitis E have been described related to fecal contamination of drinking water associated with flooding and other disruptions (Bernal et al., 1995). Hepatitis E may be the most common cause of acute hepatitis in the developing world; outbreaks have been documented in Asia, north and central Africa, and South and Central America. The incubation period is 2 to 9 weeks. The disease caused by hepatitis E is mild and usually without sequelae; asymptomatic cases outnumber icteric cases. The exception is pregnant women in whom a more severe form is seen, particularly in the third trimester where mortality has been as high as 10% to 20%. There is currently no vaccine for hepatitis E.

Hepatitis B and D

Hepatitis B is endemic worldwide and is hyperendemic in the Far East, Africa, and South America; there are an estimated 200 million cases worldwide. Hepatitis B causes an acute illness as well as chronic liver disease with cirrhosis and hepatocellular carcinoma as possible sequela. Transmission is by blood products, shared needles, sexual contacts or from mother to child. Unlike the epidemiologic pattern in the United States, in the developing world less than half of the patients with hepatitis B have a risk factor such as parenteral exposure from injection drugs (Edmunds et al., 1996). Hepatitis B should be considered prominently in the differential diagnosis of refugees or immigrants with jaundice, chronic hepatitis, or hepatoma, and appropriate serologic tests should be ordered.

Hepatitis D causes acute hepatitis in subjects who are acutely or chronically infected with hepatitis B, and the epidemiology of hepatitis D somewhat paralells that of hepatitis B and is transmitted by close contact or by the parenteral route. The areas of greatest hepatitis D prevalence are Italy, the Middle East, Central Africa, and the Amazon basin. For reasons that are not clear, hepatitis D is less common in certain hepatitis B risk groups such as medical care workers and homosexual males in Northern Europe, the United States, and in China and Southeast Asia. Hepatitis D superinfection can cause fulminant hepatic failure, and overall has a mortality of 5% to 20%.

Hepatitis C

Hepatitis C is the major cause of transfusion-associated hepatitis worldwide and accounts for 20% to 40% of sporadic hepatitis cases (Alter, 1996). The majority of cases are minimally symptomatic, although cases of fulminant hepatitis can occur. Chronic hepatitis, cirrhosis, and hepatoma are common sequelae. Hepatitis C is endemic globally with the highest prevalence in central Africa and the Far East. There is currently no vaccine available.

Human Immunodeficiency Virus

Infection with the human immunodeficiency virus (HIV) produces immune dysfunction and immunosuppression leading to opportunistic infections, increased risk for other pathogens, malignancies, and other noninfectious complications. Worldwide, it is estimated that at least 12 million persons are infected with HIV, with the majority of infected individuals residing in the countries of sub-Saharan Africa, the United States, Western Europe, the Caribbean, and South America (Gourevitch, 1996; Mastro & de Vincenzi, 1996). India, Thailand, other countries of Asia, and the countries of the former Soviet Union are seeing increasing numbers of cases (Ford, 1995; Jain, John, & Keusch, 1994). HIV is spread by sexual, parenteral, and perinatal routes; in most countries of the developing world, HIV is spread primarily by

heterosexual contact and from mother to infant. The natural history of HIV infection is variable; on average, over many years HIV infection causes progressive immune dysfunction (particularly of cell mediated immunity) leading to severe immune dysfunction, known as the acquired immune deficiency syndrome (AIDS).

There are a variety of serologic tests that can be used to diagnose HIV infection. In addition, the World Health Organization has published a clinical case definition (Albrecht, 1997). A virus closely resembling HIV and causing a similar but often milder illness has been described in West Africa and designated HIV-2. Diagnosis of HIV-2 infection may require specific serologic tests that differ from those used for HIV-1. The social and psychological impact of the diagnosis of HIV infection in a subject cannot be overestimated, and serologic testing for HIV should not be undertaken without appropriate counseling and support services.

The impact of HIV on the health and clinical presentations of infections in refugees cannot be underestimated. In general, in the United States and other Western countries, immunosuppressed HIV-infected individuals most often present with opportunistic infections that do not routinely cause disease in immunocompetent individuals. In contrast, in most of the developing world, the infectious agents that cause disease in immunosuppressed HIV patients reflect the "endogenous" microbes that cause disease less often or with a less severe clinical course in normal hosts (Morrow, Colebunders, & Chin, 1989). There are notable exceptions, but most of the disease burden in HIV-infected patients is not caused by organisms that are only opportunists. This is most true for bacterial, mycobacterial, and protozoan infections. For example, HIV infection dramatically increases the likelihood of the development of clinical tuberculosis in subjects with co-infection of HIV and *Mycobacterium tuberculosis* (Barnes, Block, & Davidson, 1991). In a patient population with a high incidence of HIV and TB, there are increased cases of active tuberculosis with important public health ramifications. Tuberculosis is the leading cause of death of HIV-infected individuals in most developing countries. Several protozoan infections such as cryptosporidiosis and isosporiasis that are frequently encountered and cause self-limited disease in immuno-competent individuals cause prolonged, severe disease in immunosuppressed subjects. Many common bacterial infections such as pneumonia due to *Streptococcus pneumonia* occur with increased frequency in HIV-infected persons, and the clinical presentation of some common bacterial infections is more severe, as evidenced by the increased risk of bacteremia in HIV-infected subjects with bacterial gastroenteritis due to *Salmonella*. The natural history of other bacterial infections, such as syphilis, is altered by HIV infection.

Many infectious syndromes that physicians encounter in patients with advanced HIV infection in developed countries are not seen or seen only rarely in the developing world. Whether this is because the organisms are not present in the surrounding environment (e.g., *Pneumocystis carinii*), or because HIV-infected patients in the developing world do not survive long enough with severe immunosuppression to develop late complications (e.g., cytomegalovirus infection) is not known. There are some unique syndromes that are seen in the developing world. A wasting syndrome known as "slim disease" is a common manifestation of advanced HIV infection in Africa and other tropical countries (Serwadda *et al.*, 1985). Slim disease is characterized by persistent diarrhea, profound weight loss, and chronic fever. Most experts believe that slim disease is due to infection with several enteropathogens (frequently co-existing) and not one single infection.

Cryptococcosis is one exception to the rule of the limited role of true opportunists in HIV in the developing world. In some series from sub-Saharan Africa, cryptococcal meningitis is the third leading cause of death in HIV-infected patients after TB and overwhelming bacterial infections (Colebunders, Perriens, & Kapita, 1988). In addition, can-

dida frequently causes mucocutaneous infection in this population. Other fungal infections are more geographically restricted; the endogenous dimorphic fungi are opportunists in the geographic locations where they are found (e.g., histoplasmosis in the United States and parts of Latin America; paracoccidiomycosis in Central and South America).

Kaposi's sarcoma was endemic in sub-Saharan Africa before the HIV epidemic, and is also seen in AIDS patients there. Other neoplasias (lymphoma) that are seen in HIV patients in the United States and are associated with advanced immunosuppression have not been as frequently recognized in developing countries.

The management of HIV infection in refugees and immigrants should focus on management of infectious and other complications, and patient education about transmission. Interruption of HIV transmission by use of condoms and treatment of genital ulcer disease is critical to limiting the spread of HIV (Ekweozor *et al.*, 1995; Gray, Dore, Supawitkul, Effler, & Kaldor, 1997; Telzak *et al.*, 1993). Where antiretroviral agents are available, consideration should be given to initiation of anti-HIV therapy. Recent data have shown that combination antiretroviral therapy can significantly decrease the amount of the HIV virus in a patient with concomitant clinical and survival benefit. The antiretroviral drugs used in these combinations are not widely available in many parts of the world, and their expense will preclude their widespread use. Specific recommendations for treatment of opportunistic infections and antiretroviral therapy are beyond the scope of this chapter; there are many excellent references available.

Bacteria

Cholera

Worldwide, there are more than a million cases of cholera per year. While most cases have been seen in Asia and Africa, there has been a historic resurgence of cholera in South

America over the past 5 years (Brandling-Bennett & Penheiro, 1996).

Cholera is an acute bacterial diarrhea caused by the gram-negative rod *Vibrio cholera*. Clinically, cholera presents as an acute, voluminous watery diarrhea that can lead to death due to dehydration. The bacterium produces a toxin that induces secretion of fluids and electrolytes by intestinal enterocytes. The incubation period is 1 to 2 days. The diarrhea can be accompanied by cramping and abdominal pain. The diagnosis of cholera can be made by isolation of the organism in the stool or serologically. Replacement of fluid and electrolytes intravenously or with oral rehydration therapy is the crux of therapy. Antibiotics shorten the course of diarrhea; therapy with the tetracyclines or floroquinolones is effective. Available vaccines have limited efficacy and provide short-lived immunity. The spread of cholera in refugee camps where conditions preclude proper sanitation and personal hygiene has been well documented. In these settings, steps should be taken to ensure proper disposal of human waste and a safe drinking water supply to control and prevent epidemics.

Salmonellosis

Salmonella typhi causes typhoid fever, a systemic bacterial infection of the reticuloendothelial system characterized by fever, abdominal pain, hepatosplenomegaly, and constipation or diarrhea. *S. typhi* is spread by the fecal-oral route. Unlike the nontyphoidal salmonella that cause enteritis, there is no animal reservoir for *S. typhi*. There are approximately 10 to 15 million cases occurring annually in most areas of the world (Edelman & Levine, 1986).

Typhoid fever has an incubation period of 8 to 28 days. Initial symptoms of headache, fever, and malaise may be mild but usually intensify as the illness progresses. Abdominal pain is common, and a characteristic rash (rose spots) consisting of erythematous blanching macules is seen in about half of all cases in light-skinned individuals. Alterations in mental status are common, as are leukopenia and anemia. Case fatality rates range from 1% to 10%. Typhoid fever can be diagnosed by blood or stool cultures, or serologically. Chloramphenicol and the fluoroquinolones are considered the first line of therapy. Resistance to a variety of antibiotics is increasing worldwide, and resistance to chloramphenicol and the fluoroquinolones may be an issue in certain regions in the future. Dependent on drug susceptibility, other effective agents include trimethoprim-sulfamethoxazole, third-generation cephalosporins, and ampicillin. Most patients have a clinical response to antimicrobial therapy within a week. One to three percent of patients may become chronic fecal carriers. Typhoid fever can be prevented by the avoidance of contamination of food and water supplies. There are several vaccines available that have an efficacy of about 60% to 80%. *Salmonella paratyphi* types A and B cause a typhoidal-like illness that is indistinguishable from *Salmonella typhi*.

Other salmonella species cause both sporadic cases and outbreaks of acute gastroenteritis throughout the world, and less often cause other extraintestinal infectious syndromes such as osteomyelitis. Unlike *Salmonella typhi,* other salmonella species have their natural reservoir in animals, and contaminated animal products such as eggs or meat are often the source of an outbreak. They cause a febrile gastroenteritis with an incubation period of 6 to 48 hours. In most patients the disease is self-limited, but in the very young, elderly, and immunocompromised, the gastroenteritis can be more severe and associated with bacteremia and may require antibiotic treatment (Levine, Buehle, & Bean, 1991). In normal hosts, antibiotic therapy has not been shown to impact the acute illness and has been shown to prolong the carrier state.

Shigellosis

Shigellosis is an invasive diarrheal disease due to infection with one of several *Shigella* species. *Shigella* cause a spectrum of enteritis from mild self-limited disease to fulminant dysentery. Shigellosis is a disease of man and primates, and there are no large animal reservoirs. Infection is spread from human to human by the fecal-oral route, and outbreaks of shigellosis are associated with crowding, poor sanitation, and inadequate water supplies. *Shigella sp.* have the smallest inoculum size (10^2 organisms) of any of the major bacterial enteropathogens. The incubation period is 24 to 48 hours. In addition to severe dysentery, hemolytic uremic syndrome, bacteremia, obtundation, and seizures are complications of shigellosis. The diagnosis can be established by isolation of the organism in stool or, less frequently, blood culture. Empiric therapy should be considered when patients have dysentery. Another common infectious etiology of dysentery syndrome in refugees and immigrants is amebiasis, which should be ruled out, particularly in adults.

Drug resistance among *Shigella sp.* is increasing around the world (Tauxe *et al.*, 1990). Ampicillin, trimethoprim-sulfamethoxazole, and the flouroquinolones are effective in the absence of antibiotic resistance. If antimicrobial resistance determination is not possible, patients who fail to respond to antibiotic therapy in 48 hours should be switched to another antimicrobial. There is currently no vaccine for *Shigella sp.*

Borelliosis (Relapsing Fever)

Relapsing fever is an acute bacterial infection of humans caused by spirochetes of the *Borrelia* genus. The epidemic form, caused by *Borellia recurrentsis,* is of particular importance in refugees and immigrants as it is seen most often in conditions of crowding and poor hygiene where body lice may be prevalent. Transmission occurs by the bite of body lice; humans are the natural host. The illness has a 4–18-day incubation period and is characterized by the abrupt onset of fever, chills, headache, fatigue, and myalgias. In addition to fever, physical signs may include conjunctival injection, hepatosplenomegaly,

and a petechial rash that is usually truncal in distribution. Thrombocytopenia and disseminated intravascular coagulation (DIC) may occur. In untreated patients, relapses occur as the spirochetes undergo antigenic variation and subsequent evasion host immune response. In louse-borne relapsing fever, the initial episode lasts approximately 6 days, with an afebrile period of 9 days, followed by one relapse which is usually of shorter duration and less severe than the initial episode. Untreated epidemic relapsing fever can have a mortality of 40%.

Endemic relapsing fever spread by ticks is caused by several other species of *Borrelia*. The illness is usually milder than the epidemic form, but generally has more relapses.

Relapsing fever can be diagnosed by the demonstration of spirochetes on smears of peripheral blood. The infection can be treated with a single 500-mg dose of tetracycline or erythromycin. Therapy may provoke a fever and hypotension (Jarisch–Herxheimer reaction) with transient clinical worsening.

Meningococcal Infections

Epidemics of meningococcal meningitis are common in sub-Saharan Africa, and are also seen in Nepal, India, and other countries (Akpede, Abiodun, Sykes, & Salami, 1994). The clinical presentation of meningococcal infections which include acute bacterial meningitis and sepsis are familiar and are not repeated here. These infections are medical emergencies and require prompt therapy. Parenteral penicillin is the therapy of choice; chloramphenicol can be used in penicillin-allergic patients or when penicillin is not available. Close contacts of patients with meningococcal meningitis should receive prophylaxis with rifampin (600 mg per day for 2 days). This may be critical in outbreaks occurring in refugee camps, where isolation of suspected cases and treatment of close contacts with rifampin is essential to attenuate an outbreak. A vaccine is available and is recommended for outbreak control as well as in all health care workers exposed to patients in areas of frequent meningococcal outbreaks.

Tuberculosis

Despite advances in diagnosis and treatment, tuberculosis (TB) continues to infect and produce illness in staggering numbers in the 1990s (Millard, 1996). It estimated that approximately 2 billion people, half the world's population, are infected. There are approximately 20 million active clinical cases (see later discussion) and 3 million deaths per year due to tuberculosis. Ninety percent of the infections occur in people in underdeveloped countries, particularly Southern Asia, Africa, and Latin America, where 40%–90% of the population is infected. A high prevalence of tuberculosis has been documented in immigrant and refugee populations.

It is obvious from the information about this incidence and epidemiology that tuberculosis is a major concern in the majority of refugee and immigrant populations (Binkin, Zuber, Wells, Tipple, & Castro, 1996). In the United States, for example, age-specific rates of bacteriologically positive cases of tuberculosis are 15 to 70 times higher for refugees than for U.S. citizens. Management in these groups should focus on detection and treatment of both active cases and asymptomatically infected individuals. Active cases are subjects with clinical illness due to tuberculosis. Infected asymptomatic individuals (usually detected by a positive PPD skin test in the absence of clinically active tuberculosis) have been exposed in the past and harbor viable bacteria that have been contained by the host immune system. These subjects are at risk for future reactivation of the infection and development of active tuberculosis. Detecting latently infected individuals is an important public health issue as they can be treated and reactivation can be prevented.

Virtually all immigrants and refugees should be screened for tuberculosis with PPD skin testing. Several issues cloud the interpretation of PPD skin testing in these groups, particularly previous vaccination with *Bacillus Calmette-Guerin* (BCG) and anergy. Vaccination with BCG has some efficacy in preventing clinical pulmonary and extrapulmonary TB and is widely used in many of the countries with a high incidence TB. Previous vaccination with BCG vaccine can bring about a positive PPD and make interpretation of a positive PPD problematic. In general, the larger the area of induration and the longer the duration since the BGC was given, the more likely that a positive PPD represents a true positive reaction in an individual with a history of BCG vaccination. In patients with a negative reaction after BCG vaccination, the possibility of immune dysfunction (particularly HIV infection) needs to be considered.

Given these caveats, PPD testing remains beneficial in detecting infections with *Mycobacterium tuberculosis*. Ninety to ninety-five percent of individuals infected with tuberculosis never develop disease, and the number that do can be minimized by prophylactic therapy with isoniazid (INH) unless drug resistance is present. Therapy with INH for 6 to 12 months is effective in preventing the development of clinical diseases. INH prophylaxis should not be given to subjects suspected of having active disease, and INH therapy should be monitored for side effects, particularly liver toxicity. It is essential to warn patients of the symptoms of liver toxicity (nausea, abdominal pain, anorexia) and instruct them to stop the medicine and consult medical attention. A PPD skin test producing induration of 5 mm should be considered positive in high-risk immunocompromised individuals, especially those infected with HIV, who are at greater risk for developing active disease (Drobniewski, Pozniak, & Uttley, 1995). Ten mm of induration is considered positive in otherwise normal hosts.

As with other bacterial infections, antibiotic resistance is an increasingly problematic issue in therapy of *Mycobacterium tuberculosis* in immigrants and refugees. In Southeast Asia and many other parts of the world INH is widely available, and inappropriate use leads to the spread of resistance.

Multidrug regimens, with three or four drugs, should be used in any patient with active TB from parts of the world with frequent resistance, and cultures and sensitivities should be done in smear-positive cases when feasible. In subjects who have been partially or incompletely treated, retreatment should always involve two new drugs that the patient has not previously been exposed to. There are a variety of treatment regimens which have been reviewed in detail (Harries, 1997). In the United States, public tuberculosis clinics can assume responsibility for monitoring therapy in patients (including directly observed therapy), and in most cases will provide the medicines to the patient at no cost.

The clinical presentation of pulmonary TB is familiar to most clinicians. Because of the low incidence of TB and rarity of extrapulmonary disease in Western countries, health care providers may not be acquainted with the many extrapulmonary presentations of TB. Tuberculosis can affect a variety of organ systems, and while these presentations are less common than pulmonary disease, they will be encountered in a population with a high incidence of infection.

Bartonellosis

Bartonellosis is a bacterial disease caused by infection with *Bartonella bacilliformis,* a gram-negative rod that parasitizes red blood cells. The organism is transmitted by the bite of the female sandfly. Bartonellosis is seen primarily in the western slopes of the Andes, and has been reported in Central America (Alexander, 1995). The illness can be mildly symptomatic to fulminant and lethal. Acute infection is characterized by fever, rigors, headache, and myalgias. Severe anemia can occur, along with hepatosplenomegaly due to erythrophagocytosis. Chronic infection is characterized by skin lesions which can be papular or nodular and can be widespread with involvement of mucous membranes. The diagnosis of bartonellosis can be made from blood or skin cultures, or from demonstration of the organism on blood smears. The disease can be treated with a number of antibiotics, including penicillin, ampicillin, tetracycline, and chloramphenicol. Acute infection is associated with decreased cell mediated immunity, which may account for the high incidence of bacteremic salmonella infection seen in patients with acute bartonellosis.

Brucellosis

There are more than half a million cases of brucellosis reported worldwide each year (Young, 1995). *Brucella* species have a reservoir in animals, and such exposure is an important historical point in suspected cases. The geographic distribution and animal reservoir vary according to the species. *Brucella melitensis* exists mainly in the Mediterranean, Latin America, and Asia. *B. melitensis* has its reservoir in sheep and goats, and among *Brucella* species causes the most severe disease in humans. *B. abortus* and *B. suis* are found in North and South America and Southeast Asia and have a reservoir in cattle and swine, respectively. *B. canis,* with a reservoir in dogs, is found in North and South America, Europe, and Japan.

Infection is acquired via infected dairy products, or occupational exposure to infected animal products with inoculation of skin or mucous membranes. The clinical presentation varies from mild subclinical infection to symptomatic acute and chronic forms. The clinical manifestations of brucellosis are protean, and include fever, malaise, fatigue, weight loss, myalgias, adenopathy, and hepatosplenomegaly. The disease may localize to one of several organs including, bone, heart, spleen, kidney, and skin. Chronic brucellosis can occur with persistent symptoms of fever, fatigue, and weight loss.

The diagnosis of brucellosis can be made by isolation of the organism in blood or body fluids, or serologically. Combination antibiotic therapy is needed for optimal outcomes and to prevent relapse, and doxycycline-rifampin is the currently recommended combination by the World Health Organization

(Solera, Martinez-Alfaro, & Espinosa, 1997). Trimethoprim-sulfamethoxazole can be used in children. Prevention and control of brucellosis relate directly to preventive programs in animals and pasteurization of milk and dairy products.

Yersinia

Yersinia pestis is a bacterium that infects humans and animals and is the etiologic agent of plague. The disease is primarily zoonotic with transmission from rodent reservoirs to humans by the bite of infected fleas. Rats are the most important host, but other rodents such as prairie dogs, squirrels, and mice can be infected. Human-to-human transmission is now unusual but can occur during epidemics of the pneumonic form. *Yersinia pestis* is endemic in central and southern Africa, the Far East, and the Americas (Butler, 1994).

The most common form is bubonic plague, characterized by regional lymphadenitis accompanied by fever, chills, weakness, and headache. Enlarged lymph nodes can swell to become tender, oval masses (buboes). The illness can be accompanied by sepsis and disseminated intravascular coagulation; sepsis occasionally occurs without lymphadenitis, and is termed septicemic plague. Pneumonia can occur due to hematogenous spread, or by aerosol from an infected patient (pneumonic plague). Meningitis can occur in the setting of bubonic plague. The diagnosis can be made by Gram's stain of aspirates from the buboes or by culture of buboes or blood. Prompt therapy is important; untreated bubonic plague has a mortality of greater than 50%. Streptomycin and tetracycline are effective antibiotics. A formalin-killed plague vaccine is available for individuals with unavoidable exposure to infected rodents.

Rickettsia

Rickettsia are small gram-negative rods responsible for a group of febrile illnesses characterized by headache, malaise, chills, and, usually, rash (Hackstadt, 1996). Rickettsia are present in mammalian reservoirs and with one exception (Q fever) are transmitted to humans by arthropod vectors. They are found worldwide, but among the rickettsia there are specific geographic distributions (Anonymous, 1982). *Rickettsia prowazekii* is the causative agent of epidemic (louse-borne) typhus. *R. prowazekii* is transmitted from human to human by the bite of infected body lice. Epidemic typhus occurs in situations of crowding and poor sanitation, and has been seen in crowded refugee camps. The illness is characterized by headache, fever, chills, myalgias, and photophobia. A rash that spares the palms and soles occurs on the 4th to 7th day and may become confluent. Neurologic abnormalities are common, and in severe cases renal failure and DIC may occur. The mortality in untreated cases is 10% to 60%. Epidemic typhus occurs worldwide.

Scrub typhus is caused by *R. tsutsugamushi* and occurs in Asia, Australia, and the Pacific islands. The illness is characterized by an eschar at the site of the initial mite bite, fever, hepatosplenomegaly, rash in 50% of cases, and in severe cases myocarditis and pneumonia.

The Rocky Mountain spotted fever (RMSF) group of rickettsial illnesses includes *R. rickettsia,* the causative agent or RMSF, seen in North America; *R. conorii,* the causative agent of Boutonneuse fever, seen in Africa, Europe, the Middle East, and India; *R. siberica,* the causative agent of North Asian rickettsialpox, seen in Siberia and Mongolia; *R. australis,* the causative agent of Queensland fever, found in Australia; and *R. africae* in sub-Saharan Africa (Brouqui *et al.,* 1997). This group of rickettsial diseases are all transmitted by tick bites and characterized by fever, rash, and varying degrees of neurologic involvement.

Coxiella burnetii is the causative agent of Q fever, the only rickettsial illness not transmitted by the bite of an arthropod vector. *C. burnetii* is found in small mammals and domestic sheep, cattle, and goats, and infection is acquired by inhalation of dried, infected animal material. The disease is found world-wide, and the most common clinical manifestation is pneumonia, although hepatitis, endocarditis (culture negative) and vasculitis are seen. Unlike other rickettsial illness, rash is rarely a feature.

The diagnosis of rickettsial illness is made by the presence of fever and rash (except Q fever) in patients with the right arthropod or animal exposure. A clinical diagnosis can be confirmed serologically. Therapy with tetracycline or chloramphenicol is successful, and early therapy is essential in improving outcomes.

Parasites

Malaria

Malaria is the leading parasitic cause of death worldwide, with an estimated 100 million cases in the world per year, and several million deaths (Olliaro, Cattani, & Wirth, 1996). In immigrants and refugees, the possibility of malaria should be considered in every patient with fever and possible exposure and diagnostic and therapeutic steps undertaken promptly. The four *Plasmodium* species that cause malaria (*P. falciparum, P. vivax, P. ovale,* and *P. malariae*) are widely distributed throughout the world in areas where the insect vector, the anopheline mosquito, thrives. The post–World War II optimism regarding the eventual elimination of malaria with control of the mosquito vector and drug therapy of human cases has long since given way to the reality of drug and insecticide resistance along with increasing resurgence in many parts of the world (Krogstad, 1996). Except for rare instances of limited outbreaks due to transmission from imported cases, malaria has been eliminated in the United States, Puerto Rico, Jamaica, Chile, Israel, Lebanon, North Korea, and Europe, but is found in varying degrees in the rest of the world where the climate is temperate or tropical (Bawden, Slaten, & Malone, 1995). In some parts of the world, notably sub-Saharan Africa, transmission occurs in both urban and rural settings, whereas in most of the Americas where malaria is found it is primarily in rural areas (Krogstad, 1996; Olliaro *et al.,* 1996).

Malaria is transmitted by the bite of the female anopheline mosquito; the parasite is transmitted during the taking of a blood meal. Sporozoites invade hepatic cells, and merozoites emerge from the liver to infect erythrocytes. Intracellular asexual reproduction takes place with eventual rupture of the erythrocyte and release of new merozoites, with the cycle repeating itself. The process of intraerythrocytoplasmic development takes 48 hours in the case of *P. falciparum, P. vivax,* and *P. ovale,* and 72 hours in the case of *P. malariae.* Fever occurs in conjunction with rupture of the infected erythrocyte, accounting for the periodicity of fever in malaria. In the case of *P. falciparum,* the merozoite is capable of infecting erythrocytes of all ages and stages of development, with the potential for massive hemolysis, severe anemia and other complications. Other forms of malaria are not capable of infecting erythrocytes in all stages of development, do not cause massive hemolysis, and are not as clinically severe as falciparum malaria. The life cycle of malaria is completed when a subpopulation of merozoites develops into gametocytes which when taken in a blood meal of a female anopheline mosquito undergo further reproduction and development into sporozoites (Miller, Good, & Milon, 1994).

In addition to anemia and hemolysis, infection with malaria leads to tissue hypoxia and immunopathological processes involving the release of inflammatory cytokines. Together these processes account for the clinical manifestations, which in falciparum malaria can be severe or fatal. The symptoms of acute malaria are variable and protean, depending on many parasite and host factors. High fevers and rigors are the hallmark of acute infection, and malaria should be considered in any individual with the right exposure and a presentation. In addition, malaise, headaches that can be severe, myalgias, and fatigue often occur. Other symptoms such as nausea, diarrhea, and cough may mimic a variety of other illnesses. Patients may not have a synchronous infection, and the classic periodicity of fever may not be present. Patients with falciparum infection in particular often present with daily spiking fevers. Hepatosplenomegaly, pallor, and mild jaundice are common clinical signs in patients with acute malaria (Wyler, 1993). Highly immune adults from endemic areas may at times be asymptomatically infected, and asymptomatic infection has been documented among refugee groups. There is a potential for transmission in this setting.

Cerebral malaria due to *P. falciparum* occurs in 0.5% to 1% of cases, but has a mortality of approximately 50%, and accounts for more than 80% of fatal cases. Patients with cerebral malaria present with seizures and stupor, as well as other neurologic symptoms. Other severe complications of falciparum malaria include acute renal failure, noncardiogenic pulmonary edema, hypoglycemia, and shock. Partially treated patients or those with partial immunity can present with relapses of falciparum malaria, which can occur for up to one year. Late relapses due to a latent phase in the liver are seen with *P. vivax* and *P. ovale.*

Diagnosis of malaria rests on the demonstration of the parasites on Giemsa-stained blood smears. Thick blood smears are used as a screening test, and thin blood smears are necessary for species identification and estimation of the percentage of erythrocytes infected, and thus the severity of the infection. The appearance of the parasites in the blood can fluctuate, and multiple smears separated by 12 hours should be done before malaria can be excluded. Even if blood smears are initially negative, if the clinical suspicion of malaria is high, treatment should not be delayed.

Therapeutic decisions are based on the suspicion for *P. falciparum,* the severity of the infection, and the potential for drug resistance. Therapy with oral quinine or pyrimethamine-sulfadoxine should be given if chloroquine-resistant falciparum malaria is suspected.

Severe infections (greater than 5% of erythrocytes infected) requires parenteral treatment with quinine or quinidine if available and close cardiac monitoring if possible. Chloroquine-sensitive falciparum malaria and infection due to other species can be treated with oral or parenteral chloroquine; cases of chloroquine-resistant *P. vivax* have been recently reported in India, Papua New Guinea, Indonesia, and Oceania. Patients with *P. vivax* and *P. ovale* should also receive sequential treatment with primaquine to eradicate the latent liver phase and prevent relapse. Resistance patterns of malaria continue to evolve, and new therapeutic agents, such as the artemeter compounds, are becoming available, and it is imperative to have updated information when treating malaria. The Center for Disease Control and Prevention malaria hotline is a source for up-to-date information (phone 404-332-4555).

Leishmania

Leishmania are protozoan parasites transmitted from animals to humans and human to human by the bite of the sand fly. *Leishmania* cause cutaneous and systemic (visceral) infection that varies according to species and geography (Hashiguchi, 1996). The usual incubation is 2 to 6 months. Visceral leishmaniasis is characterized by fever, wasting, hepatosplenomegaly, and anemia, and is frequently fatal without treatment. Visceral leishmaniasis is also known as *kala azar,* an Indian term meaning black or fatal fever. More severe cases are seen in malnourished patients and patients with HIV. Relapse and recrudescent infection have been seen many years after individuals have left endemic areas, and leishmaniasis should be considered in the differential diagnosis of a wasting febrile illness in refugees and immigrants with even a remote exposure. The differential diagnosis in acute cases includes malaria, typhoid fever, and other systemic bacterial and fungal infections. The disease is seen in Africa, South and Central America, Asia, southern Europe, and the southern countries of the former USSR. Visceral leishmaniasis can be diagnosed by demonstration of the *Leishmania* amastigotes on staining of bone marrow aspirates; splenic aspirates and liver biopsies can also be used for histologic diagnosis. Therapy with the pentavalent antimonials is effective in most cases.

Cutaneous leishmaniasis due to *Leishmania tropica* and *L. major* in the eastern hemisphere and *Leishmania braziliensis* and *L. mexicana* in the western hemisphere is common in the dry areas of the tropics. The clinical presentation is variable, but most cases begin with a papule at the site of the sandfly bite, that enlarges to a nodule with central crusting that falls off to reveal an ulcer. Multiple lesions (*L. major*) and destructive lesions of the ear (*L. mexicana*) are sometimes seen. *L. aethiopica* causes Ethiopian cutaneous leishmaniasis, which can present as a persistent nodule without ulceration. Mucocutaneous leishmaniasis is caused primarily by *L. braziliensis* and is characterized by ulceration and progressive erosion of soft tissue and cartilage or oropharynx and nasopharynx. Mucocutaneous leishmaniasis is virtually limited to South America. Cutaneous and mucocutaneous leishmaniasis can be diagnosed by demonstration of the organism on biopsy specimens. Most therapeutic protocols involve the pentavalent antimonials.

Amebiasis

Entamoeba histolytica, the causative agent of amebiasis, is an enteric protozoan parasite that is the third leading parasitic cause of death worldwide after malaria and schistosomiasis (Ravdin, 1995). Infection is highly endemic in Africa, South America, Mexico, and southern Asia. The infection is transmitted through contaminated food and water and, less frequently, by direct fecal-oral contact. While the majority of infected individuals are asymptomatic, *E. histolytica* cause a variety of intestinal and extraintestinal syndromes. The most common clinical presentation is noninvasive colitis, characterized by nonspecific abdominal pain and loose stools. Amebic colitis due to invasion of the intestinal epithelial cells by the trophozoite form is characterized by abdominal pain and tenderness with bloody stools with few or no fecal leukocytes. Fulminant amebic colitis is infrequent and is seen in malnourished patients, pregnant women, young children, or those on corticosteroids. This syndrome is characterized by fever, severe toxicity, profuse diarrhea, and occasionally by toxic megacolon and intestinal perforation. Intestinal amebiasis can be diagnosed by the identification of the parasite in the stool; at least three stool specimens should be examined before amebiasis is ruled out. In addition, *E. histolytica* must be differentiated from nonpathogenic intestinal protozoan disease.

The most common extraintestinal site of amebiasis is liver abscess. Amebic liver abscess can present acutely, with fever, abdominal pain, and weight loss, or can have a more insidious course. Amebic liver abscesses most frequently occur 2 to 6 months after exposure, and can be seen in refugees and immigrants with a relatively remote exposure. Other extraintestinal sites of infection are rare and include brain abscess and pleuropericardial, cutaneous, and genitourinary infection. Only a minority of patients with extraintestinal disease will have *E. histolytica* in the stool, and the diagnosis is based on clinical suspicion, serologies (negative in most asymptomatically infected individuals and positive in 85% of patients with invasive infection), and imaging studies such as CT or ultrasound. In some cases, needle aspiration of a liver lesion is necessary to differentiate amebic from pyogenic liver abscess.

Therapy of amebiasis depends on the site of infection and other factors. Treatment of asymptomatic cyst passers is done only in nonendemic areas and in individuals who are at high risk for colitis, such as pregnant women, HIV-infected patients, and so on. There are a variety of luminal agents available for asymptomatic cyst passers, including diloxanide, paromomycin, and diiodohydroxyquin. Colitis is usually treated with a nitroimidazole such as metronidazole, followed by a luminal agent to eradicate the carrier state. Metronidazole is the treatment of choice for extraintestinal amebiasis.

Prevention of amebiasis is an important consideration in situations of crowding and poor sanitation, conditions prevalent in many refugee backgrounds. Boiling water will eliminate cysts; treatment of drinking water with chlorine or iodine is insufficient. Other measures to improve sanitation and hygiene are important to interrupt the cycle of fecal contamination of food and water.

African Trypanosomiasis

African trypanosomiasis, more widely known as sleeping sickness, is a protozoan illness transmitted by the tsetse fly with an incidence of about 12,000 cases per year. There are two distinct forms: West African due to *Trypanosoma brucei gambiense* and East African related to *T. brucei rhodesiense.* There are differences in the clinical course, geographic distribution, and transmission between the two forms of African trypanosomiasis (Rogers & Williams, 1993). *T. brucei gambiense* occurs in the northern and western areas of sub-Saharan Africa. The disease tends to be more chronic, and infected individuals serve as a reservoir of parasites that can be transmitted to other individuals. *T. brucei rhodesiense* occurs in the eastern areas of equatorial sub-Saharan Africa and is a more acute illness; animals serve as the reservoir for infection.

In both forms of trypanosomiasis, infection begins with the bite of a tsetse fly with the injection of trypanosomes as the fly takes a blood meal. The parasites then rapidly divide and infect a variety of extracellular spaces including the vascular and lymphatic spaces, tissue fluids, and cerebral spinal fluid (CSF). Ongoing antigenic surface changes in the parasite allow the organism to evade immune responses, and fluctuations in parasite number and corresponding cycles of symptoms are seen. Clinically, both forms of the disease begin with a painful lesion at the site of the bite, followed by the development of

headache, fever, tachycardia, dizziness, and lethargy. Episodes of illness last 1 to 6 days, with relapses separated by several weeks without symptoms. In West African trypanosomiasis, posterior cervical lymphadenopathy is frequently seen. Neurologic symptoms tend to be minimal at first, but progressively worsen over 6 months to a year, with insomnia, tremor, gait disturbance, and finally coma ensuing. West African trypanosomiasis can be seen in immigrants and refugees several months after their last exposure. East African trypanosomiasis has a similar clinical picture but the clinical course is accelerated with coma and death developing in weeks (Ekwanzala *et al.,* 1996; Kuzoe, 1993; Pepin & Milord, 1994).

Diagnosis is made by examination of CSF or lymph node aspirates and identification of the parasites. CSF studies will also reveal a pleocytosis and increased protein and IgM. Therapy is important in minimizing morbidity and mortality, and specific therapy depends on organism and severity of CNS involvement. Suramin is used for East African disease, pentamidine is used for West African disease, and arsenicals are employed with central nervous system involvement. The therapy of trypanosomiasis is complicated and the drugs toxic, and health care providers should consult a reference text for details.

Helminths

Intestinal Nematodes

Intestinal nematodes are among the most common infections in the world, and in many groups of refugees and immigrants, the prevalence of intestinal nematode infection will approach 75% (Anderson & Moser, 1985; Catanzaro & Moser, 1982). Many subjects will have multiple intestinal helminths detected (Marnell, Guillet, & Holland, 1992). The incidence of intestinal nematodes may remain high for several years after immigration (Buchwald, Lam, & Hooton, 1995). Transmission of intestinal nematodes occurs via passage of eggs in stool, and infection is uncommon in areas of good sanitation. Anemia is an important clinical consequence. Common intestinal nematodes are discussed in the following paragraphs; strongyloidiasis is discussed separately.

Infection with *Ascaris lumbricoides* affects 25% of the world's population, with the highest prevalence in Asia, Africa, and Central and South America. Because moist soil is needed for egg development, ascariasis is not prevalent in arid areas. Infection is acquired by ingestion of *Ascaris* eggs that contaminate food (particularly fruits and vegetables) or fomites. Once ingested, the eggs hatch into larvae which penetrate the abdominal wall and migrate to heart and lung and pass to the alveoli, bronchial tree, trachea, and pharynx, and eventually are swallowed and reach the intestine. Mature worms in the gut then produce thousands of eggs which are passed in the stool. Eggs must mature in warm damp soil to become infectious.

Most infected individuals do not have specific symptoms and in those who do symptoms of ascariasis vary according to the stage of infection. Larvae entering the lung can invoke an inflammatory response, leading to cough, wheezing, pulmonary infiltrates, and eosinophilia. Intestinal ascariasis may contribute to malnutrition, but is not thought to produce malnutrition in individuals with adequate caloric intake and no other infections. Complications occur in less than 1% and are most often related to mass effect of the parasites, with intestinal obstruction, volvulus, and intussusception. Ascariasis involving the biliary tree can cause biliary or pancreatic obstruction. Migrating parasites can be seen in the appendix, nasopharynx, and, rarely, other organs (Holcombe, 1995; Khuroo, 1996; Wasadikar & Kulkarni, 1997).

Ascariasis can be diagnosed by identification of eggs in freshly collected stool specimens. Several antihelminthic drugs are effective in ascariasis. Antihelminthic drugs that do not kill *Ascaris* can provoke migration, and therapy of mixed infections should first begin with drugs effective against *Ascaris*.

Hookworm infection has a worldwide prevalence and geographic distribution similar to *Ascaris*. There are two major species that cause hookworm infection, *Necator americanus* which predominates in the New World and *Ancylostoma duodenale* which predominates in the Middle East, Asia, and Africa. Hookworm transmission occurs by direct penetration of infectious larvae through exposed skin, usually due to walking barefoot on contaminated soil. Once in the skin, the parasite migrates via the circulation to the lung and passes to the intestine. Adult worms attach to the mucosa of the small intestinal wall and feed on host red blood cells and plasma. Adult worms can consume 0.03 to 0.3 ml of blood per day, and hookworm infection is an important cause of iron deficiency anemia. Adult worms produce eggs that are passed in the stool and deposited in soil where they mature into larvae with the potential to cause infection. As with ascariasis, infected individuals may have symptoms related to the migration phase of the parasite. The major morbidity of hookworm infection occurs in children, in whom the iron deficiency anemia caused by hookworm is often associated with growth retardation and developmental delay. Hookworm also causes severe anemia in women of childbearing age, whose iron stores are depleted by pregnancy and menstrual losses.

Diagnosis of hookworm is made by identification of eggs in stool. Therapy with mebendazole is effective. Children in immigrant and refugee groups from high-prevalence areas, which includes most tropical developing countries, should be screened for hookworm and treated if infected. Development in children is affected by heavy nematode infection which can lead to anemia and malnutrition (Chan, Medley, Jamison, & Bundy, 1994). Proper sanitation and shoes or other protective footwear can decrease transmission.

The intestinal parasite *Trichuris trichiura*, commonly called whipworm, has a prevalence and worldwide distribution similar to *Ascaris* and hookworm. The life cycle is similar to *Ascaris,* although *Trichuris* does not require a migratory phase for development, and ingested eggs directly develop into adult worms in the gut. Coinfection with *Ascaris* is common. Unlike ascariasis and hookworm infection which are small-intestine processes, trichuriasis is a disease of the large intestine. Most cases are asymptomatic, but colitis and diarrhea can be seen in heavy infections. Malnutrition and rectal prolapse due to whipworm are occasionally seen in children. Whipworm can be diagnosed by identification of eggs in stool, and can be treated with mebendazole.

Enterobiasis, or pinworm infection is due to the intestinal roundworm *Enterobius vermicularis.* Pinworm is common in both developed and developing countries, and is most often seen in children. Infection is acquired by ingestion of eggs, which mature into adult worms in the gut without a migratory phase. Adult female worms migrate to the anus and perineum and produce eggs that cause perianal itching. Most cases are asymptomatic except for perianal pruritus; rare cases of extraintestinal infection have been reported. There is little morbidity associated with enterobiasis. The diagnosis is best made by the application of cellophane tape to the perineum which is then examined for eggs. Therapy with mebendazole or pyrantel pamoate is effective. Treatment of household contacts of cases may be required to interrupt transmission.

Strongyloides

As mentioned above, strongyloidiasis is an important helminthic infection in immigrants and refugees due to its unique ability for autoinfection and potential for persistent infection in the human host for many years (Mahmoud, 1996). In addition, immunosuppressed patients may present with a strongyloides "hyperinfection" syndrome. *Strongyloides stercoralis* infects millions of people in both developed and developing countries, with the prevalence in developed countries of 0% to 4% and in developing countries 40% to 80% in tropical areas of Africa and South America.

S. stercoralis infection begins with the penetration of infective filariform larvae through the skin (usually the feet), migration through the lungs and development in the small intestinal tract. Mature adult worms produce noninfective rhabditiform larvae which pass in the stool to the soil, then mature into filariform larvae. Unlike most other intestinal helminths which require maturation of larvae in appropriate conditions of soil, the rhabditiform larvae are capable of maturing into the infective form in the host. Penetration of intestinal mucosa or skin at the anal verge begins the life cycle again. Individuals from endemic areas can harbor infection for decades after their last exposure. Strongyloidiasis should be high in the differential diagnosis in individuals with eosinophilia and other symptoms and epidemiologic exposure.

Most patients with strongyloidiasis are minimally symptomatic. Migration of the larvae through the lung can produce cough, wheezing, pulmonary infiltrates, and eosinophilia. Colonization and invasion of the mucosa of the intestinal tract can lead to abdominal pain and diarrhea. Heavy infection can lead to malabsorption and weight loss. Eosinophilia may or may not be present in infection limited to the intestinal tract. Chronic infection may be asymptomatic or may be associated with anal itching, rash, diarrhea, and abdominal pain. The hyperinfection syndrome is seen in patients who are immunocompromised due to a variety of causes, including corticosteroids, chemotherapy, HIV infection, or chronic illness complicated by malnutrition. The clinical presentation can range from moderately severe abdominal and pulmonary complaints to septic shock, meningitis, and coma.

Strongyloidiasis can be diagnosed by identification of the larvae in stool specimens or from duodenal aspirates. Intestinal infection can be treated with thiabendazole 25 mg/kg twice a day for 3 days. Ivermectin has recently been shown to be a very effective therapy. In the hyperinfection syndrome, supportive care and broad spectrum antibiotics are also used.

Schistosomiasis

An estimated 200 million persons in the world are infected with schistosomiasis, and more than half a billion live in endemic areas (Elliot, 1996). It is estimated that more than 100,000 individuals from schistosomiasis endemic areas migrate to the United States each year. Schistosomiasis is a parasitic illness in which the adult worm lives in the venous circulation of the human host. The adult worms produce eggs which when passed into freshwater via stool or urine infects snails. In the snail the parasite matures into free-living cercarial forms; schistosomiasis is acquired when the human host is exposed to fresh water containing schistosoma cercaria, which penetrate skin. Once in the skin, the cercarial forms undergo development and migrate to the liver or lungs and are established in the venous plexus of the intestinal tract or bladder. Mature adult worms produce hundreds of eggs each day; about half of these end up in host tissues. The granulomatous response to these eggs accounts for much of the pathologic changes due to schistosomiasis.

Areas endemic for schistosomiasis have several characteristics in common: the presence of a reservoir of human infection, the availability of human hosts, and conditions that allow the contamination of water with urine and feces and exposure of humans to local bodies of water. There are several species that infect humans each of which has a unique geographic distribution and clinical presentation. *S. mansoni* is found in Africa, the Middle East, the Caribbean, and South America; *S. haematobium* in Africa and the Middle East; *S. mekongi* in southeast Asia; *S. japonicum* in Asia; and *S. intercalatum* in central and western Africa.

The earliest clinical manifestation of schistosomiasis is cercarial dermatitis, a skin eruption related to penetration of the host skin by the parasite. The migration of the worms can produce acute symptoms; Katayama fever, or acute schistosomiasis, is more common in nonimmune individuals such as travelers, and manifests as fever, eosinophilia, adenopathy,

and hepatosplenomegaly. The chronic clinical manifestations of schistosomiasis are related to the intensity of infection; in a given population, most individuals have a light infection and are relatively asymptomatic, and a few individuals have heavy infections and pass thousands of eggs. Patients may present with hematuria or diarrhea, but the major manifestations are related to inflammation, scarring, and fibrosis due to chronic deposition of eggs in host tissue and the host immune response. The adult worms of *S. haematobium* live in the venous plexus of the bladder; eggs lodge in the ureters and over many years cause scarring and obstructive uropathy. There is also an association between *S. haematobium* and bladder cancer. Other schistosome species localize to the intestinal circulation, and chronic manifestations are related to fibrosis in the liver. Patients can present with cirrhosis and portal hypertension. Other clinical manifestations are related to migration of eggs in the venous circulation and include cor pulmonale and central nervous system disorders. *Salmonella* can coinfect patients with schistosomiasis.

The diagnosis of schistosomiasis can be made by identification of eggs in urine or stool. Antischistosomal therapy should be given to all individuals with active infection, and to individuals with chronic infections who have not been treated. The current drug of choice is praziquantel. Infection can be prevented by avoiding contamination of water with stool or urine and by avoiding wading or bathing in contaminated water.

Trichinosis

Trichinosis occurs due to the ingestion of meat (usually pork) contaminated with *Trichinella spiralis* larvae. The disease has a worldwide distribution, but is most common is countries where pork is consumed. Individuals from ethnic groups that consume lightly cooked pork who immigrate to areas where transmission of disease is more common are at particularly high risk. In the United States, the incidence of trichinosis is 25 times greater in immigrants from Laos and Cambodia than in the general population (Cunningham, 1997).

Humans are an incidental host in a cycle of transmission that occurs in animals. After individuals ingest meat infected with *Trichinella* cysts, larvae attach to the intestine and mature into adult worms that produce several hundred larvae. The larvae penetrate the gut wall and migrate to muscle, where they encyst. Adult worms are eventually expelled, and the syndrome of trichinosis is limited to several weeks to months.

The clinical manifestations are primarily related to the host's response to migrating larvae, and depend on the intensity of the infections. Symptoms typically begin 1 week after ingestion of contaminated meat, and are characterized by high fever, eosinophilia, periorbital edema, conjunctivitis, and urticaria. Later encystment in muscle produces myalgias and weakness; cardiac and central nervous system involvement occurs in about 2% of cases, and is often associated with death. The diagnosis is usually made on clinical grounds in patients with appropriate exposure and clinical symptoms combined with eosinophilia. Muscle biopsy can be used if the diagnosis is in doubt, as can serologic testing. Therapy is based on limiting infection with antihelminthic agents and decreasing inflammation. Thiabendazole acts against the adult worms but not the larva, so is useful only in limiting continued larval production once trichinosis is suspected. Corticosteroids are often used to decrease inflammation in severe cases, but their benefit has not been proven. Cooking of meat to a temperature of > 82°C or freezing at −15°C for 3 weeks kills infective larvae. Immigrants and refugees whose dietary habits include eating undercooked pork should be counseled about trichinosis when moving into an endemic area.

Paragonimiasis

Paragonimiasis, due to infection with the fluke *Paragonimus westermani,* occurs worldwide but is usually reported in the Far East. The infection is acquired through the ingestion of raw or pickled freshwater crustaceans that contains metacercaria which encyst in the duodenum and migrate to the lungs where they mature into adult flukes. Patients present with eosinophilia and cough, and may also have hemoptysis, pleuritic chest pain, and rales on exam. The chest X ray may reveal cavitary lesions that look like tuberculosis. Ectopic infection in the central nervous system can occur. The diagnosis can be made by the identification of eggs in the feces or sputum. Therapy with praziquantel is effective.

Liver Flukes

Like paragonimiasis, clonorchiasis is acquired from the ingestion of undercooked freshwater crustaceans and is seen primarily in eastern Asia. Larvae of *Clonorchis sinensis* then migrate to the biliary tree, where they mature and produce eggs that are excreted in the stool. In acute infection patients present with anorexia, jaundice, hepatomegaly, and diarrhea. Chronic infection can produce biliary strictures, cholangitis, and pancreatitis. Cholangiocarcinoma may be a late complication. Therapy with praziquantel is effective. Infection with *Opisthorchis sp.* produce a clinical picture very similar to that of clonorchiasis, and is found in eastern Europe in addition to Asia. *Fasciola hepatica* and *Fasciola gigantica* are liver flukes of large mammals that occasionally infect humans. Infection is acquired by the ingestion of freshwater plants, particularly watercress, that contain *Fasciola* metacercaria. Fascioliasis is found throughout the world in sheep- and cattle-raising areas. Clinically, patients can present with prolonged right upper quadrant pain, jaundice, eosinophilia, and urticaria.

Echinococcosis

Echinococcosis is caused by the larval forms of the canine tapeworms *Echinococcus granulosus* and *E. multilocularis.* Dogs, wolves, and other canines are the definitive hosts; they pass eggs in stool which are ingested by herbaceous or omnivorous intermediate hosts such as sheep, goats, and other mammals. In the intermediate host, echinococcosis takes the form of hydatid cyst disease, which are 5–25-cm cysts containing the parasite. When ingested by a carnivore they take up residence in the intestine, and the cycle is completed. Humans are considered an accidental intermediate host. Echinococcosis is common in all sheep- and cattle-producing areas of the world, and is most common in sheep- and goat-herding people who keep dogs as working animals. *E. granulosus* is most common in northwest Kenya, Uruguay, the Mediterranean basin, and the Middle East. *E. multilocularis* is endemic in Arctic regions. Most infections are asymptomatic, but expanding cysts can cause space-occupying lesions in the liver, lungs, or other organs. Leakage from the cysts may also cause symptoms, as can bacterial superinfection.

Echinococcosis should be suspected in individuals with a history of exposure and a loculated cyst, which can be detected on ultrasound, CT scan, or other studies. The diagnosis can be confirmed serologically. Biopsy of these lesions has traditionally been considered to be hazardous, as leakage of the cysts and secondary spread can occur. Recently, success with percutaneous drainage has been reported (Khuroo *et al.*, 1997). Asymptomatic cysts do not require therapy, but should be followed for signs of enlargement. Expanding or symptomatic cysts should be removed by a surgical procedure involving instillation of a cidal agent followed by removal of the cyst. Therapy with albendazole can be attempted in nonsurgical cases or to shrink large cysts before definitive removal.

Filariasis

There are several species of nematodes whose adult forms (filaria) infect humans via the bite of specific insect vectors. In endemic areas, the distribution of filariasis closely resembles the range of the insect vector. The various filarial species follow a similar natural history following an insect bite when the parasite larva is introduced into the skin of the human host. The parasite spends months developing into a mature worm, migrating through the circulation or tissue to reach its final destination in lymph nodes, lymphatics, or subcutaneous tissues. Adult female worms produce offspring, called microfilaria, which circulate in the blood until they are ingested by the insect vector. The microfilaria undergo development in the insect and become capable of infecting human skin, thus completing the cycle. Disease manifestations derive primarily from the host response to the adult worm which produces inflammation and scarring. Adult worms can be long-lived; the disease process can take years to develop and patients may present years after the initial exposure.

Wuchereria bancrofti, Brugia malayi, and *B. timori* are transmitted by *Culicidae* mosquitoes and produce lymphatic filariasis, producing in severe cases what is commonly known as elephantiasis (Ottesen, 1993). *Wuchereria bancrofti* is found in Asia, Africa, the South Pacific, Haiti, and parts of Brazil. *Brugia malayi* is found in China, Malaysia, the Philippines, and parts of India. *B. timori* is found only in parts of Indonesia. Clinical manifestations can range from fever and lymphadenitis to chronic lymphatic disease leading to severe lymphedema. Eosinophilia may be marked during the migration of recently acquired worms, and can occur with pulmonary infiltrates due to migrating worms, producing the tropical pulmonary eosinophilia (TPE) syndrome (discussed previously).

Loa loa is a filarial parasite found in Central Africa and transmitted by flies. The adult worm resides in subcutaneous tissue, and the most common clinical manifestation is localized edema at the site of infection ("calabar" swelling). Worm migration can cause symptoms of itching and pain, and worms may be seen when they infect the conjunctiva. Eosinophilia is common and can be quite high. Heavy infections can produce cardiomyopathy, nephropathy, and encephalopathy. Other rare causes of filarial disease include

Mansonella perstans observed in Africa and *M. ozzardi* which occurs in Central and South America. The clinical manifestations are variable; eosinophilia is a consistent finding. Definitive diagnosis is based on demonstration of the microfilaria in blood. Some patients may not have sufficient microfilaraemia to allow definitive diagnosis, and a presumptive diagnosis can be made based on clinical findings and eosinophilia, particularly in the case of TPE. Therapy is aimed at controlling microfilaraemia, as there are currently no effective drugs against adult worms. Diethylcarbamazine (DEC) and ivermectin have been used. Drug therapy can be associated with acute symptoms, and health care providers should consult up-to-date reference texts before attempting therapy.

Onchocerciasis is a filarial disease that is the cause of "river blindness," the fourth leading cause of blindness worldwide (Van Laethem & Lopes, 1996). The parasite *Onchocerca volvulus* is endemic in parts of Africa, the Arabian peninsula, and parts of Central and South America. *O. volvulus* is transmitted by the bite of the black fly, and transmission is limited to areas where the fly vector can breed in fresh water. The natural history is similar to the other filarial diseases. Adult worms living in subcutaneous tissue produce thousands of microfilaria. Over months or years circulating microfilaria invoke an immune response that damages host tissues, particularly the skin and eyes. Long-term infection leads to blindness; other clinical manifestations include dermatitis, lymphadenopathy, and subcutaneous nodules. The diagnosis is made by identification of the microfilaria in superficial skin specimens. There is no safe and effective cure. The introduction of annual or semiannual suppressive therapy with ivermectin has been shown to prevent blindness.

Cystercicosis

Cystercicosis represents human tissue infection with the intermediate cyst forms of the pork tapeworm *Taenia solium* and is acquired by ingestion of *T. solium* eggs in contaminated food (Sotelo, Del Brutto, & Roman, 1996). *T. solium* is endemic in Latin America, India, Asia, Indonesia, and parts of Africa. Cystercicosis can produce life-threatening complications, and has greater clinical significance than intestinal *T. solium* tapeworm infection. The clinical manifestations depend on the location of the cyst, which are 0.5 to 2 cm and can be located anywhere in the body. Involvement of the central nervous system (neurocysticercosis) produces the greatest morbidity. Neurocysticercosis can present as acute encephalopathy, seizures, hydrocephalus, paralysis, or visual changes. Nonacute presentations of neurocysticercosis such as seizures can occur long after primary exposure. Seizures in an otherwise healthy individual from an endemic area should prompt a workup for neurocysticercosis. Diagnosis can be made by characteristic lesions observed by CT scan or MRI, and can be confirmed serologically. *T. solium* eggs or segments can be detected in stool in about 25% of cases. Definitive diagnosis can be made by biopsy. Surgery is indicated for lesions causing obstruction or significant symptoms. Drug therapy with praziquantel or albendazole can be used for lesions not amenable to surgery. Drug therapy may be associated with symptomatic worsening due to inflammation from dying *T. solium* cysts, and many experts give corticosteroids at the same time.

Summary

Infectious diseases impact significantly the health and well-being of refugees and immigrants, and have public health implications due to the importation of transmissible agents. The spectrum of infectious diseases in immigrants and refugees range from malaria, which requires acute recognition and management, to TB and HIV which are chronic illnesses with significant public health issues. The recognition and management of infectious diseases in immigrants and refugees requires knowledge of the geographic prevalence, modes of transmission, and clinical presentation of a wide variety of viral, bacterial, protozoan, and helminthic agents. Many of these infections are unfamiliar to health care providers whose clinical experience is limited to the developed world. Recent developments such as the appearance of new pathogens, changing epidemiologic patterns, and the emergence of drug resistance will continue to provide challenges to health care providers.

References

Akpede, O., Abiodun, P. O., Sykes, M., & Salami, C. E. (1994). Childhood bacterial meningitis beyond the neonatal period in southern Nigeria: Changes in organisms/antibiotic susceptibility. *East African Medical Journal, 71*(1), 14–20.

Albrecht, H. (1997). Redefining AIDS: Towards a modification of the current AIDS case definition. *Clinical Infectious Diseases, 24*(1), 64–74.

Alexander, B. (1995). A review of bartonellosis in Ecuador and Columbia. *American Journal of Tropical Medicine and Hygiene, 52*(4), 354–359.

Alter, M. J. (1996). Epidemiology of hepatitis C. *European Journal of Gastroenterology and Hepatology, 8*(4), 319–323.

Anderson, J. P., & Moser, R. J. (1985). Parasite screening and treatment among Indochinese refugees. *Journal of the American Medical Association, 253,* 2229–2235.

Anonymous. (1982). Global surveillance of rickettsial diseases: Memorandum from a WHO meeting. *Bulletin of the World Health Organization, 71,* 293–296.

Anonymous. (1996). Dengue and dengue hemorrhagic fever. *Epidemiologic Bulletin, 17*(4), 12–14.

Antal, G. M., & Causse, G. (1985). The control of endemic treponematoses. *Review of Infectious Diseases, 7,* S220–S226.

Anydia, H., Doppl, W., & Battmane, A. (1994). Opportunistic *Strongyloides stercoralis* hyperinfection in lymphoma patients undergoing chemotherapy and/or radiation: Report of a case and review of the literature. *Acta Oncology, 20,* 78–86.

Baker, J. J. (1981). Nutritional anemias: Tropical Asia. *Clinical Hematology, 10,* 843–871.

Barnes, P. F., Block, A. B., & Davidson, P. T. (1991). Tuberculosis in patients with HIV. *New England Journal of Medicine, 324,* 1664.

Bassett, M. T., McFarland, W. C., Ray, S., Mbizvo, M. T., Machekano, R., van de Wijgert, J. H., & Katzenstein, D. A. (1996). Risk factors for HIV infection at enrollment in an urban male factory cohort in Harare, Zimbabwe. *Journal of Acquired Immune Deficiency Syndromes and Human Retrovirology, 13*(3), 287–293.

Bawden, M. P., Slaten, D. D., & Malone, J. D. (1995). Falciparum malaria in a displaced Haitian population. *Transactions of the Royal Society of Tropical Medicine and Hygiene, 89*(6), 600–603.

Beck, E. J., Mandalia, S., Leonard, K., Griffith, R. J., Harris, J. R., & Miller, D. L. (1996). Case-control study of sexually transmitted diseases as cofactors for HIV-1 transmission. *International Journal of STD and AIDS, 7*(1), 34–38.

Bell, D. R. (Ed.). (1985). Fevers in general. In *Lecture notes on tropical medicine,* Oxford: Blackwell.

Bernal, M. C., Leyva, A., Garcia, F., Galan, I., Piedrola, G., Heyermann, H., & Maroto, M. C. (1995). Seroepidemiological study of hepatitis E virus in different population groups. *European Journal of Clinical Microbiology and Infectious Diseases, 14*(11), 954–958.

Binford, C. H., Mayers, W. M., & Walsh, G. D. (1982). Leprosy. *Journal of the American Medical Association, 247,* 2283–2292.

Binkin, N. J., Zuber, P. L., Wells, C. D., Tipple, M. A., & Castro, K. G. (1996). Overseas screening for tuberculosis in immigrants and refugees to the United States: Current status. *Clinical Infectious Diseases, 23*(6), 1226–1232.

Boyer, C. B., Barrett, D. C., Peterman, T. A., & Bolan, G. (1997). Sexually transmitted disease and HIV risk in heterosexual adults attending a public STD clinic: Evaluation of a randomized controlled behavioral risk-reduction intervention trial. *AIDS, 11*(3), 359–367.

Brandling-Bennett, A. D., & Penheiro, F. (1996). Infectious diseases in Latin America and the Caribbean: Are they really emerging and increasing? *Review of Infectious Diseases, 2*(1), 59–61.

Brouqui, P., Harle, J. R., Delmont, J., Frances, C., Weiller, P. J., & Raoult, D. (1997). African tick-bite fever: An imported spotted rickettsiosis. *Archives of Internal Medicine, 157*(1), 119–124.

Buchwald, D., Lam, M., & Hooton, T. M. (1995). Prevalence of intestinal parasites and association with symptoms in Southeast Asian refugees. *Journal of Clinical Pharmacy and Therapeutics, 20*(5), 271–275.

Butler, T. (1994). Yersinia infections: Centennial of the discovery of the plague bacillus. *Clinical Infectious Diseases, 19*(4), 655–661.

Catanzaro, A., & Moser, R. J. (1982). Health status of refugees from Vietnam, Laos and Cambodia. *Journal of the American Medical Association, 247,* 1303–1308.

Chan, M. S., Medley, G. F., Jamison, D., & Bundy, D. A. (1994). The evaluation of potential global morbidity attributable to intestinal nematode infections. *Parasitology, 109,* 373–387.

Colebunders, R. L., Perriens, J., & Kapita, B. (1988). Clinical manifestations and management of adults with HIV infection. In P. Piot & J. M. Mann (Eds.),

Balliere's clinical medicine and communicable diseases: AIDS and HIV infection in the tropics (pp. 51–72). London: Balliere.

Cunningham, N. M. (1997). Lymphatic filariasis in immigrants from developing countries. *American Family Physician, 55*(4), 1199–1204.

Daly, C. C., Maggwa, N., Mati, J. K., Solomon, M., Mbugua, S., Tukei, P. M., & Hunter, D. J. (1994). Risk factors for gonorrhea, syphilis and trichomonas infections among women attending family planning clinics in Nairobi, Kenya. *Genitourinary Medicine, 70*(3), 155–161.

Drobniewski, F. A., Pozniak, A. L., & Uttley, A. H. (1995). Tuberculosis and AIDS. *Journal of Medical Microbiology, 43*(2), 85–91.

Edelman, R., & Levine, M. M. (1986). Summary of an international workshop on typhoid fever. *Review of Infectious Diseases, 8,* 329–349.

Edmunds, W. J., Medley, G. F., Nokes, D. J., O'Callagham, C. J., Whittle, H. C., & Hall, A. J. (1996). Epidemiological patterns of hepatitis B virus in highly endemic areas. *Epidemiology and Infection, 117*(2), 313–325.

Ekwanzala, M., Pepin, J., Khonde, N., Molisho, S., Bruneel, H., & De Wals, P. (1996). In the heart of darkness: Sleeping sickness in Zaire. *Lancet, 348*(9039), 1427–1430.

Ekweozor, C. C., Olaleye, O. D., Tomori, O., Saliu, I., Essien, E. M., Bakare, R. A., Oni, A. A., Oyewo, O. O., Okesola, A. O., & Onyemenem, T. N. (1995). Clinico-epidemiological patterns of HIV infection in STD patients in Ibadan. *African Journal of Medicine and Medical Sciences, 24*(4), 321–327.

Elliot, D. E. (1996). Schistosomiasis: Pathophysiology, diagnosis and treatment. *Gastroenterology Clinics of North America, 25*(3), 599–625.

Feinstone, S. M. (1996). Hepatitis A: Epidemiology and prevention. *European Journal of Gastroenterology and Hepatology, 8*(4), 300–305.

Fisher-Hoch, S. P., Khan, J. A., Rehman, S., Mirza, S., Khurshid, M., & McCormick, J. B. (1995). Crimean Congo-haemorrhagic fever treated with oral ribavirin. *Lancet, 346*(8973), 472–475.

Fleming, A. F. (1987). Anemia as a world health problem. In D. J. Weatheral, J. G. G. Leadingham, & D. A. Worell (Eds.), *The Oxford textbook of medicine* (2nd ed., pp. 72–79). Oxford, England: Blackwell.

Ford, N. J. (1995, September 17–21). Responding to the AIDS epidemic in Asia and the Pacific: Report on the third international conference on AIDS in Asia and the Pacific, Chaing Mai, Thailand. *AIDS Care, 8*(1), 117–124.

Gianella, R. A. (1986). Chronic diarrhea in travelers: Diagnostic and therapeutic considerations. *Review of Infectious Diseases, 8,* S223–S226.

Glickman, L. T., & Schantz, P. M. (1981). Epidemiology and pathogenesis of zoonotic toxocariasis. *Epidemiological Review, 3,* 230.

Gourevitch, M. N. (1996). The epidemiology of HIV and AIDS: Current trends. *Medical Clinics of North America, 80*(6), 1223–1238.

Gray, J. A., Dore, G. J., Supawitkul, S., Effler, P., & Kaldor, J. M. (1997). HIV-1 infection among female commercial sex workers in rural Thailand. *AIDS, 11*(1), 89–94.

Gubler, D. J., & Clark, G. G. (1995). Dengue/dengue hemorrhagic fever: The emergence of a global health problem. *Emerging Infectious Diseases, 1*(2), 55–57.

Guillozot, N. (1980). Diagnosing myiasis. *Journal of the American Medical Association, 244,* 698–699.

Hackstadt, T. (1996). The biology of rickettsiae. *Infectious Agents & Disease, 5*(3), 127–143.

Halsey, N. A., & Job, J. J. (1990). Measles. In K. S. Warren & A. A. F. Mahmoud (Eds.), *Tropical and geographic medicine* (pp. 601–608). New York: McGraw Hill.

Halstead, S. B. (1990). Dengue. In K. S. Warren and A. A. F. Mahmoud (Eds.), *Tropical and geographic medicine* (pp. 675–701). New York: McGraw Hill.

Harries, A. D. (1997). Tuberculosis in Africa: Clinical presentation and management. *Pharmacology and Therapeutics, 73*(1), 1–50.

Hashiguchi, Y. (1996). Leishmaniasis: Its changing pattern and importance as an imported disease. *Internal Medicine, 35*(6), 434–435.

Holcombe, C. (1995). Surgical emergencies in tropical gastroenterology. *Gut, 36*(1), 9–11.

Hussey, G. D., & Klein, M. (1990). A radomized controlled trial of Vitamin A in children with severe measles. *New England Journal of Medicine, 323,* 160.

Jain, M. K., John, T. J., & Keusch, G. T. (1994). Epidemiology of HIV and AIDS in India. *AIDS* (Suppl. 8), S61–S75.

Khuroo, M. S. (1996). Ascariasis. *Gastroenterology Clinics of North America, 25*(3), 553–577.

Khuroo, M. S., Wani, N. A., Javid, G., Khan, B. A., Yattoo, G. N., Shah, A. H., & Jeelani, S. G. (1997) Percutaneous drainage compared with surgery for hepatic hydatid cysts. *New England Journal of Medicine, 337,* 881–887.

Klouman, E., Masenga, E. J., Klepp, K. I., Sam, N. E., Nkya, W., & Nkya, C. (1997). HIV and reproductive tract infections in a total village population in rural Kilimanjaro, Tanzania: Women at increased risk. *Journal of Acquired Immune Deficiency Syndromes and Human Retrovirology, 14*(2), 163–168.

Krogstad, D. J. (1996). Malaria as a reemerging disease. *Epidemiologic Reviews, 18*(1), 77–89.

Kuzoe, F. A. (1993). Current situation of African trypanosomiasis. *Acta Tropica, 54,* 153–162.

LeDuc, J. W. (1989). Epidemiology of hemorrhagic fever viruses. *Review of Infectious Diseases, 11* (Suppl.), S730.

Levine, W. C., Buehle, J. W., & Bean, N. H. (1991). Epidemiology of non-typhoidal *Salmonella* bacteremia during the HIV epidemic. *Journal of Infectious Diseases, 164,* 81.

Longfield, R. (1984). Anthrax. In G. T. Strickland (Ed.), *Hunter's tropical medicine* (6th ed., pp. 375–380). Philadelphia: Saunders.

Mahmoud, A. A. F. (1996). Strongyloidiasis. *Clinical Infectious Diseases, 23*(5), 949–952.

Mahmoud, A. A. F., & Austin, K. F. (1980). The eosinophil in health and disease (pp. 149–165). New York: Grune & Stratton.

Marnell, F., Guillet, A., & Holland, C. (1992). A survey of intestinal helminths of refugees in Juba, Sudan. *Annals of Tropical Medicine and Parasitiology, 86*(4), 387–393.

Mastro, T. D., & de Vincenzi, I. (1996). Probabilities of sexual HIV-1 transmission. *AIDS, 10* (Suppl. A), S75–S82.

Mbizvo, M. T., Machekano, R., McFarland, W., Ray, S., Bassett, M., Latif, A., & Katzenstein, D. (1996). HIV serincidence and correlates of seroconversion in a cohort of male factory workers in Harare, Zimbabwe. *AIDS, 10*(8), 895–901.

McCormick, J. B., & Fisher-Hoch, S. (1990). Viral hemorrhagic fever. In K. S. Warren & A. A. F. Mahmoud (Eds.), *Tropical and geographic medicine* (pp. 700–706). New York:McGraw Hill.

Mertz, G. J., Hjelle, B. L., & Bryan, R. T. (1997). Hantavirus infection. *Advances in Internal Medicine, 42,* 369–421.

Millard, F. J. (1996). The rising incidence of tuberculosis. *Journal of the Royal Society of Medicine, 89*(9), 497–500.

Miller, L. H., Good, M. F., & Milon, G. (1994). Malaria pathogenesis. *Science, 264*(5167), 1878–1883.

Monath, T. P. (1987). Yellow fever: A medically neglected disease. *Review of Infectious Diseases, 9,* 165–175.

Morrow, R. H., Colebunders, R. L., & Chin, J. (1989). Interactions of HIV infection with endemic tropical diseases. *AIDS, 3,* 579–587.

Musher, D. M. (1991). Syphilis, neurosyphilis, penicillin and AIDS. *Journal of Infectious Diseases, 163,* 1201.

Nunn, A. J., Kengeya-Kayondo, J. F., Malamba, S. S., Seeley, J. A., & Mulder, D. W. (1994). Risk factors for HIV-1 infection in adults in a rural Ugandan community: A population study. *AIDS, 8*(1), 81–86.

Nutman, T. B., Ottesen, E. A., Ieng, S., Samuels, J., Kimball, E., Lutkoski, M., Zierdt, W. S., Gam, A., & Neva, F. A. (1987). Eosinophils in Southeast Asian refugees: Evaluation at a referral center. *Journal of Infectious Diseases, 155*(2), 309–313.

Olliaro, P., Cattani, J., & Wirth, D. (1996). Malaria, the submerged disease. *Journal of the American Medical Association, 275*(3), 230–233.

Ottesen, E. A. (1993). Filarial infections. *Infectious Diseases Clinics of North America, 7*(3), 619–633.

Ottesen, E. A., & Nutman, T. B. (1992). Tropical pulmonary eosinophilia. *Annual Review of Medicine, 43,* 417–424.

Pepin, J., & Milord, F. (1994). The treatment of human African trypanosomiasis. *Advances in Parasitology, 33,* 1–47.

Perine, P. L. (1994). Sexually transmitted diseases in the tropics. *Medical Journal of Australia, 160*(6), 358–363.

Piot, P., & Holmes, K. K. (1990). Sexually transmitted diseases. In K. S. Warren & A. A. F. Mahmoud (Eds.), *Tropical and geographic medicine* (pp. 894–898). New York: McGraw Hill.

Plummer, F. A., D'Costa, L. J., Nsanze, H., Dyleanski, J., Karansira, P., & Ronald, A. R. (1983). Epidemiology of chancroid and *Hemophilus ducreyi* in Nairobi, Kenya. *Lancet, 2,* 1293–1295.

Ravdin, J. I. (1995). Amebiasis. *Clinical Infectious Diseases, 20,* 1453–1466.

Robinson, N. J., Mulder, D. W., Auvert, B., & Hayes, R. J. (1997). Proportion of HIV infections attributable to other sexually transmitted diseases in a rural Ugandan population: Simulation model estimates. *International Journal of Epidemiology, 26*(1), 180–189.

Rogers, D. J., & Williams, B. G. (1993). Monitoring trypanosomiasis in space and time. *Parasitology, 106* (Suppl.), S77–S92.

Ronald, A. R., & Plummer, F. A. (1985). Chancroid and *Hemophilus ducreyi. Annals of Internal Medicine, 102,* 705–707.

Serwadda, D., Mugerwa, R. D., & Sewankambo, N. K. (1985). Slim disease: A new disease in Uganda and its association with HTVL-III infection. *Lancet, 2,* 849–852.

Solera, J., Martinez-Alfaro, E., & Espinosa, A. (1997). Recognition and optimum treatment of brucellosis. *Drugs, 53*(2), 245–256.

Sotelo, J., Del Brutto, O. H., & Roman, G. C. (1996). Cysticercosis. *Current Clinical Topics In Infectious Diseases, 16,* 240–259.

Spry, C. J. F. (1980). Eosinophilia and hypereosinophilic syndromes. *Transcripts in Research of Social Tropical Medicine Hygiene, 74* (Suppl.), 3–6.

Tauxe, R. V., Puhr, N. D., & Wells, J. G. (1990). Antimicrobial resistance of *Shigella* isolates in the United States: The importance of international travelers. *Journal of Infectious Diseases, 162*(10), 1007–1011.

Telzak, E. E., Chiasson, M. A., Bevier, P. J., Stoneburner, R. L., Castro, K. G., & Jaffe, H. W. (1993). HIV-1 seroconversion in patients with and without genital ulcer disease: A prospective study. *Annals of Internal Medicine, 119*(12), 1181–1186.

Tesh, R. B. (1990). Undifferentiated arboviral fevers. In K. S. Warren & A. A. F. Mahmoud (Eds.), *Tropical and geographic medicine* (pp. 687–692). New York: McGraw Hill.

Tignor, G. H., & Hanham, C. A. (1993). Ribavirin efficacy in an in vivo model of Crimean-Congo hemorrhagic fever virus (CCHF) infection. *Antiviral Research, 22*(4), 309–325.

Trofa, A. F., DeFraites, R. F., Smoak, B. L., Kanesathasan, N., King, A. D., Burrous, J. M., MacArthy, P. O., Rossi, C., & Hoke, C. H. (1997). Dengue fever in US military personnel in Haiti. *Journal of the American Medical Association, 277*(19), 1546–1548.

Van Laethem, Y., & Lopes, C. (1996). Treatment of onchocerciasis. *Drugs, 52*(6), 861–869.

Warner, G. S. (1996). Hantavirus illness in humans: Review and update. *Southern Medical Journal, 89*(3), 264–271.

Warrell, D. A., & Shope, R. E. (1990). Rabies. In K. S. Warren & A. A. F. Mahmoud (Eds.), *Tropical and geographic medicine* (pp. 635–642). New York: McGraw Hill.

Wasadikar, P. P., & Kulkarni, A. B. (1997). Intestinal obstruction due to ascariasis. *British Journal of Surgery, 84*(3), 410–412.

World Health Organization. (1986). Acquired immunodeficiency virus (AIDS). World Health Organization/Center for Disease Control definition for AIDS. *Weekly Epidemiological Recommendations, 61*, 69–76.

World Health Organization Consultation Group in Poliomyelitis. (1985). Report to the World Health Organization. Geneva, Switzerland: World Health Organization.

Wyler, D. J. (1993). Malaria: Overview and update. *Clinical Infectious Diseases, 16*(4), 449–456.

Young, E. J. (1995). An overview of human brucellosis. *Clinical Infectious Diseases, 21*(2), 283–289.

Zaiman, H. (1995). Cutaneous larva migrans. *Tropical Doctor, 25*(3), 136.

Zuckerman, A. J. (1996). Alphabet of hepatitis viruses. *Lancet, 347*(9001), 558–559.

19

Cancer

NAHIDA H. GORDON

Introduction

Permanent changes of the domicile of peoples, considered here as immigrants, from one country or region to another country or region with very different cancer incidence and mortality rates provide an opportunity for studying the possible association of lifestyle, environmental, and cultural factors with health outcomes. This approach may yield important clues to the etiology of a variety of types of cancer; thus comparative studies of cancer incidence and mortality rates between native and immigrant populations are of interest to the researcher. Understanding cultural differences in perception of screening, hospitalization, and seeking treatment options can be important factors to the clinician in treating immigrants and improving their adherence to accepted standards of screening and treatment practices.

Cancer incidence and mortality rates vary worldwide. Variations with time have also occurred in many locations. Overall, the incidence of most cancers, with the exception of stomach cancer, increases with time. Cancer site–specific incidence rates vary within countries as well as between international regions (Tomatis *et al.,* 1990). For example, rates in Asiatic countries relative to the rates

in the United States are high for gastric cancer; low in colon cancers for both men and women; low in breast, uterine, and ovarian cancer for women; and low in prostate cancer (Dunn, 1975). Rates in rural areas are generally lower than those in urban areas. For example, interest in diet as a putative etiologic factor in breast cancer has been stimulated by the observation that incidence of and mortality from breast cancer among Japanese immigrants to the west coast of the United States are lower than those of United States Whites.

Two basic elements are necessary for undertaking immigrant cancer studies to identify etiologic factors of cancer: the movement of sufficiently large numbers of peoples who can be identified as a reasonably homogeneous population and the existence of population-based tumor registries in both the host country or region and the region of nativity. Countries or regions, presented in this chapter, which have been host to large immigrant populations and have had a long experience with population-based tumor registries are Australia, Canada, England and Wales, France, and the United States. California has been host to sizable Asiatic immigrant populations of principally Chinese and Japanese, as well as to first-generation Mexican Americans and to indigenous Mexican Americans who have been in the region for multiple generations. Other populations of immigrants described in this chapter are from Europe and Japan to Canada; immigrants from the Maghreb countries (Algeria, Morocco, and

NAHIDA H. GORDON • Department of Epidemiology and Biostatistics, School of Medicine, Case Western Reserve University, Cleveland, Ohio 44106-4945.

Handbook of Immigrant Health, edited by Loue. Plenum Press, New York, 1998.

Tunisia) to France; and English and Indian ethnic immigrants from the Indian subcontinent to England and Wales.

Accurate tumor registries and similar criteria for disease classification in the regions that are being contrasted are necessary requisites for serving as basic resources for immigrant studies. Therefore, most immigrant studies have centered about regions with long-established tumor registries such as the Surveillance Epidemiology and End Results (SEER) registries in Connecticut, Los Angeles, New York, and San Francisco in the United States. Most European countries, Canada, Australia, Japan, and China also have reasonably good tumor registries and can provide the basis for estimation of age-adjusted cancer incidence and mortality rates.

Even though the movements of populations appear to be useful natural experiments in cancer etiology, studies involving immigrant populations have significant methodological difficulties for identifying etiologic factors. These difficulties, after presenting results from four cancer sites, are enumerated in the discussion section.

Selected Cancer Site–Specific Findings

The most frequently occurring cancers are examined in some detail. They are breast cancer in females (Tables 1, 2, and 3), colorectal cancer in females and males (Tables 4 and 5), prostate cancer (Table 6), and stomach cancer in females and males (Tables 7 and 8). Breast, colon, and prostate cancer are cancer sites for which immigrant populations generally have lower risk than do persons in their host countries. In contrast, immigrant populations have a higher risk than populations in their host countries for stomach cancer. These four sites are chosen because the numbers of observed cases tend to be the highest among all the cancer sites, thus providing more accurate es-

TABLE 1. Comparison of Female Breast Cancer Age-Adjusted Incidence Rates of Populations from Regions of Nativity (N) and Host (H) with First-Generation (I) or Second-Generation (I2) Immigrant Populations

| Study dates | Population | | | Relative rates | Authors |
	Native (N)	Host (H)	Immigrant (I)		
1983–87	China: Shanghai, Tianjin, Hong Kong, Singapore	United States: San Francisco, Los Angeles, Hawaii	Chinese	N < I < H	Ziegler *et al.*, 1993
1983–87	Philippines: Manila, Rizal	United States: San Francisco, Los Angeles, Hawaii	Filipino	N < I < H	Ziegler *et al.*, 1993
1983–87	Japan: Miyagi, Osaka	United States: San Francisco, Los Angeles, Hawaii	Japanese	N < I < H	Ziegler *et al.*, 1993
1980	Puerto Rico	U.S., Connecticut	Puerto Rican	N < I < H	Polednak, 1992
1969–73	China	U.S., San Francisco Bay area	Chinese	N < I < H	Dunn, 1975
1969–73	Japan	U.S., San Francisco Bay area	Japanese	N < I < H	Dunn, 1975
1972–73	Mexico	U.S., Los Angeles	Mexican	N < I < I2 < H	Menck *et al.*, 1975

TABLE 2. Comparison of Female Breast Cancer Age-Adjusted Mortality Rates of Populations from Regions of Nativity (N) and Host (H) with First-Generation Immigrant (I) Populations

Study dates	Population Native (N)	Host (H)	Immigrant (I)	Relative rates	Authors
1979–85	Maghreb, N. Africa	France	Maghrebian	N < I < H	Bouchardy *et al.,* 1996
1984–88	U.K. and Ireland	Australia	U.K. and Ireland	H < I < N	Kliewer & Smith, 1995
1984–88	Southern Europe	Australia	Southern European	I ≤ N < H	Kliewer & Smith, 1995
1984–88	Western Europe	Australia	Western European	H ≤ N ≤ I	Kliewer & Smith, 1995
1984–88	Northern Europe	Australia	Northern European	N ≤ I ≤ H	Kliewer & Smith, 1995
1984–88	Eastern Europe	Australia	Eastern European	N < H ≤ I	Kliewer & Smith, 1995
1984–88	Japan	Australia	Japanese	N < I < H	Kliewer & Smith, 1995
1984–88	U.K. and Ireland	Canada	U.K. and Ireland	H ≤ I < N	Kliewer & Smith, 1995
1984–88	Southern Europe	Canada	Southern European	I ≤ N < H	Kliewer & Smith, 1995
1984–88	Western Europe	Canada	Western European	I ≤ N < H	Kliewer & Smith, 1995
1984–88	Northern Europe	Canada	Northern European	I ≤ N ≤ H	Kliewer & Smith, 1995
1984–88	Eastern Europe	Canada	Eastern European	N ≤ I < H	Kliewer & Smith, 1995
1984–88	Japan	Canada	Japanese	N ≤ I < H	Kliewer & Smith, 1995
1973–85	Indian subcontinent	England & Wales	Ethnic Indian	I < H	Swerdlow *et al.,* 1995
1973–85	Indian subcontinent	England & Wales	Ethnic English	H ≤ I	Swerdlow *et al.,* 1995

TABLE 3. Comparison of Female Breast Cancer Age-Adjusted Mortality Rates of Populations from Regions of Nativity (N) and Host (H) with First-Generation Immigrant (I) Populations

Study dates	Population Native (N)	Host (H)	Immigrant (I)	Relative rates	Authors
1986–90	China, Tianjin	New York City, U.S.	Chinese	N < I < H	Stellman & Wang, 1994
1964–85	Poland	Australia	Polish	N < I < H	Tyczynski *et al.,* 1994
1979–84	Mexican	Illinois, U.S.	Mexican	I < H	Mallin & Anderson, 1988
1979–84	Puerto Rico	Illinois, U.S.	Puerto Rican	N ≤ I < H	Mallin & Anderson, 1988
1969–73	United Kingdom	Ontario, Canada	British	H < I < N	Newman & Spengler, 1984
1969–73	Italy	Ontario, Canada	Italian	N ≤ I < H	Newman & Spengler, 1984
1969–73	Germany	Ontario, Canada	German	N ≤ I < H	Newman & Spengler, 1984
1969–73	Netherlands	Ontario, Canada	Dutch	I ≤ H < N	Newman & Spengler, 1984
1969–73	Poland	Ontario, Canada	Polish	N < I < H	Newman & Spengler, 1984
1970–72	Poland	England & Wales	Polish	N < I ≤ H	Adlestein *et al.,* 1979
1964–66	Poland	Australia	Polish	N < H ≤ I	Staszewski *et al.,* 1971
1959–62	Japan	United States	Japanese	N < I < H	Haenszel & Kurihara, 1968
1949–52	Japan	United States	Japanese	N < I < H	Haenszel & Kurihara, 1968
1950	Poland	United States	Polish	N < I < H	Staszewski & Haenszel, 1965

timates of incidence and mortality rates. When the number of reported cases (incidence or mortality) is small, the observed differences in the cancer incidence and mortality age-standardized rates between the host country and immigrant populations, although often substantial, are frequently not statistically significant. Lung cancer, even though it has some of the highest rates of incidence and mortality, is not considered here because of its

TABLE 4. Comparison of Colorectal Cancer Age-Adjusted Incidence Rates of Populations from Regions of Nativity (N) and Host (H) with First-Generation Immigrant (I) or Second-Generation (I2) Immigrant Populations

Study dates	Sex	Native (N)	Host (H)	Immigrant (I)	Relative rates	Authors
1980–86	F	Puerto Rico	Connecticut, U.S.	Puerto Rican	N < I < H	Polednak, 1992
1980–86	M	Puerto Rico	Connecticut, U.S.	Puerto Rican	N < I ≤ H	Polednak, 1992
1969–73	F/M	China	San Francisco Bay area, U.S.	Chinese	N < I < H	Dunn, 1975
1969–73	F/M	Japan	San Francisco Bay area, U.S.	Japanese	N < I < H	Dunn, 1975
1972–73	F	Mexico	Los Angeles, U.S.	Mexican	N < I < I2 < H	Menck *et al.*, 1975
1973–73	M	Mexico	Los Angeles, U.S.	Mexican	N < I < I2 ≤ H	Menck *et al.*, 1975

TABLE 5. Comparison of Colorectal Cancer Age-Adjusted Mortality Rates of Populations from Regions of Nativity (N) and Host (H) with First-Generation (I) or Second-Generation (I2) Immigrant Populations

Study dates	Sex	Native (N)	Host (H)	Immigrant (I)	Relative rates	Authors
1979–85	F/M	Maghreb, N. Africa	France	Maghrebian	N < I < H	Bouchardy *et al.*, 1996
1973–85	F/M	Indian subcontinent	England & Wales	Ethnic Indian	I < H	Swerdlow *et al.*, 1995
1973–85	F	Indian subcontinent	England & Wales	Ethnic English	I ≤ H	Swerdlow *et al.*, 1995
1973–85	M	Indian subcontinent	England & Wales	Ethnic English	I ≡ H	Swerdlow *et al.*, 1995
1986–90	F/M	China, Tianjin	New York City, U.S.	Chinese	N < I < H	Stellman & Wang, 1994
1964–85	F/M	Poland	Australia	Polish	N < I < H	Tyczynski *et al.*, 1994
1979–84	F/M	Mexican	Illinois, U.S.	Mexican	I < H	Mallin & Anderson, 1988
1979–84	F	Puerto Rico	Illinois, U.S.	Puerto Rican	I ≤ N ≤ H	Mallin & Anderson, 1988
1979–84	M	Puerto Rico	Illinois, U.S.	Puerto Rican	N < I ≤ H	Mallin & Anderson, 1988
1969–73	F	U.K.	Ontario, Canada	British	N ≤ I ≤ H	Newman & Spengler, 1984
1969–73	M	U.K.	Ontario, Canada	British	H ≤ N ≤ I	Newman & Spengler, 1984
1969–73	F	Italy	Ontario, Canada	Italian	I < N < H	Newman & Spengler, 1984
1969–73	M	Italy	Ontario, Canada	Italian	I ≤ N < H	Newman & Spengler, 1984
1969–73	F	Germany	Ontario, Canada	German	I < N < H	Newman & Spengler, 1984
1969–73	M	Germany	Ontario, Canada	German	I ≤ N ≤ H	Newman & Spengler, 1984
1969–73	F/M	Netherlands	Ontario, Canada	Dutch	I ≤ N < H	Newman & Spengler, 1984
1969–73	F	Poland	Ontario, Canada	Polish	N < I < H	Newman & Spengler, 1984
1969–73	M	Poland	Ontario, Canada	Polish	N < I ≤ H	Newman & Spengler, 1984
1959–62	F	Japan	United States	Japanese	I ≤ N ≤ H	Haenszel & Kurihara, 1968
1959–62	M	Japan	United States	Japanese	N < I ≤ H	Haenszel & Kurihara, 1968
1959–62	F	Japan	United States	Japanese	I ≤ N ≤ H	Haenszel & Kurihara, 1968
1949–52	M	Japan	United States	Japanese	N < I ≤ H	Haenszel & Kurihara, 1968

TABLE 6. Comparison of Prostate Cancer Age-Adjusted Incidence (Inc) and Mortality (Mort) Rates of Populations from Regions of Nativity (N) and Host (H) with First-Generation (I) or Second-Generation (I2) Immigrant Populations

Study dates	Inc/Mort	Native (N)	Host (H)	Immigrant (I)	Relative rates	Authors
1969–73	Inc	China	San Francisco Bay area, U.S.	Chinese	N < I < H	Dunn, 1975
1969–73	Inc	Japan	San Francisco Bay area, U.S.	Japanese	N < I < H	Dunn, 1975
1972–73	Inc	Mexico	Los Angeles, U.S.	Mexican	N < I < I2 ≤ H	Menck et al., 1975
1973–85	Mort	Indian subcontinent	England & Wales	Ethnic Indian	H ≤ I	Swerdlow et al., 1995
1973–85	Mort	Indian subcontinent	England & Wales	Ethnic English	H ≤ I	Swerdlow et al., 1995
1986–90	Mort	Tianjin, China	New York City, U.S.	Chinese	N < I < H	Stellman & Wang, 1994
1964–85	Mort	Poland	Australia	Polish	N < I < H	Tyczynski et al., 1994
1979–84	Mort	Mexican	Illinois, U.S.	Mexican	I ≤ H	Mallin & Anderson, 1988
1979–84	Mort	Puerto Rico	Illinois, U.S.	Puerto Rican	I ≤ N ≤ H	Mallin & Anderson, 1988
1969–73	Mort	U.K.	Ontario, Canada	British	N < I ≤ H	Newman & Spengler, 1984
1969–73	Mort	Italy	Ontario, Canada	Italian	I ≤ N < H	Newman & Spengler, 1984
1969–73	Mort	Germany	Ontario, Canada	German	I ≤ N ≤ H	Newman & Spengler, 1984
1969–73	Mort	Netherlands	Ontario, Canada	Dutch	I ≤ H ≤ N	Newman & Spengler, 1984
1969–73	Mort	Poland	Ontario, Canada	Polish	I ≤ N < H	Newman & Spengler, 1984

TABLE 7. Comparison of Stomach Cancer Age-Adjusted Incidence Rates of Populations from Regions of Nativity (N) and Host (H) with First-Generation (I) or Second-Generation (I2) Immigrant Populations

Study dates	Sex	Native (N)	Host (H)	Immigrant (I)	Relative rates	Authors
1979–85	F/M	Maghreb, N. Africa	France	Maghrebian	I < H	Bouchardy et al., 1996
1980	M	Puerto Rico	Connecticut, U.S.	Puerto Rican	H < I < N	Polednak, 1992
1980	F	Puerto Rico	Connecticut, U.S.	Puerto Rican	H < I < N	Polednak, 1992
1969–73	F/M	China	San Francisco Bay area, U.S.	Chinese	H < I < N	Dunn, 1975
1969–73	F/M	Japan	San Francisco Bay area, U.S.	Japanese	H < I < N	Dunn, 1975
1973–73	F	Mexico	Los Angeles, U.S.	Mexican	H < I < I2 < N	Menck et al., 1975
1972–73	M	Mexico	Los Angeles, U.S.	Mexican	H < I < N	Menck et al., 1975

known association with smoking history and occupational exposures for which it is difficult to control within ecological and observational studies such as immigrant studies.

The epidemiology of breast cancer is probably the most studied of all the cancers and yet continues to be one of the least understood.

The breast cancer experience of immigrant populations is considered in greater detail in this chapter than that for colorectal, prostate, and stomach cancer and is used to demonstrate both the advantages and technical difficulties encountered in utilizing immigrant studies as a tool in understanding cancer etiology.

TABLE 8. Comparison of Stomach Cancer Age-Adjusted Mortality Rates of Populations from Regions of Nativity (N) and Host (H) with First-Generation (I) or Second-Generation (I2) Immigrant Populations

Study dates	Sex	Population Native (N)	Population Host (H)	Population Immigrant (I)	Relative rates	Authors
1979–85	F/M	Maghreb, N. Africa	France	Maghrebian	N < I < H	Bouchardy *et al.*, 1996
1973–85	F	Indian subcontinent	England & Wales	Ethnic Indian	I < H	Swerdlow *et al.*, 1995
1973–85	M	Indian subcontinent	England & Wales	Ethnic Indian	I < H	Swerdlow *et al.*, 1995
1973–85	F	Indian subcontinent	England & Wales	Ethnic English	I ≤ H	Swerdlow *et al.*, 1995
1973–85	M	Indian subcontinent	England & Wales	Ethnic English	I < H	Swerdlow *et al.*, 1995
1986–90	F/M	Tianjin, China	New York City, U.S.	Chinese	H < I < N	Stellman & Wang, 1994
1964–85	F/M	Poland	Australia	Polish	H < I < N	Tyczynski *et al.*, 1994
1979–84	F	Mexican	Illinois, U.S.	Mexican	H < I	Mallin & Anderson, 1988
1979–84	M	Mexican	Illinois, U.S.	Mexican	H ≤ I	Mallin & Anderson, 1988
1979–84	F	Puerto Rico	Illinois, U.S.	Puerto Rican	H < I ≤ N	Mallin & Anderson, 1988
1979–84	M	Puerto Rico	Illinois, U.S.	Puerto Rican	H ≤ I ≤ N	Mallin & Anderson, 1988
1969–73	F/M	U.K.	Ontario, Canada	British	H < I < N	Newman & Spengler, 1984
1969–73	F/M	Italy	Ontario, Canada	Italian	H < I < N	Newman & Spengler, 1984
1969–73	F/M	Germany	Ontario, Canada	German	H ≤ I < N	Newman & Spengler, 1984
1969–73	F	Netherlands	Ontario, Canada	Dutch	H < I ≡ N	Newman & Spengler, 1984
1969–73	M	Netherlands	Ontario, Canada	Dutch	H < I ≤ N	Newman & Spengler, 1984
1969–73	F/M	Poland	Ontario, Canada	Polish	H < I < N	Newman & Spengler, 1984
1959–62	F/M	Japan	United States	Japanese	H < I < N	Haenszel & Kurihara, 1968
1949–52	F/M	Japan	United States	Japanese	H < I < N	Haenszel & Kurihara, 1968
1964–66	F/M	Poland	United States	Polish	H < I < N	Haenszel & Kurihara, 1968

Breast Cancer

Breast cancer is a leading cause of death for women worldwide; it is estimated (Miller, Feuer, & Hankey, 1991) that worldwide incidence will exceed 1 million by the end of the century. Both incidence and mortality vary widely worldwide, with the highest rates occurring in North America and northern Europe, intermediate rates in southern Europe and Latin America, and the lowest rates in Asia and Africa (Kelsey & Horn-Ross, 1993). Incidence of breast cancer for females increases rapidly beginning at the third decade of life and then levels off or increases very little after the sixth decade when most women experience menopause (Kelsey & Horn-Ross, 1993). The range for age-adjusted incidence rates in the United States is 70 to 90 per 100,000 and for industrialized countries is 60 to 90 per 100,000 with the exception of Japan; however, rates in Japan are increasing. Rates in South American and Eastern and southern

Europe are intermediate (range is 40 to 60 per 100,000) and are low (less than 40 per 100,000) in Central and tropical South America, Africa, and Asia (Tomatis *et al.*, 1990).

Important risk factors for breast cancer, in order of greatest relative risk, are gender (female sex), age, country of birth, family history, personal history of atypical epithelial cells, socioeconomic class, race-ethnicity, religion, reproductive history, and obesity (Kelsey, 1993). If a woman has a family or personal history of breast cancer, then she has a greater risk for developing breast cancer. A personal history of atypical epithelial cells also increases the risk for the disease. Earlier menarche, late first pregnancy, no pregnancies, and few pregnancies all increase the risk of breast cancer. There has been much discussion in the literature about the putative roles of estrogens and other reproductive hormones in the etiology of breast cancer. It is thought that age and reproductive history both act as surrogate markers for total exposures to estrogens and estrogen-like chemicals. Low socioeconomic class and certain religions are associated with lower risk and with reproductive lifestyle which probably explains the association of these latter two characteristics with lower incidence of breast cancer. The putative role of cigarette smoking in the etiology of breast cancer has been examined by many investigators; Palmer and Rosenberg (1993) have reviewed the literature and concluded that "it is unlikely that cigarette smoking has a net effect of reducing the risk of breast cancer" and there is "little evidence to suggest that cigarette smoking materially increases risk" (p. 154). There may be a positive association of breast cancer risk with alcohol consumption. Rosenberg, Metzger, and Palmer (1993) have reviewed the research literature concerning the role of alcohol consumption and risk of breast cancer and concluded that "confounding cannot be ruled out as an explanation of some of the observed positive association" (p. 142) of breast cancer incidence with alcohol consumption.

Unfortunately, most immigrant studies do not control adequately for the known breast cancer risk factors even though evaluation of breast cancer risk factors is crucial in their interpretation. Immigrant studies for breast cancer reported here also include studies of colon, prostate, and stomach cancer. To avoid undue duplication, the background for these studies is described in some detail in the breast cancer section and is not repeated in succeeding sections.

Four studies in the incidence of breast cancer in immigrant populations are presented in Table 1. Ziegler and colleagues (1993) compared breast cancer incidence rates during 1983–1987 of Chinese, Filipino, and Japanese women under the age of 55 with those of similar aged women from the San Francisco–Oakland, Los Angeles, and Oahu, Hawaii, areas (Table 1). They reported that for each ethnicity, incidence rates of breast cancer in the immigrating generation were higher than those in their countries of nativity and converging to the higher rates of their host country. They further reported that risk was not related to age at immigration for women who immigrated at ages less than 36 years. Similarly, Dunn

(1975) reported on rates of Chinese and Japanese immigrants using 1969–1973 data (Table 1). Their results agree with those of Ziegler and colleagues (1993).

Polednak (1992) compared breast cancer incidence rates of Puerto Rican migrants to northeastern United States with those of Whites using the Connecticut registry for the years 1980–1986 (Table 1). Immigrant rates were lower than those of Connecticut and higher than those of Puerto Rico. Menck and colleagues (1975) examined cancer incidence in Mexican Americans (residents with a Spanish surname) who were first-generation immigrants or who were American-born in Los Angeles County. Cancer rates for first-generation Mexican Americans (Table 1) and indigenous Mexican Americans both were intermediate, higher than their native and lower than their host rates. Specifically, the breast cancer incidence ratios standardized to Whites (100) in the Los Angeles County area were 59 ($p < .01$) for the first-generation immigrants and 57 ($p < .01$) for the indigenous Mexican Americans.

A review of more recent studies in breast cancer mortality rates for immigrants is presented in Tables 2 and 3. The majority of reported mortality are for host countries with rates higher than the native countries. Bouchardy, Parkin, Wanner, and Khlat (1996) compared, after controlling for social class and area of residence, cancer mortality rates for immigrants to France from North Africa (Table 2). Female immigrants from the Maghreb countries (Algeria, Morocco, and Tunisia) had lower breast cancer rates than those in France and higher than those in their native countries.

Kliewer and Smith (1995) reported on breast cancer mortality among immigrant populations in Australia and Canada (Table 2). This study is unique in that they considered immigrant populations of women migrating from geographic regions with either higher or lower levels of breast cancer risk compared with their host countries. This provided a unique opportunity to examine the impact of exposure to new environments and lifestyles on breast cancer risk. Breast cancer mortality rates among women in the majority of immigrant populations shifted from the rate observed in their country of origin toward the rate of the native-born population in the host country (Table 2).

Swerdlow, Marmot, Grulich, and Head (1995) compared the risk of cancer mortality of immigrants to England and Wales from the Indian subcontinent to the ethnically comparable native populations for the years 1973–1985 (Table 2). The rates for the British ethnic immigrants are not significantly different from those of their native counterparts. This study has value in that it controls for ethnicity. Specifically, the odds ratio for breast cancer of the British ethnic population born in India who immigrated to England and Wales when compared to the English and Welsh natives is 1.1 (95% Confidence Interval [CI]: 1.0–1.2), and the odds ratio for the Indian ethnic immigrants compared to the English and Welsh natives is 0.8 (95% CI: 0.7–0.9, $p < .01$]. These results suggest that lifestyle factors associated with ethnicity are a determinant of observed mortality.

Stellman and Wang (1994) compared cancer mortality in Chinese immigrants to New York City and in U.S.–born Whites (Table 3) with Chinese in Tianjin for the years 1986–1990. They considered all cancer types and divided them into two populations depending on whether the proportional cancer mortality ratios were higher in Tianjin or in New York. The proportional mortality ratios for the Chinese immigrants were always intermediate between those in Tianjin and in New York City which supports the concept that environmental factors are implicated in modifying the risk of cancer mortality. Specifically for breast cancer with Tianjin Chinese as a reference population, the standardized proportion breast cancer mortality ratios for New York City Chinese was 1.43 ($p < .001$) and for New York Whites was 2.89 ($p < .001$). Haenszel and Kurihara (1968) compared breast cancer mortality rates for Japanese immigrants and U.S. Whites for the years 1949–1952 and 1959–1962 (Table 3). Rates for immigrants were intermediate between the higher host and lower native coun-

tries during both time periods. Mortality rates for immigrants were lower in 1949–1952 than for 1959–1962 suggesting a further displacement toward the host country with longer stay in the host country. Specifically the standardized breast cancer mortality ratios for 1959–1962 for female immigrants were 27 (95% CI: 20–36) when U.S. Whites serve as the reference population and were 148 (95% CI: 108–198) when Japanese natives serve as the reference population. These ratios are 23 (95% CI: 15–34) and 121 (95% CI: 78–180), respectively, for 1949–1952.

Tyczynski, Tarkowski, Pakin, and Zatonski (1994) considered the risk of cancer mortality in Polish immigrants to Australia and used Poisson regression models to compare estimates of mortality in Polish immigrants relative to Australian natives and to Polish natives (Table 3). In immigrant Polish females, breast cancer mortality risk was significantly lower relative to Australian natives and significantly higher relative to Polish natives. Risk of breast cancer mortality increased from the low of native Polish women to the relatively higher rates of Australian women. Risk estimates for Polish immigrants was 0.82 ($p < .05$) and 0.71 ($p < .001$) for native Polish women.

Mallin and Anderson (1988) compared site-specific cancer mortality in Illinois Hispanics of Mexican and Puerto Rican origin and U.S.–born non-Hispanic Whites (Anglos) (Table 3). Cancer mortality for all sites was lower in both immigrant populations than in Anglos. Standardized breast cancer mortality rates for Mexican-born immigrants was 0.39 (95% CI: 0.26–0.56) and was 0.66 (95% CI: 0.42–0.98) for Puerto Rican–born immigrants. Again rates were intermediate between the host and native countries.

Newman and Spengler (1984) examined the mortality experience of British, Italian, German, Dutch, and Polish immigrant populations to Ontario, Canada, with that prevailing in Ontario and in their countries of nativity for the period 1969 through 1973 (Table 3). Cancer mortality rates intermediate between those for Ontario and their native country was most evident for the Polish immigrants. The majority of Italian, German, and Dutch immigrants had not reached the age of highest cancer risk and therefore shifts in the rates of cancer mortality were not evident at the time of the study. Specifically, the standardized breast cancer mortality ratios and their 95% confidence intervals relative to Ontario natives were 109.6 (102.3, 117.2) for the British ethnic; 65.1 (52.9, 79.2) for Italian; 61.5 (44.3, 83.2) for German; 82.9 (60.5, 111.0) for Danish; and 65.5 (51.4, 82.4) for Polish immigrants. Relative to their native countries, these standardized mortality ratios were 92.4 (86.2, 98.8) for the British ethnic; 87.9 (71.5, 106.9) for Italian; 78.7 (56.7, 106.5) for German; 76.6 (55.9, 102.5) for Danish; and 139.0 (109.1, 174.8) for Polish immigrants

Adelstein, Staszewski, and Smith (1979) compared the 1970–1972 cancer mortality of Polish immigrants to England and Wales with that prevailing in both England and Wales and in Poland (Table 3). They found rates for immigrants to be considerably higher than those found in Poland and slightly lower than those of native women in England and Wales. They reported the age-adjusted mortality ratio for Polish immigrant women of ages 40–79 to be approximately twice that of their native counterparts and slightly less than that for English ethnic women. Staszewski and Haenszel (1965) compared the age-specific cancer death rates for Polish immigrants to the United States with rates for Polish natives and U.S. native Whites (Table 3). Mortality rates for breast cancer were displaced upward from the lower rates in Poland to the higher rates in the United States. Breast cancer mortality rates of Polish immigrants to Australia were also considered by Staszewski, McCall, and Stenhouse (1971). They reported age-adjusted rates of 65.3 for Polish natives and 100.2 for Polish immigrants with Australian natives serving as reference.

Colorectal Cancer

Worldwide, cancer of the large bowel is the third most common cancer for both fe-males and males and occurs more frequently in developed and developing countries than in underdeveloped countries (Coleman, Esteve, Damiecki, Arslan, & Renard, 1993). The highest age-standardized rates are reported in the United States and are in the range of 20–33. Rates for northern and western Europe are lower than other developed regions and are in the range of 15–20. Rates in Africa, Asia, and Latin America are generally low but are increasing in places of rapid urbanization (Tomatis et al., 1990). The most important exogenous factor linked to the incidence of colon cancer is a diet low in vegetables and high in total and saturated fats, animal and total proteins, and total energy. Other exogenous factors which might be linked with incidence of colon cancer are occupational exposures (Garabrant, Peters, Mack, & Bernstein, 1984), aspects of reproductive history, and reduced physical activity (Tomatis et al., 1990).

Similarly to breast cancer, incidence and mortality age-standardized rates of colorectal cancer of immigrant populations tend to converge to those of their host countries. Mortality rates of immigrants from countries of origin with lower rates to host countries with higher rates tend to have a displacement of rates toward their host country in the first generation (Haenszel, 1982). Table 4 exhibits several studies comparing incidence rates of colorectal cancer. Polednak (1992) compared incidence rates for female and male colorectal cancers of Puerto Rican immigrants to the Connecticut, U.S., region and found that rates were intermediate between those of the higher rates found in Connecticut and lower rates in Puerto Rico. Similar results are observed when comparing incidence rates of colorectal cancer in female and male Japanese immigrants to the San Francisco Bay area, and in U.S.–born Whites (Dunn, 1975). Incidence rates of first-generation immigrant Mexicans to Los Angeles County are lower than those for indigenous Mexicans, and both rates are intermediate between those of the higher rates for Whites in Los Angeles County and lower rates in Mexico (Menck *et al.,* 1975). Specifically, the incidence ratios standardized to Whites (100) in the Los Angeles County area for colon cancer were 35 (p <.01) for the first generation female immigrants and 73 (p < .01) for the indigenous female Mexican Americans; for males these rates were 43 (p < .01) and 91 (p > .05), respectively. Rates for rectal cancer exhibited the same association with host and native rates for both females and males.

Mortality studies (Table 5) reflect the same phenomenon observed for breast cancer. Host countries reported here are Canada, England and Wales, France, and the United States. These countries all have higher mortality rates than the countries of origin of the immigrant populations. After controlling for social class and area of residence, colon cancer mortality rates for immigrants from the Maghreb countries to France were lower than those in France and higher than those in their native countries (Bouchardy *et al.,* 1996). Similarly, the odds ratio of colon cancer mortality for the years 1973–1985 of the British ethnic group born in India and who immigrated to England and Wales when compared with the English and Welsh natives was 0.9 (95% CI: 0.8–1.0), and the odds ratio for the Indian ethnic born in India compared with the English and Welsh natives was 0.5 (95% CI: 0.4–0.7, p < .001) (Swerdlow *et al.,* 1995).

Using Chinese in Tianjin as the reference population, colon cancer standardized mortality ratios of Chinese female immigrants to New York City and U.S.–born White females were 3.49 (p < .001) and 3.68 (p < .0010), respectively, for the years 1986–1990. For males, these rates were 4.35 (p < .01) and 6.00 (p < .001), respectively (Stellman & Wang, 1994). Haenszel and Kurihara (1968) compared rectal cancer mortality rates for Japanese immigrants relative to U.S. Whites and to Japanese natives for the years 1949–1952 and 1959–1962. Rates for immigrants were intermediate between the higher host and lower native countries during both time periods for males; however, rates were the lowest for immigrant females but not significantly different from either the native or host rates. Mortality rates for immigrants were lower in 1949–1952 than for 1959–1962 for males, suggesting a further displacement toward the host country with longer stay in the host country. The standardized rectal cancer mortality ratios for female immigrants for the years 1949–1952 were 65 (95% CI: 35–109) when U.S. Whites served as the reference population and 91 (95% CI: 50–153) when Japanese natives served as the reference population. For the years 1959–1962 these rates were 63 (95% CI: 37–100) and 69 (95% CI: 41–109), respectively. For males for the years 1949–1952 these rates were 80 (95% CI: 57—109) and 137 (95% CI: 98—186), respectively; and for the years 1959–1962 these rates were 95 (95% CI: 72–126) and 134 (95% CI: 101–177), respectively.

Using Poisson regression models, risk estimates for colon cancer in Polish immigrant females were 0.59 (p < .001) relative to Australian natives and were 0.26 (p < .001) relative to native Polish women (Tyczynski *et al.,* 1994). Risk estimates for colon cancer in Polish immigrant males were 0.92 (p > .05) relative to Australian natives and were 0.28 (p < .001) relative to native Polish men. Risk estimates for rectal cancer were also intermediate for immigrants; however, the rates were not significantly different from either the host or native countries for males and were significantly greater than that of their native country for females.

Using U.S.–born non-Hispanic Whites as a reference, standardized colon cancer mortality rates for female immigrants were 0.35 (95% CI: 0.19–0.60) for the Mexican-born and were 0.50 (95% CI: 0.20–1.02) for the Puerto Rican–born (Mallin & Anderson, 1988). Standardized colon cancer mortality rates for male immigrants were 0.34 (95% CI: 0.20–0.53) for the Mexican-born and were 0.84 (95% CI: 0.45–1.44) for Puerto Rican–born. Thus, again rates were intermediate between the host and home countries. Standardized rectal cancer mortality rates for female immigrants were 0.60 (95% CI: 0.16–1.53) for Mexican-born and 1.93 (95% CI: 0.63–4.51) for Puerto Rican–born. For males, standardized colon cancer mortality rates were 0.39 (95% CI: 0.13–0.91) for the Mexican-born immigrants and not reported for Puerto Rican–born immigrants due to low numbers of cases.

Age-standardized colorectal cancer mortality ratios and their 95% confidence intervals for British, Italian, German, Dutch, and Polish female immigrants to Ontario, Canada, compared with those prevailing in Ontario and in their countries of birth for the period 1969–1973 were 94.7 (88.3, 101.5) for the British ethnic; 46.0 (34.2, 60.5) for Italian; 56.5 (36.9, 82.8) for German; 62.7 (38.7, 95.9) for Danish; and 77.9 (61.6, 97.3) for Polish immigrants. Relative to their native countries, these standardized mortality ratios were 102.8 (95.8, 110.2) for the British ethnic 72.6 (53.9, 95.5) for Italian; 63.9 (41.8, 93.7) for German; 81.2 (50.1, 124.2) for Danish; and 206.3 (163.2, 257.6) for Polish immigrants. For males, the standardized colorectal cancer mortality ratios and their 95% confidence intervals relative to their Ontario native counterparts were 100.3 (93.0, 108.0) for the British ethnic; 66.6 (53.9, 81.5) for Italian; 76.1 (52.3, 107.0) for German; 68.9 (46.6, 98.4) for Danish; and 91.6 (76.2, 111.3) for Polish immigrants. Relative to their native countries, these standardized mortality ratios were 100.1 (92.9, 107.8) for the British ethnic; 94.0 (76.0, 115.1) for Italian; 78.2 (53.7, 110.0) for German; 89.7 (60.6, 128.1) for Danish; and 215.1 (178.8, 261.4) for Polish immigrants (Newman & Spengler, 1984).

Prostate Cancer

Cancer of the prostate is the fifth most common cancer in males worldwide and is estimated to be 7% of all male cancers (Coleman et al., 1993). A large variation in prostate cancer incidence and mortality, higher in developed and developing countries, is observed worldwide. The highest age-standardized incidence rates are found in northwestern Europe and in North America. For example, age-standardized rates per 100,000 for selected regions are 100.2 for U.S. Blacks and 61.3 for U.S. Whites; 45.9 for Sweden; 27.4 for France; and 1.8 for Shanghai, China (Tomatis et al., 1990).

Possible risk factors for prostate cancer are hormones, sexual activity, and diet (Tomatis et al., 1990). Prostate cancer is frequently discovered at the time of autopsy or prostatectomy for benign prostatic hypertrophy (Coleman et al., 1993) and by screening programs. Screening programs in developed countries discover latent prostate cancers and may inflate their already higher incidence rates relative to less developed countries. This phenomenon will tend to overestimate the displacement of incidence rates experienced by immigrants from lower incidence regions to higher incidence regions.

Incidence and mortality comparisons within several populations are reported in Table 6. Dunn (1975) observed incidence rates of prostate cancer in Chinese and Japanese immigrants to the San Francisco Bay area, U.S., which were intermediate between the higher U.S. rates and lower respective native rates. Prostate cancer incidence rates for first-generation Mexican Americans (Table 6) in Los Angeles County were intermediate, higher than their native and lower than their host rates. Specifically the incidence ratios standardized to Whites (100) in the Los Angeles County area were 69 (p < .01) for the first-generation immigrants and 99 (p > .05) for the indigenous Mexican Americans (Menck et al., 1975).

Because a significant proportion of discovered prostate cancer remains dormant, incidence rates may be inappropriate for the comparison of the seriousness of this cancer in various populations. Five studies of mortality in immigrant populations are reported in Table 6. The most recent study was by Swerdlow and colleagues (1995), who obtained the odds ratios for prostate cancer mortality during the years 1973–1985 among immigrants to England and Wales from the Indian subcontinent relative to the English and Welsh natives. The odds ratio for those who were British ethnic born in India was 1.2

(95% CI: 1.0–1.4) and for the Indian ethnic born in India was 1.2 (95% CI: 1.0–1.5).

Prostate cancer standardized proportion mortality ratios, using Tianjin Chinese as a reference population, were 5.19 ($p < .001$) for New York City Chinese and 13.63 ($p < .001$) for New York Whites (Stellman & Wang, 1994). Using U.S.–born non-Hispanic Whites as a reference, standardized prostate cancer mortality rates for Mexican-born immigrants to Illinois, U.S., were 0.78 (95% CI: 0.53–1.11) and 0.62 (95% CI: 0.23–1.35) for Puerto Rican–born immigrants (Mallin & Anderson, 1988). Using Poisson regression models, Tyczynski and colleagues (1994) estimated the risk of prostate cancer mortality in Polish immigrants and Polish natives relative to Australian natives to be 0.64 ($p < .001$) for Polish immigrants and 0.52 ($p < .001$) for native Polish.

Newman and Spengler (1984) estimated the age-standardized prostate cancer mortality ratios and their 95% confidence intervals for British, Italian, German, Dutch, and Polish immigrants to Ontario, Canada, relative to Ontario natives to be 95.4 (87.2, 164.1) for the British ethnic; 65.6 (48.4, 86.8) for Italian; 79.9 (46.5, 127.8) for German; 97.6 (59.5, 150.9) for Danish; and 59.8 (44.2, 79.1) for Polish immigrants. Relative to their native countries, these age-standardized mortality ratios were 110.1 (100.5, 120.1) for the British ethnic; 86.0 (63.5, 113.8) for Italian; 77.4 (45.0, 123.8) for German; 95.2 (58.0, 147.1) for Danish; and 93.9 (69.4, 124.2) for Polish immigrants

Stomach Cancer

Stomach cancer is one of the most common forms of cancer; however, there has been a decline in rates ranging between 2% and 4% annually (Howson, Hiyama, & Wynder, 1986). This decline has been attributed to dietary changes such as an increase in the consumption of fresh fruit and vegetables containing vitamins C, E, and A and a decrease in the use of salting and pickling to preserve foods due to more widespread use of refrigeration (Howson et al., 1986). The highest rates are observed in Japan, and high incidence rates have been reported for Eastern Europe and parts of Latin America (Tomatis et al., 1990). Worldwide, incidence rates for males are approximately twice those for females (Coleman, et al., 1993). Tables 7 and 8 present comparisons of incidence and mortality, respectively, of several populations.

Gregorio, Flannery, and Hansen (1992) compared incidence rates of stomach cancer for the period 1973–1988 of five immigrant populations to Connecticut from Italy, Poland, the United Kingdom, Germany, and Portugal to those of Connecticut, U.S.–born Whites. Rates were from 1.6- to 4.7-fold higher for these five immigrant populations than rates of native-born residents of Connecticut, but were 25% to 64% lower than their native countries.

Polednak (1992) compared stomach cancer incidence rates of Puerto Rican immigrants to the northeastern United States with those of Whites using the Connecticut registry for the years 1980–1986. Immigrant rates for both males and females were lower than those of Connecticut and higher than those of Puerto Rico. Menck and colleagues (1975) compared rates of first-generation and indigenous Mexicans in Los Angeles County and found rates for indigenous Mexicans to be higher than those of first-generation immigrant Mexicans. Both rates are intermediate between those of the lower rates for Whites in Los Angeles County and higher rates in Mexico. Specifically the stomach cancer incidence ratios standardized to Whites (100) in the Los Angeles County area for females were 148 ($p > .05$) for the first-generation immigrants and 192 ($p < .01$) for the indigenous Mexican Americans; for males these rates were 214 ($p < .01$) and 159 ($p < .01$), respectively. Using U.S.–born non-Hispanic Whites as a reference population, standardized stomach cancer mortality rates for Mexican-born female immigrants was 2.92 (95% CI: 1.75–4.55) and was 2.81 (95% CI: 1.13–5.79) for Puerto Rican–born immigrants. For males, these standardized stomach cancer mortality rates were 1.11 (95% CI: 0.67–1.73) for the Mexican-born immigrants and 1.16 (95% CI: 0.42–2.52) for Puerto Rican–born immigrants (Mallin & Anderson, 1988).

After controlling for social class and area of residence, stomach cancer mortality rates for immigrants to France from the Maghreb countries were lower than those in France and higher than those in their native countries (Bouchardy *et al.*, 1996). The risk, expressed as odds ratios, of cancer mortality of immigrants to England and Wales from the Indian subcontinent to the ethnically comparable native populations for the years 1973–1985 was 0.7 (95% CI: 0.6–0.8) for the British ethnic group born in India relative to the English and Welsh natives and was 0.6 (95% CI: 0.5–0.7, $p < .001$) for the Indian ethnic born in India compared to the English and Welsh natives (Swerdlow *et al.*, 1995).

Dunn (1975) observed incidence rates of stomach cancer in Japanese immigrants to the San Francisco Bay area, U.S., which were intermediate between the higher Japanese rates and lower U.S. rates for both females and males. The age-standardized ratios for stomach cancer mortality, using Tianjin Chinese as a reference population, were 0.60 ($p < .001$) and 0.44 ($p < .001$) for New York City Chinese females and males, respectively, and were 0.21 ($p < .001$) and 0.16 ($p < .001$) for New York Whites for females and males, respectively (Stellman & Wang, 1994).

Tyczynski and colleagues (1994) considered the risk of cancer mortality in Polish immigrants to Australia and used Poisson regression models to compare estimates of mortality in Polish immigrants relative to Australian natives and to Polish natives. Risk estimates of stomach cancer were 1.69 ($p < .001$) and 2.51 ($p < .001$) for Polish immigrant females and for native Polish females, respectively. For males, the stomach cancer mortality risk estimates were 2.06 ($p > .05$) and 3.13 ($p < .001$) for the immigrant and native Polish, respectively.

Age-standardized estimates of stomach cancer mortality ratios and their 95% confidence intervals for the period 1969–1973 were estimated by Newman and Spengler (1984) for British, Italian, German, Dutch, and Polish immigrant populations to Ontario, Canada. Specifically, the age-standardized stomach cancer mortality ratios and their 95% confidence intervals for females relative to their Ontario native counterparts were 182.1 (163.5, 202.1) for the British ethnic; 198.3 (146.0, 263.1) for Italian; 170.0 (98.8, 272.0) for German; 246.4 (143.3, 394.2) for Danish; and 191.8 (138.2, 259.5) for Polish immigrants. Relative to their native countries, these standardized mortality ratios were 72.8 (65.4, 80.9) for the British ethnic; 57.6 (42.4, 76.4) for Italian; 33.8 (19.6, 54.1) for German; 100.3 (58.3, 160.5) for Danish; and 49.3 (35.5, 66.7) for Polish immigrants. Specifically, the standardized stomach cancer mortality ratios and their 95% confidence intervals for males relative to their Ontario native counterparts were 158.6 (144.7, 173.5) for the British ethnic; 189.1 (155.0, 228.4) for Italian; 26.5 (17.0, 39.4) for German; 96.2 (67.2, 130.6) for Danish; and 44.3 (36.4, 53.7) for Polish Soviet immigrants. Relative to their native countries, these standardized mortality ratios were 71.4 (65.1, 78.1) for the British ethnic; 59.1 (48.4, 71.4) for Italian; 26.5 (17.0, 69.4) for German; 96.2 (67.2, 130.6) for Danish; and 44.3 (36.4, 53.7) for Polish immigrants.

Haenszel and colleagues (1968) compared stomach cancer mortality rates for Japanese immigrants and U.S. Whites for the years 1949–1952 and 1959–1962 and found rates for immigrants to be intermediate between the higher host and lower native countries during both time periods. Mortality rates for immigrants were lower in 1949–1952 than for 1959–1962 suggesting a further displacement toward the host country with longer stay in the host country. Specifically, the standardized stomach cancer mortality ratios for female immigrants were 338 (95% CI: 287–398) when U.S. Whites served as the reference population and 52 (95% CI: 44–61) when Japanese natives served as the reference population.

Discussion

The majority of results reported here demonstrate a displacement of incidence and mortality rates for immigrant populations from those of their native to their host countries. This phenomenon is observed here whether the native rates are lower as in breast, colon, and prostate cancer or higher as in stomach cancer. There are few examples of instances where the host rate for breast cancer is lower than the native rate; an exception is the population of immigrants from the United Kingdom and Ireland to Canada reported by Kliewer and Smith (1995). This population shows a rate for immigrants also intermediate between the higher rate in their nativity region and lower rate in Canada. An instance where mortality rates for colon cancer are higher (but not statistically higher) in the region of nativity than the host region (Table 5) is reported by Newman and Spengler (1984). In this instance, however, mortality rates for the immigrant population are not significantly different from the nativity rates or the host country rates. In the case of stomach cancer, Bouchardy and colleagues (1996) provided an instance where rates are higher for the host country in contrast to the majority of other immigrant populations reported in Table 8. Even so, rates for the immigrant population are intermediate between the native and host countries for all stomach cancer studies reported here. These findings for the four cancer sites reported here suggest that environmental and lifestyle factors associated with the new place of residence influence the cancer rates of immigrants and also suggest that, since most immigrants migrate as adults, the risk of cancer can be altered in later life.

The contrast of the cancer experience of immigrant populations and populations of their host countries should ideally include a comparison of lifestyle and environmental influences. Perhaps because the environment is experienced to a considerable degree by what is consumed, the major emphasis of immigrant studies has been on differences in components of diet such as fat, fiber, and red meat and to a lesser degree on differences in the constituent elements. Diet has been studied extensively as a factor in cancer and there is some evidence for its association with colon and stomach cancer. However, in the case of breast cancer according to Hunter and Willet (1993), "few if any dietary constituents can be confidently associated with" (p. 110) breast cancer. However, possible contamination of food with pesticides or other chemicals may yet be found to be associated with breast cancer incidence.

The atmospheric environment, and particularly occupational exposures and smoking histories, has been studied as contributing factors to several cancers most notably lung cancer. Little attention has been given to the putative impact of exposure to environmental chemicals on differential rates of cancer incidence and mortality among immigrants and indigenous populations. For example, investigation into differential exposures to fat-soluble environmental chemicals may reveal etiologies of breast and prostate cancers. In addition to diet and alcohol consumption, the environment is encountered through contact with skin and lungs. Numerous chemical compounds such as hair dressings, skin lotions, and contaminated water come into contact with the skin. Determination of the possible relationship of a specific pollutant with incidence of cancer is difficult as pollution is usually a mixture of chemicals. For example, ambient air content of benzene, which is associated with mammary cancer in animal models (Maltoni, Ciliberti, Cotti, Conti, & Belpoggi, 1989), is frequently higher than acceptable U.S. Environmental Protection Agency guidelines in urban areas; however, the effort to separate its putative effect from effects of other chemicals also found in the environment is daunting.

Undercounting in underdeveloped regions where tumor registries are inadequate would lead to an obvious exaggeration of the rate of convergence from the lower rate of the region of nativity to the higher rate of the host region. Furthermore, most studies of immigrant rates have utilized large registries such as the SEER, the census, or death registries which frequently do not provide a clear indication of the nativity region in the country of origin. Since it is known, for example, that rural rates are frequently below urban rates for many sites of cancer, the lack of knowledge of the region of origin from immigrants' native country may inflate the rate of convergence to the higher rates of host countries; however, in the case of stomach cancer, undercounting from the region of nativity would tend to reduce an observed rate of convergence. The work of Menck and colleagues (1975), however, utilized data from the same tumor registry in Los Angeles County and demonstrated that the incidence rates of immigrants are less than those of indigenous Mexican Americans and are both intermediate to the lower Mexican and higher U.S. rates in the case of breast (Table 1), colon (Table 4), prostate (Table 6), and conversely for stomach (Table 7) cancer. A second notable study is that by Haenszel and Kurihara (1968) which demonstrated that mortality rates for Japanese immigrants for the years 1949–1952 compared with those for 1959–1962 were lower for breast (Table 3), lower for colorectal (Table 5), and higher for stomach (Table 8) cancer, and that these rates were intermediate between the lower rates in Japan and the higher rates in U.S. Whites for both breast and colon cancer and conversely for stomach cancer. These findings give added weight to the hypothesis that environmental and cultural differences play a role in the development of cancer during the adult years.

Socioeconomic class is an important prognostic variable in cancer incidence and mortality. For example, high socioeconomic class is associated with a higher risk of breast cancer (Kelsey, 1993); however, it is associated with a lower overall survival (Gordon, Crowe, Brumberg, & Berger, 1992). Moreover, it has frequently been shown that socioeconomic class is a more important factor than race-ethnicity in affecting disease-free and overall survival (Gordon, 1995); therefore, controlling for socioeconomic class is more important than race when comparing both incidence and mortality rates of immigrant and host populations. Reproductive practices such as the number and timing of full-term pregnancies may be confounded with socioeconomic class and are important characteristics when comparing breast and ovarian cancer incidence rates. Examples of the possible effect of socioeconomic class on the findings reported by immigrant studies are the results reported by Swerdlow and colleagues (1995). The differential in the reported experience of the British and Indian ethnic groups who immigrated to England and Wales may be explained by the fact that the English ethnic group had immigrated to England and Wales at an earlier time and were for the most part of a higher socioeconomic class while the Indian ethnic immigrants had emigrated at least 10 years later and were of a mixed socioeconomic class. In addition to the longer period of exposure and higher socioeconomic class, differences in reproductive histories may be an additional factor for the slower rate of convergence of the Indian ethnic immigrants to the native rates (Swerdlow et al., 1995).

Data from death registries and the census are more readily available than incidence data; therefore, mortality studies are more prevalent. Contrasting incidence rates may be preferable as they are not influenced by differentials in seeking care and treatment; however, differentials in screening for some cancers, for example, prostate cancer, may render mortality studies more meaningful. Furthermore, surveillance and screening programs are utilized more aggressively in developed countries which may, at least temporarily, increase the apparent incidence rates of the screened cancer. This phenomenon would tend to produce higher rates in developed countries relative to developing countries, thus exaggerating the rate of convergence of immigrant incidence rates from lower incidence regions to higher incidence regions. Other important factors which would recommend using incidence rather than mortality rates are the studies of relatively indolent cancers such as breast cancer. If there are many intervening years between incidence and death from the disease, then differential factors in treatment and competing causes of death would render mortality rates unreliable compared with incidence rates. However, if the cancer has a relatively short period of time between incidence and death, such as stomach cancer, then mortality rates may be preferable as they are not susceptible to biases caused by unequal rates of screening or competing causes of death between the immigrant and host populations.

Because immigrants from a region form a self-selected sample, they do not constitute a random sample and their risk factors for cancer will not be representative of their region of nativity. In such an instance, incidence and mortality rates of their native country would be inappropriate. An example, cited previously, is that incidence and mortality rates for breast cancer as well as many other cancers tend to be lower in rural areas compared to urban areas; if the population of immigrants does not have the same representation from urban and rural areas as the tumor registry used for reference, then inferences will be biased.

Cultural differences in perception of screening, hospitalization, and seeking treatment options can be important factors in immigrant studies. Adherence to accepted standards of screening due to psychological and cultural barriers to optimal care may differ among immigrant populations and the general population of the host country and may lead to lower estimates of cancer incidence and lower rates of disease-free and overall survival relative to the indigenous population of their host country. For example, a screening program in breast and cervical cancer conducted in Brooklyn, New York, among Caribbean immigrants demonstrated lower utilization than among the U.S.–born women (Fruchter *et al.,* 1985). And in a study of knowledge, attitudes, and behavior of a sample of a culturally diverse group of community college women, Hazlewood (1994) found that knowledge about breast self-

examination and breast cancer was higher in U.S.–born women than in immigrant women. In general, screening rates for cancer tend to be lower among immigrant populations (Bloom, 1994) and in underdeveloped countries.

Neves Arruda, Larson, and Meleis (1992) investigated the role of perceived comfort for immigrant Hispanic patients and concluded that comfort is important in illness and cancer treatment and that patients' perceptions of comfort were influenced by their culture. The role of cultural differences in regard to family perceptions of hospitalization and experiences relevant to coping and problem solving with respect to a diagnosis of cancer were examined by Boston (1992). Findings suggest that within Greek, Chinese, and Italian immigrant families, fear and loneliness were predominant emotions at the onset of hospitalization and that coping strategies and the management of stress frequently differed depending on the suggestions of health personnel who may be unfamiliar with the cultural background of their patients. The impact of the family's cultural values and beliefs in their response to a diagnosis of cancer are not emphasized in health professionals' education and, consequently, may be underestimated, leading to less effective care (Boston, 1993).

Eisenbruch and Handelman (1990) also considered the issue of compliance with health care as a function of "foreign" cultures which are frequently poorly understood by clinicians. Understanding the explanation of immigrant patients, particularly those with terminal illness, is essential to adequate care and treatment. Eisenbruch and Handelman (1990) developed a team that provided cultural consultation service by a psychiatrist, an anthropologist, and several immigrant community members and demonstrated the beneficial effects of such an approach for facilitating the treatment of terminally ill immigrant patients. Once again, they demonstrated the importance of cultural differences in perceptions which may lead to differentials in treatment adherence and thus ultimately influence disease-free and overall survival from cancer. Gifford (1994) noted that Italian immigrant women to Australia use explanatory models for cancer that are linked to their changing social role as immigrants and to their grief over their lives in Australia and a home left behind. Their perceived losses are experienced physically and are thought to contribute to their vulnerability to a range of menopause-related conditions including cancer. Inadequate rates of adherence to accepted radiotherapy regimens in Latina immigrants (16%) with carcinoma of the cervix were demonstrated to be less than that of the general population of cervical cancer patients in the United States (63%) by Formenti, Meyerowitz, Muderspach, Groshen, Leedham, Klement, and Morrow (1995). These results are not surprising as the role of socioeconomic class rather than race-ethnicity has been frequently demonstrated to be associated with seeking health care and treatment.

In summary, rates of convergence, from lower rates of regions of nativity to higher rates of host regions in the case of breast, colon, and prostate cancer, may be exaggerated due to several factors: less adequate screening practices in the native country and higher rates in the host country; less adequate screening practices in immigrant populations relative to the indigenous population of their host country; and undercounting both incidence and mortality for countries of nativity from underdeveloped regions. Other factors that may bias rate estimates are different classifications of cancer in tumor registries used for comparisons, the rate of acculturation, differentials in socioeconomic class, utilization of health services, differing exposures to pollution, viral agents, occupations, and lifestyle. A minimal remedy for current immigrant studies is a thorough investigation of population characteristics that are important risk factors. Prospective studies that would also control for temporal effects in cancer incidence and mortality would be ideal though costly.

In conclusion, the contrast of the cancer experience of immigrant populations with those of their native and host countries, even though technically flawed, is suggestive of an important environmental impact on cancer incidence and mortality. Furthermore, because most immigrants are adults at the time of migration, results are suggestive of an environmental impact during adulthood. If this conclusion is correct, then knowledge of the environmental factors for the onset of cancer may be an important tool in the control of the disease.

References

Adelstein, A. M., Staszewski, J., & Muir, C. S.. (1979). Cancer mortality in 1970–1972 among Polish-born immigrants to England and Wales. *British Journal of Cancer, 40,* 464–475.

Bloom, J. R. (1994). Early detection of cancer: Psychological and social dimensions. *Cancer, 74* (Suppl. 4), 1464–1473.

Boston, P. (1992). Understanding cultural differences through family assessment. *Journal of Cancer Education, 7*(3), 261–266.

Boston, P. (1993). Culture and cancer, the relevance of cultural orientation within cancer education programs. *European Journal of Cancer Care, 2*(2), 72–76.

Bouchardy, C., Parkin, D. M., Wanner, P., & Khlat, M. (1996). Cancer mortality among north African immigrants in France. *International Journal of Epidemiology, 25*(1), 5–13.

Coleman, M. P., Esteve, J., Damiecki, P., Arslan, A., & Renard, H. (1993). Trends in cancer incidence and mortality (IARC Scientific Publications No. 121, 1–806). Lyon, France: World Health Organization and the International Agency for Research on Cancer.

Dunn, J. E.. (1975). Cancer epidemiology in populations of the United States—with emphasis on Hawaii and California—and Japan. *Cancer Research, 35*(11, Pt. 2), 3240–3245.

Dunn, J. E., Jr. (1977). Breast cancer among American Japanese in the San Francisco Bay area. *National Cancer Institute Monographs, 47,* 157–160.

Eisenbruch, M., & Handelman, L. (1990). Cultural consultation for cancer, astrocytoma in a Cambodian adolescent. *Social Science and Medicine, 31*(12), 1295–1299.

Formenti, S. C., Meyerowitz, B. E., Ell, K., Muderspach, L., Groshen, S., Leedham, B., Klement, V., & Morrow, P. C. (1995). Inadequate adherence to radiotherapy in Latina immigrants with carcinoma of the cervix: Potential impact on disease free survival. *Cancer, 75*(5), 1135–1140.

Fruchter, R. G., Wright, C., Habenstreit, B., Remy, J. C., Boyce, J. G., & Imperato, P. J. (1985). Screening for cervical and breast cancer among Caribbean immigrants. *Journal of Community Health, 10*(3), 121–135.

Garabrant, D. H., Peters, J. M., Mack, T. M., & Bernstein, L. (1984). Job activity and colon cancer risk. *American Journal of Epidemiology, 119*(6), 1005–1014.

Gifford, S. M. (1994). The change of life, the sorrow of life, menopause, bad blood and cancer among Italian-Australian working class women. *Culture, Medicine and Psychiatry, 18*(3) 299–319.

Gordon, N. H. (1995). Association of education and income with estrogen receptor status in primary breast cancer. *American Journal of Epidemiology, 142*(8), 796–803.

Gordon, N. H., Crowe, J. P., Brumberg, D. J., & Berger, N. A. (1992). Socioeconomic factors and race in breast cancer recurrence and survival. *American Journal of Epidemiology, 135*(6), 609–618.

Gregorio, D. I., Flannery, J. T., & Hansen, H. (1992). Stomach cancer patterns in European immigrants to Connecticut, United States. *Cancer Causes and Control, 3*(3), 215–221.

Haenszel, H. (1982). Immigrant studies. In D. Schottenfeld & J. F. Fraumeni, Jr. (Eds.), *Cancer epidemiology and prevention* (pp. 194–207). Philadelphia: Saunders.

Haenszel, W., & Kurihara, M. (1968). Studies of Japanese immigrants: 1. Mortality from cancers and other diseases among Japanese in the United States. *Journal of the National Cancer Institute, 40,* 43–68.

Hazlewood, P. E. (1994). Breast self-examination practice and breast cancer knowledge in community college women, age 18–35. *Dissertation Abstracts International [A], 54*(8), 2903.

Howson, C. P., Hiyama, T., & Wynder, E. L. (1986). The decline in gastric cancer: Epidemiology of an unplanned triumph. *Epidemiologic Reviews, 8,* 1–27.

Hunter, D. J., & Willett, W. C. (1993). Diet, body size, and breast cancer. *Epidemiologic Reviews, 15*(1), 110–132.

Kelsey, J. L. (1993). Breast cancer epidemiology: Summary and future directions. *Epidemiologic Reviews, 15*(1), 256–263.

Kelsey, J. L., & Horn-Ross, P. L. (1993). Breast cancer: Magnitude of the problem and descriptive epidemiology. *Epidemiologic Reviews, 15*(1), 7–16.

Kliewer, E. V., & Smith, K. R. (1995). Breast cancer mortality among immigrants in Australia and Canada. *Journal of the National Cancer Institute, 87*(15), 1154–1161.

Mallin, K., & Anderson, K. (1988). Cancer mortality in Illinois Mexican and Puerto Rican immigrants, 1979–1984. *International Journal of Cancer, 41*(5), 670–676.

Maltoni, C., Ciliberti, A., Cotti, G., Conti, B., & Belpoggi, F. (1989). Benzene, an experimental multi potential carcinogen: Results of a long-term bioassays performed at the Bologna Institute of Oncology. *Environmental Health Perspectives, 82,* 109–124.

Menck, H. R., Henderson, B. E., Pike, M. C., Mack, T., Martin, S. P., & SooHoo, J. (1975). Cancer incidence in the Mexican-American. *Journal of the National Cancer Institute, 55*(3), 531–536.

Miller, B. A., Feuer, E. J., & Hankey, B. F. (1991). The increasing incidence of beast cancer since 1982: Relevance of early detection. *Cancer Causes and Control, 2,* 67–74.

Neves Arruda, E. N., Larson, P. J., & Meleis, A. I. (1992). Comfort: Immigrant Hispanic cancer patients' views. *Cancer Nursing, 15*(6), 387–394.

Newman, A. M., & Spengler, R. F. (1984). Cancer mortality among immigrant populations in Ontario, 1969 through 1973. *Canadian Medical Association Journal, 130*(4), 399–405.

Palmer, J. R., & Rosenberg, L. (1993). Cigarette smoking and the risk of breast cancer. *Epidemiologic Reviews: Breast Cancer, 15*(1), 145–156.

Polednak, A. P. (1992). Cancer incidence in the Puerto Rican–born population of Connecticut. *Cancer, 70*(5), 1172–1176.

Rosenberg, L., Metzger, L. S., & Palmer, J. R. (1993). Alcohol consumption and risk of breast cancer: A review of the epidemiologic evidence. *Epidemiologic Reviews: Breast Cancer, 15*(1), 113–144.

Staszewski, J., & Haenszel, W. (1965). Cancer mortality among the Polish–born in the United States. *Journal of the National Cancer Institute, 35*(2), 291–297.

Staszewski, J., McCall, M. G., & Stenhouse, N. S. (1971). Cancer mortality in 1962–66 among Polish immigrants to Australia. *British Journal of Cancer, 25*(4), 599–610.

Stellman, S. D., & Wang Q. S. (1994). Cancer mortality in Chinese immigrants to New York City: Comparison with Chinese in Tianjin and with United States–born Whites. *Cancer, 73*(4), 1270–1275.

Swerdlow, A. J., Marmot, M. G., Grulich, A. E., & Head J. (1995). Cancer mortality in Indian and British ethnic immigrants from Indian subcontinent to England and Wales. *British Journal of Cancer, 72*(5), 1312–1319.

Tomatis, L., Aitio, A., Day, N. E., Heseltine, E., Kaldor, J., Miller, A. B., Parkin, D. M., & Riboli, E. (1990). *Cancer: Causes, occurence, and control.* (IARC Scientific Publications No. 100). Lyon, France: World Health Organization, International Agency for Research on Cancer.

Tyczynski, J., Tarkowski, W., Pakin, D. M., & Zatonski, W. (1994). Cancer mortality among Polish immigrants to Australia. *European Journal of Cancer, 30A*(4), 478–484.

Ziegler, R. G., Hoover, R. N., Pike, M. C., Hildesheim, A, Nomura, A. M. Y, West, D. W., Wu-Williams, A. H., Kolonel, L. N., Horn-Ross, P. L., Rosenthal, J. F., & Hyer M. B. (1993). Migration patterns and breast cancer risk in Asian-American women. *Journal of the National Cancer Institute, 85,* 1819–1827.

20

Menta   ration

A

Introduction:
Ethnopsychia

The Immigrant Experience

The immigration experience can be difficult at best. Immigrants are exposed to a variety of noxious situations in the country of arrival. Also, in their place of origin, immigrants may have been subject to traumatic experiences, as in the case of Latin American and Southeast Asian refugees to the United States. Even the best of journeys can be trying for some. But an extended voyage with many transit points and many unpleasant experiences, as with nonlegal immigrants from Mexico, can put many at risk for psychiatric disturbances in the short and long run. One must consider, as well, that immigrants are often the more vulnerable members of their respective countries of origin.

Travel itself may portend change, but after a limited sojourn, one returns to "normalcy." Immigration, on the other hand, suggests more permanent and drastic change or changes. The experience of change, which is the experience of difference, may place individuals at risk for mental problems.

ATWOOD D. GAINES • Departments of Anthropology, Psychiatry, and Biomedical Ethics, Case Western Reserve University and School of Medicine, Cleveland, Ohio 44106.

Handbook of Immigrant Health, edited by Loue. Plenum Press, New York, 1998.

hnopsychiatry

lisorders vary widely across cultures in their definition, such problems may or may not be recognized in the host country by its health professionals (or laypersons). Conversely, mental disorders as defined in the immigrant population may be unknown to the host country.

As a result of the coming together of distinct psychiatric knowledges entailed in immigration, a consideration of the mental health of immigrants, whether guest workers or those intending longer stays, is necessarily a study in cultural or ethnopsychiatry. That is, one must consider the cultural construction of (ethno)psychiatric beliefs and practices of both immigrant and host as cultural processes. Aspects of the "new ethnopsychiatry" (Gaines, 1992a, 1992b) are incorporated in the present discussion as it allows for consideration of wider issues such as disability, gender, self-concepts, and violence that are often omitted from psychiatric considerations that focus on individual biological problems.

Problem Recognition

The nature of problem recognition is a central concern in a consideration of mental disorders of immigrants because of the great variation in cultural theories of mental illness and therapy. Distinct, divergent, and even contradictory theories about etiology, symptomatology, and therapy may be held by immigrants and the lay and professional mental health workers of the host country.

The very existence of disorders of mind as distinct from those of the body is an example of a cultural theory peculiar to Western psychiatrists, not all of whom draw this distinction in quite the same way (Gaines, 1979, 1982a, 1982b, 1992a, 1992b, 1992c, 1992d; Kleinman, 1988; Kleinman & Good, 1985; Lee, 1996). Thus the notion that illnesses of emotion are distinct from illnesses of cognition fails to resonate with understandings of human psychological function in other cultures (Kleinman, 1980, 1986, 1988; Lutz, 1985).

Questions of Western Psychiatric Nosological Universality

Specific mental disorders listed in the most recent *Diagnostic and Statistical Manual of Mental Disorders* (*DSM-IV*) of the American Psychiatric Association (1994) do not appear to be universal in their incidence despite psychiatric assertions and assumptions to the contrary. Indeed, the vast majority of the disorders listed in the *DSM* are probably culture-specific (Blue & Gaines, 1992; Castillo, 1997; Kleinman, 1988). The most notable possible exceptions include schizophrenia, anxiety disorders, bipolar affective disorder, and depression, but the universality of even these highly biologized (in U.S. psychiatry) disorders is highly debatable (Blue & Gaines, 1992; Castillo, 1997; Gaines, 1991, 1992a, 1992b, 1992c, 1992d, 1995b; Gaines & Farmer, 1986; Johnson, 1987; Kleinman & Good, 1985; Marsella, 1980).

Specifically, seemingly universal psychiatric disorders found commonly in the West such as schizophrenia, depression, but also anorexia and Posttraumatic Stress Disorder are absent from other cultures (Blue & Gaines, 1992; Devereux, 1980; Lutz, 1985; Manson, Shore, & Bloom, 1985; Marsella, 1980; Obeyesekere, 1985). Indeed, there are dramatic differences even among Western nations' nosologies and we find that disorders present in one nosology may be absent in others (Blue & Gaines, 1992; Castillo, 1997;

Gaines, 1992a; Kleinman, 1988; Lee, 1996; Maretzki, 1992; Payer, 1989).

The psychiatric profession itself has been developed in strikingly dissimilar ways in various countries even within Europe (Gaines, 1992a). In some countries it is a very small profession (Orford, 1992) focused on managing the severely mentally disabled, as in England. Or psychiatry may be a total afterthought, largely imposed by outside political forces, as is the case in Greece (Blue, 1991, 1992).

Also, disorders found in other cultures, including industrialized areas such as Japan, are not to be found in the West. Two examples are *skinkieshitsu* in Japan and France's *fatigué* (Gaines, 1991; Gaines & Farmer, 1986; Kleinman, 1986; Reynolds, 1976). Commonalities of therapies also are not found. Unique therapeutic traditions exist for the alleviation of suffering, as that is locally defined, in Japan (Reynolds, 1980), Germany (Maretzki, 1992), the former Soviet Union (Blue & Gaines, 1992) and France (Gaines, 1992d; Gaines & Farmer, 1986). There are of course myriad natural and supernatural ways employed in various folk traditions for the alleviation of mental suffering.

Because of the complexities of cultural variation, it is difficult to speak in general terms about the worldwide phenomenon of immigration and mental disorder. One must remain cognizant of the variety of distinct views of what constitutes mental disorder in the various nations and cultures of the world. What U.S. or British or other professional psychiatry defines as a mental disorder is often not what members of another culture would so define. Similarly, what is defined as healthy or nonproblematic in the West may be seen as pathological by psychiatric-psychological popular or professional healers of other cultures (Pfleiderer, 1991). The application of psychiatric categories to people from whom they were not derived is an example of the "category fallacy," but it is nonetheless often found in psychiatric epidemiological studies (Gaines & Farmer, 1986; Kleinman, 1988; Obeyesekere, 1985).

From Perspective to Illness

In discussing the mental health of immigrants, then, one must consider a variety of vantage points from which mental difficulties may be defined. The view or definition of a psychiatric problem must come from *somewhere,* some specifiable vantage point. In any given case, there may be at least two sets of definitions, those of the host country and those of the country of origin of the immigrant, assuming that each country belongs to a distinct cultural tradition (see Gaines & Farmer, 1986, for a case study of an immigrant to a culturally similar country). In what follows, I discuss "deviance" from local notions of normalcy from two general vantage points—first, that of a (Western) host country and, then, those of particular immigrants to such a country. The view is largely from the United States seen as a host country, though others are also considered.

The Problem of Diagnosis in the West

A first step in considering mental illness in immigrants is to elucidate the nature of the defining frameworks, that is, the nature of psychiatric nosologies and diagnoses. An examination of nosologies and diagnostic practices reveals that U.S. and other professional psychiatries and medicines shift their major disease paradigms over time, sometimes rapidly (Castillo, 1997; Gaines, 1992a; Unschuld, 1985). Such shifts not only lead to changes in the prevalence and incidence of specific diagnoses, but they also result in the reinterpretation of the etiology of disease and, hence, the therapeutic approaches that are employed.

In U.S. psychiatry, there have been several shifts over time in the central paradigms of mental illness. In the past century, social contextual explanations were common for "alienists" (i.e., psychiatrists) (Littlewood & Lipsedge, 1982), making it sensible to develop institutions situated away from causative noxious social environments (Dwyer, 1987). Then, too, there were notions in the past century about *neurasthenia,* exhaustion of the nerves, as a cause of some psychiatric disorders (Kleinman, 1988). This explanation, which disappeared generations ago in psychiatry, has reappeared and is increasingly employed with reference to conditions formerly labeled Chronic Fatigue Syndrome (Kleinman, 1988). This diagnostic label need not be resurrected in China; there it has been the most commonly used diagnosis in Chinese professional psychiatry for several decades (Kleinman, 1986, 1988).

Psychodynamic explanations of mental disorders from a biopsychosocial perspective traceable to H. S. Sullivan and others (Gaines, 1992a) was embodied in the first *Diagnostic and Statistical Manual of Mental Disorders* (*DSM-I*) of the American Psychiatric Association (1952). *DSM-II* (American Psychiatric Association, 1968), the second *Diagnostic and Statistical Manual of Mental Disorders,* shows the beginning of a shift away from psychodynamic explanations, for which forms of talk therapy were appropriate, to an incipient biological approach. This approach begins to eschew the importance of the social and ecological factors of the biopsychosocial model.

The biological model, we find, was not actually an advance in psychiatric thinking. It was borrowed from professional German ethnopsychiatry the founding ideology of which stems from the past century (Gaines, 1992a; Young, 1991). That ideology was itself derived from German popular culture (Gaines, 1992a; Townsend, 1978). The biological stance in psychiatry gained a substantial measure of increased credibility with the development of new neuroleptics (then called "major tranquilizers") in the 1950s; their effects suggested a biological basis of mental disorders.

In *DSM-III* (American Psychiatric Association, 1980), the shift to a biological model was completed. Psychodynamic explanations were eliminated or minimalized (e.g., neurosis ceased to exist as a psychiatric disorder)

(Castillo, 1997; Gaines, 1992a). Purporting to be atheoretical and descriptive, *DSM-III* actually was intended to advance the biological perspective. This shift sought to make psychiatry more "mainstream" within medicine by advocating somatically based diagnoses and treatment methods analogous to the rest of medicine. The biological model also tends to emphasize somatic interventions and to reduce the significance of forms of talk therapy such as psychoanalysis (Gaines, 1992a; Johnson, 1985; Young, 1991). The somato-centric strategies that resulted include diagnostic (imaging) techniques such as Positron Emission Tomography, or PET scans, and extensive and often exclusively psychopharmacotherapy therapies.

DSM-III-R (American Psychiatric Association, 1987) continued in this vein, but *DSM-IV* (American Psychiatric Association, 1994) has shown some retreat from purely biological explanations. Notable is Appendix I. It represents the beginning of a serious consideration of cultural influences on the severity and form of mental illness and notes culturally specific types of mental disorders; it was written by psychiatrists, many with anthropological training, and anthropologists (Mezzich *et al.,* 1994).

The biological approach in psychiatry, as in other branches of medicine (Engel, 1977; Kleinman, 1988), often leaves aside personally and culturally relevant meanings that frame and define illness experiences. Biological definitions, then, may have little relevance to those who suffer (Gaines & Farmer, 1986; Good, 1995; Kleinman, 1980, 1988). In addition, the nature of suffering may change with the institution or psychiatrists in or to which the patient presents.

Various viewpoints, representing a virtual archeology of psychiatric perspectives, may be found in a single psychiatry program. The pluralism of psychiatric viewpoints in one locale develops because "early" ideas may not be replaced by later ones; they may coexist in tension (e.g., Gaines, 1979, 1985) because psychiatry does not develop in a unilineal fashion with new ideas replacing older ones.

As paradigms shift, diseases appear, disappear and, sometimes, reappear in the standard nosologies (e.g., neurasthenia) (Blue & Gaines, 1992; Gaines, 1992a; Kleinman, 1988; Young, 1995). The perceived uniformity and coherence of psychiatric theory and practice is largely illusory (Gaines, 1992a, 1992b, 1995a; Kleinman, 1988; Young, 1995); change is ubiquitous and such change is not necessarily representative of advances in a specific direction, toward an implicit "end of classification" where there is full knowledge of all disorders. The same notion of an end is found in all sciences where it is likewise an illusion (Baudrillard, 1994).

Changes in psychiatry are, as in Thomas Kuhn's signal study of scientific change, *The Structure of Scientific Revolutions* (1962), represented as linear events in a cumulative historical process that is the *sine qua non* of science. The various American Psychiatric Association nosologies are scientific classifications believed by advocates to represent advances, improvements over earlier nosologies (e.g., American Psychiatric Association, 1980, 1987, 1994). However, the paradigm shifts in psychiatry do not actually produce new explanatory frameworks incorporating phenomena explained and unexplained by earlier paradigms. The paradigm shifts represent the adoption of *distinct views,* not progressive ones, as we would expect with that linear (Baudrillard, 1994), cumulative process held to represent the essence of scientific progress (see Hacking, 1983; Knorr-Cetina & Mulkay, 1983; Pickering, 1992).

The conceptual variations and differences in psychiatry have implications for immigrants, some of which are explored in the following sections. The historical moment of immigration may affect the perception of problems and the diagnosis thereof for these clinical actions are themselves reflections of professional ethnopsychiatric historical moments. In the following section, the views of stress and disorder are considered from the vantage point of Western professional ethnopsychiatry.

Sources of Disorder: Views from the West

Stress and Complexity

Immigration from one country to another can produce a variety of stresses on the displaced population. In the West, certain stressors are seen as individually, or in combination with genetic or other biological vulnerabilities, causative of mental distress. Some Western psychiatrists tend to believe that mental distress afflicts immigrants to nations of the West because they come from "simple" (sometimes referred to as "primitive") societies; Western societies are "too complex" for them (Leff, 1973; and see Beeman's critique, in Kleinman & Good, 1985).

Ethnocentrism, such as that just discussed, may be found in clinical practice when culturally different patients and healers encounter one another, making appropriate assessment difficult, if not impossible (e.g., Castillo, 1997; Gaines, 1982b, 1988, 1992a, 1995a, 1995b; Gaines & Farmer, 1986; Gilman, 1985, 1988; Good, Herrera, Good, & Cooper, 1985; Kleinman, 1988; Kleinman & Good, 1985; Littlewood & Lipsedge, 1982; Lock, 1991; Mezzich *et al.,* 1994; Racy, 1980; Van Moffaert & Vereecken, 1989; Westermeyer, 1989). The strange is often seen as pathological. There are few standards by which to distinguish that which is bizarre and idiosyncratic and that which is likewise bizarre but culturally shared.

Related to the conception of complexity is the notion of change or movement and its effect on the incidence of schizophrenia. Devereux (1980) argued that multiple alterations of habitat, even within one's own country if it is diverse in its regional traditions (e.g., the United States), take a psychological toll. He suggested that individuals can adapt successfully to new roles, role expectations, and customs only a relatively few times in their lives before developing psychiatric problems, including schizophrenia (Devereux, 1980).

In terms of adaptation, the lack of familiarity of people, language, and places is disturbing to some, but an adventure to others. For those for whom dislocation is problematic, several sources can be and have been isolated that place immigrant individuals at risk for mental problems. Some difficulties, from the point of view of Western medical and sociomedical sciences, appear to be group characteristics and others appear as individual issues.

Psychological Disorder and Stigmatization

Some immigrants arrive in the host country only to find that they are seen as representatives of a despised minority group, or one that has little, if any, status. A normally positive and unquestioned sense of self is then cast against the ideology of a society that defines one in terms of his or her membership in a stigmatized group rather than on the basis of individual characteristics and abilities. One's social identity becomes a handicap, disabling the individual in his or her competition for scarce resources and a viable social identity.

One may also be scapegoated as a member of an immigrant group, as in the case of southern and eastern European ethnic immigrants to the United States at the turn of the century, who were blamed for rising rates of STDs and, as such, posed a "threat" to the "Anglo Saxon race" (Brandt, 1985).

Such "foreign" groups may be, as was the case at the end of the past century, denied the use of medical advances because the alleged distinct physical constitution of "such people" would not benefit from their use. This justification for withholding a medical advance occurred at the end of the 19th century when anesthesia was not offered to certain European immigrants (Italians, Irish) who were said not to need it even for surgery (Pernick, 1985). Eugenics' notions were behind a variety of exclusionary medical practices at the turn of the past century (Brandt, 1985; Duster, 1990)

In cases of internal migration, some of the same problems as with immigration may appear with language and custom and with so-cial status (Edgerton & Karno, 1971; Good et al., 1985; Nathan, 1986). One model of disability applies here. The newcomer may have conferred upon him or her a stigmatized identity. Such an identity forcibly applied creates a classic double bind in that the new immigrant is accepted to the host country, or the wider society, only to be despised therein.

The stigma model of disability frames dis-ability as an undesirable or unacceptable attribute that is socially ascribed. The desig-nation of stigma, or an ascribed difference (i.e., disability), results from a process of de-valuation called stigmatization (Goffman, 1963). The nature of stigmatized identities is hierarchical, and exhibits a scale of desirable to undesirable identities. The scale is depen-dent on contexts of culture and time. What is considered stigmatizing in one time and place may be desirable in another time and place (Ainlay, Becker, & Coleman, 1986). Once stigmatized, one may fall into a category con-sidered by a host society as less "normal," or less "human." Individuals, as members of groups so perceived, are so treated and, henceforth, experience their individual selves as marked, tainted, and defective. Their social self-identity becomes "an attribute that is deeply discrediting" (Goffman, 1963, p. 3).

French ethnopsychiatrist (psychoanalyti-cally trained) Nathan (1986) writes of immi-grants to France who, as the "Other," are faced with inconstant (and often negative) so-cial experiences. In response, they must ex-ternalize psychological material that is normally unconscious in order to stabilize the unpredictable external world (i.e., the social world of potential discrimination and devalu-ation). The process of externalization, how-ever, may be read by professional insiders as pathology rather than as understandable at-tempts at adjustment and defense. Such at-tempts may also appear paranoid to host country natives as the immigrant may aggres-sively seek just and fair treatment and take exception to the variety of slights, intended and unintended, that may be visited upon him or her (Nathan, 1986).

Related to the notion of identity as disabil-ity are the cases of immigrants who are actu-ally defined as disabled by state agencies such as the U.S. Department of Health and Human Services. Due to recent changes in the U.S. Supplemental Security Income pro-gram, payments would have ceased for legal immigrants who had not become citizens by September, 1997. But congressional action was taken to prevent this. This problem is particularly acute for learning disabled or de-mented persons, who also experience what I call *medical triple jeopardy* in a society such as the United States. There, society is unsure of its obligation to care for the elderly (Bin-stock & Post, 1991), the disabled (Ainlay et al., 1986; Langness & Levine, 1986) *or the immigrant.*

The common experience of leaving one's home country, where one was a member of the majority, and subsequently finding one-self a minority group member in the host country, then, can be a source of serious dis-tress. While not always negative, minority group membership is frequently disadvanta-geous psychologically as well as socioeco-nomically (Westermeyer, 1989).

Acculturation

A major source of psychological distress for immigrants is the erosion of traditional beliefs and values, often because they are dis-valued or stigmatized in the host country (Boyer et al., 1989; Hallowell, 1955; Hersk-ovits, 1958). The process of acculturation, that is, the learning of new cultural expecta-tions in the host country, itself produces psychological problems and problems of a psychiatric and behavioral nature, including drug addiction (Hallowell, 1955; Kluckhohn, 1962; Lewton, 1997).

For the United States there is strong epi-demiological evidence suggesting that accul-turation is accompanied by increased use of illicit substances, particularly among Latino immigrants (Robins & Regier, 1991). These new data, from the largest psychiatric epi-demiological study ever undertaken in the

United States, the five-site Epidemiologic Catchment Area study (ECA) (Robins & Regier, 1991), are reminiscent of the findings related to Native Americans. Studies have shown that alcohol problems may be forms of acculturation stress and are related to attempts to acculturate through emulation of European Americans (Kunitz, 1989; Lewton, 1997).

Internal migration, as noted earlier, appears to be as difficult as transnational migration. For some, such as Native Americans, the experience of moving from an isolated reservation to the urban U.S. environment as stressful, or more so, than immigration from foreign lands (Boyer *et al.,* 1989: Hallowell, 1955; Kluckhohn, 1962; Prucha, 1985). Problems may arise with or without language difficulties.

Physical Deprivation and Trauma

One short-term source of problems placing immigrants at risk is the effect of physical deprivation of the act of immigration itself on the psyche. However, the immigration process is for many a process in which deprivation is prolonged rather than transient. Prolonged deprivation may be coupled with extreme situations in the home country, such as war, catastrophe, or state terrorism, that lead or force individuals to immigrate. Individuals may arrive in states of psychological distress (Jenkins, 1991), including suffering from Posttraumatic Stress Disorder (PTSD). We note that this is a relatively newly constructed disorder in the United States, so its diagnosis is recent and appears largely in this country. It would not appear in earlier immigrants' records if they were evaluated. The concept was developed in the United States based on a new (in the late 19th century) conception of traumatic memory (Young, 1995). It is an example of a diagnosis depending on an historical moment.

Physical, as well as psychological, stress can lead to psychological dysfunction including psychotic breaks with reality. Traumatic stress is particularly common among refugees from South Asia and Central and South America. There, political turmoil has cost tens of thousands of lives and terrorized tens of thousands of others (Jenkins, 1991).

Many immigrants are set in motion because of dire economic circumstances. Poverty, in the lives of many people in the world in their home countries and those who immigrate, is a major problem and a major contributor to psychological difficulties and psychiatric illness (Dejarlais, Eisenberg, Good, & Kleinman, 1995). The increasing impoverishment of those in (under)developing countries increases their risk of developing mental disorders both as residents and as immigrants.

Problems of Communication

Language difficulties lead to uncertainty about the meaning of interactions, written and verbal instructions, and so on. Depending on one's experience in the mother country, such uncertainty may be extremely anxiety provoking for fear of dire consequences; home or host countries are often unkind to those leaving or those arriving. Language difficulties also pose problems in psychiatric evaluations as miscommunication and misunderstanding can develop based on failures of translation of terms or of specific cultural conceptions (Edgerton & Karno, 1971; Gavira & Arana, 1987; Good *et al.,* 1985).

A central issue for immigrants is the loss of support and other normal means for stress reduction, and the ability to invoke culturally appropriate means of handling illness which result from immigration to a new land. Traditional or new means of help may be sought, such as spiritual forms of treatment and religious health resources, which may be utilized more than in the home country as, for example, with Latinos (Oths, 1992). In addition, the importance of family, however defined, is cardinal for most immigrants. Self is not seen as an isolate as it is in the dominant (but minority) culture's psychology in the United States (and its source, Northern European Protestantism)

(Gaines, 1982a; 1992a, 1995a). Rather, self is an integral part of a larger kinship whole (Schweder & Bourne, 1982). The family context may serve as a buffer against a hostile outside world, but it may be also, with emotional overinvolvement (EO), be a contributor to the chronicity of severe mental disorders, as has been found in Mexican immigrants to the United States in studies of EO (Jenkins, 1992).

To this point, we have considered sources of mental disorder as seen by Western psychiatry (and psychoanalysis). In the following, I consider how cultural Others construct their own definitions of mental and physical disorder. These constructions of "clinical reality" may provoke misreadings of the sickness and health of the Other. I consider how particular immigrants' idioms of distress might be misdiagnosed by Western psychiatry.

Non-Western Constructions of Illness

Overview

In the Western psychoanalytic model, chronic anxiety is deleterious to mental health. It is implicated in a variety of mental conditions recognized in the West including depression and psychotic illnesses. A variety of other mental conditions not recognized in the West are also implicated in the immigration process, such as Fright Illness among Middle Eastern immigrants, or Spirit Possession among many groups of Polynesian, South and Southeast Asian, and African origin (Gaines, 1992b; Good & Good, 1982; Mezzich et al., 1994; Spitzer, Gibbon, Skodol, Williams, & First, 1994). Such disorders would be recast as no-diagnosis (folk beliefs) or they may suggest psychotic experiences in Western diagnostic models and be (mis)treated accordingly.

The following section considers some general classes of disorders that are found in a variety of cultures that appear in Western psychiatric settings. The discussion is not intended to be exhaustive, but rather to briefly note some specific examples of illness and

larger categories of disorder recognized in other cultures and that are likely to be missed or misdiagnosed in Western settings when immigrants present in medical or psychiatric contexts.

In order to understand the individual's particular cultural explanation of distress, *DSM-IV,* in its cultural appendix, recommends consideration of the

> predominant idioms of distress through which symptoms or the need for social support are communicated (e.g., "nerves," possessing spirits, somatic complaints, inexplicable misfortune), the meaning and perceived severity of the individual's symptoms in relation to norms of the cultural reference group, any local illness category used by the individual's family and community to identify the condition, . . . the perceived causes or explanatory models that the individual and the reference group use to explain the illness, and current preferences for and past experiences with professional and popular sources of care. (Mezzich *et al.,* 1994, pp. 843–844)

In considering some theories of illness from non–U.S. cultures, these issues are important to keep in mind.

Cultural Constructions of Disorder

The Rhetoric of Complaint

Particular styles or forms used to articulate one's place in the world can lead to problems in clinical settings where, being unfamiliar, they can be misinterpreted. An example is what Gaines refers to as the "rhetoric of complaint" found in Mediterranean and Latin American cultures (Gaines, 1982a; Gaines & Farmer, 1986). Individuals present themselves as bearing great burdens in life, as striving to overcome enormous adversity, that is, persons who suffer.

The presentation is intended to show self-worth, as one who suffers, because only the good are said to be thus "tested" by divinity. This stance of suffering can be misinterpreted as paranoid ideation in psychiatric contexts. The author observed such a case with a (California-born) Mexican-American (internal) "immigrant" to Hawaii (see Gaines, 1982b).

This ideation and its rhetoric in Latin countries also produces false positives for clinical depression when clinical diagnostic instruments are employed (see Gaines & Farmer, 1986).

A problem for many ethnic groups in the West is the tendency to somatize illness, as among the Latinos, Mediterranean groups, Chinese, Japanese, and some African and Caribbean groups (see Angel & Guarnaccia, 1989; Castillo, 1997; Gaines & Farmer, 1986; Kay, 1974; Kleinman, 1980, 1986, 1988; Kleinman & Good, 1985; Racy, 1980; Van Moffaert & Vereecken, 1989; Westermeyer, 1989). Actually, the psychologization of problems, seen as normal in psychiatry, is rather rare in the world (Kleinman, 1988; Kleinman & Good, 1985). Despite this rarity, those who somatize distress, such as that stemming from immigration, likely would be diagnosed as having a "problem," that of somatization, in addition to any other distress they might exhibit.

In Latino traditions, conditions may cause discomfort but they often represent problems expressed in a cultural idiom, not a psychiatric one. It is very easy for a misreading or misdiagnosis to occur. Such misdiagnoses recast the culturally familiar into the psychiatrically compromised (Edgerton & Karno, 1971; Good et al., 1985). Several Latin idioms of distress, noted in the following sections, are problematic for Western psychiatric diagnosticians.

Specific Disorders

Nervios. One example is *nervios,* a common disorder found among a variety of Latin ethnic groups. *Nervios,* literally, nerves, is a cultural symbol of distress, but distress not necessarily constructed as it is in Western psychological models. The term serves as a gloss, in U.S. terms, for a very heterogeneous collection of Western-defined problems including schizophrenia, depression (Jenkins, 1988; Schreiber & Homiak, 1981), and what was once termed neurosis (excluded from U.S. nosologies in 1980). In addition, we may include a range of problems "from normal expressions of distress not associated with having a mental disorder to symptom presentations associated with the diagnoses of Anxiety, Mood, Dissociative, or Somatoform Disorders" (Mezzich *et al.,* 1994, p. 845).

An *ataque de nervios* (nervous attack) is very likely to afflict those who have immigrated legally or illegally under difficult circumstances, and those who face acculturation in a hostile environment. Such a response to immigration may result because the condition is precipitated by stressors (Angel & Guarnaccia, 1989). In the Latin context, with its strong emphasis on family, in addition to the stress of dislocation, stressors also include separations from family and friends as well as from the homeland or village. Forms of *nervios* are to be found among other Mediterranean groups as well, for example, among Greek immigrants (Lock, 1991). It is also found among the French, but analyses of this local category of distress are less well developed.

Locura is a term used by Latinos at home and abroad that refers to a severe form of illness that, in *DSM-IV,* would be seen as a chronic psychotic state, not ruling out schizophrenia. Individuals thus afflicted may be unpredictable in their behavior and incomprehensible in their speech. They also may be violent. Since Latinos tend to think of this disorder as inherited (Kay, 1974), it is less likely to be associated with immigration than *susto* (described later) or *nervios.*

Mal de ojo, literally "evil eye" is a term and concept found throughout Mediterranean and Latin American cultures. Differential success of immigrants can provoke the appearance of the disorder as it is believed to be caused by the envious gaze of a person capable of casting the evil eye. Children are especially vulnerable to the gaze of such persons. Belief in the evil eye would likely lead to a psychiatric consultation if presented in a medical environment, as occurs with cases of witchcraft (Hillard & Rockwell, 1978). The misinterpretation of *mal de ojo* or witchcraft as delusional thinking occurs in U.S. psychiatric contexts despite the fact that such beliefs are widespread in the world and in the United States (Gaines, 1988). The many other ideas about unseen forces that may be espoused by immigrants or others in Western countries would also be met with disbelief in medical contexts although they are important cultural theories that explain misfortune and malaise (Gaines, 1982a; Nathan, 1986).

Susto ("fright," or "soul loss") is a folk illness prevalent among some Latinos in the United States and among Latin Americans. It is also known as *espanto, pasmo* (Finkler, 1985), *tripa ida, perdida del alma,* or *chibih* (Mezzich *et al.,* 1994; Rubel, 1964) depending on the country of origin of the speaker. *Susto* is an illness caused by the departure of the soul from the body, often occasioned by a startling or frightening event. This separation of spirit from corporal body produces unhappiness, sickness, and even death. Symptoms of the condition relevant to immigration include decline in motivation, disturbed vegetative signs, and feelings of low self-worth. The last may be caused or exacerbated by immigration to an area where self-identity is stigmatized.

For the Latin disorders mentioned, established folk healers (*curanderos*) regularly treat such problems (Finkler, 1985; Kiev, 1968). Indigenous healers are quite successful in treating conditions such as *susto* for the conditions are known to them and the signs and symptoms have symbolic meaning that they can interpret; they therefore can be helpful in an intervention. Similar expertise may be seen with afflictions of spirit possession (Kleinman, 1980; Spitzer *et al.,* 1994). The therapeutic efficiency of indigenous healers derives from their use of local meanings and idioms of distress that are both satisfying and understandable to the patients (Finkler, 1985; Ito, 1985; Kleinman, 1980; Kleinman & Sung, 1979; Rubel, 1964).

Fright Illness. Another form of illness, *fright illness,* appears in immigrants from Iran and other parts of the Middle East (Good & Good, 1982). This illness develops as individuals begin to fear for the safety of relatives left at home. The fear and anxiety can grow unchecked because the cultural custom is not to tell those far from home about bad news relating to family members. This illness is likely to be diagnosed as an Anxiety or Panic Disorder (Good & Good, 1982), or possibly a Paranoid Disorder using *DSM-IV* criteria.

Among Haitian immigrants to France or the United States, one sees *saisissement* or fright. The condition among Haitians is associated with blood disorders but may at times lead to a passing mental disturbance or *folie passagère* (Laguerre, 1981; Weidman, 1978).

From the Middle East comes *heart distress.* The center of emotion in Islamic biopsychology is the heart. It feels and responds to a variety of difficulties including those of social context, social change, role conflicts, and so on (Good, 1977), all of which appear in the context of immigration. Heart distress would likely be viewed as psychosomatic by Western physicians who would also be unaware of the typical descriptors that those from the tradition would use to describe their condition.

Falling-Out or Blacking-Out. Among southern U.S. (African and European) Americans and Caribbean peoples, *falling-out* or *blacking-out* are instances of unconsciousness subsequent to sudden physical and mental collapse. The episodes can often occur without warning, but usually follow an event such as receipt of disturbing news or an argument. As in a trance, the individual is aware, but unresponsive to, his or her surroundings. The many cases of falling-out are (mis)diagnosed as Conversion Disorder or Dissociative Disorder pursuant to *DSM-IV* criteria.

Ghost Sickness. Among some Native Americans of the Southwest, we find *ghost sickness,* described as a preoccupation with death and the deceased. The ruminations are often related to beliefs about witchcraft. A variety of symptoms are associated with ghost sickness including fatigue, anxiety, disturbed vegetative signs, and depressive, hopeless ideation (Mezzich *et al.,* 1994).

A similar problem may afflict South Asian immigrants in the West who become despondent over loss of connection to deceased relatives in the homeland. Unable to visit shrines or burial areas, they feel cut off and may experience worrisome social isolation like that of Native Americans who have been too long away from their "people" (i.e., relations) (Kluckhohn, 1962).

Shenjing Shuairuo ("neurasthenia") is the most common psychiatric diagnosis in China (Kleinman, 1980, 1986). It is both mental and physical in its manifestations. It is to be found in the *Chinese Classification of Mental Disorders,* 2nd edition (CCMD-2) (Lee, 1996). The symptoms would meet the criteria for a *DSM-IV* Mood or Anxiety Disorder but are treated largely somatically by Chinese psychiatrists. Talk therapy and psychological explanations are not seen as appropriate, or plausibly suitable, by laypersons or professionals in China (Kleinman, 1980, 1986).

El Calor ("heat") is a condition that afflicts Latin immigrants. It may develop subsequent to immigration from areas in which there is political violence, domestic violence, and the violence of poverty (Jenkins, 1991, 1994). A group of Salvadorian women studied by Jenkins presented with symptoms diagnosed as PTSD (Posttraumatic Stress Disorder) according to the criteria of *DSM-III* and *DSM-III-R* which were in use during the period of research. *El calor* "is the experience of intense heat that may rapidly spread throughout the entire body. It sometimes emanates from the head . . . neck, back, leg, stomach, chest, and hands" (Jenkins, 1994, p. 318).

The disorder and its symptoms are not known to U.S. psychiatry and appear to represent a challenge to the dichotomy between culture and emotion (also see Lutz, 1985, 1988). It appears that it is appropriate to say the *el calor* is a bodily emotion, but one which is, in fact, culturally constructed.

Conclusions

A large number of disorders, seen as psychiatric from the perspective of U.S. or other professional medicine, are to be found in countries around the world. Any and all of these may appear in the context of immigration. This article has (1) shown how Western psychiatry would perceive causes of mental disorders in immigrant populations and (2) presented some locally constructed mental disorders and how these might be (mis)interpreted by professional Western, largely U.S., psychiatrists.

Immigrants are at risk for developing mental disorders because of contact with new and often strange social realities that can produce disorders constructed in the context of the culture of the home country, as well as conditions construed as psychopathological in developed nations to which many immigrants go. It is ironic that what is deemed pathological among the immigrants may be in fact a shared cultural theory that *explains* malaise rather than manifests it.

It is useful to consider, as attempted here, that there are at least two vantage points from which any disorder may be perceived (i.e., constructed), that of the immigrant group and that of the host country. A given ethnopsychiatric construct, that is, "disease" is no less a cultural construction than another (Gaines, 1992b). Immigration, which puts individuals at risk for the development of mental disorders, may do so for very different reasons and in very different ways for specific groups. The reasons and ways may be credible in terms of one or the other, but often not both, of the perspectives involved. As a consequence, the immigrant experience may place persons at psychological risk even within helping contexts should such ever become accessible to them.

References

Ainlay, S. C., Becker, G., & Coleman, L. M. (Eds.). (1986). *The dilemma of difference: A multidisciplinary view of stigma.* New York and London: Plenum.

American Psychiatric Association. (1952). *Diagnostic and statistical manual of mental disorders.* Washington, DC: Author.

American Psychiatric Association. (1968). *Diagnostic and statistical manual of mental disorders* (2nd ed.). Washington, DC: Author.

American Psychiatric Association. (1980). *Diagnostic and statistical manual of mental disorders.* (3rd ed.). Washington, DC: Author.

American Psychiatric Association. (1987). *Diagnostic and statistical manual of mental disorders.* (3rd ed., rev.). Washington, DC: Author.

American Psychiatric Association. (1994). *Diagnostic and statistical manual of mental disorders.* (4th ed.). Washington, DC: Author.

Angel, R., & Guarnaccia, P. J. (1989). Mind, body, and culture: Somatization among Hispanics. *Social Science and Medicine, 28*(12), 1229–1238.

Baudrillard, J. (1994). *The illusion of the end.* Stanford, CA: Stanford University Press.

Binstock, R. H., & Post, S.G. (Eds). (1991). *Too old for health care?* Baltimore: Johns Hopkins University Press.

Blue, A. V. (1991). *Culture, nevra and institution: The rise of Greek professional ethnopsychiatry.* Unpublished doctoral dissertation, Department of Anthropology, Case Western Reserve University, Cleveland, Ohio.

Blue, A. V. (1992). The rise of Greek professional ethnopsychiatry. In A. D. Gaines (Ed.), *Ethnopsychiatry: The cultural construction of professional and folk psychiatries* (pp. 327–354). Albany: State University of New York Press.

Blue, A. V., & Gaines, A. D. (1992). The ethnopsychiatric répertoire. In A. D. Gaines (Ed.), *Ethnopsychiatry: The cultural construction of professional and folk psychiatries* (pp. 397–484). Albany: State University of New York Press.

Boyer, L. B., Boyer, R. M., Dithrich, C. W., Herned, H., Hippler, A. E., Stone, J. S., & Walt, A. (1989). The relation between psychological states and acculturation among the Tanaina and Upper Tanaina Indians of Alaska: An ethnographic and Rorschach study. *Ethos, 17,* 450–479.

Brandt, A. (1985). *No magic bullet.* Cambridge, MA: Harvard University Press.

Castillo, R. J. (1997). *Culture and mental illness: A client-centered approach.* Pacific Grove, CA: Brooks/Cole.

Dejarlais, R., Eisenberg, L., Good, B., & Kleinman, A. (1995). *World mental health.* New York: Oxford University Press.

Devereux, G. (1980). Schizophrenia: An ethnic psychosis. In *Basic problems of ethnopsychiatry* (pp. 214–236). Chicago: University of Chicago Press.

Duster, T. (1990). *Backdoor to eugenics.* New York: Routledge.

Dwyer, E. (1987). *Homes for the mad.* New Brunswick, NJ: Rutgers University Press.

Edgerton, R. B., & Karno, M. (1971). Mexican-American bilingualism and the perception of mental illness. *Archives of General Psychiatry, 24,* 286–290.

Engel, G. (1977). The need for a new medical model: A challenge for biomedicine. *Science, 196,* 129–136.

Finkler, K. (1985). *Spiritualist healers in Mexico: Successes and failures of alternative therapeutics.* South Hadley, MA: Bergin and Garvey.

Gaines, A. D. (1979). Definitions and diagnoses: Cultural implications of psychiatric help-seeking and psychiatrists' definitions of the situation in psychiatric emergencies. *Culture, Medicine and Psychiatry, 3*(4), 381–418.

Gaines, A. D. (1982a). Cultural definitions, behavior and the person in American psychiatry. In A. Marsella & G. White (Eds.), *Cultural conceptions of mental health and therapy* (pp. 167–192). Dordrecht, The Netherlands: Reidel.

Gaines, A. D. (1982b). Knowledge and practice: Anthropological ideas and psychiatric practice. In N. Chrisman & T. Maretzki (Eds.), *Clinically applied anthropology: Anthropologists in health science settings* (pp. 243–273). Dordrecht, The Netherlands: Reidel.

Gaines, A. D. (1985). The once and the twice-born: Self and practice among psychiatrists and Christian psychiatrists. In R. A. Hahn & A. D. Gaines (Eds.), *Physicians of Western medicine* (pp. 223–243). Dordrecht, The Netherlands: Reidel.

Gaines, A. D. (1988). Delusions: Culture, psychosis and the problem of meaning. In T. Oltmanns & B. Maher (Eds.), *Delusional beliefs* (pp. 230–258). New York: Wiley.

Gaines, A. D. (1991). Cultural constructivism: Sickness histories and the understanding of ethnomedicines beyond critical medical anthropologies. In B. Pfleiderer & G. Bibeau (Eds.), *Anthropologies of medicine: A colloquium on West European and North American perspectives* (pp. 221–258). Wiesbaden, Germany: Vieweg und Sohn Verlag.

Gaines, A. D. (1992a). From DSM-I to III-R, voices of self, mastery and the other: A cultural constructivist reading of U.S. psychiatric classification. *Social Science and Medicine, 35*(1), 3–24.

Gaines, A. D. (Ed.). (1992b). *Ethnopsychiatry: The cultural construction of professional and folk psychiatries.* Albany: State University of New York Press.

Gaines, A. D. (1992c). Ethnopsychiatry: The cultural construction of psychiatries. In A. D. Gaines (Ed.), *Ethnopsychiatry: The cultural construction of professional and folk psychiatries* (pp. 3–49). Albany: State University of New York Press.

Gaines, A. D. (1992d). Medical/psychiatric knowledge in France and the United States. In A. D. Gaines (Ed.), *Ethnopsychiatry: The cultural construction of professional and folk psychiatries* (pp. 171–201). Albany: State University of New York Press.

Gaines, A. D. (1995a). Mental illness II: Cross-cultural perspectives. In W. T. Reich (Ed.), *The encyclopedia of bioethics* (pp. 1743–1751). New York: Macmillan.

Gaines, A. D. (1995b). Race and racism. In W. T. Reich (Ed.), *The encyclopedia of bioethics* (pp. 2189–2201). New York: Macmillan.

Gaines, A. D., & Farmer, P. E. (1986). Visible saints: Social cynosures and dysphoria in the Mediterranean tradition. *Culture, Medicine and Psychiatry, 10*(3), 295–330.

Gaviria, M., & Arana, J. (1987). *Health and behavior: Research agenda for Hispanics.* Chicago: University of Illinois at Chicago Press.

Gilman, S. L. (1985). *Difference and pathology: Stereotypes of sexuality, race and madness.* Ithaca, NY: Cornell University Press.

Gilman, S. L. (1988). *Disease and representation: Images of illness from madness to AIDS.* Ithaca, NY: Cornell University Press.

Goffman, E. (1963). *Stigma.* Englewood Cliffs, NJ: Prentice-Hall.

Good, B. J. (1977). The heart of what's the matter: The semantics of illness in Iran. *Culture, Medicine and Psychiatry, 1*(1), 25–58.

Good, B. J. (1995). *Medicine, rationality and experience.* Cambridge, England: Cambridge University Press.

Good, B. J., & Good, M.-J. D. (1982). Toward a meaning-centered analysis of popular illness categories: "Fright illness" and "heart distress" in Iran. In G. White & A. Marsella (Eds.), *Cultural conceptions of mental health and therapy* (pp. 141–166). Dordrecht, The Netherlands: Reidel.

Good, B. J., Herrera, H., Good, M.-J. D., & Cooper, J.. (1985). Reflexivity, countertransference and clinical ethnography: A case from a psychiatric cultural consultation clinic. In R. A. Hahn & A. D. Gaines (Eds.), *Physicians of Western Medicine: Anthropological approaches to theory and practice* (pp. 193–221). Dordrecht, The Netherlands: Reidel.

Hacking, I. (1983). *Representing and intervening: Introductory topics in the philosophy of natural science.* Cambridge, England: Cambridge University Press.

Hallowell, A. I. (1955). *Culture and experience.* Philadelphia: University of Pennsylvania Press.

Herskovits, M. (1958). *Acculturation.* Gloucester, MA: Smith.

Hillard, J., & Rockwell, W. (1978). Disesthesia, witchcraft and conversion reaction. *Journal of the American Medical Association, 240,* 1742–1744.

Ito, K. L. (1985). Ho'oponopono, "to make right": Hawaiian conflict resolution and metaphor in the construction of a family therapy. *Culture, Medicine and Psychiatry, 9*(2), 201–218.

Jenkins, J. H. (1988). Conceptions of schizophrenia as a problem of nerves: A cross-cultural comparison of Mexican-Americans and Anglo-Americans. *Social Science and Medicine, 26*(12), 1233–1243.

Jenkins, J. H. (1991). The state construction of affect: Passion and politics among Salvadoran refugees. *Culture, Medicine and Psychiatry, 15*(2), 139–165.

Jenkins, J. H. (1992). Too close for comfort: Schizophrenia and emotional overinvolvement among Mexicano families. In A. D. Gaines (Ed.), *Ethnopsychiatry: The cultural construction of professional and folk psychiatries* (pp. 203–221). Albany: State University of New York Press.

Jenkins, J. H. (1994). Culture, emotion and psychopathology. In S. Kitayama & H. Markus (Eds.), *Emotion and culture: Empirical studies of mutual influence* (pp. 307–335). Washington, DC: American Psychological Association.

Johnson, T. (1985). Consultation-liaison psychiatry: Medicine as patient, marginality as practice. In R. A. Hahn & A. D. Gaines (Eds.), *Physicians of Western medicine: Anthropological approaches to theory and practice* (pp. 268–292). Dordrecht, The Netherlands: Reidel.

Johnson, T. (1987). Premenstrual syndrome as a Western culture-specific disorder. *Culture, Medicine and Psychiatry, 11*(3), 337–356.

Kay, M. A. (1974). Health and illness in a Mexican-American barrio. In E. Spicer (Ed.), *Ethnic medicine in the Southwest* (pp. 99–166). Tucson: University of Arizona Press.

Kiev, A. (1968). *Curanderismo: Mexican-American folk psychiatry.* New York: Free Press.

Kirmayer, L. J. (1989). Psychotherapy and the cultural concept of person. *Santé, Culture, Health, 6*(3), 241–270.

Kleinman, A. (1980). *Patients and healers in the context of culture.* Berkeley: University of California Press.

Kleinman, A. (1986). *Social origins of distress and disease: depression, neurasthenia, and pain in modern China.* New Haven, CT: Yale University Press.

Kleinman, A. (1988). *Rethinking psychiatry: From cultural category to personal experience.* New York: Free Press.

Kleinman, A., & Good, B. J. (Eds.). (1985). *Culture and depression: Studies in the anthropology and cross-cultural psychiatry of affect and disorder.* Berkeley: University of California Press.

Kleinman, A., & Sung, L. H. (1979). Why do indigenous practitioners successfully heal? *Social Science and Medicine, 13B,* 7–15.

Kluckhohn, C. (1962). American Indians in a white man's world. In *Culture and behavior* (pp. 336–349). New York: Free Press.

Knorr-Cetina, K., & Mulkay, M. (Eds.). (1983). *Science observed.* London: Sage.

Kuhn, T. (1962). *The structure of scientific revolutions.* Chicago: University of Chicago Press.

Kunitz, S. (1989). *Disease change and the role of medicine: The Navajo experiment.* Berkeley: University of California Press.

Laguerre, M. (1981). Haitian Americans. In A. Harwood (Ed.), *Ethnicity and medical care* (pp. 172–210). Cambridge, MA: Harvard University Press.

Langness, L. L., & Levine, H. G. (Eds.). (1986). *Culture and retardation: Life histories of mildly mentally retarded persons in American society.* Dordrecht, The Netherlands: Reidel.

Lee, S. (1996). Cultures in psychiatric nosology: The CCMD-2-R and international classification of mental disorders. *Culture, Medicine and Psychiatry, 20*(4), 421–472.

Leff, J. (1973). Culture and the differentiation of emotional states. *British Journal of Psychiatry, 123,* 299–306.

Lewton, E. (1997). *Living harmony: The transformation of the self in three Navajo religious healing traditions.* Unpublished doctoral dissertation, Case Western Reserve University, Cleveland, Ohio.

Littlewood, R., & Lipsedge, M. (1982). *Aliens and alienists: Ethnic minorities and psychiatry.* Harmondsworth, England: Penguin.

Lock, M. (1991). Nerves and nostalgia: Greek-Canadian immigrants and medical care in Québec. In B. Pfeiderer & G. Bibeau (Eds.), *Anthropologies of medicine* (pp. 87–103). Wiesbaden, Germany: Vieweg und Sohn Verlag.

Lutz, C. (1985). Depression and the translation of emotional worlds. In A. Kleinman & B. J. Good (Eds.), *Culture and depression* (pp. 63–100). Berkeley: University of California Press.

Lutz, C. (1988). *Unnatural emotions: Everyday sentiments on a Micronesian atoll and their challenge to Western theory.* Chicago: University of Chicago Press.

Manson, S. M., Shore, J. H., & Bloom, J. D. (1985). The depressive experience in American Indian communities: A challenge for psychiatric theory and diagnosis. In A. Kleinman & B. J. Good (Eds.), *Culture and Depression* (pp. 331–368). Berkeley: University of California Press.

Maretzki, T. (1992). Georg Groddeck's integrative massage and psychotherapy treatment in Germany. In A. D. Gaines (Ed.), *Ethnopsychiatry: The cultural construction of professional and folk psychiatries* (pp. 379–394). Albany: State University of New York Press.

Marsella, A. (1980). Depressive experience and disorder across cultures. In J. Draguns & H. Triandis (Eds.), *Handbook of cross-cultural psychology: Vol. 6. Psychopathology* (pp. 237–289). New York: Allyn and Bacon.

Mezzich, J., Hughes, C., Good, B., Fábrega, H., Kleinman, A., Gaines, A. D., Guarnaccia, P., O'Nell, T., & Lin, T.-S. (1994). Appendix I: Outline for cultural formulation and glossary of culture-bound syndromes. In American Psychiatric Association, *Diagnostic and statistical manual of mental disorders* (4th ed., pp. 843–849). Washington, DC: American Psychiatric Association.

Nathan, T. (1986). *La folie des autres.* Paris: Dunod.

Obeyesekere, G. (1985). Depression, Buddhism and the work of culture in Sri Lanka. In A. Kleinman & B.

Good (Eds.), *Culture and depression* (pp. 134–152). Berkeley: University of California Press.

Orford, J. (1992). *Community psychology.* New York: Wiley.

Oths, K. S. (1992). Unintended therapy. In A. D. Gaines (Ed.), *Ethnopsychiatry: The cultural construction of professional and folk psychiatries* (pp. 85–123). Albany: State University of New York Press.

Payer, L. (1989). *Medicine and culture.* New York: Penguin.

Pernick, M. (1985). *A calculus of suffering.* New York: Columbia University Press.

Pfleiderer, B. (1991). The development and change of health research among migrant workers in West Germany. In B. Pfleiderer & G. Bibeau (Eds.), *Anthropologies of medicine* (pp. 105–118). Wiesbaden, Germany: Vieweg und Sohn Verlag.

Pickering, A. (Ed.). (1992). *Science as practice and culture.* Chicago: University of Chicago Press.

Prucha, F. P. (1985). *The Indians in American society.* Berkeley: University of California Press.

Racy, J. (1980). Somatization in Saudi women: A therapeutic challenge. *British Journal of Psychiatry, 137,* 212–216.

Reynolds, D. K. (1976). *Morita psychotherapy.* Berkeley: University of California Press.

Reynolds, D. K. (1980). *The quiet therapies: Japanese pathways to personal growth.* Honolulu: University Press of Hawaii.

Robins, L., & Regier, D. (1991). *Psychiatric disorders in America: The epidemiological catchment area study.* New York: Free Press.

Rubel, A. (1964). The epidemiology of a folk disorder: Susto in Hispanic America. *Ethnology, 3,* 268–283.

Schreiber, J. M., & Homiak, J. P. (1981). Mexican Americans. In A. Harwood (Ed.), *Ethnicity and medical care* (pp. 264–336). Cambridge, MA: Harvard University Press.

Shweder, R., & Bourne, P. (1982). Do conceptions of the person vary cross-culturally? In A. Marsella & G. White (Eds.), *Cultural conceptions of mental health and therapy* (pp. 97–137). Dordrecht, The Netherlands: Reidel.

Spitzer, R. L., Gibbon, M., Skodol, A. E., Williams, J. B., & First, M. B. (Eds.). (1994). *DSM-IV casebook.* Washington, DC: American Psychiatric Press.

Townsend, J. M. (1978). *Cultural conceptions and mental illness.* Chicago: University of Chicago Press.

Unschuld, P. (1985). *Medicine in China: A history of ideas.* Berkeley: University of California Press.

Van Moffaert, M., & Vereecken, A. (1989). Somatization of psychiatric illness in Mediterranean immigrants in Belgium. *Culture, Medicine and Psychiatry, 13*(3), 297–313.

Weidman, H. H. (1978). *Miami health ecology project report.* Miami, FL: University of Miami School of Medicine, Department of Psychiatry.

Weidman, H. H. (1979). Falling-out. *Social Science and Medicine, 13B,* 95–112.

Westermeyer, J. (1989). *Psychiatric care of migrants: A clinical guide.* Washington, DC: American Psychiatric Press.

Young, A. (1991). Emil Kraepelin and the origins of American psychiatric diagnosis. In B. Pfleiderer & G. Bibeau (Eds.), *Anthropologies of medicine* (pp. 175–181). Wiesbaden, Germany: Vieweg und Sohn Verlag.

Young, A. (1995). *The harmony of illusions.* Princeton, NJ: Princeton University Press.

21

Occupational Injuries

A Review of Incidence and Factors Associated with Occurrence while at Work

JESS F. KRAUS, AMY S. LIGHTSTONE, AND

DAVID L. McARTHUR

Introduction and Preface

Scope of Review

This chapter encompasses a brief synopsis of information on the occurrence of occupational injury. It includes information exclusively from the United States and focuses mostly on fatalities, as opposed to nonfatal injuries. Information referenced is largely published in the 1990s but findings from reports in the 1970s and 1980s are given as needed for balance and completeness. Though sparse, information is given when it is available about occupational injuries in immigrant populations.

JESS F. KRAUS • Department of Epidemiology, School of Public Health, and Center for Occupational and Environmental Health, University of California at Los Angeles, and Southern California Injury Prevention Research Center, Los Angeles, California 90095-1772. AMY S. LIGHTSTONE AND DAVID L. McARTHUR • Department of Epidemiology, School of Public Health, University of California at Los Angeles, and Southern California Injury Prevention Research Center, Los Angeles, California 90095-1772.

Handbook of Immigrant Health, edited by Loue. Plenum Press, New York, 1998.

Limitations of the Literature Cited

The published scientific literature on workplace injury can be found in a variety of reports across such fields as public health, labor, business, and behavioral and social sciences. Information can also be found in a variety of engineering and industrial development publications. The literature reviewed is restricted to that in the English language. In some places reference is provided to more encompassing documents where in-depth treatments of the subject can be found.

In contrast, obtaining occupational health data on immigrant populations is problematic for a variety of reasons, and few long-term studies have been conducted (Mobed, Gold, & Schenker, 1992; Slesinger & Cautley, 1981). The National Center for Health Statistics has had difficulty obtaining information on migrant workers through the National Health Interview Study because of its sample design and the necessity for those surveyed to live in an established household. Additional obstacles to collecting data on the migrant population include the transient nature of the population and migration in and out of various jurisdictions; problems counting both workers who are not legal and those who meet the legal definition of migrant but are not readily classified by ethnicity, demographics, or occupation; desire of many immigrants to avoid government contact; language barriers; the seasonal nature of much of the work that many immigrants obtain; large distances between camps or farms and remote areas of work; and the lack of uniform definition of migrant and seasonal farmworkers among government agencies (Mobed *et al.*, 1992; Rust, 1990).

Special Terms and Usage

The literature on the subject at times has contained inconsistent terminology describing occurrence of injury. In some places the reference population may be all employed persons and in others the general population is used to calculate rates. In some places there is inconsistency with regard to what is meant by a work-related injury. In some studies specific kinds of injuries are precluded, for example, homicide while at work, certain transportation injuries, and injuries in the military or other special groups. To the extent possible we identify the sources of information where there is inconsistent utilization of terms and meanings. Finally, rates of occurrence are portrayed differently across the literature. In some cases rates are expressed per 100 full time equivalents (FTEs) while in others rates are given per 100,000 work hours or some other base of working time exposure. Frequently, injury counts are portrayed only as proportions. The reader should be cautious about variations over time of the meanings of terms, phrases, and data sources used in different reports.

Occupational injuries among immigrants can be problematic for a variety of additional reasons. While there are no published estimates of the number of days per year worked by immigrants, there is most likely a significant number of days without work for many of those persons, resulting in underestimations of the true size of the immigrant labor work force when counts are based on recorded work hours. The Office of Migrant

Health calculates a count of workers based on crop acreage and number of person-hours required to harvest a given crop; this is likely to undercount the farmworker population by an amount proportionate to the number of farmworkers unemployed during the harvest season (Rust, 1990). Thus, for many reasons, both counts and proportions may be inherently more uncertain for immigrant groups than for others.

Background in Occupational Fatality Data Recording

A full discussion of the development of occupational injury reporting and recording is beyond the scope of this paper but Drudi (1995) has treated this subject well in highlighting the various points in the development and advancement of injury reporting. There have been several major sources of information on fatal injuries in the United States, including the National Safety Council, the National Institute of Occupational Safety and Health, the U.S. Bureau of Labor Statistics, and the U.S. National Health Interview Survey. All of these sources have been subject to varying requirements in reporting and, while not the focus of this review, it should be kept in mind that evolution of methodology has led to better understanding of the accuracy of estimates provided by the agencies mentioned. The first dramatic change in improving accuracy of reporting work-related fatal injury came with the development of the National Traumatic Occupational Fatality System (NTOF) which is maintained by the National Institute of Occupational Safety and Health. This system relies on a single box of the death certificate labeled "Injury at work." There were limitations, however, in how fatal occupational injuries were identified because of lack of a standard classification of work-related injuries or even the definition of what is meant by "work-related." The next major advance came from the U.S. Bureau of Labor Statistics (BLS) and its Census of Fatal Occupational Injuries (CFOI). The census improved upon NTOF by using multiple sources to identify and verify a work-related connection with fatal injuries. While advances in the past 10–15 years have improved the quality of fatal injury enumeration, advances in nonfatal injury enumeration have not kept pace. In fact, the only large-scale source of information on nonfatal injuries (also collected by the BLS) is the Annual Occupational Illness and Injury Survey, which is subject to employer reporting vagaries.

Work-Related Fatal Injuries

Annual Estimates and Comparing Different Data Sources

The number of annual work-related fatal injuries in the United States is still unknown. This may be due to differences in definitions of work-related activity and work-related injury death associated with that activity. In addition, some of the differences in estimates (Table 1) can be accounted for on the basis of differing definitions of the size of the work force and the number of deaths enumerated, more particularly the process by which those deaths are identified. In 1995, work-related deaths reported by the BLS (U.S. Department of Labor, 1997) were based on a multifaceted approach to case finding and verification. The estimate of occupational injury deaths from the National Safety Council (1995) is based on multiple reporting sources including state departments of health, industrial commissions, the National Center for Health Statistics, and other sources. With all factors considered, however, the rates per 100,000 population are reasonably close to one another and suggest an annual estimate in work-related fatal injury rates between 4 and 5 per 100,000 working population per year (Table 1). This rate, in all likelihood, is an underestimate because of the vagaries in classifying certain causes of death. It is known that in some states deaths resulting from motor vehicle crashes while commuting to and from work may be counted by a coroner as work-

related. This is not a consistent pattern and the level of subscription to this practice is unknown across all coroners' jurisdictions in the United States. In addition, deaths to certain persons engaged in self-employment on a part-time or haphazard basis also may not be identified from usual reporting sources. For example, individuals who travel between jobs may not be routinely identified as traveling for that purpose. One type of exposure which is extremely difficult to identify for work-related purposes is air travel in noncommercial private aircraft, particularly helicopters. For example, developers may routinely use helicopters to examine potential building sites but whether that travel is associated with work per se or is done for other reasons is often not known. Another form of inconsistent classification of work-relatedness is to include all those on active military duty, regardless of place of occurrence of the fatality, as "work-related." An additional problem facing the classification of work-related fatalities is the practice in some regions to classify suicide as work-related. In California, it is common that such deaths are labeled work-related only because of the place of occurrence, not because of any true work-related exposure.

With respect to immigrants, the difficulties of obtaining unambigous data are magnified, because no state is required to record migrant status on the death certificate (Rust, 1990). Thus, it is not possible to determine from state records whether a work-related death was suffered by an immigrant.

TABLE 1. Number Employed, and Number and Rate of Work-Related Fatal Injuries per 100,000, United States, 1994

Data source	Number employed (millions)	Number of deaths	Rate per 100,000
Bureau of Labor Statistics	124.5	6,588	5
National Safety Council	122.4	5,000	4

Major Industrial Divisions

With these caveats in mind, the estimates of the fatal injury rates by major industrial divisions are given in Table 2. Contrasting the BLS with the National Safety Council shows concordance in the distribution of rates by the major industrial divisions. Those engaged in agriculture, forestry or fishing, mining, construction, and transportation or public utilities show much higher fatality rates than workers in manufacturing or service occupations. These findings are consistent with other reports showing higher levels of risk as-

sociated with many occupations within these broad industrial groupings.

External Causes

National data from the BLS show the percent distribution of occupational fatal injuries in the private sector by major industrial division and external cause (U.S. Department of Labor, 1982, 1992). Across all industrial divisions almost one third of all fatal injuries while at work occur in transport-related activities. Fatal injuries from falls, assaults, and electrocutions are also among the leading

TABLE 2. Number Employed, Number Fatally Injured, and Fatal Injury Rates per 100,000 by Major Industrial Divisions,[a] 1994.

Industrial divisions[a]	Bureau of Labor Statistics			National Safety Council		
	Number employed (thousands)	Number deaths	Rate/ 100,000[b]	Number employed (thousands)	Number deaths	Rate/ 100,000[b]
Agricultural	3,496	847	24	3,400	890	26
Mining	668	180	27	600	160	27
Construction	6,948	1,027	15	6,200	910	15
Manufacturing	20,050	787	4	18,100	690	4
Transport/public utilities	7,069	944	13	6,100	740	12
Trade	25,611	1,066	4	28,100	450	2
Service	40,912	956	2	41,300	640	2

[a]Limited to those divisions with similar categories for the two data sources.
[b]Rates are not adjusted by age, gender, or related factors.

TABLE 3. Percentage Distribution of Occupational Fatal Injuries, Private Sector, by Industrial Division and Cause, United States, 1990 (BLS)

Cause[a]	Total %	Agricultural	Construction	Mfg	Transport[b]	Trade	Services
Total—all causes (%)	100	100	100	100	100	100	100
Highway vehicles	31	18	15	16	52	46	32
Heart attacks	10	2	10	7	12	9	15
Industrial vehicles or equip.	9	40	13	12	2	6	2
Falls	10	7	21	9	5	4	10
Electrocutions	7	7	15	5	7	2	6
Aircraft crashes	2	1	<1	2	7	0	4
Struck by objects	6	8	8	14	4	2	1
Plant machinery operations	3	1	<1	12	<1	2	2
Assaults	6	1	<1	1	2	17	12
Explosions	4	6	2	9	4	1	2
All others	12	9	16	13	5	11	14

[a]Cause is defined as the object or event associated with the fatality.
[b]Excludes railroads and includes public utilities.

causes of fatal injury deaths. Note, however, that heart attacks are included by the BLS as occupation-related injury deaths (Table 3).

Demographics

Little information is published on gender, race, or other worker demographic-specific fatal injury rates in the United States. Data for the United States reported by the BLS (1995) show that the fatal injury rates per 100,000 population in four broad age categories increase slightly from youngest to oldest age groups. It is noteworthy that those over age 65 are routinely excluded from the analysis because of definitional parameters. However, many investigators have identified those over the age of 65 as being at increased risk of fatal injuries (Kraus, Macurda, & Sahl, 1990). The data in Table 4 are a distinct departure from those published in a mid-1980s review of fatal and nonfatal injuries in occupational settings (Kraus, 1985). While the fatal injury rates for those in age groups 16–24 and 45–54 are about the same as in Maryland in 1978, the rates among those ages 25–44 are considerably higher. Bear in mind that the contrast is for one state only and is based on data averaged over a 10-year period.

Special Concerns

The representation of fatal injuries by cause varies across major industrial divisions. For example, fatalities in occupations associ-

ated with agriculture are more likely to involve industrial vehicles or equipment, while those involved in transport-related activities are more likely to be from highway vehicle crashes. Similarly, those in trade and service occupations are more frequently involved with fatal highway crashes. The percentage distribution of work-related fatal injuries by external causes varies also from place to place. Because of the increasing occurrence of assault-related injuries in the workplace, the section "Work-Related Violent Injury" has been devoted to this topic.

Work-Related Nonfatal Injuries

Definitions and Measures

A recordable occupational injury as defined by the BLS is "an occupational death regardless of time between injury and death . . . or which involves loss of consciousness, restriction of work or motion, transfer to another job, or medical treatment other than first aid" (U.S. Department of Labor, 1992, pp. 1–4). Furthermore, an occupational injury is one that results from a work accident or from exposure involving a single incident in the work environment. Information on new cases of occupational injury for the United States comes from several sources; however, the BLS survey of about 250,000 employer units is the most comprehensive current source of information on nonfatal injuries.

The BLS reports injuries per 100 full-time workers, calculated as: $N/EH \times 200,000$, where N equals the number of injuries or lost workdays, EH means the total hours worked by all employees during the calendar year, and 200,000 is the base equivalent to 100 full-time workers (working 40 hours per week, 50 weeks per year). However, the BLS estimate is restricted to injuries occurring in the private sector and specifically excludes workers on farms with fewer then 11 employees, workers in mines and on railroads, and government workers at all levels.

TABLE 4. Number Employed, Number of Fatal Injuries, and Rate per 100,000 of Fatal Work-Related Injuries by Age, United States, 1994 (BLS)

Age group	Number employed (thousands)	Number fatally injured	Rate per 100,000
16–24	19,464	699	4
25–34	32,829	1,558	5
35–44	33,882	1,608	5
45–64	34,612	2,162	6

Annual Estimates

There were 7.5 recordable injuries per 100 full-time workers reported in the 1995 BLS survey (U.S. Department of Labor, 1997) (Table 5). The reportable injury incidence rate is highest in the construction industry followed by occupations in manufacturing, agriculture, forestry, and fisheries. The lowest work-related reportable nonfatal injury rates are found in finance, insurance, and real estate. Substantial declines in nonfatal work injury rates from 1980 to 1995 can be seen for occupations involving mining. Additional reductions in nonfatal injury rates can be seen also in construction and to a lesser extent in manufacturing and agriculture, forestry, and fisheries. It is noteworthy that the rates, although lowest in finance, insurance, and real estate, showed an increase of approximately 20% between 1980 and 1995. A similar increase was seen in the nonfatal injury rate for occupations involving services.

It has been suggested that the incidence of injuries is probably underestimated for a variety of interrelated reasons. One may be a result of recall bias of injured workers. Another may be exclusion of injured workers from the active workforce. A third may be a consequence of superiors not providing legally required transportation and workers' fear of retribution (hence the workers are hesitant to report the injury or to assert their legal rights) (Ciesielski, Hall, & Sweeney, 1991).

Language may be an important factor influencing the reporting of injuries and thus the calculation of injury incidence rates. In a report of the Joint ILO/WHO Committee on Occupational Health, the following two significant observations were made about language: (1) non-English-speaking migrants are adversely affected on the simplest aspects of everyday life, and (2) migrants are particularly affected at work, where the unintelligibility of verbal communication is exacerbated by the work environment (Corvalan, Driscoll, & Harrison, 1994).

Industries at High Risk

Injury rates per 100 full-time workers for the United States for 1995 in specific industrial subdivisions are summarized in Table 6. Changes in rates from 1980 to 1995 are also given in the table and indicate that in the subdivisions shown there has been a substantial decline in rates over the past 15 years.

TABLE 5. Number Employed in 1995, Nonfatal Injury Rates per 100 Full-Time Workers in 1995 and 1980, and Percent Change, United States, by Major Industrial Categories (BLS)

Industry	Average annual employment (1995)[a] (in thousands)	Rate per 100 full-time workers (1995)	Rate per 100 full-time workers (1980)	% Change from 1980 to 1995
Total—private sector	96,886	7.5	8.5	−11.8
Agriculture, forestry & fisheries	1,641.3	9.3	11.3	−17.7
Mining	582.4	6.0	11.0	−45.5
Construction	5,088.1	10.4	15.5	−32.9
Manufacturing	18,478.4	9.9	11.8	−16.1
Transportation & public utilities	5,857.8	8.7	9.2	−5.4
Trade	27,563.7	7.3	7.4	−1.4
Finance, insurance, & real estate	6,617.6	2.3	1.9	+21.1
Services	30,920.3	6.1	5.1	+19.6

[a]Total private sector does not add by division because of rounding.

TABLE 6. Number Employed and Nonfatal Injury Rates per 100 Full-Time Workers, United States, 1995 and 1980, and Percent Change by Industrial Categories with Highest and Lowest Rates (BLS)

Industry	Average annual employment (in thousands)	Rate per 100 full-time workers (1995)	Rate per 100 full-time workers (1980)	% Change from 1980 to 1995
Primary metal industries	708.1	14.9	14.8	+0.7
Fabricated metal products mfg.	1,438.4	14.5	18.1	−19.9
Lumber & wood products mfg.	767.0	14.2	18.0	−21.1
Transportation equipment	1,783.0	14.2	10.1	+40.6
Trucking & warehousing	1,874.7	13.6	14.7	−7.5
Transportation by air	776.0	13.1	13.0	+0.8
Food & kindred products mfg.	1,680.1	13.0	18.4	−29.3
Furniture & fixtures mfg.	508.9	12.0	15.6	−23.1
Security & commodity brokers	522.5	0.7	0.8	−12.5
Insurance agents & brokers	694.6	1.0	0.8	+25.0
Nondepository institutions	462.5	1.1	1.0	+0.1
Legal services	923.4	0.8	1.4	−42.9

Nonetheless, nonfatal injury rates in primary metal industries, fabricated metal products manufacturing, lumber and wood products, transportation equipment, trucking and warehousing, and transportation by air remain approximately 1.5 to 2 times higher than the overall rate for the private sector of 7.5 per 100 workers. The rates are consistently low for those employed in security and commodity brokerage, insurance agents and brokers, nondepository institutions, and legal services. While there has been a 12.5% to 30% decline in rates among industries with the highest rates in 1980, there was an increase among insurance agents and brokers.

Severity of Work-Related Injuries

Major Industries

Data in Tables 7 and 8 summarize 1995 BLS information (U.S. Department of Labor, 1997) on the general industrial divisions and some specific subdivisions of the industrial divisions having the highest lost-workday case rate. Data in Table 7 show that the highest lost-workday cases (reflecting serious injury) are found among workers in construction, manufacturing, agriculture, forestry and fishing, transportation, and utilities. Also in this table are changes in rates since 1980. Most subdivisions show a decline in serious injury rates with the exception of those employed in finance, insurance, and real estate. Note the substantial decline in serious injury rate (40.6%) among those employed in mining occupations. The proportion of the total nonfatal injury rate represented by lost-workday cases for 1995 is also given in Table 1. While there has been a substantial decline in the rate in occupations in mining, note that almost 82% of the cases are lost-workday cases compared with the total private sector figure of about 52%. Similar excesses in frequency of lost-workday cases can be seen for those in construction, transportation, utilities, agriculture, forestry, and fishing.

TABLE 7. Incidence Rates of Nonfatal Lost-Workday Injury Cases per 100 Full-Time Workers, 1995, Percent Change in Rate From 1980, and Lost-Workday Rate as a Percent of 1995 Overall Rate, United States (BLS)

Industry	Rate per 100 lost-workday cases (1995)	Rate per 100 lost-workday cases (1980)	% Change from 1980 to 1995	Lost-workday rate as a % of 1995 overall rate
Total—private sector	3.4	3.9	−12.8	52.0
Transportation & utilities	5.0	5.4	−7.4	62.1
Construction	4.8	6.5	−26.2	63.5
Manufacturing	4.6	5.2	−11.5	53.5
Agriculture, forestry, & fishing	4.2	5.6	−25.0	61.3
Mining	3.8	6.4	−40.6	81.7
Trade	3.1	3.2	−3.1	42.5
Services	2.7	2.3	+17.4	44.3
Finance, insurance, & real estate	0.9	0.8	+12.5	39.1

TABLE 8. Incidence Rates of Nonfatal Lost-Workday Injury Cases 1995 and 1980, and Percent Change in Rate, for Industries with Highest and Lowest Rates, United States (BLS)

Industry	Rate of lost-workday cases (1995)	Rate of lost-workday cases (1980)	% Change from 1980 to 1995
Food & kindred products	6.9	8.7	−20.7
Coal mining	6.6	8.2	−19.5
Transportation by air	6.3	8.0	−21.3
Trucking & warehousing	5.8	8.9	−34.8
Water transportation	4.8	8.3	−42.2
Lumber & wood products	4.5	9.4	−52.1
Primary metal industries	4.0	6.9	−42.0
Insurance agents & brokers	0.3	0.3	0.0
Security & commodity brokers	0.2	0.3	−33.3
Legal services	0.2	0.2	0.0

Lost Workdays and Body Region and Nature of Injuries

Data in Table 8 show rates of lost-workday cases and change of rate from 1980 for those having the highest and a sample of the lowest lost-workday case rates for 1995. Again, those employed in transportation by air, trucking and warehousing, food and kindred products production, coal mining, water transportation, lumber and wood products, and primary metal services show a lost-workday case rate in excess of the overall average in the United States of 3.4 per 100 workers. Note also the change in rate from 1980 in all of the high-

incidence rate industrial subdivisions, most notably those in lumber and wood products.

There are no published data on the distribution of lost-workday or disabling occupational injuries by nature of the injury or body part involved. For this purpose data from California from 1991 have been used to highlight findings (Table 9). As is typical in most occupational settings, sprains, strains, dislocations, and hernias account for approximately 61% of all reported occupational injuries in California. This is followed by lacerations, puncture wounds, contusions, and crushing injuries. The anatomic regions most frequently affected depend on the nature of

TABLE 9. Percentage Distribution of Disabling Occupational Injuries by Nature of Injury and Body Part Involved, California, 1991

Nature of injury	Number injured	Percent of total	Head/ eyes	Neck	Back/ spine	Trunk	Upper ext.	Lower ext.	Multi. parts	Other	Total %
Amputations	584	<1	0	0	0	0	99	1	0	0	100
Burns	7,368	2	14	6	1	3	44	17	15	<1	100
Contusions & crushing	37,556	11	0	9	4	13	24	35	15	<1	100
Lacerations & punctures	44,656	13	2	11	<1	1	68	14	4	<1	100
Abrasions & foreign bodies (eye)	12,648	4	80	1	<1	<1	7	7	4	0	99
Fractures	22,504	7	0	4	2	10	41	40	4	<1	101
Strains, sprains, dislocations, hernias	206,984	61	0	3	47	15	8	17	10	<1	100
Concussion	1,644	<1	0	100	0	0	0	0	0	0	100
All other	3,716	1	<1	16	1	9	<1	1	59	13	99
Number	337,660	99	11,976	17,308	99,744	38,288	70,512	65,428	33,324	1,080	
Percent of row			4	5	30	11	21	19	10	<1	100

the injury sustained; for example, eye injuries most frequently involve abrasions in foreign bodies, head and neck injuries involve lacerations and punctures, and back and spine injuries involve sprains, strains, or dislocations as well as injuries to the trunk.

Special At-Work Exposures

Work-Related Violent Injury

The earliest scientifically based reports on workplace violent injury appeared only a decade and a half ago: Baker and associates analyzed fatal occupational injuries in Maryland, showing that workers were being murdered on the job (Baker, Samkoff, & Fisher, 1982), and the Centers for Disease Control described homicide among work-related deaths, the first time in a U.S. federal public health publication (Centers for Disease Control and Prevention, 1985). The earliest epidemiologic reports on incidence and features of homicides in work settings were published in the public health literature in 1987 (Davis, 1987; Kraus, 1987).

By the late 1990s the literature has increased greatly. Table 10 summarizes features of several reports on work-related fatalities in relation to external causes including motor vehicle, highway, machinery, homicide, falls, electrocution, struck by or caught in objects, and others. Except for one report, motor vehicle–related crashes (including pedestrians being struck by motor vehicles) have the highest percentage of occurrence after the miscellaneous category. Homicide was the leading cause of work-related injury death in California in 1993, followed by motor vehicle–related causes (California Department of Industrial Relations, 1992–1993). Homicide as a proportion of all work-related fatalities in these same studies averaged 12% in the United States for 1980–1989 to almost 32% in California in 1993. Note that no adjustments for age, gender, or race have been made in the proportions by external cause across these studies.

Since the late 1980s, the National Institute of Occupational Safety and Health (NIOSH) has systematically collected data about occupational fatalities (Bell, Stout, & Bender, 1990; Castillo & Jenkins, 1994; Jenkins, Layne, & Kisner, 1992; U.S. Department of Health and Human Services [USDHHS], 1993a), using death certificates from all 50 states plus New York City

TABLE 10. Percent of Work-Related Fatal Injuries by External Causes, Selected U.S. Studies

External cause	Sniezek & Horiagon N.C. 1978–84 (36)	NIOSH U.S. 1980–89 (43)	CDC TX 1982 (10)	Stone S.C. 1989–90 (38)	Bell et al. U.S. 1980–85 (4)	Cal/OSHA CA (7) 1992	Cal/OSHA CA (7) 1993	Windau & Toscano U.S. 1992 (50)	Toscano[a] 1993 (40)
Motor vehicle[b]	18	23	22	32	24	28	26	24	26
Homicide	17[e]	12	14	13	14	25	31	17	17
Falls	10	10	12	11	11	9	8	10	10
Machinery[c]	9	14	15	9	7	5	3	5	5
Struck by, against	11[f]	7	—	9	6	5	5	9	9
Electrocution	8	7	11	7	6	5	4	5	5
All others[d]	27	27	26	19	32	24	23	39	28

[a] Includes only 31 states.
[b] Includes highway collisions and pedestrians struck by vehicle.
[c] BLS and California do not classify fatalities involving machinery but "caught in or compressed by equipment" is chosen as an approximate equivalent.
[d] Includes drowning, fires, water and aircraft, etc.
[e] Defined as "gun."
[f] Defined as falling object.
— Not reported

and the District of Columbia. This survey showed a homicide rate of 0.71 per 100/000 workers, the third leading cause of injury death accounting for about 12% of all occupational injury deaths. NIOSH published the "NIOSH Alert: Request for Assistance in Preventing Homicide in the Workplace" (USDHHS, 1993b), to bring workplace violence to the attention of the public, to identify high-risk persons, occupations, and workplaces, and to encourage prevention programs and future research.

The BLS has periodically assessed violent workplace injury through a review of death certificates, state workers' compensation reports, coroner and medical examination records, OSHA reports, news media, follow-up questionnaires, state motor vehicle reports, and other sources (U.S. Department of Labor, 1994). Motor vehicle (highway) and other vehicles, combined as transportation, ranked first in occurrence. The second most commonly found cause was homicide (17%), followed by falls (10%) and contact with or struck by objects and equipment (9%). The average annual rate per 100,000 persons of nonfatal work-related assaultive injuries

ranges from 0.18 in the BLS data to 2.4 in a study using different definitions and methods of case finding conducted for the Department of Justice (Bachman, 1994). The latter study reported that approximately 1 million victimizations occur annually while persons are at work; slightly less than 160,000 (16%) of these resulted in injuries, and 10% required medical care.

Work-related homicide rates are disproportionate to the percentage of the workforce by gender: work-related homicide rates are 3.1 to 5.7 times higher for males compared with females (Castillo & Jenkins, 1994; Davis, 1987; Kraus, 1987; Sniezek & Horiagon, 1989; Toscano, 1994; Windau & Toscano, 1994). However, proportionate mortality from homicide is significantly higher for females compared with males. For example, up to 57% of all female work-related fatal injury deaths are due to homicide compared with 30% or less of male work-related deaths.

Limited data are available to provide age-specific at-work homicide rates. Those reports that provide age information on work-related homicide rates show that those 65 years of age and older have the highest rates recorded (Kraus *et al.,* 1990; Sniezek & Horiagon, 1989). For those under age 65, U.S. data (USDHHS, 1993a; Windau & Toscano, 1994) show age-specific rates of 0.4 to 0.9 per 100,000 employed; for those over age 65 the rates increase appreciably to their highest points of 1.7 to 1.9 per 100,000. Especially vulnerable to assault and murder are cooks, bartenders, and security guards. Often these are people who are retired from their usual occupations and work part-time to enhance retirement income or to keep active.

Information is incomplete on the incidence (or rate ratio) of homicide in the workplace according to racial or ethnic group. NIOSH data from 1980–1985 show a rate for employed non-Whites 1.8 times higher than the rate for employed Whites (Bell *et al.,* 1990). Later data from NIOSH show that the rate for employed Blacks is 2.4 times higher than for employed Whites and slightly less than the rate for all other races (USDHHS, 1993a). Data for Texas males show that the rate was highest among employed of "other" racial or ethnic groups (Davis, 1987). Black employed persons showed a rate 1.6 times higher than for Whites and the rate for Hispanics was 1.3 times higher than the rate for "other" Whites. However, in North Carolina the rate for non-White employed was only slightly higher than for White employed (1.1 vs. 0.9 per 100,000 workers) (Sniezek & Horiagon, 1989).

Most reports show elevated homicide rates for those employed in transportation, communication, and public utilities. Homicide rates exceed the overall average in most reports for those employed in public administration (a category that includes police and protective services), while rates are consistently below average for manufacturing, finance and real estate, agriculture-forestry-fisheries-mining, and construction. U.S. findings (Castillo & Jenkins, 1994; Toscano, 1994; Windau & Toscano, 1994) show that laborers or material handlers, persons involved in sales, transportation, service of all kinds, and executive-administrative-managerial positions are at highest risk of homicide while at work. Data

from California (Kraus, 1987) show highest rates in service and laborer or material handling occupations.

Six recent reports (Castillo & Jenkins, 1994; Davis, 1987; Hales, Seligman, & Newman, 1988; Kraus, 1987; Toscano, 1994; Windau & Toscano, 1994) give specific rates for detailed occupations or workplaces. All six reports show that police and detectives have very high rates, and five of the six reports show that taxicab drivers and chauffeurs are at extreme risk. Five reports found that homicide risks are excessive for those employed in eating and drinking places. Several reports show sheriffs, bailiffs, and other law enforcement officials, security guards, service station employees, stock handlers and baggers, bartenders, and sales personnel at elevated risk of homicide. Unfortunately, specific details of exposure remain largely unknown.

In the past decade, the public health literature has suggested that working women are at the same extreme risk of homicide while at work as the elderly working. These groups are especially vulnerable because they appear to be easy targets offering no resistance, or are perceived as having less inclination to interfere in the course of a robbery. In assessing homicide rates for employed women, we recognize that on average women may work fewer hours than men; thus lower rates found for females may not properly reflect person-time exposure. The highest risk occupation for females (based on informal conversation with police agencies) is prostitution. In parts of the U.S. prostitution is a legal enterprise but consistent practice in city and county agencies investigating homicides of prostitutes has been to avoid classifying them as "work-related" or "injury at work." Thus it has been difficult to obtain accurate information. Homicide is the leading work-related external cause of death for all females in a number of reports (Bell, 1991; Davis, Honchar, & Suarez, 1987). One study showed that, except for construction, transportation, and manufacturing, homicide was the leading external cause of injury deaths for females in all industries in Texas (Davis *et al.,* 1987), and that the rates among females were exceptionally high among women involved in sales, clerking, or management of food stores, bars, and cafes. NIOSH reported that 30% of all fatal injuries at work for employed females involve homicide and are involved in three major industries: grocery stores, eating and drinking establishments, and public safety (Castillo & Jenkins, 1994).

Several studies report month, day of week, or hours of peak occurrence of fatal and nonfatal work-related assault injuries (Bell, 1991; Davis, 1987; Hales *et al.,* 1988, Jenkins *et al.,* 1992; Kraus, 1987; Richardson, 1993). Generally, homicides are distributed evenly over the months of the year, although findings on day of the week are inconsistent. One study showed that homicides were evenly distributed over the week (Sniezek & Horiagon, 1989) but another (Davis, 1987) showed that more homicides occurred between Monday and Friday. Although hours of peak occurrence are not reported in uniform time intervals, it appears that homicide or nonfatal assault is far more frequent in the afternoon and evening hours than late morning or early afternoon hours. However, a substantial proportion of all cases in these studies had no hour of occurrence reported.

The exact cause of homicide has been evaluated in numerous reports, which are consistent in one finding: in excess of 70% of all work-related homicides involve a firearm. In most studies, stabbing or cutting with sharp and piercing objects is the second most frequently reported cause. BLS data for 1992 and 1993 show that homicide while at work was a direct result of a robbery or other felony in up to 82% of the instances (Toscano, 1994; Windau & Toscano, 1994). However, findings for California and Texas are substantially less, from 37% to 48% (Davis, 1987; Davis *et al.,* 1987, Kraus, 1987). A high degree of media attention has been paid to worker-on-worker homicides committed by current or former employees, yet the actual proportion of such instances is only from 4% to 10%.

A large proportion of what is known about risk factors for homicide in the workplace is derived from studies based on convenience stores in the United States. One study (Crow & Bull, 1975) analyzed reports of 17,600 robberies of convenience stores in five southern California counties, and on-site surveys of selected stores. A number of features were proposed as important risk factors for a robbery and, by implication, murder and assault in convenience stores: amount of cash available, poor lighting levels at remote points and on-site, obstructions and reduced visibility in and around the store, lack of security devices such as mirrors, easy accessibility and escape routes, among others. Countermeasures addressing these factors, adopted by 60 experimental stores and tested against a control group of 60 similar stores chosen randomly, resulted in reduction in robberies of up to 18% over an 8-month period following their introduction.

A subsequent study of convenience store robbery asked state prison inmates, all of whom had a conviction for robbery, to provide information for ordering the attractiveness of selected factors from the robber's point of view (Crow, Erickson, & Scott, 1987). The top-rated factors were amount of money available, escape route, anonymity, and likelihood of interference. Factors judged most effective as deterrents to robbery were an armed clerk, number of clerks in the store, number of customers in the store, a camera system, and alarm system or video recording system. An intervention program was implemented for which follow-up data showed a 65% decrease in robberies. Another study (Swanson, 1986) found that the 10 factors judged "least appealing" to a robbery were: many customers, heavy traffic in front of store, two or more clerks, a back room, male clerk, one-way mirrors, limited escape routes, alarms, clear visibility into the store, and stores that sell gasoline. The factors judged most appealing for robberies were: store in remote area, only one clerk, no customers, easy access and getaway, lots of cash, female clerks, no back room, obstructed windows, type of safe, and no alarm.

After a police department study of convenience store robberies in the late 1980s, the city of Gainesville, Florida, enacted an ordinance that mandated an unobstructed view of the cash register and sales area through windows, conspicuous signs in the windows indicating less than fifty dollars on hand and that a drop-time release safe was present that could not be removed, parking lots lit with an intensity of approximately two foot candles per square foot, security cameras of a type and number approved by the city manager, and mandatory robber prevention training for all employees who work between 8 P.M. to 4 A.M. In one year Gainesville experienced a reduction in convenience store robberies of 64% and a reduction in the number of robberies from 8 P.M. to 4 A.M. of 75%. No evaluation was made, however, of the experience of surrounding communities in the same period.

Florida's Convenience Store Security Act of 1990 (Clifton & Callahan, 1991) mandated training, posting signs about limited cash, ensuring high visibility of cash registers and clerks from the exterior, a drop-safe limited access component, and improved outside lighting. Florida requires convenience stores to include silent alarms, security cameras, drop-safes and cash management devices, along with specifications for security lighting standards for parking lots, signs on limited cash availability, unobstructed views of cash registers, and prohibition against window tinting, height markers for windows and store entrances, robbery training for employees, and limited cash from 9 P.M. to 6 A.M. However, robberies, murders, and assaults continued. Further legislation was adopted in 1992 addressing businesses open between 11 P.M. and 5 A.M., especially businesses experiencing murder or robbery; the legislation addressed additional security measures such as having two or more employees on the premises at all times from 11 P.M. to 5 A.M., bullet resistant safety enclosures, security guard on the premises, and the conduct of business through an indirect pass-through window or the closing of the business at all times between the hours of 11 P.M. and 5 A.M. Studies testing the effectiveness of these pieces of legislation have not yet been published.

Table 11 summarizes factors from the literature to date that are likely to be important in formulation of specific countermeasures for workplace violence. However, most of these factors are vaguely described and provide only the weakest of platforms from which to fashion specific interventions. On the basis of these markers, factors, and circumstances, one can only be guided toward

TABLE 11. High-Risk Markers, Factors, and Circumstances for Homicide at Work

Risk markers	
Age	Older employed persons show highest rates
Gender	Rate for males is up to 6 times the rate for females, but females are more likely than males to be murdered at work
Race or ethnicity	Black and Hispanic employed persons have higher rates than White employed
Risk factors	
Manner of death	Guns are used more often than any other instrument in fatalities at work
Industry	Retail trades (sales), public administration (security, safety, protection), and transportation
Occupation and worksite	Salesclerks in food stores, liquor stores, eating and drinking places; taxi drivers; police, sheriffs, and security guards; laborers, workers, and supervisors in gas stations, hotels, and motels
Hours of greatest risk	Late afternoon, evening or late at night, especially from 10pm to 2am
Location	One state and several metropolitan statistical areas show elevated rate
Circumstances	
Type of exposure	Robbery preceding fatal injury

broader intuitive interventions. Robbery prevention programs rely on an aggregate of many simultaneous countermeasures aimed at different factors (National Safe Workplace Institute, 1987). Hence it is not possible to isolate a group of factors that is more or less important in deterring robbery and assault.

The possibilities of control and reduction of violence at work are probably better than most because of the potential to incorporate many different approaches—environmental, behavioral, training, and regulatory—to reduce risk. However, the efficacy of specific countermeasures for prevention of violence-related injury is largely unknown. While a few experimental "trials" have been undertaken, seldom have these been designed as randomized trials of specific risk factor modifications. Detailed scientific studies must be made of changes in time trends, shifts in risk among industries and occupations, and consistency of possible interventions across different work sites and businesses. Essential to further progress in injury prevention are a full assessment of risk, identification of situations and circumstances amenable to intervention, and large-scale evaluations to demonstrate effectiveness.

Low-Back Injury

Work-related back injury is one of the most serious health problems experienced by most of the world's workforce and the lower back region is the most common anatomic site involved (Frymoyer, 1990). Between 10% and 17% of the adult population in the United States more than 25 years of age experience an episode of back pain each year (Deyo & Tsui-Wu, 1989) and about three quarters of the U.S. adult population will have low-back pain at least once in their lives (Frymoyer, 1988).

Back injuries account for about one fifth of all compensable work injuries and one third of all costs for work-related injuries (Snook, 1987). Webster and Snook (1990) observed that the cost for compensable low-back pain increased dramatically in the decade of the 1980s. Frymoyer and Cats-Baril (1991) have estimated that the total

costs of low-back injuries in 1990 ranged from $25 to $100 billion.

Occupations with high reported low-back injury occurrence include nurses and hospital workers (Harber, Billet, & Gutowski, 1985), farmers (Lloyd, Gauld, & Soutar, 1986), miners (Lloyd, Gauld, & Soutar, 1986), truck drivers (Kelsey & Hardy, 1975), and material handlers (Bigos et al., 1986), among many others. Activities that appear to be associated with a back injury event include lifting (Bigos et al., 1986; Chaffin & Park, 1973; Lloyd et al., 1986) and bending or twisting (G. B. J. Andersson, 1981; Chaffin & Park, 1973) independently or in combination with one another.

The diagnosis of low-back injury is difficult because of the general absence of objective measures of anatomic damage and an insidious onset. Nonspecificity in diagnosis is reflected in the number of different terms used to describe or classify the problem. Terms used include low-back pain (Andersson et al., 1991), back sprain or strain (Klein, Jenson, & Sanderson, 1984), low-back injury (Clemmer, Mohr, & Mercer, 1991), or low-back pain syndrome (Weeks, Levy, & Wagner, 1991). Diagnoses are based largely on patient reports of symptoms; few objective diagnostic criteria are available. Lack of specificity of definitions and inconsistency in diagnostic criteria has hampered epidemiologic studies of low-back injury and generally prohibited cross-study comparison of findings.

A number of reports in the scientific literature over the past two decades have measured general exposures or risk factors associated with low-back injury. The exposures or risk factors reported to be associated with risk of back injury or pain include manual labor (Clemmer et al., 1991; Heliovaara, 1987), jobs involving vibration (Kelsey & Hardy, 1975), or repetitive tasks (G. B. Andersson, Svensson, & Oden, 1983), age (Frymoyer & Cats-Baril, 1991), gender (Heliovaara, 1989), height and weight (Garg & Moore, 1992), smoking (Heliovaara, 1989), alcohol use (Vallfors, 1985), and medical or psychological stress or both (Frymoyer & Cats-Baril, 1991).

Many of the exposures and factors related to low-back injury have yet to be consistently studied and many more issues need to be addressed, including gender-specific factors of intensity (dose) of exposure and length of experience in cohorts of workers across different occupations.

The most reliable data on risk factors for low-back injury come from a handful of occupational cohort studies conducted from 1979 to 1996 (Table 12). Many different factors have been studied with differences in case definition and case finding across studies. For example, cases have come from

TABLE 12. Design Elements, Factors Studied, and Findings in Selected Occupational Cohort Studies of Low-Back Injury (LBI) or Pain (LBP), United States, 1979–1996

Investigator and year	Study group	Cohort size	Case definition	Factors studied	Findings
Chaffin & Park, 1973	Electronic manufacturing	411	LBI complaints	Maximum wt. lifted, age, wt., ht., LBI history, isometric lift strength	Rate = 6.1/100/yr Incidence increase with wt. increase & strength decrease
Cady et al., 1979	Firefighters	1,652	WC[a] claims	Flexibility, isometric lift strength, recovery heart rate, diastolic blood pressure, energy expenditure	Rate = 0.9/100/yr Least fit had 10 times incidence rate than most fit to work
Herrin et al., 1986	5 industrial plants	6,912	Med. dept. visit for LBI and lost work time	Task type, force, posture, vertical hand location, body movement frequency, left-strength ratio	Back overexertion associated with job stress indices
Bigos et al., 1992	Aircraft assembly	3,020	LBP incident reports/claims	Anthropometry back exams, flexibility, strength, aerobic capacity, med. history, workplace factors, job perceptions, psychological factors	Rate = 2.3/100/yr LBI history, job dissatisfaction and psychosocial responses most predictive of LBI
Rossingol et al., 1993	Aircraft assembly	205	LBI claims or complaints at med. dept.	Pain, activities of daily living, LBP history, age, body mass index, smoking, sports, work satisfaction, health care	Rate = 6/100/yr History of LBP significant, 16% absent per year with LBP
Leino, 1993	Metal industry	607	Clinical exam, 4-point scale, pain/range of motion, neurological signs	Physical activity, smoking, body mass index, stress symptoms, LBI history, depression, workload	Strenuous activity had modest inverse independent effect on clinical findings
Kraus et al., 1996	Retail home improvement stores	~36,000	Cal/OSHA report forms	Age, gender, length of employment, lifting intensity, back support use	Rate = 1/100/yr LBI rate reduced 34% with back support use

[a]WC = workers' compensation.

workers' compensation claims or medical department visits. The overall rates on injury reported within the cohorts range from less than one to approximately 6 per 100 full-time workers per year. There is a consistent finding in a few reports that those who are less fit (measured by lifting or strength testing) are more likely to sustain low-back injury.

Some preventive measures have been introduced to prevent work-related back injuries with emphasis on worker training, job screening, and ergonomic modification. This last approach is currently recommended by the U.S. National Institute of Occupational Safety and Health yet objective evidence of the effectiveness of these factors either alone or in combination has been nonconclusive and subject to many methodologic problems. A recent study by Kraus and colleagues (1996) reported evidence that among home improvement retail store employees in California the use of back supports resulted in significant reduction in low-back injury claims. The application of back supports and subsequent evaluation in other occupations, different workplace settings, or various work tasks have yet to be undertaken.

Work-Related Injuries during Adolescence

Approximately 5 million teenagers worked in the United States in 1991 (Halloway, 1993), and it was estimated that, during 1993, about 2 million persons 16 or 17 years of age were employed for some hours per week. No reliable or routinely collected data exist for working adolescents less than 16 years of age. Based on 1993 *Morbidity and Mortality Weekly Reports* (USDHHS, 1996) employer reports from approximately 250,000 private industries in the United States, there were approximately 21,620 injuries involving lost days of work to employed persons less than 18 years of age.

It has long been recognized that working adolescents need to be protected by law. In 1911, the Triangle Shirtwaist Company fire in New York City took the lives of 145 young women because of blocked exits, and was the impetus for legislation leading to current workers' compensation laws. Workers compensation insurance systems were adopted in all but six states by 1920. But it was not until 1938 that the Fair Labor Standard Act (FLSA) was adopted with child labor protection laws including federal wage, hour, and safety regulations. The law as stated by the U.S. Department of Labor (1985) prohibits persons younger than 18 years of age from working in 17 hazardous nonagricultural occupational and industrial settings including the manufacturing and storing of explosives, mining, logging, excavation, demolition, manufacturing of brick and tile, slaughtering and meat packing, roofing operations, exposure to radioactive substances, driving motor vehicles, and operating selected power-driven equipment. Furthermore, the U.S. Department of Labor (1984) prohibits hazardous agriculture work on nonfamily farms for children younger than 16 years of age, although there is no age or hazard restriction for children working on family farms. At age 14, adolescents may deliver newspapers, stock supermarket shelves, ring up and bag groceries, pump gas, and wash cars. The FLSA is enforced by the Wage and Hour Division (WHD) of the Department of Labor. In addition to the federal Fair Labor Standard Act, all states have also sanctioned child labor laws. Still, work injuries among adolescents remain a significant problem. Despite fluctuations in employment, annual injury rates remain relatively constant for 14- and 15-year-olds, but have increased for 16- and 17-year-olds (Belville, Pollack, Godbold, & Landrigan, 1993).

Earlier studies have called for rates of work-related injuries in adolescents so that risk factors can be elucidated and prevention measures implemented. In particular, the nature of the injury, the mechanism of injury, and the industry in which the injury occurred were examined by various studies.

From 61% to 82% of the injury types are accounted for in the three categories of cuts and lacerations (17%–49%), contusions (9%–25%), and sprains and strains (10%–31%) (Table 13). Burns were less frequent (6%–13%), as were fractures and dislocations (with most studies reporting in the range of 3%–7% occurrence, except for the study by Belville *et al.*, 1993, that reported a 20% occurrence). Amputations and concussions were very rare (i.e., less than 2% of the time).

Adolescent workers were most often injured by cutting or piercing objects (30%–42%), followed by being struck by or against an object (12%–25%) and falls (10%–21%) (Table 14). Overexertion was considered the mechanism of injury 6–17% of the time, and hot, caustic, and corrosive substances was the mechanism of injury 7%–9% of the time.

The industry responsible for more than 50% of adolescent injuries was wholesale and retail trade (Table 15). Up to 24% of adolescent injuries happened in the services industry, and 10% or less occurred in the industries of manufacturing, agriculture, or construction.

The rates of adolescent injuries varied among studies depending on the age and sex examined (Table 16). Only two studies

TABLE 13. Percent of Adolescent Occupational Injuries by Nature of Injury in Selected Studies, United States

Injury type	Brooks *et al.* 1993 Massachusetts	MMWR 1996 U.S.	Banco *et al.* 1992 Connecticut	Parker *et al.* 1991 Minnesota	Belville *et al.* 1993 New York	Schober *et al.* 1988 U.S.
Cuts/lacerations	49.1	17	35	26.5	35.3	36.5
Contusions	12.2	13	25	8.8	9.2	12.8
Sprains/strains	9.6	31	22	27.1	17.9	17.3
Burns	6.4	8 (heat)	7	11.4 (heat) 1.7 (chem)	7.1 (heat) 0.5 (chem)	9.7
Fractures/dislocations	3	5	3	5.7	18.1 (fx) 1.5 (dis)	5.8 (fx) 0.7 (dis)
Concussion	2	N/R	N/R	N/R	0.6	N/R
Amputations	0.4	N/R	N/R	0.4	1.2	0.6
Other	17.3	26	8	18.3	8.5	16.6
Total	100	100	100	100	100	100

N/R = Not reported.

TABLE 14. Percent of Adolescent Occupational Injuries by Mechanism of Injury in Selected Studies, United States

Injury mechanism	Brooks *et al.* 1993 Massachusetts	MMWR 1996 U.S.	Banco *et al.* 1992 Connecticut
Cutting/piercing objects	41.7	N/R	30
Struck by/against object	12	17	25
Falls	9.6	21	13
Hot/caustic/corrosive	6.8	9	7
Overexertion	6.3	17	17
Other	23.6	36	8
Total	100	100	100

N/R = Not reported.

Table 15. Percent or Rate of Adolescent Occupational Injuries by Industry in Selected Studies, United States

Industry	Banco *et al.* 1992 Connecticut	Parker *et al.* 1991 Minnesota	Belville *et al.*[a] 1993 New York	Schober *et al.* 1988 U.S.
Wholesale/retail trade	79.7	61.2	33.2/100,000	53.6
Services	11.5	24.1	16.0/100,000	20.9
Manufacturing	3.5	5.8	49.0/100,000	9.1
Agriculture	0.3	2.8	46.2/100,000	6.1
Construction	0.4	2.1	32.6/100,000	3.7
Other	4.5	4	N/R	6.7

[a]Expressed as rate per 100,000 employed persons.
N/R = Not reported.

TABLE 16. Rate of Adolescent Occupational Injuries by Age and Various Study Findings, United States

Study (author & year)	Source of injury data	Age of population at risk (years)	Findings (rate[a])
Brooks *et al.* (1993)	Massachusetts emergency departments	16 & 17 males	21.9/100 FTEs
		16 & 17 females	8.9/100 FTEs
		Overall (16 & 17)	16.0/100 FTEs
Schober *et al.* (1988)	Workers' compensation reports to BLS	16 & 17 males	12.6/100 FTEs
		16 & 17 females	6.6/100 FTEs
Belville *et al.* (1993)	New York workers' compensation	16	1.1/100 FTEs
		17	1.9/100 FTEs
Parker *et.al.* (1991)	Minnesota Dept. of Labor first report of injury	12–14	0.2/100 FTEs
		15–17	0.68/100 FTEs
		12–17	1.4/100 FTEs

[a]FTE = Full-time equivalent.

(Brooks, Davis, & Gallagher, 1993; Schober, Handke, Halperin, Moll, & Thun, 1988) stratified the data by sex (although the latter does not report an overall unstratified result). Other studies reported rates by age or a range of ages not stratified by sex. Comparisons between studies cannot be evaluated.

The databases currently available from workers' compensation claims, medical records, death certificates, and the U.S. Department of Labor all are limited in scope and definition, strongly suggesting underreporting of adolescent work-related injuries.

Workers' compensation claims often are not filed as many youths are unaware of the procedure or knowledge about workers' compensation, discouraged or intimidated by their employer from making a claim, or fearful of losing their jobs, especially if working in violation of the law or if family immigration status is uncertain (Belville *et al.,* 1993; Halloway, 1993). Also, workers may not be covered by the state compensation plan, may not have missed enough days from work (some claims can be filed only after a certain number of days are lost from work), may have received compensation from another source, may be employed part-time or in a temporary position which influences whether a claim is submitted, may have been injured while working for a family business where injuries often are not reported, or may be in agricultural labor which may not be covered by workers' compensation laws (as in most states) (Halloway, 1993; Schober et al., 1988).

Adolescent work injuries are also underreported in medical records and death certificates. Physicians often do not record or even ask information related to a young patient's occupation (Halloway, 1993). Identification of work-related deaths and appropriateness of occupation and industry information on the death certificate are inadequate (Castillo, Landen, & Layne, 1994).

U.S. Department of Labor records have data only on wage and hour infractions (Halloway, 1993). The BLS does not have data stratified by age (Suruda & Halperin, 1991). The Occupational Health and Safety Administration (OSHA) maintains a database covering 47 states. OSHA investigates approximately 25% of all work-related deaths, but does not cover work-related homicides, most transportation accidents, deaths in industries regulated by other federal agencies (e.g., the Mine Safety and Health Administration, the Department of Transportation), and deaths among federal employees. OSHA death investigations are concentrated in construction and manufacturing and report few deaths in agriculture (Castillo et al., 1994). In addition, there are variations among reports from states as there is a lack of standardization of information (Belville et al., 1993) and different criteria for qualification for workers compensation. Some states submit all current claims, while others submit only closed cases (Schober et al., 1988).

In order to determine rates of occurrence, a reliable count of the population at risk is necessary. Currently, person-at-work data are known to be underreported (Belville et al., 1993; Parker, Clay, Mandel, Gunderson, & Salkowicz, 1991).

The number of adolescents employed in jobs prohibited by law has increased as enforcement of child labor laws has decreased due to budget cuts and inadequate staffing which have limited the ability of the U.S. Department of Labor to conduct sweeps. For example, in 1991, in the United States, 27,528 children were discovered in illegal jobs (an increase of 300% since 1983); the New York Department of Labor found that the number of city establishments illegally employing children rose from 19 in 1987 to 122 in 1988 (Halloway, 1993); Suruda and Halperin (1991) found that 41% (43) of the injuries occurred while doing work prohibited by FLSA, and in 70% of the deaths OSHA issued citations for safety violations.

No comprehensive statistics that encompass the total number of children working in agriculture exists. Migrant and seasonal farmworkers' average family income is $4,700, necessitating that their children work. Migrant farmworker children face additional hazards of substandard, makeshift or nonexistent housing in fields (Wilk, 1993).

The resurgence of child labor in the United States in the 1980s and early 1990s appears to reflect the convergence of four factors: (1) a strong economy with nearly full adult employment; (2) increased poverty and an increase in the number of children living below the poverty line; (3) a growing number of (illegal) immigrants (minority and low-income adolescents are more likely to be employed in hazardous occupations); and (4) relaxed enforcement of federal child labor laws (Belville et al., 1993; Halloway, 1993).

To better understand and implement prevention of adolescent work injuries and deaths in the future, better data, education, and legislation are called for. There is a need to develop better injury surveillance, at both the federal and state levels, for identification of work-related adolescent injuries and deaths as well as monitoring working adolescents. This includes an increased sensitivity by primary care providers and emergency department staff to consider a possible work-related injury when examining an injured adolescent patient. Data coding with standard definitions of industry, occupation, and source and nature of the injury is essential so that a database or registry can be accessed and epidemiologic comparisons can be made. Other factors to consider in future studies (in addition to age, gender, industry, occupation, source and nature of the injury, and number of days lost due to injury) include job training, specific types of work exposures, job supervision, work permits, time of day of incident, number of hours worked per week, and whether working while attending school (Castillo *et al.*, 1994; Schober *et al.*, 1988).

Adolescent workers must have good job health and safety training and supervision. In addition, awareness must be increased among parents, school officials, and employers about child labor laws and potential hazards for the adolescent worker (Belville *et al.*, 1993; Castillo *et al.*, 1994).

There is a need for better enforcement of and compliance with existing federal child labor laws. It is necessary to evaluate the appropriateness of FLSA, adopted in 1938, and consider a wider extension of child labor laws to cover agriculture and modify other potentially hazardous industry activities (e.g., machinery use) (Castillo *et al.*, 1994; Schober *et al.*, 1988).

Work-Related Injuries and Fatalities among Farmworkers

Agricultural workers are a population at high risk for occupational injury and death. A major problem in understanding the causes and planning for preventive measures is a lack of surveillance data. In the 1940s data sources consisted only of newspaper clippings and personal interviews. By the late 1960s, survey procedures were standardized but they are now no longer appropriate (Murphy & Huizinga, 1989). There is a lack of consistency from one study to another mainly due to the different methods used to collect the data and different definitions of the worker population at risk (Myers & Hard, 1995). Most reporting methods focus on workers who are 16 years of age and older so there is underreporting of juvenile deaths (<16 years). Also it appears that agricultural deaths are assigned to other industries because the usual industry of the victim is not stated as agricultural (Myers & Hard, 1995).

Studies have confirmed that death certificate data are not reliable when certain occupations such as farming and agriculture industries are considered (Russell & Conroy, 1991). There is a need for detailed data that address both specific farm types and farm workers at high risk.

The average annual United States fatality rate for agricultural workers, from 1980 through 1989, was 22.9 deaths per 100,000 workers compared with the average annual fatality rate for the civilian working population of 7.0 deaths per 100,000 workers (Myers & Hard, 1995). The average annual machine-related fatality rate for the U.S. civilian working population is 0.95 deaths per 100,000 workers. Agricultural production has a 10-fold higher average annual machine-related fatality rate (Myers & Hard, 1995). Mainly due to rollovers, farm tractors are the most frequent machine-related cause of death (Myers & Hard, 1995). The annual rate of occupational fatalities related to machines decreased during the 1980s, possibly because of mandates for rollover protection structures on farm tractors. The annual rate for machine-related fatalities still remains higher than the total annual fatality rate for the entire civilian work force. Occupational agricultural deaths from falling objects (primarily trees), have a sixfold higher average annual fatality rate (2.9 deaths per 100,000 workers), compared with deaths due to falling objects in the U.S. civilian working population of 0.5 deaths per 100,000 workers (Myers & Hard, 1995) (Figure 1).

There was a decrease in the annual occupational fatality rates during the 1980s. On the other hand, occupational fatality rates increased with age especially among males (Myers & Hard, 1995) (Table 17). Part of the risk for agriculture-related fatalities can be attributed to an increasing use of machinery in agricultural production and exposure to falling objects in agricultural services (Myers & Hard, 1995). From 1930 to 1980, the fatality rate from nonfarm machinery decreased by 78%, yet the fatality rate from farm machinery increased by 44% (Nordstrom, Brand, & Layde, 1992).

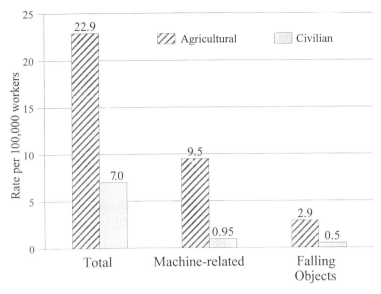

FIGURE 1. Occupational fatality rates for agricultural workers compared to nonagricultural workers in the U.S., 1980–1989, overall and for specific cases. Data derived from Myers and Hard (1995).

The highest injury rates were associated with specialty livestock operations, such as horse farms and fur farms with 12 injuries per 100 FTEs, followed by beef, hog, and sheep operations with 8.2 injuries per 100 FTEs, miscellaneous farming operations with 7.9 injuries per 100 FTEs, and nursery operations with 7.3 injuries per 100 FTEs (Myers, 1993). Family members were more likely to work on farms (63.8%) than hired workers (35.2%) and the rate of injury for a family member is 7.0 injuries per 100 FTEs compared with that of a nonfamily member of 5.5 injuries per 100 FTEs (Myers, 1993).

Currently, exposures and risk factors for agriculture-related injuries remain unknown. Since there is no mandatory reporting system for agricultural injuries and fatalities, data to guide intervention and prevention efforts are largely unavailable. This absence of data especially affects what we know about injuries among migrant workers, as noted earlier. Agricultural production and work practices are changing dramatically resulting in a substantial increase in farmers with nonfarm jobs and a greater involvement of women, seasonal workers, and youth in agricultural operations. Surveillance and epidemiologic studies are needed to identify the extent of mortality, morbidity, risk factors, and mechanisms of injury so opportunities for intervention and injury prevention can be developed.

At any one time, there are an estimated 5 million migrant and seasonal farmworkers in the United States, with about 20% of those living or working in California. The California migrant labor force is estimated to be between 600,000 and 1.1 million including dependents (Mobed *et al.,* 1992). California is the largest employer of migrant and seasonal farmworkers, more than double the next largest employers, Texas, Florida, North Carolina, and Washington (Go & Baker, 1995). More than 80% of farmwork in California is performed by hired labor (Schenker, 1996).

The Office of Migrant Health estimates that there are 3 million "migrant and seasonal farmworkers and their dependents" in the United States (Rust, 1990). The BLS noted a decline in migrant farmworkers from 400,000 in the 1960s to 200,000 in the 1970s (Rust, 1990). The numbers differ as the Office of Migrant Health's definition is "migrant and seasonal farmworkers and their

TABLE 17. Distribution of Occupational Agricultural Fatalities and Injuries by Gender, Ethnicity, Age, and Primary Causes, United States

	Fatalities 1980–1989		Injuries 1993
Average rates:	22.9 deaths/100,000 workers		6.5 injuries/200,000 hrs worked[a]
Total death:	6,727		201,081
	Percent (number)	Rate (per 100,000 workers)	Percent (number)
Gender			
Male	98.5% (6,626)	25.5	90.0% (181,070)
Female	1.5% (101)	1.5	9.7% (19,479)
Total	100.0% (6,727)		99.7% (200,549)
Race/ethnicity			
White	81.4% (5,479)	20.2	75.9% (152,544)
Black	6.9% (466)	26.4	21.8% (43,742)
Hispanic	9.8% (658)	20.7	0.7% (1,422)
Other	1.7% (112)	18.9	1.3% (2,518)
Unknown/missing	0.2% (12)		0.4% (855)
Total	100.0% (6,727)		100.0% (201,081)
Age (years)			**Age (years)**
16–24	13.6% (915)	12.9	10–19 6.4% (12,873)
25–34	17.7% (1,190)	15.9	20–29 18.9% (37,926)
35–44	13.4% (902)	15.9	30–39 24.8% (49,796)
45–54	14.6% (981)	20.3	40–49 18.2% (36,511)
55–64	18.1% (1,217)	26	50–59 15.1% (30,341)
65+	22.4% (1,506)	52.4	60–69 10.4% (21,009)
			70+ 5.9% (11,946)
Total	99.8% (6,711)		99.7% (200,402)
External cause			
Machinery	37.7% (2,538)		17.1% (34,442)
Motor vehicle	16.8% (1,131)		3.0% (6,070)
Struck by object	7.8% (522)		5.4% (10,910)
Electrocution	7.1% (479)		Not reported
Falls	5.3% (359)		21.1% (42,369)
Caught	2.0% (134)		6.2% (12,493)
Tractor	Incl. in machinery		5.4% (10,939)

[a]200,000 hours worked is equivalent to 100 FTEs.
Note: Specific rates were not available for injuries.

dependents" which is very broad and results in a large estimate in contrast to the Department of Labor and Department of Agriculture definitions which generally count only employed farmworkers 14 years of age or older, each department using different methodology (Rust, 1990). Another source estimated the total number of migrant and seasonal farmworkers plus dependents as slightly greater than 4 million, not quite 2% of the total U.S. population, but accounting for more than 2% of the United States health problems (Go & Baker, 1995). This 4 million is composed mostly of Latinos, African Americans, Haitians, Asians, West Indians, and Native Americans (Wilk, 1993). In the United States, the number of migrant and seasonal farmworkers is greater than the number of farmers and family workers (the number of people residing on farms has decreased, while there has been an increase in hired labor). This does not fully reflect the dependence of U.S. agriculture on hired workers (which varies with specific commodities and farm practices) (Schenker, 1996). For example, the average labor required for fruits and vegetables is 120 hours per acre whereas for grains it is 3 hours per acre. Labor-intensive crops are primarily farmed by migrant and seasonal laborers (Schenker, 1996).

Current estimates of the agricultural population do not have the needed accuracy or reliability to be used as the denominator in calculating morbidity and mortality (Rust, 1990). Migrant and seasonal farmworkers are not counted as a separate category from other farmworkers by most agricultural surveys; therefore, national agriculture accident statistics include all farm workers (Mobed et al., 1992). Study populations often vary and can include migrant, migrant and seasonal, or a composite of farmworkers, crew chiefs, and farm managers; also, families and dependents may or may not be included as well as unemployed farmworkers (Rust, 1990). Adding to the problem of correctly ascertaining accurate population counts is that the migrant labor season is generally from March to September with peaks in July and August (Go & Baker, 1995). In addition, reported accounts generally underestimate the dependence of agriculture on hired workers (Mobed et al., 1992). Most occupational injury categories outlined by the National Safety Council have rarely been studied in migrant and seasonal farmworkers (Mobed et al., 1992). Moreover, even when field workers are treated in the emergency room, they are seldom explicitly identified as migrant workers (Go & Baker, 1995).

No formal studies of risk of musculoskeletal and soft-tissue conditions have been examined in migrant and seasonal farmworkers, although research has shown that farmworkers are exposed to many risk factors associated with musculoskeletal injuries (Mobed et al., 1992). Data on work injuries for farmworkers compared with other industries are not readily available as workers' compensation data for agriculture are not widely available (there are numerous exclusions, exemptions, and loop-

holes) and, because agriculture is physically dispersed, collecting data about injuries would require substantial time and money (Mobed et al., 1992). Further complicating surveillance of occupational injury in migrant and seasonal workers is the difficulty in locating and identifying farmworkers and gaining their cooperation. In addition, underreporting is possible if symptoms are mild or short-lived as symptoms may be ignored for fear of losing the job or being reported to immigration authorities (Mobed et al., 1992). Migrant farmworkers may be denied access to care for occupational injuries, can be penalized for being injured, and rarely receive compensation for lost work (Ciesielski et al., 1991). Such underreporting of injuries among migrant and seasonal farmworkers may contribute to the underestimation of agricultural injuries (Schenker, 1996).

Migrant farmworkers have been characterized as being poor, marginally educated, employed at tasks requiring rigorous manual labor, and seldom members of any established community (Bleiweis, Reynolds, Cohen, & Butler, 1977). Demographically, in the United States they are predominantly young, male, foreign-born Hispanic, one half have less than 8 years of education, and about half of the migrant and seasonal farmworkers are below the poverty level as defined by the Census Bureau (Schenker, 1996). Substandard housing contributes to increased risk of accidents and sanitation-related diseases for farmworker adults and children (Wilk, 1993).

An early study of migrant farmworker injuries was conducted in three counties in northern Florida in the mid 1970s (Bleiweis et al., 1977). Locating and counting the number of people in the migrant farmwork was the first problem encountered. Three counts were conducted over 6 months; while the total size of the population did not vary, the individuals themselves changed by approximately 35%–40% in each census. Interviews were conducted with 552 people. The percentage of migrant workers who reported an injury is more than 1½ times as many as the national sample. Many acute conditions, particularly a high incidence of injuries and musculoskeletal problems, were probably related to work.

In a 1981 survey of migrant farmworkers in Tulare County, California, the relationship between work and health was examined (Mobed *et al.*, 1992). The most frequently reported work-related health problem was injuries, accounting for 56% of all health problems reported. Primary causes of farm accidents for those who worked with field crops were falling stacks of crates, overturning gondolas, and other accidents associated with farm machinery (forklifts and tractors). Tree accidents (falling down from or through ladders with bags full of fruit) resulted in fractures, sprains, contusions, lacerations, and puncture wounds.

A more recent study of injuries among migrant farmworkers was a cross-sectional study of occupational injuries among randomly selected persons living in 22 migrant camps in North Carolina (Ciesielski *et al.*, 1991). There were 24 (8.4%) injuries reported, over the previous three years, of the 287 migrant farmworkers participating in the study. Fractures, sprains, and cuts accounted for 80% of the injuries. Vehicles or machinery was the cause of 21% of the injuries which often resulted in time lost from work; 15 of 24 injuries (63%) resulted in the loss of more than one day of work.

Efforts to educate the migrant and seasonal populations should be made to increase awareness of agricultural health hazards and these efforts must be culturally and linguistically appropriate (Schenker, 1996). Farmworker Justice Fund, Inc. (FJF), a national not-for-profit Washington, DC–based organization, advocates for better wages and working conditions for migrant and seasonal farmworkers in the United States (Wilk, 1993).

Acknowledgments

Support for this work was provided by the Southern California Injury Prevention Research Center (C.D.C. grant # CCR 903622) and the UCLA Center for Occupational and Environmental Health.

References

Andersson G. B., Svensson, H. O., & Oden, A. (1983). The intensity of work recovery in low back pain. *Spine, 8,* 880–884.

Andersson, G. B. J. (1981). Epidemiologic aspects on low-back pain in industry. *Spine, 6,* 53–60.

Andersson, G. B. J., Pope, M. H., Frymoyer, J. W., & Snook, S., (1991). Epidemiology and cost. In M. H. Pope (Ed.), *Occupational low back pain: Assessment, treatment and prevention.* St. Louis, MO: Mosby-Year Book.

Bachman, R. (1994). *Violence and theft in the workplace* (U.S. Department of Justice, Bureau of Justice Statistics, No. NCJ-148199). Washington, DC: U.S. Government Printing Office.

Baker, S. P., Samkoff, J. S., & Fisher, R. S. (1982). Fatal occupational injuries. *Journal of the American Medical Association, 248,* 692–697.

Banco, L., Lapidus, G., & Braddock, M., (1992). Work-related injury among Connecticut minors. *Pediatrics, 89,* 957–960.

Bell, C. A. (1991). Female homicides in United States workplaces 1980–1985. *American Journal of Health, 81,* 729–732.

Bell, C. A., Stout, N. A., & Bender, T. R. (1990). Fatal occupational injuries in the United States, 1980 through 1985. *Journal of the American Medical Association, 263,* 3047–3050.

Belville, R., Pollack, S. H., Godbold, J. H., & Landrigan, P. J. (1993). Occupational injuries among working adolescents in New York State. *Journal of the American Medical Association, 269,* 2754–2759.

Bigos, S. J., Spengler, D. M., Martin, N. A., Zeh, J., Fisher, L., & Nachenson, A. (1986). Back injuries in industry: A retrospective study: III. Employee-related factors. *Spine, 11,* 252–256.

Bleiweis, P. R., Reynolds, R. C., Cohen, L. D., & Butler, N. A. (1977). Health care characteristics of migrant agricultural workers in three north Florida counties. *Journal of Community Health, 3,* 32–43.

Brooks, D. R., Davis, L. K., & Gallagher, S. S. (1993). Work-related injuries among Massachusetts children: A study based on emergency department data. *American Journal of Industrial Medicine, 24,* 313–324.

California Department of Industrial Relations, Division of Labor Statistics and Research. (1992–1993). Unpublished data.

Castillo, D. N., & Jenkins, E. L. (1994). Industries and occupations at high risk for work-related homicide. *Journal of Occupational Medicine, 36,* 125–132.

Castillo, D. N., Landen, D. D., & Layne, L. A. (1994). Occupational injury deaths of 16- and 17-year olds in the United States. *American Journal of Public Health, 84,* 646–649.

Centers for Disease Control and Prevention. (1985). Fatal occupational injuries—Texas, 1982. *Morbidity and Mortality Weekly Report, 34,* 130–139.

Chaffin, D. B., & Park, K. S. (1973). A longitudinal study of low-back pain as associated with occupational weight lifting factors. *American Industrial Hygiene Association Journal, 34,* 513–525.

Ciesielski, S., Hall, S. P., & Sweeney, M. (1991). Occupational injuries among North Carolina migrant farmworkers. *American Journal of Public Health, 81,* 926–927.

Clemmer, D. I., Mohr, D. L., & Mercer, D. J. (1991). Low-back injuries in a heavy industry: I. Worker and workplace factors. *Spine, 16,* 824–830.

Clifton, W., Jr., & Callahan, P. T. (1991). *Convenience store robberies: An intervention strategy by the city of Gainesville, Florida.* Gainesville: Gainesville, Florida, Police Department.

Corvalan, C. F., Driscoll, T. R., & Harrison, J. E. (1994). Role of migrant factors in work-related fatalities in Australia. *Scandinavian Journal of Work, Environment, and Health, 20,* 364–370.

Crow, W. J., & Bull, J. L. (1975). *Robbery deterrence: An applied behavioral science demonstration.* La Jolla, CA: Western Behavioral Sciences Institute.

Crow, W. J., Erickson, R. J., & Scott, L. (1987). Set your sights on preventing retail violence. *Security Management, 31,* 60–64.

Davis, H. (1987). Workplace homicides of Texas males. *American Journal of Public Health, 77,* 1290–1293.

Davis, H., Honchar, P. A., & Suarez, L. (1987). Fatal occupational injuries of women, Texas 1975–1984. *American Journal of Public Health, 77,* 1524–1527.

Deyo, R. A., & Tsui-Wu, M. S. (1989). Descriptive epidemiology of low-back pain and its related medical care in the United States. *Spine, 12,* 264–268.

Drudi, D. (1995). The evolution of occupational fatality statistics in the United States. In *Fatal workplace injuries in 1993: A collection of data analysis* (Report 891, pp. 1–5). Washington, DC: U.S. Department of Labor Statistics.

Frymoyer, J. W. (1988). Back pain and sciatica. *New England Journal of Medicine, 318,* 291–300.

Frymoyer, J. W. (1990). Magnitude of the problem. In J. N. Weinstein & S. W. Weisel (Eds.), *The lumbar spine* (pp. 32–38). Philadelphia: Saunders.

Frymoyer, J. W., & Cats-Baril, W. L. (1991). An overview of the incidence and costs of low back pain. *Orthopedic Clinics of North America, 22,* 263–271.

Garg, A., & Moore, J. S. (1992). Epidemiology of low-back pain in industry. *Occupational medicine: State of the art reviews, 7,* 593–608.

Go, V., & Baker, T. (1995). Health problems of Maryland's migrant farm laborers. *Maryland Medical Journal, 44,* 605–608.

Hales, T., Seligman, P. J., & Newman, S. C. (1988). Occupational injuries due to violence. *Journal of Occupational Medicine, 30,* 483–487.

Halloway, M. (1993). Occupational injuries among children are increasing. *Scientific American, 269,* 14–16.

Harber, P., Billet, E., & Gutowski M. (1985). Occupational low-back pain in hospital nurses. *Journal of Occupational Medicine, 27,* 518–524.

Heliovaara, M. (1987). Occupation and risk of herniated lumbar intervertebral disc or sciatica leading to hospitalization. *Journal of Chronic Diseases, 40,* 259–264.

Heliovaara, M. (1989). Risk factors for low back pain and sciatica. *Annals of Medicine, 21,* 257–264.

Jenkins, E. L., Layne, L. A., & Kisner, S. M. (1992). Homicide in the workplace: The U.S. experience, 1980–1988. *AAAOHN Journal, 40,* 215–218.

Kelsey, J. L., & Hardy, R. J. (1975). Driving motor vehicle as a risk factor for acute herniated lumbar intervertebral disc. *American Journal of Epidemiology, 102,* 63–73.

Klein, B. P., Jensen, R. C., & Sanderson, L. M. (1984). Assessment of workers' compensation claims for back strains/sprains. *Journal of Occupational Medicine, 26,* 443–448.

Kraus, J. F. (1985). Fatal and nonfatal injuries in occupational settings: A review. *Annual Review of Public Health, 6,* 403–418.

Kraus, J. F. (1987). Homicide while at work: Persons, industries, and occupations at high risk. *American Journal of Public Health, 77,* 1285–1289.

Kraus, J. F., Macurda, J., & Sahl, J. (1990). Work-related fatal injuries in older California workers, 1975–1985. *Journal of Occupational Accidents, 12,* 223–235.

Kraus, J. F., Brown, K., McArthur, D., Peek-Asa, C., Samaniego, L., Kraus, C., & Zhou, L. (1996). The effects of back supports on the occurrence of acute low back injury. *International Journal of Occupational and Environmental Health, 2,* 264–273.

Lloyd, M. H., Gauld, S., & Soutar, C. A. (1986). Epidemiologic study of back pain in miners and office workers. *Spine, 11,* 136.

Mobed, K., Gold, E. B., & Schenker, M. B. (1992). Occupational health problems among migrant and seasonal farm workers In *Cross-cultural medicine—A decade later* [Special issue]. *Western Journal of Medicine, 157,* 367–373.

Murphy, D. J., & Huizinga, M. A. (1989). A new approach to collecting farm accident data. *Journal of Safety Research, 20,* 21–29.

Myers, J. R. (1993). *Injuries among farm workers in the United States.* Washington, DC: U.S. Department of Health and Human Services, Division of Safety Research, Division of Standards Development and Technology Transfer.

Myers, J. R., & Hard, D. L. (1995). Work-related fatalities in agricultural production and services sectors, 1980–1989. *American Journal of Industrial Medicine, 27,* 51–63.

National Safety Council. (1995). *Accident facts.* (Library of Congress Catalog Card No.: 91-60648). Itasca, IL: Author.

National Safe Workplace Institute. (1987). *Understanding crime prevention.* Stoneham, MA: Butterworth.

Nordstrom, D. L., Brand, L., & Layde, P. M. (1992). *Epidemiology of farm-related injuries: Bibliography with abstracts.* Washington, DC: U.S. Department of Health and Human Services, National Institute for Occupational Safety and Health.

Parker, D. L., Clay, R. L., Mandel, J. H., Gunderson, P., & Salkowicz, L. (1991). Adolescent occupational injuries in Minnesota: A descriptive study. *Minnesota Medicine, 74,* 25–28.

Richardson, S. (1993). Workplace homicides in Texas, 1990–1991 (Report 845). Washington, DC: U.S. Department of Labor, Bureau of Labor Statistics.

Russell, J., & Conroy, C. (1991). Representativeness of deaths identified through the injury-at-work item on the death certificate: Implications for surveillance. *American Journal of Public Health, 81,* 1613–1618.

Rust, G. S. (1990). Health status of migrant farmworkers: A literature review and commentary. *American Journal of Public Health, 80,* 1213–1217.

Schenker, M. B. (1996). Preventive medicine and health promotion are overdue in the agricultural workplace. *Journal of Public Health Policy, 17,* 275–305.

Schober, S. E., Handke, J. L., Halperin, W. E., Moll, M. B., & Thun, M. J. (1988). Work-related injuries in minors. *American Journal of Industrial Medicine, 14,* 585–595.

Slesinger, D. P., & Cautley, E. (1981). Medical utilization patterns of Hispanic migrant farmworkers in Wisconsin. *Public Health Report, 96,* 255–263.

Sniezek, J. E., & Horiagon, T. M. (1989). Medical-examiner-reported fatal occupational injuries, North Carolina, 1978–1984. *American Journal of Industrial Medicine, 15,* 669–678.

Snook, S. H. (1987). The costs of back pain in industry. In R. A. Deyo (Ed.), *Occupational back pain— spine: State of the art reviews* (Vol. 2, No. 1, pp. 1–5). Philadelphia: Hanley and Belfus.

Stone, P. W., (1993). Traumatic occupational fatalities in South Carolina, 1989–1990. *Public Health Reports, 108,* 483–488.

Suruda, A., & Halperin, W. (1991). Work-related deaths in children. *American Journal of Industrial Medicine, 19,* 739–745.

Swanson, R. (1986). *Convenience store robbery analysis: A research study of robbers, victims, and environment.* Unpublished report of the Gainesville, Florida, Police Department.

Toscano, G. (1994). National census of fatal occupational injuries, 1993 (USDL No. 94, p. 384). Washington, DC: U.S. Department of Labor, Bureau of Labor Statistics.

U.S. Department of Health and Human Services, Public Health Service, Centers for Disease Control and Prevention, National Institute of Occupational Safety and Health. (1993a). *Fatal injuries to work-ers in the United States, 1980–1989. A decade of surveillance.* Cincinnati, OH: DHHS (NIOSH).

U.S. Department of Health and Human Services, Public Health Service, Centers for Disease Control and Prevention, National Institute of Occupational Safety and Health. (1993b). *NIOSH Alert: Request for assistance in preventing homicide in the workplace.* Cincinnati, OH: DHHS (NIOSH).

U.S. Department of Health and Human Services/Public Health Service Center for Disease Control. (1996). Work-related injuries and illness associated with child labor—United States, 1993. *Morbidity and Mortality Weekly Report, 45,* 464–468.

U.S. Department of Labor. (1984). *Child labor requirements in agricultural occupations under the Fair Labor Standards Act* (Child Labor Bulletin No. 102; U.S. Department of Labor Wage and Hour Pub. 1295). Washington, DC: U.S. Government Printing Office, Employment Standards Administration, Wage and Hour Division.

U.S. Department of Labor. (1985). *Child labor requirements in nonagricultural occupations under the Fair Labor Standards Act* (Child Labor Bulletin No. 101; U.S. Department of Labor Wage and Hour Pub. 1330). Washington, DC: U.S. Government Printing Office, Employment Standards Administration, Wage and Hour Division.

U.S. Department of Labor, Bureau of Labor Statistics. (1982). *Occupational injuries and illnesses in the United States by industry, 1980.* Washington, DC: Author.

U.S. Department of Labor, Bureau of Labor Statistics. (1992). *Occupational injuries and illnesses in the United States by industry, 1990.* Washington DC: Author.

U.S. Department of Labor, Bureau of Labor Statistics. (1994). *Violence in the workplace comes under close scrutiny.* Summary, pp. 94–100. Washington, DC: Author.

U.S. Department of Labor, Bureau of Labor Statistics. (1997). *Workplace injuries and illnesses in 1995.* Washington DC: Author.

Vallfors, B. (1985). Acute, subacute and chronic low back pain, clinical symptoms, absenteeism and working environment. *Scandinavian Journal of Rehabilitation Medicine, 11* (Suppl.), 1–98.

Webster, B. S., & Snook, S. H. (1990). The cost of compensable low back pain. *Journal of Occupational Medicine, 32,* 13–15.

Weeks, J., Levy, B., & Wagner, G. (Eds.). (1991). *Preventing occupational disease and injury. "Low back pain syndrome."* Washington, DC: American Public Health Association.

Wilk, V. A. (1993). Health hazards to children in agriculture. *American Journal of Industrial Medicine, 24,* 283–290.

Windau, J., & Toscano, G. (1994). *Workplace homicides in 1992.* Washington, DC: U.S. Department of Labor, Bureau of Labor Statistics.

22

Reproductive Health

LYDIA DeSANTIS

Introduction

Reproductive health is composed of four elements: (a) fertility regulation without adverse side effects; (b) risk-free pregnancy and childbirth; (c) having and raising healthy children; and (d) enjoying sexual relationships without fear of infection, unwanted pregnancy, or social and physical abuse (Doyal, 1995; Pan American Health Organization [PAHO], 1994). Reproductive health is central to health in general. Responsibility for reproductive health is borne overwhelmingly by females since males do not need to control their fertility to control their bodies and health status (Doyal, 1995; World Health Organization [WHO], 1996). Reproductive ill health is also a female burden since women must bear the biological consequences of unwanted pregnancies, unsafe abortions, reproductive tract infections, breast feeding, morbidity and mortality due to pregnancy and childbirth, and the culturally delegated responsibility for child care (PAHO, 1994; WHO, 1996). Consequently, this chapter focuses on the reproductive health of immigrant women (IW).

Due to space limitations, the discussion focuses on aspects of reproductive health especially relevant to immigrants, that is, eth-

nomedical (folk) concepts of reproductive anatomy and physiology, prenatal care, pregnancy outcomes, infectious diseases that impact pregnancy, nutritional deficiencies, contraception, and female circumcision. Cultural beliefs and practices are integrated throughout the discussion and represent those commonly attributed to the group under consideration. They cannot be generalized to all members of the group or other groups due to intra- and intergroup variations in factors such as socioeconomic status, gender, age, context, and life experiences. They are presented to assist health care providers (HCPs) to assess the cultural dimension of the reproductive health care of the individual immigrant woman.

Concepts of Reproductive Anatomy and Physiology

The reproductive care of IW necessitates HCPs understand variations in concepts of anatomy and physiology that direct immigrant decision making about conception, birth, and pre- and postnatal behavior. Concepts of anatomy and physiology are not static and vary with age, physiological and psychological states, socioeconomic status, and gender. Three conceptualizations of anatomy and physiology common to many ethnomedical (folk, popular, or traditional) belief systems are presented. For more in-depth discussion of cultural constructs of

LYDIA DeSANTIS • School of Nursing, University of Miami, Coral Gables, Florida 33124-3850.

Handbook of Immigrant Health, edited by Loue. Plenum Press, New York, 1998.

anatomy see DeSantis (1997), Good (1980), Helman (1994), Nichter and Nichter (1996a, 1996b, 1996c), and Sobo (1992).

Theories of Balance

Overview

Balance models are an ethnomedical (folk) adaptation of the humoral and balance theories underlying Hippocratic and Galenic medicine, Arabic and Unani traditional medicine, Chinese traditional medicine, and Ayruvedic (traditional East Indian) medicine. Health results from maintaining a harmonious or balanced relationship between individuals and their environment (social, physical, and supernatural). Illness results when an imbalance or disharmony of elements occurs within individuals or between individuals and their environment. Treatment consists of measures to restore balance or harmony (Anderson, 1987; DeSantis, 1997; Helman, 1994). Balance depends on internal and external forces. External forces (cosmic) include foods, fluids, and medicines ingested, supernatural entities, and environmental elements, such as climate, water, air, seasons of the year, or time of day. Internal forces (body–mind–spirit) include emotions, genetic or inherited conditions, fears, and anxieties.

Hot–Cold

Hot–cold is the most common balance theory and has been incorporated into ethnomedical systems in Latin and Central America, the Caribbean, the Middle East, Asia, and Africa. Hot and cold are conceptualized as being symbolic opposite states of the body. The normal state of the body varies on the hot–cold continuum depending on life stage and external and internal forces. Cross-culturally, pubescent girls, young adult women, and pregnant women are usually considered to be in warm to hot states while older women, and those postpartum or menstruating, are considered to be in cool to cold states (Anderson, 1987; Landerman, 1987).

Hot–cold states are symbolic classifications and have no relationship to actual body temperature. Foods, medications, herbs, and fluids are usually dicotomized into parallel symbolic classifications of hot or cold. No consistent physiological or cultural principle underlies what is hot or cold. The hot–cold power of internal and external factors can be determined only by observing their effects on the body, and people often reclassify the factors based on their own practical experience. High caloric and fatty foods, animal products, and spicy foods are classified as "hot," whereas vegetables, fruit, and foods high in water content are "cold" (Helman, 1994).

Pregnancy is a hot state and much of pregnancy behavior is directed at keeping the woman's body in balance. East Indian women attribute morning sickness to an increase in body heat. Miscarriages, premature births, burning on micturition, oliguria, and white vaginal discharge are signs and symptoms of dangerous overheating of the body (Nichter & Nichter, 1996b). Concepts of hot–cold during pregnancy exist among Malaysian, Puerto Rican, Latin and Central American, Haitian, Iranian, and Korean IW (Anderson, 1987; DeSantis, 1997; Kendall, 1987; Landerman, 1987).

Many of the same groups attribute infertility to the uterus being too cold to nourish the developing fetus. Abortions can be caused by increasing the heat in the womb, for example, abdominal massage to bring "hot blood" to the womb, intake of "hot" foods and herbal medicines, and overheating the body through excessive exercise, wrapping the body in warm clothing or blankets, confinement in an exceptionally hot room, or a combination of these practices (Kendall, 1987; Landerman, 1987).

The critical factor in dealing with hot–cold beliefs during pregnancy and postpartum is to ascertain the individual immigrant woman's concept of foods, medicines, activities, and environments that are safe. If they are contradictory to biomedical concepts, methods will need to be found to accommodate them in order to maintain adequate nutrition and other healthful self-care activities. The principle of "neutralization" can often be utilized to allow biomedically or ethnomedically contraindicated foods and medicines to be taken. Neutralization may be accomplished by giving foods or medicines classified as "neutral or intermediate" or "less cold" or "less hot." Alternative forms of medications may also be acceptable, for example, giving a liquid rather than solid form. For more information on food and medication classifications see DeSantis (1997), Helman (1994), and Nichter and Nichter (1996b, 1996c).

Blood Beliefs

The status and function of blood are central to many IW's concepts of health and reproduction, especially those from the Caribbean, African, Southeast Asian, and Middle Eastern regions and Islamic and Jewish cultures (DeSantis, 1997; Good, 1980; Siegel, 1986; Sobo, 1992). The ethnomedical properties and meanings attributed to blood focus on characteristics considered necessary to keep the person alive (e.g., volume, color, strength, temperature, viscosity, purity) rather than on biomedical concepts of blood components (e.g., cells, fluids, electrolytes). The status of blood is affected by gender and age. Women and older and younger individuals have less and weaker blood, causing them to have more illness and less energy and strength.

Restoration of the normal state of the blood can be achieved through administration of medications and herbs, diet, purging, removal of blood, modifying activity, avoiding exposure to extremes of temperature, and resolving psychosocial conflicts. Blood beliefs are especially important in reproductive health in three areas—menstruation, contraception, and hypertension. Beliefs related to contraception are discussed in the section on fertility regulation. For further information about blood beliefs see DeSantis (1997), Helman (1994), and Sobo (1992).

Menstruation

Expulsion of menstrual blood is considered as cleansing the woman's body of impurities that have built up monthly, restoring her to a healthy state, and ensuring her continued fertility. Menstruation is a cold body state and hot–cold measures are employed to keep the body in balance and maintain a balance to maintain blood flow. Of special importance are measures taken to avoid cold or sudden emotional shocks that will interfere with menstrual blood flow. A decreased flow or failure to expel "bad blood" may cause blood to accumulate in the uterus and result in cancer or blood clots. Too much blood or "high blood" will result in (a) hypertension, (b) headaches or strokes, (c) heart palpitations and "heart" conditions (emotional or psychosocial problems), or (d) hemoptysis by blood backing up in the lungs. Increased blood flow will result in too little or "low" blood, causing (a) weakness, (b) anemia, dizziness, lack of energy, and fainting, (c) premature aging, (d) infertility and loss of libido, and (e) a general vulnerability to illness (DeSantis, 1997; Good, 1980; Helman, 1994; Severy, Thana, Askew, & Glob, 1993).

Hypertension/Hypotension

HCPs doing health teaching about hypertension with IW should be aware that IW often understand the biomedical terms "hypertension" or "high blood pressure" to mean "too much blood" or "high blood" or interpret them to mean they are in a state of being "hyper-tense" due to a combination of context-related emotional and social factors. Their response is to lower or lessen the blood volume by adjusting food and fluid intake or taking herbal medicines rather than or as well as adhering to biomedically prescribed treatments. Many ethnomedical foods or fluids used to adjust blood volume or quality may be contraindicated by or potentiate biomedically prescribed medications, dietary advice, or activity levels. For example, Caribbean and African immigrant women often consider consumption of acidic foods heavy in sodium content and low in nutrients the best way to decrease blood volume. They also administer sodium-laden purgatives, such as Epsom salts, throughout pregnancy to decrease blood volume and cleanse the blood of the woman and fetus (DeSantis, 1997; Helman, 1994; Sobo, 1992).

The need of HCPs to be aware of the ethnomedical concepts related to hypertension is especially important when dealing with IW's reproductive health care. IW are often prone to hypertension (blood pressure of 140/90 or higher) due to the stress of migration, acculturation, and the adverse social and economic circumstances they face both in their country of origin and host country (Doyal, 1995; Helman, 1994; Weinstein, Dansky, & Iacopino, 1996). Multiple studies of hypertension in Asian, African, Caribbean, and Latin and Central American immigrants have demonstrated early and potentially chronic hypertension or risk factors for hypertension (Berenson, Wattigney, & Webber, 1996; Crespo, Loria, & Burt, 1996; Imazu *et al.*, 1996). Hypertension may lead to preterm births, low-birth-weight babies, and maternal strokes, renal damage, convulsions, and chronic hypertension with superimposed pregnancy-induced hypertension (Doyal, 1995; Helman, 1994). Also of concern is health teaching about hypertension for IW diagnosed with preeclampsia and eclampsia.

Confusion may also ensue over health teaching related to hypotension, "low blood pressure" or anemia, all of which may be understood by IW to mean not enough blood, "low blood," or "weak blood." Red foods, liquids, drinks, and medicines are symbolically related to strong and healthy blood. Pregnant women are encouraged to ingest red meats and other foodstuffs high in sodium content, as well as red wine, other alcoholic beverages, or red drinks to increase or strengthen their blood (DeSantis, 1997; Helman, 1994; Sobo, 1992). Concepts specifically related to anemia and the nutritional status of immigrant women are discussed under nutrition.

Prenatal Care and Pregnancy Outcomes

Early enrollment in prenatal care enhances favorable pregnancy outcomes, that is, lower infant mortality rates, fewer preterm births (<38 weeks gestation), and fewer low-birth-weight babies (<2500 gms). In a review of interdisciplinary and international research, Goldenberg, Patterson, and Freese (1992) identified demographic, situational, and psychosocial variables that influence the initiation of prenatal care. Goldenberg and colleagues stress that it is the interaction between the variables that best explains the initiation of early prenatal care. The exact combination or combinations of variables have not been adequately studied, especially in relation to pregnancy outcomes for IW.

Demographic variables consistently related to inadequate or late initiation of prenatal care are (a) maternal age of less than 20 years and greater than 35–40 years, (b) increased parity (4 or more deliveries), (c) low level of maternal education, (d) low household income often in combination with lack of health insurance, (e) lack of a stable relationship with a mate, and (f) ethnicity-race. In general, Black women receive less prenatal care than White women, but it is unclear whether race is an important predictor in and of itself or a surrogate measure of other maternal indicators.

Major situational variables are practical, external factors that cause IW not to obtain prenatal care. These are (a) lack of child care, (b) transportation difficulties, (c) distance from facilities, (d) residence in rural areas, (e) conflicts with scheduled clinic times, (f) insufficient knowledge about available resources, and (g) inability to purchase health care. Even when IW are enrolled in Medicaid, there has been a history of HCPs' reluctance to accept Medicaid payments or lack of adequate facilities to meet the need for prenatal care.

Psychosocial variables consistently affecting lack of early enrollment in prenatal care include (a) unplanned or unwanted pregnancies, (b) denial or delayed diagnosis (after the first 4 months) of pregnancy, (c) difficulty deciding whether to abort the pregnancy, (d) lack of "uncomfortable" symptoms associated with pregnancy during the first 4 months, (e) poor past experiences with HCPs, (f) a previous unfavorable pregnancy outcome, and (g) limited family or social support.

Other factors of special importance when planning prenatal care for IW are (a) access to and use of care, (b) gender of the HCP, (c) beliefs about prenatal care, (d) concerns about pelvic examinations, and (e) concerns and misperceptions about biomedical prenatal care.

Access to and Use of Prenatal Care

Many barriers affecting immigrant access to biomedical care in general also affect IW's access to and use of prenatal care. Studies in the United States, Europe, and elsewhere show that a large number of immigrants (a) suffer racial, gender, social, and political discrimination in the host country; (b) are unable to better themselves economically or socially; (c) are ineligible for many social, economic, and health care programs; (d) are reluctant to seek care due to questionable immigration status; and (e) have similar adverse health problems as indigenous minority and low-income populations in the host nation (Bollini & Siem, 1995; "Famine-Affected, Refugee, and Displaced Populations," 1992; Venema, Garretsen, & van der Mass, 1995). Such barriers will likely increase in the United States due to recent federal and state legislation affecting eligibility of legal and illegal immigrants for health care, child care, and other services combined with cutbacks in health care funding and growing societal resentment of immigrants (Trachtenberg, 1996).

Concepts of Modesty and Gender of the Provider

IW frequently express reluctance to seek prenatal care due to concepts of modesty and privacy. Hispanic, Muslim, and Southeast Asian women feel embarrassed when multi-ple persons are present during prenatal examinations, the HCP is male, or the genitalia are exposed. Southeast Asian women do not expose the area between the waist and knees even in privacy. Muslim and Hispanic women often desire the presence of another family member or their husbands if the HCP is male. Most IW are accustomed to female HCPs for reproductive care and provision of female providers will enhance their receptivity to prenatal care in a strange system (Alcalay, Ghee, & Scrimshaw, 1993; Beine, Fullerton, Palinkas, & Anders, 1995; Hutchinson & Baqi-Aziz, 1994; Mattson, 1995).

Concepts of modesty and privacy also cause IW embarrassment when discussing matters of reproductive health with HCPs if it is not culturally acceptable to discuss such topics with strangers. Concerns about privacy may be alleviated by provision of HCPs of the same gender, ethnic/racial group, and age as the IW or inclusion of appropriate family members (or both), or working through indigenous peer support persons during health assessments (Alcalay *et al.,* 1993; Beine *et al.,* 1995)

Pelvic Examinations

Pelvic examinations are among the most anxiety-producing aspects of prenatal care. They are uncomfortable, painful, may indicate pathology, and are greatly embarrassing and shameful for women who value modesty and privacy (Domar, 1986; Mattson, 1995). Many IW are reluctant to seek biomedical prenatal care due to its reliance on multiple pelvic examinations and use of male examiners. Of special concern are IW who left their countries of origin due to war, civil unrest, or ethnic violence. Many Cambodian, Rwandan, Burundi, Ethiopian, and other IW have been raped, sexually tortured, or brutally searched for items of value they had hidden in their vaginas. For such IW, pelvic examinations are physically and psychologically traumatic events and should be limited to the minimum number necessary to ensure a healthy pregnancy (Mattson, 1995; Weinstein *et al.,* 1996).

Beliefs about Prenatal Care

A common belief of Hispanic, Caribbean, African, Middle Eastern, and other IW women is that prenatal care is not necessary unless they experience some overt sign of difficulty or discomfort. Such signs are usually considered more important early in pregnancy than later (Alcalay *et al.,* 1993; Mattson, 1995).

Based on previous experiences with multiple pregnancies or lack of prenatal care, many IW consider pregnancy a natural event rather than a medical condition and fear the intrusive methods involved in biomedical prenatal care. They see little reason to obtain medical care, will seek care only when they feel "something is wrong," or will avoid initiating care until late in the pregnancy (Doyal, 1995; PAHO, 1994; Raikes, 1989).

The rise in caesarian section rates throughout the world has led many IW to avoid prenatal care for fear that the baby will be removed surgically if they do not deliver "naturally" on their due date. Caesarian sections are seen as interfering with child spacing and future "natural" (vaginal) deliveries and as being more incapacitating and dangerous than vaginal birth (Beine *et al.,* 1995; Doyal, 1995).

Pregnancy Outcomes

Singh and Yu (1996) used an interlinking combination of national databases to compare differences in adverse pregnancy outcomes (higher rates of infant mortality, low-birthweight babies, and preterm births) between U.S.–born and foreign-born women having children in the United States. Based on maternal nativity, there was considerable variation in pregnancy outcomes across the ethnicracial groups surveyed. Ethnic-racial groups included non-Hispanic Whites, Blacks, Chinese, Japanese, Filipinos, other Asians (Asian Indians, Koreans, and Vietnamese), Mexicans, Puerto Ricans (born outside the 50 states and the District of Columbia), Cubans, and Central and Latin Americans.

Data from the 1985, 1986, and 1987 birth cohorts of the Linked Birth and Infant Death data sets showed that immigrant or foreign-born (hereafter referred to as immigrant) women had better pregnancy outcomes than their U.S.–born counterparts. Substantially fewer risk factors for infant mortality and low birth weight are attached to being foreign born and having immigrant status in general and to Blacks, Cubans, Mexicans, and Chinese in particular. There is no apparent increased risk of preterm births for either immigrant or U.S.–born women as a total population, but there is a 15%–25% lower risk for infants born to Japanese, Mexican, and Black immigrant mothers.

IW had lower infant mortality rates per 1,000 live births across all ethnic groups except those from Central and Latin America. For ease of comparison, the immigrant rate is given followed by the U.S.–born, e.g., (foreign-born/U.S.–born). Chinese (5.8/7.0) and Japanese (6.1/7.1) IW had the lowest rates of infant mortality followed by Filipinos (6.9/8.9), Cubans (7.1/11.6), Mexicans (7.6/8.8), non-Hispanic Whites (7.6/8.3), Central and Latin Americans (7.8/7.5), other Asians (7.9/11.2), Puerto Ricans (10.4/11.4), and Blacks (13.5/18.5).

Except for other Asians (10.9/9.8), IW have a lower percentage rate of preterm births than their U.S.–born counterparts. Chinese (7.1/7.9) and Japanese (7.2/8.5) IW again have the lowest rates followed by non-Hispanic Whites (8.0/8.0), Cubans (9.0/10.3), Mexicans (10.0/11.8), Central and Latin Americans (10.1/10.6), Filipinos (10.8/11.5), Puerto Ricans (12.3/12.8), and Blacks (13.1/18.5).

Except for other Asians (6.4/6.3), IW have a lower percentage of low-birth-weight babies. Lowest percentages were in Chinese (4.7/6.5) and Mexican (5.0/6.6) IW followed by non-Hispanic Whites (5.2/5.5), Cubans (5.6/7.0), Central and Latin Americans (5.7/6.8), Japanese (5.9/6.5), Puerto Ricans (8.7/9.4), and Blacks (8.8/13.1).

The ethnic-nativity groups with the most favorable pregnancy outcomes have a lower prevalence of the following risk factors: (a) substantially lower adolescent births with Chinese (0.6) and Japanese (1.4) IW having the lowest percentages and U.S.–born Puerto Ricans (26.4), Central and Latin Americans (25.3), Blacks (24.4), and Mexicans (22.7) the highest; (b) fewer out-of-wedlock births with Chinese (2.8) and Japanese (5.2) IW having the least and U.S.–born Central and Latin Americans (65.1), Blacks (64.0), and Puerto Ricans (54.2) the most; and (c) residence in predominately metropolitan counties. U.S.–born groups had higher education levels with 54% of Chinese having completed 4 or more years of college followed by 42% of Filipino IW and U.S.–born (41%) and immigrant (39%) Japanese women. Regardless of country of birth, Mexican (74.6/42.3) and Puerto Rican (46.7/43.8) women were less likely to have completed 4 or more years of education. IW in general had a higher fertility level (4 or more children) and less prenatal care begun in the first trimester.

Compared with immigrant mothers, U.S.–born Hispanics (9%/3%), Blacks (14%/4%), and Asians (14%/3%) are three times as likely to smoke while non-Hispanic Whites (20%/11%) are almost twice as likely to smoke. Analysis of the 1988 National Maternal and Infant Health Survey (NMIHS) shows that U.S.–born mothers use alcohol 2.3 more times and marijuana or cocaine 3.9 more times during pregnancy than their immigrant counterparts. Exposure to environmental tobacco smoke while pregnant was likely to occur 1.3 to 1.9 times in U.S.–born non-Hispanic White and Black mothers and in Hispanic mothers than in their immigrant counterparts.

The NMIHS shows that immigrant Black and Asian mothers live with stable partners or in extended family households 6%–9% more often than their U.S.–born counterparts. Hispanic IW (10%) were more likely to live alone than U.S.–born Hispanic women (6.6%). IW breast feed at a substantially higher rate, especially Black IW who breast feed three times more than U.S.–born Blacks.

Asian (43.2%), Hispanic (21.8%), and Black (19.5%) IW are less likely to report unwanted or unplanned pregnancies than their U.S.–born counterparts.

Infectious Diseases

Infectious diseases are closely related to gender and reproductive health. The greatest incidence occurs mainly in the poorest groups with females especially vulnerable due to the political, social, and economic inequities that affect them from birth (Diaz, 1996). IW often present with a variety of infectious diseases not generally seen by HCPs in the United States in association with pregnancy. The most prominent infectious diseases found worldwide that affect pregnant women are briefly discussed. For greater detail on their gender and epidemiological characteristics, treatment, prevention, and control see Benenson (1995), Diaz (1996), and Schmunis (1993).

Leprosy

Leprosy affects 3.1 million persons worldwide. India accounts for 52% of all cases and 27% come from Bangladesh, Brazil, Indonesia, Myanmar, and Nigeria (WHO, 1996). The normal immune depressive effect of pregnancy is of concern since the disease may be exacerbated in pregnant women, resulting in sensory and motor damage by the time several pregnancies have gone to term (Schmunis, 1993).

Malaria

Malaria is suspected of having some immunosuppressive effects, making pregnant women more vulnerable to infections (Koblinsky, 1995; Schmunis, 1993). Africa accounts for more than 90% of the clinical cases of malaria, but serious malaria problems are present in Afghanistan, Brazil, India, Sri Lanka, Thailand, and Vietnam. Pregnant women with malaria have an abortion rate of up to 30% in the first half of pregnancy and increased anemia, especially if compounded by schistosomiasis (bilharziasis) and hookworm (Schmunis, 1993). Approximately 44 million women are pregnant and infected with hookworm (WHO, 1996).

Schistosomiasis

About 200 million people in 74 tropical nations are infected by schistosomiasis, and 500–600 million are at risk due to bathing, wading, or working in lakes, rivers, and irrigation canals infested by blood flukes (trematodes) (Benenson, 1995; WHO, 1996). Women are especially vulnerable since their daily routines and work put them in contact with infected water. The disease is endemic throughout most of Africa, Southeast Asia, the Middle East, South America, and the Caribbean, is becoming a rural health problem in Africa and Brazil, and is of special concern in Cambodian and other Southeast Asian refugees (Diaz, 1996; WHO, 1996).

Schistosomiasis in pregnant women causes a depressed immune system, placentitis, abortion, ectopic pregnancy, prematurity, and fetal death. Multiple gynecologic problems also occur. Granulomatous lesions throughout the reproductive tract cause pain during coitus, menstrual irregularities, menorrhagia, vulvovaginal papillomas, and oophoritis. Alterations in the hepatic system can cause hormonal problems, early menopause, amenorrhea, delayed puberty, and diminished sex drive (Diaz, 1996).

American Trypanosomiasis (Chagas' Disease)

American trypanasomiasis (Chagas' disease) occurs only in the Americas where an estimated 100 million people are at risk. More than 50% of the 16–18 million people infected are women (WHO, 1996). It is caused by the hemoflagellate protozoan *Trypanosoma cruzi* transmitted to humans primarily via insect vectors ("kissing or cone-nosed bugs"). It is also spread through blood trans-

fusions, the placenta, and contact with infected blood. Women are at special risk from delivery complications requiring transfusions of largely unscreened blood, residence in rural areas or low-income sections of large cities infested with infected vectors, and limited employment in the public or private sector where screening tests are required. In Argentina, 6% to 20% of pregnant women are infected; in Bolivia, up to 51%; in large Brazilian cities, 5.8% to 10.9%; and in Chile up to 7.4%. Chagas' disease has been linked to fetal death and prematurity. About 8% of newborns of infected mothers develop congenital Chagas' disease (Schmunis, 1993).

Chagas' disease is usually asymptomatic until irreversible chronic manifestations occur up to 20 years after infection. Irreversible sequelae include peripheral neuropathy, cardiopathy (myocardial damage, arrhythmias, and severe conduction abnormalities), gastrointestinal involvement (megacolon and megaesophagus), and diffuse meningoencephalitis with necrosis and hemorrhage in immunosuppressed individuals, including those with AIDS (Benenson, 1995; PAHO, 1994; WHO, 1996). The disease is the leading cause of cardiac death in young adults in regions of South America and generally goes undetected in women until pregnancy, if a serology for *T. cruzi* is done.

Nutrition

Nutritional deficits among IW are associated with low-birth-weight babies, stillbirths, hemorrhages, maternal deaths, vulnerability to reproductive tract infections, inability to adequately nourish the newborn when breast feeding, mental retardation in children, and limited nutrient stores in newborns and lactating mothers (Kim *et al.,* 1992; Koblinsky, 1995). Worldwide, an estimated 500 million of the 1.13 billion women ages 15 years and more are stunted in growth as a result of protein malnutrition in childhood; approximately 500 million are anemic; 100 million show the effects of iodine deficiency; and 2 million are estimated to be blind from severe Vitamin A deficiency (Koblinsky, 1995). Many are suffering from both protein-energy malnutrition and micronutrient deficiency ("Famine-Affected," 1992).

Many IW have left their countries of origin already in nutritional deficit due to (a) living under conditions of prolonged famine, (b) massive population displacement from civil unrest, war, and natural disasters, (c) being detained for long periods in countries of second asylum without adequate provisions for nutrition or health care, and (d) social and economic oppression. Prominent nutritional problems affecting IW during their reproductive years are gestational weight gain, anemia, and micronutrient deficiencies ("Famine-Affected," 1992).

Gestational Weight Gain

Optimal gestational weight gain based on Institute of Medicine recommendations is (a) 25–35 lbs. for women of normal weight, (b) 28–40 lbs. for underweight women, and (c) 15–25 lbs. for overweight women (Kim et al., 1992). Data from the United States Pregnancy Nutrition Surveillance System (PNSS) show that (a) 29% of women are overweight prior to becoming pregnant and 20% are underweight, (b) 39% of women fail to reach the recommended gestational weight, and (c) 33% gain more weight than recommended (Kim et al., 1992). Asian (27.1%) and White (22.4%) women are more likely than Blacks (16.4%) and Hispanics (14.7%) to be underweight before pregnancy. Asian (50.5%) and White (40.4%) women are also less likely to gain the recommended weight than Blacks (36.7%) and Hispanics (36.2%). Black women (32.8%) tend to be the most overweight followed by Hispanics (30.2%), Whites (27.4%), and Asians (17.3%) (Kim et al., 1992).

Excessive Gestational Weight Gain

Obesity (weight of 20% above recommended nonpregnancy weight) during pregnancy may result in large babies and difficult

births, chronic and pregnancy-induced hypertension, gestational diabetes, and postpartum weight retention with its psychoemotional and social manifestations (Gueri, Patterson, & Gonzalez-Cossio, 1993; Kim et al., 1992; PAHO, 1994). Obese women are not generally counseled to diet during pregnancy due to the risk of maternal ketosis and its threat to the fetus. Emphasis is placed instead on the quality of dietary consumption.

Obesity in IW is often a consequence of the acculturation process, for example, less active lifestyle, high unemployment and poverty, and intake of foods high in calories and fat that is accompanied by a decreased intake in indigenous foods traditionally low in fat. Obesity is of special concern in IW from Latin and Central America and the Caribbean where obesity during pregnancy has ranged from 22% to 29% (Gueri et al., 1993). Dietary and health teaching considerations when counseling about overweight and obesity in pregnancy are similar to those specified later for underweight women.

Low Gestational Weight Gain

Women 10% below their recommended weight prior to conception are at increased risk for preeclampsia and low-birth-weight infants. Based on PNSS data, the incidence of low-birth-weight infants in women gaining less weight than recommended was 10/100 live births. The incidence in women who gained more weight than recommended was 3.5/100 live births compared to 5.9/100 in women who gained the recommended amount. The incidence of low-birth-weight babies per 100 live births in women who gained less than the recommended weight was lower in Asian (7.1) than Black (15.8), Hispanic (9.4), and White (9.7) women. The incidence in women who gained more weight followed a similar pattern with the lowest incidence occurring in Asians (2.5), the highest in Blacks (5.2), followed by Hispanics (3.4) and Whites (3.3) (Kim et al., 1992).

Underweight women are usually advised to increase caloric intake by 500 kilocalories above the normal recommended daily allowance (300 kilocalories) to achieve a weight gain of the amount underweight plus 25 lbs. The latter is not often possible for IW due to a number of physical and sociocultural factors.

To assess why pregnant IW are underweight or not achieving the expected standard weight gain, HCPs must determine the factors affecting their current weight and plan interventions accordingly. Such interventions need to take into account their (a) ability to increase caloric intake in light of financial resources; (b) cultural beliefs about weight and body image; (c) family eating patterns and order; and (d) understanding of what constitutes adequate nutrition, for example, appropriate foods to consume during pregnancy, their acceptable mode of preparation, and quantities permissible. The most prominent sociocultural factors that will affect the ability of immigrant women to achieve their optimal gestational weight are discussed in the following sections.

Understanding of Gestational Weight Gain. IW often do not understand the relationship between weight gain and fetal size, thinking that every pound of gestational weight gain reflects an equal increase in fetal weight. Little is known of what contributes to gestational weight gain other than development of the fetus (Alcalay *et al.*, 1993).

Size of Baby, Ease of Delivery, and Body Image. Immigrant women may be reluctant to gain weight during pregnancy for fear that their altered body image may affect their desirability by mates or that a large fetus will cause greater pain at birth, a more difficult delivery, or damage or disfigurement of the newborn during birth. Mexican and other Hispanic women feel pressure from the baby's father not to get "too fat" (Alcalay *et al.*, 1993). Mexican American women may avoid milk and other dairy products to avoid large babies and painful deliveries (Helman, 1994). East Indian, Iranian, and Somali women often prefer a smaller baby for "ease in delivery" and "fear of pain associated with difficult delivery" (Beine *et al.*, 1995; Good,

1980; Nichter & Nichter, 1996b). Iranian women also refuse to take doctor-prescribed medications because they will produce a large baby and require a caesarean section which goes against "common sense" (Good, 1980). Nichter and Nichter (1996b) reported that nutrition teaching by HCPs described ferrous sulfate tablets as "good for health, a tonic for a big baby." Women then refused to take the tablets in order to prevent having a large baby and painful childbirth.

Iron-Deficiency Anemia

Maternal iron-deficiency anemia is defined as hemoglobin (Hgb) <11g/dL or hematocrit (Hct) <33% in the first trimester and 10.5 Hgb/dL or Hct <31% in the second trimester (Kim *et al.*, 1992). It is associated with prematurity and low-birth-weight infants, risk of maternal hemorrhage, and death during childbirth. PNSS data shows an increasing prevalence of anemia as pregnancy progresses with Black women (16.9%) showing the highest level in the first trimester. White women (6.1%) have the least anemia, followed by Hispanic (9.6%) and Asian (10.8%) women. An identical ethnic-racial sequential pattern holds true for the second and third trimesters with the percentage increasing by the third trimester to 45.8% of Black women, 31.9% of Hispanic, 26.8% of Asian, and 24.6% of White (Kim *et al.*, 1992). The increase in maternal anemia across pregnancy reflects the storage of iron in the fetal liver to help the newborn and infant compensate for lack of iron in breast milk and non-iron-fortified formulas.

The iron status of IW should be scrutinized closely by HCPs as many are iron deficient since birth or have spent considerable time in refugee status. Monitoring of iron levels should begin well before conception and continue throughout pregnancy and afterward. Worldwide, more than 50% of pregnant women are anemic with large numbers located in South Asia (75%), Southeast Asia (63%), Africa (52%), and Latin America and the Caribbean (90%) (Koblinsky, 1995). Iron-deficiency anemia may be further complicated by malaria, hookworm, previous obstetrical complications, prolonged breast feeding, and other nutrient deficiencies, such as folate and Vitamin B-12.

Ethnomedical beliefs can affect the willingness of pregnant women to increase iron intake. Many such beliefs are grounded in the concepts of hot and cold and an inability to differentiate between the functions of vitamins and iron during pregnancy. Mexican women in one study believed that iron is absorbed during the early part of pregnancy. To take iron after "the beginnings" was essentially pointless. The women (82%) associated anemia with poor nutrition, as a pregnancy risk factor, and as being bad for the baby but were unclear on how to prevent it. Vitamins were considered important for health and during pregnancy and assumed more cultural importance than iron in preventing anemia (Alcalay *et al.,* 1993). Other Mexican American women would take prescribed vitamins and minerals because they "enrich" the blood, resulting in healthy mothers and newborns. Immigrant Somali women also believed in the importance of vitamins and minerals in pregnancy, but vitamins were considered essential to give the woman energy to "push" during labor (Beine *et al.,* 1995).

Haitian immigrant women often refused to eat foods rich in iron because of the cooling effect they produced on the body during the postpartum period which is considered a cold state (DeSantis, 1997). East Indian and other Southeast Asian women considered the antenatal stage of pregnancy to be hot and refused to eat iron-rich foods classified as hot to avoid a miscarriage (Kendall, 1987; Landerman, 1987; Nichter & Nichter, 1996b). They might refuse to take deworming medications, believing that any medication strong enough to expel worms creates an exceptional amount of heat and causes the uterus to expel the fetus (Nichter & Nichter, 1996b).

Hard iron tablets were seen by East Indian women as inappropriate during pregnancy, because they compete with the fetus for space in the stomach where, based on their concept of ethnoanatomy, the womb with the developing fetus is located. Hard tablets, food, gas, and air all take up space in the stomach and "cramp" the fetus, keeping it from developing normally. Iron-containing tonics are acceptable because they are easy to digest and produce strong blood necessary for health. Ferrous sulfate tablets are hard to digest and weaken the blood (Nichter & Nichter, 1996b).

Iodine Deficiency

Iodine deficiency during pregnancy may result in irreversible mental retardation, delayed motor development, stunting, auditory, speech, and neuromuscular disorders in infants and children, miscarriage, and increased child and maternal mortality. Women with cretinism have higher rates of obstructed labor and are at higher risk for maternal mortality (Koblinsky, 1995).

Prevalence of goiter in school-age children varies throughout the world: 21% in the Middle East and North Africa, 19% in eastern and southern Africa, 14% in Latin America and the Caribbean, 13% in South Asia, 12% in Central and West Africa and East Asia and the Pacific (WHO, 1996). In the Americas, women have a higher incidence of iodine deficiency than men. Of particular concern are women from the isolated areas of the Andean region in Central America (Bolivia, Peru, and Ecuador), women from refugee camps in Pakistan and Ethiopia, and women from high mountain areas of Pakistan and Afghanistan ("Famine-Affected," 1992; Gueri *et al.,* 1993; WHO, 1996).

Vitamin A Deficiency

HCPs should establish the amount and sources of vitamin intake before prescribing additional ones. If vitamin A stores are adequate, pregnancy generally has little effect. Concern about vitamin A levels in pregnant women usually centers on the toxic effects it can have on fetal development if taken in excess, for example, cleft palate, renal abnormalities, damage to the central nervous system, and bone, ocular, and ear deformities. Such concerns are equally valid among IW due to their beliefs in the necessity of vitamins for a healthy pregnancy and energy for laboring, the easy availability of over-the-counter vitamins, and the marketing of vitamins via the media.

Deficiency of vitamin A in pregnant IW is a more common problem that should be assessed early in the prenatal period and during lactation. Such deficiency can result in corneal ulceration and blindness in the mother, poor ocular and visual development in the fetus, and increased susceptibility in both to infectious diseases, especially measles and diarrhea. Vitamin A deficiency is common in IW from Asia and sub-Saharan Africa, Haiti, isolated arid and rural areas in Bolivia, Brazil, Ecuador, El Salvador, Guatemala, and Honduras, and those from refugee camps in Thailand and Sudan ("Famine-Affected," 1992; Gueri et al., 1993; Koblinsky, 1995; PAHO, 1994).

Fertility Regulation

Women bear the bulk of responsibility for and health risks of fertility regulation since most modern methods of contraception are directed at women. Despite bearing most of the responsibility and risks, the decision to contracept, methods used, and ability to continue do not always rest with the woman. IW have encountered multiple barriers when desiring to use contraception. Some have faced sanctions from pronatalist governments while others have been forcibly sterilized or coerced into contraception by governments attempting to dramatically impact population growth. IW have been subjected to spousal or societal abuse for attempting to regulate their fertility. Many have been unable to maintain contraception due to the inability to obtain resupplies or adequate medical care for complications. Others have sustained unintended pregnancies from lack of knowledge about reproductive anatomy and physiology or the mechanism of action of the contraceptive method. HCPs counseling IW on fertility regulation will need to explore past methods used and results to adequately assess the appropriateness of contraceptive methods requested or advocated (Doyal, 1995; Hatcher, 1994; Helman, 1994; Newman, 1995). When advising on the use of any method of fertility regulation, HCPs must be certain that IW understand that while the method may protect against pregnancy, it does not necessarily protect against HIV/AIDS or other STDs.

The major contraceptive methods used by IW in their country of origin and host country are discussed in the following sections. For further information on each see Hatcher (1994).

Sterilization

Sterilization is the most prevalent contraceptive practice in the world, with female sterilization resorted to by 18% of couples. It is especially prominent among immigrants from Asia, East Asia, Latin America, and Central and Southern Africa. Tubal ligation via minilaparotomy is the dominant form (WHO, 1996).

IW from countries without adequate short-term contraceptive technologies that are accessible and which can be easily resupplied may request sterilization out of a lack of knowledge of contraceptive availability and alternatives in the host country. Others will request sterilization as a way to prevent further pregnancy without disclosing to their spouses or in-laws that they are practicing contraception (Doyal, 1995; Helman, 1994; PAHO, 1994). Sterilization is an advantageous option when women reach their later reproductive years and do not wish further children.

Beliefs about the effects of tubal ligations may affect women's willingness to undergo the procedure. Cambodian immigrants believe tubal ligation causes general weakness, visual disturbances, and the release of inappropriate sexual desires and passion, causing them to seek out other men to satisfy themselves (Kulig, 1995). East Indian women attribute the following side effects to sterilization: weakness and an inability to do work, decreased sexual desire, weight loss from decreased appetite, sensations of dizziness and imbalance, and "heavier" and more painful menses due to blockage of the flow of blood from the uterus (Nichter & Nichter, 1996c).

Alternative concepts of anatomy and physiology may cause immigrant women to expect the sterilization procedure to be self-reversible after a period of time. East Indian women believe the blood loss from sterilization renders the body too cold to conceive. Increasing the body heat through diet, activity, or other means can reverse the effects of sterilization and allow conception (Nichter & Nichter, 1996c). Others equate sterilization with tying the tubes with string which comes untied or loosened, permitting conception to occur. Other concepts of ethnoanatomy postulate that the cervix is tied shut to prevent conception, but slippage in the tautness of the "string" can occur, allowing sperm to enter (Helman, 1994; Nichter & Nichter, 1996c).

IW may consult HCPs for reversal of sterilization to restore their childbearing ability. Many IW have undergone sterilization without adequate knowledge about its permanence, due to eugenics or ethnic cleansing or forced state birth control programs to limit population growth, or to take advantage of financial inducements by the state in order to supplement income to meet basic family needs (Doyal, 1995). Counseling of such women must include particular attention to mental health issues and sensitivity to the long-term psychological effects that sterilization against one's will can have on women, especially those whose social identity is dependent on their fertility.

HCPs must proceed with caution when recommending sterilization or when counseling and educating IW who request sterilization. Every precaution should be taken to assure their right to decide and to ensure in-

formed consent has been obtained. Special caution is needed with women who are young, are suffering financially, are in unstable marriages, whose young children are ill, and who have recently been pregnant. Such candidates often regret having the procedure and desire its reversal (Hatcher, 1994).

Traditional Contraceptive Methods

Abstinence, coitus interruptus (withdrawal), fertility awareness, and lactation amenorrhea are "traditional" contraceptive practices. They remain prominent methods of birth control among IW.

Abstinence

Abstinence is predominantly a female practice since males in many societies are expected to be experienced in sexual matters in order to prove their virility and to instruct their wives upon marriage (DeSantis, Sinnett, & Thomas, 1995; Hutchinson & Baqi-Aziz, 1994; Mattson, 1995; Morris, 1992). IW who rely on abstinence as a birth control method are often from societies where their virginity is the family "badge of honor," religious practices forbid intercourse before marriage or fertility regulation after marriage, reproductive matters are simply not discussed, or accessible and affordable contraceptive services are lacking. Abstinence remains one of the most prevalent methods of contraception in the Caribbean, Central and Latin America, Asia, and the Middle East, as well as in Muslim societies (Doyal, 1995; Helman, 1994; PAHO, 1994).

Coitus Interruptus (Withdrawal)

Withdrawal is practiced by most of the same groups and for the same reasons as abstinence. It is not effective if the male cannot predict withdrawal before ejaculation or exercise the needed degree of self-control to withdraw before semen is deposited in the female's vagina or external genitalia. There is uncertainty whether preejaculation fluid can cause sperm remaining on the penis from prior ejaculation to enter the vagina (Hatcher, 1994).

Use of withdrawal decreases when the desired family size has been achieved or after several unintended pregnancies. Couples also report diminished pleasure by the necessity of interrupting the excitement phase of intercourse (Hatcher, 1994). Caribbean IW believe that withdrawal is not natural, can injure one's health, and is not effective due to the "weakness of the male"; that is, men are unable to control their sex drive once it has been aroused (Newman, 1995).

Fertility Awareness (Rhythm Method)

Fertility awareness is the basis of natural family planning methods that rely on reproductive knowledge, identification of the fertile days based on menstrual cycle signs and symptoms, and periodic abstinence during the fertile days. The most common natural signs and symptoms used to identify the fertile period are menstrual bleeding, a drop in the basal body temperature (BBT), and an increase in cervical mucous. The fertile period is generally between 7 days before ovulation to 3 days after. Depending on the length of the menstrual cycle and type of rhythm method used, abstinence from vaginal intercourse will need to occur for 10 to 14 days of the menstrual cycle. Unintended pregnancy is due mainly to sexual risk taking during the fertile days. When adhered to perfectly (no intercourse during the fertile period), unintended pregnancy rates are low. When imperfectly adhered to (unprotected sex during the fecund period), failure rates approximate the pregnancy rate of women actively trying to conceive. For a detailed discussion of fertility periods and advantages and disadvantages of fertility awareness methods of contraception see Hatcher (1994).

Successful use of fertility awareness requires immigrant couples to be aware of the female partner's menstrual cycle, to communicate with each other about sexual matters, and to have active participation on the part of the male in terms of withdrawal, periodic abstinence, or use of a condom. Knowledge of the regularity or irregularity of the menstrual cycle is generally quite good among IW (Doyal, 1995). Communication or active male participation is difficult among Caribbean, Hispanic, Moslem, and Asian couples, as well as couples from other cultures where sexual matters are not openly discussed, male virility is determined by the number of offspring, females are not instructed in sexual matters, or husbands are expected to teach their wives such matters after marriage (DeSantis *et al.,* 1995; Hutchinson & Baqi-Aziz, 1994; Mattson, 1995; Morris, 1992; Newman, 1995; Nichter & Nichter, 1996a).

HCPs counseling immigrant couples wishing to use natural family planning or rhythm methods with barrier contraception must be certain that the couple understands the anatomical and physiological basis of the fertile period since cultural constructs of anatomy and physiology can lead to misinterpretation of the "safe time." In Asian, Moslem, Middle Eastern, and Central and Latin American cultures, the "womb" (uterus) is believed to be open during menstruation which allows sperm to enter, and closed at its cessation which prevents sperm from entering. An alternative belief is that menstrual blood will wash out or otherwise prevent sperm from entering the uterus. Concepts of hot and cold and the polluting effect of menstrual blood also affect beliefs about the fertility cycle and timing of periodic abstinence or use of barrier contraception during the most fertile period, for example, menstrual blood "kills" the sperm or menstruation makes the womb too hot or cold for conception to occur or the fetus to develop (DeSantis, 1997; Helman, 1994; Newman, 1995; Nichter & Nichter, 1996a). Indonesian couples may consider the womb as dry after menstruation and therefore, not conducive to conception or the nourishing of the seed (sperm). It is considered moist and "swollen with blood" before, during, and right after menses, facilitating penetration and seeding of the sperm (Nichter & Nichter, 1996a).

Lactation Amenorrhea

The postpartum period confers a variable 4–6-week period of infertility although about one third of the first menstrual cycle is anovulatory as are 15% of the second and third cycles (Hatcher, 1994). During breast feeding, the anovulatory period is extended through the hypothalamic–pituitary–ovarian feedback system. Infant suckling stimulates the hypothalamus to reduce the level and rhythm of gonadotrophin releasing hormone which in turn suppresses the release of the follicular stimulating hormone (FSH) and the luteinizing hormone (LH). Follicular development becomes disorganized and decreased (Hatcher, 1994; Huffman & Labbok, 1994).

The lactational amenorrhea method (LAM) can be up to 98% effective as a form of postpartum contraception if three parameters are met: (a) complete or nearly complete breast feeding without supplementation, (b) less than 6 months postpartum, and (c) amenorrhea. Complementary contraceptive methods must be introduced if any of the three parameters change (Huffman & Labbok, 1994). Lactation is not adversely affected by postpartum intercourse, abstinence, withdrawal, spermicides, most methods of contraception, and tubal ligation under local or regional anesthesia. Due to the estrogen component, combined oral contraceptives have been shown to decrease lactation and should not be used before 6 weeks postpartum (Hatcher, 1994).

LAM is the leading method of postpartum contraception, child spacing, and enhancing child survival in Africa, Asia, and other developing countries (Helman, 1994; Huffman & Labbok, 1994). LAM allows women to control their own fertility, especially in areas where other contraceptive technology is unavailable. Problems may occur in the United States with IW using LAM. Employers may be unwilling to assume costs such as provision of time off for nursing breaks, part-time leave or part-time employment, and on-site child care. In many areas, breast feeding in public remains illegal or is socially discour-

aged due to taboos against public displays of the female breast. Husbands may refuse to allow breast feeding outside of the home, limiting the woman's social contacts and mobility. Increasing demands on the IW's time may decrease their ability to breast feed without supplementation which increases the risk of unplanned pregnancy. Conflicting advice is frequently received from media promotion and social marketing of infant feeding products, as well as from HCPs who believe complementary infant feeding is necessary between 4 and 6 months.

Condoms

Condoms account for about 8% of contraceptive use worldwide. More and more immigrant couples and single women have begun using condoms for contraception and safe sex, but their primary use remains as a method of pregnancy prevention rather than for safe-sex practices (WHO, 1996). Less condom use is found among women who use other contraceptive methods and couples in stable relationships, even when one or both of the partners may have sexual intercourse with multiple other persons (van Oss Marin, Gomez, & Tschann, 1993).

Condoms are moderately effective with failure rates ranging from 2% to 3% for perfect users to 12% for typical users during the first year (Hatcher, 1994). When used consistently and correctly, they provide good protection against pregnancy and infection. Major advantages of condoms are low cost, portability, availability without prescription, involvement of the male in contraception, and prevention of STDs. Major disadvantages are perceptions that they reduce glans sensitivity, interruption of foreplay to apply, interference with maintenance of an erection, breakage, embarrassment, slippage, and male involvement (Doyal, 1995; Hatcher, 1994).

Male involvement may be dangerous or impossible to obtain by IW from societies where many children are a confirmation of male fertility and virility, a source of labor for enhancing family income, and parental economic and social security in old age. Women often suffer physical and social abuse for suggesting or attempting to have male partners use condoms. Low-income IW especially are dependent on spousal income due to their lack of marketable skills and are unlikely or unable to deny sexual intercourse if the male refuses to utilize condoms (De-Santis *et al.,* 1995; Doyal, 1995; Eldridge, St. Lawrence, Little, Shelby, & Brasfield, 1995; van Oss Marin *et al.,* 1993). Due to its visibility, use of female condoms also requires the male's tolerance (Eldridge *et al.,* 1995).

HCPs will need to address a number of ethnomedical beliefs about condom use. Hispanic, African, and Asian concepts of ethnoanatomy have lead to beliefs that condoms will become dislodged, travel upward into the abdominal cavity, and cause obstruction, infection, or cancer (Helman, 1994). African, Caribbean, and Hispanic males resist condoms due to the decreased glans sensitivity factor and fear of illness or weakness from inhibiting erections or the natural act of sexual intercourse (DeSantis *et al.,* 1995; van Oss Martin *et al.,* 1993). The fear that the condom will break or "burst" also is common. HCPs need to assure immigrant couples that slippage and rupture rates are low (0.6% to 2% and 2% to 6%, respectively) (Hatcher, 1994). In multiple societies, condom use has been associated with prostitution. The social stigma of engaging in illicit sex remains, discouraging condom use or purchase for fear of guilt by association (Nichter & Nichter, 1996c).

Oral Contraceptives

More than 15% of women worldwide use the "pill" for contraception (WHO, 1996). Oral contraceptives (OCs) suppress ovulation by the combined action of progestin and estrogen. Progestin inhibits ovulation by suppression of the LH, increases production of thick cervical mucous to hamper sperm transport, alters ovum transport, decreases the capacity of the sperm to penetrate the ovum, and alters the endometrium. Estro-genic effects include inhibiting production of FSH and LH, altering uterine secretions and endometrial cell structure, and accelerating ovum transport (Hatcher, 1994). The remainder of this section discusses combined OCs. For information on progestin-only OCs see Hatcher (1994).

OCs are extremely effective with failure rates of 0.1% during the first year for perfect use and 3% for imperfect use. Most imperfect use is from discontinuation for nonmedical reasons, for example, partner influence, inability to resupply, rumors about long-term ill effects on health, or displeasure with normal side effects such as weight gain or alteration in menses (Bracher & Santow, 1992; DeClerque, Tsui, Abul-Ata, & Barcelona, 1986; Hatcher, 1994; Nichter & Nichter, 1996c).

Major advantages of OCs are their effectiveness, lessened menstrual pain, protection from pelvic inflammatory disease, prevention of ectopic pregnancy, decreased ovarian or endometrial cancer, and safety except in women 35 years of age or more who smoke more than 35 cigarettes daily. Reversibility is another advantage, but conception may be delayed 2–3 months (range 2–6 months) after discontinuation. Major disadvantages are the need to take the pill every day, the expense, the need to resupply, headaches, and depression or mood changes. Nausea and vomiting may occur mainly in the initial cycle. Cardiovascular complications, such as thrombophlebitis, pulmonary emboli, and hypertension, may occur in women already at risk for cardiovascular problems. Studies of the association of OCs and cancer have reached differing conclusions. OCs protect against ovarian and endometrial cancer, but may increase the risk of cervical cancer or of breast cancer in young, never-pregnant women. Consensus is that the risk of contraception is far less than the risk of complications of pregnancy or termination of pregnancy (Coe & Hanft, 1993; Hatcher, 1994; PAHO, 1994). The lowest dose OCs should be prescribed, especially for those at risk who desire contraception. See Hatcher

(1994) for a more thorough discussion of precautions in the use of OCs.

IW are often reluctant to use OCs because of difficulty in their acquisition, their association with medical complications, alternative conceptualizations of anatomy and physiology, or lay interpretations of their mechanisms of action. In many developing countries, OCs can be readily obtained without prescription or cost, and low-income IW are often unable to suddenly bear the cost of having to purchase OCs (Hatcher, 1994). Restricting their obtainability in the United States and other developed countries through HCP prescriptions conveys a message that they are dangerous and requires women to put their contraceptive decision making under the control of the health care establishment (Doyal, 1995; Raikes, 1989).

Alteration in menses and the side effect of weakness caused by OCs are other concerns of IW who are under social and religious restrictions when menstruating or who believe excessive loss of blood makes them susceptible to illness, promotes premature aging, or causes "heart distress" (palpations, sadness, emotional pain, worry, and weakness). "Weakness" is a constellation of symptoms, like dizziness, fatigue, or lethargy, attributed to OCs which has no biomedical basis as an illness, goes untreated, or is declared insignificant by HCPs. It is culturally grounded as an illness and is of significance in determining whether IW will start or continue with OCs. Many discontinue OC use because they cannot obtain medical treatment for "weakness." Weakness as an illness is prevalent among IW from Botswana, Egypt, Morocco, East Asia, the Middle East, Iran, the Caribbean, and Latin and Central America (Doyal, 1995; DeClerque et al., 1986; Good, 1980; Kulig, 1995; Nichter & Nichter, 1996c).

Concepts of hot–cold also relate to the effect and side effects of OCs; for example, while OCs raise the body heat or dry the uterus to prevent conception, body heat weakens the health protecting and health promoting effect of balance. Rendering the womb dry over time results in irreversible infertility. Such conceptualizations have caused never-pregnant women or those who desire additional children not to begin OCs (Kulig, 1995; Nichter & Nichter, 1996c).

A major difficulty encountered with OCs is the need to take them daily. Many IW have limited education and are at a disadvantage in understanding the relatively complicated biomedical concepts of reproductive anatomy and physiology on which OCs are based. A consequence of incomplete understanding is the tendency to self-regulate dosages or not to institute a backup contraceptive method to prevent unintended pregnancy (Bracher & Santow, 1992; DeClerque et al., 1986; Hatcher, 1994; Nichter & Nichter, 1996c).

Self-regulation is also related to the belief in the potency of OCs when taken over a long period of time. East Indian, Egyptian, Peruvian, Bangladeshi, and other immigrant women will discontinue OCs if they feel ill or will take the "pill" only when necessary, for example, just before engaging in intercourse, a few days after intercourse, or at times perceived to be those of peak fertility (DeClerque et al., 1986; Nichter & Nichter, 1996c)

Intrauterine Devices

Intrauterine devices (IUDs) are used by approximately 20% of women worldwide (WHO, 1996). IUDs are used primarily by women (a) in the later years of fertility (30–40 years), (b) in stable relationships who do not wish additional children, (c) who desire long-term contraception or who live in areas where storage of or access to shorter-term contraceptives is difficult, and (d) who must conceal contraceptive use (Doyal, 1995; Hatcher, 1994; Newman, 1995).

Major advantages of IUDs are ease of use, provision of long-term protection, usefulness as an alternative when hormonal methods are contraindicated, high level of reliability, and ability to conceal use. Major disadvantages are risk of pelvic inflammatory disease, increased dysmenorrhea, ectopic pregnancy, uterine perforation, and expulsion (Hatcher, 1994).

IW may fear IUDs because they associate them with infection, uterine perforation, cancer, forced fertility regulation by government, and death resulting from inability to access needed care when complications occur. Fears exist that the IUD will become permanently imbedded and result in infertility, illness, and death. IW may also be reluctant to utilize IUDs because their partners may detect the strings (Coe & Hanft, 1993; Doyal, 1995; Hatcher, 1994; Newman, 1995).

Alternative conceptualization of anatomy and physiology has affected IUD use throughout the world; for example, beliefs that IUDs can travel, float, or be pushed into other parts of the body, causing perforated lungs, brain hemorrhages, nerve damage, or penile injury during intercourse. East Indian women see no separation between the uterus and stomach or believe one sac opens into the other which allows the IUD to move into the stomach, requiring an operation to remove it. At greatest risk are women who engage in frequent and "vigorous sexual activity" (Doyal, 1995; Newman, 1995; Nichter & Nichter, 1996c). Women from societies with menstrual taboos or blood beliefs do not wish prolonged bleeding from IUDs during or after their insertion. Others believe the IUD increases body heat or dries out the uterus so that conception cannot occur (Doyal, 1995; Good, 1980; Nichter & Nichter, 1996c).

A common belief is that the IUD can simply fall out after insertion. East Indian women believe the IUD will fall out from heavy work or engaging in sex with several partners which causes the vagina to increase in size. If the IUD does fall out, it is interpreted as an extramarital affair (Nichter & Nichter, 1996c).

Injectibles and Implants

The major injectable progesterone contraceptives in use throughout the world are Depo-Provera and Noigest. The latter is not available in the United States. Both are administered every 3–6 months via slow-release intramuscular injection and are highly effective with a yearly failure rate of 0.3% for Depo-Provera and 0.4% for Noigest. Their primary mechanism of action is to inhibit ovulation through suppression of FSH and LH. Conception is not possible for up to 6 months after the last dose (Coe & Hanft, 1993; Hatcher, 1994).

Norplant is the major implant contraceptive in use. It is a progesterone contraceptive, is effective for 5 years, and has a 0.2% failure rate the first year, 0.5% the second year, 1.2% the third year, 1.6% the fourth year, and 0.4% the fifth year. The implant is inserted under the skin of the upper arm and consists of 6 silastic capsules that slowly release the steroid levonorgestrel. Norplant is more advantageous than progesterone injectibles because it releases a lower dose of progesterone and conception is possible within 1 month of termination (Hatcher, 1994).

Major advantages of progesterone injectibles and implants are lack of side effects associated with estrogen, reversibility, long-term effectiveness, decreased risk of ectopic pregnancy, amenorrhea, and ability to conceal its use from partners. Major disadvantages are the lack of protection against STDs, headache, weight gain, irregular bleeding, breast tenderness, and depression. Additional side effects of Depo-Provera include a fall in the level of high-density lipoprotein cholesterol and a 6–8 month delay in conception after discontinuation. Additional disadvantages of Norplant include an increased failure rate with anticonvulsant therapy, insertion-site inflammation or infection, and capsule expulsion. The greatest disadvantages of injectibles and implants is the need to be dependent on HCPs for their continued use, and the need to undergo a minor surgical procedure for implant insertion and removal (Doyal, 1995; Forrest & Kaeser, 1993; Hatcher, 1994).

HCPs should proceed with caution when advising IW on the use of implants. Because the woman must put herself totally under the control of a HCP for its insertion or removal, client education and informed decision making about risks and benefits are paramount, and medical care after insertion must be accessible. IW need to be assured the implant will be removed as requested without interference from HCPs or others who may disagree with their request. The control of removal of implants and the nature of implants have led some governments to offer financial incentives to low-income women to have them inserted or mandate their insertion without consent of the woman. In the United States, courts have offered more lenient sentences or mandated contraceptive implants for low-income women for such things as child custody, substance abuse, welfare eligibility, and probation (Doyal, 1995; Forrest & Kaeser, 1993).

Abortion

Availability of abortion as a fertility regulating mechanism varies throughout the world. Even in countries where abortion is readily available, wide regional variation in the interpretation of the same law and restrictions often apply; for example, the provision of abortion services provided only by licensed HCPs, prohibition against the use of public funding, maximum stage of gestation, parental notification or consent for minors, or both, minimum waiting period, spousal consent, and mandatory counseling. For indepth information about abortion laws and trends throughout the world see Henshaw (1990).

Due to confusion over the variety of abortion regulations that exist across the United States, IW will need considerable guidance from HCPs when an abortion is needed or being considered as a method of pregnancy termination. Equally confusing is the ever-changing state and federal eligibility requirements and funding availability for abortions, as well as the political rather than health care determination of its availability.

IW may be unaware of the availability of safe and medically sanctioned abortion services in the host country and resort instead to indigenous or clandestine sources of pregnancy termination. This is especially true of those from Latin and Central America, the Caribbean, and Africa. IW from countries where abortion services are readily available or are sanctioned as a method of birth control may not seek abortion for an unwanted or unplanned pregnancy in the United States due to the social, moral, and ethical issues raised by antiabortion groups or because they are frightened by violence directed at agencies and HCPs providing abortion services, as well as those seeking them. IW from the former Soviet Union, China, and other countries without adequate access to contraception services or where family size is state regulated often consider abortion as a method of birth control and will need to be oriented to the availability of alternative contraceptive technology in the United States.

Marital status and parity also affect IW's decisions about whether to seek an abortion. Worldwide, abortion is highest among young, unmarried teenage women, decreases to a low point among 25- to 29-year-olds, and increases with age with women 40 and older having the highest rates. Women with stable relationships who already have children have the majority of abortions for purposes of child spacing or to avoid increasing family size (Doyal, 1995; Henshaw, 1990).

IW from countries where abortions are seen as a surgical procedure done in a hospital setting and where abortions account for a large percentage of maternal deaths or pregnancy complications will need counseling as to the safety of procedures done in licensed ambulatory care settings in the United States, as well as the safety of the decreased length of stay currently advocated when having an abortion on an inpatient basis. Worldwide, approximately 20% to 25% (115,000 to 204,000) of the half million maternal deaths annually are due to complications of illegal abortions done by untrained practitioners. The majority occur in Asia and sub-Saharan Africa. In Latin America and the Caribbean, 25% of maternal deaths are due to illegal abortions and are also the main cause of death in women ages 15 to 39 (Doyal, 1995; Henshaw, 1990; PAHO, 1994).

The most frequent complications of illegal or clandestine abortions are hemorrhage, shock, pelvic infection, infertility, tetanus, bladder and intestinal damage, and reproductive organ trauma, such as uterine perforation and cervical lacerations (Doyal, 1995). HCPs should thoroughly explore with IW their knowledge about the dangers of illegal or clandestine abortions and indigenous methods of inducing abortion since the type of abortion induction can affect the kind and degree of complications. East Indian women often attempt to induce abortions with twigs or sticks coated with arsenic or phosphorous, resulting in uterine tears and requiring emergency surgery. Women in Asia, the Caribbean, Latin and Central America, Africa, and the Middle East will employ hard abdominal massage, drink herbal or medical concoctions with quinine that can cause toxic reactions in the liver or kidneys, or insert caustic substances into the cervix, causing burns, bladder or intestinal fistulae, or bleeding. Caribbean women will drink home brews of "bush" teas, castor oil, Epsom salts, or sea salts to cause abortions or douche with castor oil to "clean" themselves out (Doyal, 1995; Newman, 1995). For greater in-depth information about types of indigenous abortifacients, emmenagogues to restore normal menstruation, and mechanical methods of inducing abortions, see Newman (1995) and Wood (1979).

Female Circumcision

Female circumcision (FC) is a general term used to describe a variety of surgical procedures that include incision and often removal of portions or all of the external female genitalia. The severity of FC depends on the degree of anatomic alteration that occurs.

FC is practiced in 26 countries that form a broad east–west triangle across the horn of Africa, extending from Egypt at the northeast to Tanzania in the southeast to Senegal in the west. It is also practiced in the southern region of the Arabian peninsula, portions of the Persian Gulf, and among Muslim groups in Malaysia, Indonesia, the Philippines, Pakistan, Brazil, Peru, and Mexico, as well as by immigrants in Australia, the United Kingdom, France, Australia, Canada, the United States, and other Western countries. An estimated 100 million women have been circumcised with prevalence rates varying between 20% and 90% in West Africa, to almost 100% in Somalia and Djibouti, and 90% in Ethiopia, Mali, and northern Sudan. FC cuts across all social classes and religions, including Islam, Judaism, Christianity, and indigenous African religions (Johnson & Rodgers, 1994; Toubia, 1994).

Types of Female Circumcision

FC based on the amount of tissue removed has been medically classified as either clitoridectomies (Types I and II) or infibulations (Types III and IV) (Hicks, 1996; Toubia, 1994).

- Type I: Clitoridectomy: Removal of the prepuce or hood of the clitoris along with all or part of the clitoris. It is the mildest form of FC, has been described as being "anatomically equivalent to amputation of the penis" (Toubia, 1994), and is generally referred to as the "Sunna" or "traditional circumcision." "Sunna" is variously defined as meaning tradition in Moslem countries or as adhering to the traditions of Mohammed (Arbesman, Kahler, & Buck, 1993; Flannery, Glover, & Airhinenbuwa, 1990).
- Type II: Clitoridectomy: Excision of the clitoris and all or part of the adjacent tissue (the labia minora). The urethra and vaginal introitus remain uncovered.
- Type III: Intermediate or Modified Infibulation: Removal of the clitoris and labia minora with either removal of all or part (generally two thirds) of the labia

majora or incision of the labia majora to create a raw and rough surface. The anterior two thirds of the amputated remains of the labia majora or its roughened edges are sewn or pinned together, leaving a fairly large posterior opening for the passage of urine and menstrual blood.

- Type IV: Total Infibulation: Excision as described in Type III, but with the remnants of the roughened or partially amputated labia majora sewn together to form a hood or covering over the urethra and vaginal opening. Only a very small posterior opening about the size of a ballpoint pen is left for the passage of urine and menstrual blood. The orifice is held open by a matchstick-size reed or wood slivers. The legs of the girl are bound together until the wound heals which may take 2 to 3 weeks or more. Type IV is referred to as "Pharaonic circumcision" based on its discovery circa 200 B.C. in Egyptian mummies (Hicks, 1996; Toubia, 1994; van der Kwaak, 1992).

FC is primarily done when a girl is 7 or 8 years old but may be performed during infancy or young adulthood. The majority are performed by traditional birth attendants, midwives, or elderly women with limited knowledge of anatomy, physiology, or surgical technique. FC is usually done without anesthesia and under less than hygienic conditions. Surgical instruments include razor blades, kitchen knives, scissors, broken glass, sharpened stones, or hot rocks. The incised areas are pinned together with thorns, stitched with silk or catgut, or held together with dung or indigenous adhesives such as tree sap or eggs and sugar. Morbidity and mortality from FC is essentially unknown (Flannery et al., 1990; Hicks, 1996; Johnson & Rodgers, 1994; van der Kwaak, 1992).

Defibulation is often required for women with Types III and IV procedures prior to first sexual intercourse, first vaginal examination, or vaginal delivery. To consummate the marriage, the husband (or traditional midwife) must open the scar often using fingers, razors, knives, glass, or acid. It may take up to 8 weeks to achieve full penetration (Flannery et al., 1990).

Reinfibulation is often done on women who have given birth, who symbolically wish to re-create their virginity due to divorce or widowhood, or on wives to ensure their monogamy when their husbands are absent for long periods of time (Hosken, 1994). Two types of reinfibulation may be done: (a) loose tissue around the fourchette is stitched and the vulval area is left open to permit the flow of urine and menstrual blood and facilitate intercourse, or (b) the more common procedure where the preexisting scar tissue edges are cut, restructured to form the hood of skin over the vaginal introitus and urethra, and sewn together to make the vaginal opening smaller and tighter. Failure to do some type of reinfibulation is equivalent to not repairing an episiotomy (Toubia, 1994).

Rationale for Female Circumcision

Justification of FC lies in a variety of cultural, socioeconomic, political, and psychological explanations that are generally group-specific, complex, and vary with the culture, gender, and background of the researcher. Synopses of the major categories of explanations are given in the following sections. For more detailed discussions, see Hicks (1996), Hosken (1994), and van der Kwaak (1992).

Tradition

Older women, often grandmothers of the girls to be circumcised, insist the tradition of FC be continued as a rite of passage prior to marriage, to preserve virginity and family honor, for socialization into womanhood, to symbolize the shared heritage of the group, and to fulfill the obligation girls must meet to belong to the group or face ostracism and stigmatization (Flannery et al., 1990; Johnson & Rodgers, 1994; van der Kwaak, 1992).

Religion

FC is often incorrectly justified as being required by "religious doctrine." FC is not required by either the Bible or Koran nor advocated in the Hadith, the sayings of the Prophet Muhammad. FC has been linked to religious doctrine because chastity and modesty are highly valued virtues in African and Islamic societies, are prescribed by the Bible and Koran, and appropriate verses in religious texts have been cited to justify its use by its proponents (van der Kwaak, 1992; Winkel, 1995).

Economic

FC is considered demonstrable proof of virginity in groups were virginity is essential for marriage, inheritance of property, perpetuation of the lineage, payment of bride price, and transference of the right to the woman's labor from the bride's father to the bridegroom. Uncircumcised women are often left in social isolation and poverty since marriage and motherhood have been the only career options available to most women where FC is practiced. FC, especially infibulation, provides a valuable source of income for traditional birth attendants and others who perform it (Flannery *et al.,* 1990; Lightfoot-Klein & Shaw, 1991; van der Kwaak, 1992).

Effects on Childbirth and Fertility Enhancement

FC is believed to enhance vaginal function and the newborn's survival. Contact with the clitoris may be potentially fatal or result in symbolic or spiritual injury to the newborn. Poisonous substances contained in the clitoris are considered harmful to the husband during intercourse. An unexcised clitoris is also seen as developing or symbolizing masculine characteristics and impeding the chance for marriage (Flannery *et al.,* 1990; van der Kwaak, 1992).

Prevention of Promiscuity

FC is seen as protecting women from their own nature by reducing sexual desire and making excessive sexual demands on their husbands while still preserving their reproductive function. The need to reduce female sexual desire is a prime concern in groups where men are believed to be harmed by too much sex, in polygamous societies where reduction of wives' sexual appetites is deemed necessary, and in communities where men are absent for long periods of time. Reduction of female sexual desire also serves to assure female monogamy if husbands are incapable of meeting their wives' sexual needs (Flannery *et al.,* 1990; Hicks, 1996; Hosken, 1994; van der Kwaak, 1992)

Cleanliness, Aesthetics, and Health

The clitoris should be excised because it is "ugly." FC is necessary to counterbalance the "lumpy" male with the "smooth" female. The purifying nature of FC enhances feminine hygiene by removing "dirty" body parts, decreasing "malodorous discharges," facilitating cleanliness of the vulva, and preventing dirt and worms from entering the vagina (Lightfoot-Klein & Shaw, 1991; van der Kwaak, 1992).

Health Consequences of Female Circumcision

Precise statistical data on morbidity and mortality are difficult to obtain since (a) women often do not seek care for fear of sanctions in countries where infibulation is illegal; (b) there is a general lack of knowledge of human anatomy, physiology, and reproductive health among women who are circumcised; and (c) women often do not associate reproductive and gynecological complications experienced as adults with FC done during childhood.

Circumcised IW are concerned about seeking biomedical reproductive health care due to

(a) the unfamiliarity of HCPs with FC, its purpose, and altered genital anatomy; (b) humiliation experienced over reactions of HCPs to the circumcised perineum; and (c) fear of being subjected to painful pelvic examinations and unnecessary cesarean sections (Lightfoot-Klein & Shaw, 1991; Toubia, 1994).

Psychological and Sexual Consequences

Psychological consequences have not been extensively investigated, but several major studies indicate considerable adverse psychoemotional and sexual sequelae, especially in infibulated women. In Sudan, 80% of Pharaonically infibulated women had never experienced orgasm compared to 12% of the Sunna circumcised (Flannery et al., 1990). Similar results were found in an Egyptian study, suggesting that the extent of the operation may affect the degree of sexual pleasure experienced. Infibulated Sudanese women are reported to experience chronic anxiety and depression over worry about the state of their genitals, infertility, and dysmenorrhea (Toubia, 1994). Reports of extreme anxiety due to dyspareunia and social pressure to please one's husband are said to be common (Flannery et al., 1990; Hosken, 1994; Lightfoot-Klein & Shaw, 1991; van der Kwaak, 1992).

Physical Consequences

Physical consequences are divided into immediate and long-term effects, as well as those due to childbirth. Treatment of the gynecological complications in circumcised women are basically the same as for any surgical complication (Toubia, 1994).

Immediate Complications. Hemorrhage and excruciating pain, resulting in shock and death, may occur from doing the procedure without anesthesia and from removal of just a small amount of the neurovascular tissue concentrated in and around the clitoris. Prolonged bleeding may lead to anemia and malnourishment. Unhygienic surgical conditions can result in local or systemic infections—abscesses, wound infections, tetanus, ulcers, septicemia, delayed healing, and gangrene. Urinary retention and urinary tract infection are common due to fear, pain, tissue swelling, and narrowness of the opening left for urine. Damage to surrounding genitalia and anus may have occurred if the girl struggled or moved during the procedure (Arbesman et al., 1993; Flannery et al., 1990; Toubia, 1994).

Long-Term Complications. Infibulation rather than clitorectomy alone is responsible for the majority of long-term complications. Interference with drainage of urine and menstrual flow leads to (a) chronic urinary infection, urinary stones, and renal damage; (b) chronic pelvic infection, resulting in menorrhagia, dysmenorrhea, back and pelvic pain, and possibly infertility; and (c) leakage of urine and feces from fistulae in the tissue between the vagina and urinary tract and bowel caused by tears from calculi formed by accumulation of urine and menstrual blood in the vagina. Dermoid and keloid cysts form along the scar from suturing keratinized epithelial cells and sebaceous glands into the incision. Such cysts can lead to recurrent abscesses and separation of the scar, require excision if they become large and disfiguring, and cause extreme anxiety among women who perceive that their genitals are growing or cancer has developed. Neuromas formed along the scar may cause severe dyspareunia and painful intercourse (Arbesman et al., 1993; Johnson & Rodgers, 1994; Toubia, 1994).

The risk of circumcised women acquiring HIV/AIDS is postulated to be high from (a) use of unhygienic instruments during circumcision, (b) increased chances of tears in the circumcised vagina during intercourse, (c) presence of vaginal lesions, and (d) frequency of anal intercourse due to abnormal female anatomy and inability of the male to penetrate the small vaginal opening. The association between HIV/AIDS and FC still requires further investigation since the incidence of HIV/AIDS is high in central African countries where FC is not practiced (Flannery *et al.,* 1990, van der Kwaak, 1992).

Childbirth. A circumcised woman may deliberately decrease her nutritional intake to keep the developing fetus small to facilitate its passage through the narrowed vaginal opening and decrease the pain during childbirth. Reduction of the size of the introital opening creates difficulty in performing routine pelvic examinations due to pain or inability to penetrate, necessitating rectal examinations instead.

The majority of complications occur in infibulated women during the second stage of labor. Deinfibulation is required for each delivery and should be performed before the first vaginal examination or early in the second stage of labor to prevent mechanical obstruction of the birth process, prolonged labor, fetal death, perineal tears, fistulae, hemorrhage from rupture of scar tissue, and uterine rupture. Avascular necrosis due to prolonged pressure of the fetal head may lead to vesico-vaginal and recto-vaginal fistulae, causing urinary incontinence and possible social ostracism due to the woman's lack of "cleanliness." An episiotomy may not be necessary if deinfibulation is performed early. For detailed information on the timing and technique of deinfibulation and the delivery process see Erian and Goh (1995), Lightfoot-Klein and Shaw (1991), and Toubia (1994).

Postpartum infection risks are high from (a) the prolonged healing time required of fibrous and scar tissue and (b) tight reinfibulations that may cause urinary retention and obstruct the flow of lochia and evacuation of clots (Johnson & Rodgers, 1994; Toubia, 1994; van der Kwaak, 1992).

Ethical and Legal Issues

Multiple ethical-legal issues must be considered when caring for circumcised IW and their families. FC has been condemned and its abolition called for by multiple health care organizations. Human rights groups have condemned FC as a human rights violation. Specific legislation forbidding FC exists in Canada, Great Britain, Sweden, Switzerland, and most African countries where FC is performed. Reinfibulation is also illegal in Great Britain, Canada, and Sweden. Enforcement in African countries has become impossible or simply not attempted because FC is ingrained in cultural tradition and the practice is considered moral and reasonable by those who perform and undergo it. Others believe enforcement will drive the act underground and prevent women from seeking needed medical care. Advocates consider such legal statutes and campaigns against FC as evidence of Western cultural imperialism, racism, religious intolerance, and radical feminist rhetoric (Arbesman *et al.,* 1993; Johnson & Rodgers, 1994; van der Kwaak, 1992; Winkel, 1995).

Medico-legal problems arise in countries with large populations of immigrant parents who wish their daughters to undergo FC. Many plan to have them return to their country of origin for the procedure. Others have the procedure done clandestinely in the host nation. Most host countries forbid the act under existing child abuse statutes (Toubia, 1994). In the United States, potential FC is a legitimate reason for seeking political asylum.

Summary

Reproductive health is essential to health in general and encompasses fertility regulation, pregnancy, childbirth, raising healthy children, and having sexual relations without fear of complications or social or physical abuse. Delivering reproductive health care to IW is a special challenge to HCPs due to the broadness of the topic and the intra- and intergroup variations in cultural beliefs and practices, the immigration and acculturation experience, and the situational context in which care is delivered.

When providing reproductive health care to IW, HCPs must remember the following key points:

1. Many IW may not have had access to biomedical health care prior to immigration. They also may hold different concepts of what constitutes reproductive health or use alternative constructs of anatomy and physiology to evaluate the validity of biomedical therapies and health teaching, or both. Unless HCPs carefully assess the individual immigrant woman's explanatory model of each aspect of reproductive health care under consideration, her understanding of and willingness to adhere to therapies and health teaching will be compromised as will the HCP's ability to develop culturally acceptable health care actions that promote healthy pregnancy outcomes.

2. IW are frequently exposed to a variety of infectious diseases and nutritional deficiencies not commonly seen by HCPs in the United States. IW at special risk are (a) those who have experienced social and economic oppression in their countries of origin or in the country into which they have immigrated, or both, and (b) those who have spent long amounts of time in refugee camps or countries of second asylum without provision of adequate nutrition or health care. Such IW must be assessed for infectious diseases and nutritional deficits and carefully monitored to enhance favorable pregnancy outcomes.

3. IW and their spouses are usually aware of many traditional and biomedical methods fertility regulation. However, the use of contraception may be compromised by an inability to obtain resupplies, a failure to understand the mechanism of action of the contraceptive, or a lack of accurate knowledge about the reproductive cycle. HCPs will need to ascertain the type and result of fertility regulation used in the past to better assess the appropriateness of methods currently requested or advocated. HCPs advising on the use of any method of fertility regulation should be certain to consistently caution IW that the method may be effective in preventing pregnancy, but it might not protect them against HIV/AIDS or other STDs.

4. HCPs may encounter multiple ethical-moral-legal dilemmas when caring for the reproductive health needs of IW. Decisions about fertility regulation and reproduction often do not rest with the individual woman. Such decisions are frequently imposed on IW or, if made independently, have resulted in physical or social abuse for being contrary to spousal wishes, governmental policy, or sociocultural beliefs and practices. When confronted with such dilemmas, HCPs must act in accordance with their understanding of the sociocultural basis and function of the practice, its resultant health care complications or benefits, the relevant legal statutes concerning it, and their own values and beliefs related to it.

The discussion of reproductive health care of IW has been limited in scope due to space restrictions. Not discussed in any depth are other aspects of the reproductive health of IW, such as menarche and menstruation, menopause, maternal and infant mortality, adolescent pregnancy, childrearing practices, delivery and postpartum beliefs and practices, infant feeding and nutrition, and common gynecological conditions. The four key points mentioned earlier are also guidelines for care of IW in the areas of reproductive health not presented.

References

Alcalay, R., Ghee, A., & Scrimshaw, S. (1993). Designing prenatal care messages for low-income Mexican women. *Public Health Reports, 108,* 354–362.

Anderson, E. N. (1987). Why is humoral medicine so popular? *Social Science & Medicine, 25,* 331–337.

Arbesman, M., Kahler, L., & Buck, G. M. (1993). Assessment of the impact of female circumcision on the gynecological, genitourinary, and obstetrical health problems of women from Somalia: Literature review and case series. *Women & Health, 20,* 27–42.

Beine, K., Fullerton, J., Palinkas, L., & Anders, B. (1995). Conceptions of prenatal care among Somali women in San Diego. *Journal of Nurse-Midwifery, 40,* 376–381.

Benenson, A. S. (1995). *Control of communicable diseases manual.* Washington, DC: American Public Health Association.

Berenson, G. S., Wattigney, W. A., & Webber, L. S. (1996). Epidemiology of hypertension from childhood to young adulthood in Black, White, and Hispanic population samples. *Public Health Reports, 111* (Suppl. 2), 3–6.

Bollini, P., & Siem, H. (1995). No real progress towards equity: Health of migrants and ethnic minorities on the eve of the year 2000. *Social Science & Medicine, 41,* 819–828.

Bracher, M., & Santow, G. (1992). Premature discontinuation of contraception in Australia. *Family Planning Perspectives, 24*(2), 58–65.

Coe, G. A., & Hanft, R. S. (1993). The use of technologies in the health care of women: A review of the literature. In E. Gómez Gómez (Ed.), *Gender, women, and health in the Americas* (pp. 195–207). Washington, DC: Pan American Health Organization.

Crespo, C. J., Loria, C. M., & Burt, V. L. (1996). Hypertension and other cardiovascular disease risk factors among Mexican Americans, Cuban Americans, and Puerto Ricans from the Hispanic Health and Nutrition Examination Survey. *Public Health Reports, 111* (Suppl. 2), 7–10.

DeClerque, J., Tsui, A. O., Abul-Ata, M. F., & Barcelona, D. (1986). Rumor, misinformation and oral contraceptive use in Egypt. *Social Science & Medicine, 23*(1), 83–92.

DeSantis, L. (1997). Providing care in a transcultural environment. In J. Luckman (Ed.), *Saunders manual of nursing care* (pp. 23–66). Philadelphia: Saunders.

DeSantis, L., Sinnett, K., & Thomas, J. T. (1995). Concepts of sexuality: Haitian immigrants parents and adolescents in South Florida. In J. F. Wang (Ed.), *Health care and culture: Proceedings of the Second International and Interdisciplinary Health Research Symposium* (pp. 223–232). Morgantown, WV: University of West Virginia School of Nursing.

Diaz, J. C. P. (1996). Tropical diseases and the gender approach. *Bulletin of the Pan American Health Organization, 30,* 242–260.

Domar, A. D. (1986). Psychological aspects of the pelvic exam: Individual needs and physician involvement. *Women & Health, 10*(4), 75–90.

Doyal, L. (1996). *What makes women sick: Gender and the political economy of health.* New Brunswick, NJ: Rutgers University Press.

Eldridge, G. D., St. Lawrence, J. S., Little, C. E., Shelby, M. C., & Brasfield, T. L. (1995). Barriers to condom use and barrier method preferences among low-income African-American women. *Women & Health, 23*(1), 73–89.

Erian, M. M. S., & Goh, J. T. W. (1995). Female circumcision. *Australian & New Zealand Journal of Obstetrics and Gynecology, 35,* 83–85.

Famine-affected, refugee, and displaced populations: Recommendations for public health issues. (`1992). *Morbidity and Mortality Weekly Report, 41,* 1–25.

Flannery, D., Glover, E. D., & Airhinenbuwa, C. (1990). Perspective on female circumcision: Traditional practice or health risk? *Health Values, 14,* 34–40.

Forrest, J. D., & Kaeser, L. (1993). Questions of balance: Issues emerging from the introduction of the hormonal implant. *Family Planning Perspectives, 25*(3), 127–132.

Goldenberg, R. L., Patterson, E. T., & Freese, M. P. (1992). Maternal demographic, situational and psychosocial factors and their relationship to enrollment in prenatal care: A review of the literature. *Women & Health, 19*(2/3), 133–151.

Good, M. J. D. (1980). Of blood and babies: The relationship of popular Islamic physiology to fertility. *Social Science & Medicine, 14b,* 147–156.

Gueri, M., Patterson, A. W., & Gonzalez-Cossio, T. (1993). Women and nutrition in the Americas: Problems and perspectives. In E. Gómez Gómez (Eds.), *Gender, women, and health in the Americas* (pp. 118–130). Washington, DC: Pan American Health Organization.

Hatcher, R. A. (Ed.). (1994). *Contraceptive technology.* New York: Irvington.

Helman, C. G. (1994). *Culture, health and illness.* Oxford, England: Butterworth-Heinemann.

Henshaw, S. K. (1990). Induced abortion: A world review, 1990. *Family Planning Perspectives, 22*(2), 76–89.

Hicks, E. E. (1996). *Infibulation: Female mutilation in Islamic Northeastern Africa.* New Brunswick, NJ: Transaction.

Hosken, F. P. (1994). *The Hosken report: Genital and sexual mutilation of females.* Lexington, MA: Women's International Network News.

Huffman, S. L., & Labbok, M. H. (1994). Breastfeeding in family planning programs: A help or hinderance? *International Journal of Gynecology & Obstetrics, 47* (Suppl.), S23–S32.

Hutchinson, K., & Baqi-Aziz, M. (1994). Nursing care of the childbearing Muslim family. *Journal of Obstetric, Gynecologic, & Neonatal Nursing, 23*(9), 767–771.

Imazu, M., Sumida, K., Yamabe, T., Yamamoto, H., Ueda, H., Hattori, Y., Miyauchi, A., Hara, H., & Yamakido, M. (1996). A comparison of the prevalence and risk factors of high blood pressure among Japanese living in Japan, Hawaii, and Los Angeles. *Public Health Reports, 111* (Suppl. 2), 59–61.

Johnson, K. E., & Rodgers, S. (1994). When cultural practices are health risks: The dilemma of female circumcision. *Holistic Nursing Practice, 8,* 70–78.

Kendall, L. (1987). Cold wombs in balmy Honolulu: Ethnogynecology among Korean immigrants. *Social Science & Medicine, 25,* 367–376.

Kim, I., Hungerford, D. W., Yip, R., Kuester, S. A., Zyrkowski, C., & Trowbridge, F. (1992). Pregnancy nutrition surveillance system—United States, 1979–1990. *Morbidity and Mortality Weekly Report, 41* (SS-7), 25–41.

Koblinsky, M. A. (1995). Beyond maternal mortality— Magnitude, interrelationship, and consequences of women's health, pregnancy-related complications and nutritional status on pregnancy outcomes. *International Journal of Gynecology & Obstetrics, 48* (Suppl.), S21–S32.

Kulig, J. G. (1995). Cambodian refugees' family planning knowledge and use. *Journal of Advanced Nursing, 22,* 150–157.

Landerman, C. (1987). Destructive heat and cooling prayer: Malay humoralism in pregnancy, childbirth and the postpartum period. *Social Science & Medicine, 25,* 357–365.

Lightfoot-Klein, H., & Shaw, E. (1991). Special needs of ritually circumcised women patients. *Journal of Obstetric, Gynecologic, & Neonatal Nursing, 20,* 102–107.

Mattson, S. (1995). Culturally sensitive perinatal care for Southeast Asians. *Journal of Obstetric, Gynecologic, and Neonatal Nursing, 24*(4), 335–341.

Morris, L. (1992). Sexual experiences and use of contraception among young adults in Latin America. *Morbidity and Mortality Weekly Report, 41* (SS-4), 27–40.

Newman, L. E. (Ed.). (1995). *Women's medicine: A cross-cultural study of indigenous fertility regulation.* New Brunswick, NJ: Rutgers University Press.

Nichter, M., & Nichter, M. (1996a). Cultural notions of fertility in South Asia and their impact on Sri Lankan family planning practices. In M. Nichter & M. Nichter (Eds.), *Anthropology and international health* (pp. 3–33). Amsterdam: Gordon and Breach.

Nichter, M., & Nichter, M. (1996b). The ethnophysiology and folk dietetics of pregnancy: A case study from South India. In M. Nichter & M. Nichter (Eds.), *Anthropology and international health* (pp. 35–69). Amsterdam: Gordon and Breach.

Nichter, M., & Nichter, M. (1996c). Modern methods of fertility regulation: When and for whom are they appropriate? In M. Nichter & M. Nichter (Eds.), *Anthropology and international health* (pp. 71–108). Amsterdam: Gordon and Breach.

Pan American Health Organization. (1994). *Health conditions in the Americas.* Washington, DC: Author.

Raikes, A. (1989). Women's health in East Africa. *Social Science & Medicine, 28*(5), 447–459.

Schmunis, G. A. (1993). Infectious diseases of women: Tropical diseases and reproductive tract infections. In E. Gómez Gómez (Ed.), *Gender, women, and health in the Americas* (pp. 171–177). Washington, DC: Pan American Health Organization.

Severy, L. J., Thana, S., Askew, I., & Glob, J. (1993). Menstrual experiences and beliefs: A multicountry study of relationships with fertility and fertility regulating methods. *Women & Health, 20*(2), 1–20.

Siegel, S. J. (1986). The effect of culture on how women experience menstruation: Jewish women and *Mikvah. Women & Health 10*(4), 63–74.

Singh, G. K., & Yu, S. M. (1996). Adverse pregnancy outcomes: Differences between U.S.- and foreign-born women in major US racial and ethnic groups. *American Journal of Public Health, 86*(6), 837–843.

Sobo, E. J. (1992). "Unclean deeds": Menstrual taboos and binding "ties" in rural Jamaica. In M. Nichter (Ed.), *Anthropological approaches to the study of ethnomedicine* (pp. 101–126). Philadelphia: Gordon and Breach Science.

Toubia, N. (1994). Female circumcision as a public health issue. *New England Journal of Medicine, 331,* 712–716.

Trachtenberg, B. (1996). Emotional lives of refugees and immigrant mothers in the urban U.S.: Strategies for acculturation. In A. M. Rynearson & J. Phillips (Eds.), *Selected papers on refugee issues* (Vol. 4, pp. 174–198). Arlington, VA: American Anthropological Association.

van der Kwaak, A. (1992). Female circumcision and gender identity: A questionable alliance? *Social Science & Medicine, 35,* 777–787.

van Oss Marin, B., Gomez, C. A., & Tschann, J. M. (1993). Condom use among Hispanic men with secondary female sexual partners. *Public Health Reports, 108*(6), 742–750.

Venema, H. P. U., Garretsen, H. F. L., & van der Mass, P. J. (1995). Health of migrants and migrant health policy, the Netherlands as an example. *Social Science & Medicine, 41,* 809–818.

Weinstein, H. M., Dansky, L., & Iacopino, V. (1996). Torture and war trauma survivors in primary care practice. *Western Journal of Medicine, 165*(3), 112–118.

Winkel, E. (1995). A Muslim perspective on female circumcision. *Women & Health, 23,* 1–7.

Wood, C. S. (1979). *Human sickness and health: A biocultural view.* Palo Alto, CA: Mayfield.

World Health Organization. (1996). *The world health report 1996.* Geneva, Switzerland: Author.

23

Aging

CHARLOTTE IKELS

Introduction

In order to understand the health needs of older immigrants (those 60 or more years of age) it is especially important to appreciate the heterogeneous nature of this population. First, older immigrants differ from one another in terms of the immigration experience itself, for example, age on arrival in the United States, country of origin, and mode of immigration. Each of these differences shapes their adaptation to life in the United States, their experiences and perceptions of health and illness, and their preferences for treatment. Second, as older people, elderly immigrants are also distinct from younger immigrants from the same country. On average older immigrants are likely to be more rural in origin, less educated, and less employable than younger cohorts. These characteristics can contribute to high rates of financial and emotional dependence on the young. Finally, as older people, elderly immigrants are also likely to face an array of health problems less frequently faced by the young, for example, chronic illness, disability, and the need for long-term care. The sections that follow focus on the impact of the diversity of the older immigrant population on health care needs and on the meeting of those needs.

CHARLOTTE IKELS • Department of Anthropology, Case Western Reserve University, Cleveland, Ohio 44106.

Handbook of Immigrant Health, edited by Loue. Plenum Press, New York, 1998.

Characteristics of Older Immigrants

There are at least two broad categories of older immigrants: those who left their native country in youth or middle age and thus aged in the United States and those who left their native country already aged. Members of the first category have lived in the United States for many years, learned at least rudimentary English, spent time in the work force, become eligible for Social Security and Medicare on retirement, raised their children as Americans, perhaps become citizens themselves, and otherwise adapted to life in a new environment. Members of the second category face quite a different situation. Because most are close to or already past the age of retirement at the time of their arrival in the United States, they are unlikely to seek or obtain employment and, as a result, have fewer natural opportunities to interact with the American-born population and to learn English. They are also less likely to qualify for Social Security and Medicare benefits. Their children have often preceded them to the United States; elderly immigrants are most likely to arrive in the United States as parents of U.S. citizens. In 1995 people 60 or older accounted for 53,762 of the annual total of 720,461 immigrants while parents accounted for 48,382 though by no means all immigrant parents were elderly (U.S. Immigration and Naturalization Service, 1997).

477

Analyzing the health status and needs of older immigrants is problematic for two reasons. First, there are no statistical data available that indicate the recency of immigration of the older immigrant population, that is, that allow us to determine how many have been U.S. residents for many or only a few of their years. Yet it is likely that recency of immigration will have some impact on health-related variables, such as explanatory models of illness and therapeutic preferences. Second, many health researchers do not identify their study populations in terms of immigration status but in terms of ethnicity. Thus, for example, studies of elderly Chinese or elderly Hispanics that focus on ethnic communities might or might not include immigrants in their samples. Despite their lack of specificity I draw on such studies when I think that they illuminate the health care needs of older immigrants, especially but not exclusively of immigrants who were already elderly at the time of their arrival in the United States.

Historically older people have made up only a minority of the immigrating population. As Table 1 indicates, since 1980 people

TABLE 1. Annual Admission of Immigrants Aged 60 or More, 1980–1995

Year	Number	Percent of total immigration
1980	32,414	6.1
1981	33,893	5.7
1982	34,829	5.9
1983	29,950	5.4
1984	30,587	5.6
1985	34,303	6.0
1986	40,108	6.7
1987	39,190	6.5
1988	43,068	6.7
1989	56,055	5.1
1990	73,139	4.8
1991	73,199	4.0
1992	62,151	6.4
1993	64,524	7.1
1994	62,806	7.8
1995	53,762	7.5

Note: From *Statistical Yearbook of the Immigration and Naturalization Service* (1990, p. 70; 1995, p. 54), by U.S. Immigration and Naturalization Service, Washington, DC: U.S. Government Printing Office.

60 or older have constituted between 4.0% and 7.8% of the annual immigrant total. Generally older immigrants leave "young" societies in which they constitute a tiny fraction of the total population to enter an "old" society. For example, in 1990 people 65 or older accounted for 12.6% of the U.S. population. Coming to an old society can offer certain advantages to the elderly as local policy makers are more likely to be aware of the special needs of the elderly and to have developed programs and services to meet those needs, for example, pensions, assisted living facilities, geriatric clinics, opportunities for rehabilitation. The United States is neither the most aged society in the world nor the one offering the widest array of special services to older people—in these respects it is exceeded by the nations of Western Europe—but the United States is "older" and offers more than the nations from which the majority of older immigrants originate.

As Table 2 demonstrates, since the early 1980s immigrants 60 years of age or older have come disproportionately from Asia and Latin America with the (former) Soviet Union becoming prominent in the 1990s. These figures are, of course, based on official statistics and do not include illegal immigrants. On the one hand, given that most illegals come to the United States seeking employment and that the process of illegal entry is arduous as in the case of Mexicans crossing the border on foot, expensive as in the case of Chinese coming by boat, or both as in the case of the Vietnamese "Boat People," it is highly unlikely that the elderly make up more than the tiniest proportion of illegal entrants in any given year. On the other hand, some unknown proportion of once young illegal immigrants have entered old age and remained in the United States. Of the countries currently contributing relatively large numbers of older immigrants, Mexico stands out as a special case. Its numbers are large only because its overall number of immigrants is large. In none of the 3 years presented in Table 2 do older Mexicans exceed 3.5% of all Mexican immigrants. (The surge

TABLE 2. The Six Leading Places of Origin of Older Immigrants

Place of origin	Number	Older immigrants as a % of country total
1985		
Philippines	5,661	11.8
China (mainland)	4,401	17.8
Cuba	2,833	13.9
India	2,604	10.0
Korea	2,595	7.4
Mexico	1,428	2.3
1990		
Mexico	15,903	2.3
Philippines	6,886	10.8
China (mainland)	6,842	21.5
India	3,468	11.3
Soviet Union	3,361	13.2
Vietnam	3,131	6.4
1995		
Soviet Union	10,116	18.6
Philippines	5,128	10.1
China (mainland)	4,540	12.8
Cuba	3,285	18.3
Mexico	3,185	3.5
Vietnam	3,122	7.5

Note: From *Statistical Yearbook of the Immigration and Naturalization Service* (1985, pp. 48–55); 1990, pp. 71–73; 1995, pp. 54–56), by U.S. Immigration and Naturalization Service, Washington, DC: U.S. Government Printing Office.

figures suggest that the special needs of the aged are likely to have different salience for the various immigrant communities.

One of the major problems immigrants face in a new country is ignorance of their heterogeneity on the part of the host population. Nonimmigrant Americans are especially likely to have little knowledge of the important differences in language, culture, and history that distinguish the various Asian populations and that may be of exceptional importance to older immigrants, the cohort that best remembers the events of World War II, the Chinese civil war between the Communists and the Nationalists, the Korean War, and the Vietnam War. While younger Asian and Pacific Islander immigrants may be able to merge their identities and unite for a common cause, older ones may find it intolerable to have to associate with their former enemies. Nonimmigrant Americans are even more likely to be unaware of the great diversity that exists within the population from the same country in terms of local characteristics, such as language and customary diet, and personal characteristics, such as level of education, occupation, and social status. Failure to take note of these differences can easily lead to misunderstandings between health care providers and the people they are trying to serve.

in Mexican immigration in 1990 is an artifact of the amnesty program then in effect that allowed large numbers of illegal aliens to adjust their status to permanent resident.) In contrast to Mexico, several countries (China, the Philippines, Cuba, the Soviet Union, and India) send strikingly high proportions of older immigrants (between 10% and 21.5% of their totals) to the United States. With the exception of the Soviet Union, most of this patterning is related to family reunification efforts. Older immigrants from the Soviet Union are more likely to have come to the United States as refugees or asylees. With elders constituting roughly 6% to 8% of their immigrants, Vietnam and Korea fall between Mexico and the high-rate contributors. These

Place of Origin Effects on Health and Health Care Seeking

The longer an individual has spent in his or her place of origin prior to emigration the greater his or her exposure to local beliefs about health and aging, local medical traditions, and local expectations about access to appropriate care. (Length of stay in the place of origin also has direct effects on individual health status through exposure to local pathogens, nutritional deficits, and, in some cases, the physical demands of manual labor, but due to a scarcity of data these health effects will not be discussed here.) The closeness of a population's beliefs, traditions, and expectations to those of the host country pop-

[handwritten margin note: "close 'fit' of beliefs & behaviors = greater ease in host country"]

ulation will influence the ease with which the older immigrant engages the new health care system.

Within the American research community, medical anthropologists have long dominated the study of indigenous or non-Western medical systems under the general rubric of ethnomedicine. In its early years the subject matter of ethnomedicine was usually seen as something other than the hospital-based biomedicine familiar to most Americans. Increasingly, however, even mainstream American medicine has been contextualized and interpreted as a particular example of medicine, and even a particular example of biomedicine, and subjected to the same kinds of analysis as other forms of medicine (Gaines, 1992; Payer, 1988; Rhodes, 1996; Rubel & Hass, 1996). Early medical anthropologists focused their attention primarily on the conceptual distinctions between illness and disease (Fabrega, 1972) and on culture-bound syndromes (Foulks, 1972), explanatory models (EMs) (Kleinman, Eisenberg, & Good, 1978), patterns of resort (Obayesekere, 1978), and the therapeutics of indigenous healers (Reynolds, 1989). The unit of analysis was typically the individual whether as patient or practitioner. Later medical anthropologists have paid more attention to the system level, for example, to professionalization (Jeffery, 1988; Last, 1996; Unschuld, 1985), the interaction of diverse medical traditions (Leslie, 1975; Topley, 1975), and the impact of political and economic factors in shaping the practice of medicine (Morsy, 1996; Singer, 1989, 1992; Singer & Baer, 1995). Research focused on the individual level has continued, but new topics, such as perceptions of the body (Csordas, 1994; Lock & Scheper-Hughes, 1996), the nature and meaning of suffering (Kleinman, 1988), and the efficacy of various treatments and interventions (Anderson, 1992; Desjarlais, 1992; Etkin, 1996), have taken center stage.

The implications of these types of studies for those of us concerned with maintaining or improving the health status of older immigrants are substantial. Most important, they alert us to the existence of culturally specific interpretations of symptoms. These interpretations affect how individuals or their family members are likely to view the individual's condition, whether they are likely to seek treatment, and what kind of treatment and healer they are likely to prefer. Let us look closely at three studies that have examined health issues among the populations having large numbers of elderly immigrants in the United States: Chicanos (Mexican Americans), Koreans, and Chinese.

Health Issues among Elderly Chicanos

In an extensive review of the literature, Mayers (1989) found little consistency regarding the extent of knowledge and utilization of folk medicine (*curanderismo*) among Chicanos. *Curanderos/as* are practitioners of "formal" folk medicine; that is, they are recognized within the community as having unusual gifts of healing though they have not undergone any formal training program. It is this public recognition that distinguishes them from the legions of informal practitioners, who are simply women looking after the health care needs of their own families. *Curanderos/as* treat culturally specific illnesses such as *mal ojo* (evil eye), *empacho* (surfeit), *caida de mollera* (fallen fontanel), *susto* (magical fright), and *mal puesto* (hex), as well as more conventional disorders such as headache, anxiety, and nervousness. Mayers found that contrary to the assertions of some earlier researchers, recourse to *curanderos/as* does not usually have a negative impact on Mexican American participation in mainstream medicine for two reasons. First, both patients and *curanderos/as* recognize that folk medicine and mainstream medicine deal with different kinds of conditions, and for most illnesses, patients seek treatment from physicians. Second, the limiting factor in visiting physicians is money or the lack of medical insurance. Most physicians have set fees whereas *curanderos/as* generally do not have set fees and accept payments in kind or even none at all. Thus, the two medical systems are complementary rather than directly competitive in nature. Mayers also found that recourse to folk healers was more common among those with closer ties to Mexico, less education, and lower income status—characteristics especially common among elderly persons.

Based on his findings, Mayers made several suggestions to health care providers worried about their ability to serve elderly Mexican American patients. First, he argued that physicians should not automatically attribute the failure of such patients to follow through with medical treatments ("noncompliance") to their attachment to folk medicine; rather, they should be sure to make recommendations for treatment that their patients can realistically be expected to follow. This means making sure to explain in the clearest terms possible the nature of the instructions; it also means being aware of the environmental and financial barriers that hinder compliance. The elderly, for example, may be dependent on others for transportation or prescription pick-up. Helping patients access supportive services may be essential. Second, Mayers pointed out that the elderly may have low physical tolerance for waiting times and difficulties with English; these barriers must be reduced. Third, physicians must be aware of the possibility that their patients are treating themselves or being treated concurrently by a *curandero/a*. The biggest danger here is that of polypharmacy, that is, adverse drug reactions because the patient may be using active folk remedies (of which there are many) along with physician-prescribed drugs. To elicit this information requires great sensitivity. Mayers notes that elderly Mexican American women often do not tell even their children that they are visiting a *curandero/a* because they fear being branded "foolish" or "superstitious" by their more acculturated children. Thus, children are not necessarily the best informants or interpreters in a clinical setting.

Health Issues among Elderly Koreans

Pang (1991, 1994, 1995, 1996) has been the most prolific writer on elderly Korean women in the United States. Though Korean immigrants are concentrated in California, New York, and Illinois, Pang's study was conducted in the greater Washington, D.C., area. Utilizing concepts borrowed from Kleinman (1980), Pang explicated the nature of the traditional Korean health care system in terms of its popular, folk, and professional sectors. By popular, Pang means the stuff of everyday knowledge, that is, the beliefs, ideas, and practices characteristic of ordinary laypeople as they attempt to meet their own or their family members' health care needs. The beliefs, ideas, and practices of the popular sector derive from both the folk and professional sectors. Pang views the folk sector as primarily the realm of shamanistic healers (*mudang*), whose distinctive diagnostic technique involves communication with the spirit world. The professional sector consists of practitioners who have mastered a rich body of knowledge (theory, diagnostics, pharmacopeia, and therapeutics) through formal study or apprenticeship. Traditionally this body of knowledge was known as *hanbang,* an indigenized form of classical Chinese medicine, but in contemporary Korea professional medicine also includes biomedicine.

These two professional medicines differ substantially in all four areas previously mentioned, that is, theory, diagnostics, pharmacopeia, and therapeutics, and popular medicine is much closer to *hanbang* than to biomedicine. Older Korean immigrants, particularly those with rural backgrounds, still think largely in *hanbang* terms, in which illness is construed as an imbalance in the functioning of one or more organ systems due to an insufficiency of vital energy (*ki*). This insufficiency can reflect either depletion of *ki* or a blockage in its flow through the meridians that radiate from the spine and carry it throughout the body. Depletion and blockage can be due to a wide variety of factors: inappropriate diet, reckless living, emotional excess, or the penetration of the body by "wind." A *hanui* (practitioner of *hanbang*) diagnoses the imbalance by taking the patient's pulses, visually examining his or her tongue, eyes, and skin, and asking questions about symptoms, behavior, and sources of stress. The *hanui* then offers an interpretation of the imbalance in conceptual language readily accessible to the patient and usually prescribes familiar herbal medications designed to correct the imbalance and strengthen the affected organ systems. Sometimes acupuncture, which stimulates the flow of *ki,* will also be recommended. The patient may visit the *hanui* without appointment and normally obtains a diagnosis without the need of specialized tests.

Pang interviewed a sample of 20 elderly women over an extended period and observed numerous clinical encounters between these and other patients and ethnic Korean physicians of *hanbang* and of biomedicine. She noted that while patients seemed generally satisfied with their visits to a *hanui,* they were less satisfied with those to biomedical physicians. Several factors account for this dissatisfaction, including (1) patient reliance on the importance of the subjective experience of symptoms that the physician invalidates when he or she reports that test results indicate everything is within normal limits, thereby, in essence, telling the patient nothing is wrong; (2) distaste for the drawing of their blood which is equated with vital essence; (3) belief that by the time something can be detected by a laboratory test the disease is already well advanced; (4) belief that there is no point in submitting to tests because if something is found to be wrong, they are already too old to be cured, and (5) belief that some symptoms are signs of old age rather than of disease and cannot really be cured.

One of the important lessons of Pang's study is that shared ethnicity of patient and biomedical physician is not necessarily sufficient to ensure effective communication because the major obstacle to communication is not native language but adherence to different medical cultures. Another lesson is that despite their preference for *hanbang* for certain kinds of health problems, most elderly feel that they have little choice but to go to a biomedical physician first as this is the kind

of medicine for which their health insurer pays. Because of the expense of herbal medicine, only those with their own funds or those who have not been able to obtain relief from biomedicine *and* have children willing to pay are likely to visit the *hanui.*

Health Issues among Elderly Chinese

The kinds of issues, for example, differences in EMs, that Pang raises in connection with elderly Korean immigrants are equally relevant for elderly Chinese, but are not raised again here. Instead, in this section we look at place of origin effects on perceptions of and responses to mental difficulties, particularly dementia, among the elderly. Many writers (e.g., Elliott, Minno, Lam, & Tu, 1996; Gaw, 1975; Kleinman, 1986; Phillips, 1993) have pointed out that mental illness, particularly schizophrenia, is greatly stigmatized in Chinese societies. This stigmatization may lead to two somewhat contradictory responses; on the one hand, the family may try to conceal the fact of mental illness while on the other, it may discreetly seek out all possible means of treatment. Elliot and colleagues (1996) suggested that the more the symptoms of dementia resemble those of mental disorders such as schizophrenia, for example, paranoia, suspiciousness, disorientation, hallucinations, the greater the risk that some families will simply conceal their affected family member.

The more common symptoms of dementia, however, are much less likely to generate excitement. Ikels (1998) reported that in Guangzhou, the capital of Guangdong province, an area that sends many emigrants to the United States, older people and their family members generally do not dread the occurrence of dementia to the same degree as Americans. Impaired memory, confusion, and passivity are not viewed so much as mental illness as they are normal concomitants of aging. The elder need not be concealed, but neither is treatment likely to be sought. Elders whose mental impairment results in inappropriate behavior, that is, ag-

not language but customs as barriers

gression or stubbornness, are less easily tolerated largely because their actions are frequently believed to be voluntary.

Ikels attributed the different reactions of Americans and Chinese to dementia to the fact that the various symptoms have different effects on both the elder and his or her family members. First, most Chinese elders live in multigenerational households, usually with a married son's family, whereas most American elders live independently. Consequently the situational demands on a Chinese elder are generally less than those on an American, who must be able to carry out a host of complex tasks every day. When a Chinese elder falters, family members are already present in the same household and able to take over most of the senior member's responsibilities with relatively little inconvenience. When an American elder falters, however, he or she may have to exit the household to move in with family members or go to an assisted living facility. Thus even relatively minor cognitive impairment may be extremely threatening to the well-being of an older American. Second, the need to rely on others is likely to be less upsetting psychologically to a Chinese elder than to an American since Confucian values have long emphasized the obligation of adult children to look after elderly parents. Being cared for is a right, not an imposition though, at the same time, even Chinese parents do not wish to impose a burden on their children. Third, in the case of Chinese, a different conception of personhood probably lessens the threat dementia poses to identity. In the West, as Post (1995) put it, "we live in a hypercognitive culture" (p. 142); to paraphrase Descartes, we are because we think. Any erosion of cognitive function represents an erosion of the self. Chinese culture takes a broader view of selfhood; the self is realized in social interaction. Therefore, even if the individual is severely impaired cognitively, so long as he or she retains the capacity for social interaction, in Chinese eyes, he or she is probably still "there."

When Chinese emigrate to the United States, they encounter a health care system with distinctive assumptions about the nature of the impact of dementia on the family unit. These assumptions include a belief that caregivers experience a sense of burden, that they will benefit by support services such as day care for their demented relative and support group contacts for themselves, and that eventually they will recognize the wisdom of institutionalizing their relative. However, whether caregivers experience burden or not, they may be reluctant to seek services because they believe they must continue to provide care at home or fail in their duty as children. Furthermore, given the lack of such support services in the home country, immigrants are unlikely to be aware that such services even exist, and, finally, sending a parent or grandparent to an institution is often unthinkable as in Chinese societies this option has normally been available only to aged people without any close relatives.

The Special Health Care Needs of Older Immigrants

In the preceding sections, we considered the impact of characteristics of the culture of the place of origin on immigrant health care seeking. Here we consider the special health care needs of the older immigrant population. These needs derive from the fact that older immigrants are both old and immigrants.

Needs Related to Age

Although being old should not be equated with being sick, old people are more likely than the young or middle aged to experience a wide array of health problems. These include chronic diseases, such as arthritis, circulatory disorders, and respiratory problems; sensory impairments, such as vision and hearing loss; and various disabilities resulting from these diseases and impairments. As Verbrugge (1990) put it: "The legacy of longevity . . . is disability" (p. 71). The clinical identification of disease is one of the primary tasks of biomedicine; it is generally a straightforward task, and incidence and prevalence rates in different populations can be relatively easily estimated. The situation with disability rates is quite different; they are notoriously difficult to determine due to disagreement among researchers on the concept of disability, the most effective way to measure disability, and the range of activity domains measurement should encompass (Ikels, 1991; Jette, Crawford, & Tennstedt, 1996; Keith *et al.*, 1994; Kopec, 1995; Verbrugge, 1990).

Verbrugge (1990) argued that we need to differentiate more clearly between *intrinsic* and *actual* disability. Intrinsic refers to the ability to carry out an activity on one's own whereas actual refers to the ability to carry out an activity taking into account available supports, for example, a cane, a helper, a pain-reliever. Keith and colleagues (1994) pointed out that different cultures assign different roles to the elderly such that *in*ability to do something, for example, write a check, drive a car, perform household chores, cannot simply be equated with *dis*ability. Ikels (1991) and Kopec (1995) both pointed out that performance of an activity is not exclusively determined by physical capacity; rather, the importance of the activity to the individual must be taken into account. Highly valued and obligatory activities will be carried out even in the face of great discomfort; less valued and discretionary activities will be relinquished in the face of lesser discomfort. This last point also alludes to the temporal dimension of disability, for example, that people make accommodations over time, and that measuring disability status only once may generate false positives as well as false negatives. Finally, Verbrugge (1990) criticized researchers for their narrow focus on the more obligatory activities of daily living (ADLs), for example, dressing, toileting, and feeding, and instrumental activities of daily living (IADLs), for example, shopping, managing finances, performing household chores, at the expense of discretionary activities, for example, visiting friends, engaging in hobbies. This narrow focus, she argued, highlights only the tip of the "iceberg of disability" because it obscures the fact that many people have already had to cut back on their normal activities due to physical limitations.

Disability rates vary with ethnic status. Generally European Americans are found to have lower disability rates than members of minority groups, but precisely why this is the case is not clearly understood (Jette *et al.,* 1996). Are these differences due to differences in rates of disease and impairment, different use of external supports, different role demands, different accommodations to physical limitations, or even to different communication styles (the stiff upper lip versus the highly expressive)? Since most disability research in the United States has policy implications—the findings are used to determine the need for special programs and services—it is crucial that researchers determine the bases for whatever differentials exist.

Last, older people have higher mortality rates than the young and the middle aged and, therefore, are far more likely to encounter the need not only for long-term care but also for hospitalization and terminal care. Patients and families may have to confront issues and decisions they would never have anticipated in the place of origin, for example, filling out advance care directives or "living wills," assigning durable power of attorney for health care, withholding or withdrawing life support. Unfamiliarity with modern technology and its consequences may make it impossible for patients (or more likely their family members) to make truly informed decisions. If they come from more paternalistic health care systems, they may be puzzled and worried by a physician who waits for them to make a decision about treatment, and when they are accustomed to euphemisms in the case of cancer or other serious conditions, they may be appalled to hear the naked truth that they or their family member is terminally ill.

Murphy and colleagues (1996) carried out an investigation into knowledge of, attitude toward, and possession of advance directives among 800 elderly in Los Angeles County. The sample consisted of 200 people age 65 or older drawn from each of four ethnically defined populations: African Americans, European Americans, Korean Americans, and Mexican Americans. Only 12% and 13% of African Americans and Korean Americans, respectively, were aware of the nature of advance directives in contrast to 69% and 47% of European Americans and Mexican Americans, respectively. Familiarity with the concept of advance directives, however, did not translate directly into possession of a living will. Murphy and colleagues (1996) found that of those with knowledge only 40% of European Americans, 22% of Mexican Americans, 17% of African Americans, and no Korean Americans actually had living wills. In the case of Korean Americans and Mexican Americans, they attributed the low rates to negative attitudes related to advance planning and, here and elsewhere (Blackhall, Murphy, Frank, Michel, & Azen, 1995), to the beliefs that it is better not to inform a patient of a terminal diagnosis and that family members rather than the patient should make decisions about his or her treatment. They concluded that a focus on advance directives may be inappropriate for these populations as it too often links the need for decision making to death, and suggested their decoupling.

Needs Related to Immigrant Status

One of the inescapable facts of immigration is that no matter how desired the move to the new country, it nevertheless entails a number of losses, for example, of familiar people, places, and routines. The greater the distance and the higher the costs of travel the greater the likelihood that an immigrant will never revisit his or her homeland. This is especially true of older immigrants who are less likely to have the stamina to undertake such a trip and must, therefore, be accompanied—doubling the costs to the family of any such trip. Furthermore, by virtue of being well advanced in years, the older immigrant has less of a future in the new land. While an immigrant may highly value the move for the opportunities it offers the younger genera-

tion, he or she may also feel to some extent that his or her own life is over.

Even when an older immigrant has an optimistic view of the immigration experience and looks forward to starting a new life, he or she faces obstacles that younger ones do not. For example, younger people are more often thrust into situations, school or workplace, that require them to learn to function in the new society. Unless they live and work in an ethnically dense community, they will need to learn English, drive a car or ride public transportation, behave appropriately in public, and so on. In order to do all these things, younger adults are given priority in enrolling in most language and vocational classes. As a result, the elderly may find themselves humiliatingly dependent on their more acculturated family members to carry out even the simplest of tasks, for example, locating a clinic, communicating symptoms to a health care provider, determining how often, how many, and in what sequence to take various medications. If acculturation also undermines the elder's traditional position of authority in the family, his or her morale may plummet leading to apathy or clinical depression.

Immigrants who came inititally as refugees or asylees may also experience anxiety, insomnia, nightmares, flashbacks, or other symptoms of posttraumatic stress disorder. They may worry about the fate of loved ones left behind or endlessly relive persecution for their political or religious beliefs or their ethnic or regional identity (e.g., Omidian, 1996). They may experience a complex swirl of emotions, such as anger at being forced to leave, relief at obtaining security, and guilt that others were left behind. If left with few people to share these feelings, they may fear losing their sanity. The impact of all of these problems is magnified, of course, if the older immigrant is in the host country illegally.

Accessing Health Care Services

While on average older immigrants are more in need of health care services than the young, they have also been more likely to have financial access to them, because, until very recently, older legal immigrants have had the same rights as older citizens to participate in various government-funded programs aimed primarily at the elderly (e.g., Medicare, or, disproportionately, Medicaid).

Government-Funded Programs for the Elderly

A vast array of programs with at least some health care component is available to older people as a result of federal legislation (Gelfand, 1993). These programs include everything from hospitalization to home care, day care, long-term care, congregate meals, and nutrition counseling as well as income support (Supplemental Security Income or SSI) that makes it possible for the recipient to pay for health care services that are not subsidized directly by the government. The two most important programs for the elderly, Medicare and Medicaid, have different eligibility criteria and pay for overlapping but nevertheless different categories of service.

Medicare originated with the Older Americans Act of 1965; it has been extended and amended periodically ever since. As a part of the Social Security program, eligibility for Medicare requires recipients to have participated in the labor force in covered employment for a specified period of time or to be the spouse or widowed partner of such a participant. Recipients must be at least 65 years of age (or, if younger, suffering from end-stage renal disease). The program consists of two parts, A (hospital insurance) and B (medical insurance). All participants receive coverage under Part A at no cost and are entitled to 60 days of hospitalization per illness episode though they must pay for the first day themselves. When hospitalization exceeds 60 days, Medicare will pay for another 30, but the patient is required to meet a daily copayment.

One of the major criticisms of the Medicare program is that it is designed to meet acute care needs rather than the chronic care needs more characteristic of the older population. This bias is clearly visible in Medicare's policy toward long-term care which is directly linked with hospitalization. When a patient has been stabilized in the hospital but is still in need of medical care beyond what he or she is able to receive at home, he or she is discharged to a facility offering skilled nursing care. The expectation is that a stay of a few weeks or months should result in sufficient improvement in the patient's medical condition that eventually he or she can leave the facility and return home. Thus, Medicare pays for 20 days of care and then requires the patient to pay a substantial part of the care for the next 80 days. Medicare also pays for medically necessary home health care, that is, not custodial care or homemaker services, and for hospice care for those with a terminal condition and a life expectancy of less than 6 months.

Coverage under Part B of Medicare is not free but is obtained by meeting a monthly fee. Nearly all Medicare recipients subscribe to Part B (Gelfand, 1993) which pays for physician services though the recipient must meet an annual deductible and 20% of the normal physician charges. Part B does not pay for prescription (or over-the-counter) drugs, dental care, and various other services. According to Gelfand, Medicare meets less than 40% of the health care costs of the elderly. Consequently most Medicare beneficiaries buy additional private medical insurance (so-called "Medigap" policies) to cover the costs and services that Medicare does not. As the American population ages and as policy makers debate the future solvency of the Medicare program, advocates for older people fear that their share of health care expenses will inevitably rise both absolutely and relatively.

Unlike Medicare, Medicaid is a welfare program, that is, it is means tested and its beneficiaries must already be recipients of Aid to Families with Dependent Children or, in the case of the elderly or disabled, SSI; eligibility for Medicaid is not contingent on labor force participation. It is important to note that Medicaid is a state-administered program through which federal funds are channeled and to which states must contribute a portion themselves. To obtain these federal funds individual states must cover a certain minimum of services, but they have considerable discretion over what additional services they cover. Consequently wealthy and politically liberal states generally offer substantially more covered benefits than poor and politically conservative states. Medicaid is required to pay for the uncovered Medicare-related expenses, for example, deductibles, copayments, and Part B insurance premiums, of its recipients. States must also offer inpatient and outpatient hospital services, skilled nursing home services, and physician services as well as periodic screening services for children (Gelfand, 1993).

States have the option (among others) of covering services in an intermediate care facility, a type of facility that falls between a skilled nursing home and a residential facility. Medicaid services are not contingent on hospitalization nor must they have the objective of restoring the recipient to a higher level of functioning. A patient with irreversible dementia but no condition requiring hospitalization is not admissible to long-term care under Medicare but is under Medicaid. Furthermore Medicaid will pay for long-term care for people whose Medicare allotment has run out and whose private funds have been "spent down." As a result the bulk of Medicaid expenditures are for long-term care. Together Medicare and Medicaid have provided major benefits to older immigrants, but since the passage of the Welfare Reform Act in 1996, immigrant eligibility for Medicaid and other federal programs has come under threat.

Impact of Recent Legislation on Access to Health Care

The two acts with the greatest implications for older immigrant access are the Personal Responsibility and Work Opportunity Reconciliation Act of 1996 (the Welfare Reform Act) and the Illegal Immigration Reform and Immigrant Responsibility Act of 1996 (the Immigration Reform Act). Because these acts have similar, but not identical, objectives and provisions, their impact on older immigrants is discussed in what follows as if they were a single bill. Basically these acts disqualify legal (and illegal) immigrants (with certain exceptions) from receiving a wide range of federal, state, and local public benefits and, most unsettling, disqualify even some of those immigrants, such as healthy elderly receiving SSI, who have been legally receiving them for years.

Precisely who is eligible to continue to receive which benefits is difficult to say as there are (1) various statutory exceptions to the exclusions, for example, veterans, those who have worked and paid taxes in the United States for 40 quarters (10 years); (2) temporary exceptions to the exclusions, for example, refugees or asylees who are within 5 years of having been granted their status; and (3) ongoing federal and state legislative efforts to amend the regulations or their implementation. For example, some states are prepared to absorb, at least temporarily, the Medicaid expenses of people who are decertified for SSI or to institute their own financial assistance programs, or both. Nevertheless, within months of the bills' passage, nursing home operators, uncertain how to interpret the legislation, which positively bars immigrants who have arrived in the United States since August 22, 1996, from most public benefits, were refusing admission to legal immigrants who had been in the country many years before that date (Swarns, 1997). Sponsors of newly arriving immigrants are now subject to a more stringent enforcement of earlier rules that required them to guarantee they would assume responsibility for meeting the immigrant's expenses and would not allow him or her to become a public charge. They are now being asked to provide proof that the newcomer, if elderly or disabled, is eligible for medical coverage by the sponsor's insurer or that he or she has purchased medical insurance in the immigrant's name.

Neither long-established nor newly arrived immigrants are forever barred from access to public welfare programs as they need only become American citizens to establish eligibility. Not surprisingly, this has spurred many immigrants to apply for naturalization, a process that requires at least 5 years as a permanent resident alien and the passing of a citizenship examination. Normally the examination involves answering correctly and in English a set of questions about American history and government drawn from study materials available from government bookstores. Since the elderly are more likely than the young to have limited knowledge of English and to be illiterate, the examination can pose serious problems for them though some accommodations have been made. For example, those who are 65 or older and have been lawful permanent residents of the United States for at least 20 years may be tested in their native language and on a much smaller body of knowledge. In addition, disability waivers are available to applicants who have a medically determinable physical, developmental, or mental impairment that renders them unable to learn English and/or U.S. history and civics so long as they can understand and take the oath of allegiance. An older immigrant with dementia could under these rules be exempted from the test altogether.

Utilizing Health Care Services

Some of the issues affecting the utilization of health care services, such as place of origin effects and financing, were introduced in earlier Sections. Here we focus on the role of the ethnic community in providing or enhancing the delivery of care to the elderly.

In the 1960s Congress passed not only Medicare and Medicaid but also a variety of civil rights legislation designed to promote the greater participation of minority and ethnically diverse populations in publicly funded programs. In order to determine the extent to which minority and ethnic elderly were currently receiving health care services, a number of studies were commissioned. These early studies (Bell, Kasschau, & Zellman, 1976; Cuellar & Weeks, 1980; Human Re-

sources Corporation, 1978; Pacific/Asian Elderly Research Project, 1978) soon documented that these populations were underrepresented, particularly as recipients of long-term care. Possible reasons for their underrepresentation included (1) preference for care by the family, (2) discrimination, (3) lack of awareness of services, and (4) lack of appropriate services. Because the 1960s legislation made discrimination in service provision and in admission to nursing homes receiving federal funds illegal, advocates for the elderly have turned their attention primarily to increasing awareness of and developing culturally appropriate services.

As indicated earlier, many older immigrants are non-English speakers and, depending on the particular immigrant group, may be illiterate even in their native language. Consequently conventional outreach methods, such as posters in ethnic grocery stores or notices of service availability in ethnic newspapers, may not be sufficient to reach their targets who are more dependent on the spoken than the written word. Ikels (1986) noted the importance of natural helpers, "individuals who, although not usually employed in the helping professions, voluntarily choose to spend part of their time helping others informally" (p. 216), in providing what amounted to information and referral services to older Chinese immigrants in Boston. She observed that the ability of natural helpers to perform this function rested on several shared characteristics: (1) established reputations, (2) bilingual and bicultural expertise, (3) geographic accessibility, (4) prior managerial experience, (5) closeness in age to those being helped, and (6) a genuine belief in the importance of helping others. Because these individuals easily elicited trust and did not ask intrusive questions, such as one's immigration status, some older immigrants were more comfortable initiating contact with them than with younger agency personnel.

The importance of matching or, at a minimum, culturally sensitizing direct care providers and clients is widely acknowledged, (e.g., Padgett & Baily, 1995; Skinner, 1995). Drawing on the findings of medical anthropologist Margaret Clark, Padgett and Baily enumerated five distinctive negative responses that can occur when people of different cultural backgrounds interact: blindness, shock, conflict, imposition, and stereotyping. Some cultural differences, for example, language and food preferences, are readily detectable, but others, such as communication styles or sensitivities related to historical experiences, are not, and if not recognized for what they are can result in unresolvable tension and hostility. Skinner noted that many nursing homes appreciate the need for mutual respect and compatibility of providers and recipients of care, but the realities of the marketplace often do not allow for matching. For example, African Americans constitute only a tiny fraction of the population living in nursing homes, but almost one third of the aides, orderlies, and attendants. Residents of European American backgrounds may be fearful or resentful of being under the control of a population that historically has had subordinate status while demented residents, lacking the capacity for self-restraint, may heap racial abuse on them.

Yet shared ethnicity does not necessarily eliminate interaction problems. For example, immigrants from countries in which household servants are common may relate inappropriately to home care staff, attempting to order them to perform tasks that are not officially authorized. Similarly in China and other developing countries it is customary for family members or hired attendants to perform much of the personal care assigned to hospital or nursing home aides in the United States. This practice can easily lead to misunderstandings in ethnically oriented nursing homes in which low-ranking staff are often physicians or nurses from the same country as the residents, but who, because of difficulties with English, are not yet able to practice medicine in the United States. At the same time that they are enduring the loss of their occupational status, their charges may be pouring salt on their wounds by treating them as inferiors.

Ethnically oriented residential facilities did not originate with the passage of Medicare and Medicaid, but the introduction of these two programs, along with the expansion of the ethnic elderly population, certainly contributed to their growth or conversion into nursing homes (Folmar, 1993; Kaplan & Shore, 1993; van Steenberg, Ansak, & Chin-Hansen, 1993). In an effort to determine what factors facilitate the delivery of care to institutionalized ethnic elders, Yeo (1993) drew on a review of the literature and her own study of five ethnically oriented nursing homes serving Asian (primarily Japanese and Chinese), Jewish, Russian Orthodox, Japanese, and Chinese, and one residential care facility for Spanish-speaking elderly. She listed 11 factors thought to contribute to quality care: (1) history, ownership, and policy-making authority; (2) location; (3) selection and training of staff; (4) admission policy and process; (5) cost; (6) interaction with family; (7) language; (8) food; (9) activity program; (10) religious observances, and (11) delivery of personal and nursing care.

As this review of the literature and issues indicates, the provision of health care to older immigrants has become an increasingly common experience for health care providers in the United States. Over the past two decades much has been learned about what does and does not work, and future older immigrants (albeit increasingly at their own expense) should be more successful than their predecessors in locating providers who understand their needs.

References

Anderson, R. (1992). The efficacy of ethnomedicine: Research methods in trouble. In M. Nichter (Ed.), *Anthropological approaches to the study of ethnomedicine* (pp. 1–17). Philadelphia: Gordon and Breach Science.

Bell, D., Kasschau, P., & Zellman, G. (1976). *Delivering services to elderly members of minority groups: A critical review of the literature.* Santa Monica, CA: Rand.

Blackhall, L. J., Murphy, S. T., Frank, G., Michel, V., & Azen, S. (1995). Ethnicity and attitudes toward patient autonomy. *Journal of the American Medical Association, 274,* 820–825.

Csordas, T. J. (Ed.). (1994). *Embodiment and experience: The existential ground of culture and self.* Cambridge, England: Cambridge University Press.

Cuellar, J. B., & Weeks, J. (1980). *Minority elderly Americans: A prototype for area agencies on aging.* San Diego, CA: Allied Home Health Association.

Desjarlais, R. R. (1992). *Body and emotion: The aesthetics of illness and emotion in Nepal.* Philadelphia: University of Pennsylvania Press.

Elliott, K. S., Minno, M. D., Lam, D., & Tu, A. M. (1996). Working with Chinese families in the context of dementia. In G. Yeo & D. Gallagher-Thompson (Eds.), *Ethnicity and the dementias* (pp. 89–108). Washington, DC: Taylor & Francis.

Etkin, N. L. (1996). Ethnopharmacology: The conjunction of medical ethnography and the biology of therapeutic action. In C. F. Sargent & T. M. Johnson (Eds.), *Medical anthropology: Contemporary theory and method* (Rev. ed., pp. 151–164). Westport, CT: Praeger.

Fabrega, H. (1972). Medical anthropology. In B. J. Siegel (Ed.), *Biennial review of anthropology 1971* (pp. 167–229). Stanford, CA: Stanford University Press.

Folmar, S. (1993). A higher purpose: Jewish tradition and model long-term care in Cleveland. In C. M. Barresi & D. E. Stull (Eds.), *Ethnic elderly and long-term care* (pp. 191–203). New York: Springer.

Foulks, E. F. (1972). *The Arctic hysterias of the North Alaskan Eskimo.* Washington, DC: American Anthropological Association.

Gaines, A. (Ed.). (1992). *Ethnopsychiatry: The cultural construction of professional and folk psychiatries.* Albany: State University of New York Press.

Gaw, A. C. (1975). An integrated approach to the delivery of health care to a Chinese community in America: The Boston experience. In A. Kleinman, P. Kunstadter, E. R. Alexander, & J. L. Gale (Eds.), *Medicine in Chinese cultures: Comparative studies of health care in Chinese and other societies* (pp. 327–349). Washington, DC: John E. Fogarty International Center, National Institutes of Health.

Gelfand, D. E. (1993). *The aging network: Programs and services* (4th ed.). New York: Springer.

Human Resources Corporation. (1978). *Policy issues concerning the minority elderly: Final report executive summary.* Submitted to the Federal Council on the Aging, San Francisco.

Ikels, C. (1986). Older immigrants and natural helpers. *Journal of Cross-Cultural Gerontology, 1,* 209–222.

Ikels, C. (1991). Aging and disability in China: Cultural issues in measurement and interpretation. *Social Science & Medicine, 32,* 649–665.

Ikels, C. (1998). The experience of dementia in China. *Culture, Medicine, and Psychiatry, 22.*

Jeffery, R. (1988). *The politics of health in India.* Berkeley: University of California Press.

Jette, A. M., Crawford, S. L., & Tennstedt, S. L. (1996). Toward understanding ethnic differences in late-life disability. *Research on Aging, 18,* 292–309.

Kaplan, J, & Shore, H. (1993). The Jewish nursing home: Innovations in practice and policy. In C. M. Barresi & D. E. Stull (Eds.), *Ethnic elderly and long-term care* (pp. 115–129). New York: Springer.

Keith, J., Fry, C., Glascock, A., Ikels, C., Dickerson-Putman, J., Harpending, H., & Draper, P. (1994). *The aging experience: Diversity and commonality across cultures.* Thousand Oaks, CA: Sage.

Kleinman, A. M. (1980). *Patients and healers in the context of culture.* Berkeley: University of California Press.

Kleinman, A. M. (1986). *Social origins of distress and disease: Depression, neurasthenia, and pain in modern China.* New Haven, CT: Yale University Press.

Kleinman, A. M. (1988). *The illness narratives: Suffering, healing and the human condition.* New York: Free Press.

Kleinman, A. M., Eisenberg, L., & Good, B. J. (1978). Culture, illness, and care: Clinical lessons from anthropologic and cross-cultural research. *Annals of Internal Medicine, 88,* 251–258.

Kopec, J. A. (1995). Concepts of disability: The activity space model. *Social Science & Medicine, 40,* 649–656.

Last, M. (1996). The professionalization of indigenous healers. In C. F. Sargent & T. M. Johnson (Eds.), *Medical anthropology: Contemporary theory and method* (Rev. ed., pp. 374–395). Westport, CT: Praeger.

Leslie, C. (1975). Pluralism and integration in the Indian and Chinese medical systems. In A. Kleinman, P. Kunstadter, E. R. Alexander, & J. L. Gale (Eds.), *Medicine in Chinese cultures: Comparative studies of health care in Chinese and other societies* (pp. 401–415). Washington, DC: John E. Fogarty International Center, National Institutes of Health.

Lock, M., & Scheper-Hughes, N. (1996). A critical-interpretive approach in medical anthropology: Rituals and routines of discipline and dissent. In C. F. Sargent & T. M. Johnson (Eds.), *Medical anthropology: Contemporary theory and method* (Rev. ed., pp. 41–70). Westport, CT: Praeger.

Mayers, R. S. (1989). Use of folk medicine by elderly Mexican-American women. *Journal of Drug Issues, 19,* 283–295.

Morsy, S. A. (1996). Political economy in medical anthropology. In C. F. Sargent & T. M. Johnson (Eds.), *Medical anthropology: Contemporary theory and method* (Rev. ed., pp. 21–40). Westport, CT: Praeger.

Murphy, S. T., Palmer, J. M., Azen, S., Frank, G., Michel, V., & Blackhall, L. J. (1996). Ethnicity and advance care directives. *Journal of Law, Medicine & Ethics, 24,* 89–100.

Obayesekere, G. (1978). The impact of Ayurvedic ideas on the culture and the individual in Sri Lanka. In C. Leslie (Ed.), *Asian medical systems* (pp. 201–227). Berkeley: University of California Press.

Omidian, P. A. (1996). *Aging and family in an Afghan Refugee Community: Transitions and transformations.* New York: Garland.

Pacific/Asian Elderly Research Project. (1978). *Final report.* Los Angeles.

Padgett, D., & Baily, S. J. (1995). Culturally specific psychosocial nursing care for the ethnic elderly. In D. Padgett (Ed.), *Handbook on ethnicity, aging, and mental health* (pp. 242–264). Westport, CT: Greenwood.

Pang, K. Y. C. (1991). *Elderly Korean women in America: Everyday life, health, and illness.* New York: AMS.

Pang, K. Y. C. (1994). Understanding depression among elderly Korean immigrants through their folk illnesses. *Medical Anthropology Quarterly, 8,* 209–216.

Pang, K. Y. C. (1995). A cross-cultural understanding of depression among elderly Korean immigrants: Prevalence, symptoms, and diagnosis. *Clinical Gerontologist, 15,* 3–20.

Pang, K. Y. C. (1996). Self-care strategy of elderly Korean immigrants in the Washington, D.C. metropolitan area. *Journal of Cross-Cultural Gerontology, 11,* 229–254.

Payer, L. (1988). *Medicine and culture: Varieties of treatment in the United States, England, West Germany, and France.* New York: Holt.

Phillips, M. R. (1993). Strategies used by Chinese families coping with schizophrenia. In D. Davis & S. Harrell (Eds.), *Chinese families in the post-Mao era* (pp. 277–306). Berkeley: University of California Press.

Post, S. G. (1995). Dementia in our midst: The moral community. *Cambridge Quarterly of Health Care Ethics, 4,* 142–147.

Reynolds, D. K. (1989). *Flowing bridges, quiet waters.* Albany: State University of New York Press.

Rhodes, L. A. (1996). Studying biomedicine as a cultural system. In C. F. Sargent & T. M. Johnson (Eds.), *Medical anthropology: Contemporary theory and method* (Rev. ed., pp. 165–180). Westport, CT: Praeger.

Rubel, A. J., & Hass, M. R. (1996). Ethnomedicine. In C. F. Sargent & T. M. Johnson (Eds.), *Medical anthropology: Contemporary theory and method* (Rev. ed., pp. 113–130). Westport, CT: Praeger.

Singer, M. (1989). The coming of age of critical medical anthropology. *Social Science & Medicine, 11,* 1193–1203.

Singer, M. (1992). Biomedicine and the political economy of science. *Medical Anthropology Quarterly, 6,* 400–403.

Singer, M., & Baer, H. (1995). *Critical medical anthropology.* Amityville, N.Y.: Baywood.

Skinner, J. H. (1995). Ethnic/racial diversity in long-term care use and services. In Z. Harel & R. E. Dunkle (Eds.), *Matching people with services in long-term care* (pp. 49–71). New York: Springer.

Swarns, R. L. (1997, April 20). Confused by law, nursing homes bar legal immigrants. *New York Times,* pp. 1, 37.

Topley, M. (1975). Chinese and Western medicine in Hong Kong: Some social and cultural determinants of variation, interaction and change. In A. Kleinman, P. Kunstadter, E. R. Alexander, & J. L. Gale (Eds.), *Medicine in Chinese cultures: Comparative studies of health care in Chinese and other societies* (pp. 241–271). Washington, DC: John E. Fogarty International Center, National Institute of Health.

U.S. Immigration and Naturalization Service. (1986). *Statistical Yearbook of the Immigration and Naturalization Service, 1985.* Washington, DC: U.S. Government Printing Office.

U.S. Immigration and Naturalization Service. (1991). *Statistical Yearbook of the Immigration and Naturalization Service, 1990.* Washington, DC: U.S. Government Printing Office.

U.S. Immigration and Naturalization Service. (1997). *Statistical Yearbook of the Immigration and Naturalization Service, 1995.* Washington, DC: U.S. Government Printing Office.

Unschuld, P. (1985). *Medicine in China: A history of ideas.* Berkeley: University of California Press.

Van Steenberg, C., Ansak, M-L, & Chin-Hansen, J. (1993). On Lok's model: Managed long-term care. In C. M. Barresi & D. E. Stull (Eds.), *Ethnic elderly and long-term care* (pp. 178–190). New York: Springer.

Verbrugge, L. M. (1990). The iceberg of disability. In S. M. Stahl (Ed.), *The legacy of longevity: Health and health care in later life* (pp. 55–75). Newbury Park, CA: Sage.

Yeo, G. W. (1993). Ethnicity and nursing homes: Factors affecting use and successful components for culturally sensitive care. In C. M. Barresi & D. E. Stull (Eds.), *Ethnic elderly and long-term care* (pp. 161–177). New York: Springer.

24

Substance Use among Immigrants to the United States

L. A. REBHUN

Introduction

There are a great variety of psychoactive substances known to human beings, mostly plant-based chemicals that change perception and sensation. Some of these are relatively mild in their natural state, but can be refined into powerful drugs. For example, the coca leaf chewed by Andean peasants is a mild stimulant, but after large amounts of coca leaf have been crushed, cooked, and chemically treated to isolate and concentrate the active ingredient, the resulting cocaine powder or crack cocaine "rock" becomes a powerful and powerfully addicting substance. Similarly, while any uncooked berry or fruit juice left overnight will begin to ferment, the resultant mildly alcoholic mash is far different in nature from triple distilled Scotch whiskey, for example.

Acculturation and Substance Use

The use of psychoactive substances is a profoundly social act among human beings, and highly affected by culture. Customs determine which drugs are available, in what

L. A. REBHUN • Department of Anthropology, Yale University, New Haven, Connecticut 06511.

Handbook of Immigrant Health, edited by Loue. Plenum Press, New York, 1998.

form, how they are purchased and consumed, how their effects are interpreted, and the consequences of their consumption. In many cultures psychoactive substances are integral to religious practice, and the use of such drugs as caffeine, khat, alcohol, nicotine, and marijuana are important to socializing in many settings. Use of drugs, even drugs damaging to health (such as tobacco and alcohol) is functional in some cultural settings. Each culture demands and reinforces particular patterns of psychoactive substance use (Blatter, 1995; Boado, 1984; Oetting, 1993). The use or abuse of a psychoactive substance by an immigrant may be a form of deviance, a reaction to the difficulties of immigration and acculturation, or it may be a normal expectation of the native culture of the immigrant (Oetting, 1993, p. 51).

When people migrate from one culture to another, they bring with them the drug-use customs of their native areas. Upon arrival in their new home, they may find a social and legal setting for drug use very different from that to which they are accustomed. The term "acculturation" refers to the process by which immigrants and their U.S.–born children change their ideas and behaviors in response to the host culture (Berry, 1980). The presence of large numbers of immigrants may also cause a reverse acculturation of mainstream culture.

The process of acculturation is complex, and researchers dispute its exact nature and consequences. Any given culture will have a variety of norms around psychoactive drug use. Immigrant individuals are multifaceted with regard to acculturation, showing more acculturation in some areas than in others. Acculturation is a dynamic process changing not only over time but with context. In instruments used to measure acculturation, measures such as length of residence are too simple to capture the full picture (Mendoza, 1989, p. 374).

Some researchers use a learning (or modeling) model of acculturation which stresses the process of assimilation to local customs. In the case of substance use, if people in the immigrant's new country drink more or take more or different kinds of drugs, the new immigrant may learn the new pattern as part of assimilation.

Alternatively, many immigrants find the experience of immigration disorienting, and they may find themselves lonely, isolated, impoverished, or discriminated against in their new country, increasing their tendency to turn to the artificial comfort of chemical cheer. This is an "acculturative stress" (Thomas, 1995) model of alcohol and drug use among immigrants, which emphasizes the tendency to develop problems as a psychological reaction to the situation of immigration itself.

It is also possible to combine the two models. For example, Graves (1967), in an early study of drinking among Latino immigrants, found that Latinos were more likely to develop higher levels of alcohol consumption and to become inebriated more frequently when they attempted to imitate the drinking patterns of Anglos in the United States—and failed. Although this study had too small a sample to be widely generalizable, Graves's combination of the two models is instructive (G. Marin & Posner, 1995, p. 780).

Acculturation may exacerbate substance use because cultural practices that had a controlling, protective function may be abandoned and not replaced. This may be exacerbated by demographic patterns in immigration. For example, in groups where men immigrate alone, the lack of women, older people, and children in their social world may constitute a lack of controls on behavior considered disrespectful or uncouth such as drinking, smoking, taking drugs, acting out sexually, and so on.

When immigrants travel as family groups, if immigrant parents are not sufficiently familiar with U.S. culture, and many are not, they may not be able to socialize their children in ways that maximize resilience. Alternatively, the attempt to negotiate differences in family authority structures and other cultural aspects of social organization may be highly stressful, and breakdowns in family authority allow youth to operate in a relatively uncontrolled manner (Kurtines & Szapocznik 1995; Rodriguez, Adrados, & De la Rosa, 1993; Szapocznik, Scopetta, Kurtines, & Aranalde, 1978).

In addition, some well-established immigrant groups have developed their own patterns of drug and alcohol use and abuse in second, third, and later U.S.–born generations, and new immigrants are socialized into these subcultural patterns. There are distinct alcohol use and abuse patterns not only for different ethnic and immigrant groups but also for men and women within these groups, for different age groups, and for particular occupational groups.

Until recently, researchers have not paid detailed attention to the importance of cultural variation in drug and alcohol use and abuse in the United States; there has been comparatively little research on ethnic minorities (Glick & Moore, 1990; Yee *et al.*, 1995) and almost none on immigrants as such. Research focusing on ethnic issues in substance use in the United States has tended to spotlight U.S. census groups (African American, Caucasian, Asian, Native American, Hispanic, etc.) rather than immigrants specifically. Consequently there is more data on immigrants from Latin America than on other immigrant groups. Even this literature suffers from a tendency to lump together immigrants from dissimilar countries in Latin

America, to gloss over significant ethnic differences among Latin American immigrants, and to fail to distinguish between U.S.–born persons of Latin American descent and immigrants. This paper focuses on alcohol and drug use and abuse among immigrant Latinos and secondarily immigrant Asians, reflecting the strengths and weaknesses of the literature.

Legal Issues in Drug Use in the United States

The concept of addiction as a medical problem has developed over the 19th and 20th centuries in the United States and Western Europe. The rise of theories of addiction was related to the development of modern, urban, industrial societies; they remain controversial today with some researchers rejecting the idea that addiction is a disease in favor of the idea of substance use as a social and psychological phenomenon with health consequences (Akers, 1991; Alt, 1991; Ferentzy, 1992; Neuhaus, 1993; Spode, 1992; Truan, 1993). The theoretical controversy is not only interesting in itself, but also has implications for the cross-cultural study of substance use.

Many immigrants come from rural or tribal backgrounds into cities, and then from cities in their home countries to cities in the United States. The rural or tribal societies of their origin may not have a concept of drug addiction; it is not clear whether one can really speak of substance abuse in such societies where psychoactive substance use is contained in religious rituals and regulated by personalistic social norms. In addition, if alcoholism and drug addiction are not diseases, it is then possible that abuse of substances may manifest quite differently in different cultural settings, rather than fitting into a one-size-fits-all medical protocol as with an infectious disease like measles or smallpox.

Although there are certainly biological aspects to substance abuse, and many psychoactive drugs cause physical as well as

psychological dependence, drug use is as much a legal as a biological problem. In the United States, psychoactive drugs can be divided into those that are regulated as foods, those that are legal for recreational use, those that are legal to use only with written prescription from a licensed physician, those that are illegal for any use, and those which are not mentioned in the legal code. Every drug that is now illegal was at one time legal in the United States. Cocaine was at one time an ingredient in Coca-Cola (Walker, 1996); heroin was invented in 1898 by the German pharmaceutical company Bayer as a treatment for morphine addiction (the name refers to its nature as a "heroic cure") (Goode, 1984, p. 224).

Throughout its history, the United States has manifested a strong ambivalence to the use of psychoactive substances (Buchanan, 1992, p. 32). There have been a series of sharp changes in public attitudes to particular drugs and to drug use in general throughout U.S. history, with opinions swinging from tolerance to condemnation in cycles of approximately 50 to 100 years (Musto, 1993, p. 30). Prior to 1800, for example, U.S. attitudes toward drug and alcohol use were relatively tolerant (Buchanan, 1992; Musto, 1993). This was before the use of distilled alcoholic beverages became common. In addition, the stronger, synthesized versions of psychoactive and analgesic drugs were not invented or were not widely available until the 19th century: morphine was isolated in the beginning of the century, cocaine in 1860, heroin in 1898, aspirin in 1899, the hypodermic syringe became widely available in the 1860s, and today's large pharmaceutical industry had its start in the same era, producing and marketing drugs on a mass scale.

Because health issues were under the jurisdiction of states rather than the federal government, psychoactive drugs were less stringently regulated in the United States than in other countries (Goode, 1984; Musto, 1993; Walker, 1996). Drugs like opium, morphine, and heroin, alone or in combination with alcohol, were commonly used as analgesics (Musto 1993, p. 32). Drinking, especially among men, was associated with personal liberty, and there was strong pressure on men to drink (Buchanan 1992, p. 36).

These liberal attitudes shifted with the introduction of more powerful drugs and also with the social shifts following the U.S. Civil War (Buchanan, 1992, p. 39). Each drug now illegal has its own particular history of first disaffection and then illegalization. In many cases the movement to illegalize particular drugs arose in response to fear of drug use among immigrants or ethnic minorities (Mark, 1975). The southern states began to regulate alcohol sales following emancipation, fearing the possibility of publicly drunken Blacks (Ayers, 1984; Huggins, 1971). The illegalization of opium came about due to anti-Chinese agitation after large-scale Chinese immigration following the Civil War (in the early 20th century, opium was suppressed in China as part of resistance to Western domination) (Musto, 1993; Rubinstein, 1973). Cocaine was the subject of an illegalization campaign after it became linked in the public mind with African Americans, marijuana when it was associated with Mexican farmworkers and immigrants in the early 20th century (Musto, 1993, p. 32). The late 19th and early 20th centuries saw a variety of antidrug campaigns including the anti-alcohol temperance movement, which succeeded in regulating or outlawing the use of many psychoactive substances.

In 1905, in response to concerns over opium use in the Philippines, newly under U.S. jurisdiction, the federal government outlawed all nonmedicinal use of opium. In 1906, the Pure Food and Drug Act brought the regulation of substances under the jurisdiction of the federal government, allowing for more stringent control. A few years later, the United States launched the first of its international efforts to control drugs by convening the International Opium Commission in 1909 (Musto, 1993, p. 33).

The history of cocaine is similar to that of opium: First introduced in 1884, it became widely and inexpensively available and was hailed as a medical breakthrough before concerns over its addictive properties and effects on personal health arose. Cocaine was so well received at first that Coca-Cola, made with coca leaf extract, was introduced in 1886 as a temperance drink: stimulating, but nonalcoholic. By 1900 the cocaine was removed in response to anticocaine statutes, and by the 1930s it was no longer in widespread use (Musto, 1993, pp. 34–35), although it resurged as a street drug in the later half of the 20th century.

Marijuana was introduced into the United States from Mexico by farmworkers in the 1920s and became popular especially among musicians. In the 1960s its use became widespread among middle-class youth, and by 1970 the government had taken steps to control its sale and possession. Unlike other psychoactive substances, it did not have known medicinal uses, and it quickly became tagged as a dangerous drug likely to lead to violent acts under the influence of "reefer madness." In the 1960s, student movement leaders hailed it as a peacekeeper drug that allowed large gatherings such as the Woodstock concert to remain "mellow"—unlike alcohol, which was associated with brawling. While toleration of possession of small amounts of marijuana rose in the 1970s, concern over the drug has increased throughout the 1980s and 1990s (Musto, 1993, p. 36), and use, especially among teenagers, has increased. The 1990s are a period of increased public concern over drug use, increasingly stringent legal controls on drugs, increasing concern over the use of legal drugs such as tobacco and alcohol (as part of the "New Temperance"), as well as rising rates of illegal marijuana and heroin use and continuing high rates of illegal cocaine use.

The legal regulation of substances has responded not only to ethnic tensions but also to the growth of the pharmaceutical industry following the Civil War and to the increasing power of the federal government to regulate licensure and commerce, including licensure of those authorized to dispense drugs (Buchanan, 1992). During the 1960s, the United

States began a swing toward more extensive use of psychoactive substances including illegal substances by the middle classes (Buchanan, 1992, p. 44). A disenchantment began in the 1970s and intensified during the 1980s and 1990s. Although the use of drugs such as marijuana and tobacco continues to rise, the federal government has stepped up control efforts both domestically, through the imposition of stiff penalties for possession and sale of illegal substances, and internationally, through efforts to suppress production of drugs in other countries. This "war on drugs" has been largely unsuccessful in reducing illegal substance use, although it has markedly increased the U.S. prison population. Some researchers posit that like drug scares of the past, the contemporary drug war is intertwined with ethnic politics (Courtwright, 1991; Goode, 1990; Zatz, 1987). Goode pointed out that while social concern over drug use among minority populations is strongly influenced by prejudice, during the 1980s the incidence of heavy chronic use of cocaine and heroin increased in the United States among all populations, including minorities. While social problems are cultural constructions, they also react to objective analyses of real situations (Goode, 1990).

In the United States today, some psychoactive substances are regulated as foods rather than drugs, controlled only for cleanliness and quality, such as caffeine, found in coffee, black teas, chocolate, cola drinks and as an additive in a number of pharmaceuticals. Others, like tobacco and alcohol, are forbidden to minors, but permitted to adults in most areas of the United States, although certain aspects of their use is regulated. For example, it is illegal to operate a motor vehicle while under the influence of alcohol, and public intoxication is a misdemeanor in most jurisdictions. Sale of both alcohol and tobacco is also legally regulated. In addition there are a number of drugs which, under federal law, are either entirely illegal for any purpose (Schedule 1 drugs) or available only upon prescription by a licensed physician. In the case of Schedule 1 drugs, any use is considered abuse.

When immigrants come to the United States, they may be unaware of the details of U.S. regulation of particular drugs, or they may be accustomed to open use of drugs that are legal or tolerated in their home countries. There are also some drugs in use in some parts of the world that are not covered by U.S. regulation, are not illegal, or are not serious problems in the United States. For example, some East and North Africans chew the leaves of the *khat* (*catha edulis;* also spelled *ghatt* and *quat*) plant which has amphetamine effects. The production, use, or possible abuse of *khat* is not regulated by the United States. Although *khat* use can be studied as a health problem, and some African and Middle Eastern immigrants use the drug (Destremau, 1990; Kalix, 1988; Litman *et al.,* 1986; Nencini, Grassi, Botan, Asseyr, & Paroli, 1989), its lack of legal status has prevented it from being defined as a public health problem in the United States. In addition, its confinement to the African immigrant community means that many public health and medical officials are unaware of the drug. In Finland, the use of buprenorphine in the treatment of narcotics addicts led to such serious problems with buphrenorphine use that it was eventually reclassified as a narcotic and illegalized (Hakkarainen & Hoikkala, 1992); in the United States it is a prescription analgesic.

Differing legalities also imply differing definitions of problematic use. That is, for substances that are entirely illegal in the United States, any use is defined as abuse. For legal drugs such as alcohol, researchers use measures of quantity consumed as well as measures of negative impact on personal health (cirrhosis of the liver, for example) and on lifestyle (ability to sustain employment, impacts on marriage and family life, psychological complications) to determine whether a person is a problem drinker. Although there are relevant measures of severity of illegal substance abuse, even very moderate use of any illegal substance constitutes abuse in itself.

The discussion now turns to consideration of particular issues in drug and alcohol use and abuse among immigrants to the United States from specific areas of the world.

Alcohol Use and Tobacco Use

The use of alcohol and tobacco differs from the use of other psychoactive substances in the United States in that such use is permitted for adults. Only excessive use or use by underage individuals is considered abuse. In addition, there are a wide variety of settings in which alcohol and tobacco may be legally purchased and consumed. The details of legal regulation of alcohol sale vary by state and by county and city within states. Generally study and treatment of alcohol, tobacco, and other drug use are separate, although there is an increasing movement toward unification of anti-abuse efforts for all psychoactive substances (Weisner, 1992).

Both alcohol and tobacco use have come under fire from public health officials in the 1980s and 1990s. Historically, conditions of alohol use have been more tightly regulated than conditions of tobacco use, but increasingly, both federal law and local ordinances restrict type (pipe, cigar, cigarette) and location of tobacco use. In another result of the New Temperence, the consequences of drunken comportment (especially automobile accidents) have been redefined as criminal misbehavior in the 1980s and 1990s. For example, fatal accidents caused by inebriated drivers can now be prosecuted under manslaughter and homicide statutes as well as DWI regulations.

The age at which it is legal to purchase alcoholic beverages, dropped to 18 years of age in the 1960s, has been changed back to 21 years of age in all 50 states in response to federal pressure. It is illegal for any person under the age of 21 to purchase or consume alcoholic beverages, and it is illegal for any person to sell alcoholic beverages to persons under the age of 21.

Studies vary widely in the measures used to assess alcohol use and abuse, and are often difficult to compare (Ames & Rebhun, 1996;

G. Marin & Posner, 1995). Generally, however, alcohol researchers are interested in whether an individual has had an alcoholic beverage in the past 5 years or is an abstainer, and then among drinkers, the frequency and volume of drinking. Volume can include both average volume per drinking session and total number of drinks over a set period. Different types of beverages contain different amounts of ethanol, but there are standard equivalences among wine, beer, and distilled beverage servings. To assess problems, researchers may use some measure of "heavy" drinking, or they may focus on "problem" drinking. Heavy drinking is a volume measure; problem drinking is a measure of psychosocial and personal health impact.

Alcohol and Tobacco Use among Immigrants from Latin America

"Hispanic" and "Latino" are U.S. ethnic categories. There are no "Hispanics" south of the U.S. border because there is no need to designate Latin Americans as a special population in Latin America: they are everybody. Upon entrance into the United States, Latin Americans are transformed into an ethnic minority, and their U.S.–born children inherit the designation "Latino" which is increasingly used as a racial category in the United States. Persons of Latin American descent form part of the fastest growing ethnically defined minority in the United States. Some researchers believe that Latinos will surpass African Americans in number to become the largest U.S. ethnic minority by the first third of the 21st century. This will be a major demographic shift. In 1980, the U.S. census enumerated 61% more Hispanics than in 1970 (the U.S. population as a whole grew 11% in that same 10 years) (Glick & Moore, 1990, p. 3). Between 1980 and 1990, the Latino population increased by a further 53% (Chavez & Mora, 1994). The birth rate among Latinos is higher than that among non-Latino Caucasians and African Americans, and immigration across the U.S.–Mexican border, both legal and illegal, continues at high levels (Chavez, 1993, p. 227).

Although significant numbers of U.S. farmworkers are Mexican nationals or Mexican Americans, most Latinos live in cities; the mainland U.S. Puerto Rican population, for example, is almost entirely urban. In addition, the immigrant Latino population is young, having a larger population of school-age children than any other ethnically defined group in the United States, although it also has a higher school dropout rate than other groups (Glick & Moore, 1990, p. 4). In 1991, only 52.1% of all U.S. Latinos graduated from high school or received a GED (Chavez & Mora, 1994, p. 1079). In 1993, the median age of Mexican Americans was 23, as compared with 32 for non-Hispanic Caucasians (Chavez, 1993, p. 227).

Latinos also tend to be poor, earning an average 63% of the median income for Caucasians in 1987 (a drop of 8% from 1972) (Glick & Moore, 1990, p. 4). They have a higher unemployment rate (12.2%) than non-Latinos (7.5%) (Chavez & Mora, 1994, p. 1079). Puerto Ricans living in the U.S. Northeast are the poorest Latinos, earning on average 47% of the Caucasian median income according to the 1987 U.S. census (Glick & Moore, 1990, pp. 3–5). The 1990 census found that the Mexican American average family income ($26,000) was more than $20,000 below the non-Hispanic average family income (Chavez, 1993, p. 227). An urban, impoverished population composed largely of children and adolescents, suffering from the dislocations of immigration, the effects of racism, the unemployment of the undereducated, and the family disruptions of the urban underclass is at high risk for substance use.

U.S. Latinos are very heterogeneous in terms of generation since immigration, economic class, and national origin. Since much of the U.S. Southwest was part of Mexico until the 1840s, persons of Mexican descent living there may not be immigrants or descendants of recent immigrants at all. Some Latinos come from families that have lived in what is now the United States since the 16th-century beginnings of European colonization of the Americas; others are part of the contemporary wave of immigration especially from Mexico, the Caribbean, and Central America. The largest populations of Latinos in the United States have ancestry in Mexico, Cuba, and Puerto Rico (Glick & Moore, 1990, p. 2). Mexican Americans make up about 58% of all U.S. Latinos, and some have projected that by the year 2000 Mexican Americans will comprise a majority of persons under the age of 30 living in the Southwestern United States (Chavez, 1993, p. 227).

Latin American countries are multiethnic and immigrants may have ethnic origins in any European, African, Native American, or Asian group, or may be of ethnically or racially mixed (or both) background. The situations of Latin American immigrants of different ethnic backgrounds may be quite different (cf. Schiller, 1992). For example, members of many Mexican and Central American Native tribal groups may not speak either Spanish or English and may come from isolated, rural areas without much knowledge of cosmopolitan societies. Increasingly such persons may immigrate in search of agricultural labor, coming into contact with drug and alcohol consumption customs in the United States. Their situation is different from the situation of Spanish-speaking urban migrants.

In general, U.S. Latinos show lower rates than non-Latinos of use of alcohol, tobacco, prescription psychotherapeutics, marijuana, heroin, cocaine, and other illicit drugs. Use rates are lowest in Latino populations living along the U.S. border with Mexico, and higher for more acculturated populations to the north, despite the prevalence of drug smuggling across the border (Harrison & Kennedy, 1996). In combination with evidence of heavier drinking and drug use among U.S. Latino populations than in comparable populations in countries of origin (Gilbert, 1991; Velez & Ungemack, 1989), this suggests that the situation of being an immigrant, perhaps in combination with the transformation into an ethnic minority, increases substance abuse.

Latino drinking patterns are affected by concepts of honor mandating chastity and abstemious behavior for women and competitive behavior for men. Drinking and smoking, because they are associated with the sexual behavior of adult men, are disapproved for women except in limited, controlled settings. In general, women are associated with the domestic, private sphere and men with the extradomestic public sphere. This underlies the tendency of Latino men to drink in public gatherings and in a showy, boisterous fashion (Alaniz, 1994; Alcocer, 1982; Caetano, 1983, 1987, 1990; Caetano & Medina Mora, 1988; Canino, 1994; Corbett, Mora, & Ames, 1991; Gilbert, 1991; Gordon, 1981, 1985; Holck, Warren, Smith, & Rochat, 1984; Horowitz, 1983; Page, Rio, Sweeney, & McKay, 1985).

Drinking patterns vary as part of acculturation. Among Latinos, drinking norms are affected by nationality of origin, whether the drinkers are immigrants or native born, gender, and social class (Gilbert, 1985, p. 256). Such factors as preference for type of beverage vary by national origin, with South Americans tending to prefer wine (South American immigrants are more likely to be middle class than Mexican, Caribbean, or Central American immigrants), Puerto Ricans preferring distilled spirits, and Mexican Americans preferring beer (Canino, 1994, p. 1085). Although the word "alcoolico" exists in Spanish, heavy drinking is not widely seen as a progressive disease with distinct stages. Drinking is generally considered a problem among Latinos when it interferes with the performance of family and gender roles, and is seen as a failure of will or a reaction to family, financial, or job-related stress rather than as a medical condition (Gilbert, 1985, p. 276).

Acculturation is a very complex process in which many social, historical, economic, and personal variables interact. Gilbert (1991) saw it in terms of "interacting lifestyle alterations" including exposure to new ideas and groups, changes in economic and educational opportunity, and the acquisition of new roles,

new ways of thinking, and new norms and expectations. The young are socialized into the new culture by their peers, because their parents are too unfamiliar with it to help them. This peer acculturation is especially important in Latina women's drinking, and is a factor in the progressively heavier drinking of each generation (p. 235).

Similarly, Page and colleagues (1985) showed that since many young Cuban immigrants lost one or both parents in the immigration process, peer socialization is very important in both their drinking and drug-taking behavior (p. 329). A study of substance use among women in Canada (Adrian, Dini, MacGregor, & Stoduto, 1995) found that the amount of difference in substance use patterns between studied immigrant groups and the national norm was strongly related to both individual factors, such as the length of time a particular immigrant had been in Canada or in which generation since immigration she or he had been born, and to factors such as how long a particular ethnic group had been in Canada in significant numbers. The ethnic groups studied were mostly European (e.g., Polish, Jewish, Irish, Italian), Chinese, and "other."

Trotter (1985), in a study on the lower Rio Grande valley in southern Texas, showed how complex the relationship between acculturation and alcohol use can be in a multicultural area. He pointed out that three cultures interact in the area: (1) Mexican national, (2) Mexican American, and (3) Anglo American. Each system is itself subdivided by ethnicity, lifestyle, and economic status (p. 279). Trotter defined lifestyle as composed of economic, occupational, linguistic, and educational status and stated that it is a more accurate marker than race, class, or caste. Each subdivision has its own unique pattern of alcohol consumption including quantities consumed and drunken comportment.

Seasonal migration (in which farmworkers move into an area during harvests) and residential segregation also affect the context in which acculturation takes place (Trotter, 1985, p. 280). Alaniz (1994) found that

Latino seasonal farmworkers in California face a number of problems including low wages, lack of adequate housing, and inadequate health care. Female farmworkers have no maternity leave, are exposed to pesticides that affect their fertility and the health of their fetuses, and are subject to sexual harassment. In addition to working from sunrise to sunset in the fields, they are exclusively responsible for child care, cooking, and household responsibilities (p. 1175). Farmworker women drank significantly less than other Mexican and Mexican American women, whereas men exibited a high-frequency, high-quantity drinking pattern. This pattern of drinking among males was found to occur after work in all male groups. The drinking takes place in public areas, exposing women and children to lewd comments, public urination, and occasional violence (pp. 1184–1187). Although women themselves abstained from drinking, they were victimized by the male drinking through this exposure and also because of heightened incidents of conjugal violence perpetrated by inebriated men.

Corbett and colleagues (1991) found that Mexican American men who were born and socialized in Mexico drink less than U.S. socialized Mexican Americans, that more educated men drink more than less educated men, and that religion is a more important factor in drinking for women than for men, with women more likely to report abstaining because of religious faith (p. 218). While some studies report higher rates of problem drinking among more acculturated male immigrants (Neff, Hoppe, & Perea, 1987), others show no change or little change. One possible effect of immigration is to lower the percentage of males who report being abstinent (Neff, 1986). Gilbert adds that Mexican men in Mexico have a less frequent, high-quantity drinking pattern, but upon entering the United States, Mexican men begin to drink more frequently while maintaining the high quantity per sitting pattern. This more frequent, high-quantity pattern continues over subsequent generations and is not affected by class or educational level, according to Gilbert (1991), in contrast to the finding of Corbett and colleagues (1991, p. 235). Trotter (1985) found that Mexican American men engage in more drinking episodes per unit of time than Anglos but drink less per occasion so the total quantity consumed over time is similar (p. 286).

As indicated, gender is very important to Latino drinking patterns. While some researchers emphasize the importance of *machismo* (a Latin American male honor complex) to male drinking in Latino populations, others think that the concept of *machismo* as used by social scientists has been too stereotyped and overemphasized. Gordon (1985), for example, showed that *machismo* is not the only factor or perhaps not even the most important factor in male drinking patterns in Latino groups (p. 298). Trotter (1985) described as an "Anglo stereotype" the image of the Mexican American man who drinks up the money he should be spending on his children's food or clothing because he is the victim of uncontrolled *machismo*. Mexican American men tend to drink in public more than Anglo men; however, Trotter did not find that Mexican American men are more frequent, heavy, and boisterous drinkers than Anglo men. Rather, he found that they are more conservative drinkers in the same environment (p. 285).

Several researchers have found a conservative drinking pattern among Mexican American women in that they drink on fewer occasions and drink less per occasion than Anglo women, and have higher rates of abstention because female drinking is constrained by ideas of virtue and respectability (Alaniz, 1994; Canino, 1994; Gilbert, 1991; Gilbert, Mora, & Ferguson, 1994; B. V. Marín & Flores, 1994; Pérez-Arce, 1994). For both men and women, heavy drinking is considered a sign of lack of virtue and lack of respect for parents and other family members. Drunken comportment is also different for men and for women: Women attempt to act sober even when drunk, whereas men get expansively humorous or morosely violent. Male drunken comportment varies little with setting except that in settings where "decent" women are present, physical and verbal aggression are constrained (Corbett, Mora, & Ames, 1991; Gilbert, 1985, 1991; Gordon, 1985; Madsen, 1964; Markides, Krause, & Mendes de Leon, 1988; Neff *et al.,* 1987; Trotter, 1985).

Immigration to the United States affects the drinking patterns of Mexican men and women differently. While the drinking patterns of individual men change on immigration to the United States, Gilbert (1991) found a strong generational pattern to drinking in immigrant Mexican and Mexican American women. Immigrant women are more likely to be abstinent than women who remain in Mexico, and they remain abstinent following immigration. But their daughters and granddaughters drink more in each generation. Daughters of Mexican immigrant women are more likely to drink than their immigrant mothers, and granddaughters display a drinking pattern similar to that of non-Latino U.S. women. Drinking patterns among Mexican American women are also more clearly correlated with education, income, and employment than among men (p. 235). Other studies have also found that Mexican American women's drinking increases with degree of acculturation, presumably higher in U.S.–born daughters and granddaughters of immigrants (Corbett *et al.,* 1991; Markides *et al.,* 1988).

Latina women have particular problems including an increase in female-headed households with children (15% of Latino households in 1970, 22% in 1990). They tend to earn less than men, and are less likely to be covered by insurance (Chavez & Mora, 1994, p. 1080). They are increasingly victims of domestic violence, and rates of HIV infection are increasing among Latinas, suggesting that in addition to having their own problems with substance use they are the also the victims of the behaviors accompanying male substance use. Current research suggests the outlines of substance use problems among Latinas; much more is needed to fill out the details (pp. 1080–1081).

As with other immigrants, scholars debate the relative importance of acculturation (as a learning model) and acculturative stress as factors in alcohol abuse among Latino immigrants (Caetano, 1986; Graves, 1967; Madsen, 1964; G. Marin, 1992; Markides *et al.,* 1988). The data are indeterminate on this issue, as different studies have indicated different conclusions. Part of the problem is that different studies have used incompatible measures both of alcohol use and of acculturation, and many were based on small samples (G. Marin & Posner, 1995, pp. 780–782).

Corbett and colleagues (1991) found that drinking patterns in Mexico are similar to those of working-class Whites in the United States, in that men drink with male relatives and in public whereas women drink little and only at family gatherings (p. 221). Gilbert (1991) noted a similar pattern of extreme gender difference in drinking pattern, but labeled it a distinctive Latino pattern (p. 234). Both agree that Mexican American men are more likely to drink, drink greater quantities, and have more problems related to drinking than do women (Corbett *et al.,* 1991, p. 215; Gilbert, 1991, p. 234).

Acculturation affects the family-based pattern of Mexican American drinking, because the second and subsequent generations are likely to drink in more informal, secular settings in addition to the family celebrations, where the presence of women and children limits men's drinking (Gilbert, 1985, p. 258). A family member who persists in heavy drinking may become unable to reciprocate economic aid and risks being cut off. The attenuation of kinship bonds because of heavy drinking can be economically devastating for both the drinker and his family (p. 271).

Gilbert (1985) provided a good characterization of types of drinking establishments patronized by immigrant Mexicans and Mexican Americans which range from cantinas in which both men and escorted women may drink beer, to wet T-shirt bars serving a mixed Latino and Anglo clientele where men drink beer while ogling women competing in wet T-shirt competitions. She also described "cannery bars," which serve as a location for "respite drinking," a kind of time out after work, and cocktail lounges, where white-collar Mexican American and Anglo couples go to drink mixed drinks or wine. Drinks are weak and heavily iced, and music is provided for dancing. These different kinds of settings show that drinking norms vary widely depending on the setting and the age, sex, social class, ethnicity, and profession of the drinkers (pp. 260–264).

Trotter (1985) also found a variety of types of drinking establishments in southern Texas, classifiable according to the social reputation of women who enter them. He found that men drink beer followed by hard liquor, whereas women tend to drink diluted mixed drinks and wine. Beer is considered a masculine, disreputable drink (p. 287). In addition to bars, men may drink at *pachangas* or all-male picnics where meat and beer (sometimes accompanied by stronger distilled beverages) are served and politics are discussed. Recent middle-class attempts to include women in *pachangas* have not worked out very well because of the strong taboos on women drinking beer. Trotter found that the lower class tends to drink in settings where the primary focus is socializing whereas the middle class drinks at settings where the primary focus is drinking and socializing is secondary (pp. 287–289).

Drinking patterns are affected by labor migration because migrants tend to be single and male. In some camps, ranchers prohibit drinking at the camps and expel those who break the rules. New labor laws mandating standards for migrant families have the unintended effect of encouraging growers to have all-male camps which are cheaper to maintain but which show patterns of heavier drinking (Trotter, 1985, pp. 290–292).

These studies show the importance of gender in alcohol consumption patterns for immigrant and U.S.–born Latinos. Prevention strategies need to take gender into account and possibly utilize different messages and procedures for men and for women (G.

Marin & Posner, 1995, p. 793). Drinking patterns in the United States are also strongly affected by the rhythms of work (Ames & Rebhun, 1996), and immigrant practices respond to this. Gilbert (1985) found that Mexican American men believe that they have the right to drink as respite from working, are considered old enough to drink when they are old enough to work, and considered deviant drinkers only if they are unable to work due to drinking. As more women join the workforce, they begin to drink as well. While not as likely as men to stop off at bars after work, women will buy a sixpack after work and consume it while preparing dinner, and unlike men are likely to drink alone. Acculturation, because it allows women into the drinking area, decreases men's drinking and increases women's (pp. 262–269).

Various researchers have found differences in drinking patterns among immigrants from different Latin American countries, as well as subcultural differences among U.S. Latinos living in California, Texas, Florida, and other areas of the United States. G. Marin and Posner (1995) found that Mexican American men had a lower proportion of abstainers than Central American men, and also drank more frequently and at a greater volume (p. 791). Acculturation was especially important as a factor in the proportion of drinkers versus abstainers for both groups (p. 791).

Gilbert (1991) has found that U.S. Mexican American women have more drinking problems than do Puerto Rican women and that U.S. Puerto Rican women have more drinking problems in general than do U.S. Cuban women (p. 234). Canino (1994) similarly found differences in Latina drinking patterns by national origin.

Andrew Gordon (1985) carried out a comparative study of drinking among Dominican, Guatemalan, and Puerto Rican immigrants in New Jersey. While previous studies have complained that Hispanics in general are unlikely to seek treatment for drinking problems, Gordon found that, in fact, they seek alternative treatments, and that the type of alternative treatment sought varies by national group of origin (p. 298). Gordon found that Dominicans distinguish normative and deviant drinking patterns. They are most likely to seek help for deviant drinking from the Catholic church, especially in its charismatic form. For those immigrants separated from their families, the Church can provide a setting in which the lost companionship and support of the family is provided (p. 300).

Dominicans report that their drinking patterns change after immigration. In the Dominican Republic, they drink on weekdays, but in the United States, drinking is largely confined to Saturday nights and Sundays. They get drunk less frequently and fight less in the United States than in the Dominican Republic.

U.S. Dominican drinking reflects an interest in upward mobility. Dominicans value drinking at a measured pace without losing self-control. Dominican informants told Gordon that their suave drinking style was a marker of their superiority to Puerto Ricans whom they consider to be rough drunks. The Dominican drinking pattern is related to their immigration style: Most came with intact families, and the role of family provider along with their economic aspirations is what moderates their drinking (Gordon, 1985, p. 302).

Guatemalans are more likely than Dominicans to seek help from Spanish-language Alcoholics Anonymous (AA). They used the AA format to tell elaborate stories of their former debauched lives. This style of storytelling does not appeal to Latinos of other nationalities, who did not like to participate in AA with Guatemalans. Gordon found that although the Guatemalans are a minority within the Latino community, they completely dominate Spanish-language AA in the Northeast. Their interest in AA is influenced by the unique situation of Guatemala, because in the 1960s the Guatemalan president and vice president made public statements in favor of AA, which became very popular there (Gordon, 1985, p. 306).

Guatemalan illness narratives, adopting the AA style, show heavy drinking as a progressive disease. Unlike Dominicans, Guatemalans tend to immigrate as single men, often illegally, and they explain their heavy drinking as a function of their sadness and nostalgia for the people left behind. They like to drink while singing melancholy songs, and crying in their beer. Guatemalans tend to drink beer in all-male groups at bars, Thursday through Sunday nights (Gordon, 1985, p. 305).

Puerto Ricans constitute the single largest Hispanic group in the Northeast and are the most likely to make use of clinical services and to be members of Protestant Pentecostal groups. Church members equate drinking with other sins like homosexuality, smoking, and drug use (Gordon, 1985, p. 307).

New York Puerto Ricans are more acculturated than other immigrant Latinos in the Northeast. They are also more likely to use other drugs such as marijuana, glue, cocaine, barbiturates, and methadone, sometimes in combination with alcohol. Gordon (1985) attributed combined drug use to their frustration with inability to reach their economic aspirations. The Puerto Rican population suffers a 30% unemployment rate, although unlike other Latinos, they are U.S. citizens and eligible for U.S. welfare benefits, both in Puerto Rico and the mainland. This undermines men's ability to take on the *"padre de familia"* provider role, since welfare targets women who are single heads of households with children. The drug use, which Gordon saw as an attempt to alleviate the pain of assaulted male pride and dignity, exacerbates the problem (p. 309).

Like Guatemalan and Dominican immigrants in New Jersey, Florida Cubans tend not to present at clinics for alcohol problems (Page *et al.,* 1985, p. 315). While Cuban parents disapprove strongly of their children's use of other drugs, drinking is tolerated among young men, who show a pattern of occasional binge drinking at parties. Cuban women, like other Latinas, tend to be light drinkers.

Page and colleagues (1985) also found that while Cuban American older women tend to abstain, they do take large amounts of prescription tranquilizers (p. 327). In general, the Cuban Americans studied regarded drugs such as marijuana as a greater problem. Often they would present at clinics complaining of a son's marijuana use. Care providers would see that the father's drinking was also a problem in the family drug-taking pattern, but families would deny it, focusing on the illegal drug use (p. 329).

The other major psychoactive drug in the United States besides alcohol is tobacco. Studies of smoking among Latinos are even less common than studies of drinking. One study (Escobedo *et al.*, 1996) among Mexican Americans, U.S. Puerto Ricans, and U.S. Cubans found a relationship between depressive mood in adolescence and smoking. Depressed adults in general are more likely to smoke and less likely to quit than nondepressed adults; this study showed that depression is also related to smoking initiation in adolescence, and that depressive mood rather than major depression is a risk factor. This pattern was strongest among Mexican Americans.

Alcohol and Tobacco Use among Asian Immigrants

Immigrants from Asia include such diverse groups as university-educated elites from India and Japan and refugees from the tribal societies caught up in the U.S. involvement in the war in Southeast Asia. Some Asian Americans come from families that have been in the United States for generations; others are recent immigrants. Asian Americans are an extremely varied group that encompasses a great variety of languages, cultures, class statuses, ethnic and racially defined groups, and native drug and alcohol use patterns. Although all persons with ancestry in the eastern part of the Eurasian land mass and adjacent islands are denominated "Asian" in the United States, in Asia, they do not consider themselves to be members of the same homogeneous group, denominating themselves into distinct "races" which are not so recognized in the United States.

Very little is known about substance use patterns of immigrant Asians in the United States (Austin, Prendergast, & Lee, 1989; Chi, Lubben, & Kitano, 1989; D'Avanzo, Frye, & Froman, 1994; Trimble, Padilla, & Bell, 1987), because of a paucity of national data. Indeed, little is known about substance use patterns in the countries of origin of Asian immigrants (Chi *et al.*, 1989). As with studies of Latinos, what little literature exists on Asians suffers from a lack of attention to the class, national origin, and generational differences among persons of Asian descent in the United States. Because national surveys of alcohol use and abuse pick up Asians as a census category, slightly more is known about alcohol use among U.S. Asians in general than about use patterns of other psychoactive substances. More research has been done on acculturated, middle-class groups such as Chinese and Japanese Americans and Korean American college students than on more recent immigrant groups such as Southeast Asians (D'Avanzo *et al.*, 1994, pp. 420–421).

The reputation of Asian Americans as a "model minority" has contributed to the stereotype that there are few interesting problems of substance use or deviance to study in Asian American groups. Asians are frequently lumped together with dissimilar groups as "other" by researchers more interested in African Americans and Latinos (Joe, 1993, p. 239). In addition, some Asian American communities have been successful at concealing their activities from the prying curiosity of outsiders such as social science and public health researchers. However, researchers are increasingly aware of patterns of substance use in Asian American communities.

Literature on drinking in Asian populations in the United States has focused on the so-called Asian flush in which even light drinking brings on blushing. The literature has often ignored diversity in the prevalence of the trait and attitudes toward it in Asian populations (Ames & Rebhun, 1996; Kitano, Hatanaka, Yeung, & Sue, 1985). Less attention has been devoted to cultural patterns of alcohol consumption. There is evidence that, like Latinos, Asian Americans in general tend to drink at family and communal gatherings where food is served and social mores encourage moderation (Chi *et al.*, 1989; Kitano *et al.*, 1985). In general, persons of Chinese descent in the United States have been found to have high rates of alcohol abstention and low rates of heavy drinking (Sue, Kitano, Hatanaka, & Yeung, 1985), while persons of Japanese descent have the highest rates of both moderate and heavy drinking among Asian Americans (Chi *et al.*, 1989; Kitano *et al.*, 1985; Sue, Zane, & Ito, 1979)

Asian Americans and Asian immigrants to the United States appear to have lower rates of both problem drinking and illegal substance use than the general population (Ahern, 1989; Akutsu, Sue, Zane, & Nakamura, 1989; Chi, Kitano, & Lubben, 1988; Chi *et al.*, 1989; D'Avanzo *et al.*, 1994; Flaskerud & Hu, 1992; Johnson, Nagoshi, Ahern, Wilson, & Yeun, 1987; Kitano & Chi, 1986–1987; Maddahian, Newcomb, & Bentler, 1986; McLaughlin *et al.*, 1987; Murakami, 1989; Schwitters, Johnson, Wilson, & Mc-Clearn, 1982; Singer, 1972; Sue & Morishima, 1982; Sue & Nakamura, 1984; Sue *et al.*, 1979; Trimble *et al.*, 1987; Yu & Liu, 1986–1987). Patterns of alcohol use vary by national origin, generation since immigration, and gender.

Chinese American and Korean American women have particularly high rates of abstention (Kitano *et al.*, 1985; Sue *et al.*, 1985), while Japanese American women show higher rates of both moderate and heavy drinking than women in Japan or recent female immigrants from Japan. In contrast, recently immigrated Japanese American men have higher drinking rates than American-born men of Japanese descent (Kitano *et al.*, 1985). A comparison of U.S. Caucasians with Japanese in Japan and with three generations of Japanese Americans (Issei or migrants, Nissei or first U.S.–born generation, and Sansei or second generation) found that Japanese men had higher rates of both ab-

stention and heavy drinking than the other groups. Eighty percent of the Japanese women surveyed were abstainers or light drinkers (Tusnoda *et al.*, 1992, p. 373). This suggests that acculturation to the United States moderates male drinking patterns while increasing tolerance of drinking among women. Research on immigrant Japanese American women focusing on generation since immigration would illuminate the dynamics of this pattern (Ames & Rebhun, 1996, p. 1655).

Chi and colleagues (1989) noted that younger Asian American women in their sample drank more heavily and frequently than older Asian American women, with Koreans the most likely to be abstainers, followed by Chinese. Like Kitano and colleagues (1985), Chi and colleagues found higher rates of drinking among Japanese American women. Japanese American women were more likely to drink if they had higher education. Among Chinese American women the variable most associated with heavier drinking was religion: Those who attended weekly worship services were least likely to drink. Korean American women's drinking was not affected by religion but it was positively correlated with younger age and having a parent who drank.

As with Latinos, there are indications that more acculturated individuals drink more heavily and more frequently than more recent or less acculturated immigrants (Tsunoda *et al.*, 1992). Studies of Asian American and Asian immigrant students in the United States have shown rising rates of alcohol and tobacco consumption and use of illegal substances. Studies focusing on women have shown that, like Latinos, in general, more educated, affluent, and acculturated women are more likely to use alcohol and tobacco and to abuse prescription drugs like tranquilizers (Chi *et al.*, 1989; Lubben, Chi, & Kitano, 1989; Maddahian *et al.*, 1986; Sue *et al.*, 1979; Towle, 1988).

During the years after the end of U.S. involvement in the wars in Southeast Asia (Vietnam, Cambodia, Laos), more than a million Southeast Asian refugees have resettled in the United States (D'Avanzo et al., 1994). Although some, especially Vietnamese, came from the middle classes (Kelly, 1986), many of these refugees came from tribal groups such as the Mien and Hmong. Thrust by the war from their world of traditional swidden agriculture into the very different setting of the urban United States, these refugees have had a particularly difficult time (Nicassio, 1983; Waters, 1990). Young Southeast Asian Americans, especially males, have been found to have high rates of alcohol, tobacco, and illegal substance use (D'Avanzo et al., 1994; Nicassio & Pate, 1984; Yee & Thu, 1987). This is not surprising, given the painful experiences Southeast Asian refugees endured prior to leaving their countries, en route, in refugee camps, and following resettlement in the United States. Many may have endured torture, massacre of family members, and rape during and after the war, and culture shock, isolation, and extreme poverty upon resettlement (Bernier, 1992; D'Avanzo et al., 1994; Dunnigan et al., 1993; Kinzie & Fleck, 1987; Westermeyer, Neider, & Vang, 1984).

Southeast Asian refugee immigrants include a higher percentage of women than other immigrant groups (Rynearson & DeVoe, 1984). Studies on Southeast Asian refugee women have shown that the use of alcohol, sleeping pills, and prescription drugs, especially tranquilizers is increasingly common as a way to relieve stress and depression (D'Avanzo et al., 1994).

Although some women have found employment outside the home, many have not. Immigrant housewives are less likely to learn English, less likely to become acculturated, and are more socially isolated than their husbands and children (Arakaki & Antonis, 1978; Jenkins et al., 1996; Kitano & Daniels, 1988; Krupinski, 1967). These women, while struggling with the emotional aftermath of their war experiences and the strain of trying to locate and communicate with relatives left behind, try to live up to Buddhist ideals of uncomplaining endurance in their difficult current circumstances. Their abuse of sleeping pills and tranquilizers is a response to their emotionally difficult circumstances; women have reported that they use these drugs to "forget troubles" (D'Avanzo et al., 1994, pp. 424–425).

Alcohol and other drug use may also be affected by ethnomedicine, particularly the customary practice of drinking alcohol, especially vodka, as a treatment for menstrual pain, in the late stages of pregnancy, and for a few months after birth, among Cambodian immigrant women (D'Avanzo et al., 1994, p. 424).

Use of Illegal Substances

In addition to problems with abuse of legal substances, many immigrants suffer from problems related to their use of illegal substances. The use of some substances, for example, opium, are largely confined to particular immigrant groups (in this case, Southeast Asian refugee immigrants). Members of other immigrant groups use substances common in the troubled neighborhoods to which their low economic status confines them. In addition to the deleterious effects of the substances themselves, users suffer from the often violent milieu of illegal drug sale and use, the common association of illegal drug use and prostitution, and the effects of frequent arrest and imprisonment, if their use is caught by law enforcement.

Use of Illegal Substances among Latino Immigrants

Those who use illegal drugs suffer from many of the same problems as alcoholics, including negative effects on their personal health, greater suceptibility to accidents, difficulties in maintaining personal relationships, and difficulties in performing reliably at work and therefore trouble keeping jobs. In addition, some illegal drugs have a more powerful immediate effect than alcohol, and their illegal status means that use is not only a medical problem but a criminal offense. Some users turn to violence, property crimes, or both to support their habits; the sale of illegal drugs may be controlled by criminal syndicates that use violence to protect their markets. The use of some illegal drugs also puts users at risk of serious health problems such as AIDS and other STDs resulting from sharing needles, or reliance on prostitution to obtain drugs. This is especially institutionalized in the case of crack cocaine (Fullilove *et al.,* 1992).

Illegal drug use, in addition to being a medical and legal problem, is also an economic phenomenon. Production, distribution, marketing, and consumption of drugs constitutes an illegal, underground economy. The illegal nature of the drug industry allows traffickers to create monopolies (Alvarez-Gomez, 1995) and to use violence in the conduct of their business. This industry is also especially attractive as a source of employment for people shut out of the legitimate employment market because of illegal immigration status, lack of U.S. certifications or licenses, language barriers, and ethnic or racial prejudice (Manning & Redlinger, 1983). Many immigrants suffer from these barriers to legitimate employment.

The major world producers of cocaine are located in Latin America, as are major producers of heroin and marijuana. Many illegal drugs are sold through a network of youth gangs in cities. These gangs are organized by territories (comprising city blocks) and by ethnicity. Whereas in the 1930s and 1940s youth gangs were dominated by the then-immigrant groups of Italians and Irish, today they are dominated by African American, Latino, and increasingly immigrant Asian youth. There are well-established Latino youth gangs, especially in California and Texas, that employ large numbers of teenagers and young men in the distribution of drugs such as heroin and cocaine, among other activities (Curry & Spergal, 1992; Huff, 1990; Ianni, 1974; Jankowski, 1991; Moore *et al.,* 1983; Schwartz, 1989; Vigil, 1983; Waldorf, 1993; Zatz, 1985).

The use of illegal substances is largely a behavior of young people in all groups, espe-

cially those 15 to 25 years old. Users have higher death rates at younger ages than nonusers. In addition, those who survive drug use as youths often cease or moderate their use as they grow older, either in response to treatment, to increasing physical difficulty in maintaining a habit, or because personal situations that prompted drug use have changed. Although some individuals continue to use illegal substances throughout their lives, adolescents and young adults make up the bulk of users. Researchers have found that substance use problems are highest among Native American youth, followed by Latino and Caucasian youth, and then by African American and Asian adolescents (Wallace & Bachman, 1993, p. 167).

Although comparatively little research has focused on the specific problems of immigrant youth (or even of ethnic minority youth), what literature there is suggests that patterns of and reasons for involvement in drug use vary significantly from patterns and reasons among nonminority youth, responding to differences in cultural influence, family structures, social networks, economic situations, and so on. More research on the epidemiology of drug use patterns, factors in resilience, standards of normality and abnormality, and successful methods of outreach and treatment in minority and immigrant communities is urgently needed (Brook, 1993; De la Rosa, Adrados, & Milburn, 1993).

Qualitative descriptions of life in immigrant Latino neighborhoods have yet to be integrated with quantitative measures of deviance and normality to allow for the development of culturally appropriate measures (Rodriguez *et al.,* 1993, p. 8). Study of minority populations will not only shed light on their particular strengths and problems but could also illuminate hitherto ignored cultural aspects of drug and alcohol use and abuse in nonethnically defined populations in the United States.

Current theory on adolescent drug use posits that immigrant minority youth should be at particularly high risk. Theorists emphasize that delinquency such as drug use is often a reaction to disadvantaged status, a social environment where drug use is tolerated, failures in family bonding and authority structures, strong peer bonding, and low self-esteem among adolescents. Where more than one of these factors is present, they may interact in a synergistic way (Rodriguez *et al.*, 1993, pp. 9–10). Orlando Rodriguez, for example, posited that drug use among Puerto Rican youth in the United States is related to the interaction among these various factors. He argued that strain related to low-income status and ethnic discrimination indirectly influences deviance in adolescents because it negatively impacts bonding to both family and school, leading adolescents into a peer culture in which crime and drug use are tolerated, if not valorized. This puts Latino youth from immigrant families at particular risk (p. 10).

Evidence supports the idea that drug use is a particular problem among immigrant Latinos living in impoverished ethnic enclaves in cities. A study in northern California found that Latino high school students were more likely to engage in such behaviors as alcohol, tobacco, marijuana and other substance use, various forms of violence, drunk driving, and unmarried pregnancy than non-Latino Caucasian students; the mean number of "risk behaviors" was highest for immigrant youths, followed by U.S.–born Latino students (Brindis, Wolfe, Carter, Ball, & Starbuck-Morales, 1995). A study of young Central American immigrants found higher alcohol and illegal substance use (especially marijuana, cocaine, PCP, and hallucinogens) than among other Latinos (Tommasello, Tyler, Tyler, & Zhang, 1993).

Substance use is particularly marked among U.S. Puerto Ricans, who also have high rates of hospitalization for psychiatric diagnoses (Velez & Ungemack, 1994). In a study of New York Puerto Ricans, Velez and Ungemack found that the prevalence of drug use is higher in this population than in a comparable population in Puerto Rico. "New York Ricans," (New York–born and resident) had higher rates of drug use and reported more problems with parental authority than adolescents born in New York who had re-

turned to Puerto Rico with their parents ("P.R. migrants"), island-born Puerto Ricans residing in New York, or Puerto Rican islanders, in that order (Velez & Ungemack, 1989, 1994). This research suggests a strong effect on drug use not of migration itself but of exposure to the community of immigrant Puerto Ricans in New York City. The authors posited that acculturative stress is intensified by marginalization, discrimination, and limited opportunities, leading to increases in alienation, cultural isolation, and problems in identity formation which complicate family relationships and may encourage substance use (1994, p. 100).

Szapocznik similarly found that drug use in this population is related to problems with assimilation and the effects of immigration into a multicultural setting on family cohesiveness (Kurtines & Szapocznik, 1995). His research showed that young people in immigrant families acculturate faster and more completely than older family members, and boys faster than girls, thereby exacerbating family struggles around autonomy for adolescent members, leading to loss of family leadership roles for parents and loss of emotional support for youths (pp. 180–181).

Common problems in Cuban American families include conflict around parental jurisdiction over adolescent behavior combined with attempted coparenting from extended family members, especially grandmothers. Because it is normal for Cuban American families to be more emotionally enmeshed than Anglo families, families may measure as dysfunctional on scales that are not culturally sensitive. Measurement is not the only problem: Troubled young people may be caught between the norms of their peer culture and of their families, contributing to motivations for substance use and difficulties in controlling it in this population (Kurtines & Szapocznik, 1995, pp. 185–186).

Velez and Ungemack (1995) have identified difficulties caused by the use of adolescents as translators for non-English-speaking parents, the disintegration of patriarchal authority due to widespread male unemployment, and the breakdown of extended family ties. These factors combine with mainstream U.S. valorization of adolescent self-determination to lessen immigrant families' ability to control adolescent drug use (p. 99).

The focus on adolescents in the literature means that comparatively little is known about illegal drug use among women in general, much less women from specific ethnic or immigrant groups. An analysis of literature on drug use published in 1990 showed that researchers largely ignore gender as a variable and conduct few studies on females or with females among the subjects (Brett, Graham, & Smythe, 1995).

As with alcohol, researchers debate the importance of *machismo* in Latino male gang membership and drug use. Some emphasize the painful disjuncture between the demand that men be strong, independent financial providers and the reality of low education, unemployment, and racial discrimination faced by many Latino men as an important factor in male gang membership (Bourgois, 1995; Erlanger, 1979; Horowitz, 1982, 1983).

Youth gangs historically have been mostly male phenomena, but increasingly girls and young women are joining gangs and forming their own gangs as well (Harris, 1994; Moore, 1994). Moore argued that while traditional Latino values are generally protective against substance use for Latino girls and women, these conservative values can encourage substance use in women defined as deviant in the community. Moore studied female adolescents from families defined as *cholo* or street oriented in Los Angeles barrio neighborhoods. She critiqued earlier literature claiming that female substance use is largely initiated and maintained through relationships with men (Bowker, 1977; Bullington, 1977), showing that while this may have been true in the past, today there are multigenerational drug-using families in the *barrio* (impoverished Latino neighborhood). Because Latino values permit more freedom for males to be out on the streets, sons of parents with conventional values are at risk for gang membership and substance use more than their sisters. Female gang members tend

to be daughters of parents who themselves use drugs, have a history of gang membership, and who fail to control their children (Moore, 1990, 1991, 1994; Moore & Devitt, 1989; Moore & Vigil, 1987).

Conservative mores label girls as bad or good, and once labeled bad, girls cannot retrieve reputations. Moore (1994) argued that daughters of heavy drinking or heroin using women are born into the "bad girl" label and may find that only groups of other *tecatas* ("wild," heroin-using girls) will welcome and associate with them. Heroin-using gang girls are regarded as deviant not only by the wider *barrio* community but by male gang members as well, even those who do not regard their own drug use or gang membership as a form of deviance. Heroin-using girls were also more likely to remain involved with gangs in adulthood than non-heroin-using girls associated with gangs as adolescents, to serve time in prison, and to be intimately involved with heroin-using men throughout the life course (pp. 1121–1123).

Moore (1994) posited that conservative values "encapsulate" substance use by isolating users, serving a protective function for most girls and women by isolating them from contact with substance use. But for girls born on the "wrong" side of social barriers, or for girls who cross over, the same values serve to keep them isolated from social contacts that might help them to from escape an abusive lifestyle (pp. 1123–1124; see also Flores-Ortiz, 1994). Moore's argument also implies that the problem will become worse in the future as *barrio* communities become better established. In a process similar to the Latino female drinkers studied by Gilbert (1991), heroin use increases in each subsequent generation since immigration, increasing the size of the population caught in the cycle.

Use of Illegal Substances among Asian Immigrants

There is little accurate information on drug use among persons of Asian descent in the United States, or on drug use in contemporary Asian countries (Beroud, 1995), or on how that might translate to drug use among Asian immigrants to the United States. Historically, opium has been the psychoactive drug of choice in Asian countries, although the extent to which its use was as widespread as Western observers (mostly missionaries) reported is disputed (Newman, 1995). Countries such as China and Korea historically have been major sources of opium for the international market, and have used emigrants to market opium internationally (Jennings, 1995). There is some evidence of opium use among such Asian American populations as Southeast Asian immigrants. Both opium and heroin use have been reported among Laotians living in Laos and expatriate Laotians (Westermeyer, 1978). Treatment and prevention in this group is complicated by language barriers, especially the difficulty of translating concepts such as addiction into Southeast Asian languages, and the resistance of refugees to Western biomedical treatment (Dunnigan *et al.,* 1993; Martin & Zweban, 1993). A study of Hmong in a Thai refugee camp showed more success by traditional healers than Western drug treatment professionals in treating heroin and opium use (Jilek & Jilek-Aall, 1990).

There are ethnically based youth gangs among some Asian American and immigrant Asian communities, although researchers have found them especially difficult to study. Strong traditions of hiding anything possibly shameful from outsiders, combined with distrust of outsiders and authority figures make Asians especially reluctant to speak to researchers. Asian youth gangs are not as visible as African American and Latino gangs, eschewing public markers like special clothing or gestures. In addition, they may reasonably fear retribution from members of groups they inform on (Burke & O'Rear, 1990; Joe, 1993, p. 244; Poole & Pogrebin, 1990). In addition to youth gangs, adult organized crime groups and secretive syndicates such as the *tongs* (fraternal associations) of China-towns operate especially in Chinese neighborhoods, usually running gambling games,

protection rackets, and sometimes dealing in distribution of substances such as heroin (Kinkead, 1992).

Preliminary research indicates that Southeast Asian war refugees who immigrated as unaccompanied minors are at particular risk for substance use. Similarly, young refugees from families divided by war experiences or missing significant members due to their war and refugee experiences are at particular risk (Westermeyer, 1993, p. 315). More research is needed on the relationships between traumatic experiences, posttraumatic stress disorder (PTSD), and substance use disorders in immigrant refugee populations.

These studies suggest that alcohol and illegal substance abuse are more prevalent in Asian American populations than previously thought. Much more research is needed to delineate the patterns of substance use in these populations as well as the dynamics that underlie substance use. Outreach and prevention techniques for U.S. Asian populations are also at a very preliminary stage.

Implications for Prevention

The large literature on prevention and treatment of drug and alcohol abuse has not paid detailed attention to class and ethnic variation until recently. For example, why Latinos are less likely than Anglos to utilize drug treatment programs remains an open question (Longshore, Hsieh, Anglin, & Annon, 1992). A number of researchers have suggested ways to improve research and enhance prevention among immigrant groups.

Culturally appropriate psychotherapy may enhance bicultural skills and generational communication in immigrant Latino families (Kurtines & Szapocznik, 1995, pp. 181–182). In contrast, Rodriguez and colleagues' (1993) research among second-generation New York Puerto Rican adolescents did not find a moderating effect for biculturalism. The discrepancy may relate to subcultural and generational differences, or to problems with measurement.

More comparative, interdisciplinary research may ameliorate these problems and identify protective factors (Adrados, 1993, p. 73). Vega, Zimmerman, Gil, Warheit, and Apospori (1993) urged more detailed qualitative research to determine how acculturative strain interacts with other risk factors to impact substance use. Also, although most researchers emphasize the importance of familism, methods of measuring it and determining its role in resilience remain undetermined (p. 157). Techniques such as back translation of instruments* and the development of more culturally sensitive scales may enhance research on these issues (Kurtines & Szapocznik, 1995; Szapocznik, Scopetta, & King, 1978; Szapocznik, Scopetta, Kurtines, & Aranalde, 1978; Szapocznik, Kurtines, & Fernandez, 1980; Szapocznik et al., 1989; Szapocznik et al., 1991; these references contain examples of culturally sensitive scales).

Prevention efforts might also be enhanced by more accurate views of the nature of acculturation and its impact on substance use in immigrant populations. Oetting (1993) criticized the simplicity of acculturation models in complex, urban societies. Broad cultural designations such as "Puerto Rican" or "Catholic" interact with more narrowly defined associational groups including schools, gangs, professions, and clubs, each in turn subdivided so that the subculture of a *barrio* youth gang may include a "microculture" of *barrio* youth gang heroin users, for example (p. 41). Failure in one subculture, such as that of school, may impel an individual to seek out membership or intensify identification with an alternative subculture such as that of a drug-using peer cluster (pp. 44–48). Acculturation processes take place among all the different nested subcultures.

---

* Here the interview schedule is written out in English, translated into Spanish, and then given to a second translator to retranslate back into English in order to catch any anomalies in the translation. It is also helpful to use a translator familiar with the slang and speech patterns of the target group (Kurtines & Szapocznik, 1995, p. 172).

Vega and colleagues (1993) discussed acculturation and substance use as processes rather than static qualities, calling for broader studies on culture change and substance use and the end of the use of ethnic markers as catalogues (p. 159). In addition, the validity of self-report on substance use by immigrant and ethnic minority youth is largely untested (Mensch & Kandel, 1988). More research is needed on how immigrant adolescents think about and report on their experiences (Vega et al., 1993, p. 159).

Prevention strategies need to take into account variations in employment, acculturation, and drinking pattern found in the Latino population, as well as the variation in drinking patterns between men and women and among different nationalities of Latinos (Gilbert, 1985, p. 276). Given the importance of extended families and social networks in Latino communities, prevention efforts benefit from integration of the natural support systems among Latino immigrants (Delgado, 1995; see also Szapocznik et al., 1980, and Szapocznik et al., 1991). For example, a study of an injection drug–related AIDS prevention program in Puerto Rico showed how the use of Puerto Rican former drug users as outreach workers was successful in recruiting large numbers of addicts into the program. These workers were able to use unorthodox methods to develop and utilize social networks to draw addicts into treatment. Their insider knowledge of social organization in this community is what allowed them to be more successful than previous outreach workers in recruiting addicts for treatment (Finlinson, Colon, & Page, 1993).

Drug and alcohol research in general suffers from the lack of standard measures making many studies noncomparable. In addition, dissimilar immigrant groups are too frequently merged together by researchers. Although there are commonalities in alcohol abuse patterns among Latinos or Asians as groups, there are also important differences related to economic class, country of origin, gender, and generation since immigration, as well as by ethnicity within the group. There are also some drugs, such as *khat* and opium, that are understudied in the United States.

Although alcohol and drug research and prevention publications are dominated by the idea that substance use constitutes a biologically based medical problem, there is increasing evidence that cultural factors are an important part of the environment that contributes to substance use and that cultural sensitivity is important to prevention and treatment (Finn, 1994). Prevention efforts are more likely to succeed if they take into account not only the specific use patterns of particular immigrant groups but also the various social situations to which those use patterns respond. Prevention and treatment programs might be more succesful if they targeted specific cultural issues (Finn, 1994) as well as problems specific to the situation of immigrants. The use of immigrant outreach workers, native speaker interviewers, and the inclusion of immigrant community leaders in planning for prevention would help to make research, prevention, and therapy more culturally appropriate.

The alcohol and drug research field in general would benefit from more detailed ethnographic information on substance use and more standardized quantitative studies. The use of interviewers who are native speakers of the languages used by immigrants or members of the immigrant group under study, or both, would improve the ability of researchers to gather information on immigrant groups. This style of "privileged access interviewers" has proven useful in the study of a variety of minority groups (Abbot, Walker, & Otero, 1995; Finlinson *et al.,* 1993; Griffiths, Gossop, Powis, & Strang, 1993). The use of recovered addicts as peer counselors has also proved helpful (Levy, Gallmeier, & Weibel, 1995). Although increasingly detailed and interesting data are available, the literature on substance use among immigrants continues to suffer from lack of detailed information on the lives, experiences, and practices of members of immigrant communities. More effective prevention strategies await more abundant and detailed research.

References

Abbot, P. J., Walker, S., & Otero, C. J. (1995).The critical need for counselors in methadone programs. *Alcoholism Treatment Quarterly, 13,* 31–43.

Adrados, J.-L. R. (1993). Acculturation: The broader view. Theoretical framework of the acculturation scales. In M. R. de la Rosa & J. L. R. Receio Adrados (Eds.), *Drug abuse among minority youth: Methodological issues and recent research advances* (NIDA Research Monograph Series 130, pp. 57–77). Rockville, MD: National Institute on Drug Abuse, National Institutes of Health, U.S. Department of Health and Human Services.

Adrian, M., Dini, C. M., MacGregor, L. J., & Stoduto, G. (1995). Substance use as a measure of social integration for women of different ethnocultural groups into mainstream culture in a pluralist society: The example of Canada. *International Journal of the Addictions, 30,* 699–734.

Ahern, F. M. (1989). Alcohol use and abuse among four ethnic groups in Hawaii: Native Hawaiians, Japanese, Filipinos and Caucasians. In D. Spiegler, D. Tate, S. Aitken, & C. Christian (Eds.), *Alcohol use among U.S. ethnic minorities* (NIAAA Research Monograph No. 18, pp. 315–328). Washington, DC: U.S. Government Printing Office.

Akers, R. L. (1991). Addiction: The troublesome concept. *Journal of Drug Issues, 21,* 777–793.

Akutsu, P. D., Sue, S., Zane, N. W. S., & Nakamura, C. Y. (1989). Ethnic differences in alcohol consumption among Asians and Caucasians in the United States: An investigation of cultural and physiological factors. *Journal of Studies of Alcohol, 50,* 261–267.

Alaniz, M. L. (1994). Mexican farmworker women's perspectives on drinking in a migrant community. *International Journal of the Addictions, 29,* 1173–1188.

Alcocer, A. M. (1982). Alcohol use and abuse among the Hispanic American population. In *Alcohol and health monograph 4: Special population issues* (pp. 361–382). Rockville, MD: U.S. Department of Health and Human Services.

Alt, P. M. (1991). Disease or illness: Alcoholism as social metaphor. *Journal of Health Politics, Policy, and Law, 16,* 605–613.

Alvarez-Gomez, A. J. (1995). Politicas antidrogas y proyecto neoliberal. *Estudios Latinoamericanos, 2,* 71–87.

Ames, G., & Rebhun, L. A. (1996). Women, alcohol and work: Interactions of gender, ethnicity and occupational culture. *Social Science and Medicine, 43,* 1649–1663.

Arakaki, A., & Antonis, S. (1978). Asian/Pacific Island women and substance abuse. In D. Smith (Ed.), *A multicultural view of drug abuse: Proceedings of the National Drug Abuse Conference, San Francisco* (pp. 604–607). Cambridge, MA: Schenkman.

Austin, G. A., Prendergast, M. L., & Lee, H. (1989). *Substance abuse among Asian American youth* (Prevention Research Update No. 5). Portland, OR: Northwest Regional Educational Laboratory.

Ayers, E. L. (1984). *Vengeance and justice: Crime and punishment in the 19th century American south*. New York: Oxford University Press.

Bernier, D. (1992) The Indochinese refugees: A perspective from various stress theories. *Journal of Multicultural Social Work, 2,* 15–30.

Beroud, G. (1995). Problemes de toxicomanie en Republique populaire de Chine: Situation actuelle. *Sciences Sociales et Sante, 13,* 65–89.

Berry, J. (1980). Acculturation as varieties of adaptation. In A. Padilla (Ed.), *Acculturation: Theory, models, and some new findings* (pp. 9–25). Boulder, CO: Westview.

Blatter, A. (1995). Die Funktionen des Drogengebrauchs und ihre kulturspezifische Nutzung. *Curare, 18,* 279–290.

Boado, A. (1984). Resena historica antropologica de las drogas en distintas culturas. *RS, Cuadernos de Realidades Sociales, 24,* 131–152.

Bourgois, P. (1995). *In search of respect: Selling crack in El Barrio*. Cambridge, England: Cambridge University Press.

Bowker, L. (1977). *Drug use among American women, old and young*. San Francisco: R. and E..

Brett, P. J., Graham, K., & Smythe. C. (1995). An analysis of specialty journals on alcohol, drugs, and addictive behaviors for sex bias in research methods and reporting. *Journal of Studies on Alcohol, 56,* 24–34.

Brindis, C., Wolfe, A. L., McCarter, V., Ball, S., & Starbuck-Morales, S. (1995). The associations between immigrant status and risk-behavior in Latino adolescents. *Journal of Adolescent Health, 17,* 99–105.

Brook, J. S. (1993). Interactional theory: Its utility in explaining drug use behavior among African-American and Puerto Rican youth. In M. R. De la Rosa & J. L. R. Adrados (Eds.), *Drug abuse among minority youth: Methodological issues and recent research advances* (NIDA Research Monograph Series 130, pp. 79–101). Rockville, MD: National Institutes on Drug Abuse, National Institutes of Health, U.S. Department of Health and Human Services.

Buchanan, D. R. (1992). A social history of American drug use. *Journal of Drug Issues, 22,* 31–52.

Bullington, B. (1997). *Heroin use in the barrio*. Lexington, MA: Lexington Books.

Burke, T. W., & O'Rear, C. E. (1990). Home invaders: Asian gangs in America. *Police Studies, 13,* 154–156.

Caetano, R. (1983). Drinking patterns and alcohol problems among Hispanics in the U.S.: A review. *Drug and Alcohol Dependence, 12,* 37–59.

Caetano, R. (1987). Acculturation and drinking patterns among U.S. Hispanics. *British Journal of Addiction, 82,* 789–799.

Caetano, R. (1990). Hispanic drinking in the U.S.: Thinking in new directions. *British Journal of Addiction, 85,* 1231–1236.

Caetano, R., & Medina Mora, M. E. (1988). Acculturation and drinking among people of Mexican descent in Mexico and the United States. *Journal of Studies on Alcohol, 49,* 462–471.

Canino, G. (1994). Alcohol use and misuse among Hispanic women: Selected factors, processes, and studies. *International Journal of the Addictions, 29,* 1083–1100.

Chavez, E. (1993). Hispanic dropouts and drug use: A review of the literature and methodological considerations. In M. R. De la Rosa & J. L. R. Adrados (Eds.), *Drug abuse among minority youth: Methodological issues and recent research advances* (NIDA Research Monograph Series 130, pp. 224–223). Rockville, MD: National Institute on Drug Abuse, National Institutes of Health, U.S. Department of Health and Human Services.

Chavez, E., & Mora, J. (1994). Introduction to the international journal of the addictions special issue on substance use patterns of Latinas. *International Journal of the Addictions, 29,* 1079–1082.

Chi, I., Kitano, H. H. L., & Lubben, J. E. (1988). Male Chinese drinking behavior in Los Angeles. *Journal of Studies on Alcohol, 49,* 21–25.

Chi, I., Lubben, J. E., & Kitano, H. H. L. (1989). Differences in drinking behavior among three Asian-American groups. *Journal of Studies on Alcohol, 50,* 15–23.

Corbett, K., Mora, J., & Ames, G. (1991). Drinking patterns and drinking-related problems of Mexican-American husbands and wives. *Journal of Studies on Alcohol, 52,* 215–223.

Courtwright, D. T. (1991). Drug legalization, the drug war, and drug treatment in historical perspective. *Journal of Policy History, 3,* 393–414.

Curry, G. D., & Spergel, I. A. (1992). Gang involvement and delinquency among Hispanic and African-American adolescent males. *Journal of Research in Crime and Delinquency, 29,* 273–291.

D'Avanzo, C. E., Frye, B., & Froman, R. (1994). Culture, stress, and substance use in Cambodian refugee women. *Journal of Studies on Alcohol, 55,* 420–426.

De la Rosa, M. R., Adrados, J. L. R., & Milburn, N. (1993). Introduction and overview. In M. R. De la Rosa & J. L. R. Adrados (Eds.), *Drug abuse among minority youth: Methodological issues and recent research advances* (NIDA Research Monograph Series 130, pp. 1–7). Rockville, MD: National Institute on Drug Abuse, National Institutes of Health, U.S. Department of Health and Human Services.

Delgado, M. (1995). Hispanic natural support systems and alcohol and other drug services. *Alcoholism Treatment Quarterly, 12,* 17–31.

Destremau, B. (1990). Le qat: Planche de salut ou cancer de l'economie yemenite? *Etudes Rurales, 117,* 179–190.

Dunnigan, T., McNall, M., &Mortimer, J. T. (1993). The problem of metaphorical nonequivalence in cross-cultural survey research: Comparing the mental health statuses of Hmong refugee and general population adolescents. *Journal of Cross-Cultural Psychology, 24,* 344–365.

Erlanger, H. S. (1979). Estrangement, machismo, and gang violence. *Social Science Quarterly, 60,* 235–248.

Escobedo, L. G., Kirch, D. G., & Anda, R. F. (1996). Depression and smoking initiation among US Latinos. *Addiction, 91,* 113–119.

Ferentzy, P. (1992). Addiction, culture, and community. *Telos, 91,* 125–130.

Finlinson, H. A., Robles, R. R., Colon, H. M., & Page, B. J. (1993). Recruiting and retaining out-of-treatment injecting drug users in the Puerto Rican AIDS Prevention Project. *Human Organization, 52,* 169–175.

Finn, P. (1994). Addressing the needs of cultural minorities in drug treatment. *Journal of Substance Abuse Treatment, 11,* 325–337.

Flaskerud, J. H., & Hu, L. T. (1992). Relationship of ethnicity to psychiatric diagnosis. *Journal of Nervous and Mental Disease, 180,* 296–303.

Flores-Ortiz, Y. G. (1994). The role of cultural and gender values in alcohol use patterns among Chicana/Latina high school and university students: Implications for AIDS prevention. *International Journal of the Addictions, 29,* 1149–1171.

Fullilove, M. T., Lown, A., & Fullilove, R. E. (1992). Crack 'hos and skeezers: Traumatic experiences of women crack users. *Journal of Sex Research, 29,* 275–287.

Gilbert, M. J. (1985). Mexican-Americans in California: Intracultural variation in attitudes and behavior related to alcohol. In L. A. Bennett & G. Ames (Eds.), *The American experience with alcohol: Contrasting cultural perspectives* (pp. 255–277). New York: Plenum.

Gilbert, M. J. (1991). Acculturation and changes in drinking patterns among Mexican-American women. *Alcohol Health and Research World, 15,* 234–238.

Gilbert, M. J., Mora, J., & Ferguson, L. R. (1994). Alcohol related expectations among Mexican-American women. *International Journal of the Addictions, 29,* 1127–1147.

Glick, R., & Moore, J. (1990). *Drugs in Hispanic communities.* New Brunswick, NJ: Rutgers University Press.

Goode, E. (1984). *Drugs in American society* (2nd ed.). New York: Knopf.

Goode, E. (1990). The American drug panic of the 1980s: Social construction or objective threat? *International Journal of the Addictions, 25,* 1083–1098.

Gordon, A. J. (1981). The cultural context of drinking and indigenous therapy for alcohol problems in three migrant Hispanic cultures: An ethnographic report. *Journal of Studies on Alcohol, 9,* 217–240.

Gordon, A. J. (1985). Alcohol and Hispanics in the Northeast: A study of cultural variability and adaptation. In L. A. Bennet & G. Ames (Eds.), *The American experience with alcohol contrasting cultural perspectives* (pp. 297–313). New York: Plenum.

Graves, T. D. (1967). Acculturation, access, and alcohol in a triethnic community. *American Anthropologist, 69,* 306–321.

Griffiths, P., Gossop, M., Powis, B., & Strang, J. (1993). Reaching hidden populations of drug users by privileged access interviewers: Methodological and practical issues. *Addiction, 88,* 1617–1626.

Hakkarainen, P., & Hoikkala, T. (1992). Temgesic: Lattlurade lakare, narrande narkomaner. *Nordisk Alkohol Tidskrift, 9,* 261–274.

Harris, M. G. (1994). Cholas, Mexican-American girls, and gangs. *Sex Roles, 30,* 289–301.

Harrison, L. D., & Kennedy, N. J. (1996). Drug use in the high intensity drug trafficking area of the US Southwest border. *Addiction, 91,* 47–61.

Holck, S. E., Warren, C., Smith, J., & Rochat, R. (1984). Alcohol consumption among Mexican American and Anglo women: Results of a survey along the U.S. Mexico border. *Journal of Studies on Alcohol, 45,* 149–153.

Horowitz, R. (1982). Adult delinquent gangs in a Chicano community: Masked intimacy and marginality. *Urban Life, 11,* 3–26.

Horowitz, R. (1983). *Honor and the American dream: Culture and identity in a Chicano community.* New Brunswick, NJ: Rutgers University Press.

Huff, R. C., (Ed.). (1990). *Gangs in America.* Newbury Park, CA: Sage.

Huggins, P. (1971). *The South Carolina dispensary: A bottle collector's guide and history of the system.* Columbia, SC: Sandlapper.

Ianni, F. A. J. (1974). New mafia: Black, Hispanic, and Italian styles. *Trans-Action, 11,* 26–39.

Jankowski, M. S. (1991). *Islands in the street: Gangs and American urban society.* Berkeley: University of California Press.

Jenkins, C. N. N., Le, T., McPhee, S. J., Stewart, S., & The Ha, N. (1996). Health care access and preventive care among Vietnamese immigrants: Do traditional beliefs and practices pose barriers? *Social Science and Medicine, 43,* 1049–1056.

Jennings, J. M. (1995). The forgotten plague: Opium and narcotics in Korea under Japanese rule: 1910–1945. *Modern Asian Studies, 294,* 795–815.

Jilek, W. G., & Jilek-Aall, L. (1990). The mental health relevance of traditional medicine and shamanism in refugee camps in Northern Thailand. *Curare, 13,* 217–224.

Joe, K. A. (1993). Getting into the gang: Methodological issues in studying ethnic gangs. In M. R. De la Rosa & J. L. R. Adrados (Eds.), *Drug abuse among minority youth: Methodological issues and recent research advances* (NIDA Research Monograph Series 130, pp. 234–257). Rockville, MD: National Institute on Drug Abuse, National Institutes of Health, U.S. Department of Health and Human Services.

Johnson, R. C., Nagoshi, C. T., Ahern, F. M., Wilson, J. R., & Yuen, S. L. H. (1987). Cultural factors as explanations for ethnic group differences in alcohol use in Hawaii. *Journal of Psychoactive Drugs, 19,* 67–75.

Kalix, P. (1988). Khat: A plant with amphetamine effects. *Journal of Substance Abuse Treatment, 5,* 163–169.

Kelly, G. P. (1986). Coping with America: Refugees From Vietnam, Cambodia, and Laos in the 1970s and 1980s. *Annals of the American Academy of Political and Social Science, 487,* 138–149.

Kinkead, G. (1992). *Chinatown: Portrait of a closed society.* New York: Harper Collins.

Kinzie, J. D., & Fleck, J. (1987). Psychotherapy with severely traumatized refugees. *American Journal of Psychotherapy, 41,* 82–94.

Kitano, H. H. L., & Chi, I. (1986–87). Asian Americans and alcohol use: Exploring cultural differences in Los Angeles. *Alcohol Health and Research World, 11,* 42–47.

Kitano, H. H. L., & Daniels, R. (1988). *Asian Americans: Emerging minorities.* Englewood Cliffs, NJ: Prentice Hall.

Kitano, H. H. L., Hatanaka, H., Yeung, W. T., & Sue, S. (1985). Japanese-American drinking patterns. In L. A. Bennett & G. Ames (Eds.), *The American experience with alcohol: Contrasting cultural perspectives* (pp. 335–357). New York: Plenum.

Klein, M. W., Maxson, C. L., & Cunningham, L. C. (1991). "Crack," street gangs, and violence. *Criminology, 29,* 623–650.

Krupinski, J. (1967). Sociological aspects of mental ill-health in migrants. *Social Science and Medicine, 1,* 267–281.

Kurtines, W. M., & Szapocznik, J. (1995). Cultural competence in assessing hispanic youths and families: Challenges in the assessment of treatment needs and treatment evaluation for Hispanic drug-abusing adolescents. In E. Rahdert & D. Czechowicz (Eds.), *Adolescent drug abuse: Clinical assessment and therapeutic interventions* (National Institute on Drug Abuse Research Monograph 156, pp. 172–189). Rockville, MD: National Institutes of Health, U.S. Department of Health and Human Services.

Levy, J. A., Gallmeier, C. P., & Weibel, W. W. (1995). The outreach assisted peer-support model for controlling drug dependency. *Journal of Drug Issues, 25,* 507–529.

Litman, A., Levav, I., Saltz-Rennert, H., & Maoz, B. (1986). The use of khat: An epidemiological study in two Yemenite villages in Israel. *Culture Medicine and Psychiatry, 10,* 389–396.

Longshore, D., Hsieh, S., Anglin, M. D., & Annon. T. A. (1992). Ethnic patterns in drug abuse treatment utilization. *Journal of Mental Health Administration, 19,* 268–277.

Lubben, J. E., Chi, I., & Kitano, H. H. L. (1989). The relative influence of selected social factors on Korean drinking behavior in Los Angeles. *Advances in Alcohol and Substance Abuse, 8,* 1–17.

Maddahian, E., Newcomb, M. D., & Bentler, P. M. (1986). Adolescents' substance abuse: Impact of ethnicity, income, and availability. *Advances in Alcohol and Substance Abuse, 5,* 63–78.

Madsen, W. (1964). The alcoholic agringado. *American Anthropologist, 66,* 355–361.

Manning, P. K., & Redlinger, L. J. (1983). Drugs as work. *Research in the Sociology of Work, 2,* 275–301.

Marín, B. V., & Flores, E. (1994). Acculturation, sexual behavior, and alcohol use among Latinas. *International Journal of the Addictions, 29,* 1101–1114.

Marin, G. (1992). Issues in the measurement of acculturation among Hispanics. In K. F. Geisinger (Ed.), *Psychological testing of Hispanics* (pp. 235–251). Washington, DC: American Psychological Association.

Marin, G., & Posner, S. F. (1995). The role of gender and acculturation on determining the consumption of alcoholic beverages among Mexican-Americans and Central Americans in the United States. *International Journal of the Addictions, 30,* 779–794.

Mark, G. Y. (1975). Racial, economic, and political factors in the development of America's first drug laws. *Issues in Criminology, 10,* 49–72.

Markides, K. S., Krause, N., & Mendes de Leon, C. F. (1988). Acculturation and alcohol consumption among Mexican Americans: A three-generation study. *American Journal of Public Health, 78,* 1178–1181.

Martin, J., & Zweban, J. E.. (1993). Addressing treatment needs of Southeast Asian Mien opium users in California. *Journal of Psychoactive Drugs, 25,* 73–6.

McLaughlin, D. G., Raymond, J. S., Murakami, S. R., & Goebert, D. (1987). Drug use among Asian Americans in Hawaii. *Journal of Psychoactive Drugs, 19,* 85–94.

Mendoza, R. H. (1989). An empirical scale to measure type and degree of acculturation in Mexican-American adolescents and adults. *Journal of Cross-Cultural Psychology, 20,* 372–385.

Mensch, B. S., & Kandel, D. B. (1988). Underreporting of substance use in a national longitudinal youth cohort. *Public Opinion Quarterly, 52,* 100–124.

Moore, J. (1990). Mexican American women addicts: The influence of family background. In R. Glick & J. Moore (Eds.), *Drugs in Hispanic communities* (pp. 127–155). New Brunswick, NJ: Rutgers University Press.

Moore, J. (1991). *Going down to the barrio: Homeboys and homegirls in change.* Philadelphia: Temple University Press.

Moore, J. (1994). The *Chola* life course: Chicana heroin users and the Barrio gang. *International Journal of the Addictions, 29,* 1115–1126.

Moore, J., & Devitt, M. (1989). The paradox of deviance in addicted Mexican American mothers. *Gender and Society, 3,* 53–70.

Moore, J., & Vigil, J. D. (1987). Chicano gangs: Group norms and individual factors related to adult criminality. *Aztlan, 18,* 27–44.

Moore, J., Vigil, J. D., & Garcia, R. (1983). Residence and territoriality in chicano gangs. *Social Problems, 31,* 182–194.

Murakami, S. R. (1989). An epidemiological survey of alcohol, drug, and mental health problems in Hawaii: A comparison of four ethnic groups. In D. Spiegler, D. Tate, S. Aitken, & C. Christian (Eds.), *Alcohol use among U.S. ethnic minorities* (NIAAA Research Monograph No. 18, pp. 343–353). Washington, DC: U.S. Government Printing Office.

Musto, D. F. (1993). Opium, cocaine, and marijuana in American history. *Scientific American* [Special issue], 30–37.

Neff, J. A. (1986). Alcohol consumption and psychological distress among US Anglos, Hispanics, and Blacks. *Alcohol and Alcoholism, 21,* 111–119.

Neff, J. A., Hoppe, S. K., & Perea, P. (1987). Acculturation and alcohol use: Drinking patterns and problems among Anglo and Mexican American male drinkers. *Hispanic Journal of Behavioral Science, 2,* 151–181.

Nencini, P., Grassi, M. C., Botan, A. A., Asseyr, A. F., & Paroli, E. (1989). Khat chewing spread to the Somali community in Rome. *Drug and Alcohol Dependence, 23,* 255–258.

Neuhaus, C., Jr. (1993). The disease controversy revisited: An ontologic perspective. *Journal of Drug Issues, 23,* 463–478.

Newman, R. K. (1995). Opium smoking in late imperial China: A reconsideration. *Modern Asian Studies, 29,* 765–794.

Nicassio, P. M. (1983). Psychosocial correlates of alienation: Study of a sample of indochinese refugees. *Journal of Cross-Cultural Psychology, 14,* 337–351.

Nicassio, P. M., & Pate, J. K. (1984). An analysis of problems of resettlement of the Indochinese refugees in the United States. *Social Psychiatry, 19,* 135–141.

Oetting, E. R. (1993). Orthogonal cultural identification: Theoretical links between cultural identification and substance use. In M. R. De la Rosa & J. L. R. Adrados (Eds.), *Drug abuse among minority youth: Methodological issues and recent research advances* (NIDA Research Monograph Series 130, pp. 32–57). Rockville, MD: National Institute on Drug Abuse, National Institutes of Health, U.S. Department of Health and Human Services.

Page, J. B., Rio, L., Sweeney, J., & McKay, C. (1985). Alcohol and adaptation to exile in Miami's Cuban population. In L. A. Bennet & G. Ames (Eds.), *The American experience with alcohol: Contrasting cultural perspectives* (pp. 315–332). New York: Plenum.

Pérez-Arce, P. (1994). Substance use patterns of Latinas: Commentary. *International Journal of the Addictions, 29,* 1189–1199.

Poole, E. D., & Pogrebin, M. R. (1990). Crime and law enforcement policy in the Korean American community. *Police Studies, 13,* 57–66.

Rodriguez, O., Adrados, J.-L. R., & De la Rosa, M. R. (1993). Integrating mainstream and subcultural explanations of drug use among Puerto Rican youth. In M. R. De la Rosa & J. L. R. Adrados (Eds.), *Drug abuse among minority youth: Methodological issues and recent research advances* (NIDA Research Monograph Series 130, pp. 8–31). Rockville, MD: National Institute on Drug Abuse, National Institutes of Health, U.S. Department of Health and Human Services.

Rubinstein, A. (1973). How China got rid of opium. *Monthly Review, 25,* 58–63.

Rynearson, A. M., & DeVoe, P. A. (1984). Refugee women in a vertical village: Lowland Laotians in St. Louis. *Social Thought, 10,* 33–48.

Schiller, N. G. (1992). What's wrong with this picture? The hegemonic construction of culture in AIDS research in the United States. *Medical Anthropology Quarterly, 6,* 237–254.

Schwartz, A. J. (1989). Middle-class educational values among Latino gang members in East Los Angeles County high schools. *Urban Education, 24*(3), 323–342.

Schwitters, S. Y., Johnson, R. C., Wilson, J. R., & McClearn, G. E. (1982). Ethnicity and alcohol. *Hawaiian Medical Journal, 41,* 60–63.

Singer, K. (1972). Drinking patterns and alcoholism in the Chinese. *British Journal of Addiction, 67,* 3–14.

Spode, H. (1992). Normales und abweichendes Trinken: Entstehung und Folgen einer symbolischen Grenzziehung. *MMG—Medizin, Mensch, Gesellschaft, 17,* 108–117.

Sue, S., & Morishima, J. K. (1982). *The mental health of Asian Americans.* San Francisco: Jossey-Bass.

Sue, S., & Nakamura, C. Y. (1984). An integrative model of physiological and social/psychological factors in alcohol consumption among Chinese and Japanese Americans. *Journal of Drug Issues, 14,* 349–364.

Sue, S., Zane, N., & Ito, J. (1979). Alcohol drinking patterns among Asian and Caucasian Americans. *Journal of Cross-Cultural Psychology, 10,* 41–56.

Sue, S., Kitano, H. H. L., Hatanaka, J., & Yeung, J. T. (1985). Alcohol consumption among Chinese in the United States. In L. A. Bennet & G. Ames (Eds.), *The American experience with alcohol: Contrasting cultural perspectives* (pp. 359–371). New York: Plenum.

Szapocznik, J., Scopetta, M. A., & King, O. E. (1978). Theory and practice in matching treatment to the special characteristics and problems of Cuban immigrants. *Journal of Community Psychology, 6,* 112–122.

Szapocznik, J., Scopetta, M. A., Kurtines, W. M., & Aranalde, A. (1978). Theory and measurement of acculturation. *Interamerican Journal of Psychology, 12,* 113–130.

Szapocznik, J., Kurtines, W. A., & Fernandez, T. (1980). Bicultural involvement and adjustment in Hispanic American youths. *International Journal of Intercultural Relationships, 4,* 353–366.

Szapocznik, J., Rio, A. T., Murray, E., Cohen, R., Scopetta, M., Rivas-Vazquez, A., Hervis, O., Posada, V., & Kurtines, W. M., (1989). Structural family vs. psychodynamic child therapy for problematic Hispanic boys. *Journal of Consulting and Clinical Psychology, 57,* 571–578.

Szapocznik, J., Rio, A. T., Hervis, O. E., Mitrani, V. B., Kurtines, W. M., & Faraci, A. M. (1991). Assessing change in family functioning as a result of treatment: The structural family systems ratings scale (SFSR). *Journal of Marital and Family Therapy, 17,* 295–310.

Thomas, T. (1995). Acculturative stress in the adjustment of immigrant families. *Journal of Social Distress and the Homeless, 4,* 131–142.

Tomasello, A., Tyler, F. B., Tyler, S. L., & Zhang, Y. (1993). Psychosocial correlates of drug use among Latino youth leading autonomous lives. *International Journal of the Addictions, 28,* 435–50.

Towle, L. (1988). Japanese-American drinking: Some results from the joint Japanese–U.S. alcohol epidemiology project. *Alcohol Health and Research World, 12,* 216–223.

Trimble, J. E., Padilla, A. M., & Bell, C. S. (Eds.). (1987). *Drug abuse among ethnic minorities* (DHHS Publication No. 87-1474). Washington, DC: U.S. Government Printing Office.

Trotter, R. T., II. (1985). Mexican-American experience with alcohol: South Texas examples. In L. A. Bennet & G. Ames (Eds.), *The American experience with alcohol: Contrasting cultural perspectives* (pp. 279–296). New York: Plenum.

Truan, F. (1993). Addiction as a social construction: A postempirical view. *Journal of Psychology, 127,* 489–499.

Tsunoda, T., Parrish, K. M., Higuchi, S., Stinson, F. S., Kono, H., Ogata, M., & Harford, T. C. (1992). The effect of acculturation on drinking attitudes among Japanese in Japan and Japanese Americans in Hawaii and California. *Journal of Studies on Alcohol, 53,* 369–377.

Vega, W. A., Zimmerman, R., Gil, A., Warheit, G. J., & Apospori, E. (1993). Acculturation strain theory: Its application in explaining drug use behavior among Cuban and other Hispanic youth. In M. R. De la Rosa & J. L. R. Adrados (Eds.), *Drug abuse among minority youth: Methodological issues and recent research advances* (NIDA Research Monograph Series 130, pp. 144–166). Rockville, MD: National Institute on Drug Abuse, National Institutes of Health, U.S. Department of Health and Human Services.

Velez, C. N., & Ungemack, J. A. (1989). Drug use among Puerto Rican youth: An exploration of generational status differences. *Social Science and Medicine, 29,* 779–789.

Velez, C. N., & Ungemack, J. A. (1995). Psychosocial correlates of drug use among Puerto Rican youth: Generational status differences. *Social Science and Medicine, 40,* 91–103.

Vigil, J. D. (1983). Chicano gangs: One response to Mexican urban adaptation in the Los Angeles area. *Urban Anthropology, 12,* 45–75.

Vigil, J. D. (1988). Group processes and street identity: Adolescent Chicano gang members. *Ethos, 16,* 421–445.

Waldorf, D. (1993). Don't be your own best customer—drug use of San Francisco gang drug sellers. *Crime, Law, and Social Change, 19,* 1–15.

Walker, W. O., Jr. (1996). *Drugs in the Western Hemisphere: An odyssey of cultures in conflict.* Wilmington, DE: Jaguar Books on Latin America, Scholarly Resources.

Wallace, J. M., Jr., & Bachman, J. G. (1993). Validity of self-reports in student-based studies on minority populations: Issues and concerns. In M. R. De la Rosa & J. L. R. Adrados (Eds.), *Drug abuse among minority youth: Methodological issues and recent research advances* (NIDA Research Monograph Series 130, pp. 167–200). Rockville, MD: National Institute on Drug Abuse, National Institutes of Health, U.S. Department of Health and Human Services.

Waters, T. (1990). Adaptation and migration among the Mien people of Southeast Asia. *Ethnic Groups, 8,* 127–141.

Weisner, C. (1992). The merging of alcohol and drug treatment: A policy review. *Journal of Public Health Policy, 13,* 66–80.

Westermeyer, J. (1978). Indigenous and expatriate addicts in Laos: A comparison. *Culture, Medicine, and Psychiatry, 2,* 139–150.

Westermeyer, J. (1993). Substance use disorders among young minority refugees: Common themes in a clinical sample. In M. R. De la Rosa & J. L. R. Adrados (Eds.), *Drug abuse among minority youth: Methodological issues and recent research advances* (NIDA Research Monograph Series 130, pp. 308–320). Rockville, MD: National Institute on Drug Abuse, National Institutes of Health, U.S. Department of Health and Human Services.

Westermeyer, J., Neider, J., & Vang, T. F. (1984). Acculturation and mental health: A study of Hmong refugees at 1.5 and 3.5 years postmigration. *Social Science and Medicine, 18,* 87–93.

Yee, B. W., & Thu, N. (1987). Correlates of drug use and abuse among Indochinese refugees: Mental health implications. *Journal of Psychoactive Drugs, 19,* 77–83.

Yee, B. W., Castro, F., Hammond, W. R., John, R., Wyatt, G. E., & Yung, B. R. (1995). Risk-taking and abusive behaviors among ethnic minorities. *Health Psychology, 14,* 622–31.

Yu, E. S. H., & Liu, W. T. (1986–1987). Alcohol use and abuse among Chinese-Americans: Epidemiologic data. *Alcohol Health and Research World, 11,* 14–17.

Zatz, M. S. (1985). Los Cholos: Legal processing of Chicano gang members. *Social Problems, 33,* 13–30.

Zatz, M. S. (1987). Chicano youth gangs and crime: The creation of a moral panic. *Contemporary Crises, 11,* 129–158.

25

Intimate Partner Violence among Immigrants

SANA LOUE AND MARLENE FAUST

Introduction

Intimate partner violence in the immigrant household may have begun in the country of origin or it may have started upon arrival to the United States. Numerous problems arising in conjunction with immigration may contribute to the initiation or continuation of intimate partner violence, including unemployment, role changes between the intimate partners, disintegration of extended family networks, and lack of English-speaking ability (Jang, Lee, & Morello-Frosch, 1990).

Research in the area of intimate partner violence, however, has rarely considered the immigration status of either the victim or the perpetrator or the relevance of immigration status to the domestic violence. Consequently, this discussion focuses primarily on what we have learned about domestic violence from studies conducted in various geographic areas and across cultures and ethnicities. Data relating to domestic violence and immigration has been incorporated into the discussion where available.

SANA LOUE • Department of Epidemiology and Biostatistics, School of Medicine, Case Western Reserve University, Cleveland, Ohio 44106-4945. MARLENE FAUST • School of Medicine, Case Western Reserve University, Cleveland, Ohio 44106-4945.

Handbook of Immigrant Health, edited by Loue. Plenum Press, New York, 1998.

Background

Definition of Intimate Partner Violence

Intimate partner violence and its various component elements have been defined in various ways. Siann (1985) defined "aggression" as involving an intent to inflict hurt or appear superior to others. Such behavior does not necessarily involve physical injury and is not always negatively sanctioned. Gelles and Straus (1979) have defined violence as "an act carried out with the intention or perceived intention of physically hurting another person". Reiss and Roth (1993) defined violence as "behavior by persons against persons that intentionally threatens, attempts, or actually inflicts physical harm." This definition specifically excludes intense criticism, verbal harassment, a restraint of normal activities, and a denial of resources, which may often accompany intimate partner violence (Murty & Roebuck, 1992; National Institute of Mental Health [NIH], 1992; Walker, 1979). Kornblit (1994) has distinguished between abuse and violence:

> The former refers to actions which are harmful for the victim, both physically as well as mentally, committed or resulting from omission, carried out intentionally or not.
>
> Violence in a limited sense is used to refer to physical aggression.

Maltreatment includes abuse (physical, sexual, and/or emotional) and neglect (physical, educational, and/or affective). (p. 1181)

Brown (1992), addressing intimate partner violence directed to women specifically, has defined "wife-beating" as "a man intentionally inflicting pain on a woman, within a nontransient, male–female relationship, whether or not the partners are officially married. The subject is further restricted to physical aggression" (p. 1). Brown further distinguished between wife beating and wife battering. The former refers to a "physical reprimand," that is often culturally expected, tolerated by the recipient female partners, and not at all seen as deviant. Wife battering, by contrast, refers to extraordinary behavior that is neither usual nor acceptable within the society and that may result in serious injury, disability, or death.

The one element common to these definitions is that of physical aggression. Although these definitions are not uniform in their requirement of intentionality, legal definitions often incorporate intentionality as a critical element. Ohio law, for instance, defines domestic violence as

(a) Attempting to cause or recklessly causing bodily injury;
(b) Placing another person by the threat of force in fear of imminent serious physical harm . . . ;
(c) Committing any act with respect to a child that would result in the child being an abused child. (Ohio Revised Code [ORC] section 3113.31).

Emic and etic definitions of partner violence or domestic injury may vary, however, and definitions may vary between groups. A study of the attitudes of 50 women in Ghana found, for instance, that more than 60% did not believe that the beating of a husband by his wife constitutes domestic violence, although all 50 indicated that domestic violence encompasses a husband's beating of his wife, including hitting, slapping, and whipping (Ofei-Aboagye, 1994). Mexican American women in the United States have been found less likely than others to classify slapping, pushing, shoving, grabbing, and throwing things as physical abuse (Torres, 1991), although such acts are often encompassed in laws prohibiting domestic violence.

The issue of intimate partner violence not only calls into question the nature of the acts that constitute such violence, but the nature of the partner relationship that constitutes "intimate partner" (Murdock, 1949). Murdock has defined a family as a "social group characterized by common residence, economic cooperation, and reproduction" (p. 1), thereby eliminating the requirement of marriage as a basis for defining an intimate partnership. It is unclear, however, whether reproduction is seen as an essential element of "family"; if it were, it would eliminate many household units that, in fact, perceive themselves and are perceived by others as families. Many state laws reflect an awareness that neither marriage nor reproduction are prerequisites for intimate partner violence. Ohio's statute relating to domestic violence, for instance, refers to "family or household member[s]," which includes a "spouse, a person living as a spouse or a former spouse of the respondent." In turn, a "person living as a spouse" is defined as

a person who is living or has lived with the respondent in a common law marital relationship, who otherwise is cohabiting with the respondent, who otherwise has cohabited with the respondent within one year prior to the date of the alleged occurrence of the act in question . . . (ORC section 3113.31).

This provision has been interpreted to encompass both heterosexual and homosexual relationships.

Intimate Partner Violence: A Cross-Cultural Perspective

Prevalence and Incidence of Intimate Partner Violence

The occurrence of intimate partner violence is not infrequent. Intimate partner violence is one of the most common causes of injury to women, both inside and outside the United States. It has been estimated that in the

United States alone, each year approximately 1.8 million women (3.4%) to 4 million women are physically assaulted by their intimate partners (Novello, Rosenberg, Saltzman, & Shosky, 1992; Sorenson, Upchurch, & Shen, 1996; Straus & Gelles, 1990). One or both partners in approximately 500,000 couples sustain injuries from the violence each year (Sorenson et al., 1996). Those at highest risk of assault by intimate partners include younger persons, urban dwellers, individuals with less education, those with lower incomes, and African Americans (Sorenson et al., 1996). A study in Melbourne, Australia, found that approximately 22% of the 2,181 women surveyed through general practitioners' offices and clinics reported that they had been physically assaulted by their intimate partner during the previous 12 months (Mazza, Dennerstein, & Ryan, 1996). Thirteen percent of the women assaulted indicated that they had never disclosed the assault to others. Results from a telephone survey of women in Toronto, Canada, indicated an annual incidence of intimate partner violence of 14.4% and a prevalence rate of approximately 25% (M. D. Smith, 1987). A study of 1,000 women ages 22 through 55 in Santiago, Chile, found that more than 60% had experienced intimate partner violence and more than one quarter had experienced severe violence in their relationship during the previous 2 years (Larrain, 1993). In Malaysia, 39% of the 713 women participating in a study reported having been physically beaten by their intimate male partner during 1989 (Malaysia Women's Aid Organisation, 1992). The Metropolitan London Police in 1985 received nearly 1,500 calls per week from women experiencing violence in their homes (Edwards, 1986) and it was estimated in 1986 that there were over 750,000 incidents of domestic violence in London alone (L. Smith, 1989).

Perhaps what is most striking is the widespread occurrence of intimate partner violence across societies, cultures, and religions. Intimate partner violence has been documented across ethnic groups and socioeconomic strata (Schulman, 1979; Straus &

Gelles, 1990; Straus, Gelles, & Steinmertz, 1980) and in both developed (Bernard & Schlaffer, 1992; Bruynooghe et al., 1989; Kim & Cho, 1992; Knight & Hatty, 1992; Mullen, Romans-Clarkson, Walton, & Herbison, 1988; Schei & Bakketeig, 1989; Statistics Canada, 1993) and developing countries (D. A. Counts, Brown, & Campbell, 1992; Morley, 1994; Prasad, 1994; PROFAMILIA, 1990; Shamim, 1992; Women's AIDS Organization, 1992).

Despite the widespread occurrence of intimate partner violence, its frequency appears to vary across cultures. Wife beating is infrequent among families in the rural areas of northern Thailand (Potter, 1977) and the Mundurucu of South America (Murphy & Murphy, 1974). Wife beating among the !Kung, however, appears to be more frequent (Shostak, 1983), although it is surpassed in both frequency and severity in rural Taiwanese families (Wolf, 1972) and among the Yanomamo of northern Brazil (Chagnon, 1968). Researchers examining intimate partner violence at the societal level have found that the prevalence of wife beating tends to be higher in societies in which there is greater tolerance of homosexual relationships and where homosexual behavior is more frequent. Intimate partner violence tends to be less frequent, however, in societies in which a double standard exists with respect to premarital sexual relations (Erchak & Rosenfeld, 1994) and in societies where the need for affiliation is high (Lester, 1987).

Forms of Intimate Partner Violence

What is also striking is the range of circumstances across which intimate partner violence occurs and the forms that it may assume. Intimate partner violence has been committed by men against female partners; by women against male partners (Balakrishnan, Imell, Bandy, & Prasad, 1995; Bergman & Brismar, 1993; Bergman, Brismar, & Nordin, 1992; Duminy & Hudson, 1993; Fiebert, 1996; Straus, 1993); by same-sex intimate partners (V. E. Coleman, 1994; Letellier, 1994); and by partners against each other (Cook & Harris, 1995; Vivian & Langhin-richsen-Rohling, 1994). Intimate partner violence may take numerous forms including battering or beating (Levinson, 1989), stalking (Kurt, 1995), rape (Whatley, 1993), murder, or forced suicide (Levinson, 1989). The violence may be effectuated through the use of fists, feet (Straus, 1994), sexual organs, as in the case of rape (Hanneke, Shields, & Mc-Call, 1986; Whatley, 1993), poison, hanging, drowning, fire (Balakrishnan *et al.,* 1995; Prasad, 1994; Shamim, 1992), electrical shocks (Prasad, 1994), knives or guns (Bates, Redman, Brown, & Hancock, 1995), or another individual, pursuant to the request of the assaultive partner or his or her consent or acquiescence (Chin, 1994; Prasad, 1994; Shamim, 1992). The violence may be perpetrated for any number of proffered reasons, including economic considerations, such as the tendering of an inadequate dowry (Prasad, 1994; Shamim, 1992), religious or spiritual beliefs (Harlan, 1994; Narasimhan, 1990), or dissatisfaction with the actions or behavior of one's partner (Koss *et al.,* 1994).

Consequences of Intimate Partner Violence

Outcomes of intimate partner violence include damage to joints, partial loss of vision (Beck, Freitag, & Singer, 1996; Hartzell, Botek, & Goldberg, 1996) or hearing, burns (Balakrishnan *et al.,* 1995; Prasad, 1994), bites, hematomas, fractures, cuts or abrasions, inflammation, penetrating puncture wounds, dislocation, sprains (Bates *et al.,* 1995), and death (Browne & Williams, 1993). E. Stark, Flitcraft, and Frazier (1979) found that common locations of injuries resulting from intimate partner violence include the head, face, neck, chest, and abdomen. Balakrishnan and colleagues (1995) found that burns of the genitalia were common in male victims of intimate partner violence, such injuries often inflicted while they were sleeping. Initial responses to intimate partner violence often include shock, denial, withdrawal, confusion,

numbing, fear, and depression (Browne, 1987; M. A. Dutton, 1992; Hilberman, 1980; Symonds, 1979; Walker, 1979). Long-term effects may include fear, anxiety, fatigue, sleeping and eating disorders (Goodman, Koss, & Russo, 1993), and feelings of loss, betrayal, or hopelessness (Walker, 1979).

Comparisons across U.S. Ethnic and Immigrant Groups

In the United States, concern has been voiced with respect to variation in rates or the nature of intimate partner violence across various ethnic or racial groups. Such differences may be indicative of differential response to different groups, differential access to services, or differences in the definition or perception of intimate partner violence. (It is beyond the scope of this paper to engage in discussion regarding the existence or delineation of race-ethnicity; suffice it to indicate that this issue exists.) Yet, few studies have examined intimate partner violence in the context of specific ethnic groups. Such an examination would provide a better understanding of the factors that may differentially impact a specific group.

In one such study, Cazenave and Straus (1979) compared the rates of intimate partner violence among a nationally representative sample of African Americans and Caucasians. They found that, after controlling for race, income, and occupation, the rates of intimate partner violence were lower among the African Americans in three of the four income strata. They further found that African American women were less likely to be assaulted if they were part of a strong network of family and friends. E. Stark (1990), however, found in a study of intimate partner violence among African Americans and Caucasians that although the incidence of intimate partner violence was similar, the levels of lethal violence were higher among African Americans. Lockhart and White (1989), in their study of 155 African American women, found that although a smaller proportion of women in the upper socioeconomic strata reported intimate partner violence than did women in the middle or lower socioeconomic strata, they reported a higher median number of assaults per year.

Gondolf, Fisher, and McFerron (1988), in a secondary analysis of data obtained from 5,708 women in shelters, found no difference in the frequency of intimate partner violence between Caucasians, African Americans, and Hispanics. However, they found that Hispanic women were more likely to have been victims of violence for a longer period of time. Torres (1991) also found in interviews with 25 Mexican American women and 25 Caucasian women that the Mexican American women had been in their violent relationships for a substantially longer period of time than the Caucasian women. Torres further found that unlike Caucasian women, Mexican Americans were unlikely to classify such actions as slapping, pushing, shoving, grabbing, and throwing things at them as physical abuse.

In one of the few studies to recognize within-Hispanic differences, Sorenson and Telles (1991) found that Mexico-born Mexican Americans reported lower rates of intimate partner violence than either Caucasians or U.S.–born Mexican Americans (20.0% compared to 21.6% and 30.9%, respectively). Overall rates of sexual assault were lower for Mexican Americans. However, one third of the most recent incidents that were reported by Mexico-born Mexican American women involved the woman's intimate sexual partner and approximated rape. Sorenson and Telles further found that women's immigration status and minimal knowledge of English may be barriers to help seeking. Perilla, Bakeman, and Norris (1994) concluded from their study of 60 immigrant Latinas in southern California that stressors related to immigration status, such as prejudice and lack of English proficiency, contributed to the abuse.

In the one study of intimate partner violence in Puerto Rican families that appears to exist, Kantor, Jasinski, and Aldarondo (1994) found that Puerto Rican husbands were about twice as likely as Anglo husbands and 10 times more likely than Cuban husbands to assault their wives. Birth in the United States increased the risk of wife assaults by both Mexican and Puerto Rican husbands. They further found that Puerto Ricans had the highest rate of cultural approval of wife assaults, compared with Anglos, Mexicans, and Cubans.

Ho (1990) conducted one of the few systematic studies of intimate partner violence among Asian (Lao, Khmer, Vietnamese, and Chinese) women in the United States. Using focus group data, she found that physical violence by intimate partners was common and generally tolerated among the Lao, Khmer, and Vietnamese women. The problem of intimate partner violence is more acute and complex among first-generation Asians, compared with later generations. Ho attributed this finding to women's lack of English language ability, their often tenuous immigration status, and a lack of emotional support resulting from separation from their extended families.

Theories of Causation

However it is defined or effectuated, the causes of intimate partner violence remain obscure. Numerous theories have been offered to explain its origin. Many of these theories are briefly reviewed in the following sections; the literature is too vast to permit more than a brief summary of each. Some of these theories operate at the societal level, while others apply at the level of the individual or the couple. Some theories are more likely to address the issue of why men beat women, whereas others focus on the question of why women who are beaten stay with the partners who beat them. The applicability and relevance of a specific theory of causation to domestic violence within a particular immigrant group must be examined within the context of that group's culture, its definition of male and female roles and behaviors, and the group's experience before, during, and after the immigration experience. Individual factors may also be relevant to the occurrence of domestic violence.

Individual and Couple Level Theories

Biopsychosocial Perspective

The biopsychosocial perspective is an attempt to integrate into one model the various biological, social, and psychological factors that have been found to impact domestic violence (McHenry, Julian, Julian, & Garazzi, 1995). Biological factors to be considered in the etiology of intimate partner violence include testosterone levels in the assaultive male partners (Booth & Dabbs, 1993) and levels of alcohol (Martin, 1992; Pernanen, 1991). Social factors include the level of social stress (Gelles, 1989), the quality of the marital relationship (Rounsaville, 1978a), the extent of social support available (Gelles, 1994; Steinmetz, 1987), and available income (Gelles, 1983; Pan, Neidig, & O'Leary, 1994). Psychological styles have been implicated as a factor in the commission of antisocial behavior (O'Leary, 1993).

Exchange Theory

Gelles (1983) succinctly summarized the basic premise of exchange theory: "People hit and abuse other family members because they can" (p. 157). People's actions are essentially based on a cost-benefit analysis; they will use violence to obtain their goal as long as the benefit outweighs the cost. Nuclear family living arrangements, which tend to isolate the family, may render violence relatively cost-free to the perpetrator. This theory is somewhat challenged by the findings of Eisikovits, Guttmann, Sela-Amit, and Edleson (1993) who noted in their study of 120 Israeli couples that the social supports of men who battered and women who were battered were as many in number and as adequate as those available to men who did not batter and women who were not battered. However, the theory is supported by ethnographic findings in a number of societies. As one example, Lambeck (1992) found that the people of Mayotte consider spousal abuse wrong. Violence in the context of a spousal relationship is considered inappropriate and the battering husband is subject to social censure. The cost of battering is simply too great and, consequently, it rarely occurs.

Investment Theory

Rusbult (1980, 1983) defined commitment to a relationship as a function of anticipated relationship satisfaction, the negative function of the attractiveness of perceived alternatives, and a positive function of the amount that has already been invested in a relationship. Rusbult posited that one's willingness to stay in a relationship increases as the balance of rewards over costs from staying in that relationship exceeds the balance of the rewards over the costs involved in alternative relationships. Rusbult (1980, 1983) hypothesized that there are two types of investments: intrinsic and extrinsic. Intrinsic investments include the amount of time already invested in the relationship, the level of self-disclosure, and the amount of time spent together. Extrinsic investments include such things as the development of mutual friends and family networks, shared possessions, and shared activities.

Resource Theory

Resource theory posits that the decision-making power within a given family derives from the value of the resources that each person brings to the relationship (Blood & Wolfe, 1960). Such resources include money, property, prestige, and contacts, that is, both material and organizational. Goode (1971) has argued that the extent to which a partner is likely to use violence to maintain control is related to the extent of his or her control of resources outside the family; that is, the more external control one has, the less likely he or she will use violence as a means of control.

Social Learning Theory

Social learning theory posits that family violence arises due to a constellation of contextual and situational factors (O'Leary, 1988).

Key contextual factors include individual characteristics, couple characteristics, and societal characteristics, such as stress, violence in the family, and an aggressive personality. Situational factors, such as substance abuse or financial difficulties, will lead to violence in the presence of these contextual factors. Social learning theory has been used to explain the intergenerational transmission of child abuse (Ballard *et al.,* 1990; Davis & Leitenberg, 1987; Egeland, Jacobritz, & Stroufe, 1988; Kaufman & Zigler, 1987).

Theory of Marital Power

Cromwell and Olson (1975) hypothesized that power falls into three realms: power bases, power processes, and power outcomes. Power bases consist of the assets and resources that provide the basis for one partner's domination over the other. These bases can include not only knowledge, skill, personal assets, and connections, but also the cultural definition of which partner has the authority within the relationship. Power processes refers to the interactional techniques that an individual employs to gain control, such as negotiation, assertiveness, and problem solving. Power outcome refers to who actually makes the decision. According to this theory, those partners who lack power will be more likely to physically abuse their partners.

Serra (1993), noting that the use of violence possesses a different meaning when acted out by a man (power) than by a woman (powerlessness), extended the power base to include the moral choice to use or not to use violence:

> There is no moral code or reason for a "norm" forbidding woman's violence toward a man. Therefore, while *a man's nonaggression* toward a woman expresses *a norm inscribed in our morals and in our culture, a woman's nonviolence toward a man appears to be a form of nonpower,* a consequence of the biological fact that she is unable to overcome him. A man's *nonviolence* toward a woman takes on a sense of his "not wanting to"—*a moral choice.* A man who does not react to a woman's blows by beating her shows respect for the other sex, while a woman who—having been hit by a man—does not react by attacking him, gives only an impression of powerlessness.

> Hence, neither violence, nor nonviolence, are reciprocal. (p. 24; emphasis in original)

There is some empirical evidence to support the theory of marital power. Ganley and Harris (1978) noted in their study of batterers that many suffered from communication difficulties. Bograd (1988) found that many battering husbands commonly indicated that they resorted to violence because there was no other way to address the situation that confronted them. Babcock, Waltz, Jacobson, and Gottman (1993) found in their study of 95 couples that violence was used by battering husbands as a compensatory behavior to make up for their relative lack of power in the marriage.

Traumatic Bonding Theory

D. G. Dutton and Painter (1981, 1993) developed traumatic bonding theory to explain why beaten women remain with the men who beat them. They have identified two features that they argue are common to all such relationships: the existence of a power imbalance within the relationship, so that the battered partner perceives him or herself as dominated by the other, and the intermittent nature of the abuse. They hypothesize that over time, the power imbalance magnifies and as it does, the dominant person develops an inflated sense of his or her own power, while the subjugated partner feels more negative about him- or herself and gradually, as a result, becomes increasingly dependent on the dominator. Because the abuse occurs on an intermittent basis, and those interim periods are often characterized by positive behaviors such as attention and declarations of love and remorse, patterns of behavior result that are difficult to extinguish (Rounsaville, 1978b).

Societal Level Theories

Culture of Violence Theory

Wolfgang and Ferracuti (1967) theorized that in large, pluralistic societies, some subcultures develop norms that permit the use of physical force or violence to a greater degree than does the dominant culture. Levinson and Malone (1980) used this theory to postulate that family violence will occur more frequently in violent societies than in peaceful ones.

Ecological Theory

The ecological theory attempts to link violence in the family with the broader social environment. Bersani and Chen (1988) explained: "A person's environment can be understood as a series of settings, each nested within the next broader level, from the microenvironment of the family to the macroenvironment of the society" (p. 76).

Belsky (1980) outlined an ecological framework for the understanding of child abuse and neglect. That four-level framework, with some modifications, may be equally relevant to an understanding of intimate partner violence:

1. ontogenic—the family history of the parents [partners]
2. microsystem—the family setting in which violence occurs
3. ecosystem—the formal and informal social networks in which the family participates
4. the macrosystem—the culture

Evolutionary Theory

Evolutionary theory, originally advanced by anthropologists (Barry, Child, & Bacon, 1967; Lenski & Lenski, 1970; Naroll, 1970; Rohner, 1975) to explain child abuse, may be equally relevant to intimate partner violence. Evolutionary theory posits that, as societies have changed from the relatively simple to the more structurally and economically complex, families have become smaller and nuclear in form and social relations have, paradoxically, become both more structured and more ambiguous. In less complex societies, caretakers of children are more likely to emphasize independence and self-reliance

and, in comparison with caretakers in more complex societies, are less likely to rely on physical punishment to secure obedience. Obedience, it has been argued, is valued in societies that maintain a hierarchically organized social structure and in which a large amount of activity occurs in the context of formal social encounters outside the home. It can be hypothesized, then, that if such high value is placed on obedience, obedience may be demanded of children and intimate partners alike. Where such obedience is not forthcoming, violence may be used as a means to secure it.

Levinson's (1989) examination of the link between social change and wife beating may lend some support to this theory. He noted, for instance, that following the shift in the Macedonia, Bosnia, Serbia, Croatia, and Littoral regions of the former Yugoslavia from an extended family household model to a money economy in 1900, women's status increased, men's status decreased, and wife beating became more common.

However, Morley's (1994) study of domestic violence in Papua New Guinea appears to refute the evolutionary theory. Morley specifically failed to find a link between modernization or urbanization and an increase in the prevalence of wife beating. She did find, however, that a husband's right to control his wife through violence was no longer greeted with unconditional acceptance. In contrast, men's perceived need to control their wives may have increased due to women's increasing autonomy.

Tracy and Crawford (1992) have argued that several species close to *Homo sapiens* on the phylogenetic scale have engaged in wife-abuse-like behavior. Such behavior may have served to guard the female mate from other males, thereby ensuring the male partner's sexual dominance and, possibly, reproductive advantage. In this context, wife beating is a "natural tendency" (Tracy & Crawford, 1992).

Wilson and Daly (1993) advanced an evolutionary psychological perspective. They hypothesized that sexual proprietariness is a psychological adaptation of the human male, much as various animals lay claim to their territory. This proprietariness, they argue, is reflected in double standards of adultery, whereby a married woman commits adultery by having sex with other than her husband, but a married man faces no such charge; in legal actions that permit monetary recovery for loss of consortium; in man's violent response to a woman's desertion of the relationship and his consequent loss of control over her reproductive capacity; and in the coercive, nonviolent control of women by men through economic inequity, forced marriages, practices such as foot binding, and the requirement of chaperones for women in some cultures. They further assert that men's jealousy, and related violence, is directly tied to a woman's reproductive value, the social sanctions against men's use of violence against their partners, and the female partners' resistance to male coercive control.

Feminist Theory

There are numerous variants of feminist theory relating to intimate partner violence. Bograd (1990) has identified four elements common to all of these: (1) As the dominant class, men have differential access to material and symbolic resources and women are devalued as secondary and inferior; (2) intimate partner abuse is a predictable and common dimension of normal family life; (3) women's experiences are often defined as inferior because male domination influences all aspects of life; and (4) the feminist perspective is dedicated to advocacy for women.

General Systems Theory

Straus (1978) developed the general systems theory to explain how family violence results from a positive, complex feedback system. That system, which operates at the individual, family, and societal levels, includes such factors and processes as the level of conflict inherent in the family, high levels of violence in society, family socialization to violence, cultural norms legitimizing violence, the sexist organization of society, and the multitudinous reasons for the battered person's toleration of the violence.

Patriarchy Theory

Dobash and Dobash (1979) identified three tenets basic to patriarchy theory: (1) Wife assault is a systematic form of domination and social control of women by men; (2) assault is committed by men who believe that patriarchy is their right; and (3) violence is used to maintain male dominance is acceptable to society. Patriarchal theory addresses intimate partner violence on a societal level and seeks to explain why men beat women (Dobash & Dobash, 1979).

Wrangham and Peterson (1996) have argued that patriarchy theory is supported by numerous practices in a variety of cultures, including the veiling and sequestering of women in a number of Muslim countries; the once traditional practice of binding women's feet in China; the practice of *sati* in India; the practice of infibulation in many countries in Africa; the widespread practice of wife beating; and the excessive mortality rate among young girls as compared to boys of the same age in numerous countries, such as Pakistan (Holloway, 1994). Rigakos (1995) suggested that his findings from a recent study of the practices of 13 police officers and 8 justice officials in Delta, Canada, lend support to patriarchy theory. He found that (1) police officers felt that judges awarded restraining orders too easily; (2) police rationalized their inaction when protective orders were issued and violated by noting the many bureaucratic and technical impediments to obtaining a conviction; and (3) police often blamed the beaten woman for the violent incident or sympathized with the male partner's account or perceived the woman as a liar.

Patriarchy theory has been criticized on a number of grounds, including (1) its erroneous assumption that there is a direct linear relationship between the status of females in societies and the rates of wife assault (Campbell, 1992), (2) its failure to recognize that, even in patriarchal societies, it is a minority of men who assault their partners or who believe that such conduct is acceptable (R. Stark & McEvoy, 1970), and (3) its failure to recognize that there is no linear association between power and violence in the context of a dyadic relationship (D. H. Coleman & Straus, 1986).

Social Disorganization Theory

Social disorganization, social control, and social isolation theories are seen as complementary. Taken together, these theories hypothesize that the weaker the social bond, the higher the rate of assault on female intimate partners (Straus, 1994).

Responses to Intimate Partner Violence

Responses to intimate partner violence may take any of several forms, or a combination of forms, by the individual who has been attacked, by the perpetrator, and by the larger "audience," for example, neighbors, the police, and so on.

Response of the Actor or Perpetrator

The Account

The assailant in an intimate partner violence situation may offer an account of his or her actions at various points in time: to the partner at the time of occurrence, to the law enforcement officer who is called to the scene, to the defense attorney, and to the judge or jury. These accounts may be used in an attempt to excuse or justify the conduct or mitigate the consequences.

There is some empirical evidence to indicate that the nature of the account may, indeed, impact the consequences to the assailant. Saunders (1995) found in his study of 111 police officers' attitudes toward intimate partner violence that the officers' willingness to arrest the assailant was related to the as-

sailants' proffered justification for the assault. For instance, where assailants explained their behavior as a response to their partners' lack of sexual fidelity, the officers were much less likely to arrest the assailants.

In Brazil, the interplay between the assailant's account and the legal consequences of his actions is striking. The defendant in the 1990 spousal murder case in Apucarana was acquitted on the grounds that the murder constituted a legitimate defense of his honor because his wife had committed adultery. Brazil's highest court reversed the decision, holding that this did not constitute a defense of honor, but rather of "self-esteem, vanity, and the pride of the Lord who sees his wife as property." Despite this clear denunciation of murder as a legitimate response to adultery, the lower court again acquitted the husband on the grounds that he was defending his honor (Americas Watch, 1991, pp. 18–19).

Treatment

It is not unusual for a violent partner to participate in treatment or rehabilitation as a condition of a court order, rather than on his or her own initiative (personal communication, Cuyahoga County Task Force on Domestic Violence). Many of the treatment programs that are available to batterers in general may not be as easily accessible to or effective with individuals from communities of color, due to the programs' location, their lack of a bilingual staff, and their lack of sensitivity with regard to cultural issues (Williams & Becker, 1994). To date, there have been few well-done evaluations of treatment programs for batterers (personal communication, Cuyahoga County Task Force on Domestic Violence).

Victim Response

D. A. Counts (1992) identified six different strategies available to beaten women. Although these are based on her observations of wife beating in Papua New Guinea, many are applicable in concept across many societies. Potential responses include (1) leaving her husband and taking a lover or second husband (departure); (2) taking the dispute to the public arena and charging her husband before the village or provincial court authorities (help seeking); (3) leaving her husband and returning to her own kin if her relatives do not intervene on her behalf (departure and help seeking); (4) exposing her husband to menstrual blood to cause his illness (retribution); (5) committing suicide; and (6) fighting back (violence). Lateef (1992), based on her study of Indo-Fijian women, identified a seventh alternative strategy: acceptance.

Departure

One of the possible responses to intimate partner violence is for the abused partner to leave. Leaving, however, is often a process involving movement into and out of the abusive relationship (Limandri, 1987). Women have described changes in themselves that have allowed them to ultimately leave their abusive partner: redefinition of abuse as they become angrier about their victimization (Ferraro & Johnson, 1983) and passage through a variety of phases of response to the abuse, including binding, enduring, disengaging, and recovering (Landenburger, 1989). Numerous factors have been found conducive to leaving an abusive relationship, including the availability of economic support (Pfouts, 1978; Strube & Barbour, 1984), the availability of support services (Snyder & Scheer, 1981), previous separations (Snyder & Scheer, 1981), and concerns for one's own safety and personal growth (Ulrich, 1991). Various other circumstances have been found to constitute additional barriers to leaving, including potential economic hardship (Gondolf *et al.,* 1988), religious traditions (Ulrich, 1993), and love (Strube & Barbour, 1984).

Draper (1992), in her discussion of the responses of four !Kung women to battering by their husbands, noted that a decision to leave is frequently dependent on whether one has somewhere to go. In two of the four instances of battering described, the beating occurred away from kin. The wives had no adult children to whom they could flee and their parents were relatively poor. In contrast, the other two wives came from relatively wealthy families who could both intercede on their behalf and provide them with living accommodations.

Kerns (1992) found in her fieldwork in a Garifuna community in Belize that wife beating is quite rare because a woman who is beaten often has the means to leave and no compelling reason to stay. Unlike women in the United States, who often face numerous barriers to leaving, such as economic dependence, the absence of effective intervention or any intervention, social isolation, the lack of a reliable and accessible sanctuary, an ineffective criminal justice system, and an unsympathetic legal system, women in the Garifuna community are rarely dependent economically, can usually seek sanctuary with their families, and can generally rely on prompt and effective intervention by family members, who have the right and the duty to intervene.

Recent changes in U.S. immigration law may reduce immigrants' barriers to departure from an abusive relationship. These changes are discussed in the context of audience response.

Help Seeking

Women who have been the victims of intimate partner violence may seek help in a variety of arenas, some of them formal and some informal. Unfortunately, little research has examined either factors related to a decision to seek help or patterns of help seeking among physically abused women.

Health Care. This discussion focuses on the receipt of health care. Health consequences, such as physical injury and depression, were discussed previously in the context of forms of intimate partner violence.

Women who have been the victims of such violence have been found to utilize a large proportion of medical care, through emergency department services, clinic services such as chronic pain clinics (Bergman *et al.*, 1992; Haber, 1985; Rath, Jarratt, & Leonardson, 1989), and mental health services (Carmen, Riecker, & Mill, 1984; E. Stark *et al.*, 1979).

There are numerous barriers to the receipt of health care attention, however. A survey of 1,000 battered women found that health care practitioners were the least helpful of all professional help sources contacted (Brendtro & Bowker, 1989). Rather than addressing the totality of the situation, health practitioners may be more inclined to address only the medical signs and symptoms that are detectable (E. Stark & Flitcraft, 1988). This physician response, however, is not surprising in view of the fact that few medical schools provide instruction relating to domestic violence (Holtz, Hames, & Safran, 1989). Receipt of health care may be even more problematic for abused immigrants, who may refrain from seeking such services due to cultural beliefs (Capps, 1994; Frye & D'Avanzo, 1994; Moore & Boehlein, 1991; Uba, 1992) or fear of being reported to the Immigration and Naturalization Service (INS; Asch, Leake, & Gelberg, 1994), or both.

Law Enforcement. Help seeking in the context of law enforcement can take numerous forms, including appeals to the police (Bachman & Coker, 1995), reports to the chief of a man's village (Ofei-Aboagye, 1994), and consultation with attorneys.

Little empirical research has been conducted to explore the circumstances in which victims seek help from law enforcement and the legal system. Bachman and Coker (1995) found in their study of 1,535 female victims of intimate partner violence that victims were more likely to report a violent incident to the police if they were Black, had sustained an injury as a result of the assault, and had not been victimized previously by the offender. (These same factors were also predictive of whether the police arrested the assailant.) Hutchison, Hischel, and Pesackis (1994)

found in their study of 18,712 domestic violence calls for police services in a large southern metropolitan area, conducted over a 17-month period, that currently married and cohabiting (unmarried) couples were equally likely to rely on police services. Almost one quarter of the calls were attributable to incidents between divorced partners, ex-cohabitants, or dating but not cohabiting partners. Almost one half of the victims were between the ages of 26 and 35 and approximately 80% of the calls were from women.

Isolation

Not infrequently, women may self-isolate in an attempt to stop the violence. For instance, if her partner claims that he hit her because she came home late from work or school, she may cease those activities (Flitcraft, 1995).

Social Organization

Various women's movements have focused on violence against women. India's women's movement provides a good example of this. The women's movement there has organized rallies, protests, and mass meetings in an attempt to focus public attention on the problem of intimate partner violence (Katzenstein, 1989). Although many of the participants may not themselves have been abused, many of them have. Various autonomous women's organizations in India have staged street plays about dowry murders, rape, and other forms of domestic violence. Other organizations have provided legal help to women attempting to leave their abusive situations. Leaders in these movements have frequently used their connections to effect change, such as using governmental connections to arrange consultations regarding dowry violence.

A similar movement occurred in the United States during the 1970s. Feminist lawyers instituted numerous lawsuits against police departments for their refusal to arrest assaultive partners and against court personnel for denying battered women access to judges who could issue protective orders (Pleck, 1987). The National Organization for Women (NOW) in 1973 established the first task force on intimate partner violence. Various organizations established shelters for battered women. In 1976, there were about 20 such shelters throughout the United States; by 1982, there were approximately 300. Women's groups in Great Britain, Denmark, and Finland were also active in championing legal reforms and in establishing victims' services (Anonymous, 1985; Dwyer, 1995).

Suicide

Suicide is a not infrequent response to intimate partner violence. In South Africa, for instance, it has been estimated that violence occurs in 50%–60% of all marriages. Of the women in such relationships, approximately 25% attempt suicide (Adams & Hickson, 1993). Suicide has been recognized as a culturally acceptable way out for women in India who have reached the end of their endurance of physical and emotional abuse. It may, in fact, be the only viable alternative to eventual murder by the husband or his family (Prasad, 1994). D. Counts (1987) argued that in some Oceanic societies, such as Papua New Guinea, female suicide is a culturally recognized behavior that permits those without political power to obtain revenge against their tormentors. Mitchell (1992) found that Wape men in New Guinea may refrain from beating their wives because of the women's threats to commit suicide if their husbands shame them. Forty-one percent of Fijian Indian families in one study identified marital violence as the cause of suicide (Haynes, 1984).

Violence

A number of studies have indicated that females murder male partners at a rate that is substantially less than murders of females by their male partners (Browne & Williams, 1989; Straus, 1986). It has been suggested that the vast majority of such murders result

from self-defense, retaliation, or desperation following years of physical abuse (Browne, 1987; Browne & Williams, 1989).

Acceptance

Lateef (1992) found in her ethnographic examination of Indo-Fijian women that many not only accept a husband's right to physically discipline his wife, but also positively sanction this use of force. Men who do not beat their wives may become the subject of ridicule. The beatings generally stop when the sons are old enough to defend their mothers. Ho (1990) similarly found in her study of domestic violence among Southeast Asians that Lao, Khmer, and Vietnamese women, particularly those who were first generation, accepted familial violence as a common occurrence.

Despite this seeming acceptance of their fate, these wives may remain in their situations due to a lack of power rather than true acceptance. Few have any place to go if they leave. Most are economically dependent on their spouses. Many are concerned that they might lose their children if they leave or that they will bring shame to their families by doing so.

In the United States, women who seemingly accept their violent fate may, in fact, be caught in a cycle of emotional dependency that is difficult to break. (This pattern has become variously known as the battered women's syndrome, the Stockholm syndrome, and traumatic bonding; Graham *et al.*, 1995.) Although the woman's continued relationship with her batterer appears to be voluntary, the underlying dynamic is hardly one of true acceptance.

"Audience" Response

The Health Care Response

The response of the health care profession has taken a number of forms including (1) programs to increase health care worker awareness of domestic violence, (2) the development of screening protocols to assess whether an individual has been a victim of domestic violence, (3) the development of screening protocols to identify batterers, (4) the development of procedures for the examination of patients believed to have been the victims of domestic violence, (5) the formation of community consortia for the provision of health care to victims of domestic violence, and (6) consideration of ethical issues related to the diagnosis and treatment of domestic violence. These responses are discussed in the following sections.

Increasing Health Care Worker Awareness. Although the Surgeon General of the United States recommended in 1992 that physicians increase their awareness of domestic violence (Novello *et al.*, 1992), recent studies continue to underscore deficiencies in health care worker awareness. Chambliss, Bay, and Jones (1995) found in their survey of all residents in obstetrics and gynecology that the majority were unable to recognize at least 1 of 10 common clinical scenarios suggestive of battering. The majority also appeared to seriously underestimate the prevalence of battering in the patient population. Chambliss and colleagues concluded that medical education is failing to prepare residents to address relatively common situations that they would encounter in practice. Saunders and Kindy (1993) similarly concluded from their evaluation of residents and faculty that more extensive training of medical personnel is required to adequately detect and document the abuse.

Screening Protocols for Victims. Large numbers of health care providers have recently developed screening protocols to detect intimate partner violence among its victims. These initiatives have often been a response to heightened awareness of both the seriousness and prevalence of intimate partner violence (Quillian, 1996), the passage of legal mandates requiring the development of such protocols (Bell, Jenkins, Kpo, & Rhodes, 1994; Freeman, 1995; Mixon, 1995), or the require-

ments of the Joint Commission for the Accreditation of Healthcare Organizations that hospital emergency departments implement written policies and procedures for the identification, assessment, treatment, evaluation, and referral of victims of abuse (Joint Commission on Accreditation of Healthcare Organizations, 1992).

It is beyond the scope of this chapter to examine in detail the various screening protocols that have been developed. Numerous mechanisms have, however, been developed, including multilevel screening procedures based on prior history of abuse and presentation with injuries (Quillian, 1996), a two-question assessment tool (McFarlane, Greenberg, Weltge, & Watson, 1995), a single-item assessment tool (Freund, Bak, & Blackhall, 1996), a five-question screening instrument (Norton, Peipert, Zierler, Lima, & Hume, 1995), and a three-question screening tool focusing on past violence and perceived personal safety (Feldhaus *et al.*, 1997). The extent to which any of these tools can detect partner violence among either non-English speakers or specific immigrant groups with differing values remains unclear and uninvestigated. Although geared primarily to community workers rather than health care professionals, Wiebe's (1985) manual on violence against immigrant women and children pays particular attention to cultural factors that may impede both the detection of and intervention in intimate partner violence.

Screening for Batterers. Generally, batterers are identified through victim reports, rather than self-identification. Chelmowski and Hamberger (1994) have suggested that health care workers use a "funneling technique" to determine whether a patient engaged in violent behavior. Accordingly, questions may initially focus on the patient's relationship with his or her intimate partner and become progressively more specific about techniques for handling anger in the relationship. The extent to which such a technique would be successful with individuals whose culture does not encourage the discussion of feelings or relationships is unclear. Although there is generally no legal duty to report past abuse, Chelmowski and Hamberger (1994) cautioned that there may be a duty to notify the partner if the threat of further intimate partner violence appears high.

Examination Procedures. Examination procedures are relevant in situations where the clinician has reason to believe that physical violence against an intimate partner by the other has occurred. In conducting such examinations, the health care worker must be cognizant of the role of the family and the community and of ethical issues that may arise. Chapters 9 and 11 (this volume) should be consulted in this regard.

Most examination protocols recommend detailed documentation of the injuries, including a body chart (Mississippi State Medical Association, 1995; Sheridan & Taylor, 1993), a description of the event that produced them with photographs of the resulting injuries (Mississippi State Medical Association, 1995; Sheridan & Taylor, 1993), relevant laboratory tests (Mississippi State Medical Association, 1995), and an assessment for the risk of homicide (Sheridan & Taylor, 1993).

Community Consortia. Interagency domestic violence consortia have been proposed as a remedy for the often fragmented care and attention that domestic violence victims receive (Langford, 1990). Interagency domestic violence consortia could potentially include services from and linkages between educational programs, shelters, and health care facilities. This enhanced cooperation could potentially lead to the formulation and adoption of standardized protocols and policies, the development of quality assurance standards, and the development and implementation of surveillance strategies (Langford, 1990).

Ethical Issues. The Council on Ethical and Judicial Affairs of the American Medical Association (1992) has stated that (1) physicians should routinely inquire about domestic

violence as a part of the medical history; (2) physicians may have a duty to familiarize themselves with diagnostic and treatment protocols for domestic violence; (3) physicians should prevent societal misconceptions about domestic violence from interfering with the diagnosis and management of abuse; (4) the medical profession should demonstrate a greater commitment to eliminating domestic violence and helping its victims; and (5) physicians must be better trained to diagnose domestic violence and to work cooperatively with available community resources. Consequently, the diagnosis and treatment of physical injuries is insufficient. Rather,

> the aim of medicine is to address not only the bodily assault that disease or an injury inflicts but also the psychological, social, even spiritual dimensions of this assault. To heal is to make whole or sound, to help a person reconvene the powers of the self and return, as far as possible, to his [or her] conception of a normal life. (Pellegrino & Thomasma, 1988, p. 10)

The Criminal Justice Response

The criminal justice system in the United States has attempted to respond to intimate partner violence through increased frequency of response by the police (Hirschel & Hutchison, 1992; Polsby, 1992; Schmidt & Sherman, 1993; Tolman & Weisz, 1995), the imposition of increasingly punitive legal sanctions as a deterrent, including arrest (Grasmick, Blackwell, Bursik, & Mitchell, 1993; Jolin, 1983), and the notification of victims of their legal rights and the availability of supportive services (Hart, 1993). It is beyond the scope of this chapter to address the varied responses across the 50 states. Rather, we briefly focus on the use of arrest as a deterrent, since it is a commonly utilized strategy, and explore its implications for immigrant communities.

Abused immigrants may be particularly reticent to seek police intervention for domestic violence due to cultural norms (Ho, 1990), fear of being reported to the INS by their partner or the police, or fear of retaliation by their partner. Such fears are not unfounded. Immigration attorneys have frequently observed that an undocumented individual often comes to the attention of the INS as the result of a well-placed telephone call by his or her intimate partner.

In addition, it is unclear whether arrest actually serves as a deterrent to subsequent domestic violence. Sherman and Berk (1984) found in their Minneapolis study that arrest seemed to reduce the likelihood of future domestic assault. Tolman and Weisz (1995) reported similar findings from their study of arrest in DuPage County, Illinois. However, Sherman and Smith (1992) found that arrest had no significant effect on recidivism, while Pate and Hamilton (1992) found in their study of Dade County, Florida, that arrest significantly increased the likelihood of a subsequent assault in certain circumstances. Recent reports have documented the propensity of a substantial minority of police officers to arrest the victim of domestic violence, particularly where the assailant and the assaulted continue to argue in front of the officer (Saunders, 1995). Although our immigration laws now contain special provisions directed to abused spouses (see the next section), abused immigrants may be unaware of these provisions or may not meet the requirements. Consequently, attempts to seek police intervention may leave the abused immigrant vulnerable to subsequent domestic violence, deportation, or both.

The Response of U.S. Immigration Law

Prior to recent changes in the law, immigrant spouses were particularly vulnerable to intimate partner violence. They were often dependent on their U.S. citizen or lawful permanent resident spouse for the filing of a petition with the INS that would initiate the process of obtaining permanent residence, popularly known as having a "green card." Undocumented spouses who challenged the violence in their households or threatened to report it were not infrequently threatened by their citizen or legally resident spouse with

being turned over to the INS for deportation proceedings.

As an example, consider the case of Miriam Cruz-Wood. Miriam Cruz entered the United States from the Philippines in 1988. After a 1-year courtship, she married Christopher Wood, a U.S. citizen. Wood became abusive following their marriage. The abuse was intermittent at first, and then became routine. The abuse was well documented by police reports, restraining orders, and court transcripts. When Wood became convinced that his wife would no longer live with the abuse, he withdrew his petition to the INS to classify her as the spouse of a U.S. citizen, the basis for her application for permanent residence. He further asked the INS to deport her immediately; his wife went into hiding (Klein, 1993).

The Violence Against Women Act of 1994 attempted to address this situation by permitting both self-petitioning and a special form of cancellation of removal (a remedy to deportation) to abused spouses and children of U.S. citizens and lawful permanent residents. In addition, our interpretation of U.S. asylum law has been broadened to encompass domestic violence as a form of persecution and women as a particular social group. These critical changes are discussed in the following sections.

Self-Petitioning. Under the self-petitioning provision, abused spouses or children of U.S. citizens or lawful permanent residents may file their own petitions to commence the process of becoming permanent residents, rather than having to depend on abusive parents or spouses to file the petition. A spouse with an abused child may also file a petition for him- or herself and the child, based on the abuse suffered by the child.

In order to qualify for self-petitioning, the individual must demonstrate that he or she has been "battered" or has been the "subject of extreme cruelty," including "being the victim of any act or threatened act of violence, including any forceful detention, which results or threatens to result in physical or mental injury" (Immigration and Nationality Act section 204(a)). Acts of violence include "psychological or sexual abuse or exploitation, including rape, molestation, incest . . . or forced prostitution" and "other abuse actions . . . that, in and of themselves, may not initially appear violent but that are part of an overall pattern of violence" (Immigration and Nationality Act section 204(a)). Additional references should be consulted regarding the documentation of this abuse (Pendleton, 1997).

Additionally, the abuse must (1) have occurred during the marriage and (2) have been perpetrated by the self-petitioner's parent or spouse who was a lawful permanent resident or U.S. citizen both at the time the self-petitioner files the petition and at the time that the INS approves the petition. The marriage between the self-petitioner and the abuser must have been in good faith, that is, not entered into to avoid the usual immigration process. The self-petitioner must be residing in the United States at the time that he or she files the petition and must have resided with the abusive spouse.

Cancellation of Removal. Cancellation of removal is a remedy to deportation (removal from the United States) that is potentially available from an immigration judge in the context of a removal proceeding. The applicant must demonstrate that (1) he or she was abused by a U.S. citizen or lawful permanent resident or is the parent of a U.S. citizen's or permanent resident's child who was abused by the citizen or permanent resident; (2) the abuser was the spouse or parent at the time that the acts of domestic violence occurred; (3) at least a portion of the abuse occurred in the United States; (4) the applicant has been continuously physically present in the United States for at least 3 years; (5) the applicant has had good moral character during the 3-year period immediately preceding the date of application; and (6) deportation will result in extreme hardship (Immigration and Nationality Act section 240A).

Asylum. Asylum is potentially available to a foreign-born individual who is in the United States and is unwilling or unable to return to his or her country of nationality or, if he or she has no nationality, to his or her country of last habitual residence due to persecution or fear of persecution on account of race, religion, nationality, membership in a particular social group, or political opinion (Immigration and Nationality Act section 208). Other sources should be consulted for a detailed explanation of persecution, fear of persecution, application procedures, and the nature of the evidence that must be presented to support a claim for asylum (*Desir v. Ilchert*, 1988; Hines, 1997; *INS v. Cardoza Fonseca*, 1987; *INS v. Elias-Zacarias*, 1992; *Matter of Mogharrabi*, 1987).

A number of nonprecedential decisions by immigration judges have recognized domestic violence as a form of persecution. In *Matter of A and Z* (1994), the immigration judge granted asylum to a Jordanian woman who had suffered continual physical and verbal abuse from her husband during their 30-year marriage. The judge found that she was a member of the social group of women who challenged Jordan's traditions and government, and that she was unable to either divorce her husband or receive police protection. Similarly, the judge found in *Matter of M and K* (1995) that a woman from Sierra Leone had established her claim to asylum as a member of the social group of "women who have been punished with physical spousal abuse for attempting to assert their individual autonomy." A Bangladeshi woman was granted asylum in *Matter of Sharmin* (1996) on the basis of her husband's physical beatings in retaliation for her activities in the women's movement and her refusal to both remain indoors and to cease all communication with others.

A Guatemalan woman was granted asylum as a member of the social group of "Guatemalan women who become involved intimately with Guatemalan men who believe in male domination [and] are targeted by their male companions . . . through violence" (*Matter of A—P—*, 1996). The immigration judge specifically found that, despite horrific abuse, the Guatemalan police refused to protect her from her husband, who had been a soldier, and the courts had refused to grant her a divorce because her husband had refused to consent to one. The court described her abuse:

> He beat her often, and at many occasions, inflicting severe injury. He dislocated her jaw, nearly pushed out her eye, tried to cut off her hands with his machete, kicked her in the abdomen and vagina, and tried to force her to abort when she was pregnant with her second child by severely kicking her in the spine. He would drag her by her hair, use her head to break windows and mirrors, whip her with pistols and electrical cords, and threaten her with knives. . . . A—P— testified that she was severely sexually abused by her husband, both vaginally and anally, almost on a daily basis. . . . The sexual abuse severely injured A—P—, causing extensive hemorrhaging, excruciating abdominal pain and disease. (*Matter of A—P—*, 1996, pp. 3–4)

Summary

Relatively little research has been conducted on intimate partner violence in immigrant communities. We continue to lack basic data, including rates of such violence across groups and risk factors for intimate partner violence in immigrant groups. Little work has been done to examine what behaviors are perceived as intimate partner violence in different immigrant groups and how those perceptions change, if they do, following immigration. What little we do know indicates that, although the incidence and prevalence rates of intimate partner violence vary across cultural groups, most cultures demonstrate violence against intimate partners in some form, indicating perhaps a common thread in human relationships.

A research agenda for the future must include an examination of the incidence and prevalence of intimate partner violence in diverse immigrant groups, an examination of risk factors for intimate partner violence, and the development of culturally specific screening protocols and interventions appropriate to the varied immigrant populations in the United States.

References

Adams, I., & Hickson, J. (1993). Wife-beating among coloureds in South Africa and its impact on the marital relationship. *International Journal of Sociology of the Family, 23,* 117–137.

Americas Watch. (1991). *Criminal injustice: Violence against women in Brazil.* New York: Human Rights Watch.

Anonymous. (1985). Responses to wife abuse in four countries. *Response, 8,* 15–18.

Asch, S., Leake, B., & Gelberg, L. (1994). Does fear of immigration authorities deter tuberculosis patients from seeking care? *Western Journal of Medicine, 161,* 373–376.

Babcock, J. C., Waltz, J., Jacobson, N. S., & Gottman J. M. (1993). Power and violence: The relation between communication patterns, power discrepancies, and domestic violence. *Journal of Consulting and Clinical Psychology, 61,* 40–50.

Bachman, R., & Coker, A. L. (1995). Police involvement in domestic violence: The interactive effects of victim injury, offender's history of violence, and race. *Violence and Victims, 10,* 91–106.

Balakrishnan, C., Imell, L. L., Bandy, A. T., & Prasad, J. K. (1995). Perineal burns in males secondary to spouse abuse. *Burns, 21,* 34–35.

Ballard, D. T., Blair, G. D., Devereaux, S., Valentine, L. K., Horton, A. L., & Johnson, B. L. (1990). A contemporary profile of the incest perpetrator. Background characteristics, abuse history, and use of social skills. In A. L. Horton, B. L. Johnson, L. M. Roundy, & D. Williams (Eds.), *The incest perpetrator: A family member no one wants to treat* (pp. 54–64). Newbury Park, CA: Sage.

Barry, H., III, Child, I. L., & Bacon, M. K. (1967). Relation of child training to subsistence economy. In C. S. Ford (Ed.), *Cross-cultural approaches* (pp. 145–158). New Haven, CT: Human Relations Area Files.

Bates, L., Redman, S., Brown, W., & Hancock, L. (1995). Domestic violence experienced by women attending an accident and emergency department. *Australian Journal of Public Health, 19,* 292–299.

Beck, S. R., Freitag, S. K., & Singer N. (1996). Ocular injuries in battered women. *Ophthalmology, 103,* 148–151.

Bell, C. C., Jenkins, E. J., Kpo, W., & Rhodes, H. (1994). Response of emergency rooms to victims of interpersonal violence. *Hospital and Community Psychiatry, 45,* 142–146.

Belsky, J. (1980). Child maltreatment: An ecological integration. *American Psychologist, 35,* 320–335.

Bergman, B., & Brismar, B. (1993). Assailants and victims: A comparative study of male wife-beaters and battered males. *Journal of Addictive Diseases, 12,* 1–10.

Bergman, B., Brismar, B., & Nordin, C. (1992). Utilisation of medical care by abused women. *British Journal of Medicine, 305*, 27–28.

Bernard, C., & Schlaffer, E. (1992). Domestic violence in Austria: The institutional response. In E. C. Viano (Ed.), *Intimate violence: Interdisciplinary perspectives* (pp. 243–253). Washington, DC: Hemisphere.

Bersani, C. A., & Chen, H. (1988). Sociological perspectives on family violence. In V. B. Hasselt, R. L. Morrison, A. S. Bellack, & M. Hersen (Eds.), *Handbook of family violence* (pp. 57–86). New York: Plenum.

Blood, R. O., & Wolfe, D. M. (1960). *Husbands and wives: The dynamics of married living.* Glencoe, IL: Free Press.

Bograd, M. (1988). How battered women and abusive men account for domestic violence: Excuses, justifications or explanations? In G. T. Hotaling, D. Finkelhor, J. T. Kirkpatrick, & M. A. Straus (Eds.), *Coping with family violence: Research and policy perspectives* (pp. 60–70). Newbury Park, CA: Sage.

Bograd, M. (1990). Feminist perspectives on wife abuse: An introduction. In K. Yllo & M. Bograd (Eds.), *Feminist perspectives on wife abuse* (pp. 11–27). Newbury Park, CA: Sage.

Booth, A., & Dabbs, J. (1993). Testosterone and men's marriages. *Social Forces, 47*, 334–355.

Brendtro, M., & Bowker, L. (1989). Battered women: How can nurses help? *Issues in Mental Health Nursing, 10*, 169–180.

Brown, J. K. (1992). Introduction: Defnitions, assumptions, themes, and issues. In D. A. Counts, J. K. Brown, & J. C. Campbell (Eds.), *Sanctions and sanctuary: Cultural perspectives on the beating of wives* (pp. 1–18). Boulder, CO: Westview.

Browne, A. (1987). *When battered women kill.* New York: Macmillan and Free Press.

Browne, A., & Williams, K. R. (1989). Explaining the effect of resource availability and the likelihood of female-perpetrated homicides. *Law and Society Review, 23*, 75–94.

Browne, A., & Williams, K. R. (1993). Gender, intimacy, and lethal violence: Trends from 1976 through 1987. *Gender and Society, 7*, 78–98.

Bruynooghe, R. *et al.* (1989). *Study of physical violence against Belgian women.* Departement des Science et Humaines et Sociales, Limburgs Universitair Centrum, Belgium. Cited in A. Garcia. (1991). *Sexual violence against women: Contribution to a strategy for countering the various forms of such violence in the Council of Europe member states.* Strasbourg, France: European Committee for Equality Between Men and Women.

Campbell, J. (1992). Prevention of wife battering: Insights from cultural analysis. *Response, 80*, 18–24.

Capps, L. L. (1994). Change and continuity in the medical culture of the Hmong in Kansas City. *Medical Anthropology Quarterly, 8*, 161–177.

Carmen, E., Riecker, P., & Mill, T. (1984). Victims of violence and psychiatric illness. *American Journal of Psychiatry, 141*, 378.

Cazenave, N. A., & Straus, M. A. (1979). Race, class, network embeddedness and family violence: A search for potent support systems. *Journal of Comparative Family Studies, 10*, 280–300.

Chagnon, N. A. (1968). *Yanomamo: The fierce people.* New York: Holt, Rinehart, and Winston.

Chambliss, L. R., Bay, R. C., & Jones, R. F., III. (1995). Domestic violence: An educational imperative? *American Journal of Obstetrics and Gynecology, 172*, 1035–1038.

Chelmowski, M., & Hamberger, L. K. (1994). Screening men for domestic violence in your medical practice. *Wisconsin Medical Journal, 93*, 623–626.

Chin, K. L. (1994). Out-of-town brides: International marriage and wife abuse among Chinese immigrants. *Journal of Comparative Family Studies, 25*, 53–69.

Coleman, D. H., & Straus, M. A. (1986). Marital power, conflict, and violence. *Violence and Victims, 1*, 141–157.

Coleman, V. E. (1994). Lesbian battering: The relationship between personality and the perpetuation of violence. *Violence and Victims, 9*, 139–152.

Cook, C. A., & Harris, K. J. (1995). Attributions about spouse abuse in cases of bidirectional battering. *Violence and Victims, 10*, 143–151.

Council on Ethical and Judicial Affairs, American Medical Association. (1992). Physicians and domestic violence: Ethical considerations. *Journal of the American Medical Association, 267*, 3190–3193.

Counts, D. (1987). Female suicide and wife abuse: A cross-cultural perspective. *Suicide and Life Threatening Behavior, 17*, 194–204.

Counts, D. A. (1992). "All men do it": Wife beating in Kaliai, Papua New Guinea. In D. A. Counts, J. K. Brown, & J. C. Campbell (Eds.), *Sanctions and sanctuary: Cultural perspectives on the beating of wives* (pp. 63–76). Boulder, CO: Westview.

Counts, D. A., Brown, J. K., & Campbell, J. C. (Eds.). (1992). *Sanctions and sanctuary: Cultural perspectives on the beating of wives.* Boulder, CO: Westview.

Cromwell, R. E., & Olson, D. H. (1975). *Power in families.* New York: Wiley.

Davis, G. E., & Leitenberg, H. (1987). Adolescent sex offenders. *Psychological Bulletin, 101*, 417–427.

Desir v. Ilchert, 840 F.2d 723 (9th Cir. 1988).

Dobash, R. E., & Dobash, R. (1979). *Violence against wives.* New York: Free Press.

Draper, P. (1992). Room to maneuver: !Kung women cope with men. In D. A. Counts, J. K. Brown, & J. C. Campbell (Eds.), (1992). *Sanctions and sanctuary: Cultural perspectives on the beating of wives* (pp. 43–61). Boulder, CO: Westview.

Duminy, F. J., & Hudson, D. A. (1993). Assault inflicted by hot water. *Burns, 19,* 426–428.

Dutton, D. G., & Painter, S. L. (1981). Traumatic bonding: The development of emotional attachments in battered women and other relationships of intermittent abuse. *Victimology: An International Journal, 1,* 139–155.

Dutton, D. G., & Painter, S. (1993). Emotional attachments in abusive relationships: A test of traumatic bonding theory. *Violence and Victims, 8,* 105–120.

Dutton, M. A. (1992). *Empowering and healing the battered woman: A model for assessment and intervention.* New York: Springer.

Dwyer, D. C. (1995). Response to the victims of domestic violence: Analysis and implications of the British experience. *Crime and Delinquency, 41,* 527–540.

Edwards, S. S. M. (1986). *The police response to domestic violence in London.* London: Central London Polytechnic.

Egeland, B., Jacobritz, D., & Stroufe, A. L. (1988). Breaking the cycle of abuse. *Child Development, 59,* 1080–1088.

Eisikovits, Z. C., Guttmann, E., Sela-Amit, M., & Edleson, J. L. (1993). Women battering in Israel: The relative contributions of interpersonal factors. *American Journal of Orthopsychiatry, 63,* 313–317.

Erchak, G. M., & Rosenfeld, R. (1994). Societal isolation, violent norms, and gender relations: A reexamination and extension of Levinson's model of wife beating. *Cross-Cultural Research, 28,* 111–133.

Feldhaus, K. M., Koziol-McLain, J., Amsbury, H. L., Norton, I. M., Lowenstein, S. R., & Abbott, J. T. (1997). Accuracy of 3 brief screening questions for detecting partner violence in the emergency department. *Journal of the American Medical Association, 277,* 1357–1361.

Ferraro, K. J., & Johnson, J. M. (1983). How women experience battering: The process of victimization. *Social Problems, 30,* 325–337.

Flitcraft, A. H. (1995). Clinical violence intervention: Lessons from battered women. *Journal of Health Care for the Poor and Underserved, 6,* 187–197.

Freeman, J. (1995). Domestic violence: The law and physician liabilities. *Iowa Medicine, 85,* 70–75.

Freund, K. M., Bak, S. M., & Blackhall, L. (1996). Identifying domestic violence in primary care practice. *Journal of General Internal Medicine, 11,* 44–46.

Frye, B. A., & D'Avanzo, C. (1994). Themes in managing culturally defined illlness in the Cambodian refugee family. *Journal of Community Health Nursing, 11,* 89–98.

Ganley, A. L., & Harris, L. (1978). *Domestic violence: Issues in designing and implementing programs for male batterers.* Paper presented at the 86th annual convention of the American Psychological Association, Toronto, Canada. Cited in J. C. Babcock, J. Waltz, N. S. Jacobson, & J. M. Gottman. (1993).

Power and violence: The relation between communication patterns, power discrepancies, and domestic violence. *Journal of Consulting and Clinical Psychology, 61,* 40–50.

Gelles, R. J. (1983). An exchange/social theory. In D. Finkelhor, R. J. Gelles, G. T. Hotaling, & M. A. Straus (Eds.), *The dark side of families: Current family violence research* (pp. 151–165). Beverly Hills, CA: Sage.

Gelles, R. J. (1989). Child abuse and violence in single parent families: Parent absence and economic deprivation. *American Journal of Orthopsychiatry, 59,* 492–501.

Gelles, R. J. (1994). Research and advocacy: Can one wear two hats? *Family Process, 33,* 93–96.

Gelles, R. J., & Straus, M. A. (1979). Determinants of violence in the family. Toward a theoretical integration. In W. R. Burr, F. I. Nye, S. K. Steinmetz, & M. Wilkinson (Eds.), *Contemporary theories about the family* (pp. 549–581). New York: Free Press.

Gondolf, E. W., Fisher, E., & McFerron, J. R. (1988). Racial differences among shelter residents: A comparison of Anglo, Black, and Hispanic battered women. *Journal of Family Violence, 3,* 39–51.

Goode, W. (1971). Force and violence in the family. *Journal of Marriage and the Family, 33,* 624–636.

Goodman, L. A., Koss, M. P., & Russo, N. F. (1993). Violence against women: Physical and mental health effects: Part I. Research findings. *Applied and Preventive Psychology, 2,* 79–89.

Graham, D. L. R., Rawlings, E. J., Ihms, K., Latimer, D., Foliana, J., Thompson, A., Suttman, K., Farrington, M., & Hacker, R. (1995). A scale for identifying "Stockholm syndrome" reactions in young dating women: Factor structure, reliability, and validity. *Violence and Victims, 10,* 3–22.

Grasmick, H. G., Blackwell, B. S., Bursik, R. J., Jr., & Mitchell S. (1993). Changes in perceived threats of shame, embarrassment, and legal sanctions for interpersonal violence, 1982–1992. *Violence and Victims, 8,* 313–325.

Haber, J. (1985). Abused women and chronic pain. *American Journal of Nursing, 85,* 1010–1012.

Hanneke, C. R., Shields, N. M., & McCall, G. J. (1986). Assessing the prevalence of marital rape. *Journal of Interpersonal Violence, 1,* 350–362.

Harlan, L. (1994). Perfection and devotion: Sati tradition in Rajasthan. In J. S. Hawley (Ed.), *Sati: The blessing and the curse: The burning of wives in India* (pp. 79–91). New York: Oxford University Press.

Hart, B. (1993). Battered women and the criminal justice system. *American Behavioral Scientist, 36,* 624–638.

Hartzell, K. N., Botek, A. A., & Goldberg, S. H. (1996). Orbital fractures in women due to sexual assault and domestic violence. *Ophthalmology, 103,* 953–957.

Haynes, R. H. (1984). Suicide in Fiji: A preliminary study. *British Journal of Psychiatry, 145,* 433–438.

Hilberman, E. (1980). Overview: The "wife-beater's wife" reconsidered. *American Journal of Psychiatry, 2,* 460–470.

Hines, B. (1997). Asylum and withholding of removal. In R. P. Murphy (Ed.), *1997–98 Immigration & Nationality Law Handbook* (Vol. 2, pp. 414–466). Washington, DC: American Immigration Lawyers Association.

Hirschel, J. D., & Hutchison, I. W., III. (1992). Female spouse abuse and the police response: The Charlotte, North Carolina experiment. *Journal of Criminal Law and Criminology, 83,* 73–119.

Ho, C. K. (1990). An analysis of domestic violence in Asian-American communities: A multicultural approach to counseling. In L. S. Brown, & M. P. P Root (Eds.), *Diversity and complexity in feminist therapy*(pp. 129–150). New York: Haworth.

Holloway, M. (1994). Trends in women's health: A global view. *Scientific American, 271,* 77–83.

Holtz, H, Hames, C., & Safran, M. (1989). Education about domestic violence in U.S. and Canadian medical schools, 1987–1988. *Morbidity and Mortality Weekly Report, 38,* 17.

Hutchison, I. W., Hischel, J. D., & Pesackis, C. E. (1994). Family violence and police utilization. *Violence and Victims, 9,* 299–313.

Immigration and Nationality Act of 1952, Pub. L. No. 82-414, 66 Stat. 163, codified as amended at 8 U.S.C. section 1101 *et seq.*

INS. v. Cardoza-Fonseca, 480 U.S. 421 (1987).

INS. v. Elias-Zacarias, 502 U.S. 478 (1992).

Jang, D, Lee, D., & Morello-Frosch, R. (1990). Domestic violence in the immigrant and refugee community: Responding to the needs of immigrant women. *Response, 13,* 2–7.

Joint Commission on Accreditation of Healthcare Organizations. (1992). *Accreditation manual for hospitals.* Oakbrook Terrace, IL: Author.

Jolin, A. (1983). Domestic violence legislation: An impact assessment. *Journal of Police Science and Administration, 11,* 451–456.

Kantor, G. K., Jasinski, J. L., & Aldarondo, E. (1994). Sociocultural status and incidence of marital violence in Hispanic families. *Violence and Victims, 9,* 207–222.

Katzenstein, M. F. (1989). Organizing against violence: Strategies of the Indian women's movement. *Pacific Affairs, 62,* 53–71.

Kaufman, J., & Zigler, E. (1987). Do abused children become abusive parents? *American Journal of Orthopsychiatry, 57,* 316–331.

Kerns, V. (1992). Preventing violence against women: A Central American Case. In D. A. Counts, J. K. Brown, & J. C. Campbell (Eds.), *Sanctions and sanctuary: Cultural perspectives on the beating of wives* (pp. 125–138). Boulder, CO: Westview.

Kim, K., & Cho, Y. (1992). Epidemiological survey of spousal abuse in Korea. In E. C. Viano (Ed.), *Intimate violence: Interdisciplinary perspectives* (pp. 777–782). Washington, DC: Hemisphere.

Klein, D. (1993, October 8). Caught in a vicious, bitter trap. *Los Angeles Times,* p. A1 at col. 1.

Knight, R. A., & Hatty, S. E. (1992). Violence against women in Australia's capital city. In E. C. Viano (Ed.), *Intimate violence: Interdisciplinary Perspectives* (pp. 255–263). Washington, DC: Hemisphere.

Kornblit, A. L. (1994). Domestic violence—An emerging health issue. *Social Science and Medicine, 39,* 1181–1188.

Koss, M. P., Goodman, L. A., Browne, A., Fitzgerald, L. F., Keita, G. P., & Russo, N. F. (1994). *No safe haven: Male violence against women at home, at work, and in the community.* Washington, DC: American Psychological Association.

Kurt, J. L. (1995). Stalking as a variant of domestic violence. *Bulletin of the Academy of Psychiatry and Law, 23,* 219–230.

Lambeck, M. (1992). Like teeth biting tongue: The proscription and practice of spouse abuse in Mayotte. In D. A. Counts, J. K. Brown, & J. C. Campbell (Eds.), 1992. *Sanctions and sanctuary: Cultural perspectives on the beating of wives* (pp. 157–171). Boulder, CO: Westview.

Landenburger, K. (1989). A process of entrapment in and recovery from an abusive relationship. *Issues in Mental Health Nursing, 10,* 209–227.

Langford, D. R. (1990). Consortia: A strategy for improving the provision of health care to domestic violence survivors. *Response, 13,* 17–19.

Larrain, S. (1993). *Estudio de frecuencia de la violencia intrafamiliar y la condicion de la mujer en Chile* [Study of the frequency of intrafamilial violence and the condition of women in Chile]. Pan-American Health Organization.

Lateef, S. (1992). Wife abuse among Indo-Fijians. In D. A. Counts, J. K. Brown, & J. C. Campbell (Eds.), *Sanctions and sanctuary: Cultural perspectives on the beating of wives* (pp. 185–201). Boulder, CO: Westview.

Lenski, G., & Lenski, J. (1970). *Human societies: An introduction to macrosociology.* New York: McGraw-Hill.

Lester, D. (1987). Wife abuse and psychogenic motives in nonliterate societies. *Perceptual and Motor Skills, 64,* 154.

Letellier, P. (1994). Gay and bisexual male domestic violence victimization: Challenges to feminist theory and responses to violence. *Violence and Victims, 9,* 95–106.

Levinson, D. (1989). *Family violence in cross-cultural perspective.* Newbury Park, CA: Sage.

Levinson, D., & Malone, M. (1980). *Toward explaining human culture.* New Haven, CT: Human Relations Area Files.

Limandri, B. J. (1987). The therapeutic relationship with abused women. *Journal of Psychosocial Nursing, 25,* 9–16.

Lockhart, L., & White, B. W. (1989). Understanding marital violence in the black community. *Journal of Interpersonal Violence, 4,* 421–436.

Malaysia Women's Aid Organisation. (1992). *Draft Report of the National Study on Domestic Violence.* Kuala Lumpur, Malaysia: Author.

Martin, S. E. (1992). The epidemiology of alcohol-related interpersonal violence. *Alcohol Health and Research World, 16,* 230–237.

Matter of A and Z, A72 190 893, A72 793 219 (IJ Dec. 20, 1994) (Arlington).

Matter of A—P—, A73 753 922 (IJ Sept. 20, 1996) (San Francisco).

Matter of M and K, A72 374 558 (IJ Aug. 9, 1995) (Arlington).

Matter of Mogharrabi, 19 I. & N. Dec. 439 (BIA 1987).

Matter of Sharmin, A73 556 833 (IJ Sept. 27, 1996) (New York).

Mazza, D., Dennerstein, L., & Ryan, V. (1996). Physical, sexual, and emotional violence against women: A general practice-based prevalence study. *Medical Journal of Australia, 164,* 14–17.

McFarlane, J., Greenberg, L., Weltge, A., & Watson, M. (1995). Identification of abuse in emergency departments: Effectiveness of a two-question screening tool. *Journal of Emergency Nursing, 21,* 391–394.

McHenry, P. C., Julian, T. W., Julian, T. W., & Gavazzi, S. M. (1995). Toward a biopsychosocial model of domestic violence. *Journal of Marriage and the Family, 57,* 307–320.

Mississippi State Medical Association. (1995). Diagnostic and treatment guidelines on domestic violence. *Journal of the Mississippi State Medical Association, 36,* 331–348.

Mitchell, W. (1992). Why Wape men don't beat their wives: Constraints towards domestic tranquility in a New Guinea society. In D. A. Counts, J. K. Brown, & J. C. Campbell (Eds.), *Sanctions and sanctuary: Cultural perspectives on the beating of wives* (pp. 89–98). Boulder, CO: Westview.

Mixon, D. (1995). The Domestic Abuse Act: The physician's role. *Journal of the Arkansas Medical Society, 92,* 218–220.

Moore, L. J., & Boehlein, J. K. (1991). Treating psychiatric disorders among Mien refugees from highland Laos. *Social Science and Medicine, 32,* 1029–1036.

Morley, R. (1994). Wife beating and modernization: The case of Papua New Guinea. *Journal of Comparative Family Studies, 25,* 25–51.

Mullen, P. E., Romans-Clarkson, S. E., Walton, V. A., & Herbison, P. E. (1988). Impact of sexual and physical abuse on women's mental health. *Lancet, 1,* 841.

Murdock, G. P. (1949). *Social structure.* New York: Macmillan.

Murphy, Y., & Murphy, R. F. (1974). *Women of the forest.* New York: Columbia University Press.

Murty, K. S., & Roebuck, J. B. (1992). An analysis of crisis calls by battered women in the city of Atlanta. In E. C. Viano (Ed.), *Intimate violence: Interdisciplinary perspectives* (pp. 61–70). Washington, DC: Hemisphere.

Narasimhan, S. (1990). *Sati: Widow burning in India.* New York: Doubleday.

Naroll, R. (1970). What we have learned from cross-cultural surveys. *American Anthropologist, 72,* 1227–1288.

National Institute of Mental Health. (1992). *Family violence. National Workshop on Violence: Analysis and recommendations.* Report prepared by K. D. O'Leary & A. Browne. Rockville, MD: Violence and Traumatic Stress Research Branch, National Institute of Mental Health, National Institutes of Health, U.S. Department of Health and Human Services.

Norton, L. B., Peipert, J. F., Zierler, S., Lima, B., & Hume, L. (1995). Battering in pregnancy: An assessment of two screening methods. *Obstetrics and Gynecology, 85,* 321–325.

Novello, A. C., Rosenberg, M., Saltzman, L., & Shosky, J. (1992). A medical response to domestic violence. *Journal of the American Medical Association, 267,* 3132.

Ofei-Aboagye, R. O. (1994). Altering the strands of the fabric: A preliminary look at domestic violence in Ghana. *Signs, 19,* 924–938.

Ohio Revised Code section 3113.31.

O'Leary, K. D. (1988). Physical aggression between spouses: A social learning theory perspective. In V. B. Hasselt, R. L. Morrison, A. S. Bellack, & M. Hersen (Eds.), *Handbook of family violence* (pp. 31–55). New York: Plenum.

O'Leary, K. D. (1993). Through a psychological lens: Personality traits, personality disorders, and levels of violence. In R. J. Gelles & D. R. Loseke (Eds.), *Current controversies on family violence* (pp. 7–30). Newbury Park, CA: Sage.

Pan, H. S., Neidig, P. H., & O'Leary, K. D. (1994). Predicting mild and severe husband-to-wife physical aggression. *Journal of Consulting and Clinical Psychology, 62,* 975–981.

Pate, A. M., & Hamilton, E. E. (1992). Formal and informal deterrents to domestic violence: The Dade County spouse assault experiment. *American Sociological Review, 57,* 691–697.

Pellegrino, E. D., & Thomasma, D. C. (1988). *For the patient's good: The restoration of beneficence in health care.* New York: Oxford University Press.

Pendleton, G. (1997). Relief for women and children suffering abuse. In R. P. Murphy (Ed.), *1997–98 Immigration and nationality law handbook* (Vol. 2., pp. 482–512). Washington, DC: American Immigration Lawyers Association.

Perilla, J. L., Bakeman, R., & Norris, F. H. (1994). Culture and domestic violence: The ecology of abused Latinas. *Violence and Victims, 9,* 325–339.

Pernanen, K. (1991). *Alcohol in human violence.* New York: Guilford.

Pfouts, J. H. (1978). Violent families: Coping responses of abused wives. *Child Welfare,* 101–110.

Pleck, E. (1987). *Domestic tyranny: The making of American social policy against family violence from colonial times to the present.* New York: Oxford University Press.

Polsby, D. D. (1992). Suppressing domestic violence with law reforms. *Journal of Criminal Law and Criminology, 83,* 250–253.

Potter, S. H. (1977). *Family life in a northern Thai village.* Berkeley: University of California Press.

Prasad, B. D. (1994). Dowry-related violence: A content analysis of news in selected newspapers. *Journal of Comparative Family Studies, 25,* 71–89.

PROFAMILIA. (1990). *Encuestra de prevalencia, demografia y salud* [Demographic and health survey]. Bogota, Colombia: Author.

Quillian, J. P. (1996). Screening for spousal or partner abuse in a community health setting. *Journal of the American Academy of Nurse Practitioners, 8,* 155–160.

Rath, G. D., Jarratt, L. G., & Leonardson, G. (1989). Rates of domestic violence against adult women by men partners. *Journal of the American Board of Family Practice, 2,* 227–233.

Reiss, A. J., Jr., & Roth, J. A. (Eds.). (1993). *Understanding and preventing violence. Panel on the understanding and control of violent behavior, Committee on Law and Justice, National Research Council.* Washington, DC: National Academy Press.

Rigakos, G. S. (1995). Constructing the symbolic complainant: Police subculture and the nonenforcement of protection orders for battered women. *Violence and Victims, 10,* 227–247.

Rohner, R. P. (1975). *They love me, they love me not: A worldwide study of the effects of parental acceptance and rejection.* New Haven, CT: Human Relations Area Files.

Rounsaville, B. (1978a). Battered wives: Barriers to identification and treatment. *American Journal of Orthopsychiatry, 48,* 487–494.

Rounsaville, B. (1978b). Theories in marital violence: Evidence from a study of battered women. *Victimology, 3,* 11–31.

Rusbult, C. E. (1980). Commitment and satisfaction in romantic situations: A test of the investment model. *Journal of Experimental Social Psychology, 16,* 172–186.

Rusbult, C. E. (1983). A longitudinal test of the investment model: The development (and deterioration) of satisfaction and commitment in heterosexual involvements. *Journal of Personality and Social Psychology, 45,* 101–117.

Saunders, D. G. (1995). The tendency to arrest victims of domestic violence: A preliminary analysis of officer characteristics. *Journal of Interpersonal Violence, 10,* 147–158.

Saunders, D. G., & Kindy, P. (1993). Predictors of physicians' responses to woman abuse: The role of gender, background, and brief training. *Journal of General Internal Medicine, 8,* 606–609.

Schei, B., & Bakketeig, L. S. (1989). Gynecological impact of sexual and physical abuse by spouse: A study of a random sample of Norwegian women. *British Journal of Obstetrics and Gynecology, 96,* 1379–1383.

Schmidt, J. D., & Sherman, L. W. (1993). Does arrest deter domestic violence? *American Behavioral Scientist, 36,* 601–609.

Schulman, M. (1979). *A survey of spousal violence against women in Kentucky.* Washington, DC: Law Enforcement Assistance Administration, U.S. Department of Justice.

Serra, P. (1993). Physical violence in the couple relationship: A contribution toward the analysis of context. *Family Process, 32,* 21–33.

Shamim, I. (1992). Dowry and women's status: A study of court cases in Dhaka and Delhi. In E. C. Viano (Ed.), *Intimate violence: Interdisciplinary perspectives* (pp. 265–275). Washington, DC: Hemisphere.

Sheridan, D. J., & Taylor, W. K. (1993). Developing hospital-based domestic violence programs, protocols, policies, and procedures. *Association of Women's Health Obstetric and Neonatal Nurses Clinical Issues, 4,* 471–482.

Sherman, L. W., & Berk, R. A. (1984). The specific deterrent effects of arrest for domestic assault. *American Sociological Review, 49,* 261–272.

Sherman, L. W., & Smith, D. A. (1992). Crime, punishment, and stake in conformity: legal and informal control of domestic violence. *American Sociological Review, 57,* 680–690.

Shostak, M. (1983). *Nisa.* New York: Vintage.

Siann, G. (1985). *Accounting for aggression: Perspectives on aggression and violence.* Boston: Allen & Unwin.

Smith, L. (1989). *Domestic violence: An overview of the literature.* London: Home Office Research and Planning Unit.

Smith, M. D. (1987). The incidence and prevalence of woman abuse in Toronto. *Violence and Victims, 2,* 173–187.

Snyder, D. K., & Scheer, N. S. (1981). Predicting disposition following a brief residence at a shelter for battered women. *American Journal of Community Psychology, 9,* 559–566.

Sorenson, S. B., & Telles, C. A. (1991). Self-reports of spousal violence in a Mexican-American and non-Hispanic white population. *Violence and Victims, 6,* 3–15.

Sorenson, S. B., Upchurch, D. M., & Shen, H. (1996). Violence and injury in marital arguments: Risk patterns and gender differences. *American Journal of Public Health, 86,* 35–40.

Stark, E. (1990). Rethinking homicide, violence, race, and politics of gender. *International Journal of Health Services, 20,* 3–26.

Stark, E., & Flitcraft, A. (1988). Violence among intimates: An epidemiological review. In V. B. Van Hasselt, R. L. Morrison, A. S. Bellack, & M. Hersen (Eds.), *Handbook of family violence* (pp. 293–317). New York: Plenum.

Stark, E., Flitcraft, A., & Frazier, W. (1979). Medicine and patriarchal violence: The social construction of a "private" event. *International Journal of Health Services, 9,* 461–493.

Stark, R., & McEvoy, J. (1970). Middle class violence. *Psychology Today, 4,* 107–112.

Statistics Canada. (1993, November 16). The violence against women survey. *The Daily.*

Steinmetz, S. K. (1987). Family violence: Past, present, and future. In M. B. Sussman & S. K. Steinmetz (Eds.), *Handbook of marriage and the family* (pp. 725–766). New York: Plenum.

Straus M. A. (1978). Wife beating: How common and why? *Victimology, 2,* 443–459.

Straus, M. A. (1986). Domestic violence and homicide antecedents. *Domestic Violence, 62,* 446–465.

Straus, M. A. (1994). State-to-state differences in social inequality and social binds in relation to assaults on wives in the United States. *Journal of Comparative Family Studies, 25,* 7–24.

Straus, M. A., & Gelles, R. J. (1990). How violent are American families? Estimates from the National Family Violence Resurvey and other studies. In M. A. Straus & R. J. Gelles (Eds.), *Physical violence in American families: Risk factors and adaptations to violence in 8,145 families* (pp. 95–112). New Brunswick, NJ: Transaction.

Straus, M. A., Gelles, R. J., & Steinmertz, S. (1980). *Behind closed doors: Violence in the American family.* Garden City, NY: Anchor.

Strube, M. J., & Barbour, L. S. (1984). Factors related to the decision to leave an abusive relationship. *Journal of Marriage and the Family, 46,* 837–844.

Symonds, A. (1979). Violence against women: The myth of masochism. *American Journal of Psychotherapy, 33,* 161–173.

Tolman, R. M., & Weisz, A. (1995). Coordinated community intervention for domestic violence: The effects of arrest and prosecution on recidivism of woman abuse perpetrators. *Crime and Delinquency, 41,* 481–495.

Torres, S. (1991). A comparison of wife abuse between two cultures: Perceptions, attitudes, nature, and extent. *Issues in Mental Health Nursing: Psychiatric Nursing for the 90's: New Concepts, New Therapies, 12,* 113–131.

Tracy, K. K., & Crawford, C. B. (1992). Wife abuse: Does it have an evolutionary origin? In D. A. Counts, J. K. Brown, & J. C. Campbell (Eds.), *Sanctions and sanctuary: Cultural perspectives on the beating of wives* (pp. 19–32). Boulder, CO: Westview.

Uba, L. (1992). Cultural barriers to health care for Southeast Asian refugees. *Public Health Reports, 107,* 544–548.

Ulrich, Y. C. (1991). Women's responses for leaving abusive spouses. *Health Care for Women International, 12,* 465–473.

Ulrich, Y. C. (1993). What helped most in leaving spouse abuse: Implications for interventions. *Association of Women's Health Obstetric and Neonatal Nurses Clinical Issues in Perinatal and Women's Health Nursing, 4,* 395–390.

Violence Against Women Act of 1994, Pub. L. No. 103-322, 108 Stat. 1902-1955, 8 U.S.C. sections 1151, 1154, 1186a, 1254, 2245.

Vivian, D., & Langhinrichsen-Rohling, J. (1994). Are bi-directionally violent couples mutually victimized? A gender-sensitive comparison. *Violence and Victims, 9,* 107–124.

Walker, L. E. (1979). *The battered woman.* New York: Harper and Row.

Whatley, M. A. (1993). For better or worse: The case of marital rape. *Violence and Victims, 8,* 29–39.

Wiebe, K. (1985). *Violence against immigrant women and children: An overview for community workers.* Vancouver, British Columbia, Canada: Women Against Violence Against Women/Raoe Crisis Centre Society.

Williams, O. J., & Becker, R. L. (1994). Domestic partner abuse treatment programs and cultural competence: The results of a national survey. *Violence and Victims, 9,* 287–296.

Wilson, M., & Daly, M. (1993). An evolutionary psychological perspective on male sexual proprietariness and violence against wives. *Violence and Victims, 8,* 271–194.

Wolf, M. (1972). *Women and the family in rural Taiwan.* Stanford, CA: Stanford University Press.

Wolfgang, M. E., & Ferracuti, F. (1967). *The subculture of violence: Toward an integrated theory of criminology.* London: Tavistock.

Women's AIDS Organization. (1992). *Draft report of the National Study on Domestic Violence.* Kuala Lumpur, Malaysia: Author.

Wrangham, R., & Peterson, D. (1996). *Demonic males: Apes and the origins of human violence.* Boston: Houghton Mifflin.

26

Violence and Injury among Immigrants

An Epidemiological Review

HAIKANG SHEN AND SUSAN B. SORENSON

Introduction

The growing number of immigrants to the United States has become an important part of the social and public health structure of the nation.* In 1990, the immigrant population was about 20 million—the largest number of immigrants in U.S. history—and comprised about 8% of the total population, the highest proportion of foreign-born persons in the nation in the past 40 years (U.S. Department of Commerce, 1993). The primary countries of origin for immigrants have shifted over time from European nations to Asian countries and Mexico (Immigration and Naturalization Service, 1991a). Thus, besides coping with issues relevant to all immigrants, more recent ar-

rivals also must accommodate to being a minority in the United States. And, in turn, U.S. society is compelled to adapt to the addition of large numbers of recently arrived multilingual minority residents.

Immigrants present a mosaic of public health characteristics. Relatively little research has been dedicated to immigrant health, however. Epidemiological studies of the health of immigrants are especially scarce. Health studies of immigrants more typically focus on issues such as health concepts (Ailinger & Causey, 1995), health care utilization (Leclere, Jensen, & Biddlecom, 1994), and the importance of cross-cultural approaches in health care delivery and prevention interventions (Chigier & Nudelman, 1994). It is important to monitor the health of immigrants because their health care needs, as well as their access to care, may differ from those of persons born in the United States. Such information will satisfy more than intellectual curiosity. Immigrants' impact on public health has become an important policy consideration. National policy regarding what health and welfare benefits will be extended to legal as well as illegal immigrants has changed and will likely be a topic of controversy for some time. Data such as these are needed to develop informed policy.

*Although distinctions among the foreign born are possible—an immigrant (whether in the United States legally or illegally), refugee, amnesty applicant, foreign student, or other type of foreign-born U.S. resident—such a level of analysis is not possible given most currently available health data. The terms "immigrant" and "foreign born" will be used interchangeably herein to refer to U.S. residents who were born outside the United States.

HAIKANG SHEN AND SUSAN B. SORENSON • School of Public Health, University of California at Los Angeles, Los Angeles, California 90095-1772.

Handbook of Immigrant Health, edited by Loue. Plenum Press, New York, 1998.

National Data on the Health of Immigrants

Epidemiological investigations of disease and injury in immigrant populations are not common. Most encouraging is the work of the National Center for Health Statistics (NCHS) which, in 1985, began to gather information on the birthplace of persons 18 years of age and older as part of the National Health Interview Survey (NHIS) (Hendershot, 1988). A few years later, in 1989, the NHIS began to ask about the length of time that foreign-born persons had lived in the United States. Data such as these will help illuminate the issue of immigrant health.

The first systematic report on the general health of the foreign-born population using the NHIS data was published in 1994 (Stephen, Foote, Hendershot, & Schoenborn, 1994). According to the report: Immigrants are in better health than U.S.–born persons; recent immigrants are healthier than both U.S.–born persons and foreign-born persons who had lived in the United States 10 or more years; immigrants who had lived in the United States at least 10 years generally were healthier than U.S.–born persons although

differences were not as striking as between recent immigrants and the native-born population. The study's conclusions may be challenged, however, because several of the health indicators (number of physician visits, etc.) are linked closely to issues of health care availability and accessibility. In other words, the study may be a better measure of immigrants' use of the health care system than of the health of immigrants themselves.

Mortality Data

Survival, the essential basis of health, has received scant research attention in studies of immigrant health. Although immigrants generally are young persons, it is important to examine mortality, as it is a basic indicator of the health of a population. California disease mortality data parallel the findings of national morbidity and mortality data for immigrants. (See Figure 1.) Young immigrants are underrepresented in all major disease death groups—cancer, heart disease, HIV/AIDS, and cerebrovascular diseases.

Injury mortality patterns (deaths due to unintentional "accidental" injuries, homicide, and suicide) are directly relevant to U.S. im-

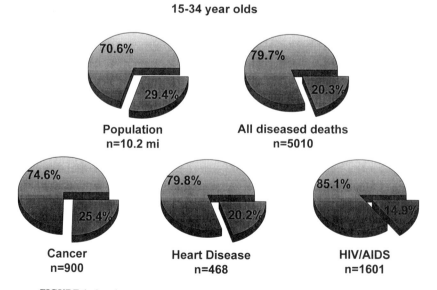

FIGURE 1. Immigrants as a percentage of Californians and selected disease deaths: 1990.

migrant health because injury-related fatalities account for 58.9% of the deaths of 15- to 34-year-olds in the United States (Kochanek & Hudson, 1995), and a substantial proportion of immigrants, especially recent arrivals, are in the 15- to 34-year-old age group (Immigration and Naturalization Service, 1991b). Unintentional injuries, homicide, and suicide rank high as causes of death among U.S. youth (Kochanek & Hudson, 1995). Many immigrants likely die of injury in that most recent immigrants to the United States are young men (Immigration and Naturalization Service, 1991b; Johnson, 1993), the group at highest risk of unintentional injury death (Kochanek & Hudson, 1995). Moreover, they are young men of color (Immigration and Naturalization Service, 1991b; Johnson, 1993), the very group at highest risk of homicide in the United States (Kochanek & Hudson, 1995).

Injury death rates differ by demographic characteristics such as gender, race, and ethnicity; reasons for the differences are not well understood. If these variables are not taken into account when comparing immigrant and native-born injury death rates, risk associated with gender, race, or ethnicity will be mistakenly attributed to nativity. For example, given that U.S. homicide rates are highest among men of color and that most recent immigrants are Asian or Latino men, one would expect homicide rates to be higher among immigrants than the native-born. In other words, the operative issue may be ethnicity, gender, or some combination thereof, rather than nativity. Thus, in order to increase the validity of the findings, analyses of immigrant health must take demographic characteristics such as gender, race, and ethnicity into account.

Violence and Injury as Causes of Death among Immigrants

Although the United States has the largest immigrant population in the world (United Nations, 1991), most of the published studies of violence and injury among immigrants have been conducted elsewhere (Burke, 1976; Burvill, Armstrong, & Carlson, 1983; Kliewer, 1994; Picot, 1992; Trovato, 1986, 1992). While such research may help inform similar investigations in the United States, study results based on these countries' data are of questionable utility for U.S. policy development because the composition of the immigrant population, the magnitude and trends in immigration, and existing immigration policies differ among nations.

In an examination of 1980 data, Kestenbaum found foreign-born persons to be at lower disease and injury mortality risk than U.S.–born persons (Kestenbaum, 1988). More recently, Shai and Rosenwaike (1988) compared injury mortality among Mexican and Cuban immigrants and Puerto Ricans who had moved to the mainland United States. They found risk to differ by country of origin: The Puerto Rican–born had the highest death rates from homicide, the Cuban-born from suicide, and the Mexican-born from accidents. Men's mortality risk was generally higher in each of these nativity groups than it was for Whites and Blacks both nationally and regionally. Sorlie, Backlund, Johnson, and Rogot (1992), investigating mortality differences between Hispanics and non-Hispanics, found Hispanics to be at higher risk of homicide, lower risk of suicide, and no ethnic differences to exist for unintentional injury deaths. Hispanics were generally at lower risk than non-Hispanics of dying of disease, even when adjusting for differences in family income. An examination of place-of-birth differences found that the foreign-born tended to have lower mortality than native-born persons. The only cited exception to this general pattern was for 25- to 34-year-old Hispanic men, where the foreign-born and U.S.–born were at similar risk.

These studies are augmented by our recent series of investigations of homicide, suicide, and unintentional injury death among young immigrants in California (Sorenson & Shen, 1996a, 1996b, in press). To our knowledge, it is the most recent systematic investigation into violent injury death among immigrants.

Injury Trends among Young Immigrants in California

According to the 1990 census (U.S. Bureau of the Census, 1991), three fourths of the immigrants to the United States reside in six states: California, New York, Florida, New Jersey, Texas, and Illinois. California is home to about one third of all the immigrants in the United States, and the 6.5 million immigrant residents in California constitute 22% of the state's population. Although California has long been a destination for immigrants to the United States, many of the immigrants now in California are relatively recent arrivals; about half of the immigrants in California moved to the United States during the 1980s (Johnson, 1993). Large numbers of both foreign- and U.S.–born persons of different ethnic backgrounds make California an ideal state in which to document mortality risks among immigrants.

Our studies addressed several core research goals:

- To examine trends in and estimate the risk of homicide, suicide, and unintentional injury death among immigrants.
- To compare the risk of these types of death for immigrants to those for the native-born.
- To determine immigrant-to-nonimmigrant risk in the four major race and ethnicity groups.
- To identify risk groups among immigrants that are associated with higher rates of homicide, suicide, and unintentional injury death.

Relevant information was abstracted from statewide mortality data tapes provided by the California Department of Health Services. Hispanics were identified using a surname linkage procedure. (A total of 2,064 names believed to be of Spanish origin was added to the census list of 12,497 Spanish surnames. This expansion was necessary because the common spelling of some names has changed since the census list was compiled in 1980 and because of the increasing practice of adopting hyphenated surnames. For more information on the compilation of the revised surname list, refer to the original work [Sorenson, 1998]). To control for the greater number of males among immigrants, rates were standardized by gender to the U.S.–born population within each year.

Immigrants and Homicide (Sorenson & Shen, 1996a)

From 1970 through 1992, 64,510 Californians died of homicide. Immigrants are overrepresented among these deaths. During the 23-year study period, immigrants were an estimated 17.4% of California's population but comprised 23.3% of the state's homicide victims. In 1990, the most recent year for which census data are available, immigrants constituted 22.8% of California's residents and 32.8% of the state's homicide victims.

In recognition of the importance of homicide during adolescence and young adulthood, analyses focused on the 38,774 homicides of 15- to 34-year-olds, who accounted for a majority of all homicide victims. The homicide of youth appears to be especially important among immigrants. A total of 73.7% of the murdered immigrants were ages 15 to 34 years, compared to 62.3% of the murdered native-born persons.

Homicide rates standardized by gender were used to compare immigrants' homicide risk and trend patterns with those of the U.S.–born population. As seen in Figure 2, immigrants were at higher risk of homicide than U.S.–born persons. Although homicide rates increased for both foreign- and U.S.–born 15- to 34-year-olds from 1970 through 1992, immigrants consistently had higher rates than U.S.–born persons.

Firearms accounted for the majority of homicide deaths each year for both immigrants and U.S.–born persons. Moreover, firearms accounted for a growing proportion of the homicide deaths of both groups. In 1970 firearms accounted for 64.1% of the homicide deaths of immigrants and 64.5% of

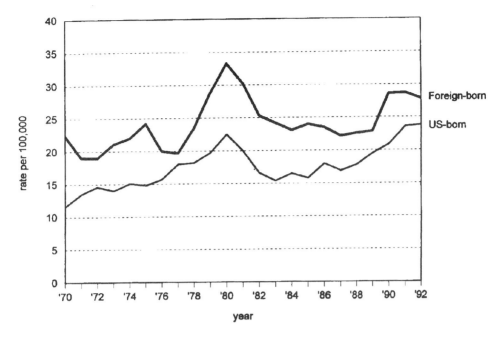

FIGURE 2. Homicide rates by nativity, 15- to 34-year-old Californians, 1970 through 1992. *Note:* Rates are standardized by gender to the U.S.–born population within each year.

the homicide deaths of U.S.–born persons; by 1992, these percentages had increased to 79.6% and 80.1%, respectively.

Immigrants' homicide risk relative to that for U.S.–born persons varied by ethnicity. As seen in the 1990–1992 data in Figure 3, the absolute rate of homicide differed substantially across the nativity and ethnic groups.

Immigrants' risk of homicide relative to U.S.–born persons differed across time as well as by ethnicity. Focusing on the most recent data (1990–1992) in Table 1, non-Hispanic Whites have the largest homicide risk ratio of the four ethnic groups, followed by an elevated risk ratio for Hispanics, a nonsignificant risk ratio for Asians, and a significant risk ratio less than one for Blacks. In other words, non-Hispanic White immigrants are 1.66 times as likely to die of homicide as non-Hispanic Whites born in the United States, and Hispanic immigrants are slightly (1.13 times) more likely than U.S.–born Hispanics to die of homicide. Foreign- and U.S.–born Asian Americans do not differ in their risk of homicide. Black immigrants were less likely

(Risk Ratio = 0.58) than U.S.–born Blacks to die of homicide. The low number of Black immigrants contributed to statistically inconsistent risk ratios across the study period and should be interpreted with caution. The general trend in each ethnic group was toward less discrepancy between immigrants' and nonimmigrants' homicide risk.

In summary, whereas young people account for a majority of all homicide victims among both immigrants and nonimmigrants, a higher proportion than expected of the homicide victims are foreign-born persons. Immigrant-to-nonimmigrant risk patterns differ by ethnicity and across time. Foreign-born Whites and Hispanics are at significantly higher risk than their U.S.–born counterparts.

Immigrants and Suicide (Sorenson & Shen, 1996b)

From 1970 through 1992, 32,928 Californians ages 15 to 34 years died of suicide. Immigrants are underrepresented among these

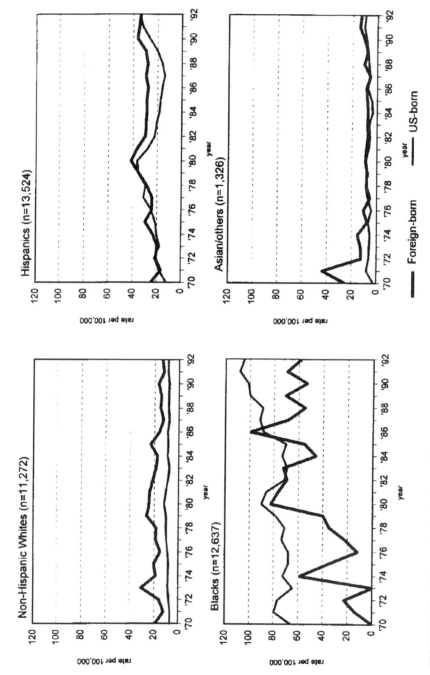

FIGURE 3. Homicide rates for foreign-born and U.S.-born 15- to 34-year-old Californians, by ethnicity, 1970 through 1992. *Note:* Rates are standardized by gender to the U.S.–born population within each year by ethnicity. From "Homicide Risk Among Immigrants in California, 1970 Through 1992," by S. B. Sorenson and H. Shen, 1996, *American Journal of Public Health, 86*(1), p. 98. Copyright 1996 by American Public Health Association. Reprinted with permission.

TABLE 1. Homicide Risk for Foreign-Born vs. U.S.–Born 15- to 34-Year-Old Californians, by Ethnicity, 1970–1992

	1970–79 R.R. 95% C.I.	1980–89 R.R. 95% C.I.	1990–92 R.R. 95% C.I.	1970–92 R.R. 95% C.I.
Non-Hispanic white	**2.29 (1.57, 3.35)**	**2.09 (1.57, 2.79)**	**1.66 (1.25, 2.21)**	**2.12 (1.55, 2.90)**
Hispanic	1.06 (0.84, 1.35)	**1.48 (1.27, 1.74)**	**1.13 (1.01, 1.28)**	**1.24 (1.05, 1.47)**
Black	0.33 (0.11, 1.00)	0.84 (0.55, 1.27)	**0.58 (0.39, 0.84)**	0.60 (0.34, 1.05)
Asian/other	**2.38 (1.26, 4.52)**	1.26 (0.74, 2.14)	1.31 (0.86, 1.99)	**1.72 (1.01, 2.93)**
All races/ethnicities	**1.42 (1.20, 1.67)**	**1.40 (1.27, 1.55)**	**1.24 (1.15, 1.35)**	**1.38 (1.23, 1.55)**

Notes: Rates are standardized by gender to the U.S.–born population within each year by ethnicity. Bold-faced risk ratios are statistically significant at $p < .05$. From "Homicide Risk Among Immigrants in California, 1970 Through 1992," by S. B. Sorenson and H. Shen, 1996, *American Journal of Public Health, 86*(1), p. 99. Copyright 1996 by American Public Health Association. Reprinted with permission.

deaths. During the 23-year study period, the foreign-born were an estimated 17.4% of California's residents but only 13.7% of California's suicides. In 1990, the most recent year for which census data are available, immigrants constituted 22.8% of California's residents yet only 17.6% of the state's suicide deaths.

Subsequent analyses were limited to 15- to 34-year-olds for several reasons in addition to increasing the comparability to the homicide data reported in the previous section. First, young immigrants are more likely than older immigrants to be more recent arrivals in the United States and, therefore, would be the best group with which to address competing hypotheses regarding suicide. For example, immigrants will have lower rates of suicide because the immigration endeavor requires good health and personal resilience; immigrants will have higher rates of suicide because they have limited resources (i.e., limited financial, linguistic, and educational resources, along with a primary social support system that is far away) with which to deal with the stresses of immigration; immigrants will have lower rates of suicide because they are mostly persons of color, groups with lower suicide rates than whites (Kochanek & Hudson, 1995; Smith, Mercy, & Warren, 1985). Second, a substantial portion of the suicides—33.5% for the foreign-born and 38.5% for the U.S.–born— were of 15- to 34-year-olds. All rates and

risk ratio comparisons reported herein are standardized by gender.

The suicide rate for 15- to 34-year-old Californians declined from 1970 through 1992. As shown in Figure 4, the youth suicide rate decreased by about one half among immigrants and by about one third among persons born in the United States. With the exception of the early 1970s, foreign-born 15- to 34-year-olds were at lower risk of suicide than U.S.–born youth during the study period.

Firearms were the most common method of suicide for both immigrants and nonimmigrants. The proportion of suicides using a firearm increased nearly 20%, from 45% in 1970 to 53% in 1992. Although there were some differences in choice of method, trends for immigrants and nonimmigrants were similar across the study period: Poisoning deaths decreased from 33% to 16% and hanging increased from 14% to 22%. The home was the most common site of suicide for both immigrants and nonimmigrants.

As seen in the 1990–1992 data in Figure 5, although the absolute rate of suicide differed substantially across the nativity and ethnic groups, suicide rates were lower among immigrants than U.S.–born persons both overall and within ethnic group.

Immigrants' risk of suicide relative to U.S.–born persons differed little across time and within ethnic group. As seen in Table 2, immigrants' risk of suicide was lower than

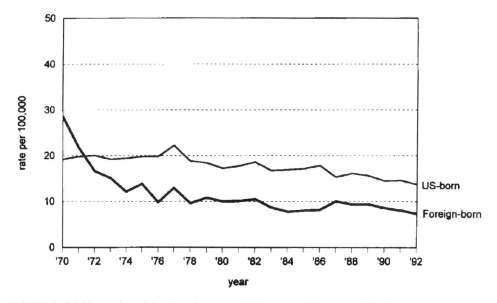

FIGURE 4. Suicide rates by nativity, 15- to 34-year-old Californians, 1970 through 1992. *Note:* Rates are standardized by gender to the U.S.–born population within each year. From "Youth Suicide Trends in California: An Examination of Immigrant and Ethnic Group Risk," by S. B. Sorenson and H. Shen, 1996, *Suicide and Life-Threatening Behavior, 26*(2), p. 148. Copyright 1996 by The Guilford Press. Reprinted with permission.

TABLE 2. Suicide Risk for Foreign-Born vs. U.S.–Born 15- to 34-Year-Old Californians, by Ethnicity, 1970 Through 1992

	1970–79 R.R. 95% C.I.	1980–89 R.R. 95% C.I.	1990–92 R.R. 95% C.I.	1970–92 R.R. 95% C.I.
Non-Hispanic White	**1.65 (1.24, 2.18)**	1.28 (1.00, 1.63)	0.94 (0.73, 1.23)	**1.41 (1.10, 1.81)**
Black	0.86 (0.22, 3.31)	0.95 (0.37, 2.46)	1.03 (0.42, 2.55)	0.91 (0.32, 2.57)
Hispanic	**0.44 (0.29, 0.66)**	**0.53 (0.41, 0.70)**	**0.57 (0.44, 0.74)**	**0.49 (0.36, 0.66)**
Asian/other	1.50 (0.79, 2.85)	0.82 (0.47, 1.43)	1.03 (0.67 1.59)	1.15 (0.67, 1.97)
All races/ethnicities	**0.70 (0.57, 0.85)**	**0.51 (0.44, 0.60)**	**0.54 (0.47, 0.62)**	**0.60 (0.52, 0.71)**

Notes: Rates are standardized by gender to the U.S.–born population within each year by ethnicity. Bold-faced risk ratios are statistically significant at $p < .05$. From "Youth Suicide Trends in California: An Examination of Immigrant and Ethnic Group Risk," by S. B. Sorenson and H. Shen, 1996, *Suicide and Life-Threatening Behavior, 26*(2), p. 149. Copyright 1996 by The Guilford Press. Reprinted with permission.

the suicide risk of U.S.–born persons from 1970 through 1992. Trends across the study period indicate relatively stable immigrant-to-nonimmigrant risk ratios by ethnicity: Foreign-born Blacks and Asians/others were at statistically similar risk of suicide as their U.S.–born counterparts whereas foreign-born Hispanics were at consistently lower risk than U.S.–born Hispanics. Foreign-born non-Hispanic Whites were at significantly higher risk

of suicide than U.S.–born non-Hispanic Whites from 1970 through 1989 when the risk differential dropped and became statistically nonsignificant.

The data suggest that the lower suicide risk for the foreign-born compared with the U.S.–born is accounted for primarily by foreign-born Hispanics. Hispanic immigrants to California come primarily from Mexico (Johnson, 1993), which reports lower rates

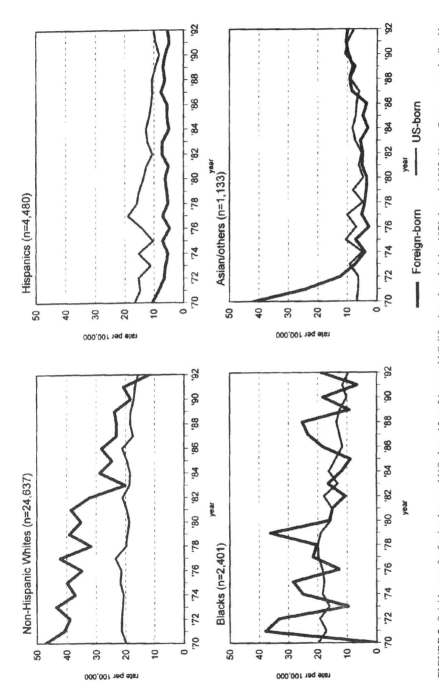

FIGURE 5. Suicide rates for foreign-born and U.S.-born 15- to 34-year-old Californians, by ethnicity, 1970 through 1992. *Note:* Rates are standardized by gender to the U.S.-born population within each year. From "Youth Suicide Trends in California: An Examination of Immigrant and Ethnic Group Risk," by S. B. Sorenson and H. Shen, 1996, *Suicide and Life-Threatening Behavior, 26*(2), p. 148. Copyright 1996 by The Guilford Press. Reprinted with permission.

of suicide for same-aged youth (World Health Organization, 1994). A comparison of 1990 data (World Health Organization, 1991) indicates that among 15- to 34-year-old males, Mexican American immigrants are at higher risk than their counterparts who stayed in Mexico but at lower risk than same-aged U.S.–born Hispanics (9.9 vs. 5.6 vs. 13.6 per 100,000, respectively). Other research indicates Mexican American immigrants have lower rates of suicide attempt than U.S.–born Mexican Americans and U.S.–born non-Hispanic Whites (Sorenson & Golding, 1988). Strong religious ties appear to be one mediator for the lower rates of suicide attempt among Mexican American immigrants (Sorenson & Golding, 1988).

In summary, foreign-born persons are consistently underrepresented in the suicide deaths of 15- to 34-year-olds in California. Hispanic immigrants, most of whom are from Mexico, appear to account for most of the discrepancy between foreign-born and U.S.–born suicide rates. It is important to note that within each ethnic group any foreign-born vs. U.S.–born difference appears to be decreasing over time.

Immigrants and Unintentional Injury

Unintentional injuries are the leading cause of death among all persons under 45 years of age (Kochanek & Hudson, 1995). In acknowledgment of the importance of unintentional injuries among youth and in order to facilitate comparison with analyses of the homicide and suicide data, analyses focused on the 104,395 15- to 34-year-olds who died of unintentional injury in the years 1970 through 1992. Immigrants appear to be represented roughly as would be expected among these deaths. From 1970 to 1992, California immigrants constituted 17.5% of the unintentional injury deaths, a proportion slightly under their 18.7% representation in the population. In 1990, the most recent year for which census data are available, 15- to 34-year-old immigrants constituted 29.4% of California's residents and 31.7% of the state's unintentional injury deaths.

The unintentional injury rate for 15- to 34-year-old Californians declined substantially over time. As shown in Figure 6, from 1970 to 1992 the unintentional injury rate for youth decreased by about 72% among immigrants and by about 47% among persons

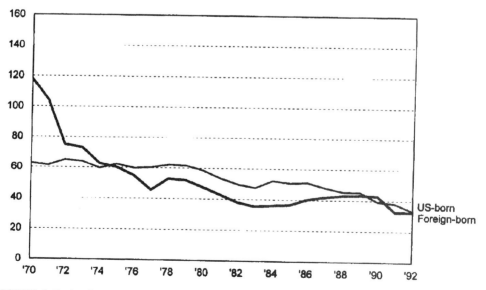

FIGURE 6. Fatal unintentional injury rates by nativity, 15- to 34-year-old Californians, 1970 through 1992. $N = 104,595$. Rate standardized by gender to the U.S.–born population within each year.

born in the United States. Foreign-born and U.S.–born 15- to 34-year-olds appeared to be at similar risk of unintentional injury death during most of the study period.

Motor vehicles, the most common external cause of unintentional injury death, accounted for a greater percentage of unintentional injury deaths among immigrants than nonimmigrants (70.2% vs. 62.4%). Poisons accounted for a lower proportion of unintentional injury deaths among immigrants than U.S.–born persons (10.2% vs. 19.7%). The remaining external causes of death accounted for a similar percentage of the deaths of foreign-born and U.S.–born persons (Sorenson & Shen, in press).

As seen in the 1990–1992 data in Figure 7, although the rate of unintentional injury death differed across nativity and ethnic groups, rates generally were similar for immigrants and U.S.–born persons both overall and within ethnic group. (Note that gender-standardized rates are presented here.) Risk ratio data (see Table 3) confirm that the risk of unintentional injury death for immigrants was similar to that of U.S.–born persons both overall and within ethnic group. The one exception to this pattern was among non-Hispanic Whites—immigrants were at higher risk than their U.S.–born counterparts until 1990–1992 when the risk differential dropped sharply from the 1970s and became statistically nonsignificant.

In summary, immigrants appear to be represented commensurate with their representation in the population in the unintentional injury deaths of 15- to 34-year-olds in California. This pattern has been stable since 1970 with one exception—non-Hispanic White immigrants were at higher risk than their U.S.–born counterparts until 1990 when the risk differential dropped sharply and became statistically nonsignificant. Of note is the observation that rates of unintentional injury deaths have decreased consistently since 1970 for both immigrants and nonimmigrants. Vehicle restraint systems, highway design modifications, changes in legal drinking age, and other technological, environmental, and policy strategies to prevent injury appear to have had positive impact on the unintentional injury deaths of both immigrants and nonimmigrants.

Additional Comparisons

Education levels are known to differ both between the U.S.– and foreign-born and within immigrant groups. Thus, education is a variable of considerable interest when examining mortality differentials by birthplace. Education data have been recorded consistently on death certificates only recently. Education effects generally were consistent across nativity and type of injury death (Sorenson & Shen, in press). Having more than a high school education, compared to being a high school graduate, was related to lower risk of homicide, suicide, and unintentional injury for both the foreign-born and

TABLE 3. Fatal Unintentional Injury Risk for Foreign-Born vs. U.S.–Born 15- to 34-Year-Old Californians, by Ethnicity, 1970–1992

	1970–79 R.R. 95% C.I.	1980–89 R.R. 95% C.I.	1990–92 R.R. 95% C.I.	1970–92 R.R. 95% C.I.
Non-Hispanic white	**1.58 (1.34, 1.87)**	**1.19 (1.02, 1.38)**	**1.17 (1.00, 1.37)**	**1.38 (1.18, 1.61)**
Black	0.52 (0.21, 1.25)	0.86 (0.50, 1.49)	0.83 (0.49, 1.40)	0.67 (0.36, 1.26)
Hispanic	1.15 (1.00, 1.32)	0.95 (0.84, 1.06)	1.06 (0.95, 1.18)	1.06 (0.95, 1.19)
Asian/other	0.98 (0.66, 1.47)	**0.69 (0.50, 0.97)**	0.94 (0.70 1.26)	0.86 (0.62, 1.20)
All races/ethnicities	**1.13 (1.03, 1.24)**	**0.81 (0.75, 0.87)**	0.98 (0.91, 1.05)	0.98 (0.91, 1.06)

Notes: Rates are standardized by gender to the U.S.–born population within each year by ethnicity. Bold-faced risk ratios are statistically significant at $p < .05$.

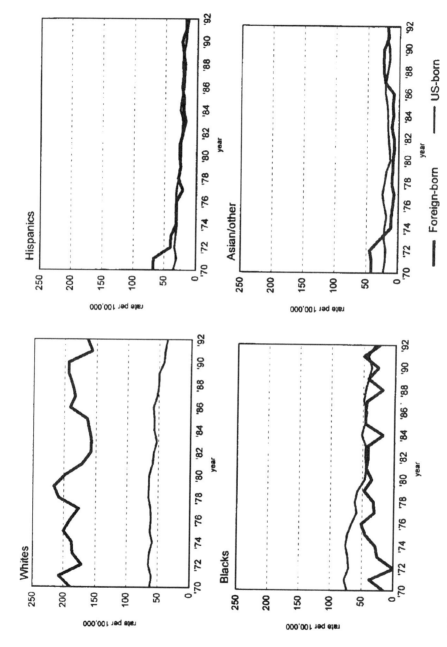

FIGURE 7. Fatal unintentional injury rates for foreign-born and U.S.–born 15- to 34-year-old Californians, by ethnicity, 1970 through 1992. Rates are standardized by gender to the U.S.-born population within each year.

U.S.–born. These findings must be interpreted with some caution given that they are based on only 1 year of data.

As shown in Table 4, the external cause of death is generally similar across injury type for foreign- and U.S.–born persons: Firearms and motor vehicles predominate in the injury deaths of both groups (Sorenson & Shen, in press). Motor vehicles, however, were the cause of a greater proportion of unintentional injury deaths among foreign-born than U.S.–born persons. Among suicide and unintentional injury deaths, the deaths of foreign-born persons were more likely to be due to submersion or suffocation and less likely due to poisoning than U.S.–born persons.

Discussion

Summary of Findings

Risk of disease, homicide, suicide, and unintentional injury death differs by birthplace. Foreign-born persons consistently are at higher risk of homicide than U.S.–born persons. Suicide rates are lower among foreign-born youth than among their U.S.–born counterparts. Unintentional injury mortality risk generally is similar for foreign- and U.S.–born persons. Risk of homicide, suicide, and unintentional injury death differs by ethnicity and birthplace in different ways; most notably, non-Hispanic White immigrants are at higher risk of homicide than U.S.–born non-Hispanic Whites, and Hispanic immigrants are at lower risk of suicide than U.S.–born Hispanics. Homicide and suicide risk differences between immigrants and nonimmigrants within ethnicity have diminished since 1970. The external cause of injury death was generally similar, mostly motor vehicles and firearms, for the foreign-born and U.S.–born. Immigrant–nonimmigrant differences in the mechanism of death have decreased since 1970. Men generally were at higher mortality risk than women for both nativity groups. This general outline of

immigrant injury risk is one of the first several steps in depicting the overall health of immigrants.

Implications

Exposure to the External Cause of Injury

A most effective prevention strategy to reduce injury death rates of both immigrants and nonimmigrants across different race and ethnicity groups would be to reduce their exposure to the mechanism of fatal injury. Motor vehicles accounted for the largest percentage of unintentional injury death among both immigrants (70%) and nonimmigrants (62%). Firearms accounted for the largest percentage of homicides (72% for immigrants, 68% for U.S.–born persons) and suicides (53% for both groups). In subsequent paragraphs we explore possible reasons for the difference in rates for immigrants and U.S.–born persons despite the similarity of the mechanisms of fatal injury.

The similarity in unintentional injury death risk for foreign- and U.S.–born persons is somewhat unexpected. Recent young immigrants, in general, tend to take manual labor or other jobs that require relatively low skills and that are associated with higher rates of on-the-job injury death. Off-the-job exposures could be expected to differ as well. For example, immigrants, most of whom are poorer than U.S.–born persons, could be expected to be more likely to drive older vehicles that would lack injury-preventing safety equipment (e.g., air bags, three-point belt restraint systems, antilock brakes). But perhaps immigrants are, for a variety of reasons (limited finances, less need or desire, etc.), less likely to drive as frequently or as far as U.S.–born persons and, thus, reduce their risk. In other words, differential exposure of immigrants and U.S.–born persons to injury-causing hazards is mostly a matter of speculation at this point. The underlying basis for the similarity in unintentional injury death risk remains unclear.

TABLE 4. Demographic Ratios for Injury Deaths, Foreign- and U.S.-Born 15- to 34-Year-Old Californians, 1989–1993

Type of injury death[a]

	Unintentional injury $n = 19,000$		Suicide $n = 6,547$		Homicide $n = 12,619$		Other injury death $n = 38,166$	
	U.S.-born	Foreign-born	U.S.-born	Foreign-born	U.S.-born	Foreign-born	U.S.-born	Foreign-born
Sex ratio								
M:F	3.24 (2.96, 3.55)[c]	4.62 (3.93, 5.44)[c]	4.22 (3.61, 4.93)[c]	3.91 (2.84, 5.40)[c]	4.45 (3.91, 5.05)[c]	9.34 (7.34, 11.90)[c]	3.74 (3.50, 4.00)[c]	5.69 (5.03, 6.43)[c]
Ethnicity ratio								
Black:White	1.11 (0.98, 1.25)	1.10 (0.64, 1.89)	0.70 (0.56, 0.88)[c]	0.84 (0.34, 2.18)	13.65 (12.1, 15.4)[c]	8.17 (4.90, 13.6)[c]	2.63 (2.46, 2.82)[c]	2.18 (1.60, 2.97)[c]
Hispanic:White	1.23 (1.12, 1.35)[c]	1.46 (1.20, 1.78)[c]	0.71 (0.60, 0.84)[c]	0.50 (0.36, 0.70)[c]	4.25 (3.70, 4.87)[c]	4.79 (3.33, 6.91)[c]	1.48 (1.39, 1.59)[c]	1.74 (1.50, 2.02)[c]
Asian/other:White	0.57 (0.44, 0.74)[c]	0.64 (0.50, 0.82)[c]	0.57 (0.39, 0.83)[c]	0.73 (0.51, 1.04)	1.27 (0.87, 1.85)	1.51 (1.00, 2.27)	0.67 (0.56, 0.80)[c]	0.80 (0.67, 0.96)[c]
Education ratio[b]								
<= 8 yr : H.S.	0.87 (0.65, 1.16)	1.06 (0.91, 1.23)	0.61 (0.36, 1.03)	0.40 (0.27, 0.61)[c]	0.95 (0.66, 1.39)	1.48 (1.22, 1.79)[c]	0.84 (0.70, 1.03)	1.11 (1.00, 1.24)
H.S. dropout : H.S.	0.96 (0.87, 1.07)	0.69 (0.58, 0.83)[c]	0.83 (0.69, 0.99)[c]	0.68 (0.47, 0.99)[c]	1.41 (1.24, 1.61)[c]	1.15 (0.93, 1.43)	1.06 (0.98, 1.14)	0.83 (0.73, 0.94)[c]
> H.S. : H.S.	0.24 (0.21, 0.26)[c]	0.33 (0.27, 0.40)[c]	0.27 (0.24, 0.32)[c]	0.46 (0.32, 0.65)[c]	0.13 (0.11, 0.15)[c]	0.19 (0.14, 0.26)[c]	0.22 (0.20, 0.23)[c]	0.30 (0.26, 0.35)[c]

[a]Several types of cases were not included: deaths outside California, deaths due to legal intervention or wars, and when type of injury was undetermined. Unadjusted rates were used in these analyses.
[b]Education rate ratios are based on 1990 data only; denominator estimates were not available for the other years.
[c]$p < .05$

Cross-National Risk and Relative Safety

During the study period 1970–1990, firearms accounted for a growing proportion of the homicide deaths of both immigrants (from 64% to 80%) and nonimmigrants (from 65% to 80%). Firearms are more available and easily accessed in the United States relative to many nations, particularly European countries, many of which have severe limits on firearm ownership and access. Relatively easy access to lethal means may be related to higher homicide rates in the United States. The role of firearms is also central in suicide in that a gun was the most common suicide method used by foreign- and U.S.–born men and women. A few cross-national studies have investigated how suicide rates are related to firearm availability; Canada–U.S. findings are equivocal on the topic (Sloan, Rivara, Reay, Ferris, & Kellermann, 1990), although U.S. research indicates that gun ownership is related to firearm suicide in the home (Brent *et al.,* 1993; Kellermann *et al.,* 1992). Population-based violence and injury prevention efforts of reducing exposure to guns aspire to reduce risk for all U.S. residents. Study findings indicate that public health efforts focusing on firearms are relevant for immigrants and nonimmigrants alike in that gunshot wounds account for a substantial majority of their homicides and suicides.

Immigrant–nonimmigrant differences and differences among ethnic groups are evident in homicide and suicide risks. Risks relative to country of origin may be an important factor. Cross-national data show that U.S. homicide rates are substantially higher than those in most developed and many developing countries (Deane, 1987; Fingerhut & Kleinman, 1990; World Health Organization, 1994). European immigrants to the United States have higher rates of homicide than both their European counterparts and U.S. counterparts. As previously noted by others, many European nations strictly regulate access to firearms and have much lower rates of homicide than the United States (Fingerhut & Kleinman, 1990; World Health Organization, 1994). Most non-Hispanic White immigrants are from these European countries; thus, their higher risk of homicide relative to their U.S.–born and European counterparts may be due, in part, to a change in exposure. By contrast, Hispanic immigrants to California primarily come from Mexico (Johnson, 1993), a country that reports higher rates of homicide than the United States (World Health Organization, 1994). As a consequence, Hispanic immigrants to California have lower rates of homicide than their Mexican counterparts (World Health Organization, 1994) but higher rates of homicide than U.S.–born Hispanics.

Suicide risks relative to the country of origin may be related to cultural factors such as religious ties and beliefs (e.g., Catholicism, Confucianism). Research on suicide attempts found Mexican Americans born in Mexico to be at lower risk of suicide with lowest rates among those who are the least acculturated and most active in institutionalized religion (Sorenson & Golding, 1988). Hispanic immigrants to California, primarily from Mexico, are at lower risk of suicide than their U.S.–born counterparts and higher risk than their Mexican counterparts (Sorenson & Shen, 1996b).

Housing Patterns

Immigrant households tend to be larger than those of the U.S.–born: 40% live in homes with four or more persons, compared to 25% of natives (Miller & More, 1994). They are more likely than natives to live in families: 76% versus 70%. This is especially true for Hispanic immigrants (85%), who have the lowest suicide rate. Recent immigrants are believed to reside primarily in relatively crowded housing units so if they attempt suicide they may be more likely to be discovered. In other words, a suicide attempt would remain an attempt rather than become a completed suicide because the person living with more people is more likely to be discovered than those living in less densely populated housing.

More than 90% of immigrants move into cities, and many live in highly visible ethnic enclaves (Miller & More, 1994). Immigrants tend to settle near other immigrants, often friends and family. According to 1990 census data (U.S. Bureau of the Census, 1991), about 28% of total immigrants over age 5 live in "linguistically isolated households," in which no member of the household over age 14 speaks English "very well." These residential housing patterns could serve as a preventive factor for suicide by reducing day-to-day social isolation in that immigrants are likely to be in frequent and close contact with others who are similarly situated in the social structure.

Study Strengths and Limitations

California's nearly 30 million residents constitute about 12% of the U.S. population and one third of all immigrants in the United States (U.S. Bureau of the Census, 1991). The large and diverse population provided the opportunity to investigate violent injury risk differentials for immigrants and nonimmigrants by ethnicity, an issue that has received relatively little scientific investigation.

We took ethnicity as well as nativity into account in our investigations in order to ascertain whether observed discrepancies in health outcomes are related to ethnicity, to birthplace, or to a combination of the two. Research that does not take nativity into account risks mistakenly attributing immigrant-to-nonimmigrant differences to ethnicity. Unfortunately, most prior research has either assumed ethnicity based on birthplace (Shai & Rosenwaike, 1988) or not examined birthplace in ethnic groups that are likely to have large numbers of recent immigrants (Becker, Samet, Wiggins, & Key, 1990). Research including the work reported herein that assesses the effects of ethnicity, gender, and nativity will help untangle their respective effects on morbidity and mortality.

Ethnicity Considerations

Ethnic differences in mortality are shaped by the method used to identify ethnicity. The identification of Hispanics, the largest immigrant group, in existing databases has relied primarily on Spanish surname linkage procedures. The most widely used list was assembled by the U.S. census in 1980 (U.S. Bureau of the Census, 1980). Census and survey data generally assume that respondents accurately report their race and ethnicity. Response discrepancies have been documented when different self-report identification methods are used with Hispanics (Sorenson, 1998). Failure to correctly identify Hispanics not only limits research on Hispanics as a separate ethnic group but also distorts studies on other ethnic groups. The 1990 census indicated that among persons self-identified as Hispanic, 46% reported their race as White, 3% as Black, Asian, or American Indian, and 51% as "other race." This distortion is potentially overwhelming in studies of immigrants, a substantial proportion of whom are Hispanic.

Our injury mortality studies improved on the standard Spanish-surname linkage procedure by excluding Asians and Blacks from the linkage and by generating a revised list of Spanish surnames based on the death certificates (Sorenson, 1998). The expanded Spanish surname list, however, is by no means exhaustive. The list is based on death certificate data from only one state in which most of the Hispanics are of Mexican heritage and, therefore, is likely to miss Hispanics of other origins. The goal was to develop a relatively accurate list for studies on California mortality data and at the same time to illustrate potential implications of the development and implementation of a new census Spanish-surname list. Future studies may be able to apply a similar method to improve the identification of Hispanics.

Native Americans, by definition, are not immigrants to the United States; analysis of these data indicates that none of the Native American decedents were born outside the

United States, and they should have been excluded from the analyses because there was no variance in nativity, the primary variable of interest. However, population projections (i.e., denominator data) were not available until 1990 when the California Department of Finance started projecting the American Indian population separately. Considering that Native Americans have high mortality rates from suicide (Indian Health Service, 1994), including them with the Asian/other group likely inflated the risk for U.S.–born decedents. Thus, we must interpret the findings for the Asian/other group with caution.

Documented and Undocumented Immigrants

The central problem in research on immigrants to the United States is the lack of data on illegal immigrants. According to census officials, questions about immigration status are not included on the census and other government surveys because they might provoke untruthful responses or reduce the participation rate and thereby affect the quality of the data (U.S. General Accounting Office, 1995). In recent years, concern about illegal immigrants in the United States has focused on their use of public benefits and their overall costs to society. Information on illegal immigrants would allow researchers to assess differentials by immigrant status as well as nativity and may be useful in developing the most appropriate violence and injury prevention strategies.

Gross estimates of the illegal immigrant population vary greatly. According to government estimates, 3.5 to 4 million illegal immigrants resided in the United States in 1994 (U.S. General Accounting Office, 1995). More than 904,000 legal immigrants were admitted to the country in 1993 alone, and as many as 300,000 illegal immigrants settled permanently in the United States that same year (Miller & More, 1994). Although the census does not exclude undocumented immigrants from its population counts, one could surmise that for a variety of reasons the

U.S. census undercounts illegal immigrants. Estimates of this possible undercount, however, are not available. Considering that there could be as many as one illegal immigrant for every three legal immigrants, a substantial undercount of illegal immigrants would spuriously inflate risk rate estimates for immigrant subgroups with a large proportion of undocumented members, as well as inflate the overall immigrant-to-nonimmigrant risk ratio.

Despite the lack of information, our mortality studies of immigrants reasonably describe immigrant-to-nonimmigrant risk using currently available data. The numerator and denominator data used in the research are comparable in that they both include legal and illegal immigrants without identifying their legal status. Analysis by immigrant type (e.g., legal, undocumented), however, is not possible, because of the lack of information about immigrants' legal status. Although it is difficult to collect data about a population that has an incentive to remain hidden from government officials, future studies would provide much-needed information if they could study some of the basic public health characteristics of the illegal immigrant population.

Misclassification of Deaths

Medical examiners and coroners have been able to document their indecision regarding manner of death through the death certification process since 1969. The "undetermined" category was introduced in the 8th revision of the *Manual of the International Statistical Classification of Diseases, Injuries, and Causes of Death* and was continued in the 9th and 10th revisions. Whether a death was an accident, a suicide, or a homicide is not always clear. Our recent findings (Sorenson, Shen, & Kraus, 1997) indicate that females and Blacks, Asians, and Native Americans are far more likely to be assigned to the undetermined manner-of-death category than males and Whites; and deaths among immigrants were less likely than those among

U.S.–born persons to be certified as undetermined. Although only about 2% of the injury deaths were classified as such, if assignment to the undetermined category is not random, as was found to be the case, implications for certain population groups can be substantial. We have no evidence that undetermined-cause-of-death fatalities may be investigated more thoroughly. Therefore, it is important to acknowledge that the injury death rates may be misestimated somewhat because some deaths are incorrectly classified into the category of undetermined.

Future Research Needs

Future research will need to take into account the differing social and cultural conditions within immigrant populations. The foreign-born population is diverse in multiple important ways. In 1990, the most recent year for which data are available about the 20 million foreign-born persons in the United States, about 33% were naturalized citizens, 45% were legal permanent residents, 13% were illegal aliens, 6% were refugees or asylees, and another 4% were other legal residents such as foreign students (Miller & More, 1994). One would not expect similar injury risk rates among wealthy immigrants who voluntarily resettled, students temporarily relocated until they finish their education, poor refugees who experienced a number of traumas before they were able to flee to the United States, and illegal aliens who are working at low-wage labor jobs and trying to hide from government officials. To further investigate specific public health issues, additional resources will be needed so as to conduct studies that target particular immigrant groups.

Archival research using death certificates, the primary and logical source of information about mortality, is an efficient way to obtain data about large numbers of homicides, suicides, and unintentional deaths. Additional resources will be necessary to investigate important variables not available in existing

mortality data. How acculturated an immigrant is to the United States is a crucial piece of information to improve our understanding of the differences between the U.S.– and the foreign-born in injury death risk. Acculturation, a progressive process, is constantly changing. For example, the lifestyle and health risks of foreign-born persons educated in American schools and living in United States society for decades can be expected to be more like those of U.S.–born persons than like those of more recent immigrants. Such differences would not be possible to note in most research, however, because only a "foreign-born" versus "U.S.–born" dichotomy is recorded. More complete depictions of health will be possible if acculturation to U.S. society is measured. Acculturation can be measured in a variety of ways: age at immigration, length of time in the United States, language used in daily life, food preferences, demographic composition of neighborhood of residence, and so forth. Future health studies will need to include acculturation measures to improve our understanding of injury risk among the foreign-born.

The racial and ethnic composition of the immigrant population has changed dramatically (Immigration and Naturalization Service, 1992). In 1994, about 80% of immigrants were from eight Asian or Latin American countries (Chavez, 1995). According to the 1990 census, Latinos are the second largest minority group and the largest immigrant group in the United States (Immigration and Naturalization Service, 1991c). Both immigration and a relatively high fertility rate contribute to the expected continued rapid growth of the Latino population. The U.S. Asian Pacific population grew from about 1 million to more than 7 million from 1960 to 1990, making it the fastest growing segment of the country ("Leadership Education for Asian Pacifics," 1996). The demographic and socioeconomic characteristics of the two largest immigrant groups differ greatly. For example, about 83% of Latin American immigrant males are in the labor force, a rate as high or higher than that of almost any group

(Chavez, 1995). Two thirds of Latin American immigrants have not completed high school (Chavez, 1995). By contrast, nearly 38% of Asian immigrants age 25 years or more hold college degrees, compared with 20% of the total U.S. population. And per capita income among foreign-born Asians in the United States was roughly the same as that of non-Hispanic Whites.

According to population projections (U.S. Department of Commerce, 1996), while the non-Hispanic White share of the U.S. population will fall steadily from 74% in 1995 to 64% in 2020, Hispanics and Asian and Pacific Islander populations will have the highest rates of increase, with annual growth rates that may exceed 2% until 2030. In comparison, even at the peak of the Baby Boom era, the total U.S. population never grew 2% each year. Growth of the Hispanic-origin population likely will be a major element of the total population growth. By 2000, Hispanics are expected to increase to 31 million persons, and to constitute the second-largest race-ethnic group by 2010. Population projections suggest that the Hispanic population will double its 1995 size to 53 million by 2020, triple to 80 million by 2040, and reach nearly 97 million by 2050. Asian and Pacific Islanders are projected to continue to be the fastest growing ethnic group with growth rates that could exceed 2.5% a year through 2020. Asian American numbers are expected to grow from 7 million in 1990 to 20–23 million by 2020, a projected increase of 300% within 30 years ("Leadership Education for Asian Pacifics," 1996). Immigration is an integral part of the growth of the Asian population. Due to the large number of immigrants and their fast-growing pace, more research attention is needed especially for Asian and Hispanic populations.

Conclusions

The health of immigrants will be a continuing topic of interest for a relatively long time. Although immigrants have become an important part of the public health structure, relatively little research has been dedicated to immigrant health. Extending public health knowledge to immigrant injury risk patterns and risk factors is more than a topic of academic curiosity. It is a matter of importance for health service delivery and public health policy.

Of particular interest is the recent controversy over whether and how to provide health care for immigrants, whether in the country legally or illegally. Whether such questions are addressed at the federal level or at the state level in the form of block grants, the health of the foreign-born is of importance to the nation whose immigrant population doubled from 1970 to 1990 (U.S. Bureau of the Census, 1994) and to states such as Florida, New Jersey, Florida, and California, where immigrants constitute 13%–22% of the population (U.S. Bureau of the Census, 1991). Public health research on immigrants can be useful to lawmakers in developing appropriate policy responses to address the differences between U.S.–born and foreign-born populations. Unfortunately, there are relatively few empirical data to guide policy makers at this time.

Population-based violence and injury prevention efforts, such as increasing motor vehicle safety and reducing exposure to handguns, aspire to reduce violence mortality risk for all U.S. residents. Study findings indicate that public health efforts focusing on motor vehicles and firearms are relevant for immigrants as well as nonimmigrants in that motor vehicles account for a majority of unintentional injuries for both groups, and gunshot wounds account for a substantial majority of the homicides and a sizable number of the suicides in both groups.

Services and programs designed specifically for foreign-born residents (e.g., churches, temples, social organizations, the Immigration and Naturalization Service) may serve as good distribution points for information about immigrants' risk of violence mortality in the United States. Such efforts would need to include information about known risk factors (e.g., keeping a gun in the home) to avoid the unintended consequence of immigrants taking counterproductive actions to reduce mortality risk in response to increased awareness.

To improve our understanding of disease and injury death in foreign-born populations, additional resources and sophisticated research will be necessary to investigate important variables not available in existing databases. Such information includes legal immigration status, acculturation levels, years in the country, and so on. Theoretical sophistication and substantial methodological precision are necessary to conduct work that will advance our understanding of the interplay of the multiple distal and proximal factors associated with violence and injury death risk among both foreign- and U.S.-born populations.

Acknowledgments

This work was supported by a grant from the California Wellness Foundation to the second author. Dr. Shen is now with the Department of Psychiatry and Biobehavioral Science, University of California, Los Angeles.

References

Ailinger, R. L., & Causey, M. E. (1995). Health concept of older Hispanic immigrants. *Western Journal of Nursing Research, 17,* 605–613.

Becker, T. M., Samet, J. M., Wiggins, C. L., & Key, C. R. (1990). Violent death in the west: Suicide and homicide in New Mexico, 1958–1987. *Suicide and Life-Threatening Behavior, 20,* 324–334.

Brent, D. A., Perper, J. A., Mortiz, G., Baugher, M., Schweers, J., & Roth, C. (1993). Firearms and adolescent suicide. A community case-control study. *American Journal of Diseases of Children, 147,* 1066–1071.

Burke, A. W. (1976). Socio-cultural determinants of attempted suicide among West Indians in Birmingham: Ethnic origins and immigrant status. *British Journal of Psychiatry, 129,* 261–266.

Burvill, P. W., Armstrong, B. K., & Carlson, D. J. (1983). Attempted suicide and immigration in Perth, Western Australia, 1979–1978. *Acta Psychiatrica Scandinavica, 68,* 89–99.

Chavez, L. (1995, May 31). Immigration not about race. *USA Today,* p. 13A.

Chigier, E., & Nudelman, A. (1994). A cross-cultural approach to health education for immigrants and refugees. *Collegium Antropologicum, 18,* 195–198.

Deane, G. D. (1987). Cross-national comparison of homicide: Age/sex-adjusted rates using the 1980 U.S. homicide experience as a standard. *Journal of Quantitative Criminology, 3,* 215–227.

Fingerhut, L. A., & Kleinman, J. C. (1990). International and interstate comparisons of homicide among young males. *Journal of the American Medical Association, 263,* 3292–3295.

Hendershot, G. E. (1988). *Health of the foreign-born population: United States, 1985–86* (Advance data from vital and health statistics, No. 157). Hyattsville, MD: National Center for Health Statistics.

Immigration and Naturalization Service. (1991a). *Statistical yearbook of the Immigration and Naturalization Service, 1990.* Washington, DC: U.S. Government Printing Office (Table 2, p. 50).

Immigration and Naturalization Service. (1991b). *Statistical yearbook of the Immigration and Naturalization Service, 1990.* Washington, DC: U.S. Government Printing Office (Chart E, p. 44).

Immigration and Naturalization Service. (1991c). *Statistical yearbook of the Immigration and Naturalization Service, 1990.* Washington, DC: U.S. Government Printing Office.

Immigration and Naturalization Service. (1992). *Statistical yearbook of the Immigration and Naturalization Service, 1991.* Washington, DC: U.S. Government Printing Office.

Indian Health Service. (1994). *Indian Health Service: Trends in Indian health—1994.* Washington, DC: Author.

Johnson, H. (1993, September). *Immigrants in California: Findings from the 1990 Census.* Sacramento, CA: California Research Bureau.

Kellermann, A. L., Rivara, F. P., Somes, G., Reay, A. T., Francisco, J., Banton, J. G., Prodzinski, J., Flinger, C., & Hackman, B. B. (1992). Suicide in the home in relation to gun ownership. *New England Journal of Medicine, 327,* 467–472.

Kestenbaum, R. (1988). Mortality by nativity. *Demography, 23,* 87–90.

Kliewer, E. V. (1994). Homicide victims among Australian immigrants. *Australian Journal of Public Health, 18,* 304–309.

Kochanek, K. D., & Hudson, B. L. (1995, March 22). Advance report of final mortality statistics, 1992. *Monthly Vital Statistics Report, 43*(6), (Suppl.). Hyattsville, MD: National Center for Health Statistics.

Leadership Education for Asian Pacifics. (1996, February). *Connections, 9*(1), 1.

Leclere, F. B., Jensen, L., & Biddlecom, A. E. (1994). Health care utilization, family context, and adaptation among immigrants to the United States. *Journal of Health and Social Behavior, 35,* 370–384.

Miller, J. J., & More, S. (1994). *The index of leading immigration indicators.* The Center for the New American Community, Manhattan Institute.

Picot, M. (1992). Recent violent deaths of immigrants in France. *Temp Modernes, 47,* 202–208.

Shai, D., & Rosenwaike, I. (1988). Violent deaths among Mexican-, Puerto Rican-, and Cuban-born migrants in the United States. *Social Science and Medicine, 26,* 269–276.

Sloan, J. H., Rivara, F. P., Reay, D. T., Ferris, J. A., & Kellermann, A. L. (1990). Firearm regulation and rates of suicide. A comparison of two metropolitan areas. *New England Journal of Medicine, 322,* 369–373.

Smith, J. C., Mercy, J. A., & Warren, C. W. (1985). Comparison of suicides among Anglos and Hispanics in five southwestern states. *Suicide and Life-Threatening Behavior, 15,* 14–26.

Sorenson, S. B. (1998). *Identifying Hispanics in existing databases: Effect of three methods on mortality patterns of Hispanics and non-Hispanic whites.* Evaluation Review, 22, 520–534.

Sorenson, S. B., & Golding, J. M. (1988). Suicide attempts in Mexican Americans: Prevention implications of immigration and cultural issues. *Suicide and Life-Threatening Behavior, 18,* 322–333.

Sorenson, S. B., & Shen, H. (1996a). Homicide risk among immigrants in California, 1970 through 1992. *American Journal of Public Health, 86,* 97–100.

Sorenson, S. B., & Shen, H. (1996b). Youth suicide trends in California: An examination of immigrant and ethnic group risk. *Suicide and Life-Threatening Behavior, 26,* 143–154.

Sorenson, S. B., & Shen, H. (in press). Mortality among young immigrants to California: Injury compared to disease deaths. *Journal of Immigrant Health.*

Sorenson, S. B., Shen, H., & Kraus, J. F. (1997). Undetermined manner of death: A comparison with unintentional injury, suicide, and homicide death. *Evaluation Review, 21,* 43–57.

Sorlie, P. D., Backlund, E., Johnson, N. J., & Rogot, E. (1992). Mortality by Hispanic status in the United States. *Journal of the American Medical Association, 270,* 2464–2468.

Stephen, E. H., Foote, K., Hendershot, G. E., & Schoenborn, C. A. (1994). Health of the foreign-born population: United States, 1989–90. *Advance Data, 14,* 1–12.

Trovato, F. (1986). A time series analysis of international immigration and suicide mortality in Canada. *International Journal of Social Psychiatry, 32,* 38–46.

Trovato, F. (1992). Violent and accidental mortality among four immigrant groups in Canada, 1970–1972. *Social Biology, 39,* 82–101.

United Nations. (1991). *Demographic yearbook, 1989.* New York: United Nations, Department of Economic and Social Affairs, Statistical Office.

U.S. Bureau of the Census. (1980). Census of Population and Housing, *Spanish surname list* [Machine-readable data file]. Washington, DC: Author [producer and distributor].

U.S. Bureau of the Census. (1991). Census of Population and Housing, 1990 [Machine-readable data files]. Washington, DC: Author [producer and distributor].

U.S. Bureau of the Census. (1994). *Statistical abstract of the United States.* Washington, DC: Author (Table 54, p. 52).

U.S. Department of Commerce. (1993, September). *We, the American foreign born.* Washington, DC: Bureau of the Census, Economics and Statistics Administration.

U.S. Department of Commerce. (1996). *Population projections of the United States by age, sex, race, and Hispanic origin: 1995 to 2050.* Washington DC.: Author.

U.S. General Accounting Office. (1995). *Illegal aliens: National net cost estimates vary widely* Washington, DC: Author.

World Health Organization. (1991). *World health statistics annual, 1990.* Geneva, Switzerland: Author.

World Health Organization. (1994). *World health statistics annual, 1993.* Geneva, Switzerland: Author.

27

Strategies for Health Education

Theoretical Models

JOHN P. ELDER, J. XAVIER APODACA,

DEBORAH PARRA-MEDINA, AND

MARIA LUISA ZUÑIGA DE NUNCIO

Health Behavior Change Theories

Modern health promotion practice emerged from models and theories such as the Health Belief model (Becker, 1974; Janz & Becker, 1984), the PRECEDE model (Green, 1984; Green & Kreuter, 1991), social cognitive theory (Bandura, 1986, 1989, 1991), the theory of Reasoned Action (Ajzen & Fishbein, 1980; Fishbein, 1980; Fishbein & Ajzen, 1975), and behavior analysis (Elder, Geller, Hovell, & Mayer, 1994; Skinner, 1953). These theories are deemed relevant to immigrant health due more to their popularity among health psychologists and public health educators in the United States and industrialized countries than to their necessary relevance to immigrant populations and their cultures.

Although cast as distinct, in practice these theories overlap to a considerable extent. For example, they generally support the notion that "intention" to perform behavior is an immediate determinant of that behavior. This line of reasoning has been extended and popularized by Prochaska and DiClemente (1983) and their own Transtheoretical or Stages of Change model. Indeed, the Stages of Change (SOC) model has become one of the most influential in health promotion, and therefore should be viewed as a sixth major contender in the array of health promotion theories.

The overlap among these six theories (which term we will from this point use for this entire category, although three are labeled models), includes an emphasis on the following variables: intentions to behave, environmental constraints impeding the behavior, skills, outcome expectations, norms for the behavior, self-standards, affect, and self-confidence with respect to the behavior. In short, the person must

1. have a strong positive intention or predisposition to perform a behavior;
2. face a minimum of environmental barriers to performing the behavior;
3. have the requisite skills for the behavior;
4. believe that positive outcomes or "reinforcement" will follow the performance of the behavior;

JOHN P. ELDER, DEBORAH PARRA-MEDINA, AND MARIA LUISA ZUÑIGA DE NUNCIO • Graduate School of Public Health, Center for Behavioral and Community Health Studies, San Diego State University, San Diego, California 92123.   J. XAVIER APODACA • SDSU–UCSD Joint Doctoral Program, Clinical Psychology, San Diego State University, San Diego, California 92123.

Handbook of Immigrant Health, edited by Loue. Plenum Press, New York, 1998.

5. believe that there is normative pressure to perform the behavior and none sanctioning the behavior;
6. believe that the behavior is consistent with the person's self-image;
7. have a positive affect regarding the behavior;
8. encounter cues or enablers to act or engage in the behavior at an appropriate time and place.

Theorists generally agree that the first three of these (positive intention, minimal environmental barriers, and skills) may be the critical predictors of any given health-related behavior.

The Health Belief Model

The Health Belief model holds that health behavior is a function of the perceptions an individual has of vulnerability to an illness and the potential effectiveness of treatment that the individual perceives with respect to his or her decision regarding whether to seek medical attention. Developers of the Health Belief model (Becker, 1974; Rosenstock, 1966, 1974) maintained that health-related behaviors are determined by whether individuals (a) perceive themselves to be susceptible to a particular health problem; (b) see this problem as a serious one; (c) are convinced that treatment or prevention activities are effective yet not overly costly in terms of money, effort, or pain; and (d) are exposed to a prompt or cue to take health action. For example, a mother may choose to take her child in for vaccinations if she (a) has seen her neighbors' children get ill from the disease being vaccinated for; (b) has seen other children remain healthy after receiving vaccinations; (c) does not have to pay much for the services; and (d) has heard over the radio that vaccinations will be offered in the coming days at a nearby clinic for reduced charge.

The PRECEDE Model

The PRECEDE model by Green (1984) has received extensive application in health programs. It focuses on examining factors that shape behavioral actions and environmental actions. Behavioral actions are shaped by predisposing, reinforcing, and enabling factors; environmental factors such as availability of preventive services and hazardous workplace conditions are influenced primarily by enabling factors. Predisposing factors provide the motivation or reason behind a behavior; they include knowledge, attitude, cultural beliefs, and readiness for change. Enabling factors make it possible for motivation to be realized; that is, they "enable" persons to act on their predisposition; they include available resources, supportive policies, and services. Reinforcing factors come into play after a behavior has begun, and provide continuing rewards or incentives; they contribute to repetition or persistence of behaviors. Social support, praise, and symptom relief might all be reinforcing factors.

Theory of Reasoned Action

The theory of Reasoned Action places relatively more emphasis on the concept of "behavioral intention," which in turn can be predicted by the person's expectancies regarding the outcomes of a behavior, or their attitudes toward the behavior, and normative beliefs a person has with respect to what "influentials" (especially peers) would do in a specific situation.

Social Cognitive Theory

Social cognitive theory emphasizes the interaction between a person's mental processes (especially knowledge, attitudes, and emotions) on the one hand, and their behavior on the other. The social cognitive emphasis is on the concepts of reciprocal determinism, outcome expectations, and self-efficacy. Outcome expectations, overlapping substantially with parallel concepts in the theory of Reasoned Action and Health Belief model, represent the expectancy that a positive outcome or consequence will occur as a function of the behavior. Self-efficacy (or self-confidence

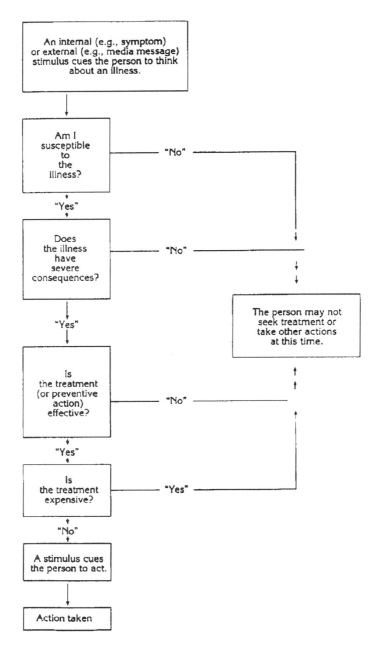

FIGURE 1. Health belief model processes.

with respect to a specific behavior) is a person's own perception of his or her skills with respect to being able to perform a behavior.

In its previous incarnation, social learning theory (Bandura, 1977), the predecessor to social cognitive theory, added "environment" to a three-part description of "person," "behavior," and "environment" interacting dynamically in a process called reciprocal determinism. This addition of the environmental element reflected the social learning theory roots in behavior analysis (the premier school of thought in the broader learning theory field). Interestingly, Bandura subsequently decided to drop the environmental element in his configuration, hence the name change from "learning" to "cognitive."

Behavior Analysis

According to behavior analysis, behaviors may or may not occur as a function of either performance or skills deficits. Performance deficits indicate that the person knows how to perform a given behavior and has the skills to do it but chooses not to engage in the behavior because (a) there are too many aversive consequences for doing so, (b) there are limited if any positive consequences for doing so, or (c) persons are receiving positive reinforcement for performing a different behavior (e.g., acceptance by peers for smoking cigarettes rather than for being physically fit), or some combination.

The notion of skill deficits, on the other hand, implies that a person might like to perform a given behavior but is prevented from doing so by a lack of ability. Remedial efforts are therefore very different for these two types of deficits. The former implies a need to do some "environmental engineering" by way of altering behavior consequence relationships in such a way as to strengthen adaptive behaviors. Skills training, in contrast, would be invoked to address problems in skills deficits.

Behavior analysts also give relatively more credence to observable behaviors and their environmental determinants* and downplay the importance of cognitive processes such as knowledge, attitudes, and emotions.

Stages of Change

The Stages of Change (SOC) model has been applied to a variety of recent health promotion and assessment efforts, including in the areas of smoking cessation and reduction

---

*Such determinants are identified inductively rather than deductively; for example, a "reinforcer" is not labeled as such until the observation is made that the environmental factor has actually strengthened the behavior.

of other addictive behaviors, promotion of condom use, and recently smoking prevention. According to Prochaska and DiClemente (1983), behavior change progresses from a person's being in the precontemplation stage (not even thinking about changing a specific behavior) to the contemplation phase (starting to consider but not yet actually acting on a behavior change course), to the action stage (making the initial steps toward behavior change), to the maintenance stage (maintaining behavior change and not even thinking about going back).

The extent to which the aforementioned theories and models emphasize intentions, barriers, skills, and other psychological variables is included in Table 1.

Critique

The aforementioned leading theories of health behavior change to a great degree emphasize the role of the individual and the individual's thought processes in the development, maintenance, and loss of adaptive health-related behaviors. Most of the theorists actually state that they consider their perspective on health behavior to be universally applicable. Moreover, they imply that for health behavior change efforts to be effective, specific efforts must be made to change these factors that contribute to the adoption of some health behaviors and the failure to adopt others.

But do these theories really apply to peoples from cultures outside of Europe, North America, Australia, and New Zealand, and elsewhere in the world where the European-rooted culture dominates? First, we must look at whether the model of the individual as a relatively autonomous being who evaluates personal potential outcomes in his or her own "self" efficacy regarding behaviors while choosing to listen to or ignore pressure from peers and relatives may be one that is not applicable to more traditional cultures. For example, in other cultures the family and community may be placed above the individual in importance. Normative pressure may

TABLE 1. Relative Emphasis Given Various Psychosocial Variables by Major
Health Behavior Theories[a]

	Health belief model	PRECEDE	Theory of reasoned action	Social cognitive theory	Behavior analysis	Stages of change
Intentions	2	2	3	1	1	2
Barriers	2	3	1	2	3	1
Skills	2	2	1	2	3	1
Outcome expectations/ reinforcement	3	3	3	3	3	2
Self-confidence	1	2	1	3	1	2
Normative pressure	1	2	3	1	2	1
Self-standards	1	2	1	2	0	2
Affect	1	1	2	1	0	1
Prompts/cues	3	3	1	1	3	1

[a]0 = none at all; 1 = little; 2 = substantial; 3 = major

not be seen as something that needs to be considered at all but is directly accepted, regardless of what specific outcome may be incurred. Fatalism may override a person's positive expectations about the benefit of engaging in a specific behavior.

The following presents an examination of the applicability of behavior theories to the American Latino population a) in the context of broader sociopolitical forces at work in American society and b) in light of the fact that roots of this population are in the traditional societies of Latin America while their physical presence is in the United States.

When considering the theoretical models of health behavior, we must keep in mind the ethnographic milieu of their origin. In most cases these models are normalized on stabilized populations; oftentimes college students are used as subjects and instruments are developed to assess White middle-class reaction. We are not bringing to question the reliability or even necessarily the validity of these models but rather their generalizability. Unique populations require unique considerations. When people emigrate from their native land they bring with them the beliefs and values associated with that past. As their new status as an immigrant becomes part of their consciousness and they go through the jolting contact with the dominant culture, they may become dis-associated from these beliefs and values or may cling to them as a source of support and self-worth. This choice, either freely committed or forced, is contextual and can only be understood within a broader health behavior framework.

The Sociopolitical Context

To support the argument that health behavior may be driven by broader societal factors than theoretical factors typically addressed in health behavior theory, we present the three most salient issues affecting immigrants: (1) socioeconomic status, (2) the geographical proximity of the homeland, and (3) the political atmosphere that new immigrants may find themselves part of.

Socioeconomic Status

Where poverty prevails, the priorities of the population are directed at survival needs such as food and shelter. How does this tie in with Mexican immigrant health, when it is reported that the Mexican immigrant's main reason for immigration to the United States is employment (Velez-Ibanez, 1994)? There is a paradox that must be considered.

Although the majority of both male and female immigrants work, they are most likely employed in low-paying jobs. Herein lies the health care paradox. Because of the high rate of employment among Mexican immigrants, they generally do not qualify for state-supported medical assistance. However, as most work at jobs that do not offer health insurance benefits, most are uninsured. Of the Latino immigrants in this country, Mexican immigrants, along with Central and South Americans, are the most likely to lack health insurance or receive state-assisted health care when compared with Cuban Americans and other Latinos. In addition, Hispanics in general are disproportionately represented when it comes to lacking health insurance when compared with Whites-Anglos and African Americans (Johnson *et al.,* 1995).

Demographically, Mexican immigrant families are younger and larger than either White or African American families. In order to obtain health care, basic needs would have to be sacrificed. With limited options, health care becomes unaffordable for most Mexican immigrants, and especially for the 25% of Mexican families living in poverty. Overall, Mexican workers have a lower per capita income than either African Americans or Whites; with earnings being 40% lower than Whites (Johnson *et al.,* 1995; Velez-Ibanez, 1994).

With poverty comes related diseases and health risks. Mexican immigrants living in lower SES communities have a higher incidence of tuberculosis and are experiencing an increase in measles among their children. Obesity is more prevalent among Mexican immigrants, as is AIDS. Further, HIV/AIDS is strongly linked to drug abuse in this population.

Specific to the Mexican immigrants' working as migrant or seasonal farmhands is the high incidence of parasitic infection, as much as 50 times greater than the general population, an infant mortality rate 25% higher than the general population, and life expectancy far below that of the general population (Johnson *et al.,* 1995; Velez-Ibanez, 1994).

These facts suggest that low SES and associated stressors are determinants of health behaviors and risks. To overlook or ignore such evidence, whether by ignorance or due to the complexity of the issues, will result in a biased approach to health care intervention and prevention. Although it is difficult to separate the effects of poverty and related stressors from race and ethnicity in health research and implementation, it is paramount that such variables be considered for results, outcomes, and interpretations to be meaningful. The development of clinically relevant instruments designed to measure these issues should be the focus of ongoing scholarship.

Proximity of the Homeland

As health providers, or individuals interested in the welfare of the migrant, we must take into consideration the unique characteristics of the specific immigrating population. One such attribute specific to Mexican immigrants is the maintenance of close ties with their homeland. The fact that Mexico and the United States share a 2,000-mile border and that one half of the immigrated population lives within 200 miles of that border creates a unique set of circumstances. The symbiotic relationship along the border includes manufacturing, processing, and labor exchange (Velez-Ibanez, 1994). Along with the economic growth, social services including hospitals and clinics have been established for the region's binational population.

An ethnographic view of this situation characterizes the effect as one where the participants freely cross from one culture to the other. This is evidenced by the number of people who live in Mexico, yet work in the United States as well as by the number of Mexicans who live in the United States but shop and maintain close family ties in Mexico. The freedom of movement and familiarity with the homeland may be affecting the utilization of these health services by the Mexican immigrant.

Due in part to the high cost of health care in the United States, the lack of health insurance, and low-wage employment, many Mexican immigrants may be seeking health care in their country of origin. In some cases this care may be traditional, meaning that individuals may seek help from an herbalist, *curandero,* or other traditional healer. In other cases home remedies may promote the use of prescription drugs to treat culturally recognized maladies. Such drugs are readily available in Mexico, often by simply purchasing them over the counter at the local pharmacy. The results of such practice may benefit as well as deleteriously impact a patient.

Political Atmosphere

The sensitivity to immigration of the public in general and the political system in particular is of concern. The new immigrant may find him- or herself in a less than positive atmosphere on arrival.

Politically, the atmosphere is as volatile for the undocumented as well as the legal Mexican immigrant. It is important to note that the difference between undocumented "illegal" and legal immigrant may be distinct in legislation but cloudy in practice. The passage of proposition 187 (Save Our State Initiative) and proposition 209 (California Civil Rights Initiative) in California, a state with a growing Mexican population, and similar legislation in other states rich in Mexican heritage, is clearly directed at curtailing the continued migration of Mexicans to the United States as well as suppressing their upward mobility in the United States.

By legislating the discontinuance of social services to undocumented immigrants and by introducing legislation that negatively affects bilingualism in the public school system, the political machine is feeding the distrust felt by Mexican immigrants toward the dominant Anglo system. The clear message is that Mexican immigrants are not to achieve the "American dream" and are considered unwelcome. The feelings of distrust engendered by such a message are certainly transferred to the social services, including health services, that are, for the most part, staffed by English-speaking Americans.

The distrust by the Mexican immigrant was made apparent when the Immigration and Control Act of 1986 offered amnesty for undocumented aliens, giving legal status if proof of residency since 1982 could be produced; less than 50% of the estimated 2 million eligible aliens applied by the beginning of 1988. Given that normative support is important in the Mexican culture, it is safe to argue that family dynamics influenced the decision to ignore the amnesty offer. The consensus among scholars is that mistrust of the system was the main impediment, with the disruption of the family unit as the greatest fear (Chilman, 1993).

It is not a great leap to extrapolate and suggest that the underutilization of health services by Mexican immigrants may, in part, be based on mistrust and fear of the dominant system—a system that on the one hand closes its eyes to the exploitation of the immigrant as cheap labor and on the other hand denigrates and socially ostracizes that citizenship.

It is imperative that the values and conditions of our growing multicultural and pluralistic population be given consideration and incorporated into mainstream wellness programs. By working with ethnic health organizations and promoting health education through community advertising considerate of language and literacy, we can enhance the utilization and effectiveness of health programs.

The overt anti-immigration sentiments of this country need to be touched on to fully understand the plight of the Mexican immigrant. Such nationwide beliefs affect the well-being of immigrants. Without an understanding of the psychological comfort level of the immigrant, health policy and treatment will miss their marks.

Nationwide there are several well-established anti-immigration organizations working with substantial budgets. The Federation for American Enterprise (FAIR) operates on an annual budget of $1.7 million and boasts 50,000 supporters. The American Immigration Control Foundation works with $2.2

million and is larger in membership than FAIR, and the National Association for the Advancement of White People, which many consider to spread the most extreme anti-immigration message, reports a membership of 40,000. The common threads that tie these and other anti-immigration organizations together include xenophobia, discrimination, and racism. The overriding erroneous belief of these organizations is that immigration negatively impacts U.S. resources; for example, immigrants will take jobs that would otherwise go to Americans or, contradictorily, that immigrants are generally illiterate, uneducated, and unskilled and are therefore unable to work, and will therefore become a drain on the education, health, and welfare systems. Many of these organizations target Mexican immigration specifically.

Positions taken by more respected, mainstream organizations may less directly reinforce relatively dangerous anti-immigration proponents. For example, the Sierra Club with a membership of 500,000 and an annual budget of $29.9 million also supports anti-immigration. The Sierra Club shares the sentiments of organizations such as Zero Population Growth, Californians for Population Stabilization, Negative Population Growth, and others that feel that immigration may negatively impact America's social stability and environment.* The aforementioned organizations have strong lobbyists in Washington, D.C., advocating anti-immigration legislation. Such legislation has resulted in more stringent immigration laws, sanctions on employers who hire undocumented workers, and an increase in border guards, and in general contribute to an overwhelming anti-Mexican sentiment. Such a sentiment would be difficult for an immigrant, whether documented or not, to ig-

nore. Further, the resultant fear and distrust transfers to all government organizations including health and educational services.

Analysis of Latin American Culture: Major Themes and Differences

A person's cultural beliefs affect the manner in which they perceive health, illness, and the prevention and treatment of illness. Within a broader social framework, community perceptions of health and illness have great potential to influence individual health beliefs and behaviors, particularly if the culture is more community or family centered than centered on the individual. U.S. mainstream culture, for example, is perceived to be more individualistic; personal preference is given priority over community preference. In contrast, traditional Latino culture is more community oriented, and individual preferences may come after family or community needs have been met. It is within this context of individual versus community-centered perceptions that we wish to explore application and appropriateness of health promotion theories for U.S. Latino populations.

According to the 1990 census, approximately 9% of the U.S. population was Hispanic. This percentage is expected to increase to 11% by the year 2000. As Latinos are the fastest growing ethnic group in the United States (Mikhail, 1994), it is of increasing relevance for public health professionals and health care providers to understand common Latino cultural beliefs and behaviors as they relate to potential health outcomes and disease patterns. An important part of the process of gaining this understanding is to appreciate the cross-ethnic differences and similarities between Latino subgroups. Persons of Mexican descent comprise the largest proportion of U.S. Latinos and represent diverse sociopolitical and religious realities based on their state of origin. Clusters of populations from other parts of Latin America (e.g.,

---

*Even though the pro-environmental stance of these groups is inherent hypocrisy in unilateral attention to population growth problems without addressing the more important issue of excessive consumerism.

Puerto Rico, Cuba, Central America) also contribute to U.S. Latino population diversity.

Latino Cultural Beliefs surrounding Illness: An Overview

Persons of Latin American origin, although in many cases culturally diverse, hold many common beliefs with respect to their views on health and illness. Latinos generally rely more on the family and community to help than on institutional health care programs (United Way of San Diego County, 1991). How an individual conceptualizes an illness depends on their ethnocultural beliefs, personal and idiosyncratic beliefs, and biomedical concepts.

An underlying belief system that influences the perceived origins of illness in many Latino cultures includes a belief in balance of hot and cold, similar to the yin–yang philosophy in Chinese culture. This theory implies that there is a "hot" and "cold" equilibrium in the body, and that an illness may be producing disequilibrium. In this theory, illness and treatments of illness may also be categorized as either hot or cold, where certain "hot" ailments should be remedied with a "cold" treatment to restore balance (Autotte, 1995). Some illnesses are recognized in the biomedical model; however, there is also a subset of illnesses that may have a spiritual or nonbiomedical origin. These illnesses are termed folk illnesses and may be defined as illnesses that are common within a cultural group, and whose explanations often conflict with that of western biomedicine (Pachter, 1994).

Religion holds an important place in Latino culture, and influences health beliefs. Although a majority of Latinos are nominal, if not practicing, Catholics, public health advocates must be aware that Protestant conversion has occurred throughout Latin America, and may impact the "traditional" Catholic belief system that influences health. Within the predominantly Catholic Latino community, however, major life events are often tied to religion or the Church (United Way of San

Diego County, 1991). Latino belief in fatalism, for example, is closely tied with the concept that "our health is in the hands of God." Prior to Spanish conquest and the imposition of Catholicism, this hemisphere's indigenous groups had their own highly developed religions and belief systems. Upon conquest, indigenous peoples sought ways to incorporate their own gods or beliefs into the imposed Catholic religion. For example, the Catholic belief in saints who hold special "powers" became a means by which indigenous gods could be incorporated into the Catholic religious structure and could continue to be worshipped (as saints). Further, as Catholicism involves a variety of rituals, native rituals were incorporated as part of the newer religion. Still today in the southeastern Mexican states of Chiapas and Oaxaca, and throughout Guatemala, indigenous rituals are performed as part of regular church worship. The *Dia de los Muertos* (Day of the Dead) celebrated on All Saints Day (November 2) by people of Mexican descent everywhere, is a product of both indigenous rituals and Catholic beliefs. Although this syncretism has evolved somewhat, it pervades the belief systems of many Latino immigrants, and is part of the oftentimes complex perception of faith, healing, and illness.

As we address health behavior and illness in Latino communities, other sociocultural forces, such as access to medical care and cultural acceptability of prevention strategies, must be addressed in order to better focus health promotion strategies in this population.

Factors Influencing Latino Health Beliefs and Practices

Health beliefs and health behaviors are also influenced by the medical or therapeutic resources available to an individual. When clinical treatment is unavailable, Latinos often turn to self-treatment. Thus home treatments are not uncommon in Latino culture. For example, a parent may first choose to treat a child's conjunctivitis with chamomile tea because this therapy is culturally acceptable, is available and inexpensive, and does not require a trip to the physician. If the condition does not improve, however, consultation with a health care provider may be the next step. Across studies, there is a tendency for families to attempt home remedies before proceeding to another form of medical care. One author stated that "most Hispanics seek medical care only when their illness is severe, relying on other systems for help and support" (Mikhail, 1994). Fishman, Bobo, Kosub, and Womeodu (1993) stated that even among persons of low socioeconomic status there are differences in health care use across ethnicity. Social isolation—low or poor interaction with the surrounding society—may also result in underutilization of health care (Fishman *et al.*, 1993). Social isolation may stem from a variety of factors such as lack of transportation or financial resources, fear of being deported due to documentation status, or geographic distance from the community. This type of isolation reduces the likelihood that the family will seek formal health services or participate in health promotion efforts geared toward the surrounding society. As a whole, social isolation, poverty, and lack of health care coverage may encourage individuals to postpone professional treatment in the hope that the illness will resolve itself (Mikhail, 1994).

Acculturation and Health

Issues

There has been a considerable amount of research examining the underlying characteristics of acculturation but an exact operational definition has yet to be established. In 1936, Redfield, Lintion, and Herskovits defined acculturation as "comprehending those phenomena which result when groups of individuals having different cultures come into continuous first-hand contact, with subsequent changes in the original cultural patterns of either or both groups" (quoted in

Cuellar, Arnold, & Maldonado, 1995, p. 278). Burnam, Hough, Teles, and Escobar (1987) simplified acculturation to mean the "changes that occur in behaviors and values made by members of a culture as a result of contact with another culture" (p. 106). In 1988, Escobar described acculturation as a process in which an individual's attitudes and behaviors shift from those of his or her culture of origin toward those of the dominant culture (cited in Orozco, Thompson, Kapes, & Montgomery, 1993). Currently, researchers call for an understanding of acculturation as a bidimensional process. It is a long-term process in which individuals learn or adapt, or both, certain aspects of the dominant culture while retaining most or some aspects of their culture of origin (Anderson *et al.*, 1993; Marin & Gamba, 1996), and may move comfortably between cultures. Thus, an individual may be acculturated to the new and dominant culture, to the native culture, or to both.

There is a growing scientific debate as to whether acculturation to the Anglicized American society presents greater socioeconomic opportunities or threatens the health and social fabric of immigrating populations. Increased acculturation is often associated with poorer health outcomes and a variety of disorders and diseases. At times, although less frequently, acculturation is a protective factor. An example of this duality can be found in studies on sexual behavior in Latinas. In studies of Latina adolescents, highly acculturated females are more likely than their low acculturated counterparts to report current sexual activity. Highly acculturated females are also more likely to have had at least one sexual partner in the previous year, to have non-Latino partners, and to have oral and anal sex (VanOss Marin & Flores, 1994). Among sexually active Latinas, highly acculturated females are also more likely to use a condom. In this example, higher acculturation is associated with increased sexual activity (risky behavior) and use of condoms (protective behavior).

The maladaptive effect of acculturation is also illustrated when examining patterns of alcohol use. Acculturation among Latinas is strongly associated with an increase in alcohol consumption and alcohol problems (Canino & Spurlock, 1994). Mexican women prior to migration are, for the most part, abstainers. Once emigrated to the United States and as the level of acculturation rises, the use of alcohol also increases (Zimmerman & Sodowsky, 1993). Diet and nutrition also seem to be adversely affected by acculturation; that is, there seems to be an association between higher levels of Latino acculturation and poorer diet, presumably because the immigrant tends to move away from the "native" healthier diet to more fast food, with lower nutrient values. The acculturation process can also work differentially within the population and varies by gender and age. For example, Marin, Perez-Stable, and Marin (1989) reported higher age-adjusted smoking rates among the *less* acculturated males and among the *more* acculturated females.

Such a contradiction of findings is not unusual in the literature's attempt to explain the role that acculturation plays in health related behaviors. As we endeavor to understand the complex relationships between acculturation and health behaviors, it is important to consider factors such as the socioeconomic and educational levels, and urban versus rural origin of the immigrant, variables that will also influence immigrant response to health promotion efforts. Moreover, as immigrants "anglicize," the American culture has also gradually shifted toward incorporating more aspects of Latino culture, as evidenced by the successful inroads of Caribbean and Andean music, Latino film stars, and most notably, Mexican cuisine. Thus, a better understanding of acculturation is vital to fully understand the role it plays in the health arena.

Acculturation Measurements

One of the challenges of introducing acculturation measurement in health behavior studies for any population is the myriad of ways in which acculturation has been defined. Because acculturation is a multidimensional phenomenon, it is a difficult construct to measure.

Variables. Currently, the measurement of acculturation is centered around behavioral variables with language as the dominant factor. Sociocultural variables, such as preferences for friends, foods, value and attitude orientations, and ethnic pride and identity, are being examined (Anderson *et al.,* 1993; Orozco *et al.,* 1993). One of the most respected and widely used instruments is the Acculturation Rating Scale for Mexican-Americans (ARSMA) developed by Cuellar, Harris, and Jasso in 1980 and revised in 1995 by Cuellar and colleagues (ARSMA-II). A factor analysis of the ARSMA conducted by Orozco and colleagues (1993) revealed five elements considered significant in the measurement of acculturation. These elements were (a) language familiarity and usage (LFU), (b) ethnic pride and identity (EPI), (c) ethnic interaction (EI), (d) cultural heritage (CH), and (e) generational proximity (GP). These variables have become the standard criteria for measuring acculturation in various health settings (Burnam *et al.,* 1987; Cuellar *et al.,* 1995; Deyo, Diehl, Hazuda, & Stern, 1985; Klonoff & Landrine, 1996; Marin & Gamba, 1996; Marin, Sabogal, VanOssMarin, Otero-Sabogal, & Perez-Stable, 1987; Markides, Ray, Stroup-Benham, & Treviño, 1990; Orozco *et al.,* 1993; Suinn, Ahuna, &Khoo, 1992).*

The ARSMA-II (Cuellar *et al.,* 1995) incorporates the same multidimensional factors as its predecessor, the ARSMA, and reflects the new perspective on acculturation by shifting from a linear representation of acculturation to a bidirectional and orthogonal view of acculturation, as does the Bi-dimensional Acculturation Scale for Hispanics (BAS; Marin & Gamba, 1996). For example, a Mexican American could be either highly

---

*The scales developed by Suinn, Ahuna, and Khoo, 1992, and Konoff & Landrine, 1996, were designed to assess acculturation in Asians and African Americans, respectively.

"Mexican" or "Anglo" in character on identification, or both.

Theory. Although the current thought is
shifting toward a bidimensional assessment
of acculturation (Cuellar *et al.,* 1995; Marin
& Gamba, 1996), the linear model of acculturation is still a commonly applied assessment concept (Norris, Ford, & Bova, 1996).
The linear representation suggests that an individual moves along a continuum with culture of origin at one endpoint and dominant
culture at the other endpoint. As an individual moves along the continuum in one direction, their cultural orientation toward the
culture of origin decreases and is accompanied by a corresponding increase in orientation to the dominant culture. The result of
such a process is that for acculturation to
occur there has to be a reduction in cultural
orientation toward the culture of origin.

The measurement of acculturation has
been developed to reflect this unidirectional
view. Items on acculturation instruments are
logically structured so that responding in one
direction automatically results in an opposite
or opposing value in orientation. Consequently, results are limited in distinguishing
variability in acculturation.

The theoretical view of acculturation as a
bidirectional process allows complex variations of acculturative types to be distinguished. Such a view is assessed through the
unidirectional measure of both orientations.
That is, the linear relationships are from low
orientation to culture of origin to high orientation to culture of origin (SO) and similarly,
from low orientation to new (dominant) culture to high orientation to new culture (DS).

The bidirectional approach of the ARSMA-
II (Cuellar *et al.,* 1995) distinguishes four acculturative types as they relate to the four
quadrants created by the orthogonal relationship of the two dimensions. This construct
can be measured only by employing two distinct sets of assessment factors, each set (or
scale) unique to the orientation of concern.
The resulting acculturative typologies include
(a) a highly integrated bicultural, as distinguished by scoring high on both the Scale of
Origin (SO) and the Dominant Scale (DS), (b)
origin-oriented bicultural distinguished by
scoring high on SO and low on DS, (c) low-
integrated bicultural as someone who scores
low on OS and low on DS,* and (d) assimilated bicultural, as indicated by a low score on
OS and a high score on DS† (Cuellar *et al.,*
1995). Although it has yet to be adequately
evaluated, it is theorized that each of these
"degrees of acculturation" is associated with a
level of health risk. Individuals scoring high
on both the SO and the DS (high-integrated
bicultural) are at least risk for negative health
behaviors and outcomes, while those scoring
low on both SO and DS (low-integrated bicultural) are most likely to exhibit negative
health outcomes or to practice high-risk
health behaviors.

Psychometrics. There was little by way of
psychometric considerations in the development of the earlier acculturation measures. In
some cases factor analysis and reliability coefficients were established after the fact, as in
the case of the very popular and still used
ARSMA (Orozco *et al.,* 1993). For the most
part, items were written that, a priori, were
considered to measure an acculturative dimension (Marin & Gamba, 1996). However,
the more recent measures are addressing this
shortcoming.

Close scrutiny of the instruments used in
the measurement of acculturation in empirical health research reveals a dependence on,
or utilization of, language related items,
stressing familiarity and usage (LFU) as a
dominant factor predictive of acculturative
level. Another factor that is often used to
measure acculturation is ethnic identity (EI).
The rationale for utilization of this variable is
based on allocentrism or collectivism. Allo-

---

*The low OS-DS person could be an immigrant who is
isolated from his or her own people. Another example
would be a mixtec or other indigenous person who integrated to the United States from Latin America but has
lived on the margins of both societies (Bade, 1994).
†The labeling is directly adapted from ARSMA-II (Cuellar *et al.,* 1995).

centrism characterizes a population as having a collective viewpoint of needs, values, and goals rather than an individualistic viewpoint that personalizes such constructs (Marin *et al.*, 1987).

Ethnic identity appears to be indicative and a strong correlate of acculturation. However, this variable has limited clinical significance, and using it as a proxy for acculturation may contribute to the confusing and at times contradictory results in health research. Language, on the other hand, appears to be both statistically and clinically important. However, one must consider whether language, as a construct, can be considered a determinant of the beliefs, values, and resources that are changing during the acculturative process.

Rigorous methodology has been exacted in translation and back-translation of instruments in order to achieve a culturally equivalent meaning in the process. Nevertheless, "language differences present a set of difficulties that go beyond simple translation; in particular, the cultural relevance of the linguistic qualifiers that are used in close-ended questions and are subsequently manipulated into scales for statistical analysis may be problematic" (Johnson *et al.*, 1995, p. 607). It is important to consider whether the basic construct of an instrument is cross-culturally relevant. As researchers are able to account for the multidimensional nature of acculturation, measurements will improve. It is important for health promotion efforts, however, to bear in mind that acculturation measurements serve as proxies to describe the cultural reality of any given immigrant group, and should be only one of the instruments employed by health professionals.

Theory Review: Immigrant Health and Health Promotion

This section addresses the applicability of theories of health behavior change to cultures other than those rooted in European American history. For example, will an AIDS prevention program that is proven successful in a White, middle-class suburb of a large, multicultural, metropolitan community be efficacious "across town" in a different cultural setting? Or, in general, can a model for health behavior change based on White, middle-class subjects cross ethnic and cultural boundaries? Specifically, these theories of change will be explored as they relate to the health behaviors of Latinos.

Rather than examine each of the five theories of health behavior this section focuses on the common factors they share. Three factors, positive intention, minimal environmental barriers, and skills, considered necessary and sufficient for producing any behavior, are reviewed and examples of their application to Latinos and especially Mexican immigrants are given. With respect to intention, five additional supporting factors (positive outcome, normative support, self-image, positive affect [emotional reaction], and perceived self-efficacy) thought to indirectly affect the strength and direction of intention are also discussed. However, it should be noted that these five factors alone or in combination may have a direct influence on health behavior.

Intention

The application of the five underlying factors of intent in the context of the Mexican immigrant is presented here. Intention can be viewed as the strength of a person's commitment to perform or try to perform a behavior. When considering the application of intention to health-related prevention and intervention, it is important to keep in mind the underlying cultural context in which such intentions occur.

Self-Image

It is often recognized that a person's perception of self may influence behavior even in the absence of an outcome expectancy. Considering the behavior consistent or inconsistent with a person's self-image is the motivating factor in performing the behavior. The more one perceives that he or she is the type to perform a specific behavior the stronger the intention to perform such a behavior becomes. When conceptually applied to health care prevention and intervention programs, understanding a population culture and how its members perceive themselves becomes vital.

For example, the Mexican immigrant imports sex practices that are culturally acceptable among Mexicans. The Mexican male distinguishes between *activo* and *pasivo* same-sex relations. In male same-sex contact, the *activo* participant inserts during anal intercourse, whereas the *pasivo* receives during anal intercourse. The distinction is important because in the role of *activo* the masculine self-image of Mexican *machismo* is not threatened. Mexicans do not consider the *activo* partner homosexual (Singer & Baer, 1995). Thus, a program focused on developing AIDS awareness and targeting Latino gays, without considering their unique self-image, may suffer in efficacy.

Cultural understanding includes awareness of values and views specific to an ethnic group. A factor that may influence self-image in Mexican immigrants is their traditional view on fatalism, the belief that all things in life are preordained. It is suggested that such a belief is based on the strong influence that Catholicism has on the Mexican population. To subscribe to Catholic tenets is to believe that (1) sacrifice is helpful to salvation, (2) charity is a virtue, and (3) one should endure wrongs. The consequences of these views for many Mexicans is a fatalistic outlook, that is, a belief that problems of events are meant to be and cannot be changed (Sue & Sue, 1990).

Such an outlook imparts a sense of disempowerment and resignation that are characteristic of depression and thought to be maladaptive in an individualistic culture. However, when fatalism and religiosity are viewed as complementary resources, the negative effects of fatalism may be offset. In a collective culture, such as the Mexican culture, a fatalistic orientation is hypothesized to be adaptive, whereas it is thought to be maladaptive in an individualistic culture, such as

the U.S. culture (Neff & Hoppe, 1995). The health behavior implications of such abdication over personal control can impact the receptivity to intervention and preventive programs. When an individual's self-image is of one who deserves to suffer, modification of negative lifestyle behaviors are less likely to occur. Nor is the importance of a healthy lifestyle as critical (Pepitone, 1995).

Normative Support

It is also important for researchers and providers to recognize the appropriate referent group of an immigrant's culture. Unlike the Anglo characteristic of seeking support, not from family but more likely from friends, neighbors, or coworkers (Gottlieb & Green, 1980), Latino immigrants bring with them a strong sense of familism. Familism has been described as a strong identification and attachment of individuals with their families, both nuclear and extended. Such an attachment promotes loyalty, unity, reciprocity, and solidarity (Sabogal, Marin, Otero-Sabogal, VanOss Marin, & Perez-Stable, 1987). Thus, when discussing health care matters with Latinos, the health care provider is either directly or indirectly discussing diagnosis and treatment recommendations with the patient's entire family (Council on Scientific Affairs, 1991). In a study of Latino immigrants by Apodaca, Woodruff, Candelaria, Elder, and Zlot, (1997), perceived family support was significant in an individual decision to participate in a heart health promotion program. An article by Sabogal and colleagues (1987) asserted that "despite changes in acculturation [family support] is the most essential dimension of Hispanic familism" (p. 397). Such collective identity is a factor that must be calculated in the development of health programs targeting Latinos in general and Mexican immigrants specifically.

Positive Outcome Expectations

Another factor governing the intention of minority immigrants to use orthodox health care systems is the belief that the benefits will outweigh the costs. Such beliefs are based on interpretation of personal experiences and knowledge and access to culturally traditional or unorthodox health care.

In the world at large, traditional medicine is practiced more often than Western medicine (Pepitone, 1995). As people migrate, they do so in the company of traditional healers with whom they can consult and receive treatment. Mexican immigrants are no different; among them in their adopted country are herbalists, spiritualists, *curanderos,* and other folk practitioners. The new immigrant, who historically is at a lower socioeconomic level, has little experience with Western medicine. Not only does this population lack knowledge and experience of Western medicine, but also they often cannot afford the cost, are less likely to have health care insurance, and may be suspicious of some treatments associated with it (Masi, Mensah, & McLeod, 1995). Too frequently, the only contact with Western medicine is the emergency room or free-clinic visit; unable to afford the costs of follow-up visits or prescribed medications the Mexican immigrant abandons Western medicine for more affordable traditional services or home remedies (Johnson *et al.,* 1995). Where poverty is the norm, limited resources are directed to meeting the basics of life, such as shelter and food. The benefits of preventive health care measures are far outweighed by the financial costs of securing such benefits.

Positive Effect

Western medicine is often perceived as a final option by the Mexican immigrant. Masi and colleagues (1995) described a five-level health care option model that was developed by Toumishey. The five-level model begins with awareness of a health problem and ends with orthodox care, with levels 2, 3, and 4 being self-care, folk or popular care, and unorthodox care, respectively. From such a model we see that there are three health care choices more familiar and acceptable to the immigrant than Western medical care, and such traditional care is perceived to be more accessible. These same factors would make culturally traditional care more emotionally satisfying, as it is familiar and trusted. According to theories of emotional responses, an environment that is perceived to be favorable or propitious is more likely to elicit a positive emotional reaction (Zimbardo, 1992).

Self-Efficacy

The final variable viewed as influencing the strength and direction of intention is self-efficacy. Self-efficacy refers to one's confidence in the ability to perform specific behaviors in particular situations. That is, one cannot say that an individual has high or low self-efficacy without reference to the specific circumstance or behavior (Bandura, 1977). It would be hard to imagine how self-efficacy could be influenced by culture, except for the four sources from which efficacy expectations are learned.

The first source of self-efficacy is through performance accomplishments. This refers to personally experiencing a situation or feared task with a consequent sense of mastery. In addition, the more an individual successfully experiences a situation or task the higher the related self-efficacy. The second source of self-efficacy is through vicarious experience which includes learning through observation of people, events, or both. For example, a recent immigrant who sees her more established counterpart successfully deal with a health clinic visit may have greater confidence in dealing with such a situation (and associated tasks) herself.

Verbal persuasion, a method with which most health caregivers are familiar, is the third source for engendering self-efficacy. However, evidence suggests that the source of exhortation is significant. Studies indicate that a message from one who is liked is more persuasive than from one who is disliked; human beings are more prone to like someone and find them more credible the more similar they are to themselves (Baron & Byrne, 1994;

Zimbardo, 1992). Thus, a health care worker who is dissimilar in appearance and language usage may attenuate the perceived self-efficacy of an immigrant patient. The final factors influencing self-efficacy are cues from one's physiological state. A highly aroused physiological state such as an anxiety reaction may impair performance, resulting in an unsuccessful experience and, thus, lead to lowered self-efficacy. That is, a highly aroused physiological state may inhibit self-efficacy (Baron & Byrne, 1994).

Considering the underlying factors it becomes clear how self-efficacy can be affected by immigrant status. For example, many new immigrants, especially those of lower socioeconomic status, may never have experienced Western-type medicine, either personally or vicariously. Furthermore, verbal persuasions by the families and friends of these people may be directed to traditional healing methods and, thus, dissuade them from using modern medicine. Finally, it would not be hard to imagine a high level of anxiety in a newly arrived immigrant when confronted with a modern clinic or hospital and the related paperwork frequently in a language foreign to the immigrant.

Environmental Facilitators and Constraints

Consistent especially with behavior analysis, but at least to some extent with the other health behavior theories as well, is the notion that reinforcement and barrier reduction will promote behavior whereas punishment and barrier imposition will impede it. Health status is integrally related to the immigrant's sociocultural environment that may have customs contrary to positive health behavior. In research conducted by Moreno and colleagues (1994) such behavior was examined. This study reported that Mexican parents who smoked involved their children significantly more often in the behavior (e.g., buying cigarettes, lighting their parents' cigarettes for them) than Anglo parents who smoked. The hypothesis that such reductions of barriers

would be predictive of future tobacco use in Latino youths was supported.

Social and economic status (a larger societal issue as well; see previous section) can also affect the health behavior of the immigrant. There is ample evidence that inequalities such as lower education, unemployment, poverty, and lower health persist in the overcrowded *barrios* to which new arrivals migrate and which they often never leave (Council on Scientific Affairs, 1991; Zambrana & Ellis, 1995). Health clinics in such areas are often found to be understaffed and in short supply, limiting availability and access to health care. Conversely, such areas are targets for promotion of alcohol and tobacco products—products associated with a high incidence of cancer and heart disease.

The literature reports numerous barriers to health care that exist for immigrants. Among the predominant ones are low income (poverty), limited access to health education due to language barriers, limited education in general, low literacy, limited health insurance, immigration status, and a single-parent family structure (Council on Scientific Affairs, 1991; Masi *et al.*, 1995; Zambrana & Ellis, 1995). Other cited barriers are institutional discrimination, a distrust of Western medicine and associated health care providers, a general suspicion of the new bureaucracy, and finally, the itinerant habits of the migrant population (Acosta, 1979; Amezcua, McAlister, Ramirez, & Espinoza, 1990; Zambrana & Ellis, 1995).

Skills

When investigating wellness behavior and methods of change, attention must be given to skills and skill deficits. We explore skills in two dimensions: (1) knowledge of the actions necessary to perform a specific behavior and the ability to perform those behaviors, and (2) intra- and interpersonal resources. Clearly, an individual who does not understand or have knowledge required or lacks the required physical or mental ability is unlikely to successfully perform a specific behavior. Similarly, if an individual lacks social negotiation skills or internal cognitive or emotional resources or both, it is unlikely that a specified behavior will occur. Elder and Stern (1986) suggested that neither of these dimensions stand alone but rather interact to strengthen behavior change.

A culturally sensitive application of a skills model requires that skills training be linguistically and culturally appropriate, taking into account the literacy level of the individual or specific population. Such a model would refrain from falling into a common trap, that of patient and provider misunderstanding, due to either lack of cultural awareness by the health provider or language deficit by the patient.

Conclusion

Although we have explored the underlying factors common to the six theories of health behavior change as they relate to the Mexican immigrant, it is plausible to extrapolate much of the above information to other Hispanics (i.e., Puerto Ricans, Cuban Americans, Central or South Americans) as well as other ethnic groups and cultures. Inasmuch as health behavior is culture bound, an ethnocentric view of health behavior intervention and prevention programs falls short of the understanding needed to design and conduct valid health behavior research and promote full utilization of resources. In addition, other sources of and restrictions on health services need to be considered. Health providers and researchers must look beyond their own horizons to better understand the complexity of the migrant's health behaviors.

References

Acosta, F. X. (1979). Barriers between mental health services and Mexican Americans: An examination of a paradox. *American Journal of Community Psychology, 7,* 503–520.

Ajzen, I., & Fishbein, M. (1980). *Understanding attitudes and predicting social behavior.* Englewood Cliffs, NJ: Prentice-Hall.

Amezcua, C., McAlister, A., Ramirez, A., & Espinoza, R. (1990). A su salud: Health promotion in a Mexican-American border community. In N. Bracht (Ed.), *Health promotion at the community level* (pp. 257–277). London: Sage.

Anderson, J., Moeschberger, M., Chen, M. S., Kunn, P., Jr., Wewers, M. E., & Guthrie, R. (1993). An acculturation scale for Southeast Asians. *Social Psychiatry, Psychiatric Epidemiology, 28,* 133–141.

Apodaca, J. X., Woodruff, S. I., Candelaria, J., Elder, J. P., & Zlot, A. (1997). Hispanic health program participant and nonparticipant characteristics. *American Journal of Health Behavior, 21*(5), 356–363.

Autotte, P. (1995). Folk medicine. *Archives of Pediatric and Adolescent Medicine, 149*(9), 949–950.

Bade, B. L. (1994). *Sweatbaths, sacrifice and surgery: The practice of transmedical health care by mixtec migrant families in California.* Unpublished doctoral dissertation, University of California, Riverside.

Bandura, A. (1977). *Social learning theory.* Englewood Cliffs, NJ: Prentice Hall.

Bandura, A. (1986). *Social foundations of thought and action: A social cognitive theory.* Englewood Cliffs, NJ: Prentice-Hall.

Bandura, A. (1989). Perceived self-efficacy in the exercise of personal agency. *Psychologist: Bulletin of the British Psychological Society, 10,* 411–424.

Bandura, A. (1991). A social cognitive approach to the exercise of control over AIDS infection. In R. DiClemente (Ed.), *Adolescents and AIDS: A generation in jeopardy* (pp. 1–20). Beverly Hills, CA: Sage.

Baron, R. A., & Byrne, D. (1994). *Social psychology* (8th ed.). Boston: Allyn & Bacon.

Becker, M. (1974). The health belief model and personal health behavior. *Health Education Monographs, 2,* 324–508.

Burnam, A. M., Hough, R. L., Teles, C. A., & Escobar, J. I. (1987). Measurement of acculturation in a community population of Mexican-Americans, *Hispanic Journal of Behavioral Sciences, 9*(2), 105–130.

Canino, I. A., & Spurlock, J. (1994). *Culturally diverse children and adolescents.* New York: Guilford.

Chilman, C. S. (1993). Hispanic families in the U.S.: Research perspectives. In H. P. McAdoo (Ed.), *Family ethnicity: Strength in diversity* (pp. 141–163). Newbury Park, CA: Sage.

Council on Scientific Affairs. (1991). Hispanic health in the United States. *Journal of the American Medical Association, 262,* 248–257.

Cuellar, I., Harris, L. C., & Jasso, R. (1980). An acculturation scale for Mexican American normal and clinical populations. *Hispanic Journal of Behavioral Sciences. 2*(3), 199–217.

Cuellar, I., Arnold, B., & Maldonado, R. (1995). Acculturation Rating Scale for Mexican Americans–II: A

Revision of the original ARSMA Scale. *Hispanic Journal of Behavioral Sciences, 17*, 275–304.

Deyo, R. A., Diehl, A. K., Hazuda, H., & Stern, M. P. (1985). A simple language-based acculturation scale for Mexican Americans: Validation and application to health care research. *American Journal of Public Health, 75*(1), 51–55.

Elder, J. P., & Stern, R. A. (1986). The abc's of adolescent smoking prevention: An environment and skills model. *Health Education Quarterly, 13*(2), 181–191.

Elder, J. P., Geller, E. S., Hovell, M. H., & Mayer, J. A. (1994). *Motivating health behavior.* New York: Delmar.

Fishbein, M. (1980). A theory of Reasoned Action: Some applications and implications. In H. Howe & M. Page (Eds.), *Nebraska Symposium on Motivation*, 1979 (pp. 65–116). Lincoln: University of Nebraska Press.

Fishbein, M., & Ajzen, I. (1975). *Belief, attitude, intention and behavior: An introduction to theory and research.* Boston: Addison-Wesley.

Fishman, B., Bobo, L., Kosub, K., & Womeodu, R. (1993). Cultural issues in serving minority populations: Emphasis on Mexican Americans and African Americans. *American Journal of the Medical Sciences, 306*(3), 160–166.

Gottlieb, N. H., & Green, L. W. (1980, Summer). Ethnicity and lifestyle health risk: Some possible mechanisms. *American Journal of Health Promotion,* 37–51.

Green, L. W. (1984). Modifying and developing health behaviors. In L. Breslow, J. A. Fielding, & L. B. Lave (Eds.), *Annual review of public health* (Vol. 5, pp. 215–236). Palo Alto, CA: Annual Reviews.

Green, L. W., & Kreuter, M. W. (1991). *Health promotion planning: An educational and environment approach* (2nd ed.). Mountain View, CA: Mayfield.

Janz, N., & Becker, M. (1984). The health belief model: A decade later. *Health Education Quarterly, 11,* 1–47.

Johnson, W. K., Anderson, B. N., Bastida, E., Kramer, J. B., Williams, D., & Morton, W. (1995). Macrosocial and environmental influences on minority health. *Health Psychology, 14,* 601–612.

Klonoff, E. A., & Ladrine, H. (1996). Acculturation and cigarette smoking among African American adults. *Journal of Behavioral Medicine, 19*(5), 501–514.

Marin, G., & Gamba, R. J. (1996). A new measurement of acculturation for Hispanics: The bidimensional acculturation scale for Hispanics (BAS). *Hispanic Journal of Behavioral Sciences, 18*(3), 297–316.

Marin, G., Sabogal, F., VanOss Marin, B., Otero-Sabogal, R., & Perez-Stable, E. (1987). Development of a Short Acculturation Scale for Hispanics. *Hispanic Journal of Behavioral Sciences, 9,* 196–198.

Marin, G., Perez-Stable, E. J., & Marin, B. V. (1989). Cigarette smoking among San Francisco Hispanics:

The role of acculturation and gender. *American Journal of Public Health, 2,* 183–205.

Markides, K. S., Ray, L. A., Stroup-Benham, C. A., & Treviño, F. (1990). Acculturation and alcohol consumption in the Mexican American population of the Southwestern United States: Findings from HHANES 1982–84. *American Journal of Public Health, 80,* 420–446.

Masi, R., Mensah, L., & McLeod, K. A. (1995). *Health cultures: Policies, professional practice and education* (Vol. 1). London: Mosaic.

Mikhail, B. I. (1994). Hispanic mothers' beliefs and practices regarding selected children's health problems. *Western Journal of Nursing Research, 16,* 623–638.

Moreno, C., Laniado-Laborin, R., Sallis, J. F., Elder, J. P., De Moor, C., Deosaransingh, K., & Castro, F. (1994). Parental influences to smoke in Latino youth. *Preventive Medicine, 23,* 48–53.

Neff, A. J., & Hoppe, S. K. (1995). Race/ethnicity, acculturation and psychological distress: Fatalism and religiosity as cultural resources. *Journal of Community Psychology, 21,* 3–20.

Norris, A. E., Ford, K., & Bova, C. A. (1996). Psychometrics of a brief acculturation scale for Hispanics in a probability sample of urban Hispanic adolescents and young adults. *Hispanic Journal of Behavioral Sciences, 18*(1), 29–38.

Orozco, S., Thompson, B., Kapes, J., & Montgomery, G. T. (1993). Measuring the acculturation of Mexican Americans: a covariance structure analysis. *Measurement and Evaluation in Counseling and Development, 25,* 149–155.

Pachter, L. M. (1994). Culture and clinical care: Folk illness beliefs and behaviors and their implications for health care delivery. *Journal of the American Medical Association, 271,* 690–694.

Pepitone, A. (1995). Foreword. In L. L. Adler & B. R. Mukherji (Eds.), *Spirit versus scalpel* (pp. xiii–xiv). London: Bergin and Garvey.

Prochaska, J., & DiClemente, C. (1983). Stages and processes of self-change in smoking: Toward an integrative model of change. *Journal of Consulting and Clinical Psychology, 51,* 390–395.

Rosenstock, I. (1966). Why people use health services. *Millbank Memorial Fund Quarterly, 44,* 94–124.

Rosenstock, I. (1974). Historical origins of the health belief model. *Health Education Monographs, 2,* 328–335.

Sabogal, F., Marin, G., Otero-Sabogal, R., VanOss Marin, B., & Perez-Stable, E. J. (1987). Hispanic familism and acculturation: What changes and what doesn't? *Hispanic Journal of Behavioral Sciences, 9*(4), 397–412.

Singer, M., & Baer, H. (1995). Critical medical anthropology. In R. H. Elling (Ed.), *Critical approaches in the health social sciences series.*

Skinner, B. F. (1953). *Science and human behavior.* New York: Macmillian.

Sue, D. W., & Sue, D. (1990) *Counselling the culturally different: Theory and practice.* New York: Wiley.

Suinn, R. M., Ahuna, C., & Khoo, G. (1992). The Suinn–Lew self-identity acculturation scale: Concurrent and factorial validation. *Educational and Psychological Measurement, 52,* 1041–1047.

United Way of San Diego County. (1991). *Herencia y futuro: Latino future scan.* San Diego, CA: Author.

VanOss Marin, B., & Flores, E. (1994). Acculturation, sexual behavior, and alcohol use among Latinas. *International Journal of the Addictions, 29,* 1101–1114.

Velez-Ibanez, C. G. (1994). Plural strategies of survival and cultural formation in US–Mexican households in a region of dynamic transsformation: The US–Mexico borderlands. In S. Forman (Ed.), *Diagnosing America: Anthropology and public engagement* (pp. 193–234). Ann Arbor: University of Michigan Press.

Zambrana, R. E., & Ellis, B. K. (1995). Contemporary research issues in Hispanic/Latino women's health. In D. L. Adams (Ed.), *Health issues for women of color: A cultural diversity perspective* (pp. 42–70). Thousand Oaks, CA: Sage.

Zimbardo, P. G. (1992). *Psychology and life.* Palo Alto, CA: Harper Collins.

Zimmerman, E. J., & Sodowsky, G. R. (1993). Influences of Mexican American drinking practices: Implication for counseling. *Journal of Multicutural Counseling and Development, 21*(1), 22–35.

28

Strategies for Health Education

Community-Based Methods

JEANETTE CANDELARIA, NADIA CAMPBELL,
GEANNE LYONS, JOHN P. ELDER, AND
ADRIANA VILLASEÑOR

Introduction and Background

For purposes of this chapter, the term "immigrants" refers to those entering a new country in order to settle there. The term "migrants" refers primarily to farmworkers who migrate in groups of individuals or groups of families within the borders of a country to seek agricultural employment. The most obvious difference between the two groups is mobility or residential status.

Important to the study of immigrant populations is the fact that there are a large number without proper documentation from the Immigration and Naturalization Service. This leads to difficulty in identifying members of this population for study or outreach who may fear deportation (Decker & Knight, 1990).

Estimates of the number of migrant workers in the United States vary considerably. The terms "agricultural population" and

"agricultural worker" encompass several groups, including farm owners and their families; migrant and seasonal workers; agricultural service workers; and persons working in the forestry, logging, and commercial fishing sectors (U.S. Department of Commerce, 1982). Migrant farm workers are "laborers who migrate to obtain temporary agricultural employment" and seasonal farm workers are "laborers who are seasonally employed in agriculture within one local area" (Martin, Gordon, & Kupersmidt, 1995). Counting migrant workers is confounded by their geographical movement and, in some cases, temporary return to their country of origin.

Migrant workers typically follow one of three paths for work: the western, midwestern and eastern streams. The western flow begins in Mexico and moves through southern Texas northwest through California to Washington state. The midwestern stream begins in Mexico and moves through Texas to Arizona, Colorado, Kansas, and Missouri to Minnesota, Wisconsin, and Michigan. The eastern stream begins in southern Florida and proceeds north to New York. The first two streams are comprised primarily of people from Mexico while the third is more diverse with African Americans from southern

JEANETTE CANDELARIA, NADIA CAMPBELL, GEANNE LYONS, JOHN P. ELDER, AND ADRIANA VILLASEÑOR • Graduate School of Public Health, Center for Behavioral and Community Health Studies, San Diego State University, San Diego, California 92123.

Handbook of Immigrant Health, edited by Loue. Plenum Press, New York, 1998.

Florida, Haitians, Puerto Ricans, and Mexicans. Given the residential instability among this group, it is estimated that between 2.7 and 5 million migrant farmworkers plant and harvest farms in the United States (Goldsmith, 1989; Lambert, 1995). The 1990 National Agricultural Workers Survey states that 62% of seasonal agricultural services workers in the United States, many of whom are migrant workers, are foreign-born and 92% of the foreign-born workers are Mexicans (Mines, Gabbard, & Boccalandro, 1991).

Until recently, many studies on health behavior did not focus on ethnic differences, much less on immigrant status (Slesinger, 1981). Factors affecting the health behaviors and needs of immigrants are complex and there is a definite need for community-based primary prevention and public health interventions that address the barriers to good health faced by migrants and immigrants (Decker & Knight, 1990). These barriers include poor living conditions, stressful working conditions, health risks associated with the working situation, language barriers, cultural barriers, educational barriers, lack of transportation, lack of health insurance, and limited office hours at clinics (Lambert, 1995). For migrant immigrant populations these problems are often compounded due to separate issues related to a migrating lifestyle. Accessing health care can be a low priority due to the pressures of being at work and not missing work hours for an office visit (McGreevy, 1993). There is a lack of primary prevention programs for immigrants (Decker & Knight, 1990) and this population is generally not targeted for mainstream prevention initiatives (National Coalition of Hispanic Health and Human Services Organizations COSSHMO], 1995).

The high level of limited English proficiency among recent immigrants to the United States is a major barrier to obtaining health services. Those unable to communicate with health care providers may become discouraged (Lamber, 1995; COSSHMO, 1995). Communication barriers may also compromise the quality and efficacy of treatment (National Conference of State Legislatures [NCSL], 1993) and may be responsible for a lack of knowledge about health services available (Decker & Knight, 1990). Immigrants who have access to a translator or those who are proficient in English will have more contact with their physicians than those who do not. Educational limitations can prevent immigrants from understanding the importance of medical intervention and how the medical care system operates (Leclere, Jensen, & Biddlecom, 1994). Estimates of educational status and literacy vary among immigrant groups, but in general, the immigrant education status and literacy levels are lower than native levels (Andrew W. Mellon Foundation, 1994; NCSL, 1993; Simon, 1995; Smart & Smart, 1995; U.S. General Accounting Office, 1994).

Many immigrants live in poverty, which can isolate them both physically and financially from health care (Andrew W. Mellon Foundation, 1994; Leclere et al., 1994; NCSL, 1993). Logistical and institutional barriers, such as limited office hours at clinics (Lambert, 1995) and an inadequate supply of providers in their communities (Goldsmith, 1989; Valdez et al., 1993) can also hinder the access to care by immigrants. Reliance on family members for transportation, lack of transportation altogether, and program eligibility requirements impede the use of health care programs (Dyck, 1992; Lambert, 1995; NCSL, 1993). Furthermore, immigrants are frequently segregated into poor neighborhoods where social services are already strapped financially. Immigrants are often employed in low-paying jobs, in stressful working conditions, without the benefit of health insurance (Valdez et al., 1993). There are often health risks associated with the work situation as well, and individuals without health insurance are less likely to pay for preventive health care. In fact, use of preventive health services is uncommon among some subgroups of immigrants and those who cannot afford insurance may neglect their health problems until an emergency medical situation arises. Accessing health care is further complicated by the fact that time taken away from work for family and medical care can confound the poverty related issues to a greater extent (Chavez, Cornelius, & Jones, 1985; Goldsmith, 1989; McGreevy, 1993; Slesinger, 1992).

Cultural differences among immigrants, including their perspective on health and how they seek help, together with stress and their perceptions of acceptance by the host country may create additional health problems or complications for new immigrants (Drachman, 1992; Frye, 1990; Hurh & Kim, 1983; Leclere et al., 1994). Use of folk medicine has also been listed as a barrier to health care, though there is some evidence to suggest that this is not necessarily so (Decker & Knight, 1990; COSSHMO, 1995). Mistrust of unfamiliar health care providers and reliance instead on social networks for health care knowledge can prevent the use of health care services or programs (Acosta, 1979; COSSHMO, 1995; Smart & Smart, 1995). Religious beliefs and customs that are linked to philosophies about what causes health problems and what methods should be employed to treat them also influence the use of health services (Frye, 1990; NCHHSO–COSSHMO, 1995).

Although urban immigrants face many of the issues just mentioned, they may have more access to medical care and other social service programs than do rural immigrants. In an urban setting, programs such as federally sponsored English as a Second Language (ESL) classes can help the immigrant adapt to the host country and provide them with a social network of immigrants in similar economic situations. Those students who seek out ESL classes are ambitious in a sociocultural sense, may be working toward a degree in this country, or may be pursuing educational enrichment for personal enrichment or to improve their communication skills. A report on student progress in California's federally funded Adult Basic Education Programs (ABE) stated that the ESL respondents had completed more years of education than the ABE sample with 53% reporting having a formal degree or diploma compared to 30% of the ABE sample (Comprehensive Adult Student Assessment System [CASAS], 1993).

On the other hand, the rural immigrant or the migrant worker may not have access to decent housing and working conditions. It is presumed that migrant farmworkers experience poor health as compared with the general population, though their health status has not been systematically measured to date (Rust, 1990). Because of poverty, living conditions, and migrant status, consistent and continuous basic medical care is not the norm and this group is at risk for, among other conditions, nutrition related disorders such as anemia, poor dental health, and malnutrition. Added to this is the problem of inadequate access to health care due to a number of factors. Migrant workers are almost universally without health insurance. The small number of migrants who are on Medicaid often find themselves without coverage when they migrate to neighboring states. Due to the cumbersome application process, many migrants are discouraged from applying in the new state (Dever, 1991; Stilp, 1994). Inadequately funded migrant health centers lack staff and often do not operate after daily prime working times and migrants may live too far from a clinic or move too often to be able to access a migrant clinic (Slesinger, 1992).

Among Hispanic migrant seasonal workers, the use of preventive medical care such as prenatal care, dental care, vision care, general physical examinations, mammography, pap smears, and other preventive tests is low compared with other groups in the United States (Slesingner, 1981). Similarly, migrant and seasonal farmworkers are likely to receive inadequate preventive health care due to a number of factors. Such individuals without medical insurance are less likely to pay for preventive care. Individuals are less likely to seek preventive care if they have to leave or take time away from work (Watkins, Larson, Harlan, & Young, 1990).

Developing Community-Based Health Education Programs for Immigrants

To reach immigrant populations and address community health problems, the barriers and issues described previously must be given attention. Community health education programs that can meet the cultural needs of immigrants, with an understanding of the issues related to migrant status and linguistic and educational limitations, and that can make available the essential resources to deal with the problems related to poverty and lack of health insurance, appear to be inconceivable. No global solution will lend itself to addressing the needs and differences of all immigrants. The theoretical applications discussed elsewhere can serve as a guide to the development of effective immigrant health programs. It is also important, however, to apply practical recommendations from past and ongoing community-based health education programs, many of which are based on these theoretical applications.

Recommendations from various organizations can provide lessons and methods to apply when developing appropriate community-based health education programs for immigrants. They include (1) identification of and collaboration with community liaisons, spokespersons, and advisory boards; (2) promotion of increased cultural competency in health institutions and among providers and employers (having culturally appropriate policy makers, fostering personalization in patient–provider relationships, gaining patient trust); (3) identification of and collaboration with community-based institutional partners; and (4) development of programs for and with the community that include strong outreach components (COSSHMO, 1995; NCSL, 1993).

Use of community spokespeople and advisory boards has proven to be a useful tool in identifying not only appropriate community-based institutional partners, but specific liaisons within those organizations who can champion the incorporation of new program components (Elder *et al.,* 1998a; Elder *et al.,* 1998b; N. Campbell, personal communication, December 10, 1996). Community-based institutional partners often have existing outreach components. The addition of a beneficial health component to their ongoing activities can enhance the attractiveness of their program. In the case of community college English as a Second Language programs, adult students are already attending English classes to improve their English skills. Instructors whom the students already trust teach those classes. To incorporate a health topic into the English classes is much more practical than asking the students to come to a health class at a time and place not part of their existing schedule for a class on a topic that is not a priority for them.

In making health outreach an additional component of the tasks of an already culturally sensitive migrant education program outreach staff, or in working with that staff to be introduced to their clients, the time required for establishing trust and an operating system to deliver a health message to a migrant population is greatly reduced (N. Campbell, personal communication, December 10, 1996). Other effective intervention components for reaching migrant groups include group education through outreach to homes or at migrant camps (especially useful when participants lack transportation), use of trained community health advisors (CHAs) (Decker & Knight, 1990), and clinic hours that can accommodate late work days (Lambert, 1995).

The community health advisor (CHA) model is based on the assumption that within every community there are formal and informal social networks through which health information is exchanged and predisposing environments are created. CHAs are indigenous lay health advisors or "subprofessionals" who exist in all communities. The model is widely believed to have originated in Latin America where CHAs (a.k.a. *promotores/as* or *consejeros/as*) have worked on various health promotion programs for many years (Werner,

1981). CHAs may be members of existing social networks such as church groups, senior groups, and other social networks, who have attributes of leadership, compassion, and familiarity with the community (Werner, 1981). They are interested in the well-being of the group to which they belong and have a well-developed sense of community. CHAs in such a setting have the capacity to create awareness, disseminate health information, and support behavior change. The formal use of these change agents in the United States is growing (Meister, Warrick, Zapién, & Wood, 1992; Watkins *et al.*, 1994). This type of approach is important to special populations such as Spanish-speaking Latinos who are generally less acculturated and do not benefit from mainstream health promotion efforts. Once trained, the CHA provides a conduit for diffusion of information and a channel for empowerment through formal and informal education sessions.

Examples of Community Health Education Programs for Immigrant Populations

Project Salsa

Project Salsa targeted an urban immigrant population and was based on components of social learning theory (covered in depth in chapter 27). The project took place in a predominantly Latino community on the U.S.–Mexico border, south of San Diego, California, targeting an urban immigrant population. The project was one of 11 projects funded by the Henry J. Kaiser Family Foundation and affiliated donors to promote health through community development. Project Salsa was constituted as a community-based nutritional health promotion project that included efforts to enhance nutritional health across the life span for residents of the community.

Project staff sought first to develop a community-owned and -operated nutritional health promotion program and second, to increase adaptive and decrease harmful nutri-

tional-related behaviors among community members. The project also endeavored to institutionalize its program, initially as a free-standing entity and subsequently through community-based organizations on a component-by-component basis.

Project Salsa was organized using the ONPRIME sequence of planning, intervention, and evaluation procedures. Particular attention was given to Rothman's (1968) category of "locality development" as part of the organizational approach. Needs and resource assessment techniques used included key informant interviews, archival research, rates-under-treatment assessment, surveys, and community forums. A community advisory council then used these data to set program priorities. Intervention components addressed skills training, education, motivation, and social marketing. Interventions included chronic disease risk factor screening; cooking classes; a newspaper column; nutritional shopping instruction; school interventions for cafeteria staff, teachers, students and parents; and CHA training on breast feeding.

Although considerable effort and expense was put into the overall promotion of the project's name and other aspects of the program, the achievement of some objectives was short-lived as many of them were irrelevant at the end of funding. Some of the elements of Project Salsa were not maintained beyond the duration of external funding. For example, the Project Salsa media efforts emphasizing program name recognition and activity promotion were no longer necessary and were discontinued at the end of the project. The nutritional column and cooking classes were too labor intensive to maintain and were dropped as well, largely because no local agency saw them as sufficiently central to its mission to adopt and continue. However, two important cooking training and media spin-off efforts continue: the Project Salsa cookbook and cooking video *El Sabor de Salsa: Cocinando Para la Salud.*

That parts of the project continue nearly 6 years beyond grant funding can be attributed to the flexibility due to true grassroots organization without a disease-specific funded mandate. Needs and resources assessment activities proved to be on target as the adoption of certain components of Project Salsa by the community and its agencies were matched with initial recommendations by community key informants. The school health program parent activities and the cardiovascular disease risk factor screenings were continued and have the following factors in common: (a) they fit closely with the mission of the adopting agency, (b) they were championed by someone within that agency, (c) they resulted in sufficient benefits for the agency, and (d) they were sustainable at minimal costs. Other components, while possibly central to the goals of the cooperating organization, were relatively costly and of no direct short-term benefit (Elder, Campbell, *et al.,* 1998).

Por La Vida

Por La Vida (For Life) was initiated to address a need for an effective model to use in conducting health education programs among low-income, minority groups. The CHA model involves training women from the community to recruit program participants from among members of their social networks and to use culturally appropriate materials to teach them about various health topics. Child care was provided while the participants attended sessions and a formal graduation was conducted when participants completed the program (Navarro *et al.,* 1995).

The program targeted low-income Anglo and Mexican American families using a locality development organizational focus. Key informant interviews and archival research were conducted to aid in the development of the intervention materials and to identify women who could serve as *consejeras* for the project. *Consejeras* were women from church groups, senior centers, or other existing networks, who were known and trusted by community members and who agreed to be trained as lay health advisors (K. Senn, personal communication, December 18, 1996). The *consejeras*

went to homes to provide bilingual and culturally appropriate educational lessons and materials to both parents and children in the family. They also served as role models and provided reinforcement to program participants. Pre- and postsurveys were administered to determine the intervention effects on the health advisors (K. Senn, personal communication, December 18, 1996).

By conducting health education programs using *consejeras* whom the target population knows, some of the issues of personalization and trust discussed previously can be addressed (Acosta, 1979; NCHHSO–COSSHMO, 1995; Smart & Smart, 1995). The fact that the *consejeras,* who were empowered by the effort, remain in the target communities after the program is over, opens the door to the possibility of addressing other health topics in the same manner. The *Por La Vida* program has been successful in providing education on a number of different health topics including tobacco use, perinatal health, cancer prevention and early detection methods, nutrition, and other topics, to nearly 2,500 Latinas (K. Senn, personal communication, December 18, 1996).

Compañeros en La Salud

Compañeros en La Salud (Partners in Health) was a church-based health promotion project targeting adult Latinas in urban areas. The goals of this project were to reduce the risk of breast, cervical, and diet-related cancers. Social planning was used as the organizational approach and the CHA model was used as an intervention method. Multiple surveys and key informant interviews with pastors, priests, and other lay leaders of the churches provided the foundation for the needs and resources assessment (Castro *et al.,* 1995).

Once churches were recruited for the program, clergy were asked to recommend women who had the capacity to act as CHAs within their congregations. These CHAs were recruited to participate in the program as *pro-*

motoras. They were trained to deliver a series of 11 educational classes on breast and cervical cancer, and other cancers related to diet. *Promotoras* received additional training regarding community resources available for referrals for medical care, social services, mental health services, and other appropriate health related services (Castro *et al.,* 1995).

Program participants were recruited from the church membership and from among relatives and friends of the *promotoras.* All classes were held on church grounds which served as convenient meeting sites, without cost to the program, and were familiar to participants (Castro *et al.,* 1995). Use of the church setting and the interaction with church leaders may also have helped to reduce some of the barriers to health care based on religious beliefs and customs (Frye, 1990; COSSHMO, 1995). The materials offered were culturally and linguistically appropriate. Modeling and reinforcement was provided by the *promotoras.* This project was successful in recruiting churches and *promotoras* who promoted cancer prevention among Latinas by teaching skills and increasing self-efficacy related to cancer screening procedures (Castro *et al.,* 1995).

En Acción Contra El Cáncer

The National Hispanic Leadership Initiative on Cancer—*En Acción Contra El Cáncer* (Action Against Cancer) was a national effort to reduce cancer risks among Hispanics. It targeted Hispanic communities in six different sites throughout the United States. This program used narrowcast and broadcast media to educate the community about cancer, with each site modifying similar interventions to the specific needs of the local population. Pamphlets and flyers produced in the target communities were distributed by project staff and volunteers. The interventions focused on cancer screening awareness (i.e., breast, lung, colon, skin, prostate). Community role models, networkers, and various media outlets such as television and radio were used to deliver the intervention

messages (Ruiz, 1996). Networkers were individuals identified by the community as leaders and they volunteered to act as liaisons between the program staff and the community. Institutional-level networkers distributed a larger number of materials and information to organizations such as churches but did not necessarily interact with the recipients of the information. Individual networkers generally interacted with a limited number of community members, and did so regularly on a monthly basis. This allowed them to be sensitive to individual needs and adjust the delivery of the intervention appropriately. In this way, a community member who expressed a special need or concern to a networker might be referred to a specific screening or media program or given addition educational materials.

Networkers reinforced ongoing positive behaviors and encouraged cancer screening behaviors that has been absent. All delivery methods stressed the importance of cancer screenings and provided information about them. Modeling of the appropriate behaviors was provided and reinforcement was given to community members by both the community role model and the community networker. In order to evaluate the project's impact, random digit dialing surveys were conducted (Talavera & Parra-Medina, 1994).

Use of such networkers to regularly interact with community members can help diminish the linguistic communication barriers for immigrants. The individualized approach can also help inform participants about the services available to them and about how the medical system works (Andrew W. Mellon Foundation, 1994; Decker & Knight, 1990; Lambert, 1995, Leclere *et al.,* 1994; COSSHMO, 1995; NCSL, 1993; Simon, 1995; Smart & Smart, 1995; U.S. General Accounting Office, 1994).

Compañeras en Acción

Compañeras en Acción (Partners in Action) was a merging of the concepts of the *Compañeros en La Salud* and *en Acción*

Contra El Cáncer programs. The project targeted Latinas using trained CHAs or *promotoras* in various community settings for the early detection of breast cancer. However, the *promotoras* began to recruit individuals from their classes to be networkers such as those used in *En Acción Contra El Cáncer.* This blending of programs created an additional referral option for community members so that networkers could now refer them to a special *promotora* class in addition to a media program or supplementary educational materials.

Key informant interviews and archival research helped project coordinators determine what materials were appropriate for this population and which women in the community could serve as *promotoras.* The project promoted breast cancer early detection through small-group classes by teaching skills and increasing self-efficacy related to cancer screening procedures. Modeling and reinforcement were provided by the *promotoras* and culturally appropriate materials were distributed. Women learned about the negative consequences of breast cancer through the testimonies and experiences of others in the small-group setting.

This project concentrated its efforts on a small number of *promotoras* who in turn recruited a large number of networkers who distributed information and interacted personally with community members. This method extended the resources of the project and addressed many of the barriers and problems (transportation, trust, inappropriate materials) that are encountered in conducting community health education programs for immigrant populations (Decker & Knight, 1990; Drachman, 1992; Dyck, 1992; Frye, 1990; Lambert, 1995; COSSHMO, 1995; NCSL, 1993; N. Campbell, personal communication, December 10, 1996).

Language for Health

Language for Health was a heart disease prevention program funded by the National Heart, Lung and Blood Institute of the Na-

tional Institutes of Health. The Language for Health project (LFH-I) was a 4-year cardiovascular disease prevention program that integrated nutrition and heart disease prevention education into English as a Second Language (ESL) classes for adults with limited English proficiency (Elder *et al.,* 1998b). The intervention was based on the principles of the social learning and operant theories.

Program staff cooperated with community college district ESL staff to identify priorities that met the goals and objectives of both the researchers and the community college district ESL program. Focus groups were conducted with teachers and students related to curriculum and procedural concepts and then staff from the two organizations developed, pilot-tested and adapted the English-language heart health education modules for use in various community college sites. To make them easier to attend, classes were offered as part of the regular English classes and taught by the students' regular teachers. The emphasis was to integrate the health promotion agenda into the priorities (becoming literate in English) of the target population. Curriculum goals included increasing the students' self-efficacy by giving them nutrition information regarding heart healthy choices that can be generalized to a supermarket, restaurant, or home setting. Furthermore, designing the curriculum to incorporate ESL guidelines and training existing ESL teachers increased the likelihood that the heart disease prevention curriculum could easily be incorporated into community college district programs at the conclusion of the project.

A total of five modules were developed following the ESL program format: warm-up and review of the previous lesson, presentation of new material (including modeling and role-playing), practice with feedback, evaluation, and application. They included lessons on nutritional heart disease risk reduction, dietary fat, cholesterol, blood pressure, healthy shopping, recipe modification, and shopping to save money. Each module was a self-contained unit that could be completed in a standard 2.5- to 3.0-hour class session. ESL activities incorporated into each module were reading, writing (healthy change goals), listening, and speaking English. Audiovisual materials and props were prepared for teachers. Students were given packets of worksheets to keep when the lessons were over. Postcards with tips reinforcing information provided in the classes were sent to students (Candelaria, Woodruff, & Elder, 1996). The sessions provided activities that reinforced the information presented and were monitored with three measurements collected at baseline, 3-month posttest, and 6-month follow-up. Measurements included physiological measures and interviews assessing blood pressure, cholesterol, body mass, smoking status, alcohol consumption, physical activity, family history of premature heart disease, and diet. A paper-and-pencil survey collected subjects' self-reports of dietary fat intake, Spanish literacy, acculturation to U.S. culture, years of education, years in the United States, income, and employment status (Elder et al., 1998b).

Hispanic students made up 87% of the participants, with the remainder being immigrants of various other ethnicities. Participants in the program were more often female (59%), in their mid-30s, and had higher education and income than nonparticipants. Program participants demonstrated stronger perceived family support and were more extroverted (Apodaca, Woodruff, Candelaria, Elder, & Zlot, 1997). Those who were less likely to comply with follow-up physical measurements tended to be male, younger, of lower income, and of lower Spanish literacy level. They also tended to drink more alcohol, to be less physically active, and to have lower dietary fat avoidance scores (Frack, Woodruff, Candelaria, & Elder, 1997).

In regard to effects of the intervention, students who attended a greater number of nutrition classes obtained significantly greater fat avoidance behavior scores at 3 months (Lamb et al., 1997). Other results indicated more long-term effects of the intervention on nutrition knowledge and fat avoidance, yet only

short-term effects on high-density lipoproteins (HDL), and total cholesterol:HDL ratio (Elder et al., 1998b).

Initial difficulties due to administrative changes within the district delayed the program onset. Several actions, however, helped to secure the acceptance of the program by community college district administration and staff. The first was the inclusion of students, teachers, and curriculum experts in the planning and implementation process which produced credible program supporters within the target organization. Second, the Comprehensive Adult Student Assessment System (CASAS) agency was contracted to prepare the Spanish literacy assessment tool. CASAS is a well-established agency that did much of the regular student assessment activities for the participating community college districts. This relationship lent further credibility to the health program. Third, interaction with participating instructors during training, in class observations, with evaluation activities, and in providing an explanation of results fostered the spirit of community college district ownership of the program.

In the end, the program was met with enthusiasm and inquisitiveness on the part of participants as well as commitment and cooperation from ESL instructors and administration from local community college districts (Elder et al., 1998b). An extremely positive working relationship with the San Diego area community college districts was fostered through these efforts. The importance of involvement of appropriate school administration, teacher, and student representation in developing and implementing the program cannot be overstated. Table 1 provides an overview of the components, development procedures, products, and lessons learned in the Language for Health program.

Sembrando Salud

Sembrando Salud (Sowing Health) was a community-based cancer risk reduction project focusing on tobacco and alcohol. The program took place in San Diego County,

TABLE 1. Language for Health Program Development and Results

Component	Development	Result or product	Lessons
Administration[a]	Student focus groups Teacher focus groups	Information to guide program staff in development of curriculum and procedures	Teacher and student input was accurate and useful for preventing problems during inter-vention and measurement
	Pilot testing[b]	Revised measurement protocols and surveys, increased knowledge regarding logistical issues at ESL school sites	Sufficient interaction with target sites before intervention can reduce the number of logistical problems during intervention
Curriculum[b]	Teacher focus groups	5 lesson, ESL appropriate CVD related nutrition curriculum, of interest to students and with with minimal demands on teachers	Using observation and feedback from target teachers to modify program materials increases useability and acceptance of materials
	Multiple stage pilot testing	Reduction of curriculum to essential components only, with flexibility for beginning and advanced level ESL students	Variations between and within ESL levels create a need for flexibility in the curriculum.
Measurements NDS[c]	Community surveillance, input modification, input standardization, interaction with NDS software staff	Standardized 24-hour dietary recall training and measurement procedures using NDS software as well as caveats and recommendations for working with Latino populations	Target population diet and recipes differed from that of other Latino populations and care should be taken to ensure that correct recipes for foods with same name among different Latino groups are used
Physical measures and written survey[d]	Use of previous questions and protocols, pilot testing	Standardized physical measurement protocols and surveys	Same as for pilot testing, above
Spanish literacy test[a]	Cooperation with recognized local instrument development organization	Spanish language reading comprehension measurement instrument	The credibility of the cooperating organization lent credibility to the project

[a] Personal communication J. Candelaria, December 20, 1996.
[b] See also Candelaria, Woodruff, & Elder, 1996.
[c] See also Lyons et al., 1996.
[d] See also Elder et al. (1998).

California, currently the second largest county in California with just under 2.5 million people, of which more than 20% of the documented population is Hispanic (U.S. Department of Defense, 1990). As a prime agricultural area, the 4,255 square miles of the county attracts large numbers of farm laborers who have recently moved into the area in search of temporary or seasonal employment in agricultural activities. Approximately 9% of the county's population is Mexican immigrants (between 200,000 and 220,000 individuals). However, just as there are inconsistencies in the numbers of migrants nationally, there are those in San Diego who are critical of these numbers and say the true number of Mexican immigrants is significantly smaller, ranging from 44,000 to

150,000. Though no consensus exists on the actual numbers, there is consensus that San Diego bears the impact of immigration more than any other region of the U.S.–Mexico border area (Eisenstadt & Thorup, 1994).

The life of these migrant workers is the same as that characterized by other authors: abject poverty, stressful working conditions, substandard housing conditions, poor health, and a lack of employee benefits. In an effort to break the cycle of poverty, the Federal Migrant Education Program emerged with the goal of graduating migrant students from high school so they could become productive citizens. It is through a collaborative relationship between the university and this locally run federal program that *Sembrando Salud* recruits its participants. The target population was students aged 12–15 years and their parents enrolled in the Migrant Education Program throughout San Diego County.

Sembrando Salud recruited parents and adolescents to participate in an 8-week-long skill training session for tobacco and alcohol. Topics covered during the 8-week sessions included effects of alcohol and tobacco, social influences of alcohol and tobacco, refusal skills training, problem solving, and development of parental support for healthy decisions and behaviors. The purpose of the program was to decrease tobacco and alcohol use in the youth. Half of recruited adolescents received the tobacco and alcohol intervention while the remaining half received an intervention package on first aid and injury prevention. Each adolescent was followed for approximately 2 years to determine maintenance effects of the program. Components of social learning theory included in the project's intervention were modeling (through refusal skills training), rehearsal (e.g., role-playing) and reinforcement (via parental support). In order to evaluate the program's impact and outcome, pre- and posttests were conducted as well as a 12- and 24-month follow-ups (N. Campbell, personal communication, December 10, 1996).

Funded by the National Cancer Institute, *Sembrando Salud* solicited possible project names from high school students similar to the target population. The selected project name was created by a 15-year-old Hispanic girl. Likewise, the logo was created by an undergraduate college student and underwent focus group testing with target group adolescents (see Figure 1). The artist depicted an Aztec-influenced, unisex worker sowing seeds of health for future children.

Sembrando Salud's primary emphasis was on the social planning model of organizational approach. This project used archival research, surveys, and limited key informant interviews for the needs and resources assessment. Project staff then collaborated with staff from the county migrant education program to set priorities, outline project intervention methods, and recruit families. Families were randomized into an intervention or control group (N. Campbell, personal communication, December 10, 1996).

The small-group format was used for the educational sessions. The intervention sessions for tobacco and alcohol use prevention focused on (1) information about the effects of tobacco and alcohol use; (2) social influences on tobacco and alcohol use (e.g., media, peers, adults); (3) training in refusal

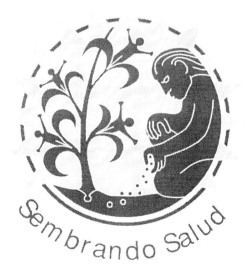

FIGURE 1. Sembrando Salud logo.

skills (e.g., modeling, practice); (4) problem solving (e.g., modeling behavioral rehearsal); and (5) development of parental support for healthy decisions and behaviors (modeling and rehearsal of effective listening, accepting messages, problem solving, norm setting). The content of these sessions included listening skills; communication skills, health effects of smoking and peer pressure, health effects of alcohol and decision making, societal influences, refusal skills, media and adult influences, and a review. The control group sessions on first aid and injury prevention focused on the following: responding in an emergency and with choking victims; first aid for fever and assembling a first aid kit, controlling bleeding and treating burns, fractures and dislocations and sudden illness, sports injury, poisoning and bites or stings, review, and household safety.

The general structure of both series of sessions was equivalent and included adolescents attending all sessions and parents attending the first, second, and eighth sessions. The structure of each session used the following format: welcome and session overview, group introductions for the first session and check-ins for the remaining sessions, review of previous session, group leader presentation of session content, break, skills demonstration and practice, homework assignments, and closure. The method of presenting the main session content varied; however, each curriculum utilized a similar mix of teaching methods including group leader–led discussions, videos, demonstrations, repetition, skills practice and role-playing. Group leaders allowed for questions and answers throughout each session. In sessions where both parents and adolescents attended, breakout groups for parents only and adolescents only were incorporated in order to facilitate discussions relevant to each group. Parental support skills such as listening, confirmation, and reassurance were developed and reinforced through behavioral methods including modeling, role-playing, and behavioral rehearsal in order to maximize maintenance and generalizability of the program (N. Campbell, personal communication, December 10, 1996).

This program addressed specific needs of this migrant population in various ways. First, sessions were facilitated by undergraduate, bilingual, and bicultural group leaders recruited from local colleges and universities. Some of these group leaders had even been enrolled in the migrant education program themselves. Parents expressed enthusiasm that their children were being exposed to these group leaders who they considered to be role models. Second, all sessions were held either on school grounds or at a nearby community center which proved to be most convenient for the families. Additionally, all sessions were conducted during evening hours which was the preferred time frame for the families. While many factors competed for the families' time (illness in the family, random checkpoints by the Immigration and Naturalization Service, homework), the project was successful at maintaining an attendance rate of 70%. Third, program staff collaborated closely with migrant education staff which gave the project credibility early on with the target population. In addition, this collaborative relationship provided the project with valuable knowledge used in designing and implementing the program.

Cardiovascular Dietary Education System Project (CARDES)

The CARDES project targeted urban African American adults and low socioeconomic (SES) communities in Washington, D.C., using primarily a social planning approach. It was a two-armed randomized evaluation trial conducted at a community-based clinic site. To determine the format and content of the education materials to be used in the intervention, project coordinators conducted archival research, focus groups, and a 6-month pilot study. The content and format of program materials were based on results of the extensive needs assessment and pilot study (S. Kumanyika, personal communication, December 18, 1996).

The primary focus of the intervention was to reduce serum cholesterol and blood pressure by encouraging a diet low in fat, cholesterol, and sodium. The intervention group received printed materials that were supplemented with a take-home audio cassette program and group counseling sessions. The control group received only self-help printed materials. Educational materials were prepared at a 5th- to 8th-grade reading level and designed specifically for African Americans. Physical measurements (i.e., blood pressure, lipid profile, height, weight, and body mass index) and a food frequency questionnaire were administered to determine the effects of the intervention (S. Kumanyika, personal communication, December 18, 1996).

This project demonstrated methods for development of programs for a specific ethnicity and a low-literate population. These methods are applicable to the cultural sensitivity and the literacy and educational issues discussed in the first section of this chapter (Andrew W. Mellon Foundation, 1994; Drachman, 1992; Frye, 1990; Hurh & Kim, 1983; Leclere *et al.,* 1994; NCSL, 1993; Simon, 1995; Smart & Smart, 1995; U.S. General Accounting Office, 1994).

Community Nutrition Education Program (CNEP)

CNEP targeted low-literate adults, primarily Mexican Americans, but inclusive of multiple ethnicities, in the Santa Clara County area in California. Participants were enrolled in vocational adult education training programs or a GED (General Education Degree) program. A social planning organizational approach was used for this project. Archival research, key informant interviews, focus groups, and pilot testing occurred prior to the delivery of the intervention. As in some of the other programs this project took advantage of existing training programs in the community to use as a channel for an educational program (M. A. Winkleby, personal communication, December 6, 1996).

Lessons were prepared for a population with a reading level at 8th grade or lower.

The intervention's primary focus was to lower dietary fat intake and consisted of six 90-min classes. These classes were highly interactive and included classroom demonstrations, small- and large-group discussions, interactive use of posters, videos, and skills practice. Activities that helped address individual needs included a goal-setting and problem-solving component. Participants were measured at baseline, immediately after the intervention was completed, and 3 months later to test for maintenance. Evaluation measures included finger stick cholesterol, body mass index, a food frequency questionnaire, and a knowledge and self-efficacy questionnaire (M. A. Winkleby, personal communication, December 6, 1996).

Comparison of Planning, Implementation, and Evaluation Strategies Used in the Community Health Education Programs

The previously reviewed studies share a variety of planning–implementation–evaluation components (p-i-e) in common, while differing in various important ways. To compare and contrast these projects, we can use a comprehensive p-i-e model such as ONPRIME, used in the development of Project Salsa. ONPRIME is an acronym representing a sequence of planning, intervention, and evaluation procedures. The seven-step process stands for *o*rganizing, *n*eeds/resources assessment, *p*riority-setting, *r*esearch, *i*ntervention, *m*onitoring, and *e*valuation (Elder, Geller, Hovell, & Mayer, 1994).

Organization or community organizing refers to development of new or mobilization and integration of existing organizations to deal with health or social issues. Strategies are used to raise awareness about the issue, to increase local capacity for problem solving, or to protect a target group considered to be vulnerable. This includes a structure, a purpose, and a mechanism for change. There are three models of community organization: (1) the social planning approach which looks at specific problems and attempts to determine appropriate solutions to them, (2) the social action approach which assumes that problems are related to inequality in a system and therefore seek changes in the system, and (3) the locality development approach which is a process oriented approach to community organization involving self-help and grassroots efforts in solving problems. The idea of locality development advocates that individuals and entire populations take charge of their own lives in order to deal with the problems at hand as well as the root causes of existing and potential problems (Elder *et al.*, 1994).

Needs and resources assessment includes research and planning activities used to determine a community's health behavior patterns. In this phase of program development, a community's health needs and priorities as well as approaches and resources that might be appropriate to meet the needs are assessed. The priority-setting process depends largely on the organizational strategy (locality development, social action, or social planning) with the priorities themselves based on the specific needs and resources assessment results (Elder *et al.*, 1994).

Research methods in the ONPRIME framework generally refer to the formative research used to guide the development of the intervention (the *R* of ONPRIME), but may include elements of needs and resources assessment and evaluation (ONPRIME's *N* and *E*). Some methods are used to plan the intervention, some are used to monitor intervention activities, and some to analyze the results. Methods can include focus groups, key informant interviews, behavioral observations, archival research, rates-under-treatment assessment, surveys, or test marketing, among others. Key informant interviews are conducted with individuals likely to be familiar with community wants, needs, and appropriate intervention approaches. Archival research utilizes existing sources of data (i.e., morbidity and mortality data) to help develop the intervention. Rates-under-treatment involves the use of

hospital or clinic records to assess treatment rates for various health problems (Elder *et al.*, 1994).

Interventions may be conducted at one of four levels: individual, group, organizational, or community. Interventions consist of educational objectives and goals, modification of existing behaviors, skills training to establish new behaviors, and social marketing and health communications. Social marketing is the "design, implementation, and control of programs seeking to increase the acceptability of a social idea or practice in a target population" (Kotler, 1984, p. 24).

In order to monitor and evaluate a program's intervention, process evaluations can be conducted during the intervention and impact and outcome evaluations can be conducted at the conclusion of the program. A process evaluation is related to how short-term objectives set during the program allow the attainment of the larger objectives of the study. The impact and outcome evaluations determine whether the program actually caused behavioral changes (Elder *et al.*, 1994). Table 2 presents a summary of the projects discussed in this chapter in the framework of ONPRIME.

Conclusions

It would be ideal for the projects described to be able to reduce the barriers to good health faced by migrants and immigrants as described in the first section of this chapter. Some of the barriers, however, are far too complex and costly to address with the limited resources of individual projects. For example, abject poverty and substandard employment, stressful working conditions, health risks associated with the working situation, and lack of health insurance would require policy and legal changes and even international diplomatic accords beyond the scope of the individual program activities.

Nevertheless, each of the projects described seeks to diminish as many barriers as possible and increase access to the health in-

TABLE 2. Community Health Education Programs in the ONPRIME Framework

Project title	Target population	Organization	Needs/resources assessment	Priority setting	Research design	Interventions
Project Salsa[a]	Predominantly Latino community on U.S.–Mexico border south of San Diego, California	Locality development	Key informant interviews, archival research, rates under treatment, surveys, community forums, behavioral observations	Established by health experts	Repeated cross-sectional surveys and other time series data	• Chronic disease/CHD risk factor screening • Cooking classes • Newspaper column on nutrition • Nutritional shopping • School cafeteria interventions health fairs, SNAC groups • *Consejera* training on breastfeeding
Por la Vida[b]	Latinas in Southern California, San Diego County	Social planning, locality development	Key informant interviews, surveys, archival research	Established by health experts in collaboration with community members	Randomized experimental-control group and others based on topic	• Multiple lessons about various topics conducted by trained *consejeras* for members of their social networks
Compañeros En La Salud[c]	Adult Hispanic women in urban areas	Social planning, locality development	Surveys, limited key informant interviews	Established by health experts	Randomized controlled trial (at church level), experimental cancer risk reduction and attention-control family mental health program	• CHAs taught series of 11 educational classes on respective health theme in churches
En Acción Contra El Cáncer	Latinos in six geographic areas throughout the U.S.	Social planning, locality development	Surveys	Established by health experts	Repeated cross-sectional surveys with a nested panel design	• Narrowcast and broadcast informational interventions, community networkers

(continued)

TABLE 2. (*Continued*)

Project title	Target population	Organization	Needs/resources assessment	Priority setting	Research design	Interventions
Compañeras en Acción	Latinas in southern California	Social planning, locality development	Surveys, limited key informant interviews	Established by health experts	Focused on process evaluation methods primarily tracking compliances of mammography referrals	• Narrowcast and broadcast informational interventions, community networkers; classes conducted by CHAs
Language for Health[f,g]	Community college adult ESL students in primarily Hispanic settings[f]	Locality development and social planning[f]	Archival research, student and teacher focus groups[g]	Established by health experts in cooperation with ESL curriculum experts and based on ESL program goals and objectives[g]	Randomized controlled trial. Experimental heart disease prevention and attention-control stress management programs[f]	• ESL instructors were trained and provided with materials to conduct the intervention activities as part of their normal ESL classes. • Five English-language hear health education modules delivered by trained ESL teachers as part of regular ESL courses[f]
Sembrando Salud[h]	Hispanic migrant teens (ages 12–15 years) and their parents	Social planning	Archival research, surveys, limited key informant interviews	Established by health experts	Randomized controlled trial	• Social skills development (e.g., refusal skills and norm setting) through the implementation of series of 8 weekly classes taught by undergraduate bilingual or bicultural students to small groups of families

Program	Target population	Approach	Methods	Standards	Design	Intervention
CARDES Project (Cardiovascular Dietary Education System)[f]	African American adults with limited literacy and communities with low SES in Washington, D.C.	Primarily social planning	Archival research, key informant interviews, focus groups, pilot testing, survey	Established by health experts	Two-armed, randomized evaluation trial	• Printed materials and take home nutrition program including an audiocassette and educational video and monthly group counseling sessions for 4 months • Self-help nutrition intervention consisting of food cards and a nutrition guide
CNEP (Community Nutrition Education Program)[g]	Low literate adults, primarily Mexican Americans, in Santa Clara County, California	Social planning	Archival data, local advisory board, key informant interviews, focus groups, pilot testing, surveys	Established by health experts	Randomized controlled trial using a cluster design with two conditions, special intervention and usual care	• Six 90-min classes focused on reducing dietary fat intake with handouts and recipes for low-literate adults • Control group received general curriculum of the California Expanded Food and Nutrition Education Program

[a] See also Elder et al., 1998b.
[b] See also Navarro et al., 1995.
[c] See also Castro et al., 1995.
[d] See also Talavera & Parra-Medina, 1994.
[e] See also Elder et al., 1998a.
[f] See also Candelaria, Woodruff, & Elder, 1996.
[g] From personal communication, S. Kumanyika, December 18, 1996.
[h] From personal communication, M. A. Winkleby, December 6, 1996.

formation and services they offer. Cultural, language, and other communication barriers, physical isolation due to poverty, as well as mistrust of unfamiliar health care providers and reliance instead on social networks are addressed in the projects described by using *promotoras, consejeras* or other change agents already linked with the target communities. The use of these change agents also helps to alleviate some of the educational barriers because the interactions are largely face-to-face, they are supported by appropriate written materials, and change agents are generally accessible on more than one occasion. Many of the projects refer the participants to further care, such as follow-up for high cholesterol, high blood pressure, or an abnormal pap smear. Therefore, many of them include information about the importance of medical intervention, how the medical care system operates, and health program eligibility requirements presented in a manner that is less intimidating and more sensitive to the situation of the participants.

Logistical and institutional barriers such as lack of transportation and health insurance, limited office hours, inaccessibility to providers in their communities, accessing health care as a low priority, and the fact that few primary prevention programs exist for this population are addressed to some degree by taking the programs to the participants. When low- or no-cost programs are offered in their communities or through high-priority channels they already access, these groups are not only more capable of participating but also much more likely to do so.

The use of community health advisors (CHAs) contributed to the success of many of the projects mentioned. They fostered credibility and trust in the program, reinforced ongoing positive behaviors, encouraged health screening, and reinforced participants for their efforts. CHAs who were empowered by the effort, and who remain in the target communities have the capacity to address other health topics in the same manner.

Finally, formative evaluation procedures such as needs and resource assessment, focus groups, key informant interviews, and pilot testing are vital to program development. They provide the key to identification of existing community agencies and individuals that lend credibility to the programs, create avenues of access for both program staff and participants, and stand to benefit in other ways through their participation. Application of formative evaluation results from appropriate representatives of community agencies increases the likelihood of participation and the ease of program implementation by the community agency and project staff when health information or program components are integrated into the agency activities.

References

Acosta, F. X. (1979). Barriers between mental health services and Mexican Americans: An examination of a paradox. *American Journal of Community Psychology, 7*, 503–520.

Andrew W. Mellon Foundation. (1994). *1994 Immigrant policy program report* [On-line]. Available: http://www.mellon.org/airp94.html.

Apodaca, J. X., Woodruff, S. I., Candelaria, J. I., Elder, J. P., & Zlot, A. (1997). Characteristics of volunteer participants and non-participants in a Hispanic health promotion program. *American Journal of Health Behavior, 21*(5), 356–363.

Candelaria, J., Woodruff, S. I., & Elder, J. P. (1996, September/October). Language for Health: Nutrition education curriculum for low-English literate adults. *Journal of Nutrition Education, 28*(5), Gem No. 266, p. 293c.

Castro, F. G., Elder, J., Coe, K., Tafoya-Barraza, H. M., Moratto, S., Campbell, N., & Talavera, G. A. (1995). Mobilizing churches for health promotion in Latino communities: Compañeros en la salud. *Journal of National Cancer Monographs, 18*, 127–135.

Chavez, L. R., Cornelius, W. A., & Jones, O. W. (1985). Mexicans immigrants and the utilization of U.S. health services: The case of San Diego. *Social Sciences Medicine, 21*(1), 93–102.

Comprehensive Adult Student Assessment System. (1993). *Student progress and goal attainment in California's federally funded ABE programs, July 1, 1992 to June 30, 1993* (Publication No. RR93ABE). San Diego, CA: Author.

Decker, S., & Knight, L. (1990). Functional health pattern assessment: A seasonal migrant farmworker community. *Journal of Community Health Nursing, 7*(3), 141–151.

Dever, A. (1991). *Migrant health status: Profile of a population with complex health problems* (Migrant Clinics Network Monograph Series). Austin, TX: Mercer University Press.

Drachman, D. (1992). A stage-of-migration framework for service to immigrant populations. *Social Work, 37*(1), 68–72.

Dyck, I. (1992). Managing chronic illness: An immigrant woman's acquisition and use of health care knowledge. *American Journal of Occupational Therapy, 46*(8), 696–704.

Eisenstadt, T. A., & Thorup, C. L. (1994). *Caring capacity versus carrying capacity: Community responses to Mexican immigration in San Diego's North County* (Monograph Series 39). San Diego: University of California, San Diego, Center for U.S.–Mexican Studies.

Elder, J. P., Geller, E. S., Hovell, M. F., & Mayer, J. A. (1994). *Motivating health behavior.* New York: Delmar.

Elder, J. P. Campbell, N., Candelaria, J. I., Talavera, G. A., Mayer, J. A., Moreno, C., Medel, Y. R., & Lyons, G. K., (1998a). Project Salsa: Development and institutionalization of a nutritional health promotion project in a Latino community. *American Journal of Health Promotion.*

Elder, J. P., Candelaria, J., Woodruff, S. I., Golbeck, A. L., Criqui, M. H., Talavera, G. A., Rupp, J. W., & Domier, C. P. (1998b). Initial results of "Language for Health": Cardiovascular disease nutrition education for Latino English-as-a-Second-Language students. *Health Education Research, 12*(6), 391–416.

Frack, S. A., Woodruff, S. I., Candelaria, J. & Elder, J. P. (1997). Correlates of compliance with measurement protocols in a Latino nutrition intervention study. *American Journal of Preventive Medicine, 13*(2), 131–136.

Frye, B. (1990). The process of health care decision making among Cambodian immigrant women. *International Quarterly of Community Health Education, 10*(2), 113–124.

Goldsmith, M. F. (1989). As farmworkers help keep America healthy, illness may be their harvest. *Journal of the American Medical Association, 261*(22), 3207–3213.

Hurh, W. M, & Kim, K. C. (1983). Adhesive sociocultural adaptation of Korean immigrants in the U.S.: An alternative strategy of minority adaptation. *International Migration Review, 18*(2), 188–216.

Kotler, P. (1989). Social marketing of health behavior. In L. W. Frederiksen, L. J. Solomon, & K. A. Brehony (Eds.), *Marketing health behavior: Principles, techniques, and applications* (pp. 23–39). New York: Plenum.

Lamb, J. K., Elder, J. P., Candelaria, J. I., Criqui, M. H., Golbeck, A. L., Rupp, J. W., & Talavera, G. A. (1997). *The effect of attendance to a nutrition intervention on fat avoidance behavior in Latino adult*

English as a Second Language students. Manuscript submitted for publication. San Diego State University, Graduate School of Public Health in California.

Lambert, M. I. (1995). Migrant and seasonal farm worker women. *Journal of Obstetric, Gynecologic, and Neonatal Nursing, 24*(3), 265–268.

Leclere, F. B., Jensen, L., & Biddlecom, A. E. (1994). Health care utilization, family context, and adaptation among immigrants to the United States. *Journal of Health and Social Behavior, 35,* 370–384.

Lyons, G. K., Woodruff, S. I., Candelaria, J., Rupp, J., & Elder, J. P. (1996). Development of a protocol to assess dietary intake among Hispanics who have low literacy skills in English. *Journal of the American Dietetic Association, 96*(12), 1276–1279.

Martin, S. L., Gordon, T. E., & Kupersmidt, J. B. (1995). Survey of exposure to violence among the children of migrant and seasonal farm workers. *Public Health Reports, 110*(3), 268–276.

McGreevy, J. C. (1993). Caring for the health and culture of migrant workers. *Pennsylvania Medicine, 96*(9), 16–17.

Meister, J. S., Warrick, L. H., Zapién, J. G., & Wood, A. H. (1992). Using lay health workers: Case study of a community-based prenatal intervention. *Journal of Community Health, 17*(1), 37–51.

Mines, R., Gabbard, S., & Boccalandro, B. (1991). *Findings from the national agricultural workers survey (NAWS) 1990: A demographic and employment profile of perishable crop farm workers* (Research Report No. 1, pp. 15–23). San Mateo, CA: U.S. Department of Labor, Office of Program Economics.

National Coalition of Hispanic Health and Human Services Organizations (COSSHMO). (1995). Meeting the health promotion needs of Hispanic communities. *American Journal of Health Promotion, 9*(4), 300–311.

National Conference of State Legislatures. (1993). America's newcomers: An immigrant policy handbook: Executive summary [On-line]. Available: http://www.ncsl.org/public/catalog/9366ex.htm.

Navarro, A. M., Senn, K. L., Kaplan, R. M., McNicholas, L., Campo, M. C., & Roppe, B. (1995). Por La Vida intervention model for cancer prevention in Latinas. *Journal of the National Cancer Institute Monographs, 18,* 137–145.

Rothman, J. (1968). Three models of social work practice. In *Social work practice: Proceedings, National Conference on Social Welfare* (pp. 1–999). New York: Columbia University Press.

Ruiz, E. (Ed.). (1996, Fall) Adapting media-based interventions to meet community needs: NHLIC-En Acción's experience. *National Hispanic Leadership Initiative on Cancer Newsletter, 2*(2). (Available from the Hispanic Cancer Control Program, Special Populations Study Branch, Division of Cancer Prevention and Control, National Cancer Institute,

EPN-240, 9000 Rockville Pike, Betheseda, MD 20892).

Rust, G. S. (1990). Health status of migrant farmworkers: A literature review and commentary. *American Journal of Public Health, 80,* 1213–1217.

Simon, J. L. (1995). Receipt of welfare and other government expenditures. *Immigration: The demographic and economic facts.* (Available from the Cato Institute and the National Immigration Forum, ISBN: 1-882577-33-7, 1000 Massachusetts Avenue, N.W., Washington, D.C. 20001.)

Slesinger, D. (1981). Medical utilization patterns of Hispanic migrant farmworkers in Wisconsin. *Public Health Reports, 96,* 255–263.

Slesinger, D. (1992). Health status and needs of migrant farm workers in the United States: A literature review. *Journal of Rural Health, 8*(3), 227–234.

Smart, J. F., & Smart, D. W. (1995). Acculturative stress: The experience of the Hispanic immigrant. *Counseling Psychologist, 23*(1), 25–42.

Stilp, F. J. (1994). The migrant health program in the United States: A personal view from the front line. *Migration World, 22*(4), 13–21.

Talavera, G. A., & Parra-Medina, D. M. (1994). *NHLIC: En Acción: A cancer prevention program for Lati-*

nos. Paper presented at the 122nd annual meeting of the American Public Health Association Conference, Washington, DC.

U.S. Department of Commerce. (1982*). 1980 census of population: Alphabetical index of industries and occupations* (Publication No. PHC80-R3). Washington, DC: U.S. Bureau of the Census.

U.S. Department of Defense. (1990). *SANDAG INFO: January 1, 1990 population and housing estimates.* Washington, DC: State Department of Transportation, County of San Diego, Tijuana/Baja Norte.

U.S. General Accounting Office. (1994). *Immigrant education—Federal funding has not kept pace with student increases* (Publication No. GAO/T-HEHS-94-146). Washington, DC: Author.

Valdez, R. B., Morgenstern, H., Brown, E. R., Wyn, R., Wang, C., & Cumberland, W. (1993). Insuring Latinos against the costs of illness. *Journal of the American Medical Association, 269*(7), 889–894.

Watkins, E. L., Larson, K., Harlan, C., & Young, S. (1994). A model program for providing health services for migrant farmworker mothers and children. *Public Health Reports, 105*(6), 567–575.

Werner, D. (1981). The village health worker: Lackey or liberator? *World Health Forum, 3*(1), 46–68.

29

Immigrant Health Care Providers in the United States

JAMES C. SPILSBURY AND MARGARET C. COONEY

Introduction

Immigrants have played a significant role in the provision of health care to Americans. The experience of immigrant physicians, nurses, and other health care providers, especially their reception by Americans, has been shaped over time by various political, social, and economic circumstances in their host country. At times they have been considered lifesavers; at other times they have been perceived as substandard practitioners (Friedman, 1979). They have been acknowledged for practicing in geographic areas and in medical specialties considered undesirable by U.S.–born citizens and have also been accused of taking jobs away from Americans. Some say that their numbers should be reduced in the United States; others say that their work is indispensable.

In this chapter, we discuss the experience of immigrant health providers in the United States since the 1950s. After first describing the current status of immigrant health care providers in the United States, we discuss the range of factors that have affected their experience in the United States: perceptions of practitioner sup-

ply, potential competition with U.S. doctors, changes in immigration law, concerns about quality, and issues of prejudice and discrimination against immigrant providers. Finally, we briefly describe actions various hospitals and private practices have taken to facilitate the assimilation of immigrant providers into American medical practices.

Immigrant Providers in the United States—The Current Picture

Physicians who were born outside the United States and graduated from non–U.S. medical schools are referred to as international medical graduates (IMGs). As of 1992, IMGs comprised 20% of the U.S. physician workforce (Mullan, Politzer, & Davis, 1995). Foreign-educated nurses (FENs) make up a much smaller percentage of the U.S. nurse workforce—only 4% in 1984 (Arbeiter, 1988). The majority of these individuals entered the United States through employment-based preferences, followed by those with an immediate relative in the United States (Immigration and Naturalization Service [INS], 1996). Looking specifically at the IMGs who entered U.S. residency programs, 38% entered the United States as exchange visitors and 29% were permanent U.S. residents ("Graduate Medical Education," 1995, p. 760).

JAMES C. SPILSBURY AND MARGARET C. COONEY • Department of Anthropology, Case Western Reserve University, Cleveland, Ohio 44106.

Handbook of Immigrant Health, edited by Loue. Plenum Press, New York, 1998.

Although foreign-educated health care providers come from all over the world, a few countries contribute large proportions of these professionals. More than 40% of IMGs come from India, Pakistan, and the Philippines (Mullan *et al.*, 1995). In 1994, a partial breakdown of the numbers of certificates granted by the Education Commission for Foreign Medical Graduates (ECFMG) was as follows: 25.9% to doctors from India, 8.1% from the Philippines, 5.9% from Pakistan, 4.2% from countries of the former Soviet Union, 3.7% from China, 2.6% from Egypt, and 4.9% to U.S. citizens who were graduates of foreign medical schools (Iglehart, 1996). U.S. citizens who receive their medical training abroad attend schools primarily in the Dominican Republic, Grenada, Mexico, and Montserrat (Mullan *et al.*, 1995). FENs come from a wide variety of countries throughout the world. However, 75% of them are natives of four countries: Ireland, Great Britain, Canada, and the Philippines (Arbeiter, 1988).

Why do they come to the United States? Cheng and Yang (1998) identified certain structural features of the United States that lead to increased immigration, particularly of skilled workers: a service-oriented economy with a demand for highly trained individuals, living conditions higher than many countries around the world, and a resource-rich educational system. Analyses of individuals' reasons for coming to America, while varied, often mirror these factors. Lack of adequate compensation or lack of jobs in the home country are often cited, particularly among women who come from cultures where women bear a large burden of responsibility for the family (Arbeiter, 1988; Phillips, 1996; Stevens, 1995; Wong, 1979). Better working conditions, including better hours and better equipped facilities and perception of greater opportunities for training and advancement also bring individuals to the United States (Jabbour, 1996; Joyce & Hunt, 1982; Mosberg, Angelides, Hayes, & Evans, 1979; Stevens, 1995). Finally, health care providers also come to the United States because of political and social instability at home (Grecic, 1995; Stevens, 1995). In fact, about 4% of

newly arrived immigrant provider arrivals are refugees (Mullan *et al.*, 1995; Zoler, 1989).

When IMGs or FENs come to the United States, they tend to locate in several geographical areas. Several states rely heavily on IMGs to provide health care to their populations, including New Jersey, New York, Illinois, Connecticut, and Michigan (Mullan *et al.*, 1995). Residency programs in New York, Illinois, Pennsylvania, and New Jersey have almost half of all IMG residents in the United States (Iglehart, 1996). FENs, on the other hand, tend to be heavily recruited to practice on both the West and East coasts, particularly in inner cities (Arbeiter, 1988).

Most IMGs fill positions in the medical system left unfilled by graduates of U.S. medical schools (USMGs) and doctors. Recent trends indicate that IMGs enter generalist specialties at a higher rate than their USMG counterparts, at 53.8% and 31.9% respectively. As generalists, IMGs today work predominantly in internal medicine (35.9%) and pediatrics (11%) (Mullan *et al.*, 1995). By contrast, they were historically concentrated in anesthesiology, general surgery, pathology, radiology, psychiatry, and obstetrics and gynecology—areas once unpopular with USMGs and areas in which IMGs are now underrepresented (Friedman, 1979; Mullan *et al.*, 1995). Despite their initial focus in internal medicine, IMGs subsequently subspecialize at a higher rate than their USMG counterparts: in 1987, 25% of IMGs in graduate medical training chose medical subspecialities compared with 16% of USMGs (Mullan *et al.*, 1995). Mullan and colleagues suggested that IMGs' choice of initial training area may be based more on availability of vacant residency slots than on personal or professional preferences or than on the fact that they fill vacant residency slots.

The Collective Experience

The General Picture

Dunn and Miller (1996) have used the image of "shifting sands" to describe the changing circumstances in which immigrant physicians receiving graduate education find themselves in this country. This image could aptly be applied to the general pattern of immigrant providers in the United States for the past 40 years. Over this time period, the number and distribution of immigrant providers, as well as the work they have performed, have changed according to the demand for health care, perceptions of oversupply and the desire to protect U.S. jobs, and the consequent changes in immigration policy that these concerns catalyzed.

Analysis of immigrant nurses' (Bernsen & Rubin, 1990; Ishi, 1988) and physicians' collective experiences (Aronson, 1996a; Mick, 1987; Page, 1994b) in the United States indicate that they have followed a similar trajectory. Initially, in a climate of great demand and short supply, immigrant providers were welcomed to this country and enjoyed a preferential immigration status. However, the growing number of immigrant providers raised concerns about oversupply and competition between U.S.–born and immigrant providers, as well as concerns about quality of care provided by immigrants. These concerns led to conservative bills in Congress (Iglehart, 1996) and more restricted immigration laws, including the introduction of mandatory examinations to obtain a visa. However, because of benefits to populations living in medically underserved areas, to employers, and to the immigrant providers themselves, immigrant providers have continued to play a significant role in the American health care system.

The remainder of this section uses the example of immigrant physicians to the United States to illustrate and to describe the complex interaction of the factors mentioned earlier that have shaped the experience of immigrant practitioners in the United States since the 1950s. The section is not intended to be a detailed review of immigration law as it pertains to immigrant providers or physician supply. Readers interested in this topic will find Aronson (1996a, 1996b) and Aronson, Domingue, and Lichtman (1997) pertinent.

Case Study: Immigrant Physicians in America

1950s–1960s: Welcome to the United States

As part of its activities to assist countries devastated by World War II, the U.S. government created the exchange visitor program (J-1 visa) to encourage foreign scholars to study in the United States (Page, 1994c). Through this program, U.S. authorities provided training to foreign physicians and were also able to "showcase" the American medical system to program participants (Page, 1994b). Opportunities soon increased for immigrant physicians. Beginning in the 1950s and continuing through the 1960s, U.S. policy makers perceived a shortage of physicians in the country. They responded by employing a two-pronged strategy to correct the problem: Increasing the number of U.S. citizens being trained as physicians and increasing and encouraging continued immigration of physicians into this country. Bolstering the medical education of U.S. citizens was accomplished through the passage of the Health Professions Educational Assistance Act in 1963. This act represented the first substantive federal assistance for undergraduate medical education, provided student loans and supported construction of medical schools (R. B. Sullivan, Watanabe, Whitcomb, & Kindig, 1996).

To boost immigration, physicians were given preferential status through the provisions of the Immigration and Naturalization Act, replacing immigration by national quotas with a system based on occupational preference (Chase, 1979). Moreover, requirements for J-1 visas and permanent residency status were relaxed, and many IMGs successfully obtained permanent visa status after completion of their residency training (Mullan *et al.*, 1995; Page, 1994c). Marriage to a U.S. citizen also proved a frequent route for IMG citizenship (Page, 1994c). Furthermore, to encourage immigration of physicians, health care institutions and training programs advertised employment opportunities in foreign journals, paid travel costs to the United States, and also worked to streamline state licensing procedures (Page, 1994b).

This two-pronged strategy worked: From 1965 to 1985, the total number of medical schools increased from 88 to 127, and the number of medical students rose from 32,835 to more than 66,600 (Mick, 1987). In the same time period, the number of practicing physicians rose from 316,457 to 511,090, and the overall ratio of physician to population increased by 50% (Mullan *et al.*, 1995). As part of this increase, the number of immigrant physicians also climbed from approximately 300 newly licensed IMGs in 1950, to 1,419 in 1960, to more than 3,000 in 1970 (Page, 1994b). Of note, the percentage of the physician workforce made up of IMGs also climbed: 10% in 1963, 18% in 1970, 19% in 1985, and 20% in 1992 (Mullan *et al.*, 1995). Moreover, one third of internships and residencies were filled by IMGs (Chase, 1979).

1970s: The Climate Changes

By the mid 1970s, however, the political climate turned less favorable to IMGs as the rising number of physicians generated concern about an oversupply (Friedman, 1979; Page, 1994b). In addition to a potential physician glut, issues such as inappropriate (to some) "conversion" of visitor exchange visas to permanent resident visas, brain drain, poor English skills, and the quality of IMG practice raised concern about the growing number of IMGs in the American medical system (Chase, 1979; Friedman, 1979; Page, 1994b, 1994c). In response, and with the endorsement of organizations such as the American Medical Association (AMA), the U.S. Congress enacted the Health Professions Educational Assistance Act of 1976, which restricted IMGs' opportunities to train or practice in the United States (Friedman, 1979). Requirements for visas tightened. More significantly, the Act required immigrant graduates of foreign medical schools coming to the United States for graduate education or to practice, and seeking either temporary or permanent residency status, to pass a professional qualifying examination. This requirement was unprecedented in U.S. immigration law—no similar requirement had been imposed by law on prospective immigrants in any other profession (Bernsen & Rubin, 1990).

In addition to the examination, IMGs seeking permanent residency status also needed to obtain labor certification from the Department of Labor attesting (1) that qualified Americans were unavailable to fill the position (usually demonstrated by the employer's having advertised the position in a relevant medical journal to no avail); and (2) that the salary offered was not lower than the prevailing wage (Bernsen & Rubin, 1990). Following these steps, an IMG could file for permanent residency as a member of a profession (third preference) or as a worker in general (sixth preference). The average time between filing the application for a visa and obtaining the third preference visa was approximately 2 years (Bernsen & Rubin, 1990).

Physicians seeking temporary employment in the United States as researchers or teachers at a nonprofit institution could apply for an H-1B visa, which did not require a qualifying exam or labor certification. Administrative processing for this type of visa usually took up to 8 weeks (Bernsen & Rubin, 1990). Physicians seeking graduate medical education and training as residents were required to pass the qualifying examination, demonstrate competence in English skills, demonstrate in writing that they would receive their training from an accredited U.S. medical school or affiliated hospital, and commit to return to their home country for 2 years before applying for permanent resident status (Friedman, 1979). Moreover, the original legislation limited a residency to 2 years, with a 1-year extension available only on request from the home government, and required the physician to demonstrate assurance from his or her home country that a position would be available on return home (Chase, 1979). The legislation also required the individual to return to her or his home country for 2 years before applying for permanent resident status.

Certain provisions of the 1976 Act were virtually impossible for immigrant physicians to meet: completion of a residency in 2 years (most took at least 3) and guarantee of a position on return home (Chase, 1979). Later amendments to the Act increased the allowed time in the United States to 7 years and required the physician to show assurance from her or his home government that it needed the skills the resident would obtain (Bernsen & Rubin, 1990). Later amendments also provided for a waiver to the mandatory return home after 2 years if (1) compliance with the law would impose exceptional hardship on a spouse or child who was a U.S. citizen; (2) a federal agency verified that the physician's work was in the national interest; (3) a return home would subject the physician to persecution; or (4) the home government issued a "no objection" letter to a longer stay, only for physicians who came to the United States to teach or conduct research (Bernsen & Rubin, 1990). Moreover, the requirement to pass the qualifying examination and the need to train at an accredited medical school or its affiliated hospital could be waived temporarily if a hospital could demonstrate that provision of health care to patients would be substantially disrupted. However, such hospitals were then required to reduce their IMG workforce (Friedman, 1979). These tightened restrictions slowed the rate of increase of IMGs in the workforce and decreased the percentage of medical residents who were IMGs from 1980 to 1990 (Mullan *et al.,* 1995).

Much of the rhetoric surrounding passage of the legislation concerned ensuring quality of health care to U.S. citizens (Bernsen & Rubin, 1990; Chase, 1979). As one administrator at the Department of Health Education and Welfare indicated, "the intent of the law is to protect U.S. patients from physicians whose training and practice have not been calibrated with U.S. medical training and standards of care" (Friedman, 1979, p. 75). However, the fear of oversupply was also a clear concern to medical authorities and gov-

ernment officials alike, with one physician summarizing bluntly, "If we take IMGs, our own citizens will go begging" (Eiseman, 1979, p. 13).

In the mid 1980s, two additional factors, besides supply and quality, also contributed to a less favorable climate for IMGs practicing in the United States. First, there was a large rise in the number of U.S. citizens attending foreign medical schools. Several of these schools were established in the Caribbean and marketed to students who failed to obtain admission to American schools. The composition of the student body, coupled with scandals in some of these schools involving the award of fraudulent degrees, raised great concern over the credentials and competence of these graduates and foreign medical schools in general (Mick, 1987). Second, concerns over the rising costs of the Medicare program led some members of Congress to attempt to reduce costs by decreasing the number of physicians generating those costs, and IMGs comprised a large proportion of this group. Some bills called for increased testing requirements for IMGs seeking visas, a freeze on Medicare payment for graduate medical education, and no funding at all to hospitals for services provided by IMGs and U.S. citizens who graduated from foreign medical schools (Mick, 1987). The bills failed.

Late 1980s–Early 1990s: Managed Care, the Need for Generalists, and Residencies as Good Business

Since the late 1980s, the number of IMG residents and practicing physicians has risen for reasons that are not entirely clear but are probably related to changes in the immigration law (described later) and, perhaps, the collapse of the Soviet Union and influx of immigrant professionals to the United States from countries of the former Soviet Union and Eastern Europe (Page, 1994b). From 1988 to 1993, the number of IMG residents increased from 12,433 to 33,706, and constituted 26.7% of all first-year residents in allopathic and osteopathic programs (Mullan *et al.,* 1995). Moreover, the total number of IMG first-year residents was 47.8% greater than the number of medical school (allopathic and osteopathic) graduates (Mullan *et al.,* 1995). By 1992, IMGs comprised 23% of the 605,000 practicing physicians in U.S. practice (Mullan *et al.,* 1995).

Mullan and colleagues (1995) reported that the likely driving force behind this increase was a fourfold increase in the number of exchange visitor residents (J-1 visa) from 1988 to 1993. Moreover, changes in immigration law made it more likely that IMG residents might remain in the United States. First, a 1991 amendment expanded the scope of the H-1B visa, formerly given only to those engaging in teaching or research, to include foreign national IMGs who desired to practice medicine in the United States, had an employment offer, and were eligible for state licensure. Second, waivers of the requirement to return home after their training were permitted if IMGs worked for a federal program or did primary care in an officially designated underserved area. Since 1990, the number of IMGs working in underserved areas has doubled to about 160 per year (Page, 1994b). In addition, a recent law permits each state to request up to 20 waivers per year for physicians completing their J-1 visa training who will practice in a shortage area (Mullan *et al.,* 1995).

What is driving the increase? Aronson (1996a) has identified several factors that are ultimately responsible for the current situation. First, and perhaps foremost, is the absence of a comprehensive national policy that determines the need for physician services. Consequently, the American health care system is characterized by unequal distributions of physicians both geographically and by specialty. Some areas face a physician oversupply while other regions are dealing with shortages, and many areas face a growing shortage in primary care. For example, although the 1994 ratios of full-time equivalent primary care physicians and non-primary care physicians to 100,000 population in

New York state are greater than the national average (69.7 vs. 69.4 for primary care physicians, and 141.3 vs. 111.8 for non-primary care physicians), the ratios vary significantly by regions within the state. Smaller areas (counties, communities) experience shortages, especially in rural areas and in inner cities (Salsberg, Wing, Dionne, & Jemido, 1996). In fact, despite the large overall supply of doctors in the state, more than 3.8 million New York residents live in 105 areas designated as federal Health Professional Shortage Areas (Salsberg *et al.,* 1996). Nationwide, approximately 50 million persons, 17% of the U.S. population, live in such shortage areas (Aronson *et al.,* 1997).

Faced with these shortages, many health care facilities have recruited IMGs to fill the gaps in some parts of the United States. The Appalachian Regional Commission, the Veterans Administration, the Department of Health and Human Services, the Department of Housing and Urban Development, the Department of Agriculture, and even the U.S. Coast Guard have taken advantage of the waivers to the J-visa requirement for IMG residents. Residents do not have to return home after training from hospitals if the waiver is requested by a federal agency and no American doctor will take the position (Anonymous, 1995; Schusterman, 1995; White, 1993). In rural America, 44% of which is medically underserved (Aronson *et al.,* 1997), as well as in many inner-city areas, it has not been difficult to demonstrate U.S. physicians' unwillingness to take the position: "When you run an ad in *JAMA* for areas like Appalachia, the typical response is no response" (White, 1993, p. 44). From 1990 to 1993, more than 570 IMGs were approved for practice in Appalachia (White, 1993). Individual states are also taking advantage of the 1994 amendment to the immigration act that allowed state health departments to sponsor up to 20 IMGs for waivers to the J-1 restrictions per year; as of 1995, 32 states had decided to participate in this program (Schusterman, 1995).

Managed care has also emerged as another major factor affecting the IMG situation by heightening the demand for generalists or primary care practitioners (Aronson, 1996a; Korcok, 1994). HMOs increasingly look to primary care physicians to serve as gatekeepers to a system of specialists. Restricted use of specialists lowers costs and keeps the HMO competitive. The U.S. system, though, has long been focused on training specialists: Currently fewer than one third of practicing American physicians are generalists and only about 20% of graduates from American medical schools state a preference for a generalist career (Aronson,1996a; D. Kindig, Cultice, & Mullan, 1993; Mullan et al., 1995).

Employers have found Canadian-trained physicians to be especially attractive candidates to fill shortages or work in HMOs. U.S. agencies have increasingly advertised in Canadian medical journals (Sullivan, 1994). Although Canadian physicians are required to take the U.S. national licensing examination to work in the United States (Korcok, 1994), Canadian medical schools' accreditation is recognized by U.S. authorities, making it easier for their qualifications to be approved in the United States. Canadian graduates are excluded from many of the restrictions of the immigration law, and more than 30 states grant licenses to Canadian-trained physicians without requiring the completion of a residency in the United States (Korcok, 1994; White, 1993). Furthermore, more than 53% of Canadian physicians are general or family practitioners, groups specifically sought by recruiters (White, 1993). In 1992, almost 700 Canadian physicians left for the United States, and at least 635 had done so by the middle of 1993; these numbers represented a 120% increase in emigrating Canadian physicians since 1986 (Korcok, 1994).

The Clinton administration's failed health reform efforts called for a 50/50 ratio of generalists to specialist physicians, but achieving this ratio by 2004 would require that 100% of all U.S. medical school graduates from 1993 on enter generalist practices (D. Kindig et al., 1993). Some authorities have suggested establishing a quota system for types of specialty, but U.S. students, a loud voice in the AMA, are displeased with such an idea, presumably because they want the opportunity to seek well-paying, prestigious specialty positions (Page, 1993, 1994b). According to them, the government should not force students into areas they do not want; rather, various incentives and enticements should be used to get physicians to practice primary care in underserved areas. While the U.S. students have resisted going to these geographic and specialty areas, IMGs apparently have not hesitated.

Another major factor affecting IMGs relates to the financial support hospitals and other provider institutions derive from graduate medical educational activities. Because the Medicare Prospective Payment System reimburses costs related to direct and indirect medical education, teaching hospitals benefit financially by using residents to provide care, especially expensive specialty services (Sullivan et al., 1996). In 1993, the mean Medicare payment to hospitals per resident was $70,000 and reimbursement reached $200,000 per resident in some states (Sullivan et al., 1996). By contrast, most residents earn a salary between $25,000 and $40,000 (Aronson, 1996a). In New York state, hospitals received over $3 billion in reimbursement for graduate medical education–related activity ($1.7 billion from state payers and $1.2 billion from Medicare), resulting in a yearly mean reimbursement of $188,000 per resident (Salsberg et al., 1996). These payments cover far more than training: they also cover uncompensated care for uninsured patients and support teaching and research activities. Thus, although organizations such as the AMA may worry about the effects of a physician oversupply, hospitals have in essence received great financial incentive to increase the number of doctors in training (Sullivan et al., 1996). Because the graduation rate of U.S. medical schools has been relatively constant the past several years, the increase in residents is accomplished by hiring more IMGs. It is perhaps not surprising that between 1988 and 1993 the number of

IMGs in graduate medical education has almost doubled from 12,433 to 22,706 and, concomitantly, the percentage of IMGs in the resident workforce has risen from 15.3% to 23.3% (Mullan *et al.*, 1995).

Although IMGs can hardly be faulted for taking advantage of the increasing number of residency slots, solutions to the problem of ballooning residency positions and physician oversupply seem to identify IMGs as a primary culprit. For example, the Council on Graduate Medical Education recently recommended reducing Medicare payments for IMGs to 25% of the 1994 level and reducing first-year graduate positions to 110% of U.S. medical school graduates (D. A. Kindig & Libby, 1996; Sullivan *et al.*, 1996). Similarly, the Pew Health Professions Commission (1995) has recommended reducing graduate medical education slots to the same percentage and has also called for tightening visa requirements to ensure that IMG residents return to their home countries after completion of training. The commission also recommended reducing the number of first-year U.S. medical students by 25%. This recommendation was hotly contested by the Association of American Medical Colleges; the president of the association pointed out that the recent annual intake of IMG residents was "equivalent to the entire graduating classes of some 56 average-sized U.S. medical schools" (Greenberg, 1996, p. 607).

In what might be considered one of the more drastic proposed solutions, Whitcomb (1995) suggested limiting the number of IMGs who can enter a residency program and eliminating Medicare payments for direct or indirect medical education for any hospital that hires IMGs beyond the regulated amount. To ensure that hospitals not lose their ability to provide health care to the underserved, Whitcomb suggested increasing federal funding for physician assistants and nurse practitioners. According to Whitcomb, the fact that two thirds of IMGs in the United States are already U.S. citizens or permanent residents makes restricting immigration laws superfluous. Critics of Whitcomb's proposal

argue that it will result in (1) the creation of a two-tiered medical system—the poor get mid-level practitioners instead of physicians; (2) the inherent "equating" of IMG physicians to physician assistants; (3) a devaluation of individual merit in the residency selection process; and (4) potential violations of the equal protection doctrine contained in the Fifth Amendment of the U.S. Constitution (DeWitt, 1995; Kellis, 1995; Vasireddi & Chowdappa, 1995; Wynia, 1995).

The effects of reducing the number of IMG physicians, particularly residents, are debated. IMGs have constituted a major provider of medical care in areas with physician shortages, especially rural and inner-city areas, as well as to specific ethnic groups in the United States (Balon & Munoz, 1996; Carmichael, 1994; Nagelberg, Schwartz, Perlman, Paris, & Thornton, 1980). Thus, reduction in IMG numbers might well seriously reduce services for the very populations that need them the most.

Other potential effects of an IMG reduction have also been suggested. For example, McNiven (1992) has noted that IMG women have historically served as a large proportion of the teachers, mentors, and role models of the growing number of U.S. women graduates. Although times have changed since 1970 (when women constituted 15% of IMGs practicing in the United States but only 6% of U.S. medical graduates), IMG women's perspectives on a variety of issues related to health care and career development might well be useful to U.S.–trained women physicians and would be missed in their absence.

Other authors (e.g., Evans, 1981; Mosberg *et al.*, 1979) suggest another potential effect of IMG reduction: During the course of their training, IMG residents become accustomed to a variety of North American products (e.g., drugs, medical supplies and equipment, publications) and tend to utilize these items on their return home (if available). Thus, reduction of these "customers-in-training" may send them to other countries' training programs and to other countries' manufacturers, resulting in decreased business for North American manufacturers.

Recent research has seemingly strengthened the argument for reducing the number of IMGs. For instance, Whitcomb and Miller's (1995) research indicates that only 77 of the country's 688 primary teaching hospitals can be considered dependent on IMG resident care to the poor. In other words, over one third of IMG resident physicians and 40% of IMG-dependent residency programs are not providing disproportionate care to the poor. Moreover, Mullan and colleagues' (1995) analysis indicated that a disproportionate percentage of IMG residents initially in primary care switch to subspecialties, so that the percentage of IMGs ultimately choosing a generalist position, 25%, is virtually identical to the percentage of U.S. medical graduates who do so. Moreover, Mullan and colleagues report that when IMG residents finish their training, they establish office practices in urban areas just as U.S. medical graduates do. Despite the migration of IMGs toward better paying, urban areas, many hospital administrators report satisfaction that they are able to get at least a few years of generalist practice out of IMGs (Page, 1994b). Results of studies such as that of Seifer, Troupin, and Rubenfeld (1996), whose analysis of advertised positions in specialty areas showed a decline in demand for physicians, especially in specialist fields, will continue to fuel the controversy.

1995 Onward: Recent Developments

Aronson and colleagues (1997) have noted a series of recent changes in the law and in federal agency procedures that will affect IMGs in the United States. To begin with, the recently passed 1996 Illegal Immigration Reform and Immigrant Responsibility Act contains several provisions that will affect IMG practice. First, the program that enables state health departments to obtain waivers of the return-home-after-residency requirement for 20 J-1 physicians per year has been extended until 2002. Second, all physicians receiving the waiver through either a state or federal agency must complete 3 years of employment in H-1B visa status before applying for permanent resident status (previously, doctors sponsored by federal agencies could apply directly for permanent residence). Third, J-1 physicians need not return to their home county to process their H-1B visa. These provisions will presumably (1) continue to enable communities with medical shortages to obtain needed care; (2) ease the procedure necessary to obtain a visa; and (3) increase the likelihood that the IMG and employer complete the terms of their contract.

Although the passage of the act reinforced state implementation of J-1 waivers, subsequent events have complicated federal implementation of the program. In late 1996, the U.S. General Accounting Office issued a review of the Exchange Visitor Program, which acknowledged the importance of the program to underserved populations and found that the vast majority of IMGs were completing the terms of their contracts. In fact, 13% of IMGs whose waivers were recommended by the Appalachian Regional Commission had remained at their facilities for more than 4 years. However, the review also found problems with implementation of the waivers; namely, no single government agency had been assigned clear responsibility for overseeing the program. As a result, activities of participating agencies were uncoordinated, nonstandardized, and at times overlapping. Moreover, the review found disagreement over program goals: Unlike other participating agencies, HHS did not view the program as a solution to medical underservice. In light of these problems, the GAO report called on Congress (1) to reevaluate how the program fits into the federal government's strategy to providing health care to underserved populations; (2) to designate a single federal agency to manage the program or delegate it to the states; and (3) to develop standardized application, placement, and monitoring procedures.

In apparent response to this report, HUD has announced an indefinite moratorium on the J-1 waiver program and has discontinued all processing of waivers, even those only awaiting signature from the Secretary (Aronson *et al.,* 1997). According to HUD officials, this action was taken to coordinate its responsibilities with other agencies and because it lacks the staff to monitor compliance. Moreover, in response to concerns about potential abuses by facilities and IMGs, the USDA now requires more stringent documentation from applicants showing additional proof that (1) the IMG's employment will provide medical care to rural populations, and (2) U.S. physicians are unavailable to fill those positions.

Finally, the Department of Health and Human Services has recently announced a Medicare reimbursement pilot program that will effectively reduce by about 20% the size of medical residency programs (Aronson *et al.,* 1997). Although the program does not target IMGs specifically, cuts will most likely affect IMGs more than U.S. medical graduates because a disproportionate percentage of IMGs provide care for Medicare patients.

The Individual Experience

In this section we examine several issues that have shaped individual experiences of immigrant health care providers. The major issues include those of quality control through examinations for licensing, beliefs about the inferiority of IMGs, and the sense of discrimination felt by many IMGs. The section concludes with a discussion of training programs devised to assist immigrant providers in their work and to help them assimilate into American society.

Testing

Quality of any health care provider is certainly a legitimate concern. From the beginning, U.S. authorities have faced the formidable task of trying to assess the credentials of individuals trained in different countries. To this end, in the mid 1950s the

Educational Commission on Foreign Medical Graduates (ECFMG) was established by the AMA, the American Hospital Association, the Association of American Medical Colleges, and the Federation of State Medical Boards (Mou, 1988). With the assistance of the National Board of Medical Examiners, the ECFMG has developed examinations to determine the competence of IMGs coming to the United States (Chase, 1979). There are four steps required to earn ECFMG certification: (1) pass an examination in basic medical science, (2) pass an examination in clinical science, (3) pass an English proficiency test, and (4) document completion of educational requirements to practice medicine in the country where they received their medical education (Sutnick, Shafron, & Wilson, 1992). Similarly, concern over the quality of immigrant nurses in the United States led to the creation in the mid 1970s of the Commission on Graduates of Foreign Nursing Schools to assesses the nursing skills and English proficiency of graduates of non–U.S. nursing schools (Ishi, 1988).

The examinations developed by these commissions typically consist of multiple sections that are taken sequentially. Concerning the physicians, as Aronson (1996a) has indicated, the history of the examination process, including the multipart examinations themselves, (e.g., Visa Qualifying Exam, administered from 1977 to 1986; the Foreign Medical Graduate Examination in the Medical Sciences, administered from 1984 to 1994; the National Board of Medical Examiners examination, used from 1989 to 1993, the Federation Licensing Examination, valid if taken before 1985, and the currently used U.S. Medical Licensing Examination) is complex and worthy of detailed study in its own right. Although discussion of the evolution of the certification process is beyond the scope of this chapter, two points are noteworthy. First, until recently, IMGs generally needed to take two separate test sequences: one to obtain a visa and another to obtain a license to practice (Aronson, 1996a). Second, attempts have been made since 1994 to simplify testing requirements by having one examination, the U.S. Medical Licensing Examination (USMLE), serve both purposes. However, as will be noted later, test requirements for licensing are ultimately a prerogative of the states.

One particular problem created by the phasing in and out of various certification examinations is that individuals over time may have taken various combinations of the tests (e.g., parts 1 and 2 of the NBME but part 3 of the USMLE). Although various state medical examining boards will accept passing test scores from parts of different tests for licensing purposes, the INS does not accept them for the purposes of obtaining a H-1B visa (Aronson et al., 1997). As Aronson and colleagues have noted, in every other professional field requiring a license to practice, the INS bases its visa eligibility criteria on the states' criteria for licensing. Doctors practicing medicine are the only exception.

Similar to the case of immigrant physicians, immigrant nurses have needed to demonstrate clinical competence through the passage of examinations. To this end, in order to obtain employment as a nurse, an alien nurse must have passed the Commission on Graduates of Foreign Nursing Schools (CGFNS) examination or be fully licensed in the state of intended employment (Bernsen & Rubin, 1990). Moreover, nurses granted a visa for temporary employment based on the CGFNS examination are admitted for one year only and must pass the first available state licensing examination to apply for a visa extension.

Quality Control, Licensing, and Discrimination

To ensure adequate and safe patient care, rigorous criteria for licensing both U.S. providers and immigrant providers are desirable. However, as with any testing process, the degree of rigor is not always clear-cut, and there comes a point when what one individual might perceive as "quality control," another might (accurately or inaccurately) interpret as discrimination.

Unfortunately, when concerns arise about competition or oversupply, quality of care may serve as a smoke screen for concerns about job preservation. This is not an unknown occurrence in the U.S. health field. For example, in the first decade of the twentieth century, midwives, many of whom were immigrants, provided prenatal and maternal care to large numbers of women, especially among immigrant populations (Kobrin, 1985; Radosh, 1986). In 1910, almost half of all recorded births were delivered by midwives, and care afforded by midwives was generally as good as or superior to that provided by physicians (Kobrin, 1985). Obstetricians, however, were concerned that their livelihoods and the growth of obstetrics in general were in jeopardy. Although many factors were at play, including bigotry aimed at immigrants and changing conceptions of womanhood and what constituted "natural motherhood," physicians' success in taking over the "birthing market" can be partly attributed to their ability to convince American women about the dangers of childbirth in the hands of immigrant midwives compared with the safety of delivery overseen by obstetricians (Radosh, 1986).

Today, it does not seem unreasonable to suspect that concerns about quality may on occasion mask economic interests. At times, treatment of IMGs under the guise of quality control can amount to discrimination. Several reports of prejudice and discrimination experienced by immigrant practitioners can be found in the medical literature (e.g., Cameron, 1993; Jabbour, 1996; Jarrahi, 1993; Myers, 1995; Page, 1994a). Immigrant nurses have reported encountering prejudice and discriminatory practices by American practitioners, including more frequent assignment to menial and onerous tasks, failure to receive real training, and difficulty in obtaining the certification necessary for employment (Joyce & Hunt, 1982). Similarly, many immigrant physicians believe that the separate treatment they receive in residency selection, licensing procedures, and obtaining hospital privileges slights their clinical abilities, reduces their ability to obtain a livelihood, and amounts to discrimination (Page,

1994a). In 1991, more than 80% of IMGs considered antidiscrimination legislation to be the critical priority for IMG organizations (Osteen, 1991). Page (1994a) reported that both medical authorities and federal officials investigating allegations of discrimination "stop short of the 'D' word, but agree that IMGs have been subject to unnecessary 'separate treatment' " (p. 3).

Varki (1992) attributed prejudice against IMGs to the tendency of physicians, patients, and policymakers to categorize physicians by the location of their primary medical training, thereby ignoring the considerable diversity in country of origin, background, training, and capabilities represented by these individuals. According to Varki, a series of generalizations commonly applied to IMGs foment prejudice and lead to discrimination: (1) IMGs have no right to be in the United States; (2) IMGs have deserted their home countries and have, therefore, contributed to the brain drain; (3) foreign medical schools are intrinsically worse than U.S. schools; and (4) IMGs are intrinsically inferior to USMGs. However, in rebuttal of these generalizations, Varki noted that most IMGs have fulfilled all legal requirements to reside in the United States and, therefore, have every right to be in the country. Moreover, accusations of abandoning the home country and "brain drain" ignore the lack of professional opportunities in some developing countries for health care providers, the fact that some IMGs have financially supported their own education in the United States, and that a significant proportion of IMGs do, in fact, return home after their training. Concerning the intrinsic inferiority of foreign medical schools, Varki noted that although U.S. medical schools are on average better than foreign schools, many IMGs have attended outstanding medical schools that are comparable with any American school.

To support the contention that IMGs are generally less effective physicians than USMGs, attention is often drawn to the tendency of IMGs as a group to perform more poorly on standardized tests than USMGs

(Page, 1994a). For example, in 1992 the pass rate of those taking parts 1 and 2 of the U.S. Medical Licensing Examination was 90% for USMGs and about 40% for IMGs (Page, 1994a). However, this observed difference may be due to factors other than presumed inferiority of foreign medical schools. IMGs usually take various standardized qualifying tests years after their medical education and their scores are often compared with those of USMGs, who are taking the examination soon after finishing medical school curricula often patterned specifically after material covered in the qualifying exams (Varki, 1992).

According to Varki (1992), the great diversity of IMGs renders meaningless any study that places IMGs into a single group and compares them with USMGs. Worse, continued publication of results that show IMGs as poorer performers on standardized tests perpetuates stereotypes about immigrant providers that *every* IMG must face. As Page (1994a) notes, concerns about IMG competence have at times reached the illogical extreme that high failure rates on standardized tests suggest that IMGs *passing* the test were low quality.

Unfair generalizations concerning IMGs may not arise only from comparisons of scores or pass rates on standardized tests. For example, Jesilow (1992) reported an overrepresentation of minority and immigrant physicians perpetrating Medicaid fraud but failed to mention that minority and immigrant physicians are overrepresented in providers giving care to Medicaid recipients (Rios, 1992). Although they later acknowledged this mistake (Jesilow, 1992), the potential damage was done: At least one major newspaper reported the original story without the subsequent correction (Price, 1991).

Some investigators have attempted to demonstrate "experimentally" the prejudice and discrimination against immigrant providers. For example, Riley, Hannis, and Rice (1996) mailed a confidential survey to 702 fourth-year U.S. medical students asking them to rank and rate hypothetical residency programs and to rate the importance of selected characteristics in the rankings. The results showed that programs with higher numbers of IMGs worsened significantly both in rank and rating, and that the proportion of IMGs in a residency program was as important a factor in selection of a residency program as was the program's reputation. However, students didn't acknowledge this factor as an important criterion in rating or ranking the programs. Although the authors were quick to note the limitations of the study (particularly the 44% survey response rate) Riley and colleagues concluded that despite the lack of acknowledgment, the proportion of IMGs may well affect perceptions of residency programs. These results seem to underscore "the unspoken bias that ranks . . . residencies according to the percentage of U.S. medical graduates in their program" (Carmichael, 1994, p. 630). In fact, published residency program evaluations frequently used a high percentage of resident IMGs as an indicator for poor quality until 1991, when the AMA contacted 6,500 program directors to correct the misconception among accreditors (Page, 1994a).

In another study, Nasir (1994) sent two sets of letters asking for information and an application to a random sample of 146 family practice residency programs. The letters were identical except that the author of the first set was self-described as a foreign medical graduate, while that of the second letter was described as fourth-year medical student from the University of Nebraska. Nasir found that the U.S. graduate received significantly more replies than did the IMG, and that in the 46 cases where programs responded to both letters, the U.S. graduate received significantly more applications and other information than did the IMG. Nasir also found that 9 of these 46 programs required IMGs to meet standards exceeding those established by the Educational Commission for Foreign Medical Graduates. Sixty-one percent of the programs failed to respond to the IMG letter and 28% did not respond to the USMG. One institution flatly refused to consider IMGs for admission to the residency program. The results

of this study corroborated IMGs' accounts of receiving program information and applications only after signing their letter with a more "Americanized" name. Nasir concluded that a significant percentage of family practice residency programs' admissions processes may discriminate against IMGs. IMGs who received letters from residency program directors stating that the program simply did not accept foreign medical graduates (described in Page, 1992, 1994a) probably would not have agreed more.

Beginning in the mid 1980s, IMG associations began lobbying the U.S. Congress to enact legislation to end unfair treatment of IMGs (Page, 1994b). Following several unsuccessful attempts from 1987 to 1991 to introduce antidiscrimination legislation, the International Association of American Physicians, an umbrella organization of IMG groups, and the AMA successfully worked together to push antidiscrimination legislation through Congress in 1992. Their efforts culminated with the amendment of the Health Professions Reauthorization Act that contained a provision to end discrimination against IMGs by terminating various sources of federal funding for residency programs that violate the law (Nasir, 1994; Page, 1992). The law also mandated the formation of a panel to investigate potential discrimination in other procedures, such as licensing.

From most accounts, treatment of IMGs, at least in applying for residency programs, has improved since amendment of the Health Professions Reauthorization Act; however, there is still great concern over differences in procedures to obtain licenses and hospital privileges, which are perceived by some as discriminatory (Page, 1994a). For example, 27 states require 3 years of graduate training for IMGs before they become eligible for licensing, but only 1 year for USMGs; another 10 states have a 2-year training requirement for IMGs but, again, a 1-year requirement for USMGs (Myers, 1995). Moreover, in Texas, to ensure that IMGs have a premedical education similar to that of USMGs, the Texas legislature mandated that IMGs have 60 se mester hours of college courses outside of medical school—a requirement that is difficult for IMGs coming from countries where they enter medical school directly after high school (Myers, 1995). Myers pointed out that the state has set up a blanket treatment for all IMGs regardless of their education or experience: Except for IMGs coming to teach in medical school, the regulations apply to all.

However, Osteen (1991) pointed out that lack of uniformity in licensing procedures has arisen from the constitutionally derived privilege of each state or other licensing jurisdiction (i.e., District of Columbia, Guam, Virgin Islands, and Puerto Rico) to determine its own rules. Such differences have provided frustrating difficulties for both IMGs and U.S. medical graduates, especially when physicians licensed in one state, assuming simple "reciprocity," attempt to obtain a license in another state. According to Osteen, "a review of the complaints made by IMGs suggests . . . that it is the differences in requirements between states that are the problem. It is not so much that state A treats U.S. medical graduates and IMGs differently, but that state A and state B have different rules" (p. 957). Movement toward uniformity among the states in licensing procedures, including use of the nationally administered USMLE, has helped rectify the problem.

One particularly onerous requirement for licensure has been presentation of all credentials, including in some cases even high school diplomas, to state medical boards (Osteen, 1991). The need to repeatedly obtain proof of graduation is burdensome to IMGs because of factors ranging from reluctance of foreign officials to provide the documentation to the uncertainty of international mail (Osteen, 1991) Moreover, half of all states' licensing boards require IMGs to provide additional information about their medical schools, sometimes including reports on the number of faculty and books in the school's library, even in situations when an IMG already has a license in one state and is applying for a license in another state (Page, 1994a). To address this problem, the AMA has established the National Physicians Credentials' Verification Service, which serves to maintain credentials for licensing purposes.

Another example of differential treatment for IMGs has recently surfaced. Reports have indicated discrimination against IMGs in awarding hospital privileges and in placement on HMOs' provider lists due to hospital administrators' beliefs that having IMGs on staff places the institution at a competitive disadvantage (Page, 1994a). Page reported that as market competition increases in provision of medical care, IMGs fear that they will be the first to lose their spots on provider lists and, therefore, IMG groups strongly support state statutes that restrict insurers from excluding physicians.

According to U.S. medical officials, the crux of the matter revolves around the U.S. medical system's need to ensure that graduates of non–U.S. medical schools, with generally unknown standards, are qualified physicians who have the necessary skills, including language skills, to practice in the United States. Thus, IMGs are usually required to provide additional documentation about their education, complete additional graduate training, and prove competence in English (Page, 1994a). Is this discriminatory? As some writers have noted, even the language issue is not "cut and dried." For instance, in some areas of the country, English proficiency may not be required because both physician and patient speak Spanish (Page, 1994a).

Training Programs

As noted earlier, one of the most common complaints regarding IMGs and FENs is that their medical training in overseas institutions is not equivalent to the training received in American or Canadian medical schools. Some of the areas in which IMGs and FENs are typically lacking include their facility with the English language, imbalance between their clinical and technical skills, and substandard general medical skills. It is important to bear in mind that these problem areas are most often related to the very different format of U.S. and foreign medical school programs (Bogdonoff & Jins, 1991). In theory the Educational Commission for Foreign Medical Graduates (ECFMG) examination provides an assessment of IMGs' clinical skills and English language competency in order to certify them to enter U.S. residency programs or fellowships. Nurses must pass the Nurse Certification Licensure Examination for Registered Nurses (NCLEX-RN) in order to practice in the United States. Recent passing rates for foreign-trained medical personnel on both of these examinations indicate that many of these individuals appear to be academically deficient. In 1992, for example, among those taking parts 1 and 2 of the USMLE, about 40% of IMGs and 90% of USMGs passed the examination (Page, 1994a). Among nurses, in 1987, only 43% of FENs passed the NCLEX-RN the first time compared with a 91% rate among U.S.–trained nurses (Arbeiter, 1988).

Training for IMGs

Because of low test scores, many have argued the need for additional training for IMGs prior to beginning graduate medical training in the United States (Berland, 1993; Sands & Jones, 1993). Levey (1992) advocated rigorous, mandatory evaluation of IMGs' clinical skills followed by additional training when necessary. Evaluation should focus particularly on deficiencies in history taking and conducting physical examinations. Those trainees with marked deficits in training would then be required to take part in preresidency training. Such training programs should include lectures, presentations, reading assignments, sessions in diagnosis, medical ethics, and patient-encounter skills. While some may argue that requiring such additional training of IMGs is discriminatory (Polavarapu, 1993; Singer, 1992), Levey argued that because IMGs and USMGs will be following the same graduate medical curriculum, they must both start out with the same knowledge base (Levey, 1992).

It seems more constructive to pinpoint the actual areas in which IMGs typically have difficulties once they enter U.S. graduate medical training than to simply criticize their lack of preparation. Pretraining programs like the one Levey describes, as well as others (Berland, 1993; Bohnen & Balantac, 1994; Burns, 1991; Dhillon, 1976; Drury, 1976), have been designed to help doctors and nurses improve their medical skills as well as feel more comfortable in the United States. Such programs focus on a number of areas: improving reasoning (Bohnen & Balantac, 1994; Drury, 1976; Romem & Benor, 1993; Sands & Jones, 1993); increasing English comprehension (Dhillon, 1976; Drury, 1976; Ferguson & Maclean, 1988; Sands & Jones, 1993); understanding of hierarchical relations—between professors and students, doctors and nurses, doctors and patients, nurses and patients—inherent in the U.S. medical system (Arbeiter, 1988; Bohnen & Balantac, 1994; Cole-Kelly, 1994); and sharing the great cultural variability of the foreign nurses and doctors who come to the United States to ease their acculturation (Antony, 1995; Chen, 1978; Cole-Kelly, 1994). The United States is not alone in offering training to foreign-trained medical personnel; supplemental medical training is also available in Canada (Nasmith, 1993), Scotland (Ferguson & Maclean, 1988), and Israel (Romem & Benor, 1993).

The importance of additional training for IMGs and its benefits have been well documented (Chen, 1978; Cole-Kelly, 1994; Ferguson & Maclean, 1988; McDermott & Martezki, 1975; Sands & Jones, 1993; and see Romem & Benor, 1993, for a training program in Israel). Training programs for IMGs focus on enhancing clinical skills, familiarizing IMGs with U.S. ethical standards, attending to the IMGs' psychoemotional needs and assimilation to American culture, respecting IMGs' cultural variability, and improving their English skills. Sands and Jones (1993), who have trained many Asian physicians, support Levey's (1992) call for additional training. In their experience, while training in the United States, these physicians often do not gain the clinical experience they need to practice medicine. This is directly related to the fact that their medical training in Asia did not emphasize inductive reasoning and making clinical judgments (Sands & Jones, 1993). Furthermore, passing a test in written English does not guarantee fluency in speaking English, a necessary skill for interacting with patients on a clinical level. Consequently, Sands and Jones stress the need for U.S. training programs to take responsibility for assisting IMGs in acquiring these skills while in the United States. Programs that train IMGs need to take a greater role in supervising and teaching these students.

An interesting program developed at the Edinburgh University in Scotland helps Kuwaiti doctors learn English (Ferguson & Maclean, 1988). The program does not teach medical terminology itself. Rather, participants in the English courses learn to improve skills in speaking, listening, reading, and writing. The program cut the time of learning English at a level of minimum proficiency from a period of 6 months to 4 months. The course consisted of small-group sessions where participants were engaged in role-playing, presenting cases and short papers, and discussing problems of diagnosis and current issues in medical practice. In addition, these Kuwaiti physicians were paired with Edinburgh families from whom they received extra practice with English as well as social support such as help finding apartments.

IMGs can benefit from programs that pay attention to their needs while they become accustomed to an American way of life. In many cases, IMGs tend to socialize almost exclusively with one another, often with those of similar national background (Chen, 1978). One program has focused on the psychosocial development of IMGs (Cole-Kelly, 1994). Cole-Kelly described a family practice residency program that pays particular attention to its residents' cultural heritage, cultural and family influences, and the role of healers in other and U.S. cultures, and how to pronounce the names of its resident physicians.

In addition they have support groups, international meals, and cultural retreats to ease residents' adaptation to U.S. life. This program also examines current issues in the United States relevant to providing health care: gender and race constructions, child abuse, and alcohol and drugs. Finally, in the survival skills seminar, IMG residents are oriented to working in a U.S. hospital and learning how to interact with attending physicians and other colleagues.

Training for Nurses

FENs have long been important health care providers in an area with frequent staffing shortages (Arbeiter, 1988). Like IMGs they often have difficulty passing certification examinations. This is not exclusively a result of poor training but because they lack other necessary skills. A study of the schools from which FENs graduated prior to being recruited by California hospitals revealed gaps in both cultural and medical realms (Bohnen & Balantac, 1994). Most nurses were unfamiliar with the U.S. cultural groups they were serving, had difficulty understanding certain medical concepts and terminology in English (as well as the vocabulary of American slang), and their training often discouraged qualities of independence and assertiveness among the nurses. Furthermore, most of the nurses had few opportunities for problem solving and critical thinking—skills required and highly valued in the United States. Consequently, any continuing education offered to FENs should be prepared to address these issues.

Drury (1976) and Dhillon (1976), nursing professors, reported on their experiences with training FENs. These authors, working nearly 20 years before Bohnen and Balantac (1994), encountered virtually identical training needs among FENs. Drury's and Dhillon's respective training programs were designed both to familiarize FENs with cultural and professional aspects of nursing in the United States and to prepare them to take their board examinations. Drury and her colleagues reviewed the clinical areas of nursing (medical, surgical, pediatric, obstetric, and psychiatric), and helped the nurses learn technical and vernacular English. In addition, they helped prepare the nurses to comprehend and work through various types of examination questions, including objective, situational, and multiple-choice formats. Also, to familiarize FENs with problem-oriented thinking, staff presented FENs with various scenarios and asked them to evaluate each scenario and develop a course of action (Drury, 1976). Dhillon's program focused on these areas, but also included teaching FENs about American cuisine and family structure (Dhillon, 1976).

Providing IMGs and FENs with additional skills through preresidency or continuing education training programs may better enable these health care providers to pass their required licensing examinations. Bergen (Anonymous, 1975) urged the medical profession to pay more attention to medical education and help those who are unable to pass their exams. Specifically, IMGs need help assimilating in the medical system through better supervision and evaluation. Furthermore, one member of the AMA's IMG council warns against wasting the talent of the many unlicensed IMGs. He proposed to liken these IMGs to Physicians' Assistants in order for them to work directly with a physician to sharpen their skills and increase their ability to pass their examinations (Page, 1994b).

Working in the United States

The experiences of individuals working as immigrant health care providers in the United States are, of course, varied. Whether one successfully completes the licensing process—including necessary examinations—is, perhaps, the major determinant of an immigrant's experience in the United States. Persons not passing the examinations do not always return to their home countries; instead, they may remain in the United States. working in low-paying positions such as health aides in hospitals, home health care, or nursing home facilities (Arbeiter, 1988; Erdmans, 1996; Page, 1994b). In some cases, they work in the health care system while they wait to pass their examinations (Erdmans, 1996; Page, 1994b). Meanwhile, a lack of credentials or a license often does not prevent these foreign-trained health care providers from practicing medicine illegally in the United States. For example, Feinstein (1986) noted that some individuals without licenses or other credentials (e.g., postgraduate internships) may decide to practice medicine, considering themselves to be fullfledged doctors simply because they have a medical degree. Estimates of the number of IMGs who are in the United States practicing medicine illegally ranged from 10,000 to 30,000 in 1994 (Page, 1994b). Many of these individuals are married to American citizens and have not yet been accepted into the U.S. medical system. A survey of IMGs applying for ECFMG certification in 1974 showed that 48% of them were already working in the health care field—73% in individual care, 64% in hospitals (Feinstein, 1986). Those individuals who practice this so-called underground medicine, whom Feinstein numbered at 50,000, include both IMGs and foreign-trained U.S. citizens.

Others may arrive in the United States on temporary visas but work illegally as health care providers. Erdmans's (1996) study in Chicago described the symbiotic relationship between Eastern Europeans working illegally as home health care aides and providing 24-hour care to elderly residents of Chicago who could not otherwise afford this level of care. Typically, these workers amass sizable savings and return home. According to Erdmans, this system works well for all except local, legal home care providers, whose efforts to obtain better compensation may be undercut by the illegal workers.

For those practicing their professions legally in the United States, the experience seems mixed. Both personal and professional expectations may be challenged. Although the economic opportunity may be rewarding, living conditions may vary widely and present unexpected circumstances. Joyce and Hunt's (1982) study of Filipino immigrant nurses found that most expressed fairly easy and pleasant adjustment to the United States. However, nurses stated that separation from family and disruption of family relations and obligations was the most difficult problem and the most frequent reason for returning home. Even persons coming from areas thought of as "similar" to the United States (e.g., Canada and Western Europe), can find the adjustment to American life difficult. Canadian doctors are able to make more money and have greater opportunities to practice medicine and utilize technically superior facilities. However, they must contend with other aspects of American life such as high crime rates and the potentially high cost of educating their children (Sullivan, 1994).

On the professional side, various aspects of the working conditions in the United States also have their positive and negative points. Certain geographic areas may be rejected by U.S.–trained physicians because of working conditions—poor local infrastructure, inadequate opportunity or facilities to use the specialized skills acquired during residency, and, in rural areas, isolation from other colleagues with whom to discuss difficult cases. However, since some countries require their health care providers to work in rural areas for a few years, when they immigrate to the United States, some report that they are already accustomed to rural conditions (White, 1993). On the negative side, foreign health care providers seem generally unprepared for the amount of paperwork required and the fear of litigation found in the U.S. health care system (Arbeiter, 1988; Sullivan, 1994). Another common criticism by Canadian physicians of the U.S. system is that millions of Americans have no health care. Although it has its own flaws, the Canadian system does provide access to care for all citizens (Sullivan, 1994).

An immigrant physician or other health care worker is faced with numerous hurdles, from licensing examinations to criticisms of their nationality or foreign education, to adapting to a foreign cultural setting when they come to train or work in the United States. These potential difficulties may be ameliorated if issues such as discrimination, evaluation of medical skills, and the implementation of training programs such as those discussed earlier are addressed seriously so that immigrant providers, American patients, and the United States health care system can all benefit from the skills and labor of immigrant providers.

Conclusion

Immigrant providers find themselves at the intersection of two powerful trends in the United States. The first is a climate that has grown generally less hospitable to immigrants over the past 15 years. Such a climate has resulted in increasing restrictions on immigration. The second trend involves the evolution of the American health care system toward managed care and the growing need for generalists. There seems to be a difference of opinion among policy and medical circles about whether the current medical system, left to its own devices, will correct the current imbalances in care. Aronson and colleagues (1997) have raised the fear that the system is not self-corrective and that reducing the numbers of immigrant providers will curtail services to people in areas with the least access to health care. While the number of U.S.–trained generalist providers is growing, it will take years to approach the needed number. In the meantime, what will the 17% of the population living in Health Professional Shortage Areas do for their medical care? Closing a source of needed practitioners may well exacerbate the inequalities in our system that are already experienced by so many people.

References

Anonymous. (1975). Turning FMGs into U.S. doctors. *Modern Healthcare, 3,* 68, 72.

Anonymous. (1995). Prospecting for primary-care docs? Foreign medical grads can ease the search. *Medical Network Strategy Report, 4,* 6–7.

Antony, S. (1995). International hero [Letter]. *American Journal of Medicine, 98,* 99.

Arbeiter, J. S. (1988). The facts about foreign nurses. *RN, 51,* 56–63.

Aronson, R. D. (1996a). Foreign physicians within the health care system: Immigration strategies and procedures: Pt. 1. *Immigration Briefings, 8,* 1–28.

Aronson, R. D. (1996b). Foreign physicians within the health care system: Immigration strategies and procedures: Pt. 2. *Immigration Briefings, 8,* 1–24.

Aronson, R. D., Domingue, G. C., & Lichtman, E. C. (1997). This year's tumultuous developments affecting the representation of international medical graduates and their employers. In R. P. Murphy (Ed.), *1997–98 Immigration and nationality law handbook* (Vol. 2, pp. 142–156). Washington, DC: American Immigration Lawyers Association.

Balon, R., & Munoz, R. A. (1996). International medical graduates in psychiatric manpower calculations [Letter]. *American Journal of Psychiatry, 153,* 296.

Berland, D. (1993). Pretraining for international medical graduates [Letter]. *Annals of Internal Medicine, 118,* 397.

Bernsen, S., & Rubin, T. M. (1990). Immigration trends affecting health care employment. *HealthSpan, 7,* 3–10.

Bogdonoff, M. D., & Jins, J. J. (1991). University medical center participation in residency training programs for graduates of foreign medical schools. *Annals of Internal Medicine, 114,* 426–427.

Bohnen, M. V., & Balantac, D. D. (1994). Basic academic preparation of foreign-educated nurses: A base for developing continuing education. *Journal of Continuing Education in Nursing, 25,* 258–262.

Burns, J. (1991). Soviet nurses help alleviate Baltimore hospital's shortage. *Modern Healthcare, 21,* 71, 73.

Cameron, V. (1993). Fighting prejudice in the profession [Letter]. *Wisconsin Medical Journal, 92,* 58.

Carmichael, L. P. (1994). Of pride and prejudice. *Family Medicine, 26,* 630–631.

Chase, R. A. (1979). How U.S. law affects FMGs. *Bulletin of the American College of Surgeons, 64,* 4–7.

Chen, R. M. (1978). The education and training of Asian foreign medical graduates in the United States. *American Journal of Psychiatry, 135,* 451–3.

Cheng, L., & Yang, P. Q. (1998). *Global interaction: Global inequality, and migration of the highly trained to the United States. International Migration Review, 23.*

Cole-Kelly, K. (1994). Cultures engaging cultures: International medical graduates training in the United States. *Family Medicine, 26,* 618–24.

DeWitt, A. L. (1995). The oversupply of specialists and graduates of foreign medical schools [Letter]. *New England Journal of Medicine, 333,* 1782.

Dhillon, G. L. (1976). Study programs for foreign nurses . . . special needs of foreign nurses. *Nursing Outlook, 24,* 43–44.

Drury, R. K. (1976). Study programs for foreign nurses . . . A university-based program. *Nursing Outlook, 24,* 41–42.

Dunn M. R., & Miller, R. S. (1996). The shifting sands of graduate medical education. *Journal of the American Medical Association, 276,* 710–713.

Eiseman, B. (1979). FMGs in transition. *Bulletin of the American College of Surgeons, 64,* 13–14.

Erdmans, M. P. (1996). Illegal home care workers: Polish immigrants caring for American elderly. *Current Research on Occupations and Professions, 9,* 267–292.

Evans, J. P. (1981). Restoring America's role in international graduate medical education. *New England Journal of Medicine, 304,* 1542–1543.

Feinstein, R. J. (1986). Underground medicine: The widening problem of unlicensed physicians in the United States. *Journal of Florida Medical Association, 73,* 459–463.

Ferguson, J. J., & Maclean, J. (1988). Introductory course in medical english and primary care for overseas doctors. *Family Practice, 5,* 260–4.

Friedman, E. (1979). FMGs, hospitals, P.L. 94-484, and the future. *Hospitals, 53,* 74–78.

Graduate Medical Education, Appendix. (1995). *Journal of the American Medical Association, 274,* 755–760.

Grecic, V. (1995). Migration of scientists and professionals from the Republic of Serbia. *Studi Emigrazione/Etudes Migrations, 32,* 117–127.

Greenberg, D. S. (1996). Cut immigration, medical schools say. *Lancet, 347,* 607.

Iglehart, J. K. (1996). The quandary over graduates of foreign medical schools in the United States. *New England Journal of Medicine, 334,* 1679–1683.

Immigration and Naturalization Service. (1996). *Table 11: Immigrants aged 16 to 64 admitted by major category of admission and occupation: fiscal years 1996.* Immigration to the United States in Fiscal Year 1996 [on line]. Available: http://www.ins.usdoj.gov/public/stats/1015.html [1997, June 24].

Ishi, T. (1988). *Politics of labor market: Immigrant nurses in the United States.* Paper presentation, American Sociological Association Annual Meeting, Atlanta, Georgia.

Jabbour, S. (1996). Training too many, training too few. *Journal of the American Medical Association, 276,* 729.

Jarrahi, S. (1993). State of affairs: The U.S.–Iran medical exchange program. *North Carolina Medical Journal, 54,* 575–576.

Jesilow, P. (1992). Physician fraud and Medicaid. *Journal of the American Medical Association, 267,* 2037.

Joyce, R. E. & Hunt, C. L. (1982). Philippine nurses and the brain drain. *Social Science and Medicine, 16,* 1223–1233.

Kellis, D. (1995). The oversupply of specialists and graduates of foreign medical schools [Letter]. *New England Journal of Medicine, 333,* 1781.

Kindig, D., Cultice, J. M., & Mullan, F. (1993). The elusive generalist physician. *Journal of the American Medical Association, 270,* 1069–1073.

Kindig, D. A., & Libby, D. L. (1996). Domestic production vs international immigration. *Journal of the American Medical Association, 276,* 978–982.

Kobrin, F. E. (1985). The American midwife controversy: A crisis of professionalization. In J. W. Leavitt & R. L. Numbers (Eds.), *Sickness and health in America: Readings in the history of medicine and public health* (2nd ed., pp. 197–205). Madison: University of Wisconsin Press.

Korcok, M. (1994). U.S. health care reforms may create heavy demand for Canada's primary care MDs. *Canadian Medical Association Journal, 150,* 1849–1854.

Levey, G. S. (1992). Internal medicine and the training of international medical graduates: A time for open discussion and new approaches. *Annals of Internal Medicine, 117,* 403–407.

McDermott, J. F., Jr., & Martezki, T. W. (1975). Some guidelines for the training of foreign medical graduates: Results of a special project. *American Journal of Psychiatry, 132,* 658–61.

McNiven, M. (1992). Study of women IMGs revealing. *Michigan Medicine, 91,* 43–44.

Mick, S. S. (1987). Contradictory policies for foreign medical graduates. *Health Affairs, 6,* 5–18.

Mosberg, W. H., Angelides, A. P., Hayes, G. J., & Evans, J. P. (1979). Preserving our international role in postgraduate medical education. *Bulletin of the American College of Surgeons, 64,* 6–7.

Mou, T. W. (1988). Impact of ECFMG examinations. *Federation Bulletin, 75,* 131–38.

Mullan, F., Politzer, R. M., & Davis, H. (1995). Medical migration and the physician workforce: International medical graduates and American medicine. *Journal of the American Medical Association, 273,* 1521–1527.

Myers, C. (1995). Different paths, same goal. *Texas Medicine, 91,* 30–32.

Nagelberg, S., Schwartz, A. H., Perlman, B. B., Paris, M., & Thornton, J. C. (1980). Providers and receivers in the private psychiatric Medicaid system. *American Journal of Psychiatry, 137,* 690–694.

Nasir, L. (1994). Evidence of discrimination against international medical graduates applying to family practice residency programs. *Family Medicine, 26,* 625–629.

Nasmith, L. (1993). Programs for international medical graduates. *Canadian Family Physician, 39,* 2549–53.

Osteen, A. (1991). Licensure and international medical graduates. *Journal of the American Medical Association, 266,* 956–958.

Page, L. (1992). Discrimination against IMGs barred. *American Medical News, 35,* 3.

Page, L. (1993). IMGs flock to match. *American Medical News, 36,* 2, 34.

Page, L. (1994a). Discrimination or discriminating? *American Medical News, 37,* 3, 7.

Page, L. (1994b). Filling the gaps. *American Medical News, 37,* 1, 7–8.

Page, L. (1994c). Immigration policy keeps door open. *American Medical News, 37,* 7–8.

Pew Health Professions Commission. (1995). Critical challenges: Revitalizing the health professions for the twenty-first century. San Francisco: University of California at San Francisco Center for the Health Professions.

Phillips, D. (1996). The internationalization of labor: The migration of nurses from Trinidad and Tobago. *International Sociology, 11,* 109–127.

Polavarapu, P. (1993). Pretraining for international medical graduates [Letter]. *Annals of Internal Medicine, 118,* 397.

Price, J. (1991, December 19). Medicaid fraud: A costly epidemic. *Washington Times,* p. A1.

Radosh, P. F. (1986). Midwives in the United States: Past and present. *Population Research and Policy Review, 5,* 129–146.

Riley, J. D., Hannis, M., & Rice, K. G. (1996). Are international medical graduates a factor in residency program selection? A survey of fourth-year medical students. *Academic Medicine, 71,* 381–386.

Rios, M. (1992). Physician fraud and Medicaid [Letter]. *Journal of the American Medical Association, 267,* 2037.

Romem, Y., & Benor, D. E. (1993). Training immigrant doctors: Issues and responses. *Medical Education, 27,* 74–82.

Salsberg, E. S., Wing, P., Dionne, M. G., & Jemiolo, D. J. (1996). Graduate medical education and physician supply in New York state. *Journal of the American Medical Association, 276,* 683–688.

Sands, C., & Jones, D. W. (1993). Pretraining for international medical graduates [Letter]. *Annals of Internal Medicine, 118,* 397.

Schusterman, C. (1995). New methods for securing J-1 physicians. *Medical Network Strategy Report, 4,* 10–11.

Seifer, S. D., Troupin, B., & Rubenfeld, G. D. (1996). Changes in marketplace demand for physicians. *Journal of the American Medical Association, 276,* 695–699.

Singer, J. (1992). Licensing of international medical graduates [Letter]. *Journal of the American Medical Association, 267,* 53–54.

Stevens, R. A. (1995). International medical education and the concept of quality: Historical reflections. *Academic Medicine, 70,* S11–S18.

Sullivan, P. (1994). Growth in number of advertisements indicates increased U.S. interest in Canadian MDs.

Canadian Medical Association Journal, 150, 1855–1856.

Sullivan, R. B., Watanabe, M., Whitcomb, M. E., & Kindig, D. A. (1996). The evolution of divergences in physician supply policy in Canada and the United States. *Journal of the American Medical Association, 276,* 704–709.

Sutnik, A. I., Shafron, M. L., & Wilson, M. P. (1992). Impact of the new United States medical licensing examination on the certification process of the educational commission for foreign medical graduates. *International Journal of Dermatology, 31,* 798–799.

Varki, A. (1992). Of pride, prejudice, and discrimination. *Annals of Internal Medicine, 116,* 762–764.

Vasireddi, S. S., & Chowdappa, J. (1995). The oversupply of specialists and graduates of foreign medical schools [Letter]. *New England Journal of Medicine, 333,* 1781–1782.

Whitcomb, M. E. (1995). Correcting the oversupply of specialists by limiting residencies for graduates of foreign medical schools. *New England Journal of Medicine, 333,* 454–456.

Whitcomb, M. E., & Miller, R. S. (1995). Participation of international medical graduates in graduate medical education and hospital care for the poor. *Journal of the American Medical Association, 274,* 696–699.

White, O. (1993). This could end the rural doctor shortage. *Medical Economics, 70,* 42–49.

Wong, J. C. (1979). An echo in other countries. *Bulletin of the American College of Surgeons, 64,* 17–18.

Wynia, M. K. (1995). The oversupply of specialists and graduates of foreign medical schools [Letter]. *New England Journal of Medicine, 333,* 1781.

Zoler, M. (1989). Rules eased for Nicaraguan MDs. *Medical World News, 30,* 53.

30

Public Health Planning and Policy Change

RUTH LYN RIEDEL

The good, the bad, the ugly. That's America. You gotta deal with it!

Bill Cosby (1996)

Introduction

In 1988 the Institute of Medicine's (IOM) Committee for the Study of the Future of Public Health identified two factors that determine problem solving in public health in the United States: (1) the level of scientific and technical knowledge, and (2) the content of public values and popular opinions. Given few would dispute the wealth of science and technical knowledge accumulated over the past century of public health practice, this chapter focuses on the more public aspects of planning, which are socioeconomic and political.

Over the years the quality of life in America has improved significantly because of public health interventions. Examples include communicable disease control, maternal and child health services, and the prevention of acute and chronic disease. However, in recent years, the effectiveness of

the American public health system has diminished. In 1988, the IOM report addressed the concern of its membership and of practitioners in all areas of the field: "this nation has lost sight of its public health goals and has allowed the system of public health activities to fall into disarray" (p. 1).

Public health professionals are, by definition, committed to using their knowledge and expertise to deal effectively with existing and emerging health problems. But decision making in public health, as in other sectors of society, is driven by the dynamics of American politics. Policies are shaped by competition, bargaining, and political influence. Technical knowledge, "analysis, and judgement must compete with other perspectives for policy attention and support," (IOM, 1988, p. 4) and play a restricted role in policy development and program planning.

This chapter begins with a description of social and political trends that have influenced the development of health policy since the 1930s, and traces two dominant interest groups, the *bureaucratic reformers* and the *market reformers,* through the market reform movement of the 1980s. As social and health problems become more interconnected and the political will to address them diminishes, the United States is left with continuing and growing problems of public health, such as limited access to health services, substance

RUTH LYN RIEDEL • Alliance Healthcare Foundation, San Diego, California 92123.

Handbook of Immigrant Health, edited by Loue. Plenum Press, New York, 1998.

abuse, and new challenges such as toxic substances and new diseases and viruses. Problems of this complexity and substance require planning approaches that are politically "rational" and acceptable to stakeholders, not just technically rational.

A critical omission in health planning for underserved groups is the absence of consumer participation in the planning process. Blum (1981) attributes this problem to the elitist tendencies of health professionals and planners who prefer to control information and to coopt consumers to the "technologic imperatives of health care," ignoring the more salient issues of "resource allocation" (p. 6). While underserved immigrants and the working poor have the most to gain from participating in program planning and system reform, planning activities usually take place during the workday in inconvenient places for these consumers. With rare exceptions, immigrant groups do not organize to, in Blum's words, "take a pressure group stance" (p. 6). Without a strong presence it is unlikely that their concerns will be taken seriously.

Background

Certainly, the U.S. health care system as a whole is flawed; it is extremely costly and incapable of addressing the needs of large segments of the population. Despite several iterations of system reform and the successful manipulation of social, physical, and environmental factors by public health professionals to reduce human suffering, gross inequities remain. As before, the allocation, distribution, and utilization of resources are determined by market forces, not need. R. E. Brown (1979) was prescient in predicting that large health care systems and organized medicine would share an overriding interest and control of social and financial resources for decades. In most sectors of the economy, dominant interests control national and local markets (Waitzkin, 1978). These interest groups tend to unite when they are threatened by an interest group from other social strata, such as diverse community groups that coalesce periodically to improve the delivery of health services (Alford, 1975).

Controlling costs is the central policy issue in the U.S. health care system. In periods of real or assumed economic scarcity, the true nature of the dominant structural interests in the U.S. political economy emerges; these interests have consistently encouraged enormous disparities among social classes and ethnic groups. While there is steady improvement in the condition of America's corporate sector, poverty and unemployment in parts of the inner city are reaching catastrophic proportions. For the first time in the 20th century, large groups of adults in inner cities are not working. Individuals and families that are currently dependent on public programs are likely to remain so until they face greater hardships under the Welfare Reform Law of 1996 (H.R. 3734). Wilson (1996) identified the consequences of the disappearance of work in inner-city neighborhoods as crime, gang violence, drug trafficking, family dissolution, and welfare. These problems "undermine social organization . . . and the social processes that regulate behavior" (p. 28).

An analysis of interest group politics can be helpful in understanding failures in planning and program development, local controversies about public health issues, conflicts within health care systems (i.e., involving boards, hospitals, and medical groups), and national health policy decisions. Variations among political–economic interests generate contradictions that can provide strategic opportunities for public sector players, sometimes to the detriment of the uninsured, and "safety net" providers of health care. For example, the private sector views public sector developments as potential sources of market expansion, as in the exponential growth of Medicaid managed care in the 1990s.

As Navarro (1975) stated, dominant groups and classes are "powerful because they sway society's value-generating systems" (p. 203). Social values are inculcated by families, communities, institutions, organizations, and the media. Social values are represented in the policy positions of subcultures, social classes, and organizations. Even within organizations, "elites . . . will take a public position consistent with the interests of their organizations. Career incentives probably require that (the organization's) collective myths be publicly stated, even if there is considerable private cynicism and disbelief" (Alford, 1975, p. 71). Value systems, elite or otherwise, assign high worth to messages that conform to their script, and reject those that are contradictory. The images or ideologies of the various interests in health care are developed through continuing efforts of "groups and organizations to construct symbolic presentations" of their own legitimacy and the legitimacy of the sectors and organizations "within which their roles are defined" (p. 16). The result is a multiplicity of social roles, coexisting within diverse professional and organizational contexts. Individuals may play multiple and even contradictory roles, functioning as "reformers" in one context, and as members of a (dominant) interest group in another (Alford, 1975).

Further analysis of the ideologies of interest groups in the U.S. health care system reveals four basic groups: (1) the procompetative *market reformers,* (2) the rationalizing *bureaucratic reformers,* (3) the *liberal* perspective, a dominant interest in the 1960s, and (4) *the equal health advocates,* a class-based perspective (Alford, 1975). *Market reformers* regard the struggle among interest groups as necessary and desirable. Because professions and organizations are created as required by a technologically and economically differentiated society, they should have considerable autonomy. Market reformers place their trust in market mechanisms, believing that competition among producers will cause the entire system to become more sensitive to cost issues. Not unlike equal health advocates, market reformers expect the quality and appropriateness of care to be regulated by consumer choice. In the late 1970s, some viewed Enthoven's proposed Consumer Choice Health Plan and subsequent developments as the clarion call of the procompetitive movement.

Health services research in the market reform tradition addresses cost issues and often uses trend analysis and econometric modeling, accepting the current market environment as a given.

Bureaucratic reformers develop complex, rational plans to coordinate the organization, financing, and distribution of health care. Practitioners in this tradition argue for the efficient use of scarce resources and increased integration of the diverse components of the delivery system. According to this view, there are no problems that cannot be managed away and solved by organization or reorganization. A coordinated system will increase access and quality. The bureaucratic reform movement engendered institutional planning, the Health Systems Agencies, Certification-of-Need legislation, the concept of health system integration and managed care. Research in this tradition is often sociological or "operations" research, addressing the delivery system, providers, organizations, or patients as the unit of analysis.

The *liberal* perspective was a dominant interest in the 1960s. "Liberal" planners and researchers, then and now, encourage change from within a geographic entity like a community, a delivery system, a profession, or an organization. Since the 1980s and 1990s, many liberal practitioners have been working within the bureaucratic or market reform traditions in order to secure a place in the action. In Alford's (1975) words, "academics, specialized journalists and liberal health professionals must assume that there is a public out there waiting for insightful analysis that combines optimism and realism" (p. 261). When liberal practitioners build coalitions they are often loosely knit, and some elements may press for change at the expense of others. "Visions of changes which go too far past the emerging consensus . . . will scare off . . . crucial elements of the coalition that are ready for 'a little change, but not too much'" (p. 261).

Finally, the *equal health advocates' perspectives* (Alford, 1975) which essentially includes the class-based and Marxist perspective, maintains that defects in the health care system are attributable to corporate capitalism, which controls all sectors of the U.S. economy. In their view, the pattern of class dominance in health care gives primacy to capitalist interests as a whole, and to selected industries (i.e., insurance and hospitals) and professions (i.e., physicians). The *class-based* perspective endorses radical change of U.S. social institutions, holding that they are in need of fundamental reconstruction. Over the years these interests have become fragmented; generally, they have advocated for community control over the supply and distribution of health care resources and facilities, often organizing to defend the rights of ethnic minorities and low-income populations. Class-based, equal health advocates are proponents of quality of care and quality of life for everyone, including good health, jobs, good nutrition, adequate housing, and safe, nontoxic communities and workplaces.

According to Blum (1981) problems in the health sector are largely determined by conditions in other sectors, but inasmuch as the health sector "is an area of high political, social and individual interest" it offers opportunities to "thrash out new and old values and work out the experimental processes of planning for significant change" (p. 8–9). Blum believed that the "dominant social-economic-political ideology . . . determines a country's posture on the desirability of deliberate social change" (p. 57), the use of planning for solving public problems, and the designation of the appropriate interest groups and technologies. These ideologies vary from country to country. For example, in Russia before the 1990s, and in China, planning was a government function; the government provided for the people. In other countries, it was commonly held that the private sector should plan, organize, and produce at will; this laissez faire, market reform position supports the private market economy. In contrast, Scandinavian countries are known for free market economic growth and government sponsored health and social programs that contribute to selected low morbidity rates and low infant mortality.

While variations can be observed over time in the United States, generally, the private market shapes the framework for public planning. According to Blum's (1981) analysis, 19th-century planning to solve public problems was a function of private sector pluralistic interests. Government assumed a guiding role, but only in the accelerated development of the western United States. In other words, there was no public planning. In this capitalist framework, private interests learned how to predict and take advantage of trends, avoiding some problems and cashing in on others; this was the beginning of the market reform tradition. The planning mode was exploitive and profit oriented.

The Early Years of Health Planning

In the 1930s when the private market was paralyzed and during World War II, government was temporarily accepted as an independent force for the common good. This marked the beginnings of the bureaucratic reform tradition, a period of "disjointed incrementalism" (Lindblom, 1965), when the government took steps to modify situations that were obviously undesirable and that affected everyone. Even then, the adjustments tended to be small changes which were not goal directed, and had minimum long-term impacts. These interventions focused on one system at a time, ignoring others, which introduced new and unanticipated problems.

After the economy rebounded, the reins were handed back to pluralist, private interests, and the first major health planning movement in the United States began (Blum, 1981). The Hill–Burton Act of 1946 financed health care facilities construction, in accordance with state plans and minimum federal guidelines. Hill–Burton was a prime example of incrementalism and partisan mutual adjustment (Lindblom, 1965); it was a compromise between government and private interests.

But when liberal interventionists and pro-government bureaucratic reform interests got close to national health insurance legislation, they were blocked. Bureaucratic reformers were also prevented from enforcing antitrust laws, or supporting prepayment systems that could have controlled costs while preserving high standards of care (Starr, 1981). The barrier was a coalition of private market interests and politically conservative forces that supported "organized" medicine, hospitals, and the insurance industry. The incentives for expansion in programs like Hill–Burton were joined with a weak regulatory component to achieve a minimal standard of public accountability. At the same time, technological breakthroughs in industry and the military led to technological approaches to social problems and the beginning of social engineering. Bureaucratic reformers explored the new frontiers of planning. In retrospect, these explorations did little to correct the continuing and unacceptable "distributive failures" of prior years, that is, high cost and inequities in access and quality.

Starr (1981) described the redistributive programs of the 1960s as the second wave of government intervention, emerging from the dynamics of the market. The economy was growing, allowing ideological shifts, and government was permitted to take an active role. By this time systems analysis had found a home in social science, and health planners and practitioners believed that "technology and specialization" could be used to "manage problems away." Blum (1981) gave this period high marks because populist goals of equal access, better quality, and improved health status pushed government forces into action. Medicare and Medicaid were initially successful in improving access to care for the medically underserved. But these very programs accelerated tendencies toward growth and inflation through generous, flexible, and uncontrolled reimbursement provisions. In addition, the 1960s was a period of monumental growth of specialization and technology in medicine, which increased costs immeasurably.

Health Planning in the 1970s

The first approximation of deliberative, long-term, goal-oriented health planning legislation in the United States was the passage of P.L. 89749 in 1966, creating the Health Systems Agencies (HSAs). Liberals and equal health advocates were given a voice, participating with government to set standards as anchors for health services planning and program development. P.L. 89749 was described as the "planning vehicle for deliberate social change in the health arena in 1966" (Blum, 1981, p. 62) because it was to ensure a consumer voice in regional decision making. Yet the legislation, as written, prevented consumers from interfering "with existing patterns of the private, professional practice of medicine, dentistry and related healing arts" (p. 62).

In 1974, P.L. 93641 was an attempt to mandate federal, regional, and local long-range planning and decision making. State and local planning bodies were forced to include a majority of consumer representatives, as well as providers. These regional planning structures were the most evolved form of health planning bodies thus far. Unfortunately, the majority of the consumer representatives were relatives of providers, upper middle class and able to convince or overrule low-income consumers. Consequently, public interests remained subservient to dominant provider groups.

Zeckhauser and Zook (1981) offered other explanations for the ineffectiveness of the "complicated, economically inefficient and hard-to-manage collection of regulatory programs" (p. 87). By the 1970s, new entitlement programs and expenditures contributed to excessive demand. Instead of creating disincentives for excessive consumption, the government regulated capital investments in new facilities through the Certificate-of-Need (CON) program, clinical practice patterns through Professional Standards Review Organizations (PSROs), and facilities expansion and location decisions through the Health Systems Agencies (HSAs). Research on HSAs and CON programs demonstrated relative ineffectiveness. Only half of the HSAs could quantify the need for hospital beds in their own planning areas, and fewer than 20% could project future needs. A study of CON programs showed no evidence of reduced capital investments in health care facilities in the aggregate (Joskow, 1981). In fact, CON engendered the development of new and expensive outpatient facilities and in-home services. PSROs, also introduced in 1972, were costly to administer and achieved minimal reductions in hospital utilization. However, as Olson (1981) reminded us, the public gets involved only when "momentous policy controversies arise," as in the passage of Medicare and Medicaid legislation. National health policy is inevitably influenced by the "discrete lobbying efforts of small groups of wealthy individuals and firms." Providers who have "incentives to preserve or increase overspending are organized, and heard," and "taxpayers and people who pay insurance premiums are not" (Olson, 1981, p. 17).

Health Planning in the 1980s

Observers of public health policy in the 1980s witnessed the magnification of social injustice and social inequality in the distribution of housing, food, education, and employment, the prerequisites of a healthy life. After the regulatory failures of the 1970s, conservatives rose to power, and national government grew fearful, refusing to address the thorny issues of health promotion and illness prevention. Looking back on the 1980s, the executive director of the American Public Health Association, William McBeath (1991) described the "abrogation of governmental responsibility in public health" (p. 1563). Instead, the federal government introduced regulatory constraints which did control costs, initially. Unable to withstand grinding pressure from conservative professional lobbies and "Reaganomic" market forces, the federal government went into a "broad scale retreat"on public health policy issues. Although state and local health departments sought funding to round out limited

budgets, there was great national reluctance to support America's public health infrastructure. Goals and objectives for national plans were developed, but without structures for implementation (McBeath, 1991). With the strengthening of market reform interests came an emphasis on individual responsibility for healthier behaviors that bordered on "victim blaming," as conservatives sought to reduce public expenditures and privatize the delivery of health services.

The 1980s witnessed more attempts at provider regulation, which paralleled the growth of competition among payers and providers. According to L. D. Brown and McLaughlin (1990), all of the activity produced "only one clear outcome: the system preaches cost containment but practices cost shifting" (p. 20). The decade of prudent buyers rewarded "economic individualism" while the costs of health care in the aggregate continued to rise. L. D. Brown and McLaughlin contrast the United States with other Western nations that experienced similar spiraling costs in the 1970s, but were able to achieve "relative restraint." Through the Medicare prospective payment system and state rate-setting "experiments," the government did achieve cost savings. Using different strategic approaches, private sector payers clung to the belief that, somehow, "market forces" would contain costs; there was no reason to infringe on "community forces" that would voluntarily and miraculously agree to manage costs and create integrated health care systems at the community level. Said "community forces" included providers, payers, and community leaders who had served the interests of American business for years. Moreover, the 1980s was an "egocentric, money-minded period," and the decade of Independent Public Offerings (IPOs) which greatly inflated the value of health care stocks in the public market.

While the battle between bureaucratic and market reformers raged on, there were a number of noteworthy developments in health planning and policy. The World Health Organization's (WHO) 1981 global strategy for Health for All by the year 2000 identified "a level of health that will permit . . . all citizens of the world" to lead socially and economically productive lives. The "essential, basic health services" should be available to everyone, and delivered in an acceptable manner to individuals, families, and communities (McBeath, 1991, p. 1564). Thereafter, the U.S. Surgeon General issued a report to guide the U.S. Public Health Service in an expanded set of health promotion and disease prevention activities for the 1980s. Published in 1979 as *Promoting Health, Preventing Disease: Objectives for the Nation,* these goals gave public health professionals something to strive for by 1990. Progress was made on about half of the objectives that were measurable and could be achieved. The initial "Healthy People" objectives survived the 1980s and were revised for the 1990s, offering broad national goals and clear objectives, and inviting public accountability.

At the same time, the Centers for Disease Control and Prevention (CDC), influenced by national health policy in Canada, published *Recommendations for a National Strategy for Disease Prevention,* a prioritization of 31 preventable health problems in the environment, lifestyles, and medical care (CDC, 1978). The CDC observed that, in America, 50% of premature mortality is attributable to unhealthy lifestyles, 20% to biology or genetics, 20% to the environment, and 10% to health care.

In 1983, the CDC in collaboration with the American Public Health Association (APHA), the National Organization of County Health Officials, and the Association of State and Territorial Health Officials developed "model standards" for community-oriented preventive health services. At the community level, the standards provided specific, quantifiable objectives for reducing existing levels of preventable morbidity and mortality (McBeath, 1991). By 1983, surveys had been conducted in 47 states, detailing the level of compliance to public health standards (Schaefer, 1985). The implementation process brought out numerous policy and program issues. State and local politics were primary obstacles to achieving objectives; secondary obstacles included scarce resources, technical deficiencies, development costs, and inadequate information systems.

Once these inadequacies were observed and proclaimed by the Institute of Medicine and government agencies, funding followed. While gains in reducing preventable morbidity and mortality in the 1980s were limited, there was much improvement in planning technology, especially in data systems and information management. Roos (1995) reminded us that there are "three types of information about populations" needed to "refocus policy on the determinants of health: health status, socioeconomic status, and health care use" (p. DS133). Without these elements information systems cannot describe the health of a population and the relationships among utilization, expenditures, and health. Planners and policy makers require data systems that can track developments and monitor the effects of interventions over time.

A good example of improved planning technology is the work of Nutting and Shorr which started in the Indian Health Service in the early 1980s. They designed new approaches to assessing the quality and continuity of ambulatory care and a new model for developing comprehensive care at the community level known as Community Oriented Primary Care (COPC). Subsequently, the IOM developed an operational COPC model that was even more carefully articulated by Paul Nutting (1987). Nutting's model contained four elements or "stages" of community program development:

1. Definition and characterization of the community
2. Identification of the community's health problems
3. Modification of the health care program or delivery system in response to identified needs
4. Monitoring the impact of program or system modifications through careful evaluation

The School of Public Health at the University of California, Berkeley, developed a manual for planners and practitioners that combined COPC with a strategic planning process for community health centers and like entities, giving them tools to cope with the extensive budgetary cutbacks of the eighties, which were aimed at reducing the overlap among categorical programs (Overall & Williamson, 1985).

The cost and quality advantages of the regionalization of medical care were rediscovered in the 1980s. Evidence for improved patient outcomes in hospitals with higher volumes of medical diagnoses and surgical procedures, was based on hospital mortality rates and posthospital morbidity and mortality data (Luft, 1985). Better outcomes were not due only to bigger volumes ("quality-of-scale effect") but could also be explained by the "referral effects" of institutions or physicians with reputations for superior performance (Maerki *et al.,*1986). Cost containment arguments for regionalization included economies of scale and more stringent criteria for performing specialized procedures (Luft, 1985).

Finally, the 1980s witnessed the gradual abandonment of health planning structures created in the 1970s by P.L. 93641. There was growing sentiment among HSA observers that consumers were neither well represented nor effective. Politically, the voices of consumers became less welcome than the voices of insurers, labor unions, and business coalitions. Funds for health planning were severely cut in the "new federalism," and planners sought alternative funding sources as the HSAs dropped out (Carpenter, 1982). The Reagan administration entered office prepared to use market incentives to control hospital costs. Research on state Certificate-of-Need (CON) programs provided clear evidence of poor performance in containing hospital cost inflation. Subsequently, market reformers withdrew support from the planning structures created by P.L. 93-641 (Simpson, 1985).

The "Wicked" Problems of Public Health

The purpose of the IOM study of the Future of Public Health (1988) was to reach a broader audience than its own membership and demonstrate that, as a nation, we had let down our public health guard. The report pointed to evidence that as a nation we were no longer capable of maintaining past progress, arresting the development of continuing problems, or preventing new and emerging health crises. The public health system was incapable of exercising its responsibilities. The applications of "fully current scientific knowledge and organizational skills" (IOM, 1988, p. 126) did not work on the "messy" (e.g., nonlinear, convoluted) health and social problems that required immediate solutions. Nor was the U.S. public health system in a position to "generate new knowledge, methods and programs" (IOM, 1988, p. 126) sufficient to justify society's assumption that public health could respond to continuing and emerging threats. Instead the United States was faced with an array of complex problems: old problems that reemerged, continued, and grew; current problems, some of which were reaching crisis proportions; and new and emerging problems with the potential for future disaster.

Continuing and Growing Problems

Substance Abuse and Injection Drug Use

A 1993 study conducted by the Institute for Health Policy at Brandeis University, and commissioned and published by the Robert Wood Johnson Foundation (1993) demonstrated that substance abuse in the United States was responsible for more deaths, illnesses, and disability than any other preventable health problem. Substance abuse places undue financial and psychological burdens on families and stretches health, education, social services, and criminal justice systems to the breaking point. Every year, approximately 500,000 individuals die from substance abuse; 20,000 of these deaths are caused by the use of illegal drugs and result from an overdose, homicide, suicide, motor vehicle crashes, or the complications of HIV/AIDS. Half of U.S. males arrested for homicide or assault test positive for illegal drugs (RWJF, 1993).

Drug-related deaths, often involving more than one illegal drug, or drugs combined with alcohol, are increasing among men, especially African Americans. African American men are more than twice as likely as Cambodian men to die from the direct effects of illicit drugs, and African American women are nearly twice as likely as Caucasian women to die from drug use. More than one third of all new AIDS cases occur in injecting drug users or their sexual partners (RWJF, 1993).

Along the United States–Mexican border, young people start using alcohol, tobacco, and other drugs before age 13. A high percentage of older teens (ages 15–24) use hospital emergency services for problems related to substance abuse. In 1991, 14% of those arrested for substance abuse in Arizona border counties were juveniles ("Border Youth and Substance Abuse," 1996).

Adolescent Pregnancy

Unintended pregnancy is widespread in the United States, representing 60% of all pregnancies (California Wellness Foundation [CWF], 1996). Each year, 1 million adolescents, or 12% of all 15–19-year-olds, become pregnant. The adolescent pregnancy rate is four to five times higher in America than in other developed countries. In America, approximately 19% of African American teens become pregnant, 13% of Hispanic teens, and 8% of White teens. In California, 60% of all adolescent births occur in Latino communities. The birth rate in young Latinas has nearly doubled in the past decade (CWF, 1996).

High numbers of teen births engender higher rates of complications including birth defects, prematurity, miscarriage, and death. Adolescent pregnancy is linked to dropping out of high school, poverty, and poor health in future years (IOM, 1988). Research ties teen pregnancy to various social, cultural, economic, and cultural issues. Educating adolescents about responsible sexual behavior does not encourage promiscuity, and learning about responsible sexual behavior can assist teens to better take charge of their lives (CWF, 1996). Studies also show that promoting abstinence alone is ineffective (CWF, 1996).

Violence

Violence affects the lives of millions of individuals in the United States, whether they are perpetrators, victims, or witnesses. In all of these situations, "individuals have a diminished capacity for healthy living, and poorer health outcomes" (Pacific Center for Violence Prevention, 1994b, p. 1). In 1991, 25,020 Americans were murdered and 11,043,600 were injured in robberies and assaults. On a typical day, 68 individuals died and 30,256 were injured from violent acts of others. Firearms were used in most homicides (Pacific Center for Violence Prevention, 1994b). Males were overwhelmingly the victims and perpetrators of violence. Young people, ages 12–24, committed about half of the 6.4 million nonfatal violent crimes in 1991. These youth are still at greatest risk for falling victim to nonfatal assault (Pacific Center for Violence Prevention, 1994b).

In 1991, the risk of nonfatal assault was three times greater for persons with family incomes below $7,500 than it was for those with family incomes above $50,000. Homicide victimization rates are highest in areas of cities where poverty is most prevalent. In America, the direct and indirect costs of violent crimes and crimes against property are $425 billion each year (Pacific Center for Violence Prevention, 1994a). Lifetime costs for all persons ages 12 and older who are injured in rape, robbery, assault, arson, murder, or several of these crimes, in a single year in the United States are estimated to be $178 billion (Miller, Cohen, & Rossman, 1993).

In metropolitan areas of California there has been a disproportionately high increase in the rate of violent crime among Latino and Asian–Pacific Islander youth less than 25 years of age. In sections of northern San Diego County, violent crimes committed by young people increased 132% between 1988 and 1992 (Burbridge, 1993). In East San Diego in the same time period, the number of

Indochinese youth arrested increased by 500%; growth in the number of refugee gang members increased from 3 to 300 documented members in 1992 (Trang,1993).

Current Problems and Crises

HIV/AIDS

The year 1995 was a grim milestone for the AIDS epidemic in the United States. According to the Centers for Disease Control and Prevention (CDC), more than 500,000 people had been diagnosed with AIDS, and more than 300,000 had died (Kaiser Family Foundation [KFF], 1996). The CDC estimated that, in addition, between 650,000 and 900,000 are HIV-infected. Each year, there are approximately 40,000 new HIV infections in America. In 1993, AIDS was the leading cause of death among adults 25–44 years of age, and in 1994, there were nearly 42,000 deaths from AIDS (KFF, 1996).

In some communities, in recent years, there has been increased incidence of HIV infection among Asian–Pacific Islander populations. In areas of California, the incidence has been explained by cultural differences and the lack of knowledge of high-risk behaviors (Loue, 1992).

The United States has more than 1.5 million IDUs (injecting drug users), the largest reported number in the world (Des Jarlais & Freedman, 1994), with half a million drug-related deaths each year. AIDS is increasing rapidly among injecting drug users and heterosexuals. More than 33% of new AIDS cases occur in IDUs, their sexual partners, and their children; 47% of all women with AIDS are IDUs (CDC, 1993a, 1993c). Communities of color have been disproportionately affected by HIV/AIDS since the epidemic began, largely through injection drug use. Women and children of color are especially affected by ethnic disparities in incidence (CDC, 1993b).

Each year, one in four new HIV infections occur in young people between the ages of 13 and 21. More young people than before are having sexual intercourse, using drugs and alcohol, and engaging in other high-risk behaviors, leaving them vulnerable to HIV (Office of National AIDS Policy, 1996). Limited access to counseling and voluntary testing, and the lack of AIDS education and prevention programs prolongs their vulnerability (Office of National AIDS Policy, 1996).

Restricted Access to Health Care

The National Perspective. The latest statistics on the uninsured show that almost 41 million people in this country have no health insurance. The future looks even bleaker. The Council on the Impact of Health System Change estimated that in the year 2002, 67 million Americans will be uninsured; these projections assume the same rate of deterioration in job-related coverage and modest constraints on Medicaid enrollment (Davis, 1996).

Traditionally, about half of America's uninsured are medically indigent, or unable to pay for health care. A plethora of research has demonstrated that the medically indigent have more illnesses and disabilities and are less likely to seek care (IOM, 1988). Half of all Americans who are uninsured are employed. This group, known as the "working poor," are also most likely to be ineligible for Medicaid. Only half of individuals and families with incomes below the poverty line are enrolled in Medicaid programs (IOM,1988).

When the poor and uninsured do seek care, they use the "safety net"—a relatively small number of hospitals and clinics that are often public providers of health services. In 1986, a Robert Wood Johnson Foundation (RWJF) study revealed that 10% of U.S. hospitals provide more than 40% of inpatient and outpatient care to the uninsured (RWJF, 1986). As a result, America's safety net providers, which include public and teaching hospitals, federally funded community health centers, and a few local health departments, have been placed in jeopardy. These organizations rely on Medicaid revenues and other public sector funding streams to cross-subsidize care for the uninsured. They also provide essential and specialized community services not offered by other providers in their communities (Lipson & Naierman, 1996). While there is no competition for indigent patients, the Medicaid managed care movement, which started in the late 1980s, brought private sector competitors into the public market. The increasing competition from private health plans forces "safety net" providers to enter into new contractual arrangements with the state, or with commercial providers who are financially driven.

The Federal Welfare Reform Law (H.R. 3734) was signed into law in August 1996, ending 61 years of guaranteed federal cash assistance to the poor. H.R. 3734 changes eligibility requirements, and cash assistance will be replaced by block grants to states. H.R. 3734 has been touted as President Clinton's answer to "re-creating the nation's social bargain with the poor." A 5-year lifetime limit will be imposed on all families that sign up for welfare. In addition, recipients must return to work within 2 years. Previously, all recipients of Aid to Families with Dependent Children (AFDC) were automatically eligible for Medicaid. Under a new program for Temporary Assistance to Needy Families (TANF), states have the option to determine eligibility status under a time-limited, cash assistance program (Shogren, 1996).

The Impacts of Welfare Reform on Documented and Undocumented Immigrants. Since 1984, 10 million people have immigrated to the United States. Forty percent of the nation's legal immigrants (noncitizens who were admitted to the United States because of job skills or strong family ties) now live in California (Shogren, 1996). The state has provided assistance to these immigrants since 1988 at an annual cost of $3.6 billion; more than 1.2 million individuals are currently served through federally funded programs. The state is also home to approximately 2 million undocumented immigrants (California Department of Social Services,

1996). H.R. 3734 will have a profound effect on both the documented and undocumented immigrant populations, as most will become ineligible for assistance. California's agricultural economy relies heavily on this inexpensive and plentiful labor force.

Documented Immigrants: Prior to the Welfare Reform Law, legal immigrants were eligible for most state and federally funded assistance programs. These included Aid to Families with Dependent Children (AFDC), Supplemental Security Income (SSI, cash assistance for the elderly and disabled), State Supplementary Payments (SSP, state-funded cash assistance for recipients of federal SSI), Medicaid, housing assistance, and food stamps. The new law creates a new category of legal residents known as "qualified aliens"; these include veterans and those honorably discharged, persons on active duty and their dependents, asylees, and those who have worked in the United States for at least 10 years (Ingram, 1996). Unless they meet these "exception criteria," legal immigrants are entitled to Medicaid for emergency medical care only. Immigrants who were receiving SSI/SSP benefits must have had their eligibility redetermined before August 22, 1997 for continuation. Unless new and current immigrant applicants for food stamps meet "exception criteria," they are ineligible as of January 1, 1997; current recipients must be recertified to continue receiving benefits. Within California, financial responsibility has been shifted to the counties, who will also be the provider of last resort for those ineligible for federal aid. In San Bernadino County, alone, the number of immigrants transferred to general relief will rise from 500 to 8,000, costing $26 million annually. The number of disenfranchised immigrants in financially troubled Los Angeles and Orange Counties will exceed 500,000 people. California counties will be severely financially strapped (Ingram, 1996).

Undocumented Immigrants: Undocumented immigrants were already excluded from most federal benefit programs. H.R. 3734 eliminates all federal benefits and mandates the termination of state and local aid, unless states pass legislation authorizing assistance. In October 1996, California's Governor Wilson issued an executive order directing state agencies to cut off public funding as soon as possible. In 1997 and 1998, legislation was passed to restore several benefits, such as food stamps. The order placed approximately 2 million undocumented immigrants who are living in California at risk for losing benefits such as unemployment, food stamps, disability payments, government grants, contracts or loans, professional and commercial licenses, welfare benefits, public housing assistance, or nonemergency health care. H.R. 3734 is viewed by legislators as "breathing life" into Proposition 187, which was overwhelmingly approved by California voters in 1994 to ban services to undocumented immigrants, but has never been enforced. The termination of reimbursement for prenatal care once more places undocumented pregnant women and their babies at risk for levels of complications and mortality not seen since 1988. Hundreds of elderly and disabled undocumented immigrants living in California's long-term care facilities can still be reclassified as emergency medical cases and transferred to public hospitals, breaking the "safety net"(McDonnell, 1996).

Emerging Threats—the "Time Bombs" of Public Health

Toxic Substances

The 1988 IOM report on the Future of Public Health identified toxic substances in the environment and the workplace as one of the new challenges for the U.S. public health and legal systems. Evidence of the impacts of toxic substances on health is growing. Whether planned or unplanned, most releases of hazardous substances occur at fixed facilities, and not during transportation. Depending on the incident, these releases can result in evacuations, morbidity, and mortality. The substances released most frequently are ammonia, pesticides, volatile organic compounds, acids, and petroleum products (Hall, Hough, Price-Green, Dhaka, & Kaye, 1996).

Most toxic substances contaminate more than one medium, and may easily transfer from air to soil, and on to food and water. By-products from industry migrate from soil to groundwater to drinking water supplies. Pesticides that contaminate foods such as tomatoes, beef, potatoes, oranges, and lettuce are carcinogenic at certain levels. Prolonged exposure to some of these chemicals and toxins may cause cancer, reproductive problems, birth defects, and neurobehavioral disorders (IOM,1988). Documented and undocumented farmworkers are routinely exposed to pesticides and chemicals in fertilizers. Many exhibit eye problems, skin rashes, and gastrointestinal disorders. In addition to pesticides, farmworkers are unduly exposed to fecal coliforms because of the lack of potable water and sanitation facilities (Waterman, 1992). An estimated 15,000 to 50,000 farmworkers (depending on the growing seasons) live in these conditions in San Diego County each year.

New Diseases and Viruses

This section would not be complete without mentioning new diseases and drug-resistant strains of diseases that have been around for a long time. Mann (1994) reported that "AIDS is trying to teach us a lesson" (p. xvi). A health threat to "any part of the world can become a health threat to" everyone. In *The Coming Plague* (1994), Garrett identified viral and bacterial infections believed to have been eradicated in the 1950s and 1960s, that are making a comeback. Commonly found strains of *Streptococcus, Staphylococcus, Escheria coli* and tuberculosis (TB) are now multiantibiotic resistant. Microbes such *Cryptosporidium* and *Giardia* can be found in water purified by "top of the line" water treatment facilities (Garrett, 1994).

United States–Mexico border communities are experiencing marked increases in reported cases of pediatric TB. San Diego County experienced a 172% increase in pediatric TB between 1987 and 1993, and children were presenting with advanced cases that were highly contagious. The proximity to the border exacerbates the problem, and adds several forms of extrapulmonary TB to the caseload; one of these is gastrointestinal, caused by eating undercooked beef and unpasteurized milk products imported by U.S. retailers and sold in southern California (Alliance Healthcare Foundation,1995).

Vector-borne disease is on the upswing, apparently due to disruption of natural habitats and other environmental imbalances. Humans have had a direct impact on the emergence of Lyme's disease, *Ebola* virus and *Hantavirus,* by destroying the natural controls (i.e., "top predators") on certain species.

Other attributions for the emergence of "new"epidemics include overpopulation and the presence of Third World conditions such as poverty, poor housing, and poor sanitation. The lack of proper surveillance and monitoring is also a contributing factor. Apparently, public health leadership does not realize that the health of Americans is integrated with the health of international populations (Garrett, 1994).

Rational Planning for the Public Good Is Not Good Enough

Blum (1981), Lindblom (1965), and Bryson and Crosby (1992) all emphasized that, to be effective, planning and policy development need to address the "wicked" (Blum, 1981) and messy "real-time" problems that are the domain of public health; this involves working with the world in all of its complexities. In his treatise on human behavior in organizations, Herbert Simon (1976), explained the theory of intended and bounded rationality as the "behavior of human beings who *satisfice* because they have not the wits to *maximize*" (p. xxviii; emphasis in original). Simon advocated for the bigger-picture rationality of economic man who selects, from a number of alternatives, the best course of action that is available to him. Economic man (the maximizer) gets involved in all of the "buzzing, booming, and confusion

that constitutes the real world" (p. xxix) in all of its complexity. His cousin, administrative man, satisfices; he settles for gross simplifications of the real world because he believes that most of the causes and consequences of the situation he is facing are irrelevant to him. He makes decisions from just a few factors that he considers to be critical and relevant. In so doing, he "treats the world as rather empty" (p. xxx) ignoring the "interrelatedness of all things (so stupefying to thought and action)" (p. xxx) and makes decisions from simple rules "that do not make impossible demands upon his capacity for thought" (p. xxx).

While there are methods for improved decision making in private organizations, Simon (1976) reminded us that public decisions are even more complex, involving both rational and nonrational components—even community values. The values and myths undergirding the American social structure are extremely powerful, with champions like the so-called Moral Majority waiting for opportunities to get things back on track.

In *Tales of a New America,* Reich (1987) identified a few of these myths that help the American public to simplify its global policy decisions. All apply perfectly to current resistance to the social integration of immigrant groups. First is the tale of the "barbarians at the gates," reminiscent of the Mongolian hordes, that are about to take over the country and destroy the American way of life. These mythical hordes may include drug lords, legal or undocumented immigrants, or advocates for reproductive rights who are trying to change American traditions or family values. Second is the tale of "the triumphant individual" who demonstrates that anyone who works hard and has "the right stuff" can make it to the top. Third is the myth of the "benevolent" American community and its tradition of philanthropy and volunteerism, touted by President Reagan who reminded us that there was always a "safety net" in place; President Bush changed this metaphor to the "1,000 points of light." In comparison to the power of these myths, the impacts of the professional tools of public health, that is, technical knowledge, analysis, and planning seem quite ineffective.

Given all of the confounding myths, realities, and constraints, how can planning help leadership understand the trade-offs and make the hard but responsible choices to develop policies and structures that will support the health of the public? Blum (1981) described planning as the "deliberate introduction of desired social change in orderly and acceptable ways" (p. 2) and in response to the desire to create a better future, or in response to perceived problems which he views as "negative pressures" for change. Blum classified religious and political movements as positive forces for change. "Failures" of the health care system stem from unmet individual needs and the inappropriate allocation of resources. Blum identified key problems in the health sector as (1) uncontrolled cost; (2) inequities in access which exclude many because of financial, cultural, and language barriers; (3) poor quality; and (4) poor health status, often associated with poverty.

In *Planning for Health* (1981), Blum offered two frameworks to health planners that he views as necessary to improving health status or the delivery of health services. First is the "Force-Field Paradigm" which encompasses environmental factors, lifestyles, genetic characteristics, and health service systems. Second is the holistic "Well-Being Paradigm" which is based on individual experience and includes the social, psychological, and physical aspects of health, as well as intrinsic and extrinsic satisfaction with one's life and involvement with the health care system. Blum also tasked health planners with managing the socioeconomic and political factors. The United States is a pluralistic society, lacks an explicit, formal, health policy, and has no institutional "champion of the public well-being." Thus, dominant interests that "can assemble the power will dictate resource allocation" (p. 4). Problem solving requires changes in organizations, health policy, and resource commitments, but historically, vested interests have resisted inter-

ventions that are technologically and substantively appropriate.

Planning in a "Shared-Power" World

Given planning must "tackle such wicked complexities" (Blum, 1981, p. 7), can it succeed? With humanity's inherent desire to work toward "desired futures," and goals that can be clearly articulated and broadly supported, Blum believed that it can. Planning allows "people to envision new possibilities," to break out of "rigid and inappropriate paradigms," and to change social values. Thus, planning "lives at the very edge of respectability," gathering momentum from "massive dissatisfactions" with current conditions (Blum, 1981, p. 6).

In the 1990s, more than ever before, we live in a world of substantive public problems and a world in which no one is in charge. No one institution, organization, or other entity has the authority or legitimacy to act alone on critical public issues for the public good. Complex public health problems such as adolescent pregnancy, violence, poor access to health care, and toxic substances are not as likely to be solved as to be "resolved, dissolved, or redefined" (Bryson & Crosby, 1992, p. 5), because there is no single entity that has or would accept complete responsibility for any of these problems. Rather, many organizations and institutions are involved and partially responsible. The technology, information, and authority required for problem solving is distributed unevenly among a number of organizations. We live in a "shared-power world, a world in which organizations and institutions must share objectives, activities, resources, power or authority in order to achieve collective gains or minimize losses" (Bryson & Crosby, 1992, p. xi).

Working in shared-power situations with fluid networks of organizations, planners need to emphasize the development of interorganizational relationships and systems of decision making. Research has demonstrated that when planners used only methods, data, and analysis, they were relatively ineffective (Cohen, 1982). In these shared-power situations, planning cannot follow the prescribed "rational" models, or any rigidly structured sequence; that is, beginning with problem definition and the identification of alternative solutions, developing proposals, and implementing the plan or program. To get results, planners and policy entrepreneurs may look to Lindblom (1965) and others who point out the advantages of trading deductive, *technical* rationality for inductive, *political* rationality in policy change environments.

Moving inductively from public issues to public policy decisions can be a slow process. The political decision-making process begins with issues or conflicts, not with consensus. Disagreements may center around philosophy, outcomes, methods, or political advantage. If efforts to resolve the issues are politically rational and acceptable to stakeholders, they can produce improved programs and policies. Eventually, specific policies related to the immediate issue may be circumscribed in more general policy frameworks that serve as agreements or "treaties" among the various stakeholders, rather than consensus. Public policies require endorsements from politicians, which slows the process further. Politicians move reluctantly and cautiously, wishing to keep other options open for as long as possible (Bryson & Crosby, 1992).

There are other reasons that a political decision making model is useful in shared-power, public arenas. The process reminds planners and leaders to make issues the core of the policy change, and to create issues that address critical public health problems. Politics and public policy are intertwined. For change to occur, leaders must be sure that the new program or policy is politically acceptable, technically feasible, and legally and ethically defensible (Bryson & Crosby, 1992).

It is easy to despair over the prospect of getting involved in political, issue-oriented planning. But public health and social problems are widespread, recurring, and severe, requiring the collaboration of multiple provider organizations, associations, and government agencies which enter into networks of relationships in order to reach common goals (Cohen, 1982). The involvement of multiple centers of power creates more opportunities for democratic change. New policies require the endorsement of coalitions that are large and powerful enough to offer protection and support (Bryson & Crosby, 1992). Planners alone could never generate all of the options available to a community, county, or state. Planning without extensive participation from those involved and affected guarantees an incomplete understanding of the issue and invites the abuses of power.

Rational Planning and Political Decision-Making Models Are Complementary

Through much of this chapter, using theory from Simon (1976), Blum (1981), Lindblom (1980) and Bryson and Crosby (1992), we have argued for a nonlinear, "messy," political decision-making model over the rational planning, ideal type. For strategic planning inside organizations, the rational planning model still works rather well. But in the shared-power environment, both are necessary, and need to be sequenced properly. Bryson and Crosby state that

> [I]n the typical sequence, political decision making is necessary to determine the issues and the politically acceptable programs and policies that resolve them. Rational planning can then be used to recast that agreement in the form of technically workable goals, policies, programs, and actions. Participants in many community-based strategies . . . are unclear about their goals. It is only as they grapple with the problems and possible solutions—the issues—that clear goals, policies, and actions emerge. (p. 10)

Community organizers have known for generations that some problems lend themselves to a rational approach and others do not. Moreover, the collective pursuit of organizational, community, or national policy change involves considerable confusion, stress, and conflict. Witness the Clinton health plan failure—the positioning and repositioning of interest groups, and the shortcomings of "the nation's leadership class" who failed to converse with each other because of ignorance, and then engaged the public in a "bizarre dialogue of the deaf" (Yankelovich, 1995, p. 8).

Bryson and Crosby (1992) describe a seven-phase policy change "cycle," which works well in community problem solving for critical public health issues. A very brief adaptation of their process model appears here.

Phase I: Initiating a Preliminary Strategy for Change. In the first phase, the leader or the group identifies key decision makers and opinion leaders and the stakeholders (i.e., people, groups, and organizations) that need to be involved. Typically, critical issues serve as catalysts to action (e.g., 26% of the population have no health insurance). Like strategic planning in one organization, stakeholders agree to work together and develop a "plan to plan." At this early stage, they may even articulate an agreement on the overall strategy and methods to be used to approach the issue that brought them together. *Phase I* is a good time to add other members to the group in order to build a strong collaborative for the future.

Phase II: Problem Identification. Although the critical issue may have been selected by the leader or planner in *Phase I,* members of the collaborative need to agree on a more precise and accurate definition of the problem. They also must determine how to frame the issue (or issues) and how to describe it publicly. For example, the problem of transmitting HIV among injecting drug users (IDUs) through used needles and "works" has different predisposing factors in different population groups. The various disease profiles and sociocultural perspectives should be understood and agreed upon by members of the collaborative in order to propose feasible solutions. In a politically conservative community, framing the HIV–IDU problem as a threat to the health and safety of the general public may be more productive than describing it as a problem of poor access

to care and clean needles for injecting drug users.

Phase III: The Search for Solutions. Basically, there are three alternatives: (1) using models or solutions that have worked elsewhere and adapting them for the problem at hand; (2) using solutions that have worked for members of the planning team; or (3) creating new models or solutions. *Phase III* is a good time to initiate a media campaign in order to bring the identified problem to the attention of the public and educate them about underlying causes and possible solutions.

Phase IV: Developing the Proposal. The plan, policy, or program designed at this stage needs to be technically, politically, and ethically viable, as well as economically feasible. Participants will propose and test out alternatives on each other within the planning group. In the lively discussion and debate of design sessions, leadership needs to be sensitive to the objectives and concerns of all group members to build a solid base of support. *Phase IV* is the ideal stage at which to elicit and work through potential problems with a design. Planners or group leaders should remain vigilant to unproductive attempts to undermine or control the group. If another leader emerges that the group prefers, at this stage the planner or policy entrepreneur can work equally effectively in a "staffer" role.

Phase V: Proposal Review and Adoption. Concerns that were not addressed and worked through in the design phase will resurface and demand resolution. At this stage, advocates for change will press for adoption and implementation of the proposal. Negotiating, bargaining, and compromising over the specifics of the proposal will dominate this part of the process. If it appears that the proposal has a high probability of endorsement, there will be a "bandwagon" effect in the group; the converse is also true (e.g., "no one loves a loser").

Phase VI: Implementation and Evaluation. Implementation kicks off yet another planning and education process as many more individuals and organizations are included. New plans or programs do not implement themselves. There is usually resistance to change based on conflicting attitudes and beliefs, commitments to other plans and programs, or scarce resources. Because of the resistance that is to be expected in this phase, it is important for the planning team to keep alive the vision of success, developed at the beginning of the process; this reenforces the original agreement. If planners think clearly about implementation, and circumstances favor adoption, the design will be implemented and the identified problem or needs will be addressed. Leaders should be prepared to function as policy entrepreneurs and champions of the designs that benefit collaborators and serve the people's deepest interests and values. Formative evaluation is a crucial component of implementation. It provides continuous feedback for improving the program and making mid-course corrections.

Phase VII: Review and Modification or Termination. Policies and programs require monitoring on a continuing basis, reassessment, and modification in order to reach the desired outcomes. In the political environment, the only constant is change. Newly elected officials may be opposed to the policy and try to undermine it. The problem itself may change making the solution obsolete. New programs or policies may be developed that conflict with the policy, or replace the need for it. Programs or policies may be starved to death as financial resources are channeled elsewhere. Wildavsky (1979) and others have described the need for reviewing the larger system of policies and weeding out individual policies that are counterproductive; this is best done in the context of large-scale, regional planning.

Think "Big", Act "Small"

Regardless of the planning model, the change process is nonlinear. Policy change includes a sequence (described previously) which can be recursive. As in the process of group development, issues that are not dealt with in earlier stages of the collaborative process come back to haunt the planner later on. While "big" change and "big" wins are tantalizing, these "big" victories are hard to attain without just the right blend of coalition support, technology, financial resources, and opportunity. "Big" wins need broad-based support and new conceptual frameworks to accommodate the massive issue or problem. It is easier to keep a collaborative educated and up-to-speed if the identified problem is broken down into smaller, more manageable "chunks." These problem "chunks" may require the development of discrete subprojects which can take on lives of their own, independent of the guiding vision. Moving several subprojects along in one direction can resemble the proverbial "herding of cats." "Big" wins are also "big" risks. They are much harder to sell. Public officials at all levels (i.e., city, county, state, and national) are usually bewildered by the complexities of public health problems and vastly prefer the risk-reducing strategies of "small" wins (Bryson & Crosby, 1992).

While there is always the option of going for a major victory, "small" wins better complement the incremental approach to problem solving. "Small" wins require smaller, marginal adjustments and less risk, so it is easier to marshal the support of individuals and organizations. Smaller wins require subdividing the problem and working on it one "chunk" at a time. However, a series of "small" wins must be guided by the larger vision of an overall plan. "If a series of small wins can be informed by a sense of strategic direction, the small wins can add up to a big win over time" (Bryson & Crosby, 1992, p. 234).

Health Planning Now and in the Future

In the 1990s the health care system is changing as never before. Policy experts such as Etheredge, Jones, and Lewin (1996) assert that these changes are driven by "socially amoral economic forces"; these include employers, providers, health plans, and consumers. All but consumers have been the key players in the market reform movement, which has evolved gradually over the past three decades. Formerly, these old and experienced players appeared in different roles. In a period of "open-ended, fee-for-service insurance payments" the system was driven by technology, hospital capacity, the physician manpower pool, demographics, and physician control. Etheredge and colleagues (1996) believed that today's dynamics are accelerated by new influences in the health care marketplace: purchasing coalitions, the managed care industry, investment capital, the scramble for market share, the assumption of insurance risk, and the "new roles" of employers and consumers.

Trends in Health Planning in the 1990s

Influenced by the "Healthy People" objectives and the APHA–CDC's model standards for health promotion at the community level, the conceptualization of Healthy Cities–Healthy Communities achieved great prominence. Leonard Duhl (1985) introduced the concept of the city as an organism in the early 1980s, identifying a city's developmental needs, its coping skills, and its "ability to modify itself to . . . meet the always emerging requirements for life" (p. 1). Health issues, broadly defined, are identified as the critical, underlying issues that citizens and their leaders must deal with to "create their healthy city" (Duhl, 1985). The excitement over this conceptual model has generated many workshops and much rhetoric and enthusiasm. But little seems to have been accomplished in terms of measuring outcomes or the overall effectiveness of Healthy Cities projects. Hancock (1993) shared his scepticism about Healthy Cities' potential for becoming a social movement, as it is a "21st century concern cut across 19th century departments" (p. 15), that is, agencies and governments that operate in shared-power arenas, which defy restructuring.

The Healthy Cities concept is appealing even to professional societies and corporate interests. In 1993 the American Hospital Association (AHA) embraced the concept through Community Care Networks. AHA argued that their version of hospital-dominated health system integration would improve health status at the community level. The Belmont Vision was articulated by a group of senior U.S. corporate executives. The Belmont group assembled loose planning guidelines for local leadership to use in creating "a community health vision" (Institute for Alternative Futures, 1993). Conceptually in tune with the 1990s, the Belmont approach invites employers, hospitals, professional associations, consumers, and government to participate in yet another elite and voluntary effort to reform the health care system at the community level. However, the Belmont Vision does accurately identify the community as the primary locus for health system change; "given the nature of health care, communities will need to be . . . courageous in developing their own approaches . . . to improve health care access and financing" (Institute for Alternative Futures, 1993, p. 1).

The Healthy Cities framework rests on the principles of health promotion and illness prevention, and makes room for the further development of promising strategies that emerged in the 1970s and 1980s. These include community health assessment, changing unhealthy behaviors through health promotion and disease prevention, and social marketing. Bor, Chambers, Inui, and Showstack (1995) described *community health assessment* as "a powerful stimulus for interdisciplinary collaboration" that "enriches the blueprint for data gathering" and choice of "methods" (p. 5). Health assessment "provides the opportunity to explore" various issues underlying health planning, and "is one step in the cycle of continuous improvement of the public's health" (p. 5). Community health assessment provides a framework with which to understand " health needs and determinants; it establishes benchmarks for achievement and builds constituencies for new programs and policies" (p. 5). In addition, this approach lays the groundwork for periodic reassessments of the impacts of programs and policies.

While most dominant interests in health care are slow to realize the benefits of health promotion and disease prevention in workplaces and at the community level, purchasers of health services are seeking to get more "value" for their dollars. In the San Francisco Bay area of California, the Pacific Business Group on Health (PBGH) is incentivizing health plans to provide "preventive care," and urging employers and consumers to select plans that include programs for smoking cessation, stress reduction, fitness, and the like (Schauffler & Rodriguez, 1996). Model standards have been developed by the PBGH purchasing alliance, and agreements negotiated with all participating health plans. PBGH routinely collects data on plan performance in providing appropriate preventive care.

Chapman-Walsh and colleagues (1993) asserted that too little is done to "persuade all Americans to make enduring changes in their personal habits and lifestyles" (p. 105). *Social marketing,* a convergence of private sector marketing and public health is recommended as a quick and effective way to improve health status. Once epidemiological research established the risk factors for cardiovascular disease and other preventable diseases, public health professionals had the platform they needed to use marketing techniques to address social problems. Philip Kotler, one of its early proponents, described social marketing as the "design, implementation, and control of programs calculated to influence the acceptability of social ideas, and involving considerations of product, planning, pricing, communication, distribution and marketing research" (Kotler & Zaltman, 1971, p. 3). On the negative side, the successful application of social marketing techniques is resource intensive, and requires considerable monitoring and follow-up.

Market Reform Is Still the Driver

By now, policy analysts and pundits have covered every aspect of the Clinton health care reform debacle. Moreover, the constraints of this chapter do not permit an analysis of the constant and eternal restructuring of Medicaid, or other significant issues that promise to make the 1990s a memorable decade. Rumblings in Washington indicate that Medicare will soon be the focus of a major health care reform effort. For now, it is preferable to return to Etheredge and colleagues (1996) for closing observations on market reform in the 1990s.

Market reform continues to drive health system change; but will the "new forces" described by Etheredge and colleagues (1996) really drive it in new directions? Regardless, patients and their providers "face years of market-driven change." As in the PBGH purchasing alliance experience, employers are trying to get more value for their dollars. In the Twin Cities, purchasers are negotiating directly with providers, obviating the need for health plans. Consumers are choosing the least expensive health plan possible. In turn, health plans are going all out to remain price competitive. Until large-scale, research-based quality assessment mechanisms can produce data for purchasers and consumers, they will not be able to make decisions on anything but stark price comparisons. In their insightful analysis, Etheredge and colleagues 1996), pointed out that providers, concerned about excess manpower and system capacity, are seeking security in partnerships and joint ventures. The investment capital behind these arrangements "seeks financial opportunity . . . not social good" (Etheredge *et al.,* 1996, p. 97).

Because networks of cross-subsidy financing will break apart from the pressures of market competition, government may be forced to take a more active role. Clearly, our leaders at the national, state, and local levels lack the courage and passion required to address the interests of the underserved and uninsured head-on. They will probably try to fight fire with fire and take advantage of the obvious buying opportunities for Medicaid and Medicare populations. In addition, there are other "systems reaching a budgetary dead end," such as the U.S. military and the Department of Veterans Affairs (Goldsmith, 1996, p. 11).

Where Did All the Planners Go?

After all is said and done, health planning is still viable in this era of public–private partnerships. If the jurisdiction of health planning is broadened only slightly, there is room in the public sector for planners to pursue private dollars, and room in the private sector for planners to pursue public markets once considered undesirable. When federal and state funds were diverted from health planning, planners found new arenas in which to apply themselves. While it seems unlikely that students in a school of public health would (or even could) choose health planning as an area of specialization, graduates often find jobs that require a planner's complex skill sets. Today's health planners have experience in epidemiology, community organization, the law, health care financing, and management; they have developed negotiating skills and are comfortable with group facilitation. Planners know how to frame policy issues and work effectively with print and broadcast media. They look for opportunities to challenge "the way things are always done," and create opportunities for assessing and reassessing the impacts of programs and policies.

Armed with these skills and resources, planners can find meaningful work in all areas of health care except in clinical capacities. Health planners are employed by all constituencies mentioned in this chapter, such as high levels of state and federal government, community health centers, commercial and public sector health plans and other aspects of managed care, the insurance industry, hospitals, health care systems, independent practice associations and other large physician groups, professional associations, and a broad array of nonprofits.

Once in a while, "mature" health planners look back longingly on the 1970s and 1980s as a time of professional opportunity and job security. But health planners, and others who do this work, have never had control of their professional destinies. They were, and are, in the words of Henrik Blum (1981) "always operating at the very edge of respectability" (p. 000)—at the behest of changing administrations and funding cycles, in the tumult of the health care marketplace, or in communities where the process is painstakingly slow but often worthwhile. But Henrik Blum did not tell us that "the edge of respectability" is a very exciting place to work.

References

Alford, R. (1975). *Health care politics: Ideological and interest group barriers to reform.* Chicago: University of Chicago Press.

Alliance Healthcare Foundation. (1995). *Triennial Report, 1992–1995* (Vol. 13). San Diego: Author.

Blum, H. (1981). *Planning for health: Generics for the eighties* (2nd ed.). New York: Human Sciences.

Bor, D. H., Chambers, L. W., Inui, T. S., & Showstack, J. A. (1995). *Community health improvement through information and action.* San Francisco: Health of the Public Program.

Border Youth and Substance Abuse. (1996, August). *Arizona: Border Health News North–South, 1*(2), 7.

Brown, L. D., & McLaughlin, C. (1990). Constraining costs at the community level. *Health Affairs, 9*(4), 5–28.

Brown, R. E. (1979). *Rockefeller medicine men: Medicine and capitalism in America.* Berkeley: University of California Press.

Bryson, J. M., & Crosby, B. C. (1992). *Leadership for the common good: Tackling public problems in a shared-power world.* San Francisco: Jossey-Bass.

Burbridge, K. (1993). *Violence prevention initiative for Escondido youth encounter.* Proposal to the Alliance Healthcare Foundation, San Diego, CA.

California Department of Social Services. (1996). *Federal welfare reform law (HR 3734)* [Fact sheet]. Sacramento, CA: Author.

California Wellness Foundation. (1996). *Preventing teenage pregnancy: An adult responsibility* [Brochure on new initiative]. Woodland Hills, CA: Author.

Carpenter, E. (1982). Consumer participation in local health planning: The beginning of the end or the end of the beginning? *Medical Care, 20*(12), 1163–1165.

Centers for Disease Control and Prevention. (1993a, September). *Facts about drug use and HIV/AIDS.* Atlanta, GA: Author.

Centers for Disease Control and Prevention. (1993b, November). *Facts about HIV/AIDS and race/ethnicity.* Atlanta, GA: Author.

Centers for Disease Control and Prevention (1993c, October). *Facts about women and HIV/AIDS.* Atlanta, GA: Author.

Chapman-Walsh, D. C., Rudd, R. E., Moeykens, B. A., & Moloney, T. W. (1993). Social marketing for public health. *Health Affairs, 12*(2), 104–119.

Cohen, P. D. (1982). Community health planning from an interorganizational perspective. *American Journal of Public Health, 72*(7), 717–721.

Cosby, W. (1996, December 28). Presentation at the 50th anniversary celebration of the publication of *Ebony,* Los Angeles.

Duhl, L. W. (1985). The healthy city: Its function and its future. *Health Promotion, 2*(2), 1–6.

Davis, K. (1996, Spring). The nation's healthcare safety net: The leadership challenge for health philanthropy. *Grant scene,* 5–6

Des Jarlais, D. C. & Friedman, S. R. (1994, February). AIDS and the use of injected drugs. *Scientific American,* 82–88.

Etheredge, L., Jones, S. B., & Legin, L. (1996). What is driving health system change? *Health Affairs, 15*(4), 93–104.

Garret, L. (1994). *The coming plague: Newly emerging diseases in a world out of balance.* New York: Penguin.

Hall, H., Hough, G. S., Price-Green, P. A., Dhaka, V. R., & Kaye, W. E. (1996). Risk factors for hazardous substance releases that result in injuries and evacuations: Data from 9 states. *American Journal of Public Health, 86*(6), 855–857.

Hancock, T. (1993). The evolution, impact and significance of the healthy cities/healthy communities movement. *Journal of Public Health Policy, 14*(1), 5–18.

Ingram, C. (1996, October 11). Welfare bill could cost state $7 billion, study says. *Los Angeles Times,* pp. A3–4.

Institute for Alternative Futures. (1993). *The Belmont vision: Creating community health visions, a guide for local leaders.* Alexandria, VA: Author.

Institute of Medicine. (1988). *The future of public health.* Washington, DC: National Academy Press.

Joskow, P. L. (1981). Alternative regulatory mechanisms for controlling hospital costs. In M. Olson (Ed.), *A new approach to the economics of health care* (pp. 219–257). Washington, DC: American Enterprise Institute for Public Policy Research.

Kaiser Family Foundation. (1996). *Where is the epidemic headed?* (AIDS Public Information Project). Menlo Park, CA: Author.

Kotler, P. & Zaltman, G. (1971). Social marketing: An approach to planned social change. *Journal of Marketing, 35,* 3–12.

Lindblom, C. E. (1965). *The intelligence of democracy.* New York: Free Press.

Lindblom, C. E. (1980). *The policy-making process* (2nd ed.). Englewood Cliffs, NJ: Prentice Hall.

Lipson, D. J., & Naierman, N. (1996). Effects of health systems changes on safety-net providers. *Health Affairs, 15*(2), 33–48.

Loue, S. (1992). *Child and adolescent health outreach project for Asian/Pacific Islander communities.* Proposal to Alliance Healthcare Foundation, San Diego, CA.

Luft, H. S. (1985). Regionalization of medical care. *American Journal of Public Health, 75*(2), 125–126.

Maerki, S., Luft, H. S., & Hunt, S. S. (1986). Selecting categories of patients for regionalization, implications of the relationship between volume and outcome. *Medical Care, 24*(2), 148–158.

Mann, J. M. (1994). Preface. In L. Garrett, *The coming plague: Newly emerging diseases in a world out of balance* (pp. xv–vii). New York: Penguin.

McBeath, W. H. (1991). Health for all: A public health vision. *American Journal of Public Health, 81*(12), 1560–1565.

McDonnell, P. J. (1996, August 31). Wilson moves to limit benefits for illegal immigrants. *The Los Angeles Times,* p. A3.

Miller, T. R., Cohen, M. A., & Rossman, S. B. (1993). Victim costs of violent crime and resulting injuries. *Health Affairs, 12*(4), 186–197.

Navarro, V. (1975). Social policy issues: An explanation of the composition, nature and functions of the present health sector of the United States. *Bulletin of the New York Academy of Medicine, 54*(1), 199–234.

Nutting, P. A. (Ed.). (1987). *Community-oriented primary care: From principle to practice* (HRSA-A-PE, 86-1). Washington, DC: U.S. Government Printing Office.

Office of National AIDS Policy. (1996). *Youth & HIV/AIDS: An American agenda* (A report to the president). Washington, DC: Author.

Olson, M. (Ed.). (1981). *A new approach to the economics of health care.* Washington, DC: American Enterprise Institute for Public Policy Research.

Overall, N. A., & Williamson, J. (1985). *Community oriented primary care in action: A practice manual for primary care settings.* Berkeley: University of California Press.

Pacific Center for Violence Prevention. (1994a). *Violence: The cost* [Fact Sheet]. San Francisco: Author.

Pacific Center for Violence Prevention. (1994b). *Violence: Facts in brief* [Fact Sheet]. San Francisco: Author.

Program & Policies Advisory Committee. (1978). *Recommendations for a national strategy for disease prevention.* Atlantac, GA: Centers for Disease Control.

Reich, R. B. (1988). *The power of public ideas.* New York: Harper Business.

Robert Wood Johnson Foundation (RWJF). (1993). *Substance abuse: The nation's number one health problem: Key indicators for policy.* Prepared by the Institute for Health Policy, Brandeis University.

Robert Wood Johnson Foundation (RWJF). (1986). *Updated report on access to care for the American people.* Princeton, NJ.

Roos, N. P. (1995). From research to policy. What have we learned from designing the population health information system? *Medical Care, 33*(12), 132–145.

Schaefer, M. (1985). Moving the "standards movement." *American Journal of Public Health, 75*(6), 645–648.

Schauffler, H. H., & Rodriquez, T. (1996). Power for preventive care. *Health Affairs, 15*(1), 73–85.

Shogren, E. (1996, August 23). Clinton's signature launches historic overhaul of welfare. *Los Angeles Times,* p. A–1.

Simon, H. A. (1976). *Administrative behavior* (3rd ed.). New York: Free Press.

Simpson, J. B. (1985). State certificate-of-need programs: The current status. *American Journal of Public Health, 75*(10), 1225–1229.

Starr, P. (1981). Commentary. In M. Olson (Ed.), *A new approach to the economics of health care.* Washington, DC: American Enterprise Institute for Public Policy Research.

Trang, K. M. (1993). *Violence prevention initiative for the Indochinese mutual assistance association.* Proposal to the Alliance Healthcare Foundation, San Diego, CA.

Waitzkin, H. (1978). A Marxist view of medical care. *Annals of Internal Medicine, 89,* 264–278.

Waterman, S. (1992). *North County safe water and sanitation project.* Proposal to the Alliance Healthcare Foundation, San Diego, CA.

Wildavsky, A. (1984). *Speaking truth to power: The art and craft of policy analysis.* Boston: Little, Brown.

Wilson, J. W. (1996, August 18). Work. *The New York Times Magazine,* pp. 26–54.

Yankelovich, D. (1995). The debate that wasn't: The public and the Clinton plan. *Health Affairs, 14*(1), 7–23.

Zeckhauser, R. & Zook, C. (1981). Failures to control health costs: Departments from first principles. In M. Olson, *A new approach to the economics of healthcare.* Washington, DC: American Enterprise Institute for Public Policy Research.

Index